Essentials of EMERGENCY MEDICINE

SECOND EDITION

EDITOR-IN-CHIEF

DOUGLAS A. RUND, MD, FACEP

Professor and Chairman, Department of Emergency Medicine,
The Ohio State University, Columbus, Ohio

ASSOCIATE EDITORS

ROGER M. BARKIN, MD, MPH, FAAP, FACEP

Vice President for Pediatric and Newborn Programs, Columbia-HealthONE;
Professor of Surgery, Division of Emergency Medicine, University of Colorado
Health Sciences Center, Denver, Colorado

PETER ROSEN, MD, FACEP

Professor of Clinical Medicine and Surgery; Director, Emergency Medicine
Residency Program; Director of Education, Department of Emergency Medicine,
University of California at San Diego Medical Center, San Diego, California

GEORGE L. STERNBACH, MD, FACEP

Clinical Professor of Surgery, Emergency Medicine Service, Stanford University
Medical Center, Stanford, California; Emergency Physician, Seton Medical Center,
Daly City, California

with 137 illustrations

M Mosby

An Imprint of Elsevier Science

St. Louis London Philadelphia Sydney Toronto

M Mosby

An Imprint of Elsevier Science

Vice President and Publisher: Anne S. Patterson
Editor: Kathryn H. Falk
Developmental Editor: Carolyn M. Kruse
Project Manager: Deborah L. Vogel
Production Editor: Jodi Willard
Layout Artist: Jeanne Genz
Designer: Pati Pye
Manufacturing Manager: Linda Ierardi

SECOND EDITION

Printed in the United States of America

Mosby, Inc.
11830 Westline Industrial Drive
St. Louis, Missouri 63146

Library of Congress Cataloging in Publication Data

Essentials of emergency medicine / editor-in-chief, Douglas A. Rund; associate editors,
  Roger M. Barkin, Peter Rosen, George L. Sternbach. —2nd ed.
      p.   cm.
    Rev. ed. of: Essentials of emergency medicine / Peter Rosen, Roger M. Barkin, George
L. Sternbach. c1991.
    Includes bibliographical references and index.
    ISBN 0-8151-7146-3 (pbk.)
    1. Emergency medicine.   I. Rund, Douglas A.   II. Barkin, Roger M.   III. Rosen, Peter,
        Essentials of emergency medicine.
    [DNLM: 1.   Emergencies.   2. Emergency Medicine.   WB 105 E78 1996]
RC86.7.R674   1996
616. 02′5—dc20
DNLM/DLC
                                                                    96-17608

    02   03   04   /   9 8 7 6 5 4 3 2

Essentials of
EMERGENCY
MEDICINE

CONTRIBUTORS

JEAN ABBOTT, MD, FACEP
Associate Professor, Department of Surgery, Division of Emergency Medicine, University Hospital, University of Colorado School of Medicine, Denver, Colorado
45: Pregnancy

TOM P. AUFDERHEIDE, MD, FACEP
Associate Professor of Emergency Medicine, Department of Emergency Medicine, Medical College of Wisconsin, Milwaukee, Wisconsin
35: Peripheral Arteriovascular Disease

STEVEN M. BARRETT, MD, FACEP
Emergency Physician—Community Practice, Emergency Department, Baptist Hospital of Southeast Texas, Beaumont, Texas
10: Respiratory Distress

WILLIAM G. BARSAN, MD
Professor and Section Head, Emergency Medicine, Department of Surgery, University of Michigan Medical Center, Ann Arbor, Michigan
50: Stroke

PHILLIP I. BIALECKI, MD, MHE
Clinical Instructor, Department of Emergency Medicine, The Ohio State University, Columbus, Ohio
55: Suicide

ROBERT A. BITTERMAN, MD, JD, FACEP
Director of Risk Management and Managed Care; Co-Coordinator of Medical Student Education, Department of Emergency Medicine, Carolinas Medical Center, Charlotte, North Carolina
15: Acute Infectious Diarrheal Disease; 41: Lower Gastrointestinal Tract Disorders

MARC BORENSTEIN, MD, FACEP, FACP
Chief, Division of Emergency Medicine; Director, Integrated Residency in Emergency Medicine; Associate Professor, Department of Surgery, University of Connecticut Health Center, Farmington, Connecticut
47: Oncologic Emergencies

MARY ANN COOPER, MD, FACEP
Associate Professor and Director, Lightning and Electrical Injury Evaluation Program, Department of Emergency Medicine; Deputy Head for Academic Affairs, The University of Illinois at Chicago, Chicago, Illinois
28: Electrical and Lightning Injuries

RITA K. CYDULKA, MD
Director, Emergency Medicine Residency Program, Department of Emergency Medicine, Metro Health Medical Center, Case Western Reserve University School of Medicine, Cleveland, Ohio
58: Endocrine Disorders

DANIEL F. DANZL, MD, FACEP
Professor and Chair, Department of Emergency Medicine, University of Louisville, Louisville, Kentucky
30: Heat- and Cold-Induced Injuries

ANN M. DIETRICH, MD
Assistant Professor, Department of Pediatrics, The Ohio State University; Attending Staff, Pediatric Emergency Medicine Department, Children's Hospital, Columbus, Ohio
66: Pediatric Emergencies

STEVEN C. DRONEN, MD

Associate Section Head and Residency Director, University of Michigan Medical Center, Section of Emergency Medicine, Ann Arbor, Michigan
5: Shock

CHARLES L. EMERMAN, MD

Associate Professor, Department of Emergency Medicine, Case Western Reserve University, Cleveland, Ohio
32: Acute Adult Asthma and Exacerbations of Chronic Obstructive Pulmonary Disease

CRAIG F. FEIED, MD, FACEP

Associate Clinical Professor of Emergency Medicine, The George Washington University Medical Center; Director, National Center for Emergency Medicine Informatics; Director of Informatics, Department of Emergency Medicine, The Washington Hospital Center; Director of Informatics, The Ronald Reagan Institute of Emergency Medicine, Washington, DC
34: Deep Venous Thrombosis and Pulmonary Embolism

JOEL GEIDERMAN, MD

Director and Co-Chair, Department of Emergency Medicine, CSMC Research Institute, Cedars-Sinai Medical Center; Associate Professor of Medicine, Department of Emergency Medicine, UCLA School of Medicine, Los Angeles, California
26: Orthopedic Injuries

W. BRIAN GIBLER, MD

Professor of Emergency Medicine; Chairman; Director—Heart ER, Department of Emergency Medicine, University of Cincinnati Medical Center, Cincinnati, Ohio
62: Parasitic Disease

DAVID A. GUSS, MD, FACP

Director, Department of Emergency Medicine; Adjunct Professor of Medicine and Surgery, UCSD Medical Center, San Diego, California
42: Disorders of the Liver, Biliary Tract, and Pancreas

GLENN C. HAMILTON, MD, MSM, FACEM, FACP

Professor and Chair, Department of Emergency Medicine, Wright State University, Dayton, Ohio
46: Hematologic Disorders

JONATHAN A. HANDLER, MD

Research Director, Department of Emergency Medicine, Northwestern University Medical School, Chicago, Illinois
8: Altered Mental Status and Syncope

ANN L. HARWOOD-NUSS, MD, FACEP

Professor, Division of Emergency Medicine, Department of Surgery, University of Florida Health Science Center, Jacksonville, Florida
43: Acute Genitourinary Disorders

STEPHEN R. HAYDEN, MD

Assistant Clinical Professor of Medicine; Associate Program Director; Emergency Medicine Residency, Department of Emergency Medicine, University of California School of Medicine, San Diego, California
38: Congestive Heart Failure

PHILIP L. HENNEMAN, MD

Vice Chair, Department of Emergency Medicine, Harbor-UCLA Medical Center; Associate Professor of Medicine, UCLA School of Medicine, Torrance, California
13: Gastrointestinal Bleeding

GREGORY L. HENRY, MD, FACEP

Clinical Associate Professor, Department of Surgery, Section of Emergency Services, University of Michigan Medical Center, Ann Arbor, Michigan
9: Headache

ROBERT S. HOCKBERGER, MD

Professor of Medicine, UCLA School of Medicine; Chair, Department of Emergency Medicine, Harbor-UCLA Medical Center, Torrance, California
21: Spinal Injury

JAMES W. HOEKSTRA, MD, FACEP

Associate Professor of Emergency Medicine; Director of Ambulatory Education, Department of Emergency Medicine, The Ohio State University, Columbus, Ohio
11: Chest Pain

D. MICHAEL HUNT, MD

Medical Director, Emergency Medical Services, Columbia/HealthOne, Englewood, Colorado
8: Altered Mental Status and Syncope

JOHN J. KELLEY, DO, FACEP

Assistant Chairman, Department of Emergency Medicine, Albert Einstein Medical Center; Associate Professor, Department of Medicine, Temple University School of Medicine; Adjunct Associate Professor, Department of Emergency Medicine, Medical College of Pennsylvania, Philadelphia, Pennsylvania
31: Acute Respiratory Tract Infection

MICHAEL T. KELLEY, MD

Associate Professor, Departments of Emergency Medicine and Pediatrics, The Ohio State University, Columbus, Ohio
64: Toxicology: General Management Principles

EUGENE E. KERCHER, MD, FACEP

Assistant Clinical Professor, Department of Medicine, University of California, Los Angeles; Chairman, Department of Emergency Medicine, Kern Medical Center, Bakersfield, California
54: Acute Psychosis

ROBERT KNOPP, MD, FACEP

Residency Director, St. Paul Ramsey Medical Center; Professor of Clinical Emergency Medicine, Department of Emergency Medicine, University of Minnesota, St. Paul Ramsey Medical Center, St. Paul, Minnesota
29: Near-Drowning

RASHMI U. KOTHARI, MD

Assistant Professor, Department of Emergency Medicine, University of Cincinnati College of Medicine, Cincinnati, Ohio
50: Stroke

JAY LANCE KOVAR, MD

Assistant Professor, Department of Emergency Medicine; Residency Program Director, Department of Emergency Medicine, The University of Texas Medical School at Houston, Houston, Texas
52: Meningitis and Encephalitis

FRANK W. LAVOIE, MD

Associate Professor, Division of Emergency Medicine, University of Texas Southwestern Medical School, Dallas, Texas
56: Violence

DAVID CHUNGSANG LEE, MD

Medical Toxicology Fellowship Director, Department of Emergency Medicine, Misericordia Hospital, Medical College of Pennsylvania, Philadelphia, Pennsylvania
17: Joint and Back Pain

NEAL LITTLE, MD, FACEP

Clinical Associate Professor, Department of Surgery, University of Michigan, Ann Arbor, Michigan
53: Special Neurologic Problems

RICHARD L. MAENZA, MD

Attending Emergency Physician, Department of Emergency Medicine, Mercy Hospital of Pittsburgh, Pittsburgh, Pennsylvania
44: Renal Failure and Dialysis

VINCENT J. MARKOVCHICK, MD, FACEP

Director, Emergency Medical Services, Denver General Hospital; Professor of Surgery, University of Colorado Health Sciences Center, Denver, Colorado
6: Multiple Trauma; 23: Cardiovascular Trauma

DANIEL R. MARTIN, MD, FACEP

Associate Professor and Program Director, Emergency Medicine Residency Program, Department of Emergency Medicine, The Ohio State University, Columbus, Ohio
25: Soft-Tissue Injuries and Lacerations

MARCUS L. MARTIN, MD, FACEP

Associate Professor and Chairman, Department of Emergency Medicine, The Medical College of Pennsylvania, and Hahneman University—Allegheny Campus, Pittsburgh, Pennsylvania
40: Upper Gastrointestinal Tract Disorders

JOHN MARX, MD

Chair, Department of Emergency Medicine, Carolinas Medical Center, Charlotte, North Carolina; Clinical Professor, Department of Emergency Medicine, University of North Carolina, Chapel Hill, North Carolina
24: Abdominal and Genitourinary Trauma

JAMES MATHEWS, MD, FACEP

Professor of Medicine and Chief, Division of Emergency Medicine, Department of Medicine, Northwestern University Medical School, Chicago, Illinois
37: Hypertension

MICHAEL G. MIKHAIL, MD

Assistant Residency Director, Department of Emergency Medicine, University of Michigan, St. Joseph Mercy Hospital; Emergency Medicine Residency Program, St. Joseph Mercy Hospital, Ann Arbor, Michigan
53: Special Neurologic Problems

LINDSAY MURRAY, MB, BS, FACEM

Senior Fellow, Center for Clinical Toxicology, Vanderbilt University Medical Center, Nashville, Tennessee; Staff Specialist, Emergency Department, Prince of Wales Hospital, Randwick, New South Wales, Australia
65: Specific Toxins

BRUCE K. NEELY, MD
Clinical Instructor, Department of Emergency Medicine, The Ohio State University, Columbus, Ohio
48: Rheumatology and Connective Tissue Diseases

RICHARD N. NELSON, MD, FACEP
Associate Professor, Department of Emergency Medicine, The Ohio State University, Columbus, Ohio
27: Thermal and Chemical Injuries

RICHARD M. NOWAK, MD, MBA, FACEP
Vice Chairman, Department of Emergency Medicine, Henry Ford Health System, Detroit, Michigan; Clinical Assistant Professor, Emergency Medical Services, Department of Surgery, University of Michigan Medical School, Ann Arbor, Michigan
32: Acute Adult Asthma and Exacerbations of Chronic Obstructive Pulmonary Disease

JONATHAN S. OLSHAKER, MD
Associate Professor of Surgery; Program Director; Emergency Medicine Residency Program, University of Maryland Medical Center, Baltimore, Maryland
51: Vertigo

DAVID W. OLSON, MD, FACEP
Assistant Professor, Department of Surgery, University of Texas Medical School, San Antonio, San Antonio, Texas
52: Meningitis and Encephalitis

NORMAN A. PARADIS, MD
Director, Resuscitation Research Laboratory, Department of Medicine, Columbia University College of Physicians and Surgeons, New York, New York
4: Cardiac Arrest

EDWIN CARY PIGMAN, MD
Medical Director, World Access Group; Acting Medical Director, Department of Emergency Medicine, Winter Haven Hospital, Winter Haven, Florida
36: Ischemic Heart Disease

PETER PONS, MD
Emergency Department, Denver General Hospital; Associate Professor of Emergency Medicine, Division of Emergency Medicine, Department of Surgery, University of Colorado Health Sciences Center, Denver, Colorado
19: Head Trauma; 33: Aspiration and Foreign Bodies

JOEL J. REICH, MD, FACEP
Chairman, Department of Emergency and Ambulatory Care Services, Manchester Memorial Hospital, Manchester, Connecticut; Clinical Assistant Professor, Department of Surgery, Division of Emergency Medicine, University of Connecticut School of Medicine, Farmington, Connecticut
59: Bacterial Infections

GERALYNN S. RENNER, MD, FACEP, FAAEM
Assistant Professor, Department of Emergency Medicine, Georgetown University Medical Center, Washington, DC
68: Disorders of the Eye

LINDA A. ROBINSON, MD, FACEP
Department of Emergency Medicine, Jackson Memorial Hospital, Miami, Florida
60: Viral Infections

PETER ROSEN, MD
Professor of Clinical Medicine and Surgery; Director, Emergency Medicine Residency Program; Director of Education, Department of Emergency Medicine, University of California at San Diego Medical Center, San Diego, California
2: General Approach to the Emergency Patient

DOUGLAS A. RUND, MD, FACEP
Professor and Chairman, Department of Emergency Medicine, The Ohio State University, Columbus, Ohio
1: Emergency Medicine: An Introduction; 20: Facial and Oral Trauma; 48: Rheumatology and Connective Tissue Diseases; 61: Human Immunodeficiency Virus Infection and AIDS

RICHARD JOSEPH RYAN, MD
Assistant Professor, Department of Emergency Medicine, University of Cincinnati; Mills, Sherman, Githam, and Goodwin, PSC, Cincinnati, Ohio; Department of Emergency Medicine, St. Elizabeth Medical Center, Edgewood, Kentucky
62: Parasitic Disease

ROBERT E. SCHNEIDER, MD
Residency Director, Department of Emergency Medicine, Carolinas Medical Center, Charlotte, North Carolina; Clinical Assistant Professor, Department of Emergency Medicine, University of North Carolina at Chapel Hill, Chapel Hill, North Carolina
24: Abdominal and Genitourinary Trauma

DONNA SEGER, MD, FACEP, ABMT
Assistant Professor of Medicine and Emergency Medicine; Medical Director, Middle Tennessee Poison Control Center; Department of Medicine and Emergency Medicine, Vanderbilt University Medical Center, Nashville, Tennessee
65: Specific Toxins

COREY M. SLOVIS, MD, FACP, FACEP
Professor of Emergency Medicine and Medicine; Chairman, Department of Emergency Medicine, Vanderbilt University Medical Center, Nashville, Tennessee
57: Fluids and Electrolytes

THOMAS OSBORNE STAIR, MD
Professor, Department of Surgery, University of Maryland, Baltimore, Maryland
67: Otolaryngologic Emergencies

J. STEPHEN STAPCZYNSKI, MD, FACEP
Chair and Associate Professor, Department of Emergency Medicine, University of Kentucky, College of Medicine, Lexington, Kentucky
39: Dysrhythmias

GEORGE L. STERNBACH, MD, FACEP
Clinical Professor of Surgery, Emergency Medicine Service, Stanford University Medical Center, Stanford, California; Emergency Physician, Seton Medical Center, Daly City, California
49: Dermatologic Problems

GARY L. SWART, MD, FACEP
Assistant Professor of Emergency Medicine; Residency Program Director; Department of Emergency Medicine, Medical College of Wisconsin, Milwaukee, Wisconsin
14: Vomiting

HAROLD THOMAS, JR., MD
Chief, Emergency Medical Services, Portland V.A. Medical Center; Residency Director, Department of Emergency Medicine, Oregon Health Science University, Portland, Oregon
7: Fever

MICHAEL CHARLES TOMLANOVICH, MD
Chairman, Department of Emergency Medicine, Henry Ford Hospital, Detroit, Michigan; Clinical Associate Professor, Department of Surgery, Division of Emergency Medical Services, University of Michigan, Ann Arbor, Michigan
18: Seizure

ALEXANDER TROTT, MD
Professor of Emergency Medicine; Director, Clinical Practice Improvement, University Hospital, University of Cincinnati College of Medicine, Cincinnati, Ohio
12: Abdominal Pain

THOMAS W. TURBIAK, MD, FACEP
Director, Department of Emergency Medicine, The Reading Hospital and Medical Center, West Reading, Pennsylvania; Clinical Assistant Professor, Department of Surgery, Division of Emergency Medicine, University of Connecticut School of Medicine, Farmington, Connecticut
59: Bacterial Infections

LEONARD F. URBANSKI, DO
Attending Physician, St. Francis Hospital Emergency Department; Program Coordinator, Internal Medicine/Emergency Medicine Residency; Assistant Professor of Emergency Medicine, Medical College of Pennsylvania—Allegheny Campus, Department of Emergency Medicine, Allegheny General Hospital, Pittsburgh, Pennsylvania
40: Upper Gastrointestinal Tract Disorders

MICHAEL L. VORBROKER, MD
Clinical Assistant Professor, Department of Emergency Medicine, The Ohio State University, Columbus, Ohio
63: Tickborne Illnesses

DAVID J. VUKICH, MD
Associate Professor and Chief, Division of Emergency Medicine, University of Florida Health Science Center, Jacksonville, Florida
22: Chest Trauma

RON M. WALLS, MD, FRCPC, FACEP
Chairman, Department of Emergency Medicine, Brigham and Women's Hospital; Associate Professor, Harvard Medical School, Boston, Massachusetts
3: Airway Management

JOANNE WILLIAMS, MD
Diplomate, American Board of Emergency Medicine; Board Certified Forensic Examiner; Assistant Professor and Assistant Residency Director, Department of Emergency Medicine, Martin Luther King, Jr./Charles R. Drew Medical Center, Los Angeles, California
61: Human Immunodeficiency Virus Infection and AIDS

ALLAN B. WOLFSON, MD, FACEP, FACP
Program Director, Affiliated Residency in Emergency
Medicine; Associate Professor of Emergency Medicine, University of Pittsburgh, Pittsburgh, Pennsylvania
44: Renal Failure and Dialysis

GARY P. YOUNG, MD, FACEP, FACP
Chair, Department of Emergency Medicine, Highland
Hospital, Oakland, California; Associate Professor,
University of California, San Francisco, California
*16: Pelvic Pain, Vaginal Bleeding, and Genital Infec-
tion*

PREFACE

This second edition of *Essentials of Emergency Medicine* revises and expands its predecessor. While renewing the goal of providing a "core" of knowledge in emergency medicine for the medical student and other practitioners who wish to learn about emergency medicine, the second edition includes contributions from the most authoritative educators in our field. Most chapters present a set of *key considerations* to help focus the student on the most critical elements of patient management for a specific condition or situation.

This revised edition draws on but does not duplicate the encyclopedic *Emergency Medicine: Concepts and Clinical Practice, third edition,* which presents in-depth coverage of the concepts of the clinical practice and pathophysiology of emergency medicine.

Essentials of Emergency Medicine includes sixty-eight succinct chapters that are arranged into six parts: general concepts, signs and symptoms, trauma, environmental emergencies, systemic disorders, and special problems. The symptoms, signs, and conditions discussed include common emergency conditions, serious emergency conditions, and situations in which appropriate emergency treatment makes a critical difference in outcome.

It is our hope that this book will introduce, provide a focus for, overview, and review the most salient features of critical emergency medicine.

ACKNOWLEDGMENTS

We thank the authors of this text as well as the contributors to *Emergency Medicine: Concepts and Clinical Practice* for helping to establish and clarify the body of knowledge on which we base our teaching of emergency medicine.

Special thanks to Kathy Sturgeon at The Ohio State University for her dedication to this project and for the many hours she has devoted to the preparation of this text.

We thank Carolyn Kruse, Kathy Falk, and Laurel Craven at Mosby-Year Book, Inc., for outstanding assistance and encouragement throughout the project.

Finally we offer our deepest thanks to our families, who have tolerated long hours and our many pages of manuscript. We are forever grateful to Ann Rosen; Suky, Adam, and Michael Barkin; Joshua and Rebecca Sternbach; and Sue, Carie, Emily, and Ashley Rund.

DOUGLAS A. RUND, MD
ROGER M. BARKIN, MD
PETER ROSEN, MD
GEORGE L. STERNBACH, MD

To students of Emergency Medicine, because clinical learning never ends;

and to our patients, because your care is our trust and our mission.

CONTENTS

Part *I*

GENERAL CONCEPTS

1 *Emergency Medicine: An Introduction, 3*
   DOUGLAS A. RUND
2 *General Approach to the Emergency Patient, 7*
   PETER ROSEN
3 *Airway Management, 16*
   RON M. WALLS
4 *Cardiac Arrest, 29*
   NORMAN A. PARADIS
5 *Shock, 50*
   STEVEN C. DRONEN
6 *Multiple Trauma, 60*
   VINCENT J. MARKOVCHICK

Part *II*

SIGNS AND SYMPTOMS

7 *Fever, 71*
   HAROLD THOMAS, JR.
8 *Altered Mental Status and Syncope, 80*
   JONATHAN A. HANDLER AND D. MICHAEL HUNT
9 *Headache, 94*
   GREGORY L. HENRY
10 *Respiratory Distress, 106*
   STEVEN M. BARRETT
11 *Chest Pain, 120*
   JAMES W. HOEKSTRA

12 *Abdominal Pain, 131*
   ALEXANDER TROTT
13 *Gastrointestinal Bleeding, 142*
   PHILIP L. HENNEMAN
14 *Vomiting, 153*
   GARY L. SWART
15 *Acute Infectious Diarrheal Disease, 165*
   ROBERT A. BITTERMAN
16 *Pelvic Pain, Vaginal Bleeding, and Genital Infection, 174*
   GARY P. YOUNG
17 *Joint and Back Pain, 187*
   DAVID CHUNGSANG LEE
18 *Seizure, 201*
   MICHAEL CHARLES TOMLANOVICH

Part *III*

TRAUMA

19 *Head Trauma, 219*
   PETER PONS
20 *Facial and Oral Trauma, 231*
   DOUGLAS A. RUND
21 *Spinal Injury, 243*
   ROBERT S. HOCKBERGER
22 *Chest Trauma, 254*
   DAVID J. VUKICH

23   *Cardiovascular Trauma, 264*
    VINCENT J. MARKOVCHICK

24   *Abdominal and Genitourinary Trauma, 272*
    JOHN MARX AND ROBERT E. SCHNEIDER

25   *Soft-Tissue Injuries and Lacerations, 283*
    DANIEL R. MARTIN

26   *Orthopedic Injuries, 294*
    JOEL GEIDERMAN

Part *IV*

ENVIRONMENTAL EMERGENCIES

27   *Thermal and Chemical Injuries, 333*
    RICHARD N. NELSON

28   *Electrical and Lightning Injuries, 342*
    MARY ANN COOPER

29   *Near-Drowning, 345*
    ROBERT KNOPP

30   *Heat- and Cold-Induced Injuries, 349*
    DANIEL F. DANZL

Part *V*

SYSTEMIC DISORDERS

SECTION 1   RESPIRATORY SYSTEM

31   *Acute Respiratory Tract Infection, 361*
    JOHN J. KELLEY

32   *Acute Adult Asthma and Exacerbations of Chronic Obstructive Pulmonary Disease, 379*
    RICHARD M. NOWAK AND CHARLES L. EMERMAN

33   *Aspiration and Foreign Bodies, 391*
    PETER PONS

SECTION 2   CARDIOVASCULAR SYSTEM

34   *Deep Venous Thrombosis and Pulmonary Embolism, 395*
    CRAIG F. FEIED

35   *Peripheral Arteriovascular Disease, 410*
    TOM P. AUFDERHEIDE

36   *Ischemic Heart Disease, 421*
    EDWIN CARY PIGMAN

37   *Hypertension, 433*
    JAMES MATHEWS

38   *Congestive Heart Failure, 445*
    STEPHEN R. HAYDEN

39   *Dysrhythmias, 455*
    J. STEPHEN STAPCZYNSKI

SECTION 3   GASTROINTESTINAL SYSTEM

40   *Upper Gastrointestinal Tract Disorders, 472*
    MARCUS L. MARTIN AND LEONARD F. URBANSKI

41   *Lower Gastrointestinal Tract Disorders, 480*
    ROBERT A. BITTERMAN

42   *Disorders of the Liver, Biliary Tract, and Pancreas, 491*
    DAVID A. GUSS

SECTION 4   GENITOURINARY SYSTEM

43   *Acute Genitourinary Disorders, 507*
    ANN L. HARWOOD-NUSS

44   *Renal Failure and Dialysis, 520*
    ALLAN B. WOLFSON AND RICHARD L. MAENZA

45   *Pregnancy, 547*
    JEAN ABBOTT

SECTION 5   HEMATOLOGIC AND ONCOLOGIC DISORDERS

46   *Hematologic Disorders, 556*
    GLENN C. HAMILTON

47   *Oncologic Emergencies, 572*
    MARC BORENSTEIN

SECTION 6   CONNECTIVE TISSUE DISEASES AND DERMATOLOGY

48   *Rheumatology and Connective Tissue Diseases, 577*
    BRUCE K. NEELY AND DOUGLAS A. RUND

49   *Dermatologic Problems, 584*
    GEORGE L. STERNBACH

SECTION 7   NEUROLOGIC PROBLEMS

50   *Stroke, 600*
    RASHMI U. KOTHARI AND WILLIAM G. BARSAN

51   *Vertigo, 608*
    JONATHAN S. OLSHAKER

52   *Meningitis and Encephalitis, 617*
     DAVID W. OLSON AND JAY LANCE KOVAR
53   *Special Neurologic Problems, 628*
     NEAL LITTLE AND MICHAEL G. MIKHAIL

SECTION 8   *EMERGENCY PSYCHIATRY*

54   *Acute Psychosis, 647*
     EUGENE E. KERCHER
55   *Suicide, 656*
     PHILLIP I. BIALECKI
56   *Violence, 660*
     FRANK W. LAVOIE

SECTION 9   *METABOLIC DISORDERS*

57   *Fluids and Electrolytes, 664*
     COREY M. SLOVIS
58   *Endocrine Disorders, 688*
     RITA K. CYDULKA

SECTION 10   *INFECTIOUS DISEASES*

59   *Bacterial Infections, 698*
     THOMAS W. TURBIAK AND JOEL J. REICH
60   *Viral Infections, 716*
     LINDA A. ROBINSON

61   *Human Immunodeficiency Virus Infection
     and AIDS, 726*
     JOANNE WILLIAMS AND DOUGLAS A. RUND
62   *Parasitic Disease, 733*
     RICHARD JOSEPH RYAN AND W. BRIAN GIBLER
63   *Tickborne Illnesses, 748*
     MICHAEL L. VORBROKER

SECTION 11   *TOXICOLOGY*

64   *Toxicology: General Management Principles,
     762*
     MICHAEL T. KELLEY
65   *Specific Toxins, 771*
     DONNA SEGER AND LINDSAY MURRAY

Part VI

SPECIAL PROBLEMS

66   *Pediatric Emergencies, 791*
     ANN M. DIETRICH
67   *Otolaryngologic Emergencies, 822*
     THOMAS OSBORNE STAIR
68   *Disorders of the Eye, 827*
     GERALYNN S. RENNER

Part I
GENERAL CONCEPTS

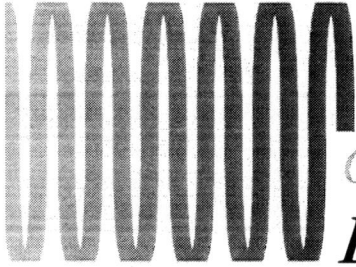

Chapter *One*
EMERGENCY MEDICINE: AN INTRODUCTION

DOUGLAS A. RUND

Emergency medicine is an exciting specialty. The emergency physician is a specialist whose breadth and depth of knowledge and skills spans a wide range of medical conditions in patients of all ages. The effective practice of emergency medicine requires a thorough comprehension of the urgent and emergent assessment and management of conditions that threaten life and limb; the ability to provide immediate care is fundamental.

HISTORY OF THE SPECIALTY

The history of emergency medicine as a distinct medical discipline encompasses the past 50 years, although we question why the specialty did not develop earlier after the Civil War, which demonstrated the need for emergency medical care for battlefield causalities. The genesis of emergency medicine involved several elements and stemmed from a recognition of the unique nature of trauma care and emergency transport, increasing mobility of the population, increased physician medical specialization, and improvements in emergency cardiac care and resuscitation.

During World War II the creation of field hospitals staffed by specialized trauma teams significantly improved the timeliness and effectiveness of field care for combat casualties. Blood transfusions and improvements in the surgical care of the wounded soldier represented innovations that could ultimately be applied in civilian hospitals. During the Korean conflict, the development of radio communication, the battalion aid station, and timely helicopter evacuation to a mobile field hospital (MASH) provided the impetus for future improvements in the medical care of the civilian trauma victim.

Trauma care was further developed during the Vietnam conflict, and the experience produced a cadre of physicians dedicated to improving cardiac casualty care at home. It was widely felt that preventable trauma deaths were occurring needlessly because known improvements in the care of the trauma victim were not being applied uniformly throughout the country. Reflecting this sentiment, the National Academy of Science published the monograph entitled "Accidental Death and Disability: The Neglected Disease of Modern Society" in 1966. In 1972, a group of surgically trained physicians who had been appointed chief of emergency service at various university hospitals recognized the need for scientific and professional exchange and for the development of programs. These physicians formed the University Association for Emergency Medical Services in 1972, which became the Society for Academic Emergency Medicine (SAEM) in 1989.

As trauma care improved, so did emergency cardiac care. The development of external electric cardiac defibrillation in 1956 and the discovery of medications to restore an effective rhythm to the fibrillating heart led eventually to the development of mobile coronary care units such as the "Flying Squad" in Belfast in 1966 and the "Heart Mobile" in Columbus, Ohio in 1969. Such units were originally staffed by physicians and ambulance personnel, which included specially trained firefighters in Columbus and who practiced under specific protocols.

In 1973, Congress enacted the EMS System Act, which established demonstration projects that provided up-to-date emergency medical services throughout the United States. The establishment of prehospital care provided by EMTs and paramedics led eventually to a critical examination of the facilities and medical staffing of the hospital-based "emergency rooms" to which patients were delivered after being resuscitated and temporarily stabilized in the field. Hospital emergency facilities typically consisted of a single treatment room, held one or two stretchers, and were often located on the ground floor of the hospital. These facilities bore little resemblance to those now described as comprehensive emergency *departments*.

The typical medical staff member of a university-based hospital "emergency room" before the 1970s was the intern, who was the most junior member of the hospital's house staff. Thus the paradox developed that the most junior and least experienced physician was caring for probably the sickest and most unstable patients in the hospital. In private hospitals, the situation was almost equally deficient, with staffing being provided on rotation by the medical staff members who took calls from home or within the hospital. If such staff members were specialists in areas remote from emergency pa-

tient care, such as radiology or pathology, the variation in the quality of care provided could be substantial. Alternate staffing may have been provided by "moonlighting" residents who typically worked during evenings and nights for hourly wages.

After 1950, emergency department visits increased dramatically. This pattern reflected a nationwide decrease in general practitioners, increased mobility of the population, a greater need for indigent care, the use of the emergency department by many patients with minor illness as access improved, and better insurance and Medicare coverage for hospital-based emergency treatment in comparison with that paid for office-based care.

One of the first full-time physician groups to staff an emergency department was developed by Mills in Alexandria, Virginia. The success of this arrangement encouraged the development of similar groups throughout the country. In 1968, Wiegenstein and his colleagues founded the American College of Emergency Physicians and in the mid 1970s began working actively toward the establishment of an EM specialty board certification process.

The American Board of Emergency Medicine (ABEM) became the twenty-third medical specialty following its approval by the American Board of Medical Specialties in September of 1979. The first board certification examination in emergency medicine was offered in 1980. The Board to date has certified more than 14,000 emergency physicians. Candidates for certification must successfully pass a written examination, which is followed by an oral examination. Diplomates must recertify every 10 years by successfully completing a recertification examination.

RESIDENCY TRAINING

The first residency program in emergency medicine began with a single resident (Dr. Janiak) at the University of Cincinnati in 1969. Residency training programs soon followed at the University of Southern California, the University of Louisville, the Medical College of Pennsylvania, and the University of Chicago.

There are now well over 100 residency programs throughout the United States and Canada, and these programs graduate 800 emergency medical specialists each year. In the United Kingdom, a separate facility in emergency medicine has been recognized by the Royal College of Surgeons in London and in Edinburgh.

In the United States, residents must complete a minimum training requirement of 36 months in an approved emergency medicine residency program before they can take the ABEM certification examination. A typical residency curriculum includes the following clinical assignments: emergency medicine, intensive care units, pediatrics, trauma surgery, toxicology, orthopedics, neurology/neurosurgery, obstetrics and gynecology, emergency medical services, and electives.

The necessary technical skills and knowledge are acquired during residency training and in practice and are published in texts that outline relevant procedures. Such skills include, but are not limited to, airway control, venous access, diagnostic procedures, and pericardiocentesis/thoracocentesis.

MEDICAL STUDENT EDUCATION

In medical schools, emergency medicine faculty members typically teach topics in emergency resuscitation, basic trauma care, and toxicology. Students taking required or elective courses in emergency medicine usually obtain their clinical experience in the emergency department and gain at least some exposure to the prehospital emergency medical services system. The Macy Foundation Report of 1994 emphasized the importance of coursework in emergency medicine for all medical students.

RESEARCH

Research in emergency medicine focuses on the pathophysiology of acute disease processes and effective intervention, the epidemiology of acute medical events and illnesses seen in the emergency department, and the creation of efficient emergency medical care systems. Researchers in the discipline have substantially advanced the knowledge regarding cardiac and cerebral resuscitation following cardiac arrest, as well as toxicology, shock, wound management, environmental emergencies, emergency airway management, acute infection illnesses, pediatric emergency care, emergency medical services systems, and behavioral emergencies. The publication of research findings in the emergency medicine literature has contributed to the unique body of knowledge encompassed by emergency medicine and demonstrates a universal growth of knowledge in recent years.

INTERFACES

Perhaps more than any other specialty, emergency medicine interfaces with outside agencies and specialties; management is always based on a team approach to care. The emergency medical services system, which is typically headed by emergency physicians, interfaces with police, firefighters, news media, transportation authorities, disaster planning agencies, and others. Within the emergency department, patient care is provided by a team of professionals, including nursing staff; phlebotomists; ECG, respiratory, and radiologic technicians; pharmacists; blood bank and clinical laboratory personnel; social workers; and psychiatric nurses. The emergency physician must also rely on medical colleagues for consultation, postadmission care, and postdischarge follow-up care. Such colleagues include internists, surgeons, gynecologists, pediatricians, family physicians, psychiatrists, and subspecialists in all disciplines.

The overall orchestration of personnel and resources for the immediate care of the acutely ill or injured patient is the responsibility of the emergency physician until an evaluation shows that the patient can be formally transferred to another physician or service.

SUMMARY

The skilled practice of emergency medicine rewards the practitioner with a sense of helping patients requiring urgent or emergent intervention to reduce immediate and long-term problems, relieve pain, and prevent loss of life or limb.

These rewards are sufficient trade off for the satisfaction gained from the continuous care of one's patients over many years. However, experienced emergency physicians do note that a relationship often does develop with patients whose chronic diseases necessitate relatively frequent hospitalizations. The ability to manage several ill patients simultaneously, mobilize and direct a team approach, and prioritize needs for immediate care are skills that provide the emergency physician a long and rewarding career.

Recommended Reading

Rosen P: "History of Emergency Medicine." In *The role of emergency medicine in the future of American health care,* Proceedings of a Conference sponsored by the Josiah Macy, Jr Foundation, Williamsburg, Va, April 17-20, 1994. Published by the Josiah Macy, Jr Foundation, New York, pp 59-79.

Rund DA: *Essentials of Emergency Medicine,* ed 2, Appleton-Century-Crofts, Norwalk, Conn, 1986.

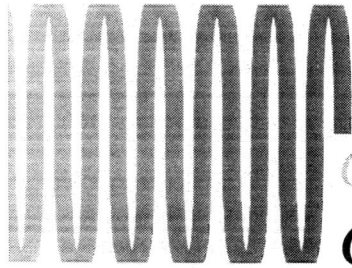

Chapter Two
GENERAL APPROACH TO THE EMERGENCY PATIENT

PETER ROSEN

Emergency medicine is a team sport. Without a constructive design of the emergency system, the patient finds help difficult to obtain. Efficient design requires a full aggregate of communications and transportation personnel, emergency medicine technicians, triage personnel, clerks, nurses, physicians, and ancillary personnel. This design also requires primary treatment areas and referral centers that are committed to providing the facilities and support necessary to the effective practice of emergency medicine. Without good laboratory and radiology facilities, intensive care units, operating suites, inpatient facilities, and follow-up outpatient facilities, it is not possible to practice safe and competent emergency medicine.

At times the potential diseases and disasters may appear to be overwhelming, even when working in an effectively designed and supported system. Therefore the specialty of emergency medicine has evolved as an autonomous medical discipline. In this chapter, we track the patient through an emergency department encounter and describe the generic responses. We assume that the patient has been able to communicate and has been transported to the emergency department. We do not attempt to discuss field considerations and responsibilities; this in no way implies that they are not important but instead reflects this book's focus on the activities of the emergency department itself. Similarly, we spend little effort in defining inpatient or operative treatments.

INITIAL PRIORITIES

The conventional approach to patient problems involves taking a careful history; performing a physical examination; and obtaining laboratory, radiologic, and other diagnostic results to lead to the proof of a specific diagnosis. This approach does not work well in the emergency department because the immediate problem does not involve achieving a specific disease diagnosis but rather managing a final common pathophysiologic derangement that may be identical for many different diseases. For example, respiratory failure is no different if it is caused by pneumonia or fatigue in a patient with asthma. The emergency physician should make a diagnosis if possible and if helpful, but the emergency team has more important priorities than establishing a precise diagnosis (see the box on p. 8).

The first responsibility is to determine which emergency patient is most ill. A billing clerk cannot do this. Patients must be assessed by someone who is not only skilled in the recognition of serious but subtle illnesses but who also has the capacity to avoid becoming involved with the

INITIAL APPROACH TO THE PATIENT

Assess severity of illness or injury
Assign patient to a room
Help patient disrobe
Obtain vital signs

details of care. This assessment has become known as triage.* Although conventionally assigned to a nurse or a technician trained for the task, triage should also be part of the expertise of the emergency physicians.

The next task is to assign the patient to a physical location within the department. Emergency personnel must learn and relearn that placing the patient in a room usually assigned to trivial problems does not mean that the patient cannot harbor serious disease. Unfortunately, once a problem is labeled as trivial, rethinking the case in a more serious fashion is difficult. Nevertheless each member of the emergency department must constantly reassess patients to acquire more than one point on the curve of their disease.

Emergency personnel should help the patient disrobe for examination. There is an unfortunate habit of either not examining patients at all or of confining the examination to only the area of chief complaint. Although a total body physical examination is not necessary for every patient with a sprained finger, it is wise to perform one on all patients with serious complaints.

Obtain the vital signs (blood pressure, pulse, respirations, and temperature) on every patient without exception. We cannot stress enough

---

*Triage is a French battlefield concept and means to sort into three groups: dead or dying, wounded and incapable of fighting, wounded and capable of returning to combat. In modern usage, the three groups are life- or limb-threatened (true emergencies), need treatment within a couple of hours to avoid becoming a life or limb threat (urgent problems), and nonemergencies.

the need for accurate temperature determination, especially in children. Physicians often overlook temperature determination in adults, which results in serious delays in perceiving the magnitude of their problems or in beginning appropriate interventions. With children, take a rectal temperature. Axillary and oral temperatures are simply too inaccurate in children as well as in uncooperative, drugged, drunken, or confused adults.

We find it hard to understand why so many physicians pay little attention to vital signs and then face the unhappy task of trying to explain away abnormalities that should have provided clues to the seriousness of the patient's problems. Although a patient can be seriously ill with what appears to be normal vital signs and may not be seriously ill with abnormalities of the same, it is best to believe abnormal vital signs and search for a serious rather than a trivial cause. Remember also to repeat vital signs in patients who appear ill, because changes in vital signs may provide clues to a worsening of the patient's condition.

KEY QUESTIONS

What is the Life Threat?

Perhaps the most important principle of emergency medicine is to search for and assume to be present the most potentially serious problem for each patient, even if it is statistically improbable.

Thus the first key question will lead you away from an untimely focus on diagnosis. This question is: What is the life threat? Always ask: Are there any life threats, and am I missing anything?

For example, if a patient comes to the emergency department with chest pain, you should attempt to prevent a dysrhythmic arrest, extension of the infarction, or worsening of the patient's disease instead of ordering an immediate ECG to prove the diagnosis of acute myocardial infarction. Therefore your first response must be to place an intravenous line, start the patient on oxygen, and consider antidysrhythmic drugs before proving or disproving the diagnosis.

Does the Patient Need Admission?

The second key question (again before diagnosis) is: Does this patient need admission? Or the question might be phrased: How ill does this patient appear? If you start with the perception that the patient is very ill, not only do you increase the diligence of the search for a cause, but you are also prevented from reaching through tunnel vision for a specific diagnosis that in fact may be incorrect. For example, a patient may look nearly normal after receiving replacement intravenous fluids, but if the patient was in shock in the prehospital setting, more time will be needed to recover than you can arrange in the emergency department. Moreover, you need to communicate to the physician who will be responsible for the in patient care of the patient the perception that the patient is truly ill. You must overcome any work aversion on the part of technicians or physicians who must be called into action in the middle of the night.

Can the Diagnosis Be Supported by the Evidence Available?

A third key question is: Can the diagnosis be supported by the evidence available? One normal ECG tracing does not eliminate the diagnosis of an acute myocardial infarction, nor does a normal white blood cell count rule out a diagnosis of appendicitis. Can you prove what you believe the patient has, or will the diagnosis require other tests that are not available within the emergency department? For instance, more than one patient has been diagnosed as having reflux esophagitis as an explanation for the "indigestion" that was actually a reflection of an inferior wall myocardial infarction. A barium-swallow upper GI x-ray study is not readily available in most emergency departments, but an ECG is. Also surprisingly common are cases in

which all the evidence to support a serious diagnosis and mandate admission is present but is ignored in favor of a trivial diagnosis that cannot be supported but is compatible with the discharge of the patient. An example is sending the patient home with a diagnosis of gastroenteritis when the patient has no nausea, vomiting, or diarrhea but does have a tender abdomen and absent or diminished bowel sounds and is in the age group most common for appendicitis.

What is the Most Serious Diagnosis?

The previous step leads to the fourth key question: What is the most serious diagnosis that could apply to the patient's condition, and have I safely ruled it out? Many physicians appear to have an unwillingness to recognize serious disease, but unless they constantly search for it, it will never be found. Many patients are much sicker than they initially appear, which deceives even experienced physicians who are used to seeing patients late in the course of their disease rather than early on. Wishing that bad diseases would not occur in anyone is human nature, but the ability to be suspicious is integral to the safe and effective practice of emergency medicine.

Have I Arranged a Satisfactory Disposition?

The next key question asks: Have I arranged a satisfactory disposition for the patient? In no other phase of medicine is it so critical to consider the circumstances under which a patient's disease is going to evolve and to obtain more than one point on a curve to determine if a patient is getting worse or better. Physicians have a proclivity for making a definitive diagnosis in instances wherein it would be preferable to beg the question and see the patient again after some evolution of the disease process has occurred. At this point many emergency medicine disasters could be avoided. To either arrange to see the patient again personally, to ensure that the patient will see an appropriate consultant the next morning, or to observe the patient over some time prevents the all too common occurrence of the patient being sent home to die or decompensate into a terrible outcome.

Many times the diagnosis, management, and predicted good outcome of a disease state are foiled by the failure to arrange an appropriate disposition; for example, sending a child with a fracture caused by nonaccidental trauma back to the same environment that produced it in the first place. This example may seem extreme, but it occurs because the physician either does not recognize the child abuse or is content to report it to an appropriate agency and not pursue the next step of trying to assess the environment.

Physicians also appear to have difficulty using a hospital environment for something other than sophisticated diagnosis and treatment. This difficulty, of course, has been compounded by the health planners, various insurance plans, and restrictions on admission. However, some patients need the help of a hospital to recover, and we must overcome our reluctance to use the hospital for sociologic necessities. For example, you may be able to prescribe adequate analgesia for an elderly patient with a stable pelvic fracture, but if that patient lives alone and must climb stairs, discharge is not going to be a satisfactory disposition for that patient. Similarly, a young adult can usually recover from pneumonia when treated as an outpatient, but if that patient is a mother with three small children, she will not have any rest without being placed in the hospital.

Have I Performed a Pertinent and Thorough Work-up?

The next key question is: Have I performed an adequate and pertinent work-up to fit the particular case? Along with getting fooled by the early subtleties of disease, physicians tend to take shortcuts when they become busy in the emergency department. For example, if the patient has not completely disrobed, you may attempt a modified physical examination. If a language barrier exists, you may not persist in finding an

interpreter or in acquiring the historical information that is so often key to good medicine. Moreover, you simply may become lazy. You may conclude that the patient is not seriously ill and neglect to perform the rectal or pelvic examinations that would provide useful information and perhaps steer you in the direction that the patient needs to have you take for safety. You cannot practice perfect medicine, but if you use safe diligence, rarely will a problem remain unrecognized and unidentified.

Why is the Patient Here? Have I Made Him or Her Feel Better?

Another pair of useful questions to ask are: Why is the patient here, and have I made the patient better—both subjectively and objectively? It is often difficult to determine what has changed to make a patient enter an emergency department. Many patients, of course, overestimate the magnitude of their illness, but more commonly, many people underestimate the level of seriousness of their problems. The frustration of trying to deal with illness over a day's time may drive some people to seek attention that night. They usually can tell you what is bothering them, and with a little patience, you can usually find out what they fear. Remember that nobody comes to an emergency department for the same reason they would go out to buy something they want. No emergency department is without inconvenience, pain, and expense, and to be there means that the patient has a need that is acute and requires satisfaction. You may take great pride in your department, but with any honesty, you will be forced to admit that all patients would prefer to be somewhere other than in an emergency department and at your mercy. Keeping this in mind helps to overcome the easy reach for the simple, not serious (and probably wrong) diagnosis.

The second question—Have I made the patient feel better?—addresses something that physicians do poorly in emergency medicine. It may relate to the fact that emergency physicians do not often see patients more than once. A patient may return to the same emergency department but probably will be seen by a totally different team. Many times physicians may be content with making a diagnosis such as viral syndrome and forget that knowing what is wrong does not help a patient feel better. Instead physicians should ask: Can I lower a temperature, restore some fluids, relieve some pain, and provide some reassurance? These things are often overlooked in the pressure to "treat'em and street'em."

On an inpatient service, physicians spend much less time with individual patients than do nurses and in general are unaware that a large part of recovery from any illness is independent of invasive procedures. Physicians are also often fooled by subjective improvements in the patient. It is well known that a ruptured appendix may cause a patient relief from the intense agony that he or she experienced while that organ was under bursting pressure. The patient may therefore describe a feeling of improvement, but objective findings will not support this. Again, physicians should ask. Have the patient's vital signs improved; have the positive physical findings that were so well described by the triage nurse and the initial physical examination improved; do I have an acceptable explanation for why the patient is better? These are the types of facts that physicians need to determine rather than merely breathing a sigh of relief that the patient is no longer a problem.

One source of poor or erroneous decision making that is not recognized is the physical condition and the frame of mind of the emergency physician. Although our specialty has a reputation for nice work schedules, in reality the only nice thing about them is their predictability. Emergency physicians work more nights, late evenings, weekends, and holidays than almost any other medical specialty, and the knowledge about when they are coming to pass does not make them any easier to bear. Night shift fatigue is responsible for many poor decisions and for failure to obtain useful dispositions or consultations because of a misguided desire

to avoid being a burden to other physicians. Although emergency physicians must not abuse their colleagues they must be the advocate for what the patient needs, which often means insisting that the CT scan technician come in from home to do a procedure in the middle of the night or convincing a sleep-protecting colleague that it is not prudent or possible to say that it is safe to send home a patient after only a telephone conversation.

Nor is it only fatigue that plagues effective patient care. A physician, of course, is much more irritable when tired, and it becomes easier to deal with difficult consultants by simply sending the patient out rather than putting up with chronic second guessing. Trying to fix the system by correcting negative behavior in advance of a specific case is worthwhile but can often be a problem when the consulting service is unwilling to address the problems.

Was I Angry When I Made My Decision?

Anger is an emotion that almost always guarantees faulty decision making. It is therefore wise to try to understand the sources of the anger before committing the patient to a final disposition. At times, anger originates from personal life circumstances rather than the professional workplace. Nevertheless, the outcome of the anger can be devastating as professional decisions become incomprehensible. Sometimes an irritating co-worker inspires rage. We have all had the experience of disliking a paramedic, nurse, physician, or other colleague who tells us what is wrong with the patient. We mentally set out to prove that person wrong, but the patient may suffer unnecessarily.

At times, the patients themselves produce the rage. Not all patients are lovable, as we are taught in medical school. They smell bad, they act worse, they do not care about themselves, they produce many of the difficulties for which they seek our care and do not listen to our advice, and they do not treat us with the respect and gratitude we think we deserve.

You do not need to love or even like a patient to deliver professional and competent care, but you must rid yourself of anger and frustration to accomplish this. The goals of emergency medicine are to relieve suffering and to prevent untimely death. All patients are entitled to those goals even if they were themselves the cause of much of that suffering. Learn to reserve judgments on the patients in the emergency department. Let society protect its interests, and let the emergency physician protect the patients' interests. In this way, you will not fail to care for a patient simply because he or she appears to be a drunken derelict. More than one patient who was thought to have simple alcoholic intoxication has harbored something far more serious or was not drunk at all.

Does the Chart Reflect My Thinking?

Charting in the emergency department is a burden. There are too many patients, there are few departments that have a convenient or useful technical system, and there is the plaintiff bar ready to define our medical care by what is written. "Not written, not done" is not a true vision of a busy emergency department. It is not possible to record every phase of a patient's stay in the emergency department. Nevertheless, charting has a purpose and does not need to be as dismal as it often is. The purpose of charting is to provide the points on the curve that measure the natural history of a patient's disease. If you have taken more than a single measurement, you can predict the shape and the slope of the curve. Even if you do see the patient yourself on a return visit, it is unlikely that you will remember any useful details of the previous visit.

The chart must focus on the present problem; you do not need to know if the patient with a finger laceration had chickenpox as a child. However, you should know what the neurovascular function of that finger was before injection of the local anesthetic. The emergency department record is not the junior medical student internal medicine work-up. It is terse and

pointed and contains important negatives and positives. These points vary for each condition. The best way to remember what is important is to ask, What am I seeing, and am I communicating this to someone else in the future? For example, in the infant with diarrhea, how can you indicate the state of hydration without describing the general appearance of the baby, the presence or absence of tears, diaper wetting, skin turgor, fontanelle appearance, and mucous membrane moisture? This description does not take much space or time and when combined with the number of estimated stool productions will help you realize the degree of hydration, if present, and the need for admission.

There is no excuse for the execrable handwriting that physicians think is their due. It truly requires little extra time to produce a legible document. An illegible chart is more a reflection of undesirable arrogance than a heavy workload.

An error that many physicians fall into is to list every possible item in a differential diagnosis, to be "complete." List only those significant diseases that must be considered, as well as how you ruled them out in your mind. Only in this way can you draw a reasonable picture of what you are seeing and thinking. For example, gastroenteritis is a real disease, and patients do come to the emergency department with this. Because it can easily be mistaken for appendicitis, how do you chart to provide information that you considered this? Provide the data that support the diagnosis of gastroenteritis—nausea, vomiting, diarrhea, malaise, increased bowel sounds—as well as why you don't think appendicitis is present, such as no localized or rebound tenderness and a normal rectal examination. This does not mean that you will not occasionally be wrong, but if you have observed the above admonition to ensure an adequate disposition, you will have provided adequate and competent care to the patient. Even if you are wrong, the patient will have a means of being seen in time to correct the error. Your record can certainly help that process if it contains information that depicts an accurate reflection of how the patient appeared during the visit.

The box below summarizes key questions to consider with each patient.

DEALING WITH GRIEF

One of the responsibilities that the emergency physician finds the most difficult is dealing with the grief that is constantly being generated by the difficult problems of emergency medicine. Each specialty has its own unique failures, but for emergency medicine it almost certainly is the sense of failure that develops when the physician is not capable of preventing death. Physicians are so conditioned to thinking that because they can prevent some untimely deaths, they can prevent all deaths. Therefore they may think that the failure to do so is attributable to poor practice, lack of knowledge, or weaknesses of the team.

Physicians also are not taught how to manage grief properly, and therefore the task is uncomfortable. They tend to avoid it by saying they are too busy or that it appropriately is the job of pastors, social workers, nurses, or anyone other than themselves.

However, emergency physicians do have the responsibility, and they can ensure that the grieving process will be healthy if they approach it

correctly. If they shun the responsibility, not only do they increase the risks of making the grieving process a pathologic one but also increase their own sense of failure, raise the prospects that their care will be held responsible for the outcome (even if it were outstanding), and produce problems where they need not exist.

Many people will not believe the details of care, nor will they have an ability to form a realistic impression of how their relative or friend has died if they have not talked to a physician involved in the care. The suddenness of the illness; the lack of prior contact with the emergency staff; and the emotional turmoil of needing to deal with sudden, undesired, and intense loss conspire to produce a delicate balance between sadness and rage. That balance can too easily shift toward rage when the process is not understood or dealt with effectively.

The emergency physician's first responsibility is to come to terms with one's own mortality. This task is much easier for older physicians who may have experienced serious personal disease. The younger person who cannot conceive of personal mortality is much less willing to accept the reality that not all death is preventable with appropriate medical care. Especially with the improvements in prehospital care and the rapid transport times now being achieved, many gravely ill or injured patients are being brought to the emergency department in a critical state. They have not completed the act of dying, and because they appear to be serious but salvageable, much anger and guilt are induced in the emergency staff.

Each physician has particular areas of emotional vulnerability; for some it may be mutilating injury, for others death in childhood. Whatever your vulnerabilities, you can be sure to encounter them in a busy emergency department. It does help to think about those problems; to realize that other members of the team are probably experiencing similar feelings; and to realize that the hardened, cynical, apparently sophisticated facade that the more experienced members of the team seem to possess is proba-

---

KEY QUESTIONS

1. What is the life threat?
2. Does the patient need admission?
3. Can the diagnosis be supported by the evidence available?
4. What is the most serious diagnosis?
5. Have I arranged a satisfactory disposition?
6. Have I performed a pertinent and thorough work-up?
7. Why is the patient here? Have I made him or her feel better?
8. Was I angry when I made my decision?
9. Does the chart reflect my thinking?

bly a defense against emotions that threaten to be overwhelming.

If time permits, discuss emotionally troublesome cases, as well as medically difficult ones. Even if you cannot do this immediately because of the work demands of a busy shift, you usually can accomplish this discussion within the next few shifts. Even a few minutes of ventilation about a particularly stressful death will be helpful, and other team members will almost certainly appreciate a chance to ventilate their own feelings. It is sad that more emergency departments do not have a structure that permits such discussion on a regular basis.

Realizing that you can anticipate a common response to death among the patient's friends and relatives can help you approach them with confidence. The first response to sudden death of a close relative or friend is an emotional shock comparable to a sudden overwhelming physical pain. The whole world disappears except for that pain, and it is truly incapacitating. We have called this the psychic pain spike and have found that we can lessen its amplitude with even brief preparation for the event. Thus during a cardiac arrest resuscitation attempt, we have found it helpful for the nurse, or if possible, a physician, to talk to the relatives and inform them of the gravity of the situation. Even if relatives are not reached until after the death, attempt to prepare them by starting the transmission of the bad news by saying, "I have some very bad news for you." Even a few moments of preparation is better than none.

We prefer to inform people in person rather than over the telephone. However, this is not always possible, such as when we are calling out-of-state relatives. We do always try to have someone present at the remote site who can help with the grief.

There is no good way to attenuate the pain other than to be direct and clear in the communication. Avoid euphemisms for death; they are not always understood, and relatives have left emergency departments not realizing that death has occurred. We recommend a direct state-

ment such as, "I have very bad news. Your father (alternatively the patient's name) is dead."

The psychic pain spike never appears to be absent, even when the patient has died from a long-term and very debilitating illness. In such a case, the end point of death may represent an emotional relief, but the psychic pain spike still occurs. It occurs even when the relative was not close and appears to be an almost universal human response to death.

One of the additional initial emotional responses to death is guilt, and may well play a strong role in the production of the psychic pain spike. Not only do we all have unfinished emotional business with relatives and friends, we have a human need to believe that death or other undesirable events are within our control. We think that if we had just taken an appropriate action, we could have prevented all this from happening. This belief apparently is more tolerable than feeling at the mercy of an indifferent universe. Deal directly with this guilt so that it will not become misdirected at other members of the family or at the emergency personnel. We have found that the most effective approach is to tell the relatives that they were not responsible for what happened, and neither was the emergency team. Tailor the facts to each situation.

Guilt can be particularly difficult to overcome in cases in which the person actually had some responsibility for what occurred, such as child abuse. However, because the emergency team can rarely know the circumstances of the patient's environment, we suggest being nonjudgmental and trying to assuage this relative's guilt as with any other patient.

Often in such a case, guilt is displaced into anger. Although this need not be directed against the emergency medicine personnel, anger may easily be misinterpreted by the emergency department medical teams. By not understanding the above mechanisms and by reacting to the relatives anger with personal anger, the physicians or nurses may cause the relatives' grief and anger to be directed toward themselves. Partially to blame is their own guilt and sense of failure at having been unsuccessful at preventing death or achieving a successful resuscitation. In this case the physician should help the relatives express their anger by allowing some time for ventilation and by carefully reinforcing the impression that medical tasks were carried appropriately.

In most cases, the relatives will wish to view the body. We feel that this can be done after cleaning up some of the mess of the resuscitation. We have been very unwilling to have relatives in the resuscitation room and believe that sending messengers to talk to the relatives during the resuscitation is far more productive and helpful than having close relatives watch an emergency department thoracotomy.

We do not give sedatives except under unusual circumstances that would in our minds define a pathologic grief response. In such a case, we would involve our psychiatric consultation service and might use pharmacology at their advice. In general, however, sedation merely prolongs the grieving process. There is no "normal" response to grief; some people will experience insomnia, whereas others will need to sleep more. Some people will experience great hunger, and others will be anorectic. Reassure all those concerned that no set pattern can be expected but that whatever is experienced will be part of the grieving process.

More resources exist for the immediate hours and days surrounding a death than there will be after some time has passed. At that later time, relatives may well experience some major depression. We always give relatives a contact phone number for such an eventuality.

The immediate postdeath time is not the time for making major life decisions. Tell people to delay the work of reorganizing their lives until they have gotten through some grieving. Suggest that they make a connection with a family pastor, attorney, or close relative or friend who can provide the emotional and practical support that the immediate postdeath period requires.

Most relatives need some advice regarding the appointment of an undertaker, but you need

not specify more than that one need be appointed and that the undertaker will transfer the body from the morgue or coroner's office.

Relatives often express a fear that a relative who is not present is too ill to hear "bad news." We always offer to break the news if someone will bring that relative to the emergency department. If that person is hospitalized, we inform the other relatives that one cannot hide a death forever and that the best place to hear about it would, in fact, be the hospital.

Some families are large and appear to have almost a competitive grieving process, with victory apparently being awarded to the loudest and most visibly affected person. In these situations, we try to see who is the focus of leadership in the family, often a grandparent. We suggest that everyone help each other, but especially that family leader. Often this suggestion ends the competition and produces a more manageable family group. When appropriate, we try to break up incipient fights between feuding family factions by pointing out the opportunity for making peace.

The more you accept this responsibility of emergency medicine, the easier it will become to perform the task well. Emergency medicine has many challenges and emotional burdens. By preparing properly to approach these responsibilities, you can develop the sense of confidence that is imperative to react quickly, effectively, and without fear.

Recommended Reading

Aries P: *The hour of our death,* New York, 1981, Alfred A Knopf.

Dailey RH: Approach to patient in emergency department. In Rosen P et al, editors: *Emergency medicine: concepts and clinical practice,* ed 2, St Louis, 1988, Mosby.

Kubler-Ross E: *On death and dying,* New York, 1969, MacMillan.

Rosen P, Honigman B: Life and death. In Rosen P et al, editors: *Emergency medicine: concepts and clinical practice,* ed 2, St Louis, 1988, Mosby.

Schoenberg B et al, editors: *Loss and grief,* New York, 1970, Columbia University Press.

Chapter *Three*
AIRWAY MANAGEMENT

RON M. WALLS

Airway management is a crucial skill in emergency medicine. There are few areas in emergency practice in which the potential to help the patient is so great and the risks of failure are so high. Airway management is both a technical and a cognitive skill. When working with the patient with a failing airway, often too much focus is placed on the acquisition of technical prowess at the expense of the equally important and far more challenging concepts of decision making. Often the actual technical performance of intubation is the least challenging aspect of the airway intervention because it is usually easier to intubate than to decide whether, exactly when, and by what method to achieve the intubation. Failure to control the airway in a timely fashion can greatly jeopardize a patient who is deteriorating. Procrastination, indecision, and delay can be lethal to the patient with impending airway compromise. A thorough knowledge of the various techniques for airway management, including their indications and contraindications, must be matched by an equally exquisite sense of the timing of intervention and the decisiveness and confidence to act when action is indicated. This chapter will focus on the decision making and methods related to emergency airway management.

DECISION MAKING: INDICATIONS FOR EMERGENCY AIRWAY MANAGEMENT

Two basic approaches can be taken in decision making in the context of emergency airway management. One method is to attempt to generate a list of conditions or circumstances that mandate, or usually mandate, immediate or early airway intervention. The second method involves attempting to construct a thought process or analysis that a clinician can apply at the bedside to reach a rational and reproducible decision to intubate. It is the latter approach that we will stress in this discussion. We will attempt to elaborate on the decision rules that will provide guidance in *all* situations. When one is presented with a case of cardiorespiratory arrest, the decision to intubate is easy; it is obvious that the patient needs intubation. The same can be said of the comatose patient who has a gunshot wound to the head. We would also all agree that it is appropriate to intubate a patient with intracranial hemorrhage and a Glasgow Coma Scale (GCS) score of eight or less, as well as a patient with coma and seizures as a result of cyclic antidepressant overdose. But why? Although these cases are uncontroversial and can build great consensus, what can we learn from them

<table>
<tr><td>

THREE ESSENTIAL QUESTIONS IN ACTIVE AIRWAY MANAGEMENT

1. Is there a failure to maintain or protect the airway?
2. Is there a failure of ventilation or oxygenation?
3. Is there a condition present or a therapy required that by itself mandates airway management?

</td></tr>
</table>

that will help us to decide whether to intubate a patient with a less obvious presentation? What is the cognitive process that is underlying our feeling that it is just *right* to intubate these patients? The solution to the problem lies in three essential questions, which are listed in the box above.

If the answer to any of these questions is "yes," and if the problem cannot be reversed or mitigated by other, simpler means, then intubation is indicated. For example, in the patient with intravenous opioid overdose, the answers to the first two questions may well be "yes," but the administration of intravenous naloxone may correct the problem and obviate the need for active airway management. On the other hand, the comatose patient who is breathing but who has lost protective airway reflexes requires intubation even though ventilation and oxygenation may be perfectly adequate. Clearly the most difficult to answer of these three bedside questions is the third one because it requires a sophisticated knowledge of the natural course of the condition. Does this question require one to generate a list of indications as suggested earlier? The answer is yes and no. Asking the three essential questions at the bedside of the emergency patient is the first stratum of emergency airway decision making. There is a second stratum of decision making—time. After one has asked each of the three questions in the present situation, they must be asked again in the context of what is expected to happen over the next time period. That is, one must ask the following questions:

1. Is there *likely to be* a failure to maintain or protect the airway *over the next 20 minutes?*
2. Is there *likely to be* a failure of ventilation or oxygenation *over the next 20 minutes?*
3. Is there *likely to be* a condition present or a therapy required *over the next 20 minutes* that by itself mandates airway management?

The answers to these time-related questions begin to provide the answer to the third question in the first stratum, because it is precisely those conditions that lead to predictable deterioration or intervention that, *by themselves,* are considered indications for intubation. Consider the patient who has recently taken a severe cyclic antidepressant overdose but who is somnolent, protecting the airway, and breathing adequately. One would assert that this patient mandates intubation because he or she will require gastric lavage in the context of a deteriorating mental status, diminishing airway reflexes, and increasing likelihood of seizure. The knowledge of the natural course of the condition and the required interventions *over time* makes the answer clear.

Of course one could envision circumstances in which the second stratum of questions would be asked with a different time parameter, such as one hour, "the time that it will take to complete the CT scan," or "the time that it will take to transfer the patient by helicopter to the receiving hospital." The incorporation of this second stratum into the decision making prevents the tragic circumstance that arises when a patient has impending airway compromise (e.g., from adult epiglottitis) but is not intubated because of adequate ventilation, oxygenation, and airway maintenance and protection at the time of the evaluation. If the clinician would only ask and answer the question, What is likely to happen over the next 30 minutes? The need for intubation will be established, and the wisdom of performing an early intubation rather than facing a much more difficult later intubation will be evident. An additional benefit of reaching an early decision is that it allows more time to secure assistance in managing the airway, such as by calling in an anesthesiologist. This situation is preferable to being forced into a difficult, flailing intubation 45 minutes later when the predictable airway compromise and patient deterioration have occurred and mandate immediate intubation. Examples of conditions that mandate emergency airway management are shown in the box below. Although the details regarding the precise reasons for intubation in each of these conditions are dealt with in their respective chapters, an application of the analysis above to each of the conditions should clarify the indication.

In most traumatic conditions, intubation is done to take control of an airway that, if not presently compromised, will be compromised as soon as traumatic edema forms. Intubation also relieves the patient of the massive work of respiration. Thus any condition that involves anatomic distortion (e.g., a gunshot wound to the neck) should indicate immediate intubation. If one awaits airway compromise, one will not have the luxury of choosing among the many different techniques of intubation but will instead be struggling to save the compromised patient.

Epiglottitis falls into the category of mandatory airway management. Early in the course of the disease, the patient may appear to have an uncompromised airway. It is difficult for the emergency physician to decide to intubate such a patient aggressively because he or she is spontaneously breathing and because sedation or anesthesia is almost always required. However, to wait for deterioration is unwise. The airway will become increasingly difficult to manage. Having a cricothyroidotomy tray or an intubation set at the bedside does not mean that one will be able to use them appropriately. This is one time in emergency medicine in which the conservative approach is to actively manage the airway before the patient is in trouble.

The patient with multisystem trauma presents a particularly challenging problem. Again, applying the test of time and the knowledge of the natural history of the condition and the interventions will help solve the conundrum. The multisystem trauma patient is often in shock with accumulating metabolic acidosis that is aggravated by a respiratory acidosis as a result of pulmonary parenchymal injury; injury to the chest wall; abdominal distension inhibiting respiration; or decreasing respiratory effort caused by the metabolic acidosis, hypotension, and perhaps head injury or drug or alcohol ingestion. The patient will need multiple interventions, including thoracostomy, peritoneal lavage, and fluid resuscitation. The patient may also go to the CT scanner, where more trouble awaits, or to the operating room for a general anesthetic.

INDICATIONS FOR MANDATORY AIRWAY MANAGEMENT

Trauma

Massive facial injuries (see Chapter 20)
Head injury with Glasgow Coma Scale ≤ 8 (see Chapter 19)
Penetrating injury to the cranial vault (see Chapter 19)
Missile penetrating injury to the neck (see Chapter 21)
Blunt injury to the neck with expanding hematoma or alteration of the voice (see Chapter 21)
Bilateral missile penetrating injuries of the thorax (see Chapter 22)
Multisystem trauma with persistent shock (see Chapter 6)

Nontrauma

Epiglottitis (see Chapters 31 and 66)
Status epilepticus (see Chapter 18)
Cardiac arrest (see Chapter 4)

When one asks at the outset, What is going to happen to this patient? virtually all of the unfolding scenarios support a decision to intubate early because later intubation is clearly inevitable and because early intubation will enhance the patient's chance for survival through correction of hypoxemia, protection against aspiration, reversal of respiratory acidosis (which is particularly detrimental in the context of severe head injury), and facilitation of overall management of the patient.

AIRWAY ASSESSMENT

Airway assessment is the first step in the evaluation and stabilization of every seriously ill or injured patient. The assessment of airway and respiratory integrity can be thought of as two distinct steps: (1) assessment of the airway itself, and (2) assessment of the gas exchange function of the lungs. These two steps are appropriately assigned the "A" and "B" respectively of the well-known "ABCs" of resuscitation. We stated earlier that the decision to intubate is partly predicated on the determination of whether there is a failure to maintain or protect the airway. This focus cannot be overstressed. A patient's inability to maintain or protect the airway carries dire consequences. Failure to maintain the airway leads to obstruction and rapid demise. Failure to protect the airway can permit aspiration of gastric contents, which carries a very significant morbidity and mortality, especially in patients with comorbid conditions or multisystem injury.

Evaluation of the airway consists of determining the structural integrity of the airway and assessing the patient's ability to protect against aspiration. The most valuable first assessment of airway integrity is the quality of the respirations and of the patient's voice. A moment spent determining whether the air is freely traversing the upper airway as the patient breathes and whether there are sounds to indicate the presence of interfering secretions or narrowing air passages establishes with high reliability the functional quality of the airway.

Stridor is a harsh, often musical sound that is produced by the disruption of airflow through a distorted, narrowed upper airway. Stridor is audible without a stethoscope and indicates a severe degree of airway obstruction and the potential for complete loss of the upper airway. Stridor may be caused by obstruction of the oropharynx, such as by retropharyngeal abscess or hematoma; supraglottic area, such as by epiglottitis or allergic edema; the glottis itself, such as from vocal cord edema as a result of infection, trauma, inhalation injury, or allergy; or the subglottic trachea, such as a subglottic hematoma as a result of a stab wound to the lower neck or bacterial tracheitis. Stridor should always be considered an acute airway emergency, and appropriate steps should be taken to deal with the cause of the stridor, to actively manage the airway or, most often, to do both.

Upper airway secretions can also cause noisy breathing, which is often resolved by suctioning and repositioning the patient. A frequent and reversible cause of upper airway obstruction is the patient's own tongue, which the patient is not able to keep from interfering with breathing because of depressed mental status. In this case, repositioning the patient's mandible using the jaw thrust maneuver will reestablish the integrity of the airway. However, the patient has demonstrated his or her inability to protect the airway, and active airway management is indicated. Similarly, the patient who is unable to clear his or her own secretions is at risk for aspiration. Swallowing is a highly integrated function that requires intact protective airway reflexes. The absence of spontaneous swallowing or the inability to perform a coordinated swallowing maneuver on demand indicates a loss of protective airway reflexes.

A second valuable assessment of upper airway integrity is the quality of the patient's voice. A voice that is readily audible and normal in quality argues very strongly for an intact, nearly normal upper airway.

After the quality of the breathing and voice have been assessed, the airway should be visually inspected. The nares should be inspected for edema, foreign bodies, traumatic destruction, hemorrhage, or thermal or inhalation injury. The patient should be instructed to open the mouth to permit inspection of the teeth, tongue, and oropharynx. The patient should extrude the tongue, if possible, for assessment of oropharyngeal access for oral intubation if necessary, as well as for better inspection of the uvula and pharynx for edema, abscess, hematoma, foreign body or injury. The anterior side of the neck should be palpated to determine the integrity of the airway; the presence of subcutaneous air, which indicates direct airway injury; or the presence of extrinsic abscess or hematoma that might compromise the airway.

After the airway is assessed, attention should be turned to the gas exchange capabilities of the lungs. One of the most rapid initial assessments is that of the patient's color. *Color* is a quick clue to ventilatory inadequacy. When the patient exhibits cyanosis, immediate action is mandated. Unfortunately, the absence of cyanosis is no assurance of adequate ventilatory function. The presence of *labored respirations* indicates ventilatory abnormality and should always be considered indicative of respiratory compromise or of serious metabolic derangement, such as acidosis. One must avoid concluding that the patient is demonstrating psychogenic hyperventilation until more serious conditions are excluded. More than one patient with hypoxemia,

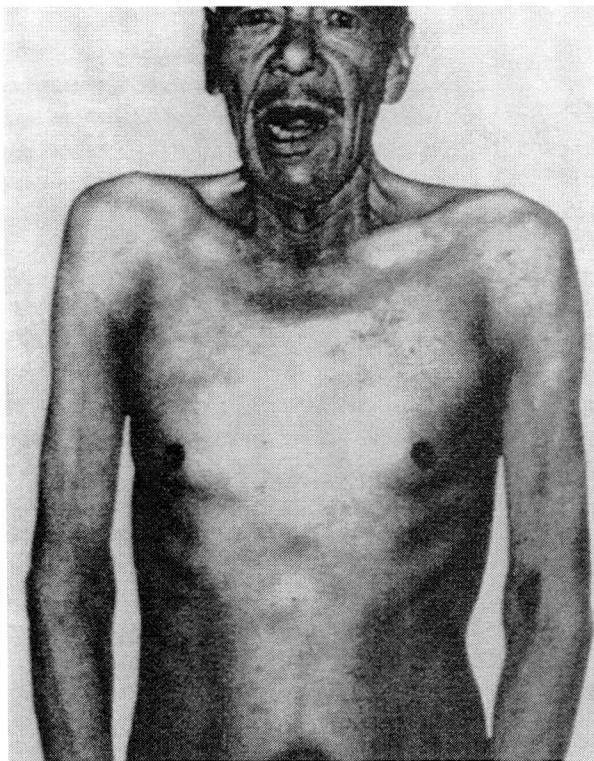

Fig. **3-1**   Pink puffer, type A emphysema.

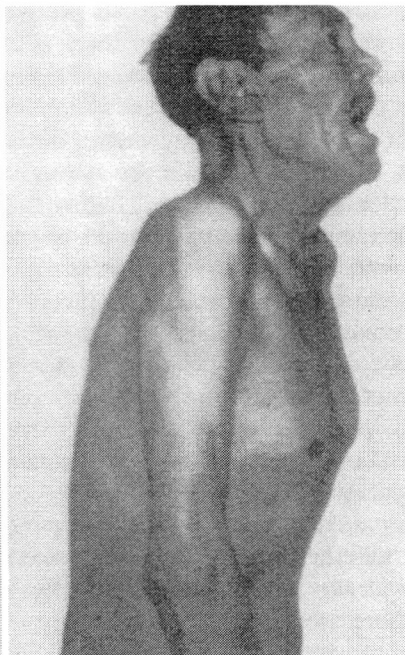

toxin-induced hyperventilation, or profound metabolic acidosis has been given a paper bag to breathe into on the basis of this misguided and dangerous assumption. It is safest to overestimate the hysterical patient as someone who is ill and to proceed to exclude serious underlying conditions.

Retractions, whether intercostal or supraclavicular, are indicative of severe airflow obstruction, and immediate assessment and intervention is mandatory. Although *auscultation* may be misleading, it can be very informative even in a noisy emergency department. If breath sounds are markedly diminished or absent on one side, and if the patient does not have the physical appearance of severe emphysema (Fig. 3-1), one must conclude that the patient has a pneumothorax. Severe respiratory distress with hemodynamic compromise in this setting mandates immediate tube thoracostomy for tension pneumothorax. It is rare for tension pneumothorax to be a bilateral problem, and the absence of breath sounds bilaterally is more suggestive of severe asthma with maximum air trapping and bronchospasm.

Wheezing is an important clinical finding. In general, wheezing refers to the high-pitched sounds that are caused by small airway obstructions and that are audible without a stethoscope. The auscultatory equivalent of wheezing is rhonchi. It is erroneous to assume that all wheezing and rhonchi are caused by reactive airway disease. Wheezing must be interpreted in the context of the patient's situation. For example, a 65-year-old patient who is wheezing for the first time probably has pulmonary edema rather than bronchial asthma.

IMMEDIATE AIRWAY MANAGEMENT

For most conditions that require active airway management, the first decision is whether the patient merely needs oxygen supplementation or whether more active invasive procedures are necessary. In the meantime, appropriate therapy is initiated to relieve the acute respiratory failure. The answer is usually quickly apparent in the adult, except for the patient with chronic respiratory failure and superimposition of an acute failure. In this particular crisis, the patient should be treated with low-flow oxygen while his or her mentation and ability to cough are assessed. If the patient cannot be roused easily and cannot cough, it must be assumed that the patient has achieved dangerous levels of hypoxemia and CO_2 narcosis that require immediate intubation. In this instance, determination of arterial blood–gas tensions is not indicated and will delay the intubation.

Determination of the Route and Method of Intubation

After it has been determined that intubation is needed, the next step is to determine the optimal route and method of intubation. Intubation should be undertaken in a way that maximizes success and minimizes the potential for adverse consequences. The practitioner's own experience and expertise is an important determinant of the route of intubation. One should generally choose a method of intubation with which one is familiar and confident. The patient's condition and anatomic attributes must also be considered. The first choice to be made is between an awake technique, such as nasotracheal intubation or awake oral intubation, and a technique that requires the patient to be unconscious. Blind nasotracheal intubation (BNTI) was enormously popular in the 1970s and 1980s, mainly because of lack of familiarity with neuromuscular blocking agents in the emergency department. However, BNTI is rapidly falling out of favor because of its high complication and failure rates when compared with rapid sequence intubation (RSI). Nevertheless, BNTI remains an important airway technique, and emergency physicians and prehospital providers should be familiar with it.

Awake oral intubation refers to the technique in which the patient is lightly sedated so that airway maintenance and ventilation are preserved; intubation is then performed using generous topical airway anesthesia. This technique is particularly desirable when the patient's anatomic attributes or presenting condition predicts a difficult intubation. By performing the intubation while the patient is awake, the physician avoids the (predicted) circumstance in which a patient has been paralyzed for intubation but cannot be intubated.

Rapid sequence intubation refers to the virtually simultaneous administration of a potent sedative and a neuromuscular blocking agent for the purpose of intubation. With this technique, special steps are taken to protect the patient against adverse events, especially aspiration of gastric contents, and the intubation is achieved promptly after administration of the agents. In general one must decide whether to intubate the patient while awake or to use a rapid sequence technique. The practice of administering potent sedatives (e.g., diazepam or midazolam) to render the patient unconscious for intubation without neuromuscular blockade carries all of the risks of losing airway reflexes and adequate spontaneous ventilation without achieving optimal intubating conditions. Therefore this technique is not recommended. Although it has been asserted that avoiding neuromuscular blockade is "safer," this assertion has never been demonstrated, and studies have shown that neuromuscular blockade affords safer, more rapid intubating conditions.

The primary determinant of whether a patient should be intubated with an awake technique or with RSI is the patient's condition and anatomic attributes. It is essential to assess the patient for difficulty of intubation before deciding whether the patient should be paralyzed for intubation. It should be determined whether the patient has ever had a general anesthetic or any problems with a general anesthetic, is allergic to any medications, or has any serious underlying conditions, such as rheumatoid arthritis, that would confound attempts at intubation. The awake patient often is able to provide this important information, which takes just a few seconds to obtain. The patient should be asked to open the mouth wide, to stick out the tongue, and to move the head and neck around if possible. These movements allow the physician to determine the accessibility to the airway through the mouth and to anticipate problems with cervical or mandibular mobility. Other patient attributes that may predict difficult intubation are listed in the box below. The prediction of a difficult intubation is not a contraindication to RSI, but the emergency physician must be assured of being able to ventilate the lungs in the event of a failed intubation. Difficult intubation combined with anticipated difficult ventilation by bag and mask should lead to a serious consideration of awake intubation as a superior technique for that patient.

The patient's condition may also dictate the appropriate airway approach. In general, a good rule of thumb is "distorted anatomy equals awake intubation." For example, the patient with a hematoma to the neck may be intubated awake in anticipation of difficulty in the event of paralysis for RSI. However, these decisions are not always easy, because the superior con-

---

INDICATIONS OF DIFFICULT INTUBATION

Immobilized trauma patient
Combative patient
Children, especially very small children
Short neck
Prominent upper incisors
Receding mandible
Limited jaw opening
Limited cervical mobility
Upper airway conditions
Facial trauma
Laryngeal trauma

trol of the patient that is afforded by RSI may minimize the likelihood of struggling with increased hemorrhage. Individual judgment is paramount. Some conditions are thought by some to be indications for BNTI over RSI. It is often asserted that patients with pulmonary edema cannot tolerate lying down so should be intubated upright, awake, and with BNTI. Although this facile rationale may have some merit, a contrary position can be stated. The patient with pulmonary edema is generally a poor candidate to tolerate the surge in systemic blood pressure and pulse that attend BNTI, and the incipient hypoxemia may be worsened by BNTI, which usually takes several minutes and precludes the administration of supplemental oxygen. An RSI can be performed in a semisitting position, and drugs can be used to control the sympathetic response to intubation and result in a controlled, rapid attainment of the airway. In addition, the patient usually requires mechanical ventilation, often with positive end-expiratory pressure (PEEP), and so is deeply sedated and often paralyzed after the intubation anyway. Again the driving element in the decision should be a simultaneous consideration of the patient's condition and the experience and capabilities of the physician.

Another condition for which BNTI is often advocated is acute asthma with respiratory failure. BNTI should be avoided with these patients because they are so near death when intubated and cannot tolerate prolonged attempts to secure the airway without supplemental oxygenation and because mechanical ventilation is mandatory after intubation in these cases. The administration of ketamine, which is a dissociative anesthetic agent with bronchodilating properties, and succinylcholine achieves optimal intubating conditions rapidly, assists with direct bronchodilatation, allows oral intubation with an endotracheal tube large enough to facilitate bronchoscopy, and permits administration of additional longer-acting agents to permit long-term mechanical ventilation. Even in the case of

a patient who has overdosed, which has long been the quintessential indication for BNTI, arguments can be made in favor of RSI on the basis of success rates, complication rates, and ease of intubation. Again the individual abilities and experience of the attending emergency physician are central in the decision.

Rapid Sequence Intubation

As previously discussed, RSI is a special technique in which the patient receives virtually simultaneously a potent sedative to induce unconsciousness and a potent neuromuscular blocking agent to induce maximal relaxation for intubation. The technique includes a deliberate preoxygenation phase, in which the patient receives 100% oxygen to allow the apnea induced by the sedative and neuromuscular blocking agent to occur without the need for positive pressure ventilation, which increases the risk of aspiration of gastric contents. Rapid sequence intubation establishes optimal intubating conditions and is a powerful tool in the airway management armamentarium. Familiarity with the indications, contraindications, and nuances of the technique is essential. The emergency physician should be well versed with the pharmacology of the various pretreatments, sedatives, and neuromuscular blocking agents that are required to perform RSI. The basic technique of RSI can be thought of as five steps performed in sequence:
1. Preparation
2. Preoxygenation
3. Pretreatment
4. Paralysis (with sedation)
5. Placement (of the endotracheal tube)
A summary of RSI is presented in the box on pp. 24-25, and the reader is encouraged to seek more detailed information from the relevant sources.

Despite the reluctance by many to use paralyzing agents in the emergency department, the use of such agents is far preferable to fighting with uncooperative and combative patients, es-

RAPID SEQUENCE INTUBATION

1. Preparation.

Assess the patient for difficulty of intubation and bag/mask ventilation. Ensure adequate intravenous access. Test suction. Load the endotracheal tube with a stylet, and test the cuff. Assemble all necessary equipment, and draw up all drugs. Initiate preoxygenation. Establish cardiac and blood pressure monitoring. Initiate pulse oximetry. Establish a plan to execute in the event of an unsuccessful intubation.

2. Preoxygenation.

Apply 100% oxygen by mask for 5 minutes of normal tidal volume breathing. This crucial step replaces the nitrogen reserve in the lungs with oxygen and allows for at least 3 minutes of apnea without significant desaturation in a reasonably healthy adult. It is this step that allows the administration of the succinylcholine and sedative to a spontaneously breathing patient, which allows paralysis and unconsciousness to ensue, then intubation *without interposed mechanical ventilation.* If time does not permit 5 minutes of preoxygenation, approximately 80% of the effect can be achieved by administration of 100% oxygen for three vital capacity breaths (largest breaths that the patient can take).

3. Pretreatment.

In most cases, no pretreatment medication is necessary. In all children under 10 years of age, administer **atropine 0.01 mg/kg IV,** which will prevent the bradycardia induced by succinylcholine in this age group. This step is not necessary in adults. In patients with severe reactive airway disease, consider **lidocaine 1.5 mg/kg IV,** which may reduce the adverse response of the small airways to intubation. **Lidocaine 1.5 mg/kg IV** is also recommended in patients with proven or presumed elevation in intracranial pressure (ICP). Lidocaine in this setting is thought to reduce the ICP response to intubation that would otherwise occur. Also in cases of elevated ICP, administer a precurarizing dose of a competitive neuromuscular blocking agent such as pancuronium or vecuronium. The dose is **pancuronium 0.01 mg/kg IV** or **vecuronium 0.01 mg/kg IV.** This dose is thought to reduce the ICP response to succinylcholine.

4. Paralysis.

Approximately 2 minutes after the administration of the last pretreatment drug, administer a sedative agent and the succinylcholine. The choice of sedative agents is highly individual and might include **thiopental sodium 3 mg/kg IV** or **midazolam 0.1 to 0.3 mg/kg IV** among others. In general, only a single sedative agent should be used, and the agent should be administered rapidly. Immediately following the sedative, administer **succinylcholine 1.5 mg/kg IV.** This potent, depolarizing neuromuscular blocking agent induces intubation-level paralysis universally in 45 to 60 seconds. As soon as the patient begins to lose consciousness and ventilation, have an assistant perform the Sellick maneuver, which is firm posterior displacement of the cricoid cartilage to occlude the esophagus and prevent gastric regurgitation. The Sellick maneuver should remain in place until the endotracheal tube has been placed with the cuff inflated and the position confirmed by auscultation and CO_2 detection. Do not ventilate the lungs during this brief phase of paralysis unless the patient was severely hypoxic before the intubation sequence was begun and the benefits of oxygenation are believed to outweigh the risks of aspiration.

RAPID SEQUENCE INTUBATION—cont'd

5. Placement.

Approximately 45 seconds after administration of the succinylcholine, check the mandible for flaccidity and proceed with intubation. After intubation is achieved, confirm tube placement, release the Sellick maneuver, secure the tube, and obtain a chest radiograph. In addition to auscultation of both lung fields and the epigastric area, a carbon dioxide detection device must be used to confirm tube placement. After intubation is achieved, consider the administration of long-acting neuromuscular blocking agents and sedatives to facilitate ongoing therapy. If the intubation attempt is unsuccessful, continue with the Sellick maneuver and ventilate and oxygenate the lungs with a bag and mask for 30 to 60 seconds before undertaking a second attempt. Continue in this manner until the airway is secured. If neither intubation nor ventilation is successful, a surgical airway or needle cricothyrotomy should be performed immediately.

Warning: Do not use a paralyzing agent if you are not prepared to surgically manage the patient's airway!

pecially when they are intoxicated or drugged and cannot protect their airways. All procedures have complications, and the use of neuromuscular blocking agents is no exception, but the complications of not using them are much greater.

Intubation of the Traumatized Patient

The traumatized patient is often harder to intubate than the nontraumatized patient because one must worry about the integrity of the spinal cord. For 20 years we have been operating under the hypothesis that oral intubation in the multiple trauma patient is unsafe in the presence of cervical spine fracture or when the status of the cervical spine is unknown. There now appear to be data to support a new hypothesis—oral intubation is safe as long as hyperflexion, hyperextension, and distraction at any potential fracture site are avoided. Numerous studies have been published that support the safety and effectiveness of RSI in seriously injured trauma patients, including patients with injured cervical spinal columns. In fact, properly performed RSI may be safer than BNTI in patients with unstable cervical columns. Al-

though BNTI was originally assumed to result in less spinal movement than oral intubation, this belief has not withstood scrutiny, and the superior patient control afforded by RSI is preferable. Again the individual abilities and experience of the attending emergency physician must be considered along with the patient's injuries and attributes.

Complications of Oral Intubation

The most common complication of intubation is failure to place the tube in the right location, which is often caused by placing the tube in the right main stem bronchus. More disastrous is an esophageal intubation. Breath sounds are often not helpful to distinguish the latter, and the use of a CO_2 detection device is mandatory. In cardiopulmonary arrest, CO_2 detection is unreliable, but a positive detection of CO_2 is always meaningful. It may sometimes be necessary to reinsert the laryngoscope to make sure that the tube has in fact passed through the vocal cords. To avoid right main stem intubation, note the centimeter measurements on the tube. The 24 cm mark should be at the lips of an average

COMPLICATIONS OF ORAL INTUBATION

During tube placement

Positioning—cervical strain, dislocation, fracture, neurologic deficit

Dislocation of mandible

Airway trauma
  Dental injury and tooth aspiration
  Oral cavity bleeding
  Epiglottic injury
  Vocal cord injury, including avulsion of arytenoids
  Piriform sinus perforation with pneumomediastinum and pneumothorax
  Tracheal or bronchial rupture with pneumothorax

Induction of vomiting and aspiration

Esophageal intubation with perforation and gastric distension

Right main stem bronchial intubation with hypoxemia and atelectasis

Laryngospasm, hypertension, tachycardia, dysrhythmia

While tube is in place

Tube obstruction (blood, mucus, kinking)

Cuff leakage

Aspiration

Endobronchial intubation

Esophageal intubation

Extubation

Increased airway resistance

"Bucking"—modified coughing with increased intrathoracic, intracranial, and intraocular pressures

Tracheal mucosa ischemia, ulceration

Vocal cord ulceration

Fistula formation (tracheo-innominate, tracheoesophageal)

Pneumothorax, pneumomediastinum

Infection (pneumonia, abscess, mediastinitis)

Following extubation

Laryngospasm—hypoxemia

Aspiration

Pharyngitis

Laryngitis

Laryngeal or subglottic edema

Laryngeal ulceration with or without granuloma formation

Tracheitis

Stenosis (tracheal), subglottic pseudomembrane formation, cord adhesions

Vocal cord paralysis (unilateral or bilateral)

Arytenoid cartilage dislocation

---

adult patient. Careful auscultation and early chest radiography are mandatory to detect main stem bronchus intubation. Other complications are listed in the box above.

PEDIATRIC AIRWAY MANAGEMENT

The pediatric airway has special problems because of its anatomy and the need for special equipment. In most instances, children can be successfully assisted with an appropriate bag. However, adult bags are too large to fit a child's

face well and can generate pressures that cause pneumomediastinum, pneumothorax, and often extreme pressures in either location. In children, it is especially easy to place the tube in the right main stem bronchus. As soon as possible, the location of the tube should be confirmed by listening for breath sounds bilaterally, assessing the color and heart rate of the child, and watching for movement of the chest wall. A portable chest x-ray study should also be obtained as soon as possible to accurately assess the location of the tube.

Blind nasotracheal intubation is difficult to

achieve in most children because of their large tonsils and adenoids and because one must use such a small tube, which makes it difficult to suction and ventilate adequately. Cricothyrotomy is not possible in small children because of the inadequate size of the cricothyroid space and of the airway itself. Needle cricothyrotomy may be an option if one has the appropriate equipment and if there is not total upper airway obstruction, which is a contraindication to this procedure. In general, cricothyroidotomy should not be considered for children under 8 years old unless they are unusually large for their age. With small children, it is safer to perform a careful oral intubation than to attempt a surgical airway. Performing a tracheostomy on a small child is not a simple task. It requires much skill and experience and is fraught with major complications. Table 3-1 shows the recommended endotracheal tube sizes for children from birth to age 12 years, as well as for adults.

Table 3-1

ENDOTRACHEAL TUBE SIZES

Age	Endotracheal Tube Internal Diameter (mm)*
Premature	2.5-3.0
Newborn	2.5 or 3.5
6 months	3.5-4.0
1 year	4.0-4.5
2 years	4.5-5.0
4 years	5.0-5.5
6 years	6.0
8 years	6.5
10 years	7.0
12 years	7.5
Adult	
Men	7.5-9.5
Women	7.0-8.5

*Guideline for age greater than 2 years (up to adult): [Age (yr) + 16] ÷ 4.

KEY CONSIDERATIONS

WHAT IS THE LIFE THREAT?

Loss of airway poses an *immediate* life threat.

DOES THE PATIENT NEED ADMISSION?

Intubated patients require admission to the intensive care unit or the equivalent, where mechanical ventilation and monitoring are available.

WHAT IS THE MOST SERIOUS DIAGNOSIS?

Loss of airway as a result of trauma, cardiac arrest, coma, aspiration, foreign body, epiglottitis, as well as an unrecognized esophageal intubation following an intubation attempt, are the most serious diagnoses.

HAVE I PERFORMED A THOROUGH WORK-UP?

Consider intubation to maintain the airway in cases of trauma, cardiac dysrhythmia, drug overdose, altered mental status, or coma.

Measure pulse oximetry and arterial blood gases as needed to monitor oxygenation.

Consider all routes for intubation and the need for rapid sequence induction.

Perform the Sellick maneuver during intubation.

Assemble all equipment necessary for endotracheal intubation, including preparation for surgical airway if anticipated; preoxygenate; intubate; listen for breath sounds bilaterally over thorax and stomach; and evaluate end tidal CO_2.

Obtain a postintubation chest radiograph and evaluate oxygenation and ventilation with pulse oximetry, arterial blood gases, and ease of ventilation.

Recommended Reading

Hauswald M et al: Cervical spine movement during airway management: cinefluoroscopic appraisal in human cadavers, *Am J Emerg Med* 9:535-538, 1992.

Morris IR: Airway management. In Rosen P et al, editors: *Emergency medicine: concepts and clinical practice,* ed 3, St Louis, 1992, Mosby.

Walls RM: Cricothyroidotomy, *Emerg Med Clin North Am* 6:725-735a, 1988.

Walls RM: The multiple trauma patient. In Dailey RH et al: *The airway: emergency management,* St Louis, 1992, Mosby.

Walls RM: Airway management. In Marx JA, editor: Advances in trauma, *Emerg Med Clin North Am* 11:53-60, 1993.

Walls RM: Rapid sequence intubation in head trauma, *Ann Emerg Med* 22:1008-1013, 1993.

Walls RM: The airway. In Wolfe RE, Moore GP: Pearls, pitfalls, and updates in emergency medicine, *Emerg Clin North Am,* 1997 (in press).

Chapter *Four*
CARDIAC ARREST

NORMAN A. PARADIS

ETIOLOGY

Clinical death is defined as the apparent cessation of ventilation and the loss of pulse and blood pressure. Brain death is the irreversible loss of CNS function and usually occurs within minutes of clinical death. Hypothermia may extend the interval between clinical death and brain death. Four interrelated processes generally lead to clinical death: lack of oxygenation, inadequate oxygen carrier, inadequate cardiac pump, and CNS damage. Cardiopulmonary resuscitation (CPR) and advanced cardiac life support (ACLS) protocols are intended to reverse clinical death before brain death.

Lack of Oxygenation

The failure of oxygen to reach the bloodstream, or hypoxemia, can lead to both cardiac dysrhythmias and CNS damage. Hypoxemia is commonly caused by one or more of the following:

1. Ventilatory insufficiency. This condition is the failure of the mechanics of breathing. Common causes include CNS and neuromuscular disorders that are either intrinsic or caused by trauma, drugs, or metabolic abnormalities. Structural abnormalities of the thorax, such as flail chest and pneumothorax, may also lead to ventilatory insufficiency.
2. Airway obstruction. The most common cause of airway obstruction is the tongue. Other causes include trauma, foreign bodies, inflammation (e.g., laryngeal edema and epiglottitis), tumors, drowning, or inadvertent esophageal intubation (see Chapter 3).
3. Pulmonary dysfunction. This condition involves intrinsic pulmonary disease such as chronic obstructive or interstitial pulmonary diseases, pulmonary edema or embolism, and acute infectious disease processes.

Inadequately Functioning Hemoglobin

An inadequate quantity of oxygen carriers or an inadequate oxygen-carrying capacity may result in end-organ dysfunction and clinical death. Anemia and carbon monoxide poisoning are examples.

Inadequate Cardiac Pump

The most common cardiac event that leads to clinical death is the onset of a sustained dysrhythmia. The most common dysrhythmia that causes sudden death is ventricular fibrillation. Other dysrhythmias are hemodynamically significant bradycardia, ventricular tachycardia, asystole, or pulseless electrical activity (previously called electromechanical dissociation). The likelihood of successfully treating such dysrhythmias during cardiac arrest decreases with time.

Central Nervous System Dysfunction

Primary CNS dysfunction may itself cause ventilatory and cardiac dysfunction and result in clinical death. Causes of CNS dysfunction include trauma, infection, vascular catastrophe, and drugs or toxins.

BASIC CARDIAC LIFE SUPPORT

The techniques of CPR provide ventilatory and circulatory support for the patient who has had a loss of cardiopulmonary function. Delay in initiating CPR decreases the likelihood of neurologically intact survival. *Basic life support* (BLS) refers to the resuscitative techniques used to manage the airway, breathing, and circulation. ACLS refers to the use of special equipment to manage the airway, breathing, and circulation, as well as the provision of definitive care, including defibrillation and pharmacologic therapy to improve organ perfusion and to treat dysrhythmias and acid-base disturbances.

Airway

In treating any unconscious patient, initially establish a patent airway. Airway obstruction is most commonly caused when the base of the relaxed tongue collapses against the posterior pharyngeal wall (Fig. 4-1). Use simple airway maneuvers to relieve this obstruction before using any airway adjuncts. These maneuvers may be all that are necessary to establish airway patency and restore normal respiration.

The most important airway maneuver is the head-tilt (Fig. 4-2), which elevates the tongue from the posterior pharynx. However, it is important to avoid cervical hyperextension in patients with suspected cervical spine injury.

Additional airway maneuvers include forward displacement of the tongue and mandible with the chin-lift or jaw thrust. The jaw thrust (Fig. 4-3) requires the least amount of cervical hyper-

extension. Therefore it is probably the safest maneuver to use on a patient with a suspected neck injury if intervention is necessary before excluding injury with an x-ray study.

Several adjuncts are available to maintain a patent airway. Two of these adjuncts are the oropharyngeal and nasopharyngeal airways (Fig. 4-4). Both are designed to hold the base of the tongue forward and away from the posterior wall of the pharynx.

Breathing

Confirm breathlessness by listening for ventilation while observing the chest from a position above the patient's head. Give two breaths followed by 10 to 12 breaths/minute. Ventilations should last 1 to 1½ seconds, and complete expiration should occur between ventilations.

Mouth-to-mouth and mouth-to-nose ventilation

Establish an airtight seal by placing your mouth around the patient's open mouth. Seal the patient's nose by pinching the nostrils with the thumb and index finger of one hand (Fig. 4-5); the other hand maintains the position of the neck. Mouth-to-nose and mouth-to-stoma ventilations are effective alternatives to mouth-

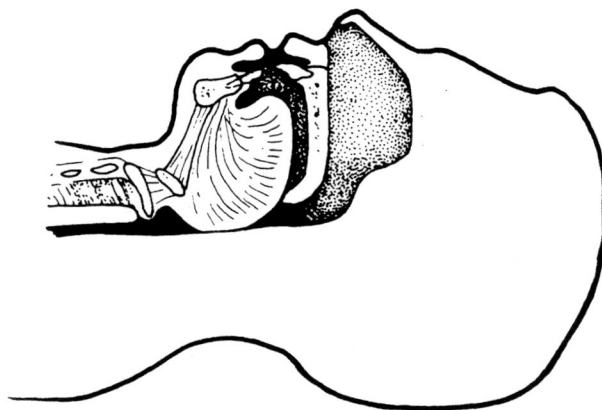

Fig.4-1 Base of relaxed tongue rests against posterior pharynx, causing airway obstruction.

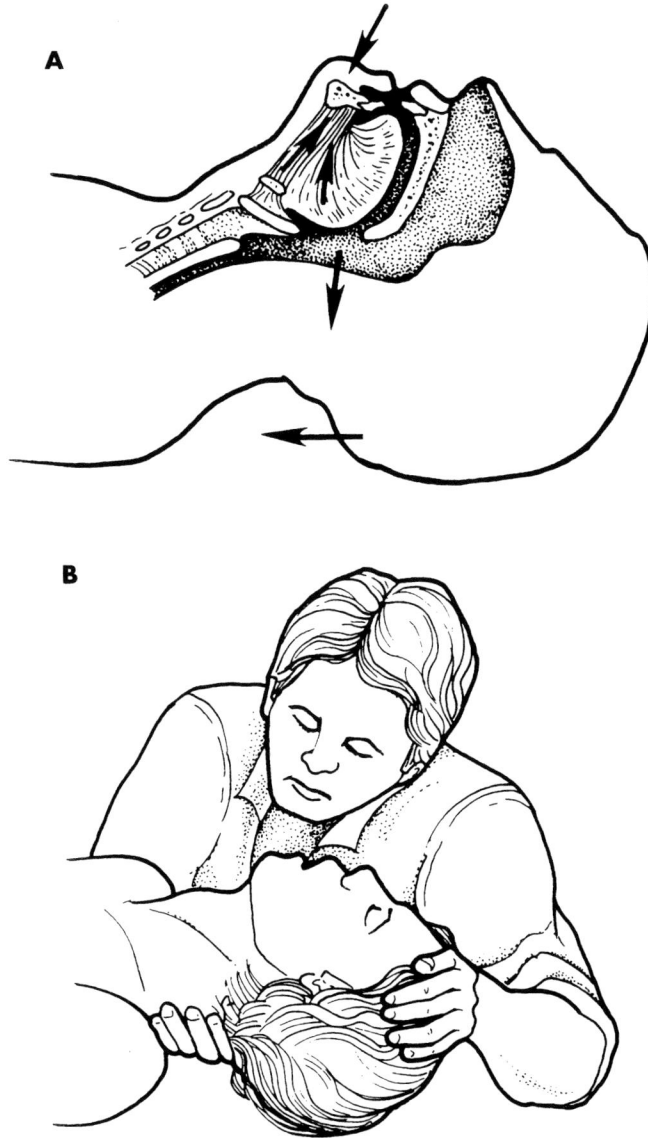

Fig. *4-2*   **A,** Head-tilt lifts tongue from posterior pharynx, opening airway. **B,** Head-tilt method of opening airway. Note position of hands.

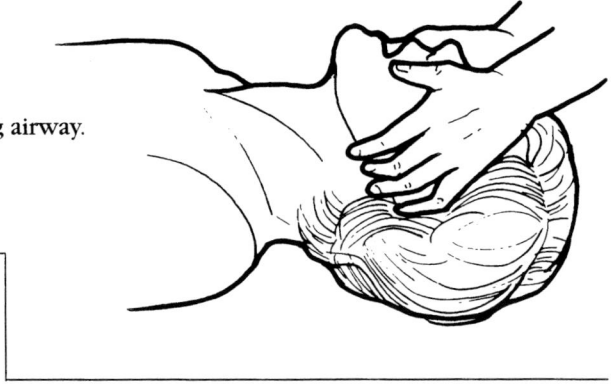

Fig. 4-3   Jaw-thrust method for opening airway.

A

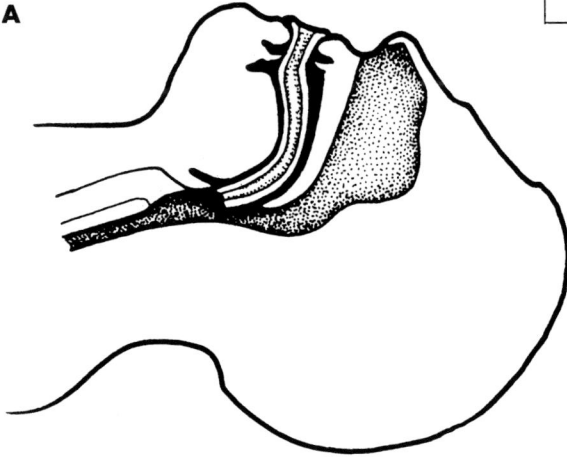

Fig. 4-4   **A,** Oropharyngeal airway. **B,** Nasopharyngeal airway.

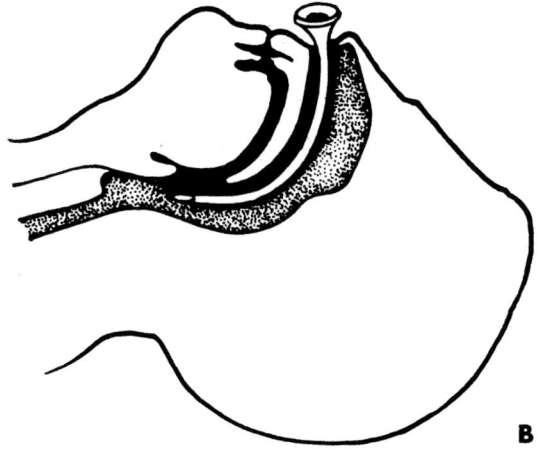

B

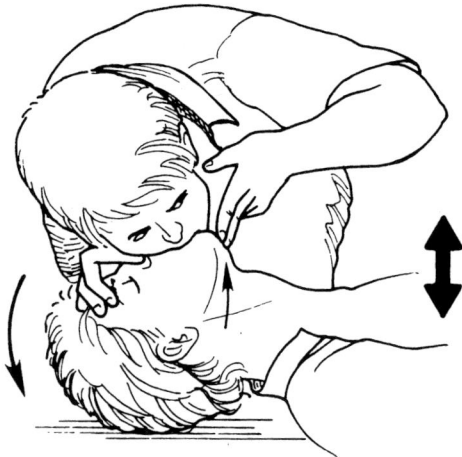

Fig. 4-5   Rescuer performing mouth-to-mouth ventilation. Airway opened with head-tilt/chin-lift maneuver.

to-mouth. Protective barriers are available and
may lower the risk of infection.

Mouth-to-mask ventilation

Mouth-to-mask ventilation provides an alternative to the direct contact with the patient that
the preceding techniques require. An advantage
of mouth-to-mask ventilation is the ability of
some masks, such as the Laerdal pocket mask,
to incorporate high-flow oxygen and provide
the victim with an FiO_2 of 50% or more.

Bag-valve-mask system

The bag-valve-mask (BVM) system consists of
a self-inflating bag with a volume of 1 to 1.5 L, a
nonrebreathing valve, and a mask. This system is
capable of delivering gas mixtures with high
FiO_2. With an oxygen reservoir, the bag-valve-
mask system can provide an FiO_2 of 95% to
100%.

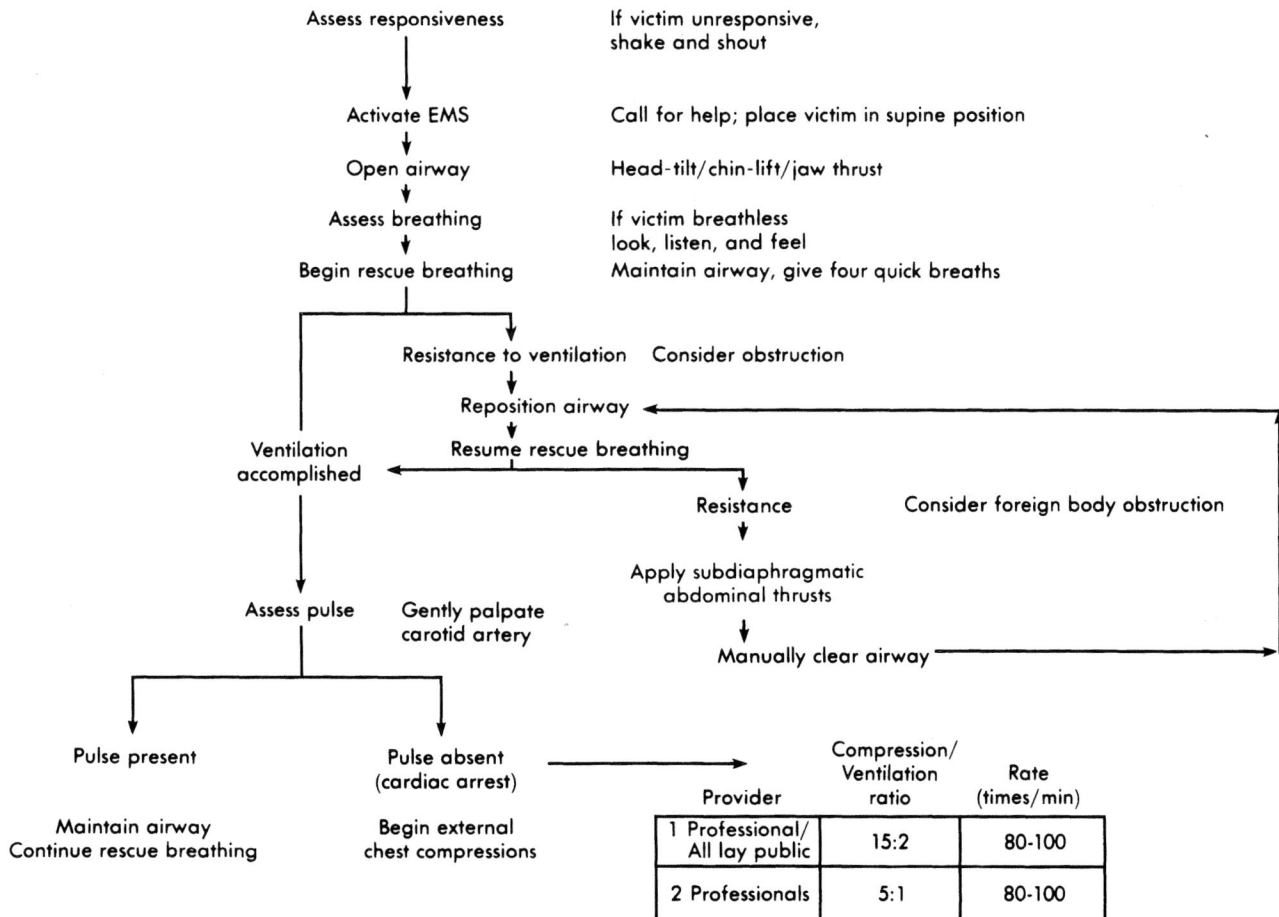

Fig.4-6   Cardiopulmonary resuscitation—basic life support sequence.

Circulation

After establishing the airway and ventilating the lungs, palpate the carotid pulse. If the pulse is absent, start external chest compressions. Fig. 4-6 summarizes the BLS sequence. Position yourself beside the patient's chest. Position the heel of your hand on the patient's sternum. Identify the compression point by locating the xiphisternal junction and measuring two finger breadths cephalad. Place the heel of your second hand directly over your first hand. You may interlock your fingers (Fig. 4-7).

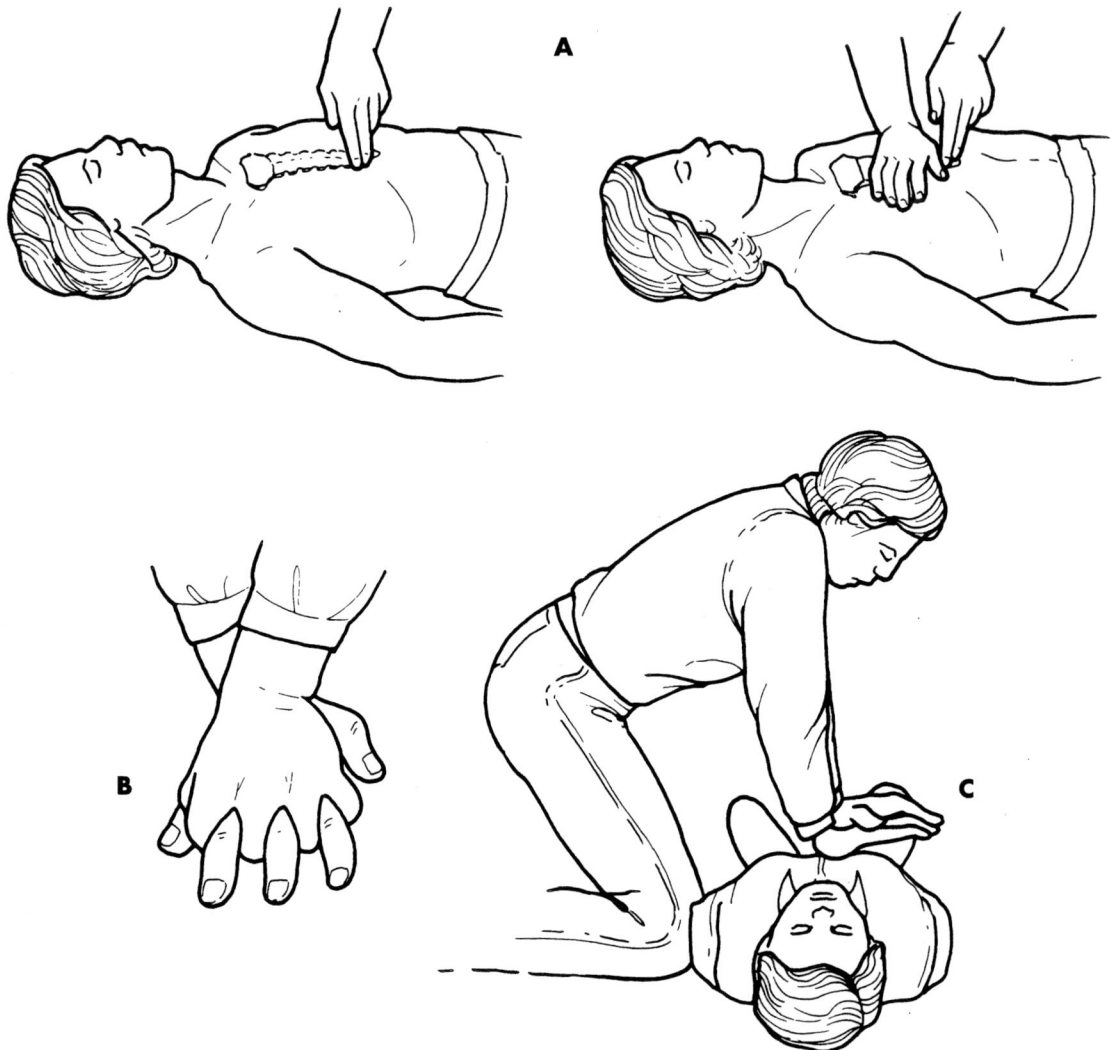

*Fig.*4-7 **A,** Determination of correct hand placement by measurement from xiphoid process. **B,** Technique of interlocking fingers. **C,** Correct position of rescuer. Note rescuer's shoulders directly over patient's sternum.

When providing chest compressions, place your center of gravity over the patient so that the weight of your upper body assists with the compressions for a normal-sized adult, use a depth of compression of 1½ to 2 inches. The duration of compression is half the cycle. During the remainder of the cycle, release sternal pressure completely while retaining correct hand position on the sternum.

The ratio of compressions to ventilations is 5:1 in two-rescuer CPR and 15:2 in single-rescuer CPR. The recommended rate of compressions is 80 to 100 per minute. Palpate for the carotid pulse periodically to determine continued pulselessness.

Perfect technique is not as important as providing forceful compressions. Some authorities believe that applying force in excess of that commonly recommended may improve organ perfusion. It is not uncommon for rib fractures to occur during chest compressions, especially in older patients. Do not interrupt CPR. Under no circumstances should chest compression be performed from an off-center location, because it will not be possible to apply adequate force.

Choking

Recognizing choking is the first step toward successful management of airway obstruction by foreign bodies. The classic signs of foreign body obstruction in the conscious patient include a sudden inability to talk associated with labored respiratory efforts and progressive cyanosis. The patient may also clutch his or her neck.

Current American Heart Association guidelines recommend using the subdiaphragmatic abdominal thrust as the primary method to relieve airway obstruction in all patients above the age of 1 year (Fig. 4–8). In patients with partial obstruction, do not perform abdominal thrusts but instead assist the patient's own ventilatory efforts with back blows. Complete airway obstruction may be distinguished from partial ob-

RELIEVING AIRWAY OBSTRUCTION CAUSED BY FOREIGN BODIES

1. Identify complete airway obstruction.
2. Repeatedly apply subdiaphragmatic abdominal thrusts (see Fig. 4–8) until successful or until the patient becomes unconscious.

If the patient becomes unconscious:

3. Perform jaw thrust followed by finger sweep.
4. Open the airway and attempt rescue breathing.
5. If unable to ventilate, repeat up to 5 subdiaphragmatic abdominal thrusts.
6. Repeat steps 3 and 4.
7. Repeat steps 3, 4, and 5 in sequence and persist as long as necessary.

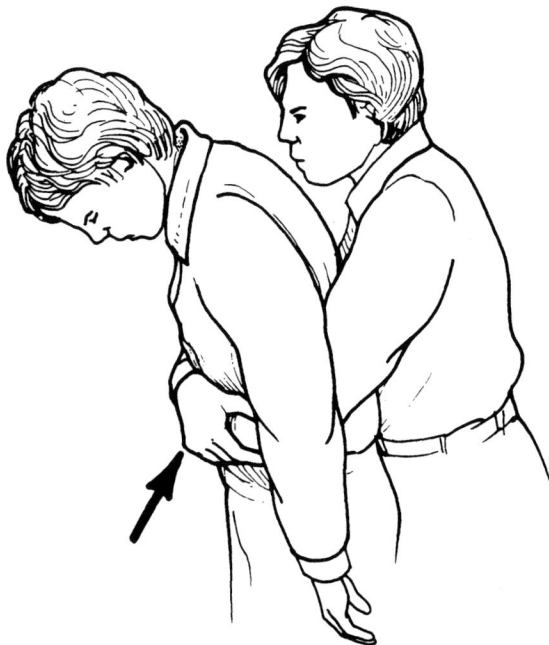

Fig. **4-8**   Subdiaphragmatic abdominal thrust recommended for conscious patient with obstructed airway.

struction by the absence of upper airway sounds with complete obstruction. The box on p. 35 outlines the recommended procedure.

ADVANCED CARDIAC LIFE SUPPORT

After the rescuer has initiated BLS for the patient who is in cardiopulmonary arrest, definitive care requires ACLS therapy. ACLS includes (1) performing endotracheal intubation; (2) establishing intravenous access; (3) using drugs to support vital organ perfusion, suppress dysrhythmias, and correct acidosis; (4) using electrical cardioversion and defibrillation; (5) having the ability to perform certain invasive procedures when necessary, such as pacemaker placement, pericardiocentesis, relief of tension pneumothorax, and open-chest cardiac massage.

Endotracheal Intubation

The airway must be secured by advanced airway management, including endotracheal intubation as discussed in Chapter 3.

Intravenous Access

Always establish intravenous access early in ACLS. However, for the patient who is in ventricular fibrillation, first attempt defibrillation. If possible, assign multiple persons to attempt venous cannulation. Because rescuers usually can start antecubital or other percutaneous peripheral lines rapidly and without complications during a resuscitation, these types of lines are preferred. However, delivery of drugs to the arterial circulation may be less rapid by the peripheral vein route compared with central venous administration. Bolus medications may need to be followed by a flush if they are to reach the central circulation rapidly.

If you cannot establish intravenous access early in the resuscitation, consider the endotra-cheal route for drug delivery. Epinephrine, atropine, lidocaine, and naloxone can be administered effectively with this technique. The technique of intratracheal administration consists of diluting the medication with saline to a volume of 10 ml, instilling it into the endotracheal tube, and facilitating delivery and absorption with five to ten forceful ventilations.

Drug Therapy

Drugs are administered to patients in cardiac arrest to control heart rhythm, elevate blood pressure, improve cardiac output, or treat acid-base imbalances. Current drug therapy does not appear to be as effective as defibrillation, ventilation, or early-bystander CPR. Table 4-1 lists details regarding the most commonly used ACLS drugs.

Recommended Protocols for Defibrillation and Pharmacotherapy

Unmonitored arrest

Perform a precordial thump after confirming apnea and pulselessness. Initiate BLS. As soon as defibrillation equipment becomes available, use direct-reading ("quick-look") paddles to identify the rhythm. If you cannot read the rhythm because of CPR artifact, you can stop CPR for 5 seconds to permit identification of the rhythm. Initiate ACLS.

Ventricular fibrillation

Resuscitation success in patients with ventricular fibrillation (VF) mainly depends on how rapidly effective countershock is applied. Accordingly, current recommendations are for prompt defibrillation before other interventions. The box on p. 38 shows the recommended management sequence.

Appropriate use of the defibrillator as noted in the box requires the following steps:
1. Apply electrode paste.
2. Turn on the defibrillator.

Table 4-1

DRUGS USED IN ADULT CARDIOPULMONARY RESUSCITATION

Drug	Administration	Remarks
Epinephrine	1.0 mg IV push every 3–5 min	Doses as high as 0.2 mg/kg may be effective; may be given intratracheally, but dose may need to be increased significantly
Sodium bicarbonate	1 mEq/kg IV push initially, followed by 0.5 mEq/kg every 10 min as guided by arterial blood gases (ABGs)	May not be effective; ventilation is first-line therapy for acidosis
IV Fluids	As needed to keep lines open	Volume and glucose contraindicated in cardiac arrest
Atropine	For hemodynamically significant bradycardia: 0.5 mg IV push q 5 min; total not to exceed 2 mg For cardiac arrest with bradycardia or asystole: 1 mg IV push repeated in 5 min if needed	Doses of less than 0.5 mg may have paradoxic parasympathomimetic effect; may be given intratracheally in a dose of 1 mg; to be used cautiously in presence of known myocardia ischemia or infarction (to avoid excessive cardiac acceleration)
Lidocaine	For ventricular ectopy and ventricular tachycardia: 1-1.5 mg/kg IV push; additional doses every 5-10 min to a total of 3 mg/kg; with return of perfusion, 1-4 mg/min range For ventricular fibrillation: 1.5 mg/kg IV push	Ventricular fibrillation and ventricular tachycardia refractory to defibrillation, multiform ventricular ectopy, and refibrillation; no longer recommended for all patients with acute myocardial infarction; may be given intratracheally in a dose of 100-200 mg
Bretylium	For refractory ventricular tachycardia: 5-10 mg/kg diluted to 50 ml in D_5W infused over 8-10 min; once loading dose is given, continuous infusion at 1-2 mg/min For refractory ventricular fibrillation: 5-10 mg IV push, may be repeated at 5 min intervals; total loading dose not to exceed 30 mg/kg; follow loading dose with 1-2 mg/min maintenance infusion	Use for treatment of ventricular fibrillation refractory to lidocaine and defibrillation; also for treatment of ventricular tachycardia refractory to lidocaine and procainamide
Procainamide	20 mg/min until dysrhythmia is controlled, hypotension is produced, QRS widens by 50%, or total of 17 mg/kg is given	Recommended when lidocaine is contraindicated or fails to suppress ventricular ectopy; safe in undifferentiated wide-complex tachycardia; may cause hypotension
Calcium chloride	2-4 mg/kg of a 10% solution; repeat in 10 min if needed	Should not be used except in the presence of hyperkalemia, hypocalcemia, and calcium-channel-blocker toxicity.
Dopamine	Initial infusion rate 2-5 μg/kg $\times$ min; pure alpha effect when infused at a rate >20 μg/kg $\times$ min	Drug of choice in treatment of hemodynamically significant hypotension

RECOMMENDED THERAPEUTIC SEQUENCE FOR VENTRICULAR FIBRILLATION

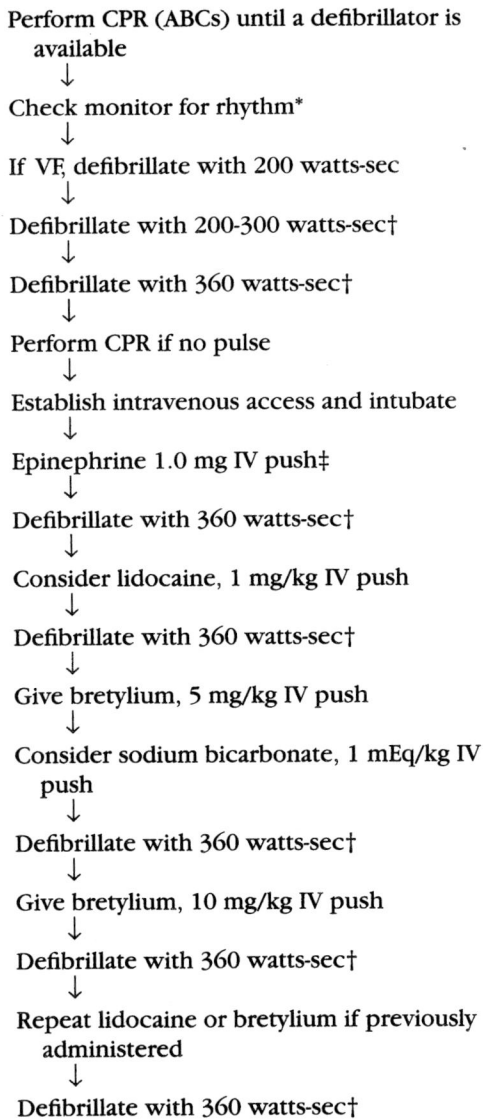

Perform CPR (ABCs) until a defibrillator is available
↓
Check monitor for rhythm*
↓
If VF, defibrillate with 200 watts-sec
↓
Defibrillate with 200-300 watts-sec†
↓
Defibrillate with 360 watts-sec†
↓
Perform CPR if no pulse
↓
Establish intravenous access and intubate
↓
Epinephrine 1.0 mg IV push‡
↓
Defibrillate with 360 watts-sec†
↓
Consider lidocaine, 1 mg/kg IV push
↓
Defibrillate with 360 watts-sec†
↓
Give bretylium, 5 mg/kg IV push
↓
Consider sodium bicarbonate, 1 mEq/kg IV push
↓
Defibrillate with 360 watts-sec†
↓
Give bretylium, 10 mg/kg IV push
↓
Defibrillate with 360 watts-sec†
↓
Repeat lidocaine or bretylium if previously administered
↓
Defibrillate with 360 watts-sec†

---

*Treat pulseless VT identically to VF.
†Check pulse and rhythm after each shock.
‡Repeat epinephrine infusion every 3-5 minutes.

3. Select the energy level.
4. Charge the paddles.
5. Confirm that all personnel are clear.
6. Apply paddles to the patient's chest with 25 pounds of pressure.

Initial countershocks in adults are 200 to 300 watts-sec and 2 watts-sec in children. If VF persists after the initial countershocks, ensure effective CPR, intubate the patient, and ventilate the lungs with 100% oxygen. Establish intravenous access. Epinephrine is the preferred drug in the pharmacotherapy of VF. Repeat the countershock at levels not to exceed 360 watts-sec. In the therapy of refractory ventricular fibrillation, consider lidocaine (1 mg/kg IV bolus) or bretylium (5 to 10 mg/kg IV bolus), followed by repeated attempts at electrical defibrillation.

Postresuscitation antidysrhythmic therapy does not have the primacy it once had, but consider lidocaine after any successful defibrillation unless a specific contraindication exists. Substitute a procainamide or bretylium infusion if you have used either agent successfully during the resuscitation.

Ventricular tachycardia

The box on p. 39 outlines the recommended sequence for the management of ventricular tachycardia (VT). In the hemodynamically stable patient with VT, the preferred intervention is lidocaine therapy. If lidocaine does not control VT, use procainamide. Sustained VT that is unresponsive to pharmacologic measures requires sedation with diazepam, midazolam, or a short-acting barbiturate, as well as synchronized cardioversion starting with an energy level of 100 watts-sec. This level will be successful in approximately 95% of the patients.

Sustained VT, especially when rapid or in the setting of underlying heart disease, may be associated with findings of hemodynamic instability, including hypotension, congestive heart failure, chest pain, respiratory distress, or a deteriorating level of consciousness. In such a patient, perform emergency synchronized cardioversion

---

RECOMMENDED THERAPEUTIC SEQUENCE FOR VENTRICULAR TACHYCARDIA

No pulse→treat as VF

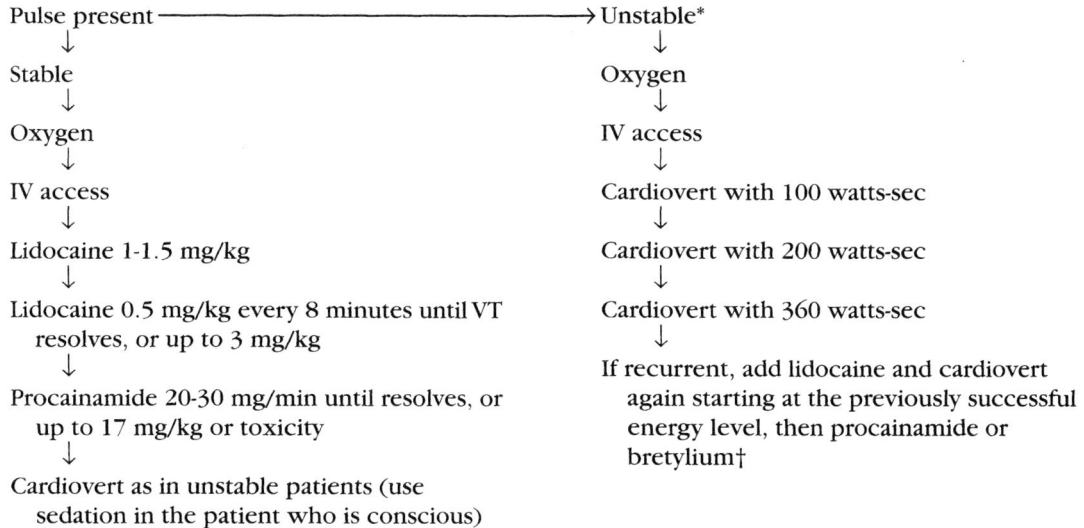

Pulse present ─────────────────────────────→ Unstable*
    ↓   ↓

Stable   Oxygen
  ↓   ↓

Oxygen   IV access
  ↓   ↓

IV access   Cardiovert with 100 watts-sec
  ↓   ↓

Lidocaine 1-1.5 mg/kg   Cardiovert with 200 watts-sec
  ↓   ↓

Lidocaine 0.5 mg/kg every 8 minutes until VT   Cardiovert with 360 watts-sec
  resolves, or up to 3 mg/kg   ↓
  ↓

Procainamide 20-30 mg/min until resolves, or   If recurrent, add lidocaine and cardiovert
  up to 17 mg/kg or toxicity   again starting at the previously successful
  ↓   energy level, then procainamide or
                                       bretylium†

Cardiovert as in unstable patients (use
  sedation in the patient who is conscious)

---

*Unstable—presence of chest pain, hypotension, congestive heart failure, myocardial ischemia or infarction.
†Once VT has resolved, begin an intravenous infusion of the antidysrhythmic agent that aided the resolution.

---

immediately, beginning at 100 watts-sec and increasing as needed.

Any VT that initiates cardiopulmonary arrest is an unstable rhythm that usually degenerates into VF in 1 to 2 minutes. Immediately give the patient who is in cardiopulmonary arrest with VT a countershock of 200 watts-sec, unsynchronized to avoid any delay, with repeat countershocks as for VF.

Asystole

Asystole in cardiopulmonary arrest is usually the result of prolonged VF and global myocardial injury. It is almost invariably fatal, with few patients surviving long enough to be discharged. Rapid control of the airway, adequate ventilation and oxygenation, and well-performed external chest compressions are the mainstays of initial therapy for asystole. As soon as you have established intravenous access, give epinephrine (1.0 mg IV push) to raise peripheral vascular tone and to improve coronary artery perfusion pressure. Accomplish endotracheal intubation, preferably simultaneously with the above interventions. Then administer atropine (1.0 mg IV push) if desired. If asystole persists, attempt cardiac pacing as shown in the box on p. 40.

Various techniques for emergency cardiac pacing have been described but are rarely, if ever, effective. Capture does not commonly result in effective mechanical activity.

RECOMMENDED THERAPEUTIC SEQUENCE FOR ASYSTOLE

Begin CPR
↓
Confirm asystole in two leads
↓
Establish IV access
↓
Epinephrine 1.0 mg IV push*
↓
Endotracheal intubation
↓
Atropine 1.0 mg IV push
↓
Attempt pacing
↓
Stop CPR

---

*Should be repeated every 3-5 minutes.

RECOMMENDED THERAPEUTIC SEQUENCE FOR PULSELESS ELECTRICAL ACTIVITY

Begin CPR
↓
Epinephrine 1.0 mg IV push*
↓
Endotracheal intubation
↓
Give atropine 1 mg IV; repeat every 3-5 minutes
↓
Attempt to treat reversible causes such as hypoxemia, hypovolemia, cardiac tamponade, tension pneumothorax, hyperkalemia, and pulmonary embolism
↓
Give sodium bicarbonate, especially in suspected hyperkalemia
↓
Attempt pacing bradycardic rhythms

---

*Should be repeated every 3-5 minutes.

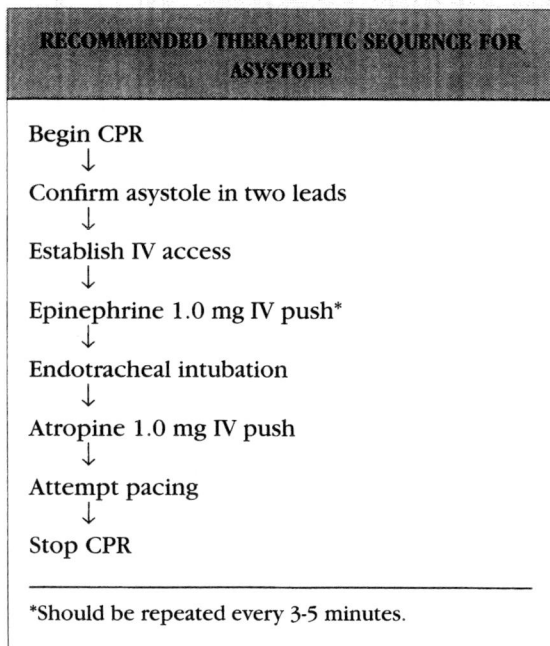

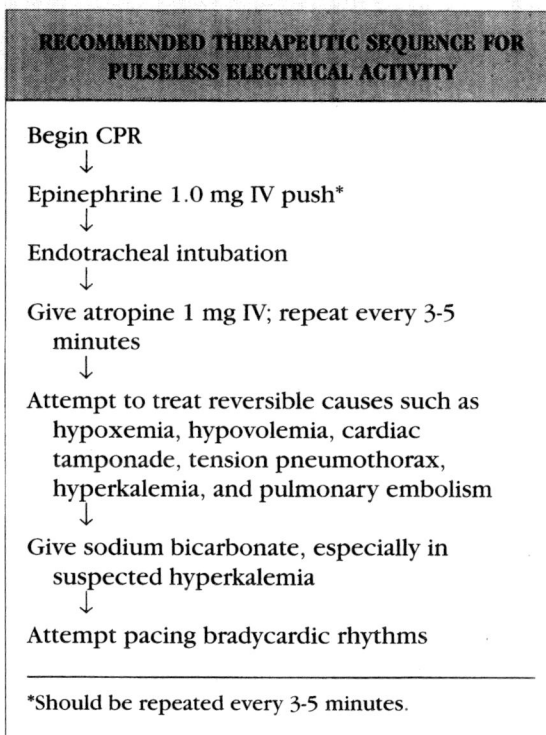

Pulseless electrical activity

Previously called electromechanical dissociation (EMD), pulseless electrical activity (PEA) is characterized by the presence of organized electrical activity on the ECG but without a palpable pulse. The box above, right shows the recommended sequence for resuscitation of PEA. When PEA occurs in cardiac arrest, the prognosis for survival is extremely poor, with few patients surviving to hospital discharge. To avoid overlooking potentially lifesaving therapy, first rule out extracardiac causes. Important reversible causes to consider include hypoxemia, hypovolemia, tension pneumothorax, and cardiac tamponade. Attempt appropriate therapeutic interventions before abandoning CPR.

Treat suspected hypovolemia in the adult with fluid boluses of 300 to 500 ml infused rapidly, and repeat as necessary with careful monitoring of clinical parameters. Empiric placement of a venting catheter or thoracostomy tube is warranted in selected cases.

Do not overlook the possibility of cardiac tamponade during resuscitation of the patient with PEA because pericardial aspiration is a simple and potentially lifesaving procedure. If tamponade is likely to be present, perform pericardiocentesis early in the course of the resuscitation.

After excluding correctable causes, treat PEA by performing CPR, giving the patient 100% oxygen, and establishing IV access. Epinephrine is the mainstay of pharmacologic therapy. If the underlying rhythm is bradycardic, administer atropine.

POSTRESUSCITATION CARE

If the patient who has been resuscitated from cardiac arrest is to have the best chance for a good outcome, there must be a coordinated transition from ACLS to critical care. Patients must be closely monitored during the immediate postresuscitation period, because additional ischemic episodes preclude a good outcome.

Insert an arterial catheter for accurate measurement of intravascular pressure. Obtain blood gases at frequent intervals, and adjust ventilatory parameters to maintain adequate oxygen content and acid-base status. Administer bicarbonate as indicated. Immediate laboratory studies should include ABGs, a complete blood count (CBC), electrolytes, and chest x-ray studies. Administer dopamine or place an aortic counterpulsation balloon to maintain adequate hemodynamics. Attempt to determine the etiology of cardiac arrest, and consider specific therapy such as thrombolytics. Some authorities believe that a brief period of hypertension immediately after the return of spontaneous circulation may improve the outcome in some patients.

The patient's neurologic status during the first few hours after resuscitation does not accurately predict eventual level of function. During this time, full critical care support should be applied unless a terminal preexisting condition is established. Patients who cannot be aroused after the first few days of care have a dismal long-term prognosis, and withdrawal of futile life-sustaining treatment is ethical.

NEONATAL AND PEDIATRIC CARDIOPULMONARY RESUSCITATION

The majority of cardiac arrests in previously healthy infants and children are secondary to ventilatory failure or hypovolemia. Trauma and intoxication are also important causes. Primary cardiac dysrhythmias are rare except in infants and children with congenital cardiac abnormalities. This different etiology results in a different presentation than that seen in adults. Asystole, bradydysrhythmias, supraventricular tachycardia, and PEA are the most common presenting rhythms in infants and children, whereas fewer than 10% develop ventricular tachydysrhythmias. Early recognition of predisposing factors is critically important so that steps can be taken to *prevent* cardiac arrest before it occurs.

Optimal resuscitation of infants and children requires preparation. All personnel must be trained in pediatric life support. Equipment of all sizes must be readily available and stored so that the components needed for a child of a certain size are grouped together.

Resuscitation of infants and children is particularly challenging but very rewarding in successful cases. Variability in the size of infants and children makes medication dosing and the performance of procedures such as intravenous cannulation difficult. The emotional overlay resulting from the sudden deterioration in a child's health status challenges medical personnel. All personnel must make every effort to function as a coherent team or it will be extremely difficult to deliver optimal resuscitation.

Newborn Resuscitation

Neonates who are at a special risk for birth-related asphyxia and apnea include those of less than 36 weeks gestation, small-for-gestational-age neonates, those with heart rate or acid-base abnormalities appearing during fetal monitoring, and those who are born with meconium-stained fluid. Maternal conditions, including hypertension, diabetes, and drug or alcohol abuse, also place the neonate at higher risk. Events during labor and delivery such as prolonged labor, abnormal presentation, and cord compression may precipitate neonatal asphyxia and require resuscitative measures.

Suction the pharynx if necessary. After delivery, rapidly dry the neonate, place him or her under a radiant heat source that maintains a skin temperature of 36.5° C, and ensure tactile stimulation. Administer naloxone if maternal opiate intoxication is suspected.

Airway

After delivery, place the neonate in a slight Trendelenburg's position, with the head and neck in a neutral position. Avoid hyperextending the head, because this can lead to airway obstruction.

After positioning the neonate, gently suction the mouth and nares with a bulb syringe, DeLee catheter, or 8F suction catheter if needed. Vigorous catheter suctioning of the pharynx during the first 5 minutes of life can induce severe bradycardia.

In most neonates, the tactile stimulation of drying and suctioning is sufficient to induce spontaneous and effective respirations. If it does not, provide further stimulation by gently slapping the soles of the feet, and give the neonate oxygen through a face mask. If tactile stimulation and oxygen do not lead to spontaneous ventilation, or if the neonate's respiratory efforts do not maintain a heart rate greater than 100 beats/minute, give the neonate several puffs with an oxygenated bag-valve-mask (BVM), which will usually initiate spontaneous respirations. The first breaths into the nonaerated lung of the neonate may require a pressure of 30 to 40 cm of water to overcome surface tension and displace fetal lung fluid. After expansion, ventilation pressures should be decreased to 10 to 20 cm of water. Visualizing chest expansion and auscultating the breath sounds remain the best guides in assessing the adequacy of ventilation.

If spontaneous breathing remains inadequate, continue to give the neonate assisted ventilation at a rate of 40/minute with a BVM and supplemental oxygen. Warm and humidify the oxygen, and deliver it at an initial flow rate of 5 to 10 L/minute. If this action does not induce spontaneous breathing, perform endotracheal intubation with an appropriately sized, noncuffed endotracheal tube and positive-pressure ventilation.

Endotracheal intubation is the definitive means of securing the airway. However, if you cannot achieve intubation, you can effectively ventilate the neonate's lungs for prolonged periods with a BVM.

Circulation

Heart rate is the primary determinant of cardiac output in the neonate. Initiate chest compression if the heart rate drops below 80 beats/minute and if the neonate does not respond to effective ventilation and oxygenation. Perform closed-chest massage by encircling the thorax with both hands, interlocking the fingertips over the infant's back, and compressing the chest with the thumbs positioned on the sternum just below an imaginary horizontal line between the nipples (Fig. 4-9). This method is preferable if a second person is available to attend to the airway. If only one rescuer is present, perform compressions with the middle and ring fingers on the sternum one fingerbreadth below the nipple line, and place your free hand under the neonate's shoulders to maintain the "sniffing" position (Fig. 4-10). With either method, compress the neonate's sternum ½ to ¾ inch at 120 compressions/minute, and give a breath after every 3 to 5 compressions. Evaluate the adequacy of the cardiac compressions by palpating the brachial or femoral pulse and by observing for improvement in color.

Vascular access

The preferred route for emergency access in the neonate is the umbilical vein. Using sterile technique, this procedure involves trimming the umbilical cord with a scalpel blade approximately 1 cm above the skin, placing a loose tie of umbilical tape around the base of the cord,

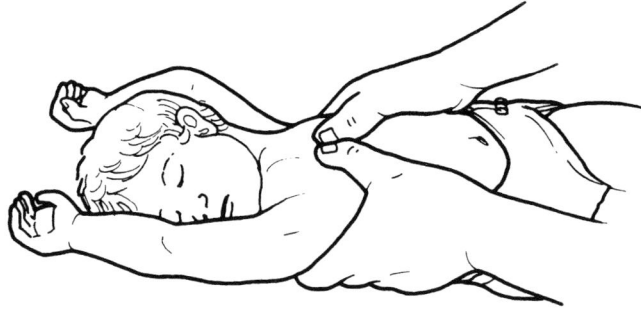

*Fig.*4-9   Chest-encircling technique for neonatal external chest compressions.

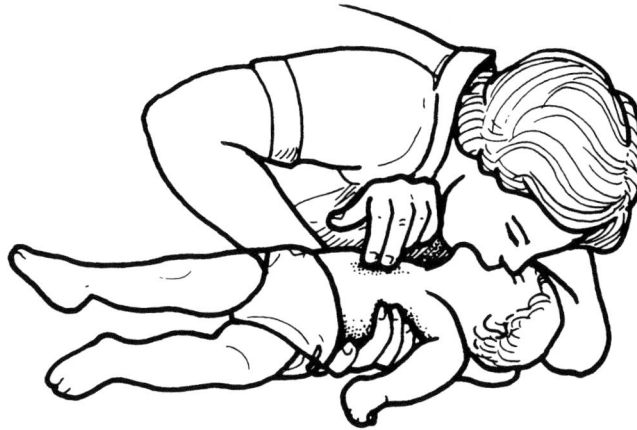

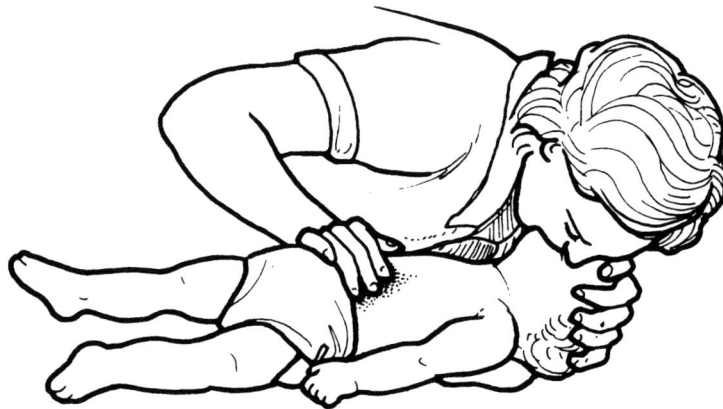

*Fig.*4-10   One-person method of CPR in infants.

and picking up the edge of the thin-walled single vein with iris forceps. Insert a 3.5F or 5F catheter that has been prefilled with saline and fitted with a three-way stopcock into the vein until you obtain a free flow of blood, usually 1 to 2 cm past the abdominal wall. Flush all medications through the catheter because no flow exists through this vessel after cord separation.

Rapidly establishing peripheral intravenous access in infants can be difficult. Attempt cannulation of antecubital, dorsal hand, dorsal feet, external jugular, or scalp veins. Femoral vein cannulation is useful for immediate short-term access. If intravenous cannulation is not rapidly achieved, interosseous access can be rapidly performed under emergency conditions. Insert a spinal, bone marrow, or interosseous needle aseptically into the anterior tibial marrow, and enter the midportion of the bone 1 cm inferior to the tibial tuberosity.

Drug therapy

Myocardial dysfunction and shock in the neonate are usually the result of profound hypoxemia. Therefore initially concentrate on oxygenation and ventilation to correct hypoxemia and acidosis. Administer fluids and medications if the heart rate remains less than 80 beats/minute after initiating chest compressions and adequate ventilation with 100% oxygen.

Table 4-2

DRUGS USED IN NEONATAL CARDIOPULMONARY RESUSCITATION

Drug	Administration	Remarks
Sodium bicarbonate	1-2 mEq/kg slow IV (3-5 min) push initially, then 0.5 mEq/kg q 10 min if needed as guided by pH measurements	Use discouraged in brief arrests; must be diluted 1:1 with D_5W
Epinephrine	0.01-0.03 mg/kg (0.1-0.3 ml/kg of a 1:10,000 solution) IV push q 5 min as needed	May be given intratracheally, 0.02 mg/kg; indicated in asystole or for a spontaneous heart rate of <80 beats/min despite adequate ventilation with 100% O_2 and chest compression
Glucose	2-4 ml/kg of 25% glucose (250 mg/ml) or 0.5 g/kg of a 50% solution IV push followed by infusion of $D_{10}W$, 4 ml/kg/hr	Rapid glucose determination essential in all neonatal resuscitations
Volume expanders	Normal saline: 10-20 ml/kg Whole blood: 10 ml/kg 5% albumin: 10 ml/kg Any may be infused over 5-10 min	Indicated in the presence of hypovolemia
Naloxone	0.1 mg/kg IV push; to repeat 2 to 3 times as needed; can also be given IM, subcutaneously, or intratracheally	Indicated for reversal of narcotic-induced respiratory depression; ventilatory assistance should precede administration; can induce withdrawal in an infant of a narcotic-addicted mother

Table 4-2 summarizes the drugs commonly used in neonatal resuscitation. Avoid using sodium bicarbonate in brief arrests without documentation of metabolic acidosis.

Infant and Child Resuscitation

Cardiac arrest in infants and children has diverse causes such as sudden infant death syndrome, hypovolemia, sepsis, foreign body aspiration, intrinsic airway disease, congenital heart disease, drug ingestion, and drowning. A primary respiratory arrest is the cause in the majority of cases, with subsequent hypoxemia and acidosis leading to cardiovascular collapse.

Airway

Establishing airway patency and providing adequate ventilation is often all that is needed to resuscitate most children and infants. First, open the airway; use the head-tilt/chin-lift maneuver in both infants and children. Begin rescue breathing if opening the airway does not initiate spontaneous breathing or if the child exhibits poor air exchange.

Perform rescue breathing with either a BVM device or mouth-to-mouth ventilation. If you use a BVM, it should consist of a self-inflating bag with a reservoir and, ideally, an in-line manometer to monitor airway pressures. With mouth-to-mouth ventilation, your mouth covers both the nose and mouth of the infant to make a seal. Give older children mouth-to-mouth ventilation in a manner similar to adults. Initially deliver two slow breaths (1 to 1½ seconds/breath), ventilating enough to raise the chest. If you need to continue rescue breathing, use a rate of 20 breaths/minute in both infants and children. Be especially careful to avoid gastric distention; ventilatory volume or force should not exceed that required to visibly raise the chest.

Foreign body aspiration

To remove an aspirated foreign body, deliver six to ten subdiaphragmatic thrusts in rapid se-

quence without preceding back blows until the foreign body is expelled. In children under 1 year, the preferred method is the combination of back blows and chest thrusts, with the infant in a head-down position. Blind finger sweeps are not performed in infants or in children because of the risk of pushing the foreign body back into the airway. Remove the foreign body only after it can be seen.

Endotracheal intubation

Definitive management of the pediatric airway may require endotracheal intubation. However, do not waste time repeatedly attempting to intubate at the expense of continued and correct performance of other methods of ventilatory support. Most children can be adequately ventilated using the BVM system. Precede all intubation attempts with hyperventilation using 100% oxygen.

Correct positioning of the airway is essential, with the "sniffing" position being appropriate for neonates, infants, and small children. Use the head-tilt/chin-lift for the older child. Use straight laryngoscope blades in neonates, infants, and children under 5 years old; use curved blades for older children. Correct endotracheal tube sizes correspond roughly to the diameter of the child's little finger. In children, the narrowest portion of the airway is found below the glottic opening. For this reason, use uncuffed tubes in children under 8 years of age.

Circulation

Opening the airway and administering rescue breathing may be sufficient to initiate spontaneous breathing in the child or infant. However, if spontaneous breathing does not occur, continue rescue breathing and assess the heart rate and pulse by feeling for the carotid pulse in the child or the brachial pulse in the infant. If you cannot obtain the pulse, or if it remains inadequate after you institute respiratory resuscitative efforts, begin cardiac compressions.

Accomplish closed-chest cardiac compres-

Table *4-3*

DRUGS USED IN PEDIATRIC CARDIOPULMONARY RESUSCITATION

Drug	Administration	Remarks
Epinephrine	0.01 mg/kg IV/IO or 0.1 mg/kg ET; subsequent doses 0.1 mg/kg	Doses as high as 0.2 mg/kg may be considered; lower dosage in neonates; be aware of preservative when using large cumulative amounts
Atropine	0.02 mg/kg IV/IO push q 5 min to a total of 0.5 mg in a child and 1 mg in an adolescent; minimum dose 0.1 mg	Used to treat asystole or symptomatic bradycardia; may be given intratracheally
Sodium bicarbonate	1 mEq/kg or $0.3 \times$ kg $\times$ base deficit	To be used in presence of documented metabolic acidosis despite adequate ventilation
Dopamine	2-20 μg/kg $\times$ min	Low-dose (<10 μg/kg) infusions produce beta-adrenergic actions; higher doses produce more alpha effects; indicated for treatment of hypotension or poor perfusion following restoration of circulation in cardiac arrest; indicated in treatment of postresuscitative hypotension and poor peripheral perfusion
Dobutamine	5-20 μg/kg $\times$ min	Inotropic; indicated in child with diminished cardiac output caused by poor myocardial function
Calcium chloride	20 mg/kg IV (0.2 ml/kg of 10% calcium chloride solution); may be repeated in 10 min if needed	Indicated for documented hypocalcemia, hyperkalemia, hypermagnesemia, and calcium-channel–blocker overdose; administer slowly
Lidocaine	1 mg/kg IV push initially, then 20-50 μg/kg/min	Consider in VF, VT, and ventricular ectopy accompanied by hypotension or poor perfusion
Bretylium	5 mg/kg IV; subsequent dose is 10 mg/kg for VF, 5 mg/kg for VT	Indicated in VF and VT that is resistant to defibrillation or cardioversion and lidocaine therapy; rapid IV

sions in infants with either the two-handed chest-encircling method (both thumbs are positioned on the sternum just below the nipple line while a second rescuer attends to the airway) or by compressing the sternum with two or three fingers positioned one fingerbreadth below the nipple line while supporting the infant's shoulders with the free hand (see Figs. 4-9 and 4-10).With either method, compress the infant's sternum ½ to 1 inch at a rate of 100 compressions/minute, with a compression phase equal to at least half of the cycle. In children under 8 years of age, perform cardiac compressions with the heel of one hand placed on the sternum and in a similar position as for adults. Compress the chest 1 to 1½ inches at a rate of 100 compressions/minute. With both infants and children, give a 1- to 1½-second breath after every fifth compression. In children older than 8 years, perform cardiac compressions as in adults.

Defibrillation cardioversion

VF is less common in children than in adults. However attempt defibrillation if you identify VF during the course of resuscitation. Defibrillation in children requires a smaller paddle size, with a 4.5 cm paddle recommended for infants and an 8.0 cm paddle recommended for older children. The recommended energy level for the initial defibrillatory attempt is 2 watts-sec/kg. If this attempt is unsuccessful, make subsequent attempts at double this original level. For cardioversion, the suggested initial energy is 0.2 to 1 watts-sec/kg. Increase the energy level as needed.

Vascular access

Establish access to the circulation as rapidly as possible, using whatever technique is most comfortable. If possible, assign more than one person to attempt vascular access because this procedure can be difficult in small children and neonates. Do not continue with one approach for longer than 90 seconds. Try a percutaneous

Table 4-4

A GUIDE TO ESTIMATING WEIGHT BY AGE IN CHILDREN

Age (yr)	Kg
Neonate	3-4
1	10
3	15
5	20
8	25
10	30
15	50

approach to the veins in the upper or lower extremities, the femoral veins, and the external jugular veins. Attempt a cutdown over the distal saphenous vein if these approaches are not successful. The interosseous route is an excellent approach in children who are less than 6 years old if percutaneous and cutdown procedures do not rapidly establish vascular access.

Drug therapy

Table 4-3 lists the drugs used in ACLS in infants and children. Estimating the approximate weight of the pediatric patient is essential to administering the correct drug dosage. Table 4-4 provides a guide to estimating weight by age.

Nonstandard therapies

Open chest cardiac massage and cardiopulmonary bypass have had only limited use in children and cannot be demonstrated to improve outcome. They may be beneficial in certain situations such as hypothermia. Institutions capable of providing these therapies should prospectively define criteria for their use.

Termination of therapy

The nature of pediatric sudden death invariably makes it difficult for clinicians to terminate therapy. Special situations such as hypothermia may result in good outcomes after prolonged resuscitation. However, the vast majority of normothermic children who remain in cardiac arrest after initial advanced life support therapy have poor outcomes.

In determining whether to continue therapy, look for signs of good end-organ perfusion and viability. Spontaneous ventilations or pupillary reactivity indicate that continued resuscitative efforts are warranted. Consider placement of an arterial catheter to detect cardiac mechanical activity.

Once a poor outcome appears inevitable, attempt to inform the family before actually terminating therapy. However, the decision to stop resuscitation is a medical decision. Do not allow a family's pain to prolong hopeless therapy.

Postresuscitation care

The same principles that govern the management of postresuscitative care in adults apply in children and infants. Because children occasionally make a remarkable recovery after severe insults, initial aggressive care is indicated in all cases.

• • •

The treatment of sudden death is difficult. Diagnosis and treatment most often occur simultaneously and under conditions of extremely limited time and information. In most patients, standard ACLS provides the best available therapy. Physicians must be prepared to individualize therapy if the best possible outcomes are to be obtained. Our current knowledge about the pathophysiology of global ischemia and reperfusion is limited. With a better understanding, our care of these patients may improve.

KEY CONSIDERATIONS

WHAT IS THE LIFE THREAT?

Cardiac arrest is an *immediate* threat to life.

Clinical death or irreversible loss of CNS function occurs within 5 to 10 minutes after the onset of untreated cardiac arrest. A higher survival rate is seen in hypothermic patients.

DOES THE PATIENT NEED ADMISSION?

The patient is admitted to an intensive care unit following successful resuscitation from cardiac arrest.

WHAT IS THE MOST SERIOUS DIAGNOSIS?

The most serious diagnoses are asystole, ventricular fibrillation, pulseless electrical activity, and pulseless ventricular tachycardia. Common causes include myocardial infarction, pulmonary embolism, hypoxemia, acidosis, electrolyte imbalance, hypovolemia, and poisoning.

Search for respiratory impairment in the infant or child who develops cardiac arrest.

HAVE I PERFORMED A THOROUGH WORK-UP?

Use paddles to obtain an early "quick-look" at rhythm on monitor; Use immediate defibrillation if needed

Establish airway by intubation, ensure ventilation and oxygenation, continue mechanical chest compressions, administer medications according to ACLS protocol, and perform electrical cardioversion or defibrillation as needed.

Consider reversible causes of pulseless electrical activity, including hypoxemia, hypovolemia (bleeding), acidosis, pulmonary embolism, cardiac tamponade, or tension pneumothorax.

Recommended Reading

Guidelines for cardiopulmonary resuscitation and emergency cardiac care, JAMA 268(16):2171-2334, 1992.

American Heart Association: *Textbook of advanced cardiac life support,* Dallas, 1994,

American Heart Association, American Academy of Pediatrics: *Textbook of pediatric advanced life support,* Dallas, 1990, The Association.

Baker FJ II, Strauss R, Walter JJ: Cardiac arrest. In Rosen P et al, editors: *Emergency medicine: concepts and clinical practice,* ed 2, St Louis, 1988, Mosby.

Paradis NA, Koscove EM: Epinephrine in cardiac arrest: a critical review, *Ann Emerg Med* 19:1288-1301, 1990.

Chapter *Five*

SHOCK

STEVEN C. DRONEN

PATHOPHYSIOLOGY

Shock is defined as a state of impaired tissue perfusion that occurs secondary to circulatory failure. Although shock has numerous causes, its etiologies are commonly categorized as hypovolemic, cardiogenic, and vasogenic. This schema is based on the three primary sites of circulatory dysfunction: the blood volume, the heart, and the vascular tone. Inadequate blood volume, or hypovolemic shock, may be secondary to acute blood loss or excessive fluid loss through the gastrointestinal tract, kidneys, or skin. Pump failure, or cardiogenic shock, occurs most often as a result of acute myocardial ischemia with secondary loss of cardiac contractility or valvular dysfunction. Other conditions such as tension pneumothorax, cardiac tamponade, pulmonary hypertension, and pulmonary embolus produce cardiogenic shock as a reflection of vascular events that impair cardiac filling or emptying. Shock caused by loss of vascular tone (vasogenic shock) may be produced by sepsis but may also result from injuries to the spinal cord or from anaphylaxis.

Although there are numerous etiologies of shock (see the box on p. 51) and the clinical presentations are quite varied, they all have in common a state of cellular hypoperfusion. This condition may or may not be manifest by hypotension, and it is a common mistake to equate the two conditions. Although hypotension is commonly present, it is an extremely crude index of the state of cellular metabolism. Not all hypotensive patients are in shock; perhaps more importantly, not all patients who are in shock are hypotensive.

The first cellular response to hypoperfusion is an alteration of the cell membrane potential and an increase in sodium influx. Adenosine triphosphate (ATP) is used to maintain the function of the Na-K pump, but during periods of low flow, it cannot be regenerated in sufficient quantities through the normal oxygen-dependent pathway. As the supply of oxygen and energy substrates diminishes, the cells revert to anaerobic metabolism to generate ATP, which results in the accumulation of lactic acid. As ATP availability decreases, sodium continues to enter the cells, which causes progressive swelling of first the cytoplasm, then the endoplasmic reticulum, and finally the mitochondria. Eventually the cells undergo clumping of mitochondria, loss of membrane integrity, and death.

The myriad of physiologic compensatory mechanisms seen with the various forms of shock are all designed to preserve cellular perfusion and prevent cell death. Compensatory mechanisms vary to a certain extent depending on the etiology of shock but commonly involve the cardiovascular, respiratory, renal, and neuroendocrine systems. These mechanisms are

ETIOLOGIC CLASSIFICATION OF SHOCK

Hypovolemic

Hemorrhage
  External: laceration
  Internal: ruptured spleen or liver, vascular injury, fracture (in neonate: intracerebral/intraventricular hemorrhage)
  Gastrointestinal: bleeding ulcer, ruptured viscus, mesenteric hemorrhage
Plasma loss
  Burn
  Inflammation or sepsis: leaky capillary syndrome
  Nephrotic syndrome
  Third spacing: intestinal obstruction, pancreatitis, peritonitis
Fluid and electrolyte loss
  Acute gastroenteritis
  Excessive sweating (cystic fibrosis)
  Renal pathologic condition
Endocrine
  Adrenal insufficiency, adrenal-genital syndrome
  Diabetes mellitus
  Diabetes insipidus
  Hypothyroidism (myxedema coma)

Distributive (vasogenic)

High or normal resistance (increased venous capacitance)
  Septic shock
  Anaphylaxis
  Barbiturate intoxication
Low resistance, vasodilatation: CNS injury (e.g., spinal cord transection)

Cardiogenic

Myocardial insufficiency
  Acute myocardial infarction: critical loss of left ventricular muscle mass
  Structural lesion
  Cardiomyopathy: congestive, hypertrophic, restrictive
  Dysrhythmia: bradycardia, atrioventricular (AV) block, ventricular tachycardia, supraventricular tachycardia
  Drug intoxication
  Postcardiopulmonary bypass
  Myocardial depressant effects of shock
  Hypothermia
Filling or outflow obstruction
  Pericardial tamponade
  Pneumopericardium
  Valvular disease
  Tension pneumothorax
  Pulmonary embolism
  Congenital heart disease, including patent ductus arteriosus (PDA), dependent lesion such as coarctation of the aorta, or critical pulmonary stenosis

presented in greater detail during the discussion of each type of shock. It is important to recognize that although shock is commonly categorized as compensated or uncompensated, this distinction is an artificial dichotomy that is often based on whether the patient is normotensive or hypotensive. There is in fact a somewhat pre-dictable and orderly progression of pathophysiologic events through which the patient passes as cellular perfusion deteriorates. A key to successful management is recognition of the shock state early in its course if possible and before the classical manifestations of hypotension, altered mentation, and acidosis become apparent.

EVALUATION AND MANAGEMENT

The clinical presentation and progression of the disease depend to a great extent on the underlying condition responsible for the shock state. Because of the urgency of the situation and the fact that treatment varies considerably depending on the etiology, a very rapid and well-focused evaluation must be performed, often simultaneously with resuscitation. Evaluation includes not only an assessment of the need for immediate resuscitative measures but also a determination of the cause of shock. In addition to monitoring vital signs, it is routine to monitor a number of parameters such as mentation, skin temperature, capillary refill, and urine output. Laboratory tests that may be appropriate depending on the clinical situation include arterial blood gases, a complete blood count, serum electrolytes, blood urea nitrate (BUN), creatinine, blood sugar, and a urinalysis (see the box below). More sophisticated procedures, such as catheterization of the right side of the heart, are not routinely performed in the emergency department but may be essential in determining both the etiology of shock and the response to therapy.

LABORATORY EVALUATION OF THE PATIENT IN SHOCK

Chemistry: electrolytes, glucose, BUN, creatinine, liver function test, calcium, phosphorus

Hematology: complete blood count (CBC), platelets, coagulation studies (prothrombin time, partial thromboplastin time; if DIC, fibrinogen, fibrin-split products)

ECG, chest x-ray film

Urinalysis

Cultures: blood, urine

Type and crossmatch

Hypovolemic Shock

Hypovolemic shock is caused by a reduction in the circulating blood volume secondary to either acute hemorrhage; excessive loss of fluid through the gastrointestinal tract, kidneys, or skin; impaired fluid intake; or third spacing of fluids. Common clinical features of hypovolemic shock include tachycardia; tachypnea; a narrow pulse pressure; decreased urine output; cool, clammy skin; poor capillary refill; low central venous pressure; and, in the later stages, hypotension and altered mentation. Hypovolemia is perhaps the most easily identifiable etiology of shock because there is often a clinically apparent source of volume loss.

Hemorrhagic shock most often accompanies blunt or penetrating trauma and is generally the presumed cause of shock in the trauma patient. However, as previously stated, alternative causes of shock include cardiac tamponade (distinguished by elevated central venous pressure), tension pneumothorax (distinguished by unilaterally diminished breath sounds), and spinal cord injury (distinguished by the presence of neurologic deficits, warm skin, and a lower-than-expected pulse rate). Nontraumatic sources of hemorrhagic shock that are relatively common and may be overlooked include a ruptured aortic aneurysm and a ruptured ectopic pregnancy.

Patients with shock secondary to excessive loss or impaired intake of fluid also tend to have a characteristic history and physical examination features. Features of the history that suggest fluid imbalance may include vomiting, diarrhea, abdominal pain, excessive thirst, and increased or decreased urine output. There may be a prior history of diabetes, diuretic use, neurologic disorders such as stroke or dementia, or psychiatric disorders such as anorexia or bulimia. Common clinical features include tachycardia, a narrow pulse pressure, dry skin and mucous membranes, a normal or elevated hematocrit, and an elevated BUN.

Standard treatment of hypovolemic shock includes maintenance of ventilation and oxygenation, correction of the underlying disease, control of the source of volume loss, placement of large-bore intravenous lines, and rapid volume replacement with crystalloid or blood. Items that should be monitored often or continuously include vital signs, mentation, skin temperature, capillary refill, pulse oxymetry, and urine output. Central venous pressures may be of some value in judging the response to therapy. Catheterization of the right side of the heart is usually not necessary during the early management of hypovolemic shock except in elderly patients who may have significant myocardial disease.

Initial fluid therapy of hypovolemic shock is rapid infusion of 20 to 40 ml/kg of crystalloid. A prompt response to crystalloid infusion is characteristic of hypovolemic shock. Therefore a failure to respond may indicate the need for rapid surgical intervention (in the case of acute hemorrhage), red cell replacement, and correction of concurrent electrolyte abnormalities. A failure to respond may also lead to a consideration of other diagnoses.

A blood transfusion is indicated early in the treatment of acute hemorrhage for patients in extremis (systolic blood pressure of 60 or less, CNS dysfunction, ventilatory failure), those with evidence of ongoing rapid blood loss, and those who fail to respond adequately to a 30 ml/kg infusion of crystalloid. A judgment is commonly required whether to administer O-negative blood or type-specific blood or to wait for a full type and crossmatch. O-negative blood is generally reserved for the patient in extremis who truly cannot wait for type-specific blood to arrive. This decision must be tailored to the efficiency of the local blood bank in providing type-specific blood. The 5-minute delivery time that is commonly advertised often becomes 10 or 15 minutes in actual practice. Type-specific blood is indicated in patients who are profoundly hypotensive on their initial presentation, those who remain hypotensive after crystalloid infusion, and those who demonstrate rapid ongoing hemorrhage. The safety of type-specific blood for the treatment of acute hemorrhage has been well documented in clinical studies. Transfusion of autologous blood to patients with a massive intrathoracic or intraperitoneal hemorrhage is an option in centers that possess the appropriate equipment and expertise. To prevent a precipitous drop in core body temperature, blood warmers should be used whenever possible in patients receiving more than 4 units of blood.

A number of commercially available asanguinous colloid solutions can be used to treat hypovolemic shock, including albumin, dextran 70, and hydroxyethyl starch. These are excellent volume expanders, and with the exception of albumin, they remain in the intravascular compartment for a prolonged period. There is, however, no evidence that colloid administration improves outcome over standard crystalloid resuscitation, and there are no well-defined indications for the use of colloids in the acute resuscitation of hypovolemic shock.

The combination of 7.5% hypertonic saline and dextran 70 (HTS/Dex) is an agent that has shown considerable promise in animal studies of acute hemorrhage. When given in small amounts, this agent causes a prompt and long-lasting shift of fluid from the interstitial to the intravascular compartments. Thus HTS/Dex may be an ideal agent for the early treatmetn of acute hemorrhage. Clinical studies have not yet demonstrated an improvement in outcome with this agent, but there may be particular injury patterns (such as combined hypovolemia and head injury) in which a benefit may exist.

Fresh-frozen plasma and platelets may be indicated to rapidly correct coagulation defects in patients who are receiving massive transfusions (equivalent to one blood volume, or 70 to 80 ml/kg). One unit of fresh-frozen plasma and five platelet packs are often administered for every 5 to 10 units of whole blood. However, these are general guidelines, and transfusion of these agents is based ideally on clinical evidence of impaired homeostasis and frequent monitoring of coagulation parameters.

The application of military antishock trousers (MAST pants) were once considered standard therapy in the treatment of hypovolemic shock, but their use has not been shown to be of any benefit. The use of MAST pants has been abandoned at most centers.

Cardiogenic Shock

Cardiogenic shock is most often caused by a loss of contractile force of the myocardium, which results in a decreased ejection fraction and cardiac output. Cardiogenic shock is primarily the result of ischemic heart disease and acute infarction of the myocardium. A vicious cycle of myocardial hypoperfusion and impaired contractility (Fig. 5-1) ensues, which has a mortality rate of approximately 70%. It is generally agreed that cardiogenic shock does not occur until 40% or more of the ventricular mass has been damaged. Therefore it is not surprising that cardiogenic shock occurs most often in patients who have had one or more prior infarc-

tions and in those with disease of the left anterior descending coronary artery. Autopsies commonly demonstrate involvement of the left ventricle and myocardial apex.

Although most patients develop cardiogenic shock as a result of impaired contractility, a small percentage do so because of mechanical abnormalities caused by infarction, such as papillary muscle dysfunction or rupture of the ventricular septum or wall. Shock may also occur with right ventricular infarction because the injured ventricle is unable to generate sufficient flow through the pulmonary circuit to the left ventricle.

Patients with cardiogenic shock often have chest pain or other symptoms that suggest acute myocardial ischemia. Often they initially present without evidence of shock and deteriorate rapidly while in the emergency department. Clinical features of the patient in cardiogenic shock include hypotension; a narrow pulse pressure; tachycardia; tachypnea; cool, clammy skin; agitation or confusion; peripheral cyanosis; a gal-

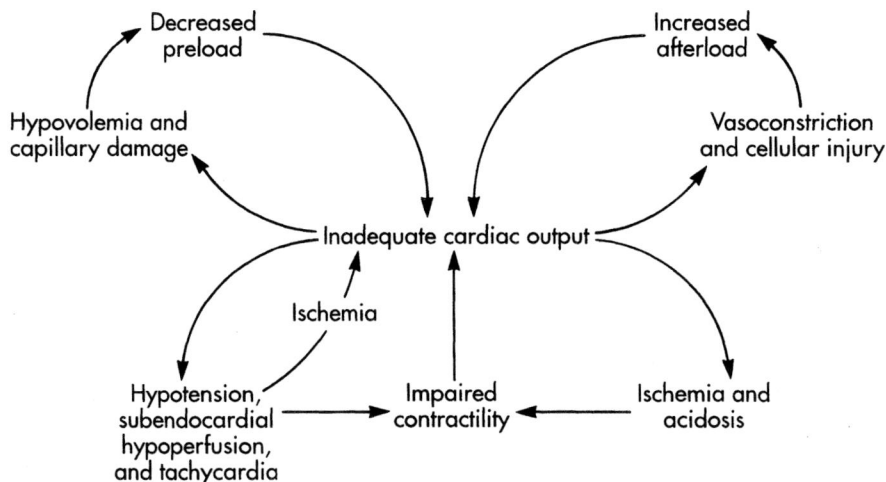

Fig.5-1 Pathophysiology of the effect of shock on cardiac function. (Modified from Shine KI, Kuhn M, Young LS, Tillisch JH: *Ann Intern Med* 93:723, 1980.)

lop rhythm; jugular venous distention; pulmonary rales; and decreased urine output. A chest x-ray study often shows cardiomegaly and signs of pulmonary venous congestion. ECG abnormalities are quite common and may include standard findings of acute infarction, nonspecific ST-segment and T-wave changes, dysrhythmias, and conduction abnormalities. A catheter placed in the right side of the heart will reveal an elevated pulmonary capillary wedge pressure and decreased cardiac output. In the setting of right ventricular infarction, signs of left ventricular failure such as cardiomegaly and pulmonary edema are likely to be absent. Ischemic changes may be seen on the ECG in the inferior or right chest leads. Both cardiac output and pulmonary capillary wedge pressure are decreased.

Because of the complexity of the variables involved, it is essential that patients in cardiogenic shock receive careful and continuous monitoring. Items routinely monitored include vital signs, pulse pressure, mental status, pulse oxymetry, and urine output. Insertion of an arterial line permits continuous assessment of blood pressure, oxygenation, and pH. Central venous pressure lines provide little useful information about left ventricular function and should not be inserted for monitoring purposes. On the other hand, a pulmonary artery catheter is essential for accurate assessment of the response to therapy and should be placed early in the course of management. If it is not practical to insert a pulmonary artery catheter in the emergency department, expeditious transfer to a critical care unit should be arranged. In the interim, therapy must be judicious and largely guided by careful observation of the patient's clinical response.

Goals in the treatment of cardiogenic shock include optimization of oxygen delivery and myocardial preservation. Oxygen delivery is optimized by assessing and possibly supporting ventilation, providing supplemental oxygen, and improving cardiac output. Myocardial preservation is directed at reducing the is-

chemic zone between necrotic and normal muscle and is determined by the balance between myocardial oxygen supply and demand. Preserving the ischemic zone requires careful regulation of preload and afterload, control of dysrhythymias, and relief of pain and anxiety. Prompt evaluation by a cardiologist and consideration of thrombolytic therapy or coronary angioplasty is essential. Reperfusion may dramatically reverse the cycle of hypoperfusion and poor contractility.

As a first priority, all patients in cardiogenic shock should be placed on high-flow oxygen by mask. Oxygenation should be continuously monitored, and by pulse oxymetry if possible. The need for intubation is indicated by persistent hypoxemia, cyanosis, deteriorating mental status, or evidence of respiratory fatigue. Positive end-expiratory pressure (PEEP) is essential if the PaO_2 does not rapidly respond to oxygen alone. Start with a PEEP of 3 to 6 cm H_2O and titrate upward, using an adequate PaO_2 as the end point.

The second priority in management is reversal of hypotension. Fluid therapy generally has a very limited role in the management of cardiogenic shock, and even small amounts may be detrimental. However, 10% to 20% of those patients with acute myocardial infarction are hypovolemic and have a low left ventricular end diastolic pressure secondary to vomiting, diuretic use, or decreased oral intake. Right ventricular infarction may also cause low left ventricular filling pressure. Some of these patients respond to fluid, and therefore it is often recommended that hypotensive patients receive a trial dose of 100 to 200 ml crystalloid boluses before initiating more aggressive therapy. Hypovolemia can be excluded as the cause of shock if the pulmonary artery wedge pressure rises above 18 mm Hg in the presence of a persistently low cardiac output.

In most cases, vasopressors are required to reverse the hypotension associated with cardiogenic shock. Dopamine and dobutamine, alone

Table 5-1

VASOPRESSOR EFFECTS

Agent	Receptor Stimulation	Primary Clinical Effect
Dobutamine	β_1	Increases cardiac contractility
Dopamine	Dopaminergic (0.5-2 µg/kg/min)	Dilates mesenteric, renal vasculature
	β_1 (2-15 µg/kg/min)	Increases cardiac contractility
	α (>10-15 µg/kg/min)	Peripheral vasoconstriction
Epinephrine	α, β_1, β_2	Increases cardiac rate and contractility; peripheral vasoconstriction
Isoproterenol	β_1, β_2	Increases cardiac rate and contractility; dilates peripheral vasculature
Norepinephrine	α	Constricts peripheral vasculature

or in combination, are most commonly used as first-line therapy (Table 5-1). Dopamine is primarily a beta-adrenergic agent at dosages less than 10 µg/kg/minute and an alpha-adrenergic agent at increasingly higher dosages. At lower dosages, it increases heart rate and contractility and dilates mesenteric and renal vasculature. A reasonable starting dosage is 2 to 5 µg/kg/minute, with incremental increases until blood pressure improves. Dosages above 15 to 20 µg/kg/minute produce significant peripheral vasoconstriction and may increase myocardial oxygen demand.

Dobutamine is a beta$_1$ agonist without significant alpha-adrenergic activity. Its primary effects are to increase cardiac contractility and stroke volume and to slightly decrease systemic vascular resistance. Compared to dopamine, dobutamine is less likely to increase heart rate or afterload and, secondarily, myocardial oxygen demand. Dobutamine is the preferred agent in the treatment of right ventricular infarction because it reduces pulmonary artery resistance and improves left ventricular contractility. The

usual dosage range of dobutamine is 2.5 to 10 µg/kg/minute, and it is often given in combination with low dose dopamine.

Other drugs that can selectively be used in the treatment of cardiogenic shock include vasodilators (nitroglycerin, nitroprusside), loop diuretics (furosemide), and analgesics (morphine). Vasodilators can be used to reduce both preload and afterload and are often used in conjunction with vasopressors. Amrinone is a relatively new drug that possesses both inotropic and vasodilator effects. All of these drugs can have significant adverse hemodynamic effects and are best administered after placement of a pulmonary artery catheter.

Intraaortic balloon (IAB) counterpulsation devices reduce afterload and improve coronary perfusion by augmenting aortic pressure in diastole and decreasing it in systole. The devices are useful early in the treatment of a serious acute myocardial infarction that is complicated by cardiogenic shock and unresponsive to normal therapy but that has surgically correctable structural lesion. Severe aortic regurgitation, aneurysm, and dysrhythmias preclude the effective use of the device.

Distributive or Vasogenic Shock

The hallmark of distributive shock is profound arterial and venous dilation and, consequently, a marked reduction in systemic vascular resistance. Cardiac output, which is universally depressed with other forms of shock, may actually increase at times with distributive shock. Sepsis, anaphylaxis, spinal cord injuries, and drug effects are the most common causes of distributive shock. This section focuses on septic shock, the most serious of these disorders.

Septic shock is most commonly caused by bacteremia with gram-negative rods, although other organisms can also cause the disease. Predisposing factors to septic shock include immunosuppression, malignancy, autoimmune disorders, and instrumentation of the genitourinary or respiratory tracts. The infectious disorders that most commonly lead to septic shock are pyelonephritis and pneumonia. Other causes that should be considered include peritonitis, cholangitis, perirectal abscesses, indwelling vascular catheters, soft tissue infections, meningitis, and pelvic inflammatory disorders. Septic shock has its peak incidence in the seventh decade of life. Mortality rates range from 30% to 50% and is greatly affected by the patient's underlying medical condition.

The clinical presentation of sepsis is commonly divided into two phases: an early high-output phase followed by a more typical low-output phase. The early phase is marked by vasodilatation. Clinical findings include agitation; warm, red skin; temperature abnormalities (elevated or depressed); and an increased rate and depth of respiration. Cardiac output may be elevated or normal during the early phase of sepsis. The late phase is more typical of the low-flow states seen with other forms of shock. Hypoten-

sion, confusion, poor capillary refill, and low urine output are characteristic symptoms. In addition, evidence of impaired clotting may be seen in the form of bruising, bleeding at puncture sites, or uncommonly, frank hemorrhage.

Laboratory abnormalities include an early leukopenia followed by leukocytosis and a left shift. Respiratory alkalosis occurs early and gradually gives way to a metabolic acidosis. The urinalysis often reveals signs of infection because it is the most common source of sepsis. Coagulation abnormalities are common, including thrombocytopenia; decreased fibrinogen; and elevated prothrombin time, partial thromboplastin time, and fibrin-split products. A chest x-ray study may reveal pneumonia.

The primary goals in the management of septic shock are restoration of cardiac output and control of the source of infection. Many patients in septic shock have been ill for several days, with fever, decreased oral intake, and vomiting. Therefore volume replacement is first-line therapy for restoration of blood pressure and cardiac output. However, crystalloid should be infused carefully because of the potentially tenuous state of the cardiovascular system. Placement of a pulmonary artery catheter is required unless there is a prompt response to crystalloid infusion. Vasopressors are indicated if shock persists despite adequate fluid therapy. Dopamine is the vasopressor of choice because it improves cardiac output, preserves renal blood flow, and, at higher doses, increases systemic vascular resistance.

Control of the infection requires a rapid and diligent search for its source, drainage of any pus collections, and initiation of antibiotic therapy. Antibiotic therapy should be started as soon as possible after blood and urine cultures have been obtained. The choice of antibiotic depends on the source of the infection, the patient's immune status, and to a certain extent on institutional or physician preference. Broad coverage is generally preferable until a specific infecting organism has been identified. Aminoglycosides or third-generation cephalosporins are commonly used to provide gram-negative coverage when the urinary tract is the suspected source of infection. An antistaphylococcal agent such as vancomycin is commonly used for infections of cutaneous origin. Immumocompromised patients require broad coverage, with multiple drugs directed against both gram-negative and gram-positive organisms.

COMPLICATIONS

Complications of shock are common and reflect the type and stage of shock, the rapidity of response, the underlying disease process, and the problems attributable to therapy. Possible complications include acute respiratory distress syndrome (ARDS); acute tubular necrosis (ATN), with renal failure caused by impaired renal blood flow, myocardial dysfunction with failure; and stress ulcers with gastrointestinal bleeding and ileus. Ultimately a prolonged low-flow state may lead to multiple-organ failure, respiratory failure, cardiopulmonary arrest, and death.

KEY CONSIDERATIONS

WHAT IS THE LIFE THREAT?

Cellular hypofusion, if severe enough, results in cell death. Sufficient cell death within critical organs, such as the brain and the heart, lead to death of the organism.

Shock associated with rapid loss of blood or massive impairment of cardiac function tends to pose the most immediate threat of life.

Septic shock is associated with an overall mortality rate of 30% to 50%.

DOES THE PATIENT NEED ADMISSION?

Patients with mild hypovolemia as a result of vomiting, diarrhea, or decreased fluid intake may have orthostatic changes in blood pressure and pulse that correct with intravenous or oral fluids and other measures. Such patients are usually able to be discharged with good follow-up instructions.

Patients with persistent shock are evidenced by acute cellular hypofusion require admission, evaluation, and aggressive treatment.

WHAT IS THE MOST SERIOUS DIAGNOSIS?

Hypovolemia (blood loss, third-space loss), myocardial infarction, pulmonary embolism, rupture of thoracic or abdominal aneurysm, sepsis, or spinal trauma are the most serious diagnoses.

HAVE I PERFORMED A THOROUGH WORK-UP?

Evaluate the patient for bleeding, fluid loss, mechanical heart failure, hypoxemia, trauma, pulmonary embolism, acute vascular rupture, sepsis, and neurogenic shock.

Recommended Reading

Bickell WH et al: Immediate versus delayed fluid resuscitation for hypotensive patients with penetrating torso injuries, *N Engl J Med* 331(17):1105-1109, 1994.

Schmidt RD, Wolfe RE: Shock. In Rosen P et al, editors: *Emergency medicine: concepts and clinical practice,* ed 3, St Louis, 1992, Mosby.

Stern S et al: The effect of blood pressure on hemorrhage volume and survival in a near-fatal hemorrhage model incorporating a vascular injury, *Ann Emerg Med* 22:155-163, 1993.

Chapter Six
MULTIPLE TRAUMA

VINCENT J. MARKOVCHICK

Few causes of untimely and, in many instances, preventable, death are more significant than major multiple-system trauma. Every year in the United States, more deaths are caused by trauma than occurred during the Vietnam War. It is unknown how many of these deaths can be prevented, but the formation of trauma systems has made a positive impact on the outcome of trauma patients.

TRAUMA TEAM

Trauma requires the coordinated efforts of many medical and nonmedical personnel. Quality in the following elements is essential:

1. A finding mechanism (usually the state highway patrol or a citizen with a cellular phone)
2. A communication system both to summon help and to prepare for appropriate treatment in a health care facility
3. A transport mechanism, such as an ambulance or helicopter, staffed by appropriately trained and equipped prehospital-care providers
4. Emergency medicine capabilities, because the patient must have good initial resuscitation and stabilization to be able to progress to definitive repair
5. Trauma surgery
6. Intensive care
7. Laboratory and radiology capabilities
8. Rehabilitation to achieve the most complete restoration to preinjury levels of function

Therefore trauma is seen as the coordinated effort of a team that consists of many players. The team members are as follows, and each is briefly discussed in the sections that follow:

1. Prehospital-care team
2. Team captain
3. Adjunct physicians (i.e., consultants)
4. Nurses
5. Hospital attendants
6. Technicians

Prehospital-Care Team

The initial field assessment of the trauma patient by emergency medical technicians (EMTs) should include the mechanism of injury and the initial evaluation of the patient. The initial evaluation includes vital signs and a Glasgow Coma Scale score. Treatment and stabilization should begin in the field and continue enroute to a receiving hospital best suited to manage trauma, such as a trauma center. If no trauma center is available, the patient should be transported to the nearest hospital emergency department.

Communication with the hospital includes a report of the initial assessment, mechanism of injury, vital signs, field treatment, response to initial therapy, and estimated time of arrival. Such communication maximizes the ability of the trauma team to prepare for the patient's arrival. In preparation for the patient's arrival, the trauma captain can summon members of the team, assign their roles, ready equipment, and call for available blood for transfusion if necessary.

Team Captain

The trauma team must have a leader, and all orders must be given either by or through this leader. The role of the team captain is to assess and supervise the overall care of the patient. It is generally unwise for the captain to become involved in the individual tasks of care because someone needs to be aware of the larger issues involved and to coordinate all the efforts. If the captain is needed to perform a task, such as intubation or a cricothyrotomy, then the overall leadership role should be given (if possible) to another member of the team.

The captain is also responsible for performing the initial and secondary surveys, which are discussed later in this chapter. These surveys are performed efficiently and according to an established protocol. Some of the tasks of physical examination can be assigned to other team members, but the results must be reported to the captain so that a complete picture is available for proper decision making.

Adjunct Physicians

Ideally the team includes physicians other than the captain who can perform the technical tasks. In smaller hospital and rural emergency departments, this may not be possible. It then becomes necessary for nurses and paramedics to perform some of the technical tasks usually performed by the physician. The team captain must perform or supervise lifesaving procedures in order of their importance to the resuscitation, such as endotracheal intubation or thoracostomy for decompression of a tension pneumothorax.

Nurses

Not only do nurses possess the technical skills needed for many tasks, but also they are usually well informed about the location and function of the equipment needed for proper care. They also supervise the administration of medications and fluids and record the events of the resuscitation. Their expertise is most important in the ongoing monitoring of the trauma victim and the early recognition of changes in parameters that may indicate deterioration of a patient's hemodynamic and respiratory status.

Hospital Attendants or Aides

Hospital attendants and aides are key players in the safe movement of the patient, not only with the original transfer from the field stretcher to the hospital gurney, but also within the hospital itself. In addition, hospital attendants and aides perform such vital tasks as the complete undressing of the patient, the placement of urinary catheters and restraints, the transporting of specimens to the laboratory, and the delivery of blood and blood products as needed.

Technicians

The value of technicians in their particular area of expertise is unlimited. For example, an experienced radiology technician can take high quality portable films and make them available to the trauma captain within minutes to expedite the decision making and treatment of the trauma victim. A respiratory technician is capable of assuming responsibility for the mechanical ventilation of the patient.

ASSESSMENT

The first step after the patient arrives is to assign the trauma patient to an appropriate location, or to perform triage. Major trauma is best treated in a major trauma resuscitation room.

For those patients placed in the minor trauma category, many variables are evaluated to ensure proper placement.

One general principle of trauma management is to treat life-threatening injuries first and leave definitive diagnostic procedures until later. It is important to consider the mechanism of injury, because a young, otherwise healthy trauma patient may not show signs of significant internal injury until some time after the accident. Treat the patient as seriously injured whenever there is a significant mechanism of injury, as judged by such variables as the amount of damage to a vehicle that was involved, the height of a fall, whether someone died in the accident, and how old and how large or small the patient is. At extremes of age, much less trauma is required to achieve a high degree of injury.

RESUSCITATION

Airway

As soon as the patient is safely transferred to the emergency department gurney, the trauma team captain assesses the airway (see Chapter 3). At the minimum, the patient should receive supplemental oxygen via a nonrebreather bag reservoir mask.

The mandatory indications for active airway management are listed in the box above. Remember the protocol for traumatic airway management: If the cervical spine has been injured or cannot be declared normal, maintain inline stabilization of the neck and perform orotracheal inbutation, preferably with rapid sequence induction. If this is not possible, or if paralysis of the patient is contraindicated, then a cricothyrotomy should be performed. For estimates of the weight of children and the corresponding tube sizes, see Table 6-1.

Breathing

To assess breathing, the patient must be undressed completely and the chest is examined.

RATIONALE FOR AIRWAY MANAGEMENT
To ensure airway patency
To facilitate suctioning and pulmonary hygiene
To prevent aspiration
To actively regulate ventilation
To administer drugs

Look for possible evidence of trauma; be sure to logroll the patient and examine the posterior side of the thorax, especially when there is evidence of penetrating trauma. Tangentially look at the chest wall to assess the rate and depth of respirations, and note any paradoxical chest-wall motion. Gently palpate the chest for subcutaneous emphysema, localized tenderness, and bony crepitus. Auscultate to determine the quality of breath sounds. A tube thoracostomy should be performed on any patient with hypotension, tachycardia, and absent breath sounds before obtaining a chest x-ray radiograph. It is also unnecessary to delay performing a thoracostomy on unstable patients with penetrating injuries to the thorax and decreased breath sounds or labored respirations.

Intravenous Lines and Bleeding

If you are satisfied that an adequate airway exists, turn your attention to venous access and bleeding concerns. An external hemorrhage should be controlled with direct pressure or tourniquets. With a good prehospital-care system, the patient often already has two large-bore intravenous lines placed; if not, place these immediately. We prefer to use peripheral catheters, but with extensive bleeding this may not be possible. A principal advantage to having lines started by the prehospital-care team is that the patient may not have completely lost accessible veins as a result of the hemorrhage, and the veins will be easier to cannulate. In addition, the paramedics can draw blood samples as part

Table 6-1

VITAL SIGNS AND ANCILLARY VENTILATORY SUPPORT

Age	Weight (kg)	Heart Rate (average/min)	Respiratory Rate	Blood Pressure (mean ± 2 SD)		ET Tube		Suction Catheter (Fr)	Chest Tube (Fr)	Laryngoscopy Blade
				Systolic	Diastolic*	ID† (mm)	Length (cm)			
Premature	1	145	<40	42 ± 10	21 ± 8	2.5	10	6	10	0 straight
Newborn	1-2	135		50 ± 10	28 ± 8	3.0	11	6-8	10-12	1 straight
Newborn	2-3	125		60 ± 10	37 ± 8	3.0	12			
1 mo	4	120	24-35	80 ± 16	46 ± 16	3.5	13	8		
6 mo	7	130		89 ± 29	60 ± 10	3.5	14			
1 yr	10	125	20-30	96 ± 30	66 ± 25	4.0	15	8-10	16-20	1 straight
2-3 yr	12-14	115		99 ± 25	64 ± 25	4.5	16	10	20-24	
4-5 yr	16-18	100		99 ± 20	65 ± 20	5.0-6.0	17		20-28	2
6-8 yr	20-26	100	12-25			6.0-6.5	18			
10-12 yr	34-42	75				7.0	20	12	28-32	2-3
>14 yr	>50	70	12-18			7.5-8.5	24		32-42	3

Modified from Nadas A: *Pediatric cardiology*, ed 3, Philadelphia, 1976, WB Saunders; Vesmond HT et al: *Pediatrics* 67:607, 1981.

*Point of muffling (Nadas).

†Variability of 0.5 mm is common. Estimate: $\dfrac{16 + age\ (yr)}{4}$

of the initial intravenous line placement and save a significant amount of time in getting a specimen to the laboratory for type and cross-match procedures. However, because not all laboratories accept specimens from the field, this protocol must be established.

Place central venous lines judiciously. If the patient's condition will not easily tolerate the complications of central line placement, you must decide if the information to be acquired is worth the risk. For example, if the patient has cirrhosis or a history of hemophilia, the risks of central line placement far outweigh the benefits. With children, special equipment is needed and is not readily available everywhere; therefore it is preferable to place intraosseous or femoral lines. It is also less likely that a child will have large quantities of fluid infused.

The prevention or treatment of shock is of paramount concern. Start an immediate infusion of lactated Ringer's or normal saline solution. If the patient does not respond to 40 ml/kg, begin intravenous volume replacement with type-specific or O-negative blood. In the child, first give a bolus of 20 ml/kg. If there is no response or only a partial response, infuse 10 ml/kg of packed RBCs.

Two intravenous lines may not be sufficient for a patient who is hemorrhaging briskly. Place additional lines both above and below the diaphragm, even though the possibility of vena caval injuries is slight. Saphenous cutdowns are easily performed in the adult and larger child. Because in children under 2 years of age such cutdowns are technically difficult, intraosseous and femoral lines are preferred. Saphenous cutdowns in the groin are difficult and time consuming; therefore percutaneous femoral lines are preferable.

After intravenous lines have been established and fluids are running satisfactorily, investigate the need for blood and blood products. Unless the patient is in cardiac arrest or arrests shortly after coming to the emergency department, administer 40 ml/kg of crystalloid. Give O-negative blood immediately to the patient

who is in cardiac arrest. Because the outcome of blunt trauma is so poor once arrest has occurred, use a maximum of two units for such patients unless true progress has been made in the resuscitation. Immediately give blood to patients with unstable pelvic fractures because of the massive retroperitoneal blood loss associated with this injury. Early orthopedic and angiographic consultations should be sought for these injuries for placement of external fixation devices and possible embolization to control massive hemorrhage.

Because it is the blood form required of blood banks, use reconstituted packed red blood cells (RBCs). With whole blood no longer available, add normal saline solution to the RBC packs to facilitate administration. Many trauma centers also routinely administer fresh frozen plasma after every 10 units of RBCs and give an ampule of calcium chloride with every 5 units of RBCs.

Monitoring

In addition to monitoring the blood pressure of the trauma patient, monitor the pulse, respiratory rate, urinary output, and O_2 saturation. If a central venous line is in place, monitor the central venous pressure. Routinely attach the patient to a cardiac monitor and insert a urinary catheter. Monitor all patients with major trauma for urinary output, even if they do not show signs of shock. For patients in shock, automatic blood-pressure–monitoring equipment does not function as accurately as central hemodynamic monitoring, arterial line pressure, and measurement of urine output. Carefully monitor the respiratory rate, because an increasing respiratory rate may be the first sign of ventilatory failure.

INITIAL INJURY SURVEY

After the trauma team captain has ensured that the ABCs of resuscitation are under control, there is usually time to conduct an initial head-to-toe survey of the extent of the patient's injuries. This survey includes a quick neurologic and rectal examination. To assess posterior injuries, it is necessary to roll over the patient while controlling the cervical spine; neurologic status should be known before turning the patient. The rectal examination assesses sphincter tone and sensation; this may be the only clue to spinal cord injury. Locate the prostate gland in male patients to evaluate the possibility of urethral injury and unstable pelvic fractures. Occult blood testing is unnecessary because any rectal injury will produce gross, not occult, bleeding. In addition, obvious fractures should be splinted.

DIAGNOSTIC TESTS

Once the initial survey is complete, obtain diagnostic studies as needed. These tests include radiologic studies of the lateral cervical spine, an anteroposterior AP chest study, and a pelvic film. Ensure that all seven cervical vertebrae are seen on the cervical spine film. Exposure of all cervical vertebrae may be enhanced by having someone pull down on the patient's arms. If the patient's condition does not allow for the time needed to obtain quality films (e.g., because of a ruptured spleen), immobilize the spine with a rigid cervical collar and deal with the life-threatening injuries first. Obtain the following initial laboratory studies:

- Type and crossmatch for at least 2 units of packed RBCs. Order prothrombin and partial thromboplastin times
- Complete blood count (CBC)
- Urine dipstick for blood with microscopic examination if positive for blood
- Electrolytes
- Blood urea nitrogen (BUN) and creatinine
- Glucose
- Serum amylase
- Blood alcohol as indicated
- Toxicology screen as indicated
These laboratory tests supply a baseline

against which to measure subsequent results. Follow the protocols regarding such things as the number of units of blood to be requested for your particular institution.

MANAGEMENT

When the initial diagnostic tests have been completed and if the patient's condition permits, perform a more detailed secondary survey. This survey includes a medical history and a more in-depth physical examination. In addition, if the patient's condition has not deteriorated, carry out more formal diagnostic maneuvers. Do a peritoneal lavage now, if indicated. Obtain or complete radiologic studies of the head, spine, chest, and extremities, as well as special procedures such as an angiography, intravenous pyelogram (IVP), and a CT scan. Do not subject a patient whose condition has not stabilized or is deteriorating to studies outside of the resuscitation suite. Request the presence of a trauma surgeon early because he or she will be responsible for coordinating the overall care of the patient and for performing the earliest life-saving definitive procedures. Notify other subspeciality consultants when it is obvious that their expertise will be needed.

SPECIAL CONCERNS

Children

Important differences in management must be emphasized in the case of children:
1. Few children younger than age 3 survive a cervical spinal cord injury. Therefore invest your time in checking the integrity of the thoracic and lumbar spines rather than the cervical spine. Children require the same immobilization for this procedure as do adults.
2. Intravenous lines are more difficult to place; give fluids judiciously and in bolus amounts with reassessment of vital signs and clinical status after each bolus.

3. The airway is much harder to manage for physicians who are not familiar with the technical details of pediatric intubation. Because of the small size of the cricothyroid space, a cricothyrotomy is contraindicated in children younger than 8 years of age unless they are very large. A tracheostomy is required to establish a surgical airway in small children and is performed in the operating room. An acceptable temporary method is a needle cricothyrotomy if the proper equipment is available; this procedure is contraindicated with an upper airway obstruction. The child may need to be intubated orally.

4. Although temperature is important even in adults, it is most important in children, who have relatively a much larger surface area than adults. Hypothermia can occur rapidly in children and lead to fatal consequences. Give all trauma victims prewarmed intravenous fluids, and infuse all blood through a blood warmer. In addition, do not leave the child uncovered any longer than it takes to complete the physical examination and use warm blankets to prevent hypothermia, even during the summer.

Pregnant Women

During the first trimester of pregnancy, the fetus is well protected within the uterus against all but penetrating injuries. However, as the pregnancy progresses, the placenta is at great risk for injury from even minor degrees of blunt trauma. Because of this risk of injury, admit all third-trimester mothers with abdominal trauma for fetal monitoring. In this way, early complications of abruptio placentae can be detected, and a cesarean section can be performed to save the lives of both mother and child.

Because of the expanded blood volume during pregnancy, the mother may not show signs of hypovolemia until 30% to 40% of her blood volume has been lost. Therefore when a major mechanism of injury is involved, search dili-

gently for an occult hemorrhage.

Because the uterus can cause obstruction of the inferior vena cavae in late pregnancy, do not transport the mother or perform resuscitation with her in the supine position. Instead turn her abdomen to a more lateral position. Even though this position may cause problems in immobilizing the lumbar spine, it should permit immobilization of the cervical and thoracic spines.

Although diagnostic peritoneal lavage is not contraindicated during pregnancy, the size of the uterus mandates an open technique or a supraumbilical incision.

Perform all the radiologic procedures needed to accurately diagnose the mother's condition unless she is in the first trimester, in which case x-ray studies of the abdomen should be avoided. However, if the mother appears to have an unstable pelvic injury, pelvic x-ray studies should be performed, even during the first trimester.

If shock can be avoided in the mother and if there are no penetrating injuries of the uterus or abruptio placentae, the fetal outcome should be good. Therefore it is especially important to aggressively diagnose and manage the mother's injuries. It is always wise to have an early obstetric consultation and to carry out fetal monitoring in patients with a gestation of at least 20 weeks.

SETTING PRIORITIES IN MULTIPLE TRAUMA

The final considerations in trauma care are the responsibilities of setting priorities among the diagnostic studies and the treatment needed when there are multiple major organ systems involved. As already stated, treat the immediately life-threatening injuries first and then approach the diagnostic studies that appear to be necessary. For example, in a patient with head, chest, and abdominal injuries, perform a laparotomy if the peritoneal lavage is grossly positive; after the patient's condition has stabilized, perform an angiography or a CT scan to evaluate the other injuries. In the case of a patient with clinical or CT scan evidence of brain herniation, a neurosurgeon may need to surgically approach the head injury without a CT scan at the same time that the laparotomy is being performed. These multiple needs are rare but possible with trauma. One guideline that can be offered is to treat abdominal injuries before thoracic artery injuries on the basis of the greater window of opportunity that exists to diagnose and repair the aorta.

TRANSFER OF PATIENTS

A smooth transition of care is needed between the emergency department and the operating room or intensive care unit. If the patient re-quires definitive therapy that is not available within the primary institution, arrange this therapy quickly and use the safest and fastest mode of transportation available. Ideally, protocols for transfer to higher level trauma centers should already be in place to minimize the time needed to arrange such transfers.

SUMMARY

Trauma care requires the commitment and expertise of the entire area in which the trauma may occur. It is truly a "team sport" that requires the smooth coordination of prehospital and inhospital personnel to prevent untimely death and ensure the best possible outcome for the injured patient.

KEY CONSIDERATIONS

WHAT IS THE LIFE THREAT?

Airway obstruction from direct trauma to the larynx, trachea, mouth, or nose constitutes a life threat. Intraoral bleeding can lead to airway obstruction.

Major intrathoracic injury includes a ruptured aorta, myocardial contusion, myocardial rupture, tension pneumothorax, massive hemothorax, a ruptured bronchus, cardiac tamponade, or other major vascular hemorrhage.

Bleeding and shock caused by internal or external bleeding can be associated with pelvic fractures and intraabdominal bleeding from a lacerated spleen, liver, or mesenteric blood vessels.

DOES THE PATIENT NEED ADMISSION?

Transfer to the operating room is usually indicated for a gunshot wound to the abdomen or thorax, uncontrollable internal bleeding associated with trauma, bronchial disruption, or cardiac laceration or tamponade. Open fracture and traumatic amputation usually require surgical treatment in the operating room.

Epidural and acute subdural intracranial hemorrhage usually require neurosurgical treatment and a transfer to the operating room.

Admission and observation is advisable in cases in which the mechanism of injury or the initial presentation suggests serious injury. Examples of such mechanisms are falls from heights greater than 15 feet, a victim ejected from vehicle, a high-speed collision, someone else killed in the accident, or a prolonged extraction time.

Examples of worrisome initial presentation are hemodynamic instability (blood pressure less than 90 systolic, pulse greater than 130 beats/minute), respiratory distress, altered level of consciousness, major burns, open fractures, or an unstable pelvic fracture.

WHAT IS THE MOST SERIOUS DIAGNOSIS?

Airway obstruction, massive hemothorax, tension pneumothorax, cardiac tamponade, aortic disruption, myocardial tear, intraabdominal hemorrhage, intracranial bleeding, massive retroperitoneal hemorrhage secondary to unstable pelvic fractures, and spinal cord injury are the most serious diagnoses.

HAVE I PERFORMED A THOROUGH WORK-UP?

Do not attribute hypotension and tachycardia to a head injury; look for internal blood loss (usually intraabdominal or intrathoracic).

In major trauma, perform a thorough assessment of airway integrity and oxygenation through pulse oximetry or arterial blood gases.

Explain any decrease in the level of consciousness by an examination and a CT scan of the head if needed.

Recommended Reading

Alexander RH, Proctor HJ: *Advanced trauma life support course for physicians,* ed 5, Chicago, 1995, American College of Surgeons.

Feliciano DV et al: *Trauma,* ed 3, Stamford, Conn, 1996, Appleton & Lange.

Jorden RC, Barkin RM: Multiple trauma. In Rosen P et al, editors: *Emergency medicine: concepts and clinical practice,* ed 3, St Louis, 1992, Mosby.

Moore EE: Resuscitation and evaluation of the injured patient. In Zuidema GD, Rutherford R, Ballinger W, editors: *The management of trauma,* ed 4, Philadelphia, 1985, WB Saunders.

Zuidema GD, Cameron JN, Sabatier HS: Initial evaluation and resuscitation of the injured patient. In Zuidema GD, Rutherford R, Ballinger W, editors: *The management of trauma,* ed 4, Philadelphia, 1985, WB Saunders.

Part II

SIGNS AND SYMPTOMS

Chapter Seven
FEVER

HAROLD THOMAS, JR.

Fever is the oldest and most widely recognized hallmark of disease and accounts for a substantial percentage of both adult and pediatric visits to the emergency department.

THERMOREGULATION AND NORMAL BODY TEMPERATURE

Body temperature is regulated by a thermoregulatory center, which is located in the anterior hypothalamus. This center receives input from central receptors that sense the temperature of the blood perfusing the brain and from peripheral receptors that sense skin temperature. The thermoregulatory center has an inherent set point, which it maintains at a relatively constant temperature of 37° C ± 1° C. This narrow range is maintained by the regulation of heat production and heat loss.

The rectal temperature is usually approximately 0.7° C greater than the oral temperature and is thought to be a more accurate reflection of the core temperature of the body. Oral temperature can vary by more than 1.6° C, depending on the position of the thermometer in the mouth. Respiratory rate also affects the oral temperature. For each increment of 10 breaths/minute in the respiratory rate, the oral temperature decreases by almost 0.5° C. Axillary temperature would be expected to be 0.7° C below the oral temperature, but this type of temperature measurement is inconsistent, and its use is not recommended. Tympanic temperatures provide a rapid measurement in adults. In children under 6 months of age, tympanic temperatures have limited reliability. Certain other conditions, such as impacted cerumen, also limit the reliability of this method of temperature measurement. If the clinical presentation is inconsistent with the tympanic measurement, an oral or rectal temperature should be obtained.

Fever is a disorder of thermoregulation in which the hypothalamic set point is raised. The patient with a fever subjectively feels cold, has increased muscular activity (such as a chill), and exhibits peripheral vasoconstriction. Various patterns of fever correlate with certain diseases.

ASSESSMENT

The emergency patient with a chief complaint of fever can have an illness that ranges in severity from an acute life-threatening disease to a benign disorder that requires no treatment. The exact cause of the fever may be readily apparent or may remain undiagnosed even after a lengthy evaluation. A logical, organized approach is extremely important in assessing the patient with a fever. In such an evaluation, consider five questions:

1. Is the fever from an infectious or noninfectious cause?
2. If infectious, is the cause bacterial or nonbacterial?
3. What is the anatomic location of the febrile process?
4. Does the patient require pharmacologic treatment for the temperature?
5. Does the patient require hospitalization for the underlying disease process?

It is particularly important to address correctly the need for urgent hospitalization. Perform a systematic, thorough history and physical examination. These steps often provide all the information needed to decide whether to hospitalize the patient, particularly an adult.

Include the following specific aspects in the history:
1. Symptoms other than fever, such as headache, cough, dysuria, or sore throat
2. Duration and magnitude of the fever
3. Close contacts with people who have a similar illness
4. Travel history and occupational or recreational exposure
5. Past medical history, especially that of chronic medical illness such as diabetes mellitus, renal failure, cardiac valvular lesions, chronic obstructive pulmonary disease, alcoholism, blood dyscrasias, malignancy, and immunosuppression
6. Use of medications, especially antibiotics and antipyretics
7. Drug abuse

Physical Examination

The most important aspect of the physical examination is the patient's general appearance: Assess how ill the patient looks and how well he or she appears to be tolerating the fever. Critically evaluate a complete set of vital signs. Fever ordinarily increases the heart rate by approximately 10 beats/minute for each 0.55° C increase in temperature. Certain diseases (e.g., typhoid fever and Legionnaire disease) often lead to a relative bradycardia. Tachycardia that is inappropriate for the degree of fever is often the earliest sign of septic shock. An elevated blood pressure caused by increased intracranial pressure may occur with CNS infection. Sustained profound hyperventilation is often associated with gram-negative bacteremia, pneumonia, or acidosis.

Note these points during the physical examination:
1. Mental status. Altered mental status is often the only sign other than fever to indicate the presence of overwhelming sepsis or a CNS infection.
2. Skin rashes. Skin eruptions usually suggest a viral origin for fever but may also represent evidence that a fever is caused by a drug reaction, meningococcemia, Rocky Mountain spotted fever, toxic shock syndrome, or other illness.
3. Lymphadenopathy. Generalized lymphadenopathy may be a systemic response to an infection or may indicate lymphoreticular abnormalities that render the patient susceptible to infection. Infectious mononucleosis is the most common cause of acute generalized adenopathy. Localized lymphadenopathy may represent an infection in the region drained by the involved nodes. The initial infection with HIV may be manifest as a febrile illness with generalized lymphadenopathy.
4. Bulging fontanelle. In an infant, a bulging fontanelle mandates consideration of meningitis.
5. Pharyngeal erythema and exudate.
6. Abnormalities of the tympanic membranes.
7. Localized rales, rhonchi, or findings of consolidation during examination of the chest.
8. Heart murmur. A murmur may indicate the possibility of endocarditis. However, a functional murmur may increase greatly in intensity because of fever-associated tachycardia.
9. Splenomegaly. Splenomegaly may occur with severe acute infections or as part of a chronic infection or blood dyscrasia.

Laboratory Evaluation

The physical assessment often suggests the need for further laboratory evaluation. Although results of definitive tests such as cultures may not be immediately available, a number of laboratory tests may be helpful in the emergency evaluation of the patient with fever.

White blood cell count

The white blood cell (WBC) count and differential is the test most commonly used to identify serious bacterial infection. Such infection is often associated with an absolute leukocytosis and an increase in polymorphonuclear leukocytes (PMNs) and band forms. Elevation of the WBC count has been found to be most useful in evaluating children with fever. The combination of a WBC count greater than 15,000/mm and an erythrocyte sedimentation rate (ESR) greater than 30 mm/hour appears to be most sensitive in identifying bacteremia in children under 2 years of age. Table 7-1 lists several noninfectious causes of alterations in the WBC.

Changes in neutrophil morphology are also associated with bacterial infection. Toxic granulation (the presence of small, dark, cytoplasmic particles in neutrophils) occurs in three fourths of all patients with bacteremia. This condition may also be present in patients with vasculitis and neoplasms. Cytoplasmic vacuolization has a high correlation with bacteremia. Dohle bodies (blue, cytoplasmic inclusions) appear in patients with bacteremia, as well as those who are pregnant and those with burns or neoplasms.

Cultures

Specific cultures can provide tremendous information about the potential focus and etiology of the condition. Blood cultures and the examination of urine and spinal fluid are particularly useful.

Gram stain

The Gram stain is one of the most useful laboratory techniques available in emergency medicine. It can confirm the diagnosis of certain bacterial infections and suggest specific antimicrobial therapy. With this technique, the specimen should contain many inflammatory cells,

Table 7-1

NONINFECTIOUS CAUSES OF ALTERATIONS IN WBC COUNT

Cause	Effect on WBC Picture	Comment
Epinephrine, stress, strenuous activity, trauma	Leukocytosis with increased neutrophils; no left shift	Increase in WBC count immediate and lasts 2 to 3 hours
Corticosteroids, Cushing syndrome	Leukocytosis with increased neutrophils, left shift, and eosinopenia	Increase occurs 18 hours after oral administration and lasts 24 hours after last dose
Addison disease	Neutropenia; lymphocytosis; eosinophilia	
Diabetic ketoacidosis	Leukocytosis with left shift as high as 25,000/mm^3	
Burns, crush injury, fractures	Leukocytosis with increased neutrophils; no left shift	

usually PMNs. A slide without inflammatory cells generally reflects an inadequate specimen. A Gram stain that reveals bacteria without leukocytes should be interpreted with caution. These bacteria may be representing colonization rather than an invasive infection.

DISPOSITION

The ultimate disposition of the patient with a fever is determined by three factors:
1. Underlying medical illness
2. Toxicity
3. Potential morbidity and mortality (Fig. 7-1)

The otherwise healthy patient who has a readily apparent source of fever and who is not acutely ill can be managed as an outpatient with specific therapy. The healthy patient with an acute febrile illness and no obvious cause often has a self-limited viral infection and can be discharged without extensive evaluation. The emergency physician arranges follow-up care and can initiate specific tests, such as cultures, for the benefit of the referral physician.

The patient who appears toxic or who has a serious underlying illness requires admission. An extensive search for a source of infection is needed for a seriously ill individual. Make every effort to obtain cultures from all appropriate sources (blood; urine; and cerebrospinal, pleural, synovial, and ascites fluid) before initiating antibiotic treatment.

In the patient with impaired immunologic

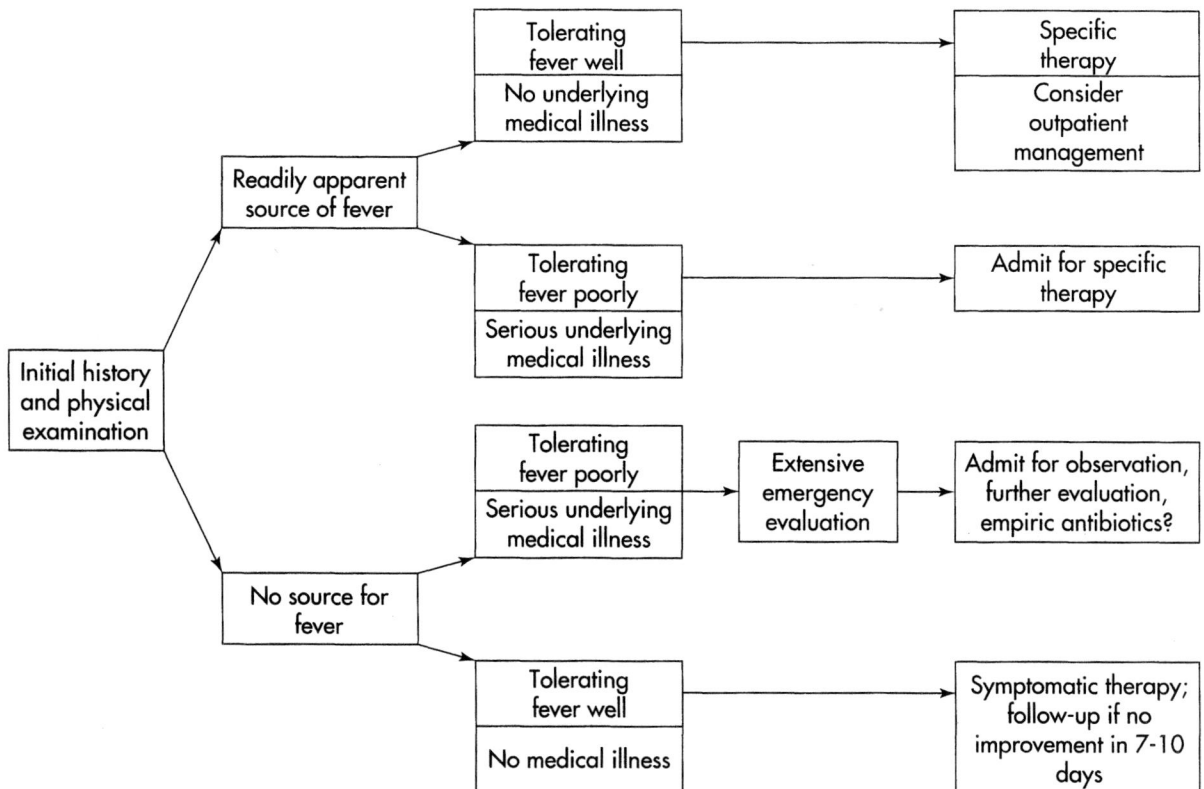

Fig. 7-1 Approach to febrile patients in the emergency department.

defenses, fever is always cause for concern. These patients (including those on high-dose steroids; those undergoing chemotherapy; those who have had a splenectomy; and those with lymphoreticular malignancy, HIV infection, sickle cell disease, diabetes mellitus, or chronic alcohol abuse) are at constant risk for developing an overwhelming infection and often fail to manifest localized findings. Fever, often of low grade, may be the only sign of significant infection. The patient with immunosuppression and fever requires intense evaluation and hospital admission. If the patient appears toxic and no source of infection can be found, initiate broad-spectrum antibiotic coverage, usually with a combination of agents.

Two groups of patients that are not always recognized as being immunosuppressed are those with alcoholism or diabetes mellitus. Such patients have several mechanisms of immune dysfunction, and their host defenses can vary greatly. These patients require admission for infections that are usually managed on an outpatient basis in a healthy population. This fact is especially true for urinary tract and lower extremity infections in patients with diabetes and for pneumonia in patients with alcoholism.

The patient with asplenia is at risk of clinically inapparent bacteremia, usually caused by *Streptococcus pneumoniae* or *Haemophilus influenzae*. Even when these patients receive prompt diagnosis and begin an appropriate therapeutic regimen, substantial mortality occurs. Obtain a culture from these patients and treat them with intravenous antibiotics promptly.

FEVER IN CHILDREN

The child with fever presents a special diagnostic challenge (see Chapter 66). Fevers, even high fevers, are common in children. Several serious febrile illnesses, most notably meningitis, have their peak occurrence in the pediatric age group.

Clinical diagnosis of the young febrile child is notoriously difficult (Fig. 7-2). After the child reaches 2 years of age, clinical assessment is more reliable, and the child is at a decreased risk for having an inapparent serious illness. Pulmonary infection is easy to miss in a small, rapidly breathing, and irritable child. The risk of inapparent bacteremia correlates closely with the degree of fever. The child with a temperature of less than 38.9° C is at minimal risk, whereas 7% of those with a temperature of 40° C and 23% of those with an initial temperature greater than 41° C can be expected to have bacteremia.

An important part of the history and physical examination is the technique of "optimal observation." After lowering the temperature with antipyretics, observe the child at rest on the parent's lap. Six observation parameters (quality of cry, reaction to parent stimulation, level of consciousness, color, hydration, and response to social overtures) have been found to be indicative of serious disease. Table 7-2 shows an observation scale that has been developed to aid in the assessment of children with fever.

Fever during the first 8 weeks of life is always cause for alarm. Patients brought to the emergency department with a rectal temperature of more than 38° C may have bacteremia, most often caused by group B streptococcus. The physician often cannot distinguish neonates with bacteremia on the basis of the degree of fever, WBC counts, or the presence or absence of a localized source of infection. Any neonate who has a fever during the first 28 days of life should undergo a complete septic work-up (CBC, blood culture, chest x-ray examination, urinalysis, and lumbar puncture) and be admitted to the hospital. In older neonates with fever, obtain a pediatric consultation. Some pediatricians advocate outpatient management after a complete septic work-up and administration of antibiotics if follow-up can be arranged in 12 to 24 hours.

Generally an older child with a fever, a viral syndrome, and no apparent complications can

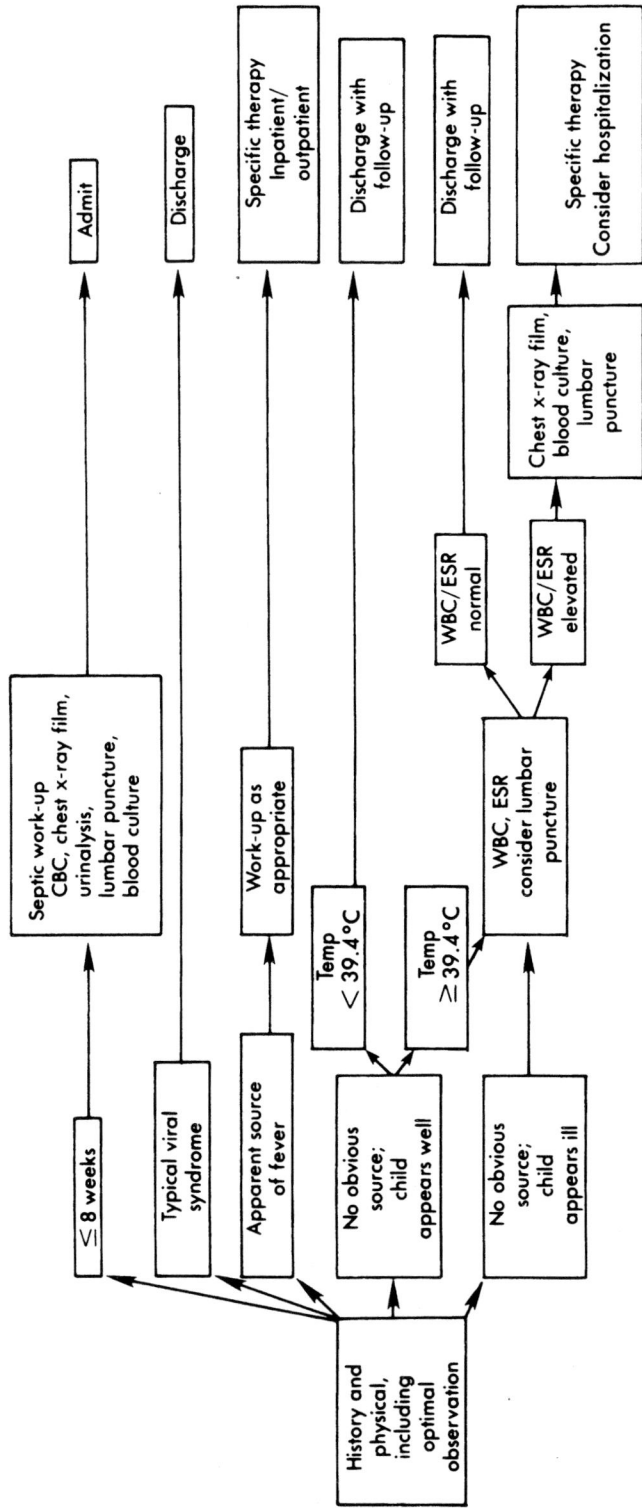

Fig. 7-2 Approach to febrile child younger than 24 months.

Table *7-2*

OBSERVATION SCALE FOR FEBRILE CHILDREN*

Observation Item	1 Point (Normal)	3 Points (Moderate Impairment)	5 Points (Severe Impairment)
Quality of cry	Not crying or strong cry with normal tone	Sobbing or whimpering	Weak, moaning, high-pitched, or continual cry
Reaction to parent stimulation	Content and not crying or cries briefly and stops	Cries intermittently	Barely responds or cries continuously
Level of consciousness	If awake, stays awake; if asleep, wakes quickly	Awakens with prolonged stimulation	Falls asleep or will not arouse
Color	Pink	Extremities pale or acrocyanosis	Pale, cyanotic, mottled, or ashen
Hydration	Skin and eyes normal, mucous membranes moist	Skin and eyes normal; mouth slightly dry	Skin doughy or tented, mucous membranes dry, and eyes sunken
Response to social overtures	Smiles (or startles[†])	Brief smile (or startles briefly[†])	Face anxious, dull, expressionless (or does not startle[†])

From McCarthy PL: Observation scales to identify serious illness in febrile children, *Pediatrics* 70:802, 1982.
*Likelihood of serious infection based on score:
   Score 10 or less: small
   Score 11-16: intermediate
   Score greater than 16: high
[†]Age 2 months or younger.

be discharged, and follow-up can be arranged. A recognizable bacterial infection requires further work-up and therapy. The child who appears well, who is without a worrisome history or focal findings on examination, and who has only recently developed a fever of 39.4° C or less has a minimal chance of having a serious infection. This child can generally be discharged if you can arrange follow-up in 12 to 24 hours. The child who appears ill or has a rectal temperature above 39.4° C requires laboratory evaluation with a CBC and ESR. If these results are normal, discharge the child and arrange for follow-up. If the screening test results are abnormal, obtain a chest x-ray study, blood culture, and other relevant studies.

If these additional studies are not decisive and if the child does not appear toxic after defervescence, discharge may be considered after the administration of antibiotics parenterally (ceftriaxone 50 mg/kg IM) or orally (amoxicillin 50 mg/kg/day or cefaclor 20 to 40 mg/kg/day). Close follow-up, including checking the culture results, in 6 to 12 hours should be arranged.

The decision to perform a lumbar puncture rests primarily on the results of optimal observation and on the child's responsiveness, mental status, and neck movement. Remember that younger children often do not have a stiff neck with meningitis. Rarely are laboratory data decisive. Children with a temperature above 41° C are at an increased risk of meningitis. Obtain a urinalysis as part of the septic work-up in a child less than 2 years of age and in the child who has a history of frequency, dribbling, or abdominal pain without signs of upper respiratory tract infection.

Follow-up within 12 to 24 hours is essential for patients with high fever and whom the emergency physician has deemed appropriate for discharge because of a negative emergency department work-up. The follow-up visit should include a check of the blood culture and an evaluation of the child's appearance.

MANAGEMENT

Acetominophen (e.g., Tylenol, Tempra, Datril, Liquiprin) is the agent of choice for fever reduction. It is well tolerated, has few side effects, and is very effective. Acetaminophen is available in liquids, tablets, and suppositories. It is rapidly absorbed, with peak levels occurring in 1 to 2 hours and a half-life of approximately 3 hours. The dosage of acetaminophen is 10 to 15 mg/kg every 4 to 6 hours. At least initially, there is a dose response curve, with higher doses being more effective. Some physicians routinely administer 20 mg/kg for initial fever control.

Aspirin is an effective antipyretic but cannot be recommended, particularly in children because of its association with Reye's syndrome. Ibuprofen is also an effective antipyretic and may lower a fever that is resistant to acetaminophen. Ibuprofen is now available in liquid form. Peak serum levels are attained 1 hour after administration, and ibuprofen has a half-life of 1.8 to 2 hours. Peak reduction of fever occurs 2 to 4 hours after the dose has been given. The dose is 5 mg/kg for temperatures less than 39° C or 10 mg/kg for temperatures greater than 39° C. Fevers resulting from serious bacterial infections are at least as responsive to antipyretics as benign viral syndromes; thus the fact that a fever has lowered with antipyretics should not be used as evidence for a viral syndrome.

External cooling is also an effective method of reducing temperature. A combination of antipyretic therapy and sponging of the skin with tepid water in the presence of a fan produces the most rapid lowering of fever. Do not use ice water bathing or alcohol sponging with a pediatric patient.

Avoid using antibiotics without a defined source of infection. The indiscriminate use of antibiotics confuses the clinical picture and may encourage the emergence of resistant organisms.

KEY CONSIDERATIONS

WHAT IS THE LIFE THREAT?

Fever may be caused by a life-threatening infection such as meningitis or urosepsis in the immune-competent host. Fever may be caused by sepsis, pneumonia, encephalitis, meningitis, brain abscess, pyelonephritis, and a wide variety of opportunistic infections in the immunocompromised host.

DOES THE PATIENT NEED ADMISSION?

Admit the patient who appears toxic, who has a serious underlying illness, or who is immunocompromised. Immunocompromised patients include those undergoing chemotherapy (especially those with a diminished absolute neutrophil count); those who have had a splenectomy; and those with AIDS, diabetes mellitus, sickle cell disease, or chronic alcohol abuse.

WHAT IS THE MOST SERIOUS DIAGNOSIS?

Meningitis, sepsis, pneumonia, and neuroleptic malignant syndrome are the most serious diagnoses.

HAVE I PERFORMED A THOROUGH WORK-UP?

Evaluate for occult infection, especially in the patient who appears toxic or is immunocompromised.

Evaluate patients for urinary tract infection; obtain a urinalysis.

With a fever of undetermined origin, obtain adequate cultures, including throat, sputum, urine, and blood.

Consider meningitis and obtain cerebrospinal fluid for cell count and culture.

Recommended Reading

Baker MD, Fosareli PD, Carpenter RO: Childhood fever: correlation of diagnosis with temperature response to acetaminophen, *Pediatrics* 80:315, 1987.

Bonadio WA et al: Efficacy of a protocol to distinguished risk of serious bacterial infection in the outpatient evaluation of febrile young infants, *Clin Pediatr* 32:401, 1993.

Dinarello, CA, Wolff SM: Pathogenesis of fever in man, *N Engl J Med* 298:607, 1978.

McCarthy PL et al: Temperatures greater than or equal to 40° C in children less than 24 months of age: a prospective study, *Pediatrics* 59:633, 1977.

McCarthy PL et al: Observation scales to identify serious illness in febrile children, *Pediatrics* 70:802, 1982.

Mellors JW et al: A simple index to identify occult bacterial infections in adults with acute unexplained fever, *Arch Intern Med* 147:666, 1987.

Chapter Eight

ALTERED MENTAL STATUS AND SYNCOPE

JONATHAN A. HANDLER AND D. MICHAEL HUNT

ALTERED MENTAL STATUS

The physician who is encountering the patient with an altered mental status may feel a sense of discomfort. The patient may not be able to give an adequate history, but the underlying problem may well be life-threatening. An organized approach to such patients, combined with knowledge about the common causes of altered mental status, can lead to a rapid diagnosis and life-saving therapy. Remember that homeostasis protects the brain at all costs. Therefore if an altered mental status is manifested, a severe physiologic problem may be occurring, and a timely diagnosis is important for such patients.

Many terms are used to describe mental status changes. The following three terms are examples: *Obtundation* is a state of reduced alertness accompanied by extreme sleepiness. A more severe state is *stupor,* which refers to a state of unresponsiveness; the patient can be roused with vigorous stimulation but quickly relapses into unresponsiveness. *Coma* is a state of complete unresponsiveness or an inappropriate response to stimuli. An example of an inappropriate response to stimulation is extension of the arms and legs after a sternal rub. *Lethargy* is a special type of altered mental status in which

there is decreased or lack of attention to surroundings, although the patient may still be awake. This term is particularly important in infants, who often manifest lethargy with extreme illness.

Etiology

The differential diagnosis for mental status change is broad. A mnemonic device has been developed to assist developing clinicians (see the box on p. 81). The most likely etiology of a patient's altered mental status changes dramatically with age. In the elderly, likely causes of such changes are stroke, sepsis, and dehydration. In the young adult, a toxin (especially alcohol), the postictal state, and trauma are the common causes of an altered mental status. In the child, infection, dehydration, and trauma are common causes.

The etiologies of mental status changes fall into two broad categories: intracerebral processes and extracerebral processes. Intracerebral processes affect the brain both locally and globally. Tumors, infarcts, and hemorrhages can affect neurologic function by affecting the surrounding brain and can cause focal neurologic defects such as an aphasia or unilateral weak-

---

MENTAL STATUS CHANGE ETIOLOGY MNEMONIC DEVICE

P = Psychiatric disorder
E = Eclampsia
T = Temperature problem (hypothermia or hyperthermia)

V = Vascular problem (hematomas, cerebrovascular accident, hypertensive encephalopathy, shock)
 I = Intoxication (medications, drugs, alcohol)
C = Cancer (brain tumor)
T = Trauma
 I = Inflammatory process (infection, collagen vascular disease)
M = Metabolic (thiamine, glucose, sodium, calcium, uremia, hepatic encephalopathy)
 S = Seizure (active, postictal state)

---

ness. Lesions in the brainstem or a large part of the reticular activating system can result in alterations in consciousness. Intracerebral processes can also affect neurologic function by increasing intracranial pressure (ICP). Large tumors, infarcts with edema, large hemorrhages, hydrocephalus, or contusions with edema can cause increased ICP, which leads to a diffusely decreased blood flow to the brain and an altered mental status. The brain is enclosed by rigid structures (the skull and dural folds such as the falx cerebri and the tentorium). When the pressure increases enough, part of the brain may herniate out of its compartment, which usually results in death. Infections of the brain or meninges can cause altered mental status through both local and global effects.

Extracerebral processes cause mental status changes through their effects on neuronal function. For instance, toxins, a lack of oxygen, or an overabundance of sodium (which causes a hyperosmolar state) may directly inhibit proper neuron function. Sepsis can cause neuronal dysfunction by forming toxins and metabolites that inhibit neuronal function and by inducing shock, which decreases cerebral blood flow.

Approach to the Patient With an Altered Mental Status

Establish unresponsiveness

Because the patient with an altered mental status may well have a life-threatening disease process, evaluation and treatment should occur simultaneously. First, check for unresponsiveness by asking the patient a question such as, "What is your name?" or by giving a command such as, "Open your eyes." If there is no response, attempt a painful or noxious maneuver, which is described later in this chapter, and check for movement.

Manage the airway and cervical spine

Assessment and management of the airway is of primary importance in *all* patients. Note the presence of any vomitus in the mouth, look for evidence of upper airway obstruction (e.g., stridor), and check for a gag reflex. Determine whether the patient's decreased level of consciousness is profound enough to require active airway control, such as endotracheal intubation. Concomitantly, determine the status of the cervical spine. Trauma may have caused the mental status change, or the mental status change may have led to the trauma (e.g., the patient was confused and fell out of bed). If an injury is suspected, take precautions to protect the cervical spine. Any trauma patient with a Glasgow Coma Scale (GCS) score of less than 8 or with signs of increased ICP needs active airway management. Of particular concern are patients with signs of impending herniation, such as a dilated and unresponsive pupil, worsening mental status, and unilateral hemiplegia. The technique used to control the airway is critical because maneuvers that increase ICP, especially gagging, must be avoided. Nasotracheal intubation is not appropriate because it increases ICP. The anesthetic technique used to prevent increased ICP is known as rapid sequence induction. This technique uses pretreatment with intravenous lidocaine to blunt such a response. Next, a rapid-acting paralytic agent and a rapid-acting anesthetic agent are given successively, after which the endotracheal tube is placed. Be sure to use agents that do not significantly increase ICP.

Breathing

After the airway has been secured either through intubation, cricothyrotomy, or assurance by examination that the patient can protect the airway, breathing is assessed. If the patient has been intubated because of increased ICP, the next maneuver is to hyperventilate the patient to bring the Pco_2 to approximately 25 mm Hg. Hyperventilation is the most rapid way to lower ICP. In the patient who is spontaneously breathing, the pattern of breathing can be a clue to the problem. *Apnea* and *bradypnea* are often seen in drug overdoses. The *Kussmaul* pattern of respiration (very deep, regular breathing) is classically seen with diabetic ketoacidosis. *Cheyne-Stokes respirations* involve a recurring pattern of apnea followed by an accelerating pattern of deeper and faster breaths that gradually slow down and become more shallow until apnea resumes. This pattern is often seen in patients with congestive heart failure, increased ICP, and other forms of brain

injury. A pattern characterized by a deep gasp, a pause, a heavy sigh for exhalation, and another pause is called *apneustic breathing* and is often seen in lesions of the pons. *Biot's breathing* involves periods of apnea that are interrupted at irregular intervals by episodes of regular respirations; this condition is often associated with meningitis. *Agonal respirations* are seen just before death or impending respiratory failure and are characterized by ineffective, shallow, weak, and irregular breaths. When any pattern of ineffective ventilation is noted, the airway should be actively managed *immediately.*

Circulation

To assess the circulation, evaluate the pulses and the capillary refill while another member of the team simultaneously checks the vital signs, including pulse and blood pressure. For cases in which the cause of the mental status change is not known to be relatively benign (such as mild alcohol intoxication), an intravenous line should be established, and the patient should be placed on a cardiac monitor. Blood should also be drawn for laboratory analysis.

Any abnormality in circulation (e.g., an abnormal pulse or blood pressure) may cause an altered mental status or may be a manifestation of the underlying cause. Correct the problem and, if the mental status does not improve, continue the work-up.

Immediate tests and therapies

Clinical and historical data alone cannot predict which patients will have hypoglycemia and respond to a dextrose infusion. Furthermore, hypoglycemia can mimic any neurologic condition. Because withholding dextrose from patients with hypoglycemia can be harmful, this condition should always be checked immediately. *Every* patient with an acute mental status abnormality should have oxygenation checked with a *pulse oximeter* and serum glucose checked with a *fingerstick glucose* test. If these tests are unavailable, the patient should be empirically given oxygen and 50 ml of a 50% dextrose solution. Children should receive 1 ml/kg of 25% dextrose. If the oxygenation and serum glucose tests are available, treat any patient with a lowered oxygen saturation (<92%) or with a measured glucose level <60. Empiric dextrose should not be given for patients with signs of an acute stroke because there is evidence that glucose may worsen the outcome in this situation. Although hypoglycemia can mimic stroke with hemiplegia, this is rare. Therefore when a patient shows the classic signs of an acute stroke, it is prudent to avoid dextrose infusion unless there is documented hypoglycemia.

In patients with a history of alcoholism or in those who appear malnourished, 100 mg of thiamine should be immediately administered intravenously. This treatment may reverse an acute Wernicke syndrome. Because a dextrose infusion given to a patient with a thiamine deficiency may precipitate Wernicke syndrome, thiamine should be administered *prior* to dextrose.

Finally, consideration should be given to administration of 2 mg of naloxone. Limit the administration of naloxone to patients who meet one or more of the following criteria: pinpoint pupils, respirations of 12 or less, or a suspicion of narcotic use. Remember that many patients with cancer are on long-acting oral narcotics such as MS Contin or long-acting topical narcotics such as a Fentanyl patch, which should be removed during the course of the evaluation.

The four vital interventions can be remembered with the mnemonic device "*DON'T*," as in "DON'T forget these!": D = dextrose, O = oxygen, N = naloxone, and T = thiamine.

History

Because it may be difficult to obtain accurate histories from patients with an altered mental status, try to find information from other sources. If the patient arrived by ambulance, interrogate the paramedics. Look in the waiting room or call the patient's home for helpful family members, or try to reach the patient's private physician, if known and available. Check the patient's pockets and wallet or purse for information. Perhaps most importantly, call for the patient's old records on arrival to the emergency department. If the patient has visited your institution before, these records will be a valuable source of information.

A full history should be taken from anyone available, and care should be taken to note several aspects of the history. Inquire about medication use and drug or alcohol abuse. Ask about the medical history, especially diabetes mellitus, other metabolic or endocrine disorders, kidney diseases, neurologic diseases (e.g., stroke or dementia), seizure disorders, cancer, and psychiatric diseases. Ask whether the patient has been ill recently, particularly with regard to symptoms of infection (e.g., fever or cough), complaints of headache or other pain, thoughts of suicide, manifestations of a worsening psychiatric disorder, or transient neurologic complaints.

Physical

Check vital signs. A careful physical examination brings valuable clues to the underlying problem. Most important to this examination are the vital signs. As noted earlier, an abnormal vital sign may be the direct cause of the mental status alteration or may be a valuable clue to the cause. A *full* set of vital signs must be documented for every patient. Extreme hyperthermia (40° C or more) or extreme hypothermia (less than 32° C) can cause mental status changes. Less severe fever or hypothermia is commonly a sign of sepsis. To obtain the patient's temperature, a rectal temperature is preferable. Hypotension can cause a mental status change via hypoperfusion and often reflects a severe underlying disease process (e.g., sepsis or an acute overdose). Similarly, hypertension can cause a hypertensive encephalopathy or may be a manifestation of the underlying disorder (e.g., an acute stroke). Changes in the pulse or the respiratory rate or pattern can also provide valuable clues to the problem. Tachycardia or bradycardia may cause hypotension and poor cerebral perfusion or may be a sign of the underlying disorder. Increased respirations can be a sign of sepsis, salicylate intoxication, or a pulmonary embolus, among other causes. Decreased respirations are often seen with opiate overdose.

Assess the level of responsiveness. Assessing the patient's level of responsiveness is best done using the Glasgow Coma Scale score for responsiveness (see the box below). If the patient is verbally unresponsive, rub your knuckles on the sternum or press vigorously with a fingertip on the supraorbital notch to cause deep pain. To check for pain response in an extremity, place the handle of a reflex hammer across a fingernail or toenail and perpendicular to the finger or toe. Squeeze the handle on the nail and observe for withdrawal or pain localization. Be certain to maintain respect for the patient and demonstrate care when performing these maneuvers.

GLASGOW COMA SCALE

Eye opening
  4 = Spontaneous
  3 = To verbal command
  2 = To pain
  1 = No response
Motor response
  6 = To verbal command
  5 = Localizes pain (e.g., moves hand to push yours away)
  4 = Withdraws
  3 = Flexor response
  2 = Extensor response
  1 = No response
Verbal response
  5 = Oriented
  4 = Confused conversation
  3 = Inappropriate words
  2 = Incomprehensible sounds
  1 = No response

Examine the eyes and head. The eyes can be a window to the brain—both literally and figuratively. Funduscopy allows the examiner to directly visualize one sign of increased ICP—papilledema. An assessment of the pupillary reactions and extraocular movements can be informative. Reactive pupils indicate at least some integrity of the second and third cranial nerves. A unilateral fixed, dilated pupil is often a sign of impending or completed brain herniation and death as a result of increased ICP. Extraocular movements should be tested in the cooperative patient. For a patient in a coma and whose cervical spine is not injured, the oculocephalogyric (or "Doll's eye") maneuver can be tested. To perform this maneuver, the patient's head is quickly but gently turned to one side and then the other. If the reflex is present, the eyes of the patient who was lying down looking at the ceiling will remain looking at the ceiling when the head is turned. If the patient's eyes move with the head, this reflex is not present. If the reflex is not present, one can assume that there is a serious lesion involving the brainstem at least at the level of the pons. If there is concern about cervical spine injury, cold calorics can be tested. Cold water is carefully poured in the ear, which should stimulate nystagmus away from the ear. Nystagmus direction is defined as the direction of the *fast* phase. The fact that cold calorics cause nystagmus in the direction opposite the ear with the water can be remembered by the mnemonic device *COWS: c*old = *o*pposite; *w*arm = *s*ame.

Examine the head for signs of trauma. If there is not a possibility of neck fracture, examine the patient for meningeal signs. Note that in the elderly, the neck commonly has very poor range of motion secondary to degenerative arthritis.

Note the respiratory pattern and the smell of the breath. Checking the patient's respiratory pattern may help localize the cause of the mental status change. Smell the breath for a sweet acetone odor (diabetic ketoacidosis) or an odor of alcohol. Because these two smells can be similar, be sure to check a serum glucose level and a blood alcohol level, or use a breath analyzer for alcohol.

Perform a neurologic examination. The neurologic examination should search for signs of focality. Cranial nerves II, III, IV and VI are tested via the pupillary reactions and extraocular movements. The fifth and seventh cranial nerves can be tested with the corneal reflex, which involves lightly touching a tissue or wisp of cotton to the cornea and which causes the patient to blink if the reflex is intact. Examine the face for unilateral droop of an eyelid or a corner of the mouth as a nerve lesion sign. Check the gag reflex to evaluate cranial nerves IX and X. See if the patient moves all the extremities, either spontaneously to command or in response to pain. If there appears to be a unilateral deficit, check the tone on that side. Quickly check for the Babinski reflex. Note the patient's Glasgow Coma Scale score because this measure is an objective way to follow the patient's neurologic status and is reflective of prognosis.

Perform a mental status examination. Finally, a mental status examination should be performed to determine whether a psychiatric cause of the mental status change is likely. Table 54-1, p. 648 provides a mnemonic for differentiating between organic and functional psychoses; the box on p. 650 illustrates the steps of the mini-mental state examination.

Tests

Standard laboratory tests in the patient with a severely altered mental status include a complete blood count (to look for evidence of severe anemia or infection), electrolytes, blood urea nitrogen (BUN), creatinine, and a serum glucose, in addition to fingerstick glucose. Check the calcium level in patients who are at risk for abnormalities (e.g., cancer or dialysis patients) or who are very ill. If appropriate, order any of the following: a urinalysis, a magnesium

level (e.g., for those on diuretics), an ammonia level (e.g., for those with liver disease), drug levels for patients on medications that can cause mental status changes, and an arterial blood gas in any seriously ill patient. Consider a toxicology test to screen for drugs of abuse.

An ECG should be obtained for all patients. Obtain a chest x-ray examination if pulmonary disease is suspected. Routine chest x-ray examinations in those patients without pulmonary signs are often abnormal in patients who have an acute alteration of mental status and therefore should be obtained, especially if the patient will be admitted. CT scans of the brain should be obtained if there is trauma with an associated mental status change; if there are focal findings on the physical examination; or if the history, physical, and first-line tests do not produce an explanation for the problem. There is a controversy in the literature over whether a CT scan is required for minor head trauma with brief loss of consciousness and a normal neurologic examination. A growing body of evidence suggests that a CT scan may be indicated in all such cases because patients with significant intracranial injury can show minimal or no signs of serious injury. Intoxicated patients are probably at an increased risk for an intracranial injury. In addition, children less than 2 years old with a mild head injury are considered to be at least at a moderate risk for intracranial injury simply because they are so difficult to examine and evaluate. Therefore serious consideration should be given to CT scanning in such populations.

In the patient with HIV, there is some evidence that adding contrast enhancement is beneficial in the acute setting only if the noncontrast head CT scan is not absolutely normal. In the non-HIV population, contrast enhancement almost never contributes to acute management.

If not clinically contraindicated, a lumbar puncture should be performed in all cases of suspected meningitis, subarachnoid hemorrhage, or unexplained seizures. Any patient with HIV and a mental status change who has a nondiagnostic work-up, including laboratory tests and a head CT scan, needs a lumbar puncture as well. Evidence suggests that in the elderly patient with a fever and a mental status change, a lumbar puncture should be performed only if there is no other source of infection found or if meningitis may be a concomitant infection.

Therapy

Therapy is tailored to the presumed cause of the altered mental status. Any patient who is being observed for clinical improvement in the emergency department (e.g., the intoxicated patient or the postictal patient) needs frequent neurologic examinations. If the patient deteriorates or does not improve as expected, immediate intervention is required. Admission is indicated for cases in which the altered mental status: (1) remains unexplained, (2) is acute and persists despite treatment, (3) may be expected to relapse, or (4) is caused by serious underlying disease (see Table 54-1, p. 648).

SYNCOPE

Syncope has been described in several ways, but the most complete definition is that of a transient loss of consciousness that is characterized by unresponsiveness and loss of postural tone with spontaneous recovery (usually within seconds to minutes) and that does not require specific resuscitative intervention. Conditions in which syncope develop may be situational or a result of an underlying disease process that may be recently developed, gradually acquired, or congenital. Regardless of the etiology or speed of development, all fainting is manifest through a final common physiologic pathway: inadequate cerebral perfusion. The brain is exquisitely sensitive to fluctuations in the provision of oxygen and glucose, and it requires a minimum perfusion pressure to supply these metabolic substrates.

Epidemiology

Each year, 600,000 people complain to their physicians about syncope or near-syncope. This figure is underscored by the fact that patients with syncope account for up to 3% of all emergency department visits. The incidence of syncope varies with age. Although as many as 15% of all children will experience syncope before the end of adolescence, more than 20% of all adults report syncope during their lifetime. The elderly population as a whole has an even higher incidence, which approaches 6% *every year.* In addition, after one syncopal episode, the recurrence rate among the elderly is 30%.

Etiology

Neurogenic

The specific etiologies of syncope vary in their categorization (see the box on p. 87). The most commonly encountered event, regardless of age, results from a vasovagal episode. Also referred to as vasodepressor or neurally mediated syncope, this condition has more recently been labelled as neurocardiogenic syncope. This condition involves the activation of myocardial mechanoreceptors (C fibers), which leads to decreased efferent sympathetic tone and increased efferent parasympathetic tone. Unless the reflex arc is interrupted, peripheral vasodilation, hypotension, and syncope occur. Cardiac vagal tone is known to decrease with age, which probably explains the fact that a neurocardiogenic mechanism accounts for as much as 50% of all cases of syncope in the pediatric population and less than 10% of those in the geriatric population. Events that produce pain, fear, apprehension, or direct vagal stimulation (as can be seen with surgical instrumentation) are required antecedents for this diagnosis.

ETIOLOGIC CLASSIFICATION OF SYNCOPE

Neurogenic

Neurocardiogenic
Orthostatic
  Dehydration
  Acute hemorrhage
  Anemia
  Third spacing
Carotid sinus disease
Seizure
Glossopharyngeal neuralgia

Metabolic

Hypoglycemia
Hyponatremia
Hypercalcemia

Psychiatric

Central nervous system

Situational

Cough
Micturition (defecation)

Cardiogenic

Dysrhythmias
  Bradydysrhythmias
  Tachydysrhythmias
  Asystole
Prolonged QT interval
Valvular disease
Mechanical obstruction

Vascular

Drugs

Beta blockers
Nitrates
Digitalis
Hypnotics
Vasodilators
Diuretics
Antidysrhythmics
Antidepressants
Phenothiazines

Orthostatic syncope is manifest by a relative decline in systolic blood pressure of more than 25 mm Hg or an absolute fall to below 90 mm Hg after standing from a recumbent posture. Assuming a standing position usually involves a "loss" of 300 to 800 ml of blood that is normally available to the central circulation as a result of redistribution in the lower extremities. The usual physiologic response to the decreased central venous return and concomitant lowered cardiac output is vasoconstriction, tachycardia, and increased myocardial contractility and cardiac output, which results in an increased diastolic and mean arterial pressure. As people age, the ability to respond efficiently to transient de-creases in venous return is somewhat diminished. Orthostatic syncope is also seen in cases of relative (third spacing) or absolute (hemorrhage, anemia, dehydration) volume loss. Orthostatic syncope can occur in individuals who have been standing immobile for extended periods (e.g., military personnel at attention). In such cases the leg muscles are unable to contract regularly and contribute to the restoration of blood to the central circulation.

Carotid sinus syncope represents a third major category of neurogenic syncope and is characterized by hypotension with or without bradycardia or ventricular asystole. It is due to hypersensitive stretch receptors in the carotid bodies and is seen most often in males; the elderly; and those with diabetes, hypertension, or ischemic heart disease. The fainting may be induced by head turning, neck flexion, shaving, or tight collars.

Seizure disorders represent a special subclass of neurologic conditions that produce a loss of consciousness. Although generalized seizures can satisfy the previously described definition, many clinicians would not classify epileptic or alcohol-withdrawal seizures as syncope. Seizures are often not self-limited and do not necessarily result in loss of muscle tone. With seizures, recovery to the premorbid state tends to take longer than seconds to minutes. Confounding the diagnosis is the fact that many patients experiencing syncope exhibit several seconds of mild opisthotonoid activity that may appear seizure-like but is, in fact, unrelated to any seizure. Unfortunately, even neurologists can find it difficult to distinguish between the two conditions.

Finally, glossopharyngeal neuralgia, which is a condition of intense paroxysmal pain in the head and neck and is thought to be triggered by some irritative lesion, can trigger a reflex arc that results in a neurocardiogenic response as described previously.

Cardiogenic

Although neurogenic causes predominate in frequency, cardiogenic causes are notable for their prognostic implications. When syncope can be attributed to a cardiogenic cause, the 1-year mortality rate of such patients ranges between 18% to 33%, and the 1-year incidence of sudden death is 24%. This rate compares remarkably with the 6% 1-year mortality rates and 3% to 4% 1-year sudden death rates of patients in whom the syncopic etiology is either noncardiac or undefined.

Dysrhythmias can be a more common cause of fainting than neurocardiogenic events, especially in older populations, and accounts for 5% to 30% of all syncopes. Either bradydysrhythmias in the form of second- or third-degree atrioven-

tricular block, ventricular standstill, or sick sinus syndrome, or tachydysrhythmias such as supraventricular tachycardia or sustained ventricular tachycardia can induce loss of consciousness. Other abnormalities may be seen on ECGs (e.g., bundle branch blocks, unsustained ventricular tachycardia, Wolff-Parkinson-White syndrome, a prolonged QT interval) that may not directly cause syncope but may suggest investigation into the possibility that some type of dysrhythmia is responsible for the event.

Mechanical dysfunction constitutes the other major cause for cardiogenic syncope. Left ventricular outflow can be reduced by aortic stenosis or hypertrophic subaortic stenosis. Pulmonary flow can be compromised by pulmonic stenosis, pulmonary hypertension, or pulmonary embolism. Global output is restricted by cardiac tamponade, and either or both ventricles may be involved in large myocardial infarctions, which leads to pump failure and syncope. Structurally, an atrial myxoma or ball-valve thrombus may transiently reduce cardiac output to the limits of cerebral tolerance.

Vascular

For consciousness to be lost secondary to an arterial obstruction, either simultaneous bilateral cerebral occlusion (in the form of carotid obstruction) or vertebrobasilar ischemia must occur. This latter scenario may be rarely seen with the subclavian steal syndrome or vertebrobasilar transient ischemic attacks (TIAs). Up to 25% of all patients with a leaking aortic aneurysm have a syncopal episode, and such an episode can also be seen with aortic dissection.

Metabolic

Blood chemistry disturbances account for syncope in only 2% to 3% of all cases, and even this figure may be a generous estimate because almost all of these episodes are hypoglycemic in nature. Like seizures the inclusion of hypoglycemia as a syncopal etiology is open to debate, because patients who lose consciousness as a result of low blood sugar do not recover spontaneously but require the administration of exogenous glucose. If these cases are excluded, the remainder are almost always a result of hypercalcemia or hyponatremia, both of which should be suspected after a history and physical examination have been obtained.

Pharmacologic

Numerous medications have been implicated as a cause of syncope: beta blockers, digitalis, nitrates, vasodilators, hypnotics, antidysrhythmics, diuretics, antidepressants, and phenothiazines. The mechanisms are varied but may be a result of orthostatic, dysrhythmic, or central nervous system interactions. Elderly adults are especially likely to faint under the influence of medication because they commonly take several prescription drugs at the same time and are subject to certain age-related physiologic changes, which makes them susceptible to the side effects of a particular drug.

Psychosomatic

Occasionally patients faint as a result of hysteria or a conversion reaction, but other potential underlying causes must be ruled out before resorting to this diagnosis.

Central nervous system

Insults to the central nervous system may occur spontaneously (subarachnoid hemorrhage) or as a result of trauma (closed head injury that produces a concussion or intracranial hemorrhage). It would be unusual and incorrect to refer to a loss of consciousness secondary to a blow to the head as "syncope." Although many mild head injuries result in only temporary unconsciousness with spontaneous return to a cognizant state, more serious head injuries result in a persistent loss of consciousness. The diagnostic and therapeutic priorities for CNS events deviate significantly from the procedures followed for more "traditional" forms of syncope.

Situational

Included within this category are certain conditions that are notoriously associated with loss of consciousness in susceptible individuals. Micturition syncope typically occurs in men who experience nocturia after ingesting alcohol. Defecation syncope probably occurs as a function of performing a Valsalva maneuver in the sitting position. Loss of consciousness may occur by a similar mechanism when either the bowel or obstructed bladder are evacuated by disimpaction or catheterization.

Cough syncope, also known as laryngeal vertigo, is seen primarily in men and occasionally in the pediatric population but almost never in women. In adults, cough syncope begins with vigorous, unrelenting coughing that ultimately terminates in syncope of short duration. Children who experience this phenomenon often have undiagnosed asthma, which requires adequate management before the recurrence of syncope can be eliminated.

Swallowing syncope is rare and usually occurs in patients who have an underlying esophageal abnormality or cardiac conduction malady. Some individuals have an aberrant reflex arc, in which the act of swallowing triggers bradycardia and atrioventricular block, occasionally to the point of inducing fainting.

Diagnostic Evaluation

The particular etiology of the syncopic event can often, though by no means always, be determined by a thorough and thoughtful emergency department work-up. Up to 47% of all cases remain undiagnosed in spite of both inpatient and outpatient study.

History

The key element in an emergency department evaluation is obtaining a complete historical account of the syncopic event. Accounts of the event should be sought from the patient, available witnesses, and prehospital personnel, if involved. First determine whether loss of consciousness actually occurred or if the patient in fact experienced dizziness, vertigo, or some other symptom that suggests a broader list of differential diagnoses. Once the true nature of syncope has been established, specific questions should be asked regarding the events occurring immediately before, during, and after the episode. As with any patient, a complete medication history should be obtained.

The patient should be questioned about the conditions under which the event occurred. Syncope during periods of exertion suggests a dysrhythmic or vascular cause. A patient with a history of syncope after isolated arm use may be a member of the small group of those with subclavian steal syndrome. Fainting in an emotionally charged situation suggests a psychogenic or possible neurocardiogenic event. Patient position can be a key to determining a diagnosis. Prolonged standing, especially in warm, crowded environments predisposes a patient to venous pooling and orthostatic syncope. Orthostatic syncope does not occur in the supine position but should be a consideration for patients who are upright or have recently assumed an upright posture. Conversely, individuals who experience unheralded fainting in the seated or recumbent position should be considered as having a cardiac source until proven otherwise. Head turning, or any situation that puts pressure on the neck, should prompt an investigation for carotid sinus syncope.

The presence or absence of premonitory symptoms can also provide a clue to the diagnosis. Although nausea, diaphoresis, and lightheadedness are nonspecific symptoms, they are common to neurocardiogenic episodes. Patients should be questioned about antecedent chest pain, a rapid heartbeat, or skipped beats that may be associated with cardiac syncope. The presence of an aura or of focal sensory or motor disturbances is more an indication of seizures than of syncope. Fainting without warning does occur in some benign situations, including tussive (cough) and micturition syncope, but this

type of fainting should always raise suspicion for an underlying dysrhythmia.

A few key questions should be asked regarding the event and the immediate postsyncopic period: How long was the period of unconsciousness? If it lasts for more than a few minutes, other considerations must be entertained. Did the patient recover in rapid fashion? Were there focal neurologic signs or incontinence? A brief period of myoclonic jerking is common, but anything prolonged or lateralizing indicates a seizure.

A general history that complements the directed interview should be obtained, and particular attention should be devoted to recent illnesses (e.g., a fever with vomiting and diarrhea may have induced significant dehydration), changes in the chronic health picture (e.g., melena may suggest otherwise asymptomatic anemia), or a pattern of prior syncope.

Physical examination

The initial impression formed by the emergency physician when first encountering the patient often provides a general assessment of whether the patient is in imminent danger— either "sick" or "not sick." However, caution should be reserved for the apparently well individual who has an intermittent manifestation of a life-threatening dysrhythmia.

A complete set of vital signs should be obtained, including orthostatic pulse and blood pressure. An orthostatic cause of syncope should be considered for patients with a position-induced decline in systolic pressure that is greater than 20 mm Hg; an absolute decline to less than 90 mm Hg; or with the development of dizziness, presyncope, or syncope when assuming the sitting or standing position. If the patient's history suggests vertebrobasilar ischemia, comparative upper extremity blood pressures should be obtained. Look for a 20 mm Hg difference, which is indicative of subclavian steal syndrome.

The carotid arteries should be examined for bruits, which is suggestive of stenosis, or for evidence of a lag time from the apical pulse, which is indicative of significant aortic stenosis. Cannon a waves are a sign of atrioventricular block. The possibility of carotid sinus hypersensitivity should be explored only under carefully monitored clinical conditions and never in patients who are elderly or who have known or suspected extracranial or cerebrovascular disease. The cardiac examination should focus on the presence of murmurs, especially those of systolic nature, which suggests aortic stenosis or hypertrophic obstructive conditions. A rectal examination should be performed to look for occult gastrointestinal hemorrhage, which can contribute to anemia and hypovolemia. Finally, a neurologic examination is needed to investigate the possibility of seizure or cerebrovascular contributions to the syncopic event.

Tests

Routine laboratory studies are rarely helpful in explaining the cause of syncope and are generally not indicated. Requesting a complete blood count and electrolyte panel as part of a general screening evaluation is not necessary when a bedside fingerstick glucose evaluation and a simple hematocrit measurement will suffice. If a particular condition is suspected on the basis of the history and physical examination, focused studies can be ordered.

Conversely, because of its demonstrated diagnostic power and implications for a diagnosis of cardiac syncope, a 12-lead ECG should be obtained for every patient unless the syncopic etiology is clearly noncardiac. Patients with a suspected cardiac source should be placed on continuous cardiac monitoring until a disposition is determined. Although the initial ECG only provides a diagnosis in 2% to 6% of all cases, other abnormalities may be detected that prompt a further work-up.

Under certain conditions, the patient may be a candidate for outpatient Holter monitoring. Patients meeting the criteria are found to have positive studies approximately 60% of the time. Echocardiography should be reserved for patients who have undiagnosed, recurrent events but can be instrumental in discovering structural anomalies such as atrial myxomas, aortic stenosis, hypertrophic cardiomyopathy, or mitral valve prolapse.

Treatment

Because syncope is defined as a self-limited condition, most events will have resolved by the time the patient arrives at the emergency department. After the patient has been stabilized, attention can be directed toward the detection

SERIOUS CONDITIONS MANIFESTED AS SYNCOPE

Subarachnoid hemorrhage	Heat illness
Pericardial tamponade	Stroke
Toxic ingestion	Gastrointestinal hemorrhage
Abdominal aortic aneurysm	Angina
Pulmonary edema	Carbon monoxide poisoning
Pulmonary embolism	Myocardial infarction
Aortic dissection	Addisonian crisis
Ectopic pregnancy	Pheochromocytoma
Anaphylaxis	Epistaxis
Hypocalcemia	

From Hunt DM: Syncope. In Rosen P et al, editors: *Emergency medicine: concepts and clinical practice,* ed 3, St Louis, 1992, Mosby.

of any injuries associated with the syncope. Hemodynamic precariousness should be addressed with crystalloid infusion and, unless the event is clearly not heart related, a cardiac monitor should be applied. It is important to remember that syncope is not a diagnosis but rather a symptom. Numerous serious conditions may be manifested as syncope (see the box on p. 91), and it remains a priority of the treating physician to rule out the life threat.

Disposition

Young patients with an isolated syncopic event that has been determined to be noncardiac in nature and patients who return to a normal state of good health in a rapid fashion after the episode can be safely discharged with appropri-

ate arrangements for outpatient follow-up. As long as the patient does not have a serious, uncorrected, and underlying precipitant and is not at risk for recurrence, it is not crucial that a final diagnosis of syncopic cause be made. Any patient suspected of having or proven to have a cardiac source should be admitted for monitoring and treatment. This group of patients would include those with documented abnormalities on the basis of physical examination, ECG or cardiac rhythm aberrancy, or a suggestive history (e.g., unheralded event, seated or supine posture, older patient, known cardiac disease). Cardiology consultation and hospital admission remain the most prudent course for those patients who cannot safely be determined to have a noncardiac etiology.

KEY CONSIDERATIONS

WHAT IS THE LIFE THREAT?

Coma suggests a profound dysfunction in both cerebral hemispheres or in the brainstem. The underlying process causing such a dysfunction (e.g., poisoning or intracranial hemorrhage) may be immediately life threatening.

The comatose patient cannot protect the airway and may aspirate, causing life-threatening impairment of ventilation.

DOES THE PATIENT NEED ADMISSION?

A persistent coma requires in-hospital evaluation. Patients previously in an unresponsive state who may be discharged include the following: following a seizure in an awake and asymptomatic patient with a known seizure disorder and subtherapeutic anticonvulsant level, or a patient with diabetes and hypoglycemia who is not suicidal, fully awake, and able to eat.

Patients with acute alteration of mental status often require medical or psychiatric evaluation and hospitalization.

WHAT IS THE MOST SERIOUS DIAGNOSIS?

Intracranial hemorrhage, stroke, sepsis, dehydration, poisoning, head injury, hypothermia, hyperthermia, and hyperglycemia are the most serious diagnoses.

HAVE I PERFORMED A THOROUGH WORK-UP?

Evaluate the patient for serious causes of syncope, including cardiac dysrhythmia, myocardial infarction, pulmonary embolism, ectopic pregnancy, subarachnoid hemorrhage, aortic dissection or aneurysm, poisoning, heat illness, gastrointestinal bleeding, hypoglycemia, or new-onset seizure.

Recommended Reading

Frame DS, Kercher EE: Acute psychosis, *Emerg Med Clin North Am* 9(1):123-135, 1991.

Gillis JH, Marshall SA, Ruedy J, editors: *Confusion. On call: Principles and protocols,* Philadelphia, 1989, WB Saunders.

Hunt DM: Syncope. In Rosen P et al, editors: *Emergency medicine: concepts and clinical practice,* ed 3, St Louis, 1992, Mosby.

Jeret JS et al: Clinical predictors of abnormality disclosed by computed tomography after mild head trauma. *Neurosurgery* 32(1):9-16, 1993.

Kapoor WN: Evaluation and management of the patient with syncope, *JAMA* 268(18):2553-2560, 1992.

Peterson J: Coma. In Rosen P et al, editors: *Emergency medicine: concepts and clinical practice,* ed 3, St Louis, 1992, Mosby.

Sra JS et al: Neurocardiogenic syncope: diagnosis, mechanisms, and treatment, *Cardiol Clin* 11(1):183-191, 1993.

Chapter *Nine*
HEADACHE

GREGORY L. HENRY

MECHANISMS OF HEADACHE

The neural tissue of the brain itself has no sensory pain fibers. Consequently, headache is produced by the stimulation of efferent pain fibers in other tissues within the cranium or from elsewhere.

There are three mechanisms that affect pain-sensitive structures of the head and neck to produce headache. Headaches may represent a combination of these mechanisms. Muscular contraction of the neck and scalp musculature is the primary cause of tension headache. Vascular headaches depend on the dilatation and distension of vascular structures. Headaches produced by this mechanism include migraines; severe hypertension headaches; and vasodilator headaches associated with medications, drugs, and various toxic substances. Pain of vascular origin has a throbbing quality.

The final major mechanism of head pain is inflammation of the peripheral nerves and vessels of the head and neck, which may produce severe pain. In addition, inflammatory processes may directly involve the meninges at the base of the brain.

The many causes of headache are listed in the box on p. 95. Most patients seen in the emergency department with this chief complaint have muscle contraction or vascular headaches.

ASSESSMENT

History

Patient type

Three major categories of patients come to the emergency department with complaints of headache. The first category includes patients with their first severe headache. Such patients have not had a previous examination or diagnostic work-up and have the highest risk of having serious intracranial disease.

The second group includes patients who have chronic headaches but in whom there has been a change in the character, quality, or intensity of head pain.

The third group comprises those who have a chronic headache problem that has been previously evaluated and who come to the emergency department not because of a change in headache pattern but for pain control.

Temporal relationship

The speed of onset and the relationship to other signs and symptoms are important. The point at which the maximum pain intensity occurs and a history of the frequency, duration, and mitigating factors of headache should be obtained. A headache that recurs regularly over a number of years is most likely either tension or vascular. A severe headache with a rapid onset, particularly with alteration of consciousness or focal neurologic deficit, is much more likely to suggest intracranial hemorrhage, infarct, or meningitis.

Migraine and tension headaches usually begin before the fourth decade of life; therefore headache appearing for the first time in the elderly should not be considered to be one of these types. The relationship to any prodromal symptoms (such as visual or auditory symptoms) or a correlation with the menstrual cycle or with the ingestion of food and medications should also be noted.

Site

The location of a headache may be important in indicating cause. Approximately two thirds of all migraine attacks are unilateral but will vary from one side of the head to the other in different attacks. If recurring, throbbing headaches are always localized to the same side, the possibility of an intracranial mass, aneurysm, or vascular malformation should be considered. Cluster headaches, trigeminal neuralgia, and focal disease of pain-sensitive structures of the head and neck are also in the differential consideration.

The site of pain is not necessarily reliable in localizing space-occupying lesions. Intracranial masses may cause pain by the displacement of pain-sensitive blood vessels distant from the lesions themselves. Focal masses may cause bilateral head pain if the flow of cerebrospinal fluid is obstructed.

Quality

The quality of the pain is often difficult for patients to articulate. A pulsatile headache is generally of vascular origin and may be caused by vasodilatation, hypertension, or fever. The discomfort of trigeminal neuralgia is almost always a transient stabbing of shocklike facial pain. Headache associated with brain tumors may have a steady, aching quality. Cluster headache patients almost always complain of a

COMMON CAUSES OF HEADACHE

Intracranial

Vascular

Migraine
Fever
Hypoxemia
Hypertension
Anemia
Effort
Aneurysmal dilatation

Traction

Subarachnoid hemorrhage
Meningitis
Encephalitis
Cerebral abscess
Intracranial hematoma
Cerebral tumor
Pseudotumor cerebri
Postlumbar puncture

Extracranial/systemic

Muscle Contraction

Tension

Inflammation

Temporal arteritis
Other vasculitis

Toxic Substances

Carbon monoxide
Cyanide
Solvents

Medications

Oral contraceptives
Nitrates
Histamine

Craniofacial Disease

Acute glaucoma
Sinusitis
Temperomandibular joint dysfunction
Cervical spine lesions
Trigeminal neuralgia

deep, intense, periodically recurrent pain that lasts 20 minutes to 2 hours.

Intensity

In general, the intensity of a headache is not a reliable indicator of the underlying pathologic conditions. For example, patients who have severe anxiety may complain bitterly of pain and yet manifest little objective evidence of severe distress. Patients with trigeminal neuralgia, glossopharyngeal neuralgia, and cluster headaches generally experience severe pain.

Associated symptoms

Associated symptoms may be helpful in diagnosis. Although nausea, vomiting, and anorexia commonly accompany migraine headaches, such headaches may be seen in any disease process that raises intracranial pressure. In patients with cluster headaches, the distinctive autonomic findings (flushing of the forehead, conjunctival injection, lacrimation, and nasal congestion) are diagnostic.

The most serious of the associated symptoms is loss or significant diminution of consciousness. An abrupt onset of headache, particularly when accompanied by neck stiffness, often indicates subarachnoid hemorrhage.

Precipitants

Factors that precipitate or aggravate the headache should be sought. Any recent head or neck trauma is an obvious cause for headache. Increasing intensity produced by jarring or rapid movements, coughing, sneezing, or walking may indicate either vascular head pain or an inflammatory process. Ingestion of certain foods that contain tyramine (cheese, red wine, bananas) may trigger migraine headaches.

Medical history

The use of certain medications may be associated with headache. Oral contraceptives are known to increase migrainous headaches in susceptible patients. Nitrates used by those with coronary artery disease may produce severe, throbbing head pain. Other systemic diseases such as anemia, severe hypertension, and recent withdrawal from various medications may cause head pain.

Family history

Of all patients with migraine headache, 80% have a family history of the disease. Other vascular headaches also have at least a partial inherited disposition. When multiple family members simultaneously have a headache, the home environment should be investigated for toxins such as carbon monoxide.

Physical Examination

Although the historical aspects of a headache are often the most important factors leading to the determination of cause, abnormal findings during a physical examination are perhaps more indicative of the need for an emergent as opposed to a routine medical work-up. The majority of life-threatening conditions causing headache have demonstrable physical findings.

The vital signs are important. Blood pressure may be elevated in any condition that causes pain, but a true hypertensive headache generally does not occur until the diastolic pressure is approximately 130 mm Hg. Because the pulse may be elevated with any severe pain, tachycardia is not particularly helpful in distinguishing the cause of a headache.

The patient with a markedly elevated respiratory rate may have an anoxic basis for the head pain. Carbon monoxide poisoning, cyanide exposure, decreased oxygenation caused by anemia, pulmonary embolus, and exacerbation of chronic obstructive pulmonary disease (COPD) may all produce significant headache with tachypnea.

Fever is commonly accompanied by headache, and it requires the clinical judgment of the emergency physician to determine whether further studies for meningitis, encephalitis, or brain abscess are indicated in the patient with fever and headache. Always view with concern any serious alteration of mentation accompanying severe headache and fever.

The majority of pain-sensitive structures of the head and neck can be either viewed directly or palpated. Eliciting palpable tenderness over discrete areas, including the calvaria, sinus processes, and neck muscles may indicate the source of head pain. In elderly patients, palpation of the superficial temporal arteries is useful because these may be tender in cases of temporal arteritis.

In suspected trigeminal neuralgia, stimulating the fifth cranial nerve by tapping inside the mouth and on the face may reproduce the pain. In patients with headache located in the midface, palpate the teeth and gums to diagnose a periapical abscess.

Inspect the eyes for the redness and ciliary flush of iritis or for the corneal haziness seen in glaucoma. When glaucoma is suspected, tonometry is indicated. Chronic ear infection associated with the onset of headache may represent a cerebral abscess.

Examination of the neck may be crucial in diagnosing serious causes of headache. Nuchal rigidity requires careful evaluation. Although muscular tension can cause some mild stiffness, true meningismus is rarely caused by a muscular tension problem. Severe cervical spondylosis, meningitis, encephalitis, or subarachnoid hemorrhage may all cause meningismus. The rigidity associated with meningeal irritation is almost always flexion rigidity. Rotary movements of the neck are generally not painful.

A basic neurologic examination is required of all headache patients. The patient's mental status is of the utmost importance and needs careful documentation. Any evidence of depressed mentation, altered speech, or specific deficits should raise the question of an intracranial pathologic condition. Headache associated with lethargy signals a medical emergency that requires immediate evaluation. Serious disorders, including subarachnoid hemorrhage, stroke, tumor, abscess, subdural hematoma, encephalitis, and meningitis, are possible causes of headache in such patients.

Cranial nerve abnormalities are most likely to be discovered during the eye examination. The presence of ptosis, dysconjugate gaze, alterations in extraocular movement and pupillary reactivity, or diminution of visual acuity or fields should be viewed as requiring more extensive evaluation.

A funduscopic evaluation is important in all patients with headache. Papilledema may be present in instances of increased intracranial pressure. Acute hemorrhages and exudates may be seen in patients with hypertensive encephalopathy. Subhyaloid and retinal hemorrhages are uncommon but when present are essentially diagnostic of acute subarachnoid hemorrhage. Visualization of spontaneous venous pulsations within the fundus of the eye essentially ensures a low intracranial pressure.

Whenever a headache is accompanied by a motor deficit, it is imperative to rule out a vascular lesion. Examination of gait, tandem walk, and finger-to-nose testing may yield the only clues to the presence of posterior fossa masses. Hemiplegic migraine may be diagnosed in its early phases with the classic headache syndrome and muscular weakness.

Sensory examination and testing of deep tendon reflexes are usually of only minor help in obtaining a diagnosis when the remainder of the neurologic examination is normal.

Laboratory Examination

In a limited number of patients with underlying medical problems or other abnormalities found on general physical examination, certain tests such as serum glucose levels, arterial blood gas measurements, hemoglobin, and white blood cell count may be indicated. The erythrocyte sedimentation rate is virtually always elevated in symptomatic temporal arteritis and should be performed on all patients in whom the diagnosis is suspected. Carboxyhemoglobin levels may be useful in the appropriate setting. The emergency physician may want to order various other toxicologic studies, depending on the history.

The indication for an emergent lumbar puncture is suspected meningoencephalitis. If focal neurologic findings are noted, the lumbar puncture is delayed (but commence antibiotics) until a head CT scan can be performed.

Lumbar puncture is also used to detect blood from a subarachnoid hemorrhage that may be too small to be noted on a CT scan. In virtually all instances of subarachnoid hemorrhage, lumbar puncture reveals bloody or xanthochromic cerebrospinal fluid.

MANAGEMENT

The aim of emergency evaluation is to establish a working diagnosis and to determine how rapidly the definitive therapy must be initiated. The headache that should raise the greatest concern is one that is accompanied by an alteration of consciousness, focal neurologic findings, papilledema, or meningismus. Another worrisome presentation is in the patient who is having "the worst headache ever." Such presentations often signal the presence of an acute intracerebral event. After stabilization and rapid physical examination, such patients generally require a CT scan. If no intracranial pathologic condition is demonstrated in this study, a lumbar puncture may be performed. Perform an immediate puncture in those patients in whom meningitis or encephalitis is suspected. If subarachnoid hemorrhage is the principle concern and if there are no clinical findings to suggest increased intracranial pressure (e.g., papilledema or focal deficits), the head CT scan should be omitted and the emergency physician should proceed directly to lumbar puncture.

Begin treatment in the emergency department in patients with less severe headache and no focal neurologic findings and in whom the diagnosis can be made on the basis of history and physical examination. For patients with longstanding headache, appropriate referral for follow-up and monitoring is essential because it is not ideal for the patient with chronic headaches to receive continued care in the emergency department at the expense of ongoing care by a neurologist or primary care physician.

VASCULAR HEADACHE

Migraine

Migraine headaches are defined as recurrent attacks of headache that vary widely in intensity, frequency, and duration. The attacks are usually unilateral in onset and are often associated with anorexia and sometimes with nausea and vomiting. In some patients they are preceded by or associated with conspicuous sensory, motor, and mood disturbances. There may be a familial history of similar headaches. Migraine headaches are usually subdivided into classic migraine, common migraine, cluster headache, ophthalmoplegic migraine, and hemiplegic migraine (see the box below).

MIGRAINE SYNDROMES

Classic migraine
Common migraine
Cluster headache
Ophthalmoplegic migraine
Hemiplegic migraine
Migraine equivalents
   Tachycardia
   Edema
   Vertigo
   Chest pain
   Abdominal pain
   Pelvic pain

Migraine often begins in childhood but may not start until after puberty. Although it may begin later in life, such occurrences are unusual. For women, a relationship often exists between attacks of headache and menstruation. During pregnancy most women who suffer from migraines are symptom free after the first trimester.

All the migraine syndromes seem to have a phase of intracranial arterial vasoconstriction followed by a vasodilatation phase (involving primarily the extracranial arteries) during which the headache occurs. It is postulated that the sudden opening of arteriovenous shunts in the head produces a steal syndrome from the cortical areas, which may cause many of the symptoms characteristic of migraine.

Types of migraine syndromes

Classic migraine.   Classic migraine occurs in only approximately 12% of all patients with migraine headaches. In this subtype, the prodromal phase is sharply defined. The aura of classic migraine usually occurs up to 1 hour before the onset of the head pain. The majority of patients develop a temporary scintillating scotoma or homonymous hemianopsia that begins centrally and spreads toward the periphery. Nausea, vomiting, photophobia, and sonophobia may be concomitant features.

Common migraine.   Common migraine is the most prevalent type of migraine and occurs in approximately 80% of all patients. The prodromes are generally vague and precede the actual headache by widely varying amounts of time. Photophobia and sonophobia are noted along with anorexia, nausea, vomiting, and general malaise. Specific visual findings usually do not appear.

Cluster headache.   Cluster headache (also known as histamine headache or migrainous neuralgia) consists of unilateral facial pain of excruciating intensity that rarely lasts longer than 2 hours. This type of headache is commonly seen in conjunction with nasal congestion, lacrimation, and conjunctival injection on the same side as the pain. These headaches tend to occur several times each day for a period of weeks or months, separated by long intervals of complete freedom from the pain.

Considerably more men than women are affected by cluster headaches. The syndrome almost always begins in midadulthood. Those suffering from cluster headaches are especially susceptible to attacks following the ingestion of alcohol and the use of nitroglycerin or histamine-containing compounds. Stress may also be a factor. Climatic changes and attacks of allergic hay fever may also trigger the cluster mechanism.

Ophthalmoplegic migraine.   Ophthalmoplegic migraine is a rare syndrome that is usually seen in young adults and consists of headache and ophthalmoplegia. The pain is generally less intense than in a classic migraine. The pain is on the same side as the ophthalmoplegia, which is usually an extraocular muscle palsy that involves the third cranial nerve. Pupillary dilatation may be found in conjunction with the typical motor palsy.

Hemiplegic migraine.   The hemiplegic migraine is characterized by neurologic deficits that range from hemiparesis to full hemiplegia. The deficit may persist for some time after the headache resolves. In all patients with first-time hemiplegia, hemiplegic migraine should be a diagnosis of exclusion.

Migraine equivalents.   Probably 10% of all migraine sufferers have other forms of autonomic attacks. Migraine equivalents may include bouts of tachycardia, edema, vertigo, chest pain, abdominal pain, or pelvic pain. These episodes may occur with little or no headache.

Management

Various agents are available for the treatment of migraine syndromes. Those agents that produce vasoconstriction include the ergotamine derivatives. A second major group consists of the serotonin inhibitors (including methysergide, seroheptadine, and pizotifen). Another group is the beta-blocking agents, of which propranolol is the prototype. Recent research has shown that when released at nerve endings, the central neurotransmitter 5-hydroxytryptamine, or 5-HT, (serotonin) causes an inflammatory response, which releases vasodilatory neuropeptides and leads to edema. Sumatriptan, the first 5-HT receptor agonist to be synthesized, has been found to block the effects of the naturally occurring serotonin with much fewer side effects. Patient-injected sumatriptan has been found to be up to 75% effective in aborting attacks of migraine headache. This area of neurotransmitter investigation is currently the principal focus of migraine research.

Other types of medications have been tried with varying degrees of success. These medications include the tricyclic antidepressants, sedatives, calcium channel blockers, tranquilizers, muscle relaxants, lithium, and corticosteroids. In a subset of patients with abnormal platelet aggregability, the number of migraine headaches may be reduced through the use of nonsteroidal antiinflammatory medications. The beta blockers, serotonin inhibitors, and tricyclic antidepressants are useful for interval treatment and prophylaxis but have little effect during an acute attack.

Many patients find that the ergotamine derivatives may be useful in aborting a headache if taken during the preheadache aura. A number of preparations are available that may be taken orally, sublingually, rectally, or by inhalation. Combinations of ergotamine with caffeine, belladonna alkaloids, and various analgesics are available. Ergotamine tartrate is the prototypic preparation, and 2 mg may be given orally or sublingually initially and repeated every ½ hour to a maximum of six tablets (12 mg) per attack. Ergotamine should not be used with pregnancy, coronary artery disease, severe peripheral arterial disease, or hypertension.

Several approaches can be attempted in patients with an established headache. Dihydroergotomaine (DHE 45) 1 mg may be given intramuscularly or intravenously. Other medications that have been found useful in the acute attack are chlorpromazine 1 mg/kg intramuscularly or metoclopramide (Reglan) 10-20 mg IV. Finally, the administration of a parenteral narcotic (such as meperidine) along with an antinausea medication may be useful in breaking the pain cycle. The patient treated in the emergency department for an acute headache should be referred to a neurologist or primary care physician for further care.

In patients with recurring migraines and cluster headaches, a course of oral steroids may prevent or reduce the severity of subsequent attacks. Prednisone 40 mg/day may be prescribed and the dose tapered over the course of 21 days.

Nonmigrainous Vascular Headache

Fever headache

Fever is an extremely common cause of headache. Most patients with headache and fever have other symptoms that may define the source of the fever. The possibility of meningeal infection needs to be considered in patients with headache and fever.

Anoxic headache

Anoxia. Anoxia from any cause can be a source of severe headache. In patients with chronic obstructive pulmonary disease and carbon dioxide retention, small shifts in blood-gas levels may result in large changes in functional state. Headache in these situations may be dull with a slight throbbing quality. The headache may be worse in the morning rather than later in the day because of decreased ventilation in the recumbent position. This fact may be particularly true of extremely obese patients with Pickwickian syndrome.

Hypertensive headaches. Hypertension is generally not a cause of head pain until diastolic pressures of approximately 130 mm Hg are reached. Modestly elevated blood pressures are commonly seen with all types of headaches as a reaction to pain, but it is wrong to ascribe the cause of headache to hypertension unless there is a significant elevation.

Anemia headache. Patients with severe anemia often experience severe head pain as a result of a relative lack of oxygen and pronounced vasodilatation. This type of pain particularly occurs with acute anemia, such as may be seen in hypovolemic shock.

Other vascular headache syndromes. A number of foods and chemical agents are ascribed as causes of severe head pain. Excessive intake of caffeine and other methylated xanthine foods may cause headache. Vascular-type headaches may occur in patients who are withdrawing from corticosteroids. Chronic use and overuse of nonprescription sympathomimetics is a relatively common cause of rebound head pain.

Management

Treatment of nonmigrainous vascular-type headache with aspirin or acetaminophen is usually adequate. The nonsteroidal antiinflammatory drugs (NSAIDs) are gaining acceptance as an effective therapy in both migraine and nonmigrainous vascular headaches. Large doses of NSAIDs early in the course of a headache can be both a safe and effective form of therapy. Sedatives, tranquilizers, and small amounts of narcotic medication such as codeine can be added to the regimen as necessary.

MUSCLE CONTRACTION HEADACHES

The principal source of pain in muscular contraction headaches is related to contraction of muscles of the head and neck. Although migraine headaches represent the largest group of headache patients who come to the emergency department, muscle contraction headaches are probably the most common type of chronic recurring head pain in the general public. These headaches are usually bilateral and have no prodrome. The discomfort is located in the back of the head and neck, but all regions of the head may be involved. Such pains are usually described as squeezing and viselike. There is often a paucity of physical findings, although the muscles of the neck and the occiput may be tender to palpation.

The treatment for muscular contraction headaches and those of psychogenic origin is essentially the same. It may be difficult to differentiate psychogenic from muscular tension head pain. Aspirin or acetaminophen is a practical choice for mild pain. When such treatment is not effective, a mild sedative or tranquilizer may be added to the regimen. Butalbital (Fiorinal) or acetaminophen with codeine (Phenaphen) combinations are often used. Again, NSAIDs are being used more often and with greater success with these types of head pain.

TRACTION HEADACHE

Intracranial mass lesions produce pain by distending or stretching the arteries and other pain-sensitive structures inside the calvaria. In the clinical course of most brain tumors, headache is produced relatively late. By the time the typical patient with an intracranial tumor comes to the emergency department, other significant findings are present on the basis of which the diagnosis is suspected. Tumors developing in the posterior fossa rarely cause early pain referred to the occipital region. Tumors developing within the ventricular system may produce headache of sudden onset by producing a ball-valve obstruction of cerebrospinal fluid outflow.

Arteriovenous Malformations

Arteriovenous malformations (AVMs) are generally located in the parieto-occipital region and usually do not cause symptoms until they have reached substantial size. Bleeding from AVMs may produce the sudden onset of pain. Neurologic signs are usually present as well, and a bruit may be heard over the cranium. In later stages, AVMs may bleed into the subarachnoid space, which leads to rapid neurologic deterioration and coma.

Cerebral Aneurysms

Aneurysms of the circle of Willis may produce intermittent headache, but unlike migraines, the headache is generally in the same location each time it occurs. Persistence of neurologic deficit, hemianopsia, or third-nerve palsy should suggest the possibility of an expanding intracranial aneurysm. As the aneurysm expands, headaches may become more intense. When aneurysms bleed, the cerebrospinal fluid fills with blood, and the patient rapidly develops meningismus.

Subarachnoid Hemorrhage

Subarachnoid hemorrhage classically causes the acute onset of severe headache. The most common age for subarachnoid hemorrhage is between 20 and 40 years. Patients often describe the headache as "the worst ever." Signs of meningismus usually develop rapidly, and the patients may exhibit severe pain, diaphoresis, tachypnea, tachycardia, and photophobia.

Rapid neurologic assessment is necessary so that therapy may begin. The diagnosis of subarachnoid hemorrhage is made by demonstrating blood in the cerebrospinal fluid. High-resolution CT scanners show such bleeding 90% to 95% of the time. If the CT scan is diagnostic, no further studies are necessary in the emergency department. If subarachnoid hemorrhage is the principle concern and if there are no clinical findings to suggest increased intracranial pressure (e.g., papilledema or focal deficits), the head CT scan should be omitted, and the emergency physician should proceed directly to lumbar puncture. Request a neurosurgical consultation to decide on the timing of arteriography and surgical management if indicated.

Pseudotumor Cerebri

Also known as benign intracranial hypertension, pseudotumor cerebri produces headaches that may be extremely severe. The syndrome is often associated with transient visual loss and papilledema. Chronic increased intracranial pressure may cause permanent vision loss.

The usual patient with pseudotumor cerebri is a young obese woman with abnormal menstrual cycles. Vitamin A or B_{12} intoxication, iron deficiency, disorders of the adrenal cortex, and parathyroid and estrogen imbalances have been associated with the disease. Outdated tetracyclines, corticosteroids, and oral contraceptives have also been implicated in the pathogenesis.

The CT scan in pseudotumor cerebri may be normal. Diagnosis of pseudotumor cerebri is by measurement of cerebrospinal fluid (CSF) pressure. Therapy consists of lowering intracranial pressure by removing CSF by means of a lumbar puncture.

Intracerebral Abscess

A brain abscess may act like any other expanding intracranial lesion. Headache usually occurs early in the course, and there may be nausea, vomiting, and alteration of mental status. Diagnosis often requires a CT scan with contrast. A lumbar puncture is not needed to diagnose intracerebral abscess and may be dangerous if the abscess has produced a mass effect. The CSF is often culture negative.

Subdural Hematoma

Headache may be the presenting complaint in chronic subdural hematoma, which is usually seen in the elderly. Changes in personality or mental status may be noted along with other signs of increased intracranial pressure.

Post–Lumbar Puncture Headache

Approximately 10% to 15% of all patients suffer headaches within hours of a diagnostic lumbar puncture. Symptoms are usually worse when the patient sits up, and the pain diminishes in the recumbent position. The headache is usually frontal.

The cause of post–lumbar puncture headache relates to persistent leakage of CSF from the dural puncture site. This leakage produces CSF hypotension, with resulting traction placed on vessels, meninges, and other pain-sensitive structures at the base of the brain. Factors that have been proposed to contribute to the headache include the size of the puncture needle, the amount of fluid withdrawn, and repeat punctures.

Treat post–lumbar puncture headaches with rest, increased fluid intake, and administration of analgesics. There is no proof that position after lumbar punctures affects these headaches. In a patient whose headache is refractory to such management, an autologous epidural blood patch may be indicated.

INFLAMMATORY CAUSES OF HEAD PAIN

Temporal Arteritis

The vessels most commonly involved in temporal arteritis are the superficial temporal, vertebral, ophthalmic, and internal carotid arteries. This condition should be suspected in patients over 50 years of age with a new headache or a change in headache pattern. Women are affected four times more often than men. During the attack, the patient may have a low-grade fever, mild meningeal signs, and diminution of vision. Headache is usually unilateral.

The patient is usually in significant distress. Examination of the head and scalp may show in-

tense tenderness over the site of the inflamed artery. Temporal arteries may be tender and warm. The erythrocyte sedimentation rate is virtually always substantially elevated. The clinical elements that distinguish temporal arteritis from other types of head pain are scalp tenderness and a unilateral decrease in vision. A definitive diagnosis is based on arterial biopsy, but treatment should not be delayed if suspicion is high on clinical grounds.

Failure to diagnose temporal arteritis and begin treatment may result in permanent neurologic loss. Visual impairment is the most common sequela of temporal arteritis, but basilar and cerebellar infarcts may also occur.

Begin corticosteroids (prednisone, 100 mg/day) to attempt to prevent progression of the vision loss; the dose can be tapered from there during follow-up. Analgesia is also an important part of therapy. Antiinflammatory agents such as aspirin and nonsteroidal agents may also be used.

Other Inflammatory Causes

Temporal arteritis is the prototype of the inflammatory diseases that cause headache. However, vasculitis from many causes, including systemic lupus erythematosus, carcinomatosis, chronic meningitis (caused by tuberculous, fungal, or parasitic infection) can cause the same degree of inflammation.

MISCELLANEOUS HEADACHE SYNDROMES

Trigeminal Neuralgia

Trigeminal neuralgia is a condition that may be disabling by virtue of intense pain. The stabbing pains are in the distribution of the trigeminal nerve and are usually unilateral. Any stimulation of the involved area heightens the patient's discomfort. Even the acts of chewing or speaking may provoke severe pain.

Patients with trigeminal neuralgia are usually in excruciating discomfort during their attacks.

Facial movements may be limited, and palpation of the areas involved may produce lancinating pain, which is essentially diagnostic.

Administer parenteral analgesics such as morphine or meperidine in the emergency department. Carbamazepine 100 mg twice daily may be initiated. Patients can usually be managed on an outpatient basis, but during the initial painful episodes, some patients require admission for pain management.

Glaucoma

An attack of acute angle-closure glaucoma may cause a headache with a boring type of pain. Severe nausea and vomiting may accompany the attack. Patients commonly complain of visual haziness or vision loss. Physical examination generally reveals an injected eye with diminution in visual acuity. The pupil is in midposition, and the cornea may have a slightly hazy appearance.

Sinus Headache

The paranasal sinuses may be a source of pain as a consequence of trauma, tumor, infection, or allergy. Pain is in the distribution of the ophthalmic and maxillary divisions of the trigeminal nerve. Pain as a result of sinusitis is usually dull but may be pulsatile. Discomfort is commonly felt in the teeth and in the orbit. Sphenoid sinus involvement may cause visual disturbances, proptosis, or disconjugate gaze. Because of the close proximity of the sinuses to intracranial structures, an alteration in mental status and an elevated temperature along with sinusitis should be viewed as representing central nervous system involvement. Admission to the hospital and parenteral antibiotics should be considered as indicated.

Headaches of Cervical Origin

Head pain may be the initial complaint in diseases of the spinal column. Head or neck pain may be caused by cervical spondylosis, trauma, and rheumatoid arthritis, as well as by cervical and foramen magnum tumors.

Head pain of cervical origin is usually unilateral and referred to the back of the head and nuchal region. Such pain is usually dull but may occasionally have a throbbing quality. It is usually increased by neck movement. Treatment of the underlying condition is the most effective way to relieve the pain.

▌▌▌▌▌▌▌*KEY CONSIDERATIONS*

WHAT IS THE LIFE THREAT?

Subarachnoid hemorrhage, subdural hemorrhage, intracerebral hemorrhage, meningitis, encephalitis, cerebral abscess, hypertensive encephalopathy, and carbon monoxide poisoning may be immediately life threatening.

DOES THE PATIENT NEED ADMISSION?

Patients with life-threatening causes of headache require admission.

WHAT IS THE MOST SERIOUS DIAGNOSIS?

Intracranial hemorrhage, CNS infection, tumors, and carbon monoxide poisoning are the most serious diagnoses.

HAVE I PERFORMED A THOROUGH WORK-UP?

Obtain a history of onset (e.g., sudden or gradual), previous treatment, severity compared to previous headaches, and associated symptoms (e.g., syncope or neurologic deficit).

Recommended Reading

Henry GL: Headache. In Rosen P et al, editors: *Emergency medicine: concepts and clinical practice,* ed 3, St Louis, 1992, Mosby.

Smith R et al: Effect of substance P in serotonin-induced pain in serotonin mechanisms. In Olesen J, Saxena P, editors: *The role of serotonin (5-hydroxytryptamine) mechanisms in primary headaches,* vol 2, New York, 1992, Raven Press.

Chapter *Ten*
RESPIRATORY DISTRESS

STEVEN M. BARRETT

The term *dyspnea* means difficult or impaired breathing and is the cardinal symptom of respiratory distress. Dyspnea, a symptom, must be differentiated from tachypnea and hyperpnea, which are signs that represent an increased respiratory rate and increased minute ventilation, respectively. The hyperventilation associated with metabolic acidemia (e.g., as a result of uremia or diabetic ketoacidosis) may not be accompanied by a sensation of dyspnea. On the other hand, patients with apparently normal breathing patterns may complain of shortness of breath.

Respiratory distress is the clinical state characterized by an abnormal respiratory rate or by increased work of breathing. Respiratory distress may progress to respiratory failure, which is defined as an impairment of oxygen absorption adequate for the body's metabolic requirements or an impairment of adequate carbon dioxide excretion. Hypoxemia and hypercapnia result from one or more of three mechanisms: (1) inadequate alveolar ventilation, (2) mismatching of alveolar ventilation and pulmonary perfusion, or (3) abnormal diffusion of gases across the alveolar-capillary interface. Some patients in respiratory failure (e.g., from certain neuromuscular disorders or from respiratory muscle exhaustion) may show little or no evidence of respiratory distress, such as tachypnea or other clues of increased respiratory effort.

The sternocleidomastoid and scalene muscles are the only accessory muscles currently believed to have important ventilatory functions. The scalene muscles are sometimes active during eupneic (normal, resting) breathing; thus using the term *accessory* to describe them may not be completely accurate. The sternocleidomastoid muscles function as muscles of respiration only during strenuous breathing.

A series of sensory receptors channels feedback from the respiratory system to the central nervous system by way of specific nerves, primarily the vagus nerve. Peripheral chemoreceptors include the carotid bodies and to a lesser extent the aortic bodies. Carotid bodies and aortic bodies are small nests of cells located bilaterally at the bifurcation of the common carotid arteries and on the aorta, respectively. The carotid bodies account for 100% of the hypoxemic stimulatory drive of ventilation in humans. This hypoxemic ventilatory drive is blunted with advancing age; in high-altitude dwellers; and in the pathologic states of chronic bronchitis, morbid obesity, and sleep apnea. Dyspnea may not be present in some patients with hypoxemia.

Central chemoreceptors in the medulla of the brainstem increase ventilation when the arterial P_{CO_2} is increased. These chemoreceptors actually respond to increased hydrogen ion concentrations induced by increased levels of carbon dioxide, which is readily diffusible into the cerebrospinal fluid. In normal individuals, ventilation increases approximately 1 L/minute for every 1 mm Hg increase in arterial P_{CO_2} above 40 mm Hg. The ventilatory response to metabolic acidosis is comparatively delayed because hydrogen ions are not so readily diffusible across the blood-brain barrier. Conditions that may attenuate the central nervous system ventilatory response to carbon dioxide include advancing age, chronic obstructive pulmonary disease (COPD), and pharmacologic central nervous system depressants.

Various receptors in the lung and upper airway also send information concerning ventilatory status to the central nervous system. A normal person at rest breathes from 8 to 16 times/minute, with a tidal volume of 400 to 800 ml. The pattern is quite regular except for an occasional slow, deep breath, and the respiratory movements appear effortless. An increase in respiratory rate usually accounts for much of the increase in ventilatory effort in patients with dyspnea, particularly in patients with stiff lungs (e.g., as a result of acute pulmonary edema). However, the patient who feels dyspneic may not be capable of augmenting ventilations in response to the increased neural drive to breathe. For example, increased impedance of the respiratory system (increased resistance to airflow or decreased lung or chest compliance) or respiratory muscle weakness or fatigue may cause a decreased ability to ventilate at a given level of neural drive. Furthermore, there is a common dissociation between tachypnea and dyspnea. For example, in the patient with chronic mitral stenosis, marked tachypnea is often unassociated with breathlessness. This discrepancy indicates that adaptation may occur to the sensation of dyspnea when the stimulus for increased ventilation is sustained.

The upper airways in infants and children are small and more easily obstructed by foreign bodies, local swelling, or the tongue than is the case in adults. In addition, an upper respiratory infection or rhinitis may cause significant respiratory compromise in an infant who is less than 4 months old and who is an obligate nose-breather. The lower airways in children are also smaller and have incompletely developed supporting cartilage. Therefore alveolar ventilation may be easily compromised if the lower airways become obstructed by mucus, blood, pus, edema, or as a result of bronchoconstriction.

DIFFERENTIAL DIAGNOSIS

The causes of dyspnea can be considered according to the pathologic origins of the symptom (see the box on p. 108). Pulmonary and cardiac disorders are the most common causes of respiratory distress in emergency patients. Upper airway obstruction is one of the most urgent.

Congestive Heart Failure

Congestive heart failure (CHF) is discussed in Chapter 38. The most common causes of CHF are coronary artery disease, valvular disease, uncontrolled hypertension, cardiomyopathy, and renal failure, but other disorders may also lead to CHF. As left-sided CHF progresses over the course of months to years, dyspnea that is present only on exertion is succeeded by dyspnea that is present at rest. A decrease in exercise tolerance over a short period of time suggests heart failure, whereas dyspnea on exertion that develops gradually suggests lung disease. Other symptoms of CHF include orthopnea and paroxysmal nocturnal dyspnea. However, orthopnea is not specific for CHF. The patient with COPD or asthma may also find it easier to breathe with the head and thorax elevated, partly because the abdominal organs are lowered away from the thoracic cavity and therefore interfere less with diaphragmatic movement.

In some patients, bronchospasm may develop because of pulmonary congestion. This "cardiac asthma" with wheezing may occur only on exertion, paroxysmally at night, or as an

COMMON CAUSES OF ACUTE DYSPNEA

Upper airway

Foreign body obstruction
Epiglottitis
Croup
Bacterial tracheitis
Angioedema
Tumor

Pulmonary

Asthma
COPD exacerbation
Pneumothorax
Noncardiogenic pulmonary edema
Adult respiratory distress syndrome
Aspiration
Pneumonia
Bronchiolitis
Toxic gas inhalation
Pleural effusion
Malignancy
Chest trauma

Cardiovascular

Congestive heart failure
Cardiogenic pulmonary edema
Myocardial infarction
Unstable angina
Cardiac dysrhythmias
Pulmonary embolism
Cardiac tamponade
Cardiomyopathy

Neuromuscular

CNS respiratory depression
Guillain-Barré syndrome
Myasthenia gravis
Polyneuropathy
Polymyositis
Botulism
Hypokalemia
Coral snake bite
Tick paralysis

Metabolic/Systemic

Hypoxemia
Hypercapnia
Metabolic acidosis
Sepsis
Shock
Drug toxicity or overdose
Anaphylaxis
Anemia
Hyperthyroidism

Psychogenic

Hyperventilation syndrome

early manifestation of pulmonary edema. Compared with bronchial asthma, patients with cardiac asthma usually have overt clinical evidence of heart disease, such as an S_3 gallop and equal inspirations and expirations.

Signs of left ventricular failure, including jugular venous distension, peripheral edema, hepatomegaly, and gallop rhythm are helpful in establishing a cardiogenic cause of dyspnea. The chest x-ray study is often diagnostic of left-sided CHF because it shows cardiomegaly, apical blood flow redistribution, and Kerley A and B lines. The primary radiographic evidence of cardiogenic pulmonary edema is consolidation (alveolar infiltrates), either diffusely or concentrated in the perihilar or bibasilar regions. Cardiomegaly may not be present in patients with acute left ventricular failure as a result of acute myocardial infarction or a ruptured papillary muscle. Pulmonary edema in a patient with emphysema can assume a patchy distribution that simulates pneumonia on the chest x-ray study.

Noncardiogenic Pulmonary Edema

Most types of noncardiogenic pulmonary edema can be classified as permeability edema and result from damage to the alveolar epithelium, the pulmonary capillary walls, or both. Fluid accumulates in interstitial and alveolar spaces without left ventricular failure. Severe permeability edema results in adult respiratory distress syndrome (ARDS). Drugs, medications, toxins, infection, near-drowning, inhalation injury, hypotension, hypoxemia, central nervous system trauma or disease, and high-altitude illness are some causes of permeability edema. Tachypnea is present, although dyspnea and rales may not be as severe as in acute cardiogenic pulmonary edema. Cyanosis and wheezing may occur, but findings typical of CHF are absent. The pulmonary parenchymal changes on the chest x-ray study are similar to those in CHF, but cephalad redistribution of blood flow in the upright patient, cardiomegaly, and pleural effusions do not develop.

High-altitude pulmonary edema (HAPE) is a type of noncardiogenic pulmonary edema that occurs most often in unacclimatized individuals who ascend rapidly to altitudes above 8000 feet (2440 meters) and promptly engage in strenuous physical activity such as skiing, hiking, or climbing. Initial symptoms of dyspnea, fatigue, and cough begin within 12 to 72 hours of ascent and are usually worse at night. Orthopnea, which is common in cardiogenic pulmonary congestion, occurs in only 5% to 10% of all patients with HAPE.

Rapid reexpansion of a collapsed lung after drainage of a large pleural effusion or pneumothorax may cause a unilateral noncardiogenic pulmonary edema. Both increased capillary permeability and a rapid rise in negative intrapleural pressure may be responsible for this problem, which is unlikely to occur unless the lung has been collapsed for a number of days or longer.

ARDS is a severe form of noncardiogenic pulmonary edema that results from diffuse alveolar injury, which is caused by a wide variety of insults. Damage to the alveolar epithelium, capillaries, or both causes a capillary leak which, along with impairment of surfactant activity, leads to edema, atelectasis, an inflammatory reaction, and hyaline membrane formation.

Radiographically, an interstitial edema pattern is followed by a patchy, then confluent, alveolar edema with diffuse volume loss that occurs hours to days after the insult. A ground-glass pattern with homogeneous, smooth opacities and scattered lucencies often appears and is more distinctive than consolidation. Clinical correlation and measurement of pulmonary capillary wedge pressure (PCWP) can help distinguish cardiogenic from noncardiogenic pulmonary edema because the radiographic appearance of the two disorders can be similar. Clinical symptoms and hypoxemia occasionally may be present before radiographic abnormalities are identified.

Chronic Obstructive Pulmonary Disease

Emphysema is defined as an abnormal increase in the size of the air spaces distal to the terminal bronchioles and is caused by dilatation or destruction of air-space walls. Chronic bronchitis is diagnosed in patients who have coughed up sputum on most days for periods of at least 3 months during the last 2 consecutive years in the absence of other possible causes such as tuberculosis or bronchiectasis. The severity of exacerbation of COPD symptoms may vary from that of a minor respiratory tract infection to that of impending respiratory failure.

Dyspnea most often leads the patient with chronic bronchitis or emphysema to seek medical attention. The patient in whom emphysema predominates generally has a history of exertional dyspnea with minimal cough. The patient with predominant chronic bronchitis has a history of productive coughing, and exertional dyspnea often begins later in the disease process. Exertional dyspnea generally correlates with the degree of airflow obstruction. As a broad guideline, activity is only minimally limited until the value for forced expiratory volume in 1 second (FEV1) falls below 65% of normal. As airflow obstruction progresses, dyspnea develops with more moderate levels of exertion, such as climbing stairs. When the FEV1 value decreases below 35% to 40% of normal, the patient may become breathless during simple activities of daily living such as making a bed or bathing.

For patients with chronic bronchitis and emphysema, the maximum breathing capacity becomes impaired. These patients often work more in breathing at rest than the normal individual does during moderate exercise. Total ventilation at rest in these patients is often only slightly greater than in the normal person but occupies an abnormally large fraction of the maximum breathing capacity. Progressive disability as a result of dyspnea accompanied by a decreasing maximum breathing capacity is the usual course for the "pink puffer," (i.e., the gaunt patient with dyspnea and emphysema predominant). For the "blue bloater," or the overweight or edematous patient with cyanosis and chronic bronchitis predominant, dyspnea is less troublesome than for the patient with emphysema who has a similar degree of impairment of maximum breathing capacity.

With COPD, medullary chemoreceptors may become less responsive to chronic hypercapnia (e.g., in the "blue bloater") so that the drive to breathe is diminished and thus the sensation of dyspnea becomes less intense. In fact, there is a wide range of responsiveness to hypoxemia and hypercapnia in the general population. Considerable COPD may be present with relatively little dyspnea sensed by the patient. Insults such

as a superimposed respiratory infection, pneumothorax, atelectasis, or myocardial infarction or ischemia may precipitate a sudden exacerbation of otherwise minimal dyspnea in these patients.

Although each can occur independently, chronic bronchitis and emphysema are often present concurrently. The patient with emphysema displays progressive dyspnea, scant sputum production, a hyperresonant chest, and distant breath sounds. The classic radiographic manifestations of advanced emphysema are diffuse air trapping and lung hyperinflation, an increased anteroposterior diameter, depression of the hemidiaphragms, decreased pulmonary vascularity, and bullae. The patient with chronic bronchitis experiences more intermittent episodes of dyspnea with copious cough and sputum production. Auscultation of the chest may reveal wheezes and rales, and cyanosis may be present. Uncomplicated chronic bronchitis without emphysema produces no specific abnormalities on plain chest x-ray studies.

Episodes of exacerbation of COPD symptoms are most commonly associated with bronchopulmonary infection. These episodes are characterized by increased coughing, increased sputum production, or a change in the character of the sputum from clear to purulent. Such episodes may progress to respiratory failure.

Alpha$_1$-antitrypsin deficiency disease should be considered in the differential diagnosis when emphysematous changes predominate radiographically in the lower lung fields, especially in a young person. Congenital lobar emphysema can appear as a life-threatening problem during the first year of life. It is more common in boys than in girls and usually involves the right upper lobe or right lower lobe. Symptoms include cough, tachypnea, respiratory distress, and cyanosis. Radiographic signs of congenital lobar emphysema include marked hyperinflation of the abnormal lobe and compression of the adjacent lobes. Definitive therapy involves surgical resection of the abnormal lobe.

Asthma

The major abnormality in asthma is widespread, reversible narrowing of the airways that results in partial airflow obstruction. Unlike the predictable exertional dyspnea of COPD, the dyspnea typical of asthma is episodic, with exacerbations and remissions, and it correlates primarily with the severity of airflow obstruction. Chest tightness or "congestion" can precede or follow the onset of shortness of breath during acute asthma episodes and is occasionally mistaken for the chest discomfort of myocardial ischemia. Most patients with asthma associate their chest tightness with the sensation of being unable to take in a full breath. During severe asthma attacks, the patient may insist on remaining in a sitting or standing position because the dyspnea worsens in the supine position. A dry cough can precede and accompany dyspnea and wheezing, or it may be the only manifestation of an asthma episode.

The patient with an acute asthma episode typically experiences dyspnea, coughing, and wheezing. The absence of wheezing in a patient with asthma and dyspnea should be considered an ominous sign that indicates that bronchial air flow is so diminished that wheezing is not produced. A chest x-ray study is ordered only to detect complications associated with the disorder and to recognize other causes of wheezing. The chest x-ray study is useful for patients with an acute asthma attack accompanied by fever, when a patient fails to respond to therapy, in a patient with dyspnea and a quiet chest, or with physical findings that suggest a pneumothorax or pneumomediastinum. Other clinical findings and treatment details for asthma are discussed in Chapter 32.

Pulmonary Embolism

Pulmonary embolism can be a subtle diagnosis to consider because of the nonspecific nature of many of the signs and symptoms. The most common symptom of pulmonary embolism is the sudden onset of dyspnea. Other symptoms include apprehension, cough, weakness, syncope, and an oppressive substernal chest discomfort that may be indistinguishable from the pain of myocardial infarction or ischemia. Pleuritic chest pain implies the development of pulmonary infarction; common signs of pulmonary embolism include tachypnea and tachycardia. Rarely, pulmonary embolism can simulate asthma by causing a sporadic, recurrent dyspnea associated with wheezing.

A concurrent or previous condition that predisposes the patient to pulmonary embolism or deep venous thrombosis may exist. These conditions include estrogen use, heart disease, cancer, obesity, previous pulmonary embolism or deep venous thrombosis, trauma, pelvic and lower extremity fractures, immobilization, pregnancy, hereditary clotting disorders, and postoperative status. As will be discussed in Chapter 34, the diagnosis of pulmonary embolism should be considered when sudden dyspnea occurs in patients who are in the postoperative or postpartum period or who have chronic CHF. Pulmonary embolism is often most subtle in the elderly patient.

Spontaneous Pneumothorax

A pneumothorax is a collection of air between the visceral and parietal pleura. Spontaneous pneumothorax can occur after coughing or straining, is often recurrent, and may be associated with a small hemothorax. The patient with a spontaneous pneumothorax is typically a thin young man who is above average in height. The cause of the pneumothorax is usually the rupture of a subpleural bulla that is usually apical. Most patients with a spontaneous pneumothorax experience the sudden onset of dyspnea and pleuritic chest pain. The dyspnea is more severe when the pneumothorax is large and when there is significant underlying lung disease (i.e., secondary spontaneous pneumothorax). For example, disorders such as asthma, staphylococcal pneumonia, metastatic disease, and pulmonary fibrosis are associated with pneumothorax. Unilateral diminution of breath sounds with increased percussion tympany may be present.

A tension pneumothorax develops if a ball-valve effect occurs so that air continues to enter the pleural space during inspiration but cannot escape during expiration. A tension pneumothorax should be suspected if severe air hunger, cyanosis, hypotension, or a mediastinal shift (as seen on a chest x-ray study) occurs. This situation is life threatening because function of the involved lung, the heart and great vessels, and eventually the contralateral lung is compromised by the expanding pleural air-space mass and the increasing intrathoracic pressure. Immediate therapy (needle followed by chest tube decompression of the pneumothorax) may be required before chest x-ray studies are even obtained.

With a pneumothorax, the visceral pleura line can be visualized radiographically between the lung and pleural air space because air is less dense than the collapsed lung. Furthermore, no pulmonary bronchovascular markings can be identified in the areas of pleural air space. Demonstration of a small pneumothorax may be enhanced on an upright x-ray study taken during expiration. The collapsed lung decreases in volume during expiration, whereas the pleural air-space volume remains constant. Therefore the lung draws away from the chest wall and renders the pneumothorax more easily visible. A small pneumothorax may also be more detectable on a lateral decubitus x-ray study, but it may be impossible to detect on a supine x-ray study if air migrates into the anterior (uppermost) pleural space. Therefore a negative supine chest x-ray study does not exclude the diagnosis of pneumothorax. The x-ray study of a tension pneumothorax (a medical emergency) reveals a collapsed lung, a mediastinal (aortic arch, right heart border) and tracheal shift away from the pneumothorax, a depressed ipsilateral hemidi-

aphragm, and a relative increase in the size of rib interspaces compared to the contralateral side. However, the x-ray study cannot define the clinical severity of the pneumothorax.

Pneumonia

In patients with pneumonia, the severity of dyspnea is influenced by the extent of lung involvement, the presence of underlying lung disease, and pleural involvement with disease (e.g., effusion). Dyspnea is more likely to occur in patients with pneumonia than in patients with acute bronchitis. Dyspnea in patients with tuberculosis may be secondary to pleural effusion, pulmonary parenchymal involvement, or an associated anemia. The onset of dyspnea on exertion in a patient with AIDS often signifies the presence of *Pneumocystis carinii* pneumonia.

Upper Airway Obstruction

Obstruction of the upper airway may be the result of diverse entities, including foreign body aspiration, epiglottitis, croup, angioedema, tumor, and peritonsillar or retropharyngeal abscess. The presenting symptoms depend on the site and the completeness of the obstruction and on the underlying cause. Dyspnea, stridor, anxiety, and retraction of the supraclavicular fossae with inspiration are cardinal manifestations of partial upper airway obstruction. Cough, aphonia, or hoarseness may also be present. If the site of the partial obstruction is supraglottic, stridor is commonly inspiratory; expiratory stridor usually results from tracheal obstruction. Upper airway obstruction can cause life-threatening hypoxemia, and partial obstruction can rapidly become complete in certain disorders. The establishment of a patent airway is vital in cases of airway compromise.

Epiglottitis is an infectious inflammation of the glottic and supraglottic tissues and occurs most often in children between 2 and 4 years old. The onset of epiglottitis is characteristically abrupt, with a mild upper respiratory infection that progresses within hours to high fever, lethargy, a difficulty swallowing oral secretions, drooling, respiratory distress, and stridor. Restlessness, tachycardia, and an unwillingness to lie down are also commonly present. In adults, the presentation of epiglottitis is typically less dramatic. Fever and sore throat are the most common complaints, and dyspnea may be minimal or absent. An inspiratory, upright, lateral neck soft tissue x-ray study may demonstrate an enlarged, edematous epiglottis (the "thumb sign"). Unstable patients may require airway stabilization before radiographic evaluation.

The most common cause of stridor in the child with fever is croup. Laryngotracheobronchitis, or croup, is a viral infection that causes inflammatory narrowing of the tracheobronchial tree. The most severe narrowing occurs in the subglottic trachea. Most anteroposterior and lateral radiographic neck studies are normal, but they may disclose either ballooning of the hypopharynx or a "church steeple" airway effect, which is caused by edema of the vocal cords and subglottic trachea. A small percentage of children will have bacterial tracheitis distinguished by high fever and a more toxic appearance.

Miscellaneous Disorders

Patients with angina may interpret their substernal discomfort as breathlessness or as an inability to take a deep breath. Severe dyspnea may accompany prolonged episodes of variant or unstable angina that cause left ventricular dysfunction and marked increases in pulmonary capillary pressure. Myocardial infarction in elderly patients appears in the classic manner in less than one half of the cases; a common initial manifestation is sudden dyspnea or exacerbation of chronic CHF.

Dyspnea and easy fatigability are common symptoms in patients with dilated, hyper-trophic, or restrictive cardiomyopathies. Dyspnea is a result of increased left ventricular end-diastolic pressures, which induce elevated pulmonary venous pressures and pulmonary congestion. Dyspnea on exertion is often a rapidly progressive symptom.

Dyspnea in congenital heart disease patients is usually related to hypoxemia caused by a right-to-left shunt. The young child may experience episodes of breathlessness with deepening cyanosis. In the older child, dyspnea is usually effort related, and sudden unconsciousness may occur during the terrifying episodes.

Dyspnea may be the presenting symptom in the patient with a pleural effusion and is often more severe if the effusion is large or has collected rapidly. A large effusion can compress the lung and thus cause a restrictive ventilatory impairment.

In patients with lung carcinoma, sudden dyspnea may be caused by an acute obstructive atelectasis or pneumonia. If the carcinoma is metastatic to the thorax, dyspnea is often related to ventilatory restriction as a result of a lung mass effect or pleural implants or effusions. Furthermore, dyspnea may be severe in patients with lymphangitic spread of carcinoma in the lung. Bronchial adenomas may induce sudden dyspnea because of acute bronchial obstruction and lobar atelectasis.

Psychogenic breathlessness as a result of anxiety is a diagnosis of exclusion in the patient with dyspnea; tachypnea and anxiety are the predominant findings. In patients with anxiety-related hyperventilation, shortness of breath often occurs at rest and may be relieved during exertion, whereas the opposite is usually true in patients with dyspnea resulting from an organic disorder. Other manifestations of the hyperventilation syndrome may be present, including fatigue, weakness, palpitations, chest pain, numbness and tingling (especially of the hands, arms, and lips), carpal spasms, lightheadedness, an "unreal" cloudy mental sensation, and even syncope. The chest pain is usually described as

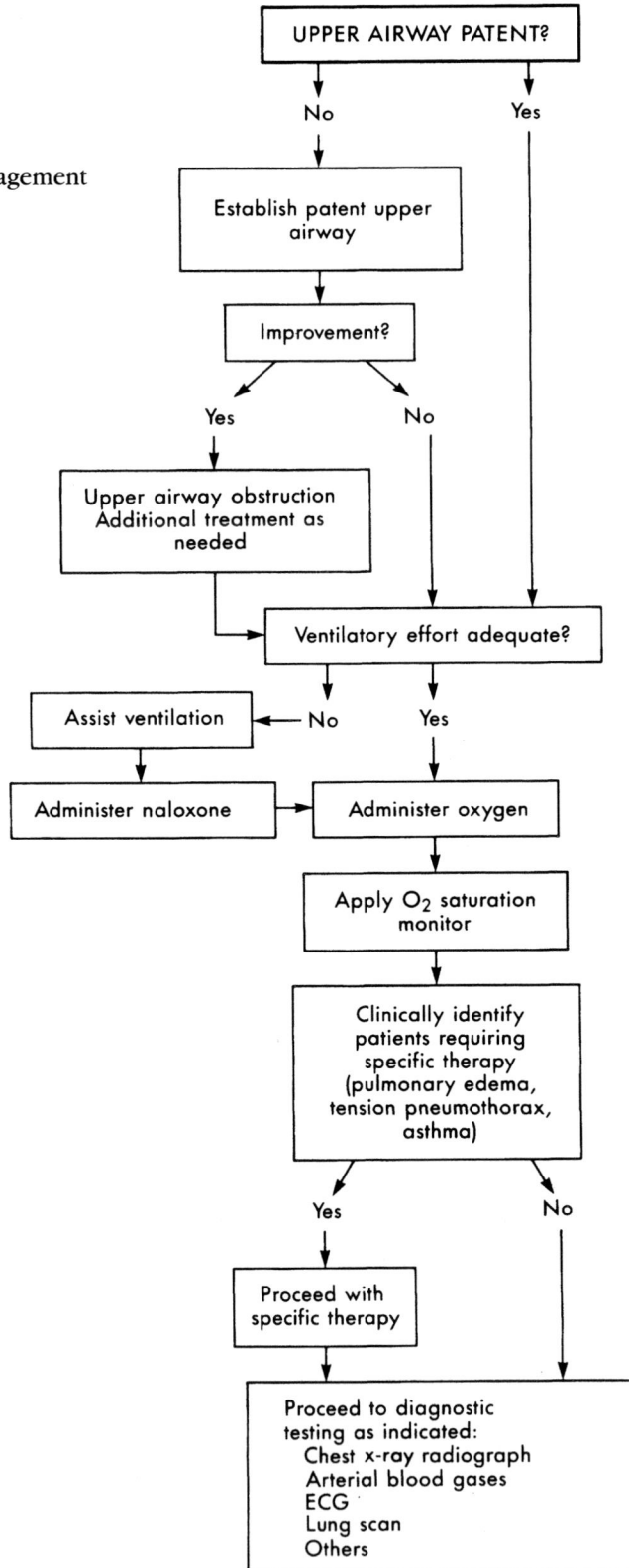

Fig. *10-1* Algorithm for management of respiratory distress.

fleeting, sharp "sticks" in various locations or as a dull precordial aching. T-wave inversions are sometimes noted on the ECG. The presence of respiratory alkalosis without hypoxemia on arterial blood-gas analysis, as well as a normal alveolar-arterial oxygen gradient, is characteristic. Other disorders that may produce respiratory alkalosis should also be considered, such as salicylate toxicity and pulmonary embolism. To complicate matters, psychogenic dyspnea may be present in patients with symptomatic pulmonary, cardiac, or other organic disorders.

DIAGNOSTIC APPROACH

Initial Evaluation

A suggested algorithm for approaching patients with respiratory distress is displayed in Fig. 10-1. The patient should receive an efficient and appropriate history and physical examination. The history should include details of the rapidity of onset of dyspnea; any possible inciting event (e.g., allergen exposure or toxic inhalation); recent respiratory illness; and other symptoms such as cough, fever, sputum production, or chest pain. Sudden onset of dyspnea occurs in patients with pulmonary embolism, spontaneous pneumothorax, toxic gas inhalation, and acute pulmonary edema. Dyspnea may develop over a period of hours with pneumonia, asthma, and CHF. Onset and progression of dyspnea over days to weeks may indicate pleural effusion, interstitial lung disorders, or bronchogenic carcinoma.

Certain interventions may take precedence over further patient evaluation. For example, airway establishment, assisted ventilations, or oxygen administration may be required immediately or may become necessary during the course of initial patient management. Evidence of respiratory failure includes severe respiratory distress in an agitated or anxious patient or inadequate air exchange in an obtunded patient.

Tachypnea and the use of accessory neck muscles indicate respiratory distress. In children, intercostal, subcostal, lower sternum, or supraclavicular retractions; nasal flaring; and paradoxical chest or abdominal wall motion represent increased work of breathing. Physical findings such as tympany and diminished breath sounds or bronchial breathing, rales, and egophony may suggest specific clinical entities. Diffuse crackles or rales may be heard in COPD, CHF, and pulmonary edema. Wheezes, which generally signify airflow obstruction, can occur in asthma, COPD, CHF, pulmonary embolism, foreign body aspiration, anaphylaxis, aspiration pneumonia, and bronchiolitis. Stridor is a particular type of wheeze with a characteristic crowing or musical sound of fixed pitch and is associated with partial obstruction of the larynx, trachea, or main stem bronchus. A harsh, brassy cough, particularly when associated with inspiratory stridor, suggests the presence of laryngeal or subglottic obstruction (e.g., foreign body or croup). Jugular venous distension and gallop rhythm support the diagnosis of CHF.

Diagnostic Studies

A chest x-ray study should be obtained in most patients with respiratory distress and may confirm the diagnosis in certain disorders such as pneumonia, pulmonary edema, and pneumothorax. However, the presence of chronic radiographic changes such as in COPD may render the appearance of a superimposed acute process, such as CHF, less apparent. Chest radiographic findings may also be minimal in certain conditions (e.g., aspiration or toxic inhalation) when the study is obtained during the initial evaluation. Special views of the chest may be helpful in certain circumstances. The lateral decubitus x-ray study can confirm the presence of a pleural effusion. With inspiratory and expiratory chest views, a bronchial foreign body is suspected if the affected lung remains more inflated relative to the unaffected lung on the expiratory radiograph.

Transcutaneous pulse oximetry is very useful in measuring hemoglobin oxygen saturation. A sensor can be applied to a digit or earlobe. A saturation level of 95% or above generally indicates adequate oxygenation, whereas a saturation level below 91% corresponds to a PO_2 of less than 60 mm Hg. However, hypercapnia, acidosis, or hyperthermia shift the oxygen-hemoglobin dissociation curve to the right so that a saturation of 91% then correlates with a PO_2 greater than 60 mm Hg. Furthermore, patients with toxic carboxyhemoglobin levels may have falsely elevated oximetry saturation readings.

Patients with severe respiratory distress and patients with chronic cardiac or respiratory disease who have acute or worsening dyspnea should have arterial blood gas measurements performed. Respiratory failure is present if the PCO_2 is greater than 55 mm Hg (assuming that there is no preexisting lung disease with chronic CO_2 elevation) in the presence of acidosis or if the PO_2 is less than 50 mm Hg (assuming that there is no cyanotic congenital heart disease) in a patient breathing room air.

The alveolar-arterial oxygen difference $P(A-a)O_2$ can be estimated in a patient with normal cardiac output who is breathing room air (ideally at sea level). In this situation, the alveolar O_2 tension added to the alveolar CO_2 tension equals approximately 145 mm Hg. Assuming intact diffusion of blood gases at the alveolar-capillary interface, the alveolar CO_2 tension is essentially the same as the measured arterial CO_2 tension. Therefore the alveolar O_2 tension is approximately equal to 145 minus the measured arterial PCO_2. The measured arterial PO_2 is now subtracted from the calculated alveolar O_2 tension to yield $P(A-a)O_2$. A $P(A-a)O_2$ value of less than 20 mm Hg is normal; 20 to 30 mm Hg represents mild pulmonary dysfunction, 30 to 50 mm Hg represents moderate dysfunction, and greater than 50 mm Hg implies severe respiratory decompensation. Hypoxemia with a normal $P(A-a)O_2$ results from hypoventilation, which might occur, for example, in patients with drug overdose or neuromuscular disease. An intrapulmonary shunt, a low ventilation-perfusion ratio (V/Q mismatch), or a diffusion impairment at the alveolar-capillary membrane level causes hypoxemia with an increased $P(A-a)O_2$. This condition might occur, for example, in patients with pulmonary edema, pneumonia, or a large pulmonary embolism.

If the patient is breathing oxygen, the PO_2/FiO_2 ratio can be calculated. The normal value for this ratio is approximately 500 to 600. A ratio of 200 (e.g., an arterial PO_2 of 80 mm Hg with an FiO_2 of 40% or 80/0.4), corresponds to an intrapulmonary shunt of approximately 20% and generally indicates a need for ventilatory support. Further information may be gained by administering 100% O_2 to the patient with hypoxemia. If the arterial PO_2 value increases to more than 100 mm Hg, either a low V/Q ratio or a diffusion impairment is present; if the arterial PO_2 value remains below 100 mm Hg, an intrapulmonary shunt is the cause of hypoxemia.

Spirometry may be useful in assessing the severity of airflow obstruction, particularly in the patient with an acute asthma episode. For example, FEV1 is normally 3000 to 4000 ml but is reduced to between 1000 and 2000 ml by moderately increased airway resistance. In patients with severe asthmatic episodes, the FEV1 is less than 1000 ml. The forced vital capacity (FVC) can also be measured at the bedside, and an FEV1/FVC ratio provides a volume-independent measure of expiratory airflow obstruction. A ratio of less than 70% indicates airway obstruction; the ratio may be less than 50% in severe acute asthma. Although wheezing may be present, the FEV1/FVC ratio is usually greater than 70% in pulmonary edema.

Respiratory distress with tachypnea may be present in patients with disorders that are not primarily related to the respiratory system, such as sepsis, congenital heart disease, or metabolic acidosis (e.g., as a result of salicylate toxicity, diabetic ketoacidosis, or gastroenteritis with dehydration). Therefore other laboratory tests may be indicated, such as a complete blood count, an extensive chemistry profile, a drug screen, and appropriate cultures. An ECG is indicated if angina or acute myocardial infarction is suspected. Other diagnostic studies should be ordered if clinically indicated.

MANAGEMENT

The goals of management of the patient with respiratory distress include reestablishing adequate gas exchange in the lung and oxygen delivery to the tissues. The clinical gravity of the situation for the patient with dyspnea dictates the order of activity. For example, a patient in obvious distress from an upper airway obstruction needs urgent, definitive therapy after the cause of dyspnea has been quickly determined. Patients may require one or more of the following treatments to stabilize ventilation and oxygenation: opening and clearing the airway, an oropharyngeal or nasopharyngeal airway, a nasal cannula or face mask for oxygen administration, assisted ventilation with a bag-valve-mask device, orotracheal or nasotracheal intubation, or (rarely) cricothyrotomy. If initial respiratory support efforts prove inadequate, endotracheal intubation and mechanically assisted ventilation are often indicated. In the breathless patient with a history or physical signs of COPD, low-flow oxygen at 2 L/minute can be administered initially and the flow rate increased later if the adequacy of oxygenation is in question. All COPD patients who receive oxygen must be observed closely at all times for the development of hypoventilation and the resulting need for respiratory support secondary to a diminished drive to breathe.

Urgent airway control is indicated in the patient who is comatose with an unprotected airway or who is deteriorating from cardiac, respiratory, or other serious disease complications. Therapy for hypotension, bronchospasm, cardiac dysfunction, and other specific problems may be required.

To achieve adequate oxygenation, the arterial PO_2 should be maintained at greater than 60 mm Hg and ideally greater than 80 mm Hg. However, in some patients with advanced COPD, a PO_2 of more than 50 mm Hg may be acceptable. A continually high FiO_2 can eventually cause oxygen toxicity in the lung, but the duration necessary to produce toxicity is uncertain, and patients vary in susceptibility. Furthermore, the use of positive pressure ventilation itself may play a role in the production of lung damage.

Concerns about oxygen toxicity should not prevent adequate oxygenation of the patient, and a high FiO_2 is occasionally necessary for temporary periods. However, the overall management protocol should allow for reduction of the FiO_2 to 60% or lower as soon as it is practical. There is no absolute level of hypercapnia that automatically indicates the need for endotracheal intubation. The patient's overall clinical status and response to specific therapy, as well as the arterial PCO_2 level, should be considered to determine the need for intubation.

Disorders that lead to respiratory distress or failure may be progressive, sometimes with acute deterioration. Patients may demonstrate impending respiratory failure, or they may be at risk for respiratory compromise. These patients must be examined repeatedly for evidence of developing respiratory distress so that respiratory failure can be anticipated and possibly prevented with timely medical management decisions. The patient's upper airway patency, respiratory rate and effort, level of consciousness, vital signs, and skin color should be initially assessed and repeatedly monitored. Available monitoring devices include continuous pulse oximetry, indwelling arterial catheters, and other techniques. Serial measurements of arterial blood gases and pH may also be indicated. The cause of the symptoms should be identified and the patient monitored so that the course of the disease process and the adequacy of therapy can be followed.

SUMMARY

An understanding of the pathophysiology and appropriate initial assessment and management of acute respiratory distress and failure enables these patients to receive optimal care. Because dyspnea may be a symptom of a variety of illnesses that require diverse management, efficient differentiation on the basis of clinical presentation and a limited group of diagnostic tests is essential. Some causes of respiratory symptoms are rapidly reversible with prompt recognition and proper therapy. Other disorders follow a prolonged course to eventual improvement and recovery or to progressive deterioration and mortality despite optimal management decisions. Because decompensation in these patients can occur rapidly, continual reevaluation and continuous monitoring is critical.

KEY CONSIDERATIONS

WHAT IS THE LIFE THREAT?

Airway obstruction, pulmonary embolism, myocardial infarction, asthma, congestive heart failure, exacerbation of chronic obstructive pulmonary disease, pneumothorax, hemothorax, and rapidly forming pleural effusion may be immediately life threatening.

DOES THE PATIENT NEED ADMISSION?

Admit for pulmonary embolism, myocardial infarction, new onset CHF, pneumothorax, and hemothorax.

Asthma patients who respond well to beta-agonist treatment and corticosteroids can be discharged if peak flow returns to normal and pulse oximetry is baseline or normal.

WHAT IS THE MOST SERIOUS DIAGNOSIS?

Myocardial infarction, pulmonary embolism, severe asthma (status asthmaticus), and severe CHF are the most serious diagnoses.

HAVE I PERFORMED A THOROUGH WORK-UP?

Look for airway obstruction. Stabilize patient by ensuring ventilation and providing oxygen. Examine lungs and obtain a chest x-ray examination. Assess oxygenation by pulse oximetry or arterial blood gases. Monitor asthma treatment with peak flow measurements. Explain all abnormal vital signs.

Recommended Reading

Baker MD, Ruddy RM: Pulmonary emergencies. In Fleisher GR, Ludwig S, editors: *Textbook of pediatric emergency medicine,* Baltimore, 1988, Williams & Wilkins.

Barrett SM, Johnson TH: Shortness of breath. In Rosen P et al, editors: *Diagnostic radiology in emergency medicine,* St Louis, 1992, Mosby.

Barrett SM: Dyspnea and shortness of breath. In Rosen P et al, editors: *Emergency medicine, concepts and clinical practice,* ed 3, St Louis, 1992, Mosby.

Seidel JS: Respiratory emergencies and cardiopulmonary arrest. In Barkin RM et al, editors: *Pediatric emergency medicine: concepts and clinical practice,* St Louis, 1992, Mosby.

Stokes DC: Respiratory disorders. In Ehrlich FE, Heldrich FJ, Tepas JJ III, editors: *Pediatric emergency medicine,* Rockville, Md, 1987, Aspen.

Wilson RF: Blood gases: pathophysiology and interpretation. In Tintinalli JE, Krome RL, Ruiz E, editors: *Emergency medicine, a comprehensive study guide,* ed 3, New York, 1992, McGraw-Hill.

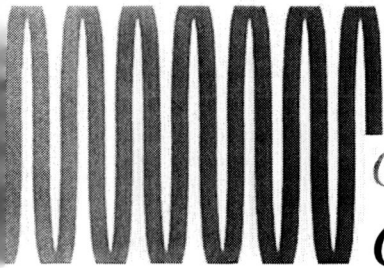

Chapter Eleven
CHEST PAIN

JAMES W. HOEKSTRA

Chest pain is a common complaint in the emergency department and represents 2% to 7% of the presenting symptoms in emergency department patients. It continues to be problematic for emergency physicians because of the wide range of conditions that cause chest pain, the overlap of presenting symptoms, the paucity of objective physical and laboratory findings, and the enormous potential for patient morbidity and mortality. The emergency physician must take an aggressive stance with regard to diagnosing patients with chest pain. Emergent conditions must be anticipated, preventive therapy must be instituted early to avoid cardiovascular complications, and serious and critical causes of chest pain must be considered and appropriately evaluated before making a patient diagnosis and disposition.

Because the differential diagnosis of chest pain is extensive and the consequence of misdiagnosis can be catastrophic, evaluating chest pain can be difficult in the emergency setting, where the history, physical examination, and various limited laboratory and imaging capabilities must be used to establish a working clinical impression.

DIFFERENTIAL DIAGNOSIS

Included in the differential diagnosis are both life-threatening and trivial conditions. The emergency physician must be especially familiar with the presentations, risk factors, and treatments for the life-threatening conditions. Diagnosing a particular cause of chest pain sometimes comes down to pattern recognition. For example, the pattern of substernal crushing chest pain in a 65-year-old smoker with hypertension, diaphoresis, and shortness of breath suggests acute myocardial infarction (AMI); the pattern of sudden onset of sharp pleuritic chest pain and shortness of breath in a 28-year-old woman who is taking oral contraceptives and whose leg has been immobilized in a cast suggests pulmonary embolism.

One way to organize the differential diagnosis of chest pain is to consider the possibilities anatomically (Table 11-1). The principal organs in the chest are the heart, the great vessels, the esophagus, the lungs and bronchi, and the chest wall. The serosal surfaces of the pleura, pericardium, and mediastinum can cause chest pain, and disorders of extrathoracic structures and abdominal organs can cause chest pain as well.

CLINICAL ASSESSMENT

History

The chest and its contents receive sensory innervation from both somatic and visceral afferent nerves. When stimulated, somatic afferents

*Table*11-1

ANATOMIC DIFFERENTIAL DIAGNOSIS OF CHEST PAIN

Organ System	Life Threatening	Non–Life Threatening
Heart	Myocardial infarction Unstable angina Prinzmetal angina Myocarditis Pericarditis	Mitral valve prolapse Stable angina
Great vessels	Thoracic aortic dissection	
Lungs/bronchi	Pulmonary embolus Mediastinitis Tension pneumothorax	Pleurisy Pneumomediastinum Pneumothorax Pneumonia Bronchitis Tracheitis Carcinoma Pleural effusion
Esophagus	Boerhaave syndrome	Esophagitis Esophageal ulcers Hiatal hernia Esophageal spasm Achalasia
Chest wall		Costochondritis Rib fractures Rib contusions Intercostal muscle strain Herpes zoster Thoracic radiculopathies Fibromyalgia Metastatic disease to ribs
Psychogenic		Hyperventilation Anxiety disorders Malingering
Extrathoracic	Abdominal aortic aneurysm	Splenic disease Cervical radiculopathies Peptic ulcer disease Biliary disease Subdiaphragmatic abscess

of thoracic spinal nerves cause pain that is localized to precise dermatomal distributions. Such nerves predominately innervate the chest wall and pleura but not the heart, lungs, esophagus, or major vessels. The major thoracic organs receive most of their sensory innervation from visceral afferents, which enter the spinal cord at levels from T1 to T6. Visceral afferents have many interconnections across and up and down the spinal column; such interconnections cause visceral pain to be perceived as dull, achy, diffuse, midline, and poorly localized. As a result, similar types of chest pain can be produced from multiple anatomic sites. For instance, the midline substernal squeezing pain of myocardial infarction can be very similar to the pain of esophageal spasm. When questioning a patient about chest pain, it is imperative to obtain a complete and accurate description of the pain. Such a description includes the character, location, radiation, chronology, associated symptoms, and aggravating and alleviating factors for the pain. Only when all these pieces are put together can an accurate pattern of chest pain be established.

Character of pain

Pain that is described as squeezing, tight, or oppressive is consistent with myocardial ischemia or myocardial infarction. Such pain tends to be severe and incapacitating; patients often describe it as a heavy weight pushing on their chest. Pain resulting from pleural or pericardial inflammation, as well as pain resulting from chest wall pathology, tends to be sharp or knifelike. Included in this category are the diagnoses of pericarditis, pneumonia, pleural effusion, and pulmonary embolism; such conditions produce sharp or "pleuritic" pain that typically becomes worse with inspiration. The pain of esophagitis tends to be gaslike, aching, or burning, whereas the pain of aortic dissection is classically described as a severe tearing sensation.

There is much overlap of the character of chest pain and the many conditions that cause

it. For instance, esophageal spasm often produces a squeezing type of pain, which is very similar to angina pectoris. Pleuritic pain can be produced by chest wall problems such as costochondritis as well as by lung problems such as pulmonary embolism, but AMI can produce both pleuritic pain and squeezing pain. Patients often have difficulty describing chest pain. For instance, "sharp" pain may mean "knifelike" to the physician when the patient actually means to describe the pain as "severe."

Location and radiation

The location and radiation of pain can often give clues to the origin of the pain. For example, AMI tends to produce pain that is located in the substernal or precordial area, with radiation to the left arm or jaw. It is less commonly located on the right side of the chest, back, or epigastric areas. Some patients with myocardial infarction experience only arm pain, not chest pain. Esophageal disorders tend to produce substernal or high epigastric pain without radiation. Aortic dissection classically causes pain in the substernal area, with radiation to the area between the shoulder blades. Because the heart, esophagus, and great vessels are mainly innervated by visceral afferents, there is considerable overlap in pain location and radiation; the pain tends to be diffuse or midline in location.

In contrast, the pleura and chest wall are innervated by somatic afferents and therefore produce pain that is much better localized than the visceral pain produced by the heart, esophagus, and great vessels. Pleuritic pain tends to lateralize to one side of the chest and localize to dermatomes. For this reason, the site of pneumonia, pleural effusions, pleurisy, and rib pathology can usually be well localized by the patient.

Chronology of pain

The timing and duration of chest pain is especially important in the evaluation of myocardial infarction. Squeezing substernal pain of 5 to 30 minutes duration is consistent with myocardial ischemia; similar pain that lasts longer than 1 hour is consistent with myocardial infarction. Patients with pain of AMI that is less than 6 hours in duration may be eligible for thrombolytic therapy, whereas patients with pain of longer durations usually are not. Constant pain that lasts longer than 48 hours and pain of extremely short duration are often not myocardial in origin. An insidious onset of pain and longer chest pain durations are more consistent with chest wall or lung disease, whereas the acute onset of pain is consistent with vascular catastrophes such as pulmonary embolism or dissecting aneurysm. The relationship between the pain onset and certain instigating events is also important. For instance, the onset of pain following vomiting is consistent with Boerhaave syndrome, whereas pain after exercise is consistent with myocardial ischemia.

Associated symptoms

It is important to consider associated symptoms when evaluating chest pain. For example, myocardial ischemia often produces diaphoresis, nausea, vomiting, and shortness of breath and less commonly produces weakness, fatigue, and syncope. The majority of patients with pulmonary embolism have an associated shortness of breath and apprehension; cough, fever, and hemoptysis are less common. Dissecting aortic aneurysms often produce diaphoresis, shortness of breath, and apprehension. Pneumonia and bronchitis are classically associated with cough, fever, sweating, and sputum production. A complete review of the associated symptoms is very helpful in determining the cause of chest pain.

Aggravating and alleviating factors

The cause of chest pain often can be further narrowed by eliciting a history of increasing or decreasing pain with certain maneuvers. For instance, the chest pain of angina pectoris is often aggravated by exercise and alleviated by rest or nitrates. Esophageal pain is often aggravated by eating, vomiting, eructation, and lying supine but is alleviated to some degree by antacids. Pleuritic pain from pulmonary embolism, pleural effusion, or pneumonia is aggravated by deep inspiration or coughing. Musculoskeletal pain is reproduced by chest wall movements, deep inspiration, or palpation of the chest wall.

Bedside diagnostic tests include palpation of the chest wall to aggravate pain and the administration of sublingual nitrates and antacids and topical anesthetics orally to alleviate pain. However, such tests are nonspecific, and the results of these tests are considered as only part of the overall clinical picture. For example, chest pain produced by palpation tends to support the diagnosis of chest wall pain, but some clinical studies report that as many as 25% of all patients with AMI report at least some pain when the chest wall is palpated for tenderness. Sublingual nitrates usually alleviate angina pectoris to some degree, but they also relieve esophageal spasm. Oral antacids may help distinguish esophageal pain in a minority of cases, but antacids may also give patients with AMI some relief from their pain. Because there is often a significant placebo effect with such therapeutic maneuvers in the emergency department evaluation of chest pain, these maneuvers should be used only as confirmatory tests to solidify clinical impressions. They cannot absolutely confirm or refute the clinical decision arrived at by the total patient assessment regarding patient diagnosis or disposition.

Risk factors

The major risk factors for AMI include hypertension, diabetes mellitus, smoking, hypercholesterolemia, and a family history of myocardial infarction at a relatively young age. Minor risk factors include an age greater than 35 years, male gender, obesity, and a "type A" personality (see the box on p. 124). Such factors should be

RISK FACTORS FOR VARIOUS CAUSES OF CHEST PAIN

Acute myocardial infarction

Major

Hypertension
Diabetes mellitus
Smoking
Hypercholesterolemia
Family history of AMI at a relatively young age

Minor

Age >35 years
Male gender
Obesity
Type A personality
Use of drugs causing or exacerbating
   myocardial ischemia (e.g. cocaine or
   sympathomimetics)

Pulmonary Embolism

Prolonged immobilization
Obesity
Peripartum state
Oral contraceptives
Hypercoagulable states
Congestive heart failure
Polycythemia
Neoplastic disease

Aortic dissection

Severe hypertension
Atherosclerosis
Marfan syndrome
Blunt chest trauma

Pneumothorax

Penetrating or blunt chest trauma
Prior spontaneous pneumothorax
Emphysematous bullae
Cocaine inhalation
Intravenous drug abuse (injection into
   subclavian vessels)
Pneumocystis carinii pneumonia

documented in any patient with chest pain that is possibly of myocardial origin, and they can help guide the physician's evaluation. Obtaining a history of consumption of drugs that can cause or exacerbate myocardial ischemia (e.g., cocaine or sympathomimetics) can also be helpful.

Risk factors for pulmonary embolism include prolonged immobilization, obesity, peripartum state, oral contraceptive use, hypercoagulable states, congestive heart failure, polycythemia, and neoplastic disease. Patients with severe hypertension, atherosclerosis, Marfan syndrome, or blunt chest trauma are at risk for aortic dissection. Patients at risk for pneumothorax include those with chest trauma, a prior spontaneous pneumothorax, emphysematous bullae, a history of drug inhalation (e.g., cocaine and marijuana), a history of intravenous drug abuse by injecting the subclavian vessels (pocket shooters), and *Pneumocystis carinii* pneumonia.

Physical Examination

In patients with chest pain the history is often more productive than the physical examination in terms of diagnosis and disposition. Nevertheless, a thorough examination should always be performed to assess for major and subtle physical findings that can alter patient care.

Any patient assessment should begin with the ABCs. Maintaining a patent airway; adequate breathing, including oxygenation and ventilation; and adequate circulation to ensure tissue perfusion is imperative. Beyond such initial assessments, vital signs can often give clues to the severity of disease. Blood pressure, pulse, respirations, and temperature should be assessed and documented. Patients with an AMI can display a wide spectrum of vital signs from hypotension to hypertension, bradycardia to tachycardia, and normal respirations to tachypnea. In this case the vital signs do not help make the diagnosis as much as they guide therapy. Tachypnea is seen in the majority of cases of pulmonary embolism and therefore can help distinguish pulmonary embolism from benign causes of pleuritic pain such as pleuritis or costochondritis. Fever is often seen with pneumonia but can also be present in pulmonary embolism, pericarditis, and Boerhaave syndrome. Severe hypertension is seen in the majority of patients with traumatic aortic dissection, but hypotension as a result of hemorrhagic shock can be seen after dissection has occurred. Hypotension and tachycardia can be seen with tension pneumothorax or cardiac tamponade.

A thorough physical examination in the patient with chest pain includes an extrathoracic examination. In the head and neck, signs of right-sided heart failure such as jugular venous distension or hepatojugular reflux can help guide therapy for certain causes of chest pain. Lymphadenopathy can be seen with inflammatory conditions such as mycoplasmal pneumonia, pneumocystis pneumonia, or tuberculosis, as well as with neoplastic conditions such as lung cancer. Examination of the extremities can reveal edema from right-sided heart failure, unilateral leg swelling from deep venous thrombosis as a source of pulmonary emboli, signs of peripheral emboli from endocarditis or atrial fibrillation, or signs of peripheral vascular occlusive disease as seen in patients with severe atherosclerosis. It is important to obtain the blood pressure in both arms to detect any difference in measured mean arterial pressure as a result of subclavian artery occlusion because of aortic dissection. Palpation of the abdomen can reveal epigastric tenderness in cases of peptic ulcer disease and biliary disease.

Examination of the lungs and heart is often nondiagnostic in patients with chest pain, especially with regard to the diagnosis of AMI, in which pallor, diaphoresis, and anxiety often tend to be more diagnostic than any specific adventitious lung or heart sound. However, certain physical findings can be helpful in managing patients with myocardial infarction. Auscultation of a new murmur can be diagnostic for papillary muscle dysfunction or rupture, which can lead to congestive heart failure and require surgical valve replacement. Basilar rales suggest congestive heart failure, which can complicate myocardial infarction.

In addition to tachypnea (97% of all cases) and tachycardia (43% of all cases), patients who have pulmonary embolism have a unilateral leg swelling of associated deep venous thrombosis in 35% of all cases. The chest examination is usually normal, but a wide spectrum of findings can be detected, including dullness produced by pleural effusions, findings of pulmonary consolidation, or a pleural friction rub. Pleural friction rubs are rare but are very specific for pulmonary embolism. Auscultation of the heart may reveal a split S_2, but this finding is very nonspecific.

The chest examination is occasionally diagnostic for other causes of chest pain. Decreased breath sounds can be heard with a pneumothorax. The addition of tracheal deviation, distended neck veins, and hypotension confirms a tension pneumothorax. With a pneumomediastinum, subcutaneous air can often be palpated in the neck or auscultated with the heartbeat (Hamman sign). Pneumonia can be detected by auscultation of rales or other signs of consolidation in the lungs. Rib fractures can be palpated, and musculoskeletal chest pain can usually be reproduced by palpation of the chest wall. Pericarditis can sometimes be detected by the auscultation of a pericardial friction rub, which may be heard better with the patient sitting forward. Cardiac tamponade can be manifested as decreased heart sounds, distended neck veins, and hypotension or a pulsus paradoxus greater than 10 mm Hg. Mitral valve prolapse is diagnosed by the auscultation of a midsystolic click, with or without a heart murmur.

DIAGNOSTIC TESTS

Depending on the cause of chest pain, diagnostic tests can either be very helpful or of limited value (see the box on p. 126). The emergency

DIAGNOSTIC TESTS FOR CHEST PAIN

Pulmonary embolism

Chest x-ray examination
Arterial blood gases
Ventilation perfusion scanning
Pulmonary angiogram

Aortic dissection

Chest x-ray examination
Transesophageal echocardiography
Chest computed tomography scan
Aortography

Unstable angina

ECG
Stress testing

Myocardial infarction

ECG
Serum markers
　Myoglobin
　Creatine phosphokinase-MB (CPK-MB)
Echocardiography
Nuclear medicine

Other conditions

Chest x-ray examination (pneumonia,
　pneumothorax, pneumomediastinum, lung
　carcinoma, pleural effusions, Boerhaave
　syndrome, chest wall trauma, cardiac
　tamponade)
Rib detail films (rib fractures)
Gastrografin swallow (Boerhaave syndrome)
Echocardiogram (pericardial effusion)
White blood cell count (pneumonia,
　bronchitis, endocarditis, pericarditis)
Pulse oximetry (shortness of breath, elevated
　respiratory rate)
Arterial blood gases (shortness of breath,
　elevated respiratory rate)

physician must weigh the usefulness of the test in terms of its ability to change patient diagnosis and management.

Myocardial Infarction

The ECG has always been helpful in diagnosing AMI. It is especially helpful in detecting acute transmural infarction, which produces ST-segment elevation of at least 1 mV in at least two contiguous leads. Subendocardial myocardial infarction can be detected by ST-segment depression in at least two contiguous leads. In addition, new ECG changes such as inverted T waves and new bundle branch blocks can be indicative of AMI if previous ECGs are available for comparison. Unfortunately, the ECG is an insensitive test because it is diagnostic for myocardial infarction in only 50% of all cases. A normal ECG can confirm a clinician's suspicion that the patient's chest pain is not a result of myocardial infarction, but if the patient's history is consistent with AMI, a normal ECG cannot eliminate the diagnosis of an evolving AMI.

Various serum markers for myocardial infarction have been investigated to provide more objective diagnostic data in the emergency department. Myoglobin, which appears in the serum within 3 hours after the onset of chest pain, is the earliest available serum indicator of AMI. It is 62% sensitive for myocardial infarction at the initial patient presentation and 100% sensitive 3 hours later. Unfortunately, it is only 84% specific. The value of a myoglobin test lies in its high negative predictive value for AMI. Creatine phosphokinase-MB (CPK-MB), an enzyme specific for myocardial muscle, is elevated in the serum of patients with AMI. Elevated CPK-MB, as measured by immunochemical techniques, has become the standard indicator for myocardial damage caused by ischemia. The CPK-MB levels increase within 4 hours after the onset of chest pain and peak 12 to 24 hours after the initiation of the infarction. In the emergency department, CPK-MB levels are not usually elevated at the initial patient presentation because patients with AMI come to the emergency department an average of 2 hours after chest pain has begun. However, 3 hours after the initial patient presentation, CPK-MB is 79% sensitive and 94% specific for AMI in patients with nondiagnostic ECGs. Elevated CPK-MB is not only diagnostic for AMI but also can predict who may be at risk for cardiovascular complications. Other serum markers such as Troponin-T, Troponin-I, myosin light chains, and CPK-MB isoforms, all of which are more specific for myocardial tissue, are presently under investigation and show some promise in the diagnosis of AMI in the emergency department.

Echocardiography and nuclear medicine imaging techniques have also been advocated as methods of detecting AMI in the emergency department. New wall-motion abnormalities or perfusion defects can often be diagnostic of myocardial infarction or ischemia, but such modalities are often not readily available in the emergency department.

Unstable Angina

Unfortunately, the diagnosis of unstable angina is difficult from an objective laboratory study standpoint. The ECG can provide the most objective findings. Depression of the ST segment, inverted T waves, or a strain pattern on the ECG can be helpful in diagnosing unstable angina, especially if the changes appear only with pain or are new compared to a previous ECG. However, a normal ECG does not rule out unstable angina. Serum markers are not elevated in unstable angina, which makes them diagnostically useless except for evaluating for associated myocardial infarction.

Stress testing, either by simple electrocardiographic methods or by nuclear medicine imaging techniques, has recently become popular in the emergency department evaluation of patients with presumed angina. Stress testing has been advocated to detect significant coronary artery disease in a low-risk, otherwise healthy patient once a patient is pain free and once AMI has been "ruled out" in the emergency department. Positive stress testing is often followed by admission to a monitored bed for further testing, including cardiac angiography.

Pulmonary Embolism

Multiple diagnostic modalities are used to detect pulmonary embolism, and their appropriate use is imperative to avoid misdiagnosis. The chest x-ray study can be positive for a number of findings, including elevation of the hemidiaphragm, localized atelectasis, pleural effusion, peripheral wedge-shaped infiltrate (Hampton hump), or localized vascular paucity (Westermark sign). However, these findings are nonspecific, and more than 50% of all chest x-ray examinations are nondiagnostic. Similarly, the ECG can demonstrate tachycardia, right axis deviation, the S_1-Q_3-T_3 pattern, atrial fibrillation, or right atrial enlargement, but most commonly the ECG is normal or shows sinus tachycardia.

Arterial blood gases can be used as a screening test for pulmonary embolism. The vast majority of patients show some evidence of hypoxemia on arterial blood gases. Even given a normal chest x-ray study, an arterial-to-alveolar (A-a) gradient of >15 mm Hg suggests the possibility of pulmonary embolism. However, a normal A-a gradient does not by itself rule out pulmonary embolism because as many as 5% of such patients will have a normal A-a gradient. Similarly, because of its inability to detect variation in oxygen saturation in relation to the carbon dioxide level, pulse oximetry cannot be used to exclude pulmonary embolism.

Ventilation/perfusion (V/Q) scanning is a nuclear medicine imaging technique used to detect pulmonary embolism. A normal V/Q scan can rule out pulmonary embolism, whereas low, intermediate, or high probability scans can be variably diagnostic when combined with the clinical picture. For instance, a low probability scan with a low clinical probability is associated with a 4% incidence of pulmonary embolism, whereas the same scan with a high clinical probability is associated with a 40% incidence. High probability V/Q scans are associated with pulmonary embolism in 56% to 96% of all cases, depending on the degree of clinical likelihood.

Pulmonary angiography is the "gold standard" test for the diagnosis of pulmonary embolism. In patients with low, intermediate, or high probability V/Q scans, the angiogram is used to confirm pulmonary embolism before committing the patient to long-term anticoagulation. An alternative to pulmonary angiography is Doppler plethysmography of the lower extremities to rule out deep venous thrombosis. Because deep venous thrombosis is present in more than 90% of all patients with pulmonary embolism, patients with low probability V/Q scans and normal lower extremity Doppler studies can be considered as "ruled out" for pulmonary embolism.

Aortic Dissection

The chest x-ray study is useful for the detection of aortic dissection in a significant portion of patients. With aortic dissection, wide mediastinum, pleural cap, left pleural effusion, depression of the left main stem bronchus, deviation of the esophagus, indistinct aortic knob, or tracheal deviation to the right can all be seen. Previous chest x-ray studies help determine whether such changes are new or old. The ECG is not useful in the diagnosis of aortic dissection except for a small subset of patients in whom the coronary arteries are involved and myocardial ischemia results.

Transesophageal echocardiography and chest CT scans have developed into good screening studies for the presence of aortic dissection. However, they are not as useful as aortography in delineating the extent of the dissection, the major vessels involved, or the location of the intimal disruption. Aortography remains the most useful test for the diagnosis of aortic dissection.

Other Conditions

The chest x-ray study is especially useful in the diagnosis of pneumonia, pneumothorax, pneumomediastinum, lung carcinoma, and pleural effusions. In patients with chest wall trauma, the chest x-ray study is more helpful in determining whether there is a secondary pneumothorax, hemothorax, or pulmonary contusion than whether there are rib fractures. Rib detail films are better for delineation of rib fractures, but the demonstration of a fracture may not change therapy unless there is underlying pulmonary damage. Patients with Boerhaave syndrome may show left pleural effusions or pneumomediastinum on the chest x-ray study, but the definitive diagnosis is best made by Gastrografin swallow to delineate any esophageal leak. Patients with cardiac tamponade as a result of bleeding, pericarditis, or malignant pericardial effusion often show an enlargement of the cardiac silhouette in a "water bag" shape or a double density on the left lateral aspect of the heart on the chest x-ray study. The definitive diagnosis of a pericardial effusion is best accomplished by acute echocardiogram, either transcutaneously or transesophageally.

An elevation of the white blood cell count, especially with a shift to the left, suggests infectious conditions such as pneumonia, bronchitis, endocarditis, or pericarditis. However, this test is nonspecific and must be used in conjunction with other clinical and laboratory findings.

Pulse oximetry and arterial blood gases should be used liberally to assess oxygenation in any patient with chest pain who either complains of shortness of breath or has an elevated respiratory rate. For example, the difference in disposition between admission and discharge for patients with pneumonia is often determined by their arterial blood gases. Patients with significant hypoxemia should not be sent home. Pulse oximetry is a good screening tool for hypoxemia but does not yield as much information as an arterial blood gas, especially with regard to the patient's A-a gradient or acid-base status.

PATIENT MANAGEMENT

On the basis of the results of the initial assessment and physical examination, certain critical actions are required before laboratory or ancillary test results can be obtained. All patients who come to the emergency department, especially those with chest pain, require assessment of their ABCs. If this assessment requires action in terms of airway control by means of endotracheal intubation, mechanical ventilation and supplemental oxygenation, or hemodynamic support, it needs to be undertaken rapidly and efficiently. Most patients with chest pain do not require immediate intervention for the ABCs, but when conditions such as AMI are present, the potential exists for rapid deterioration in the patient's condition. For this reason, preventive treatment and stabilization should be initiated early in patients with chest pain.

Supplemental oxygen administration is indicated in any patient with chest pain who complains of shortness of breath or has an elevated respiratory rate. An arterial blood gas or pulse oximetry reading can often be obtained before oxygen administration to determine the patient's baseline room-air oxygenation. The blood gas measurement is especially useful for determining the A-a gradient for patients with presumed pulmonary embolism. Any patient who has presumed end-organ ischemia, including patients with presumed myocardial infarction, unstable angina, or pulmonary embolism, should also be placed on supplemental oxygen.

Patients with presumed myocardial ischemia or hemodynamic instability should undergo continuous cardiac monitoring to watch for dysrhythmias. Patients with AMI are at risk for sudden death from ventricular fibrillation at any time, especially during the first 6 hours. Prompt treatment of ventricular fibrillation with electrical countershock is most effective if instituted within a few minutes, which makes early detection of dysrhythmias imperative. Warning dysrhythmias such as premature ventricular contractions, bigeminy, trigeminy, couplets, and runs of ventricular tachycardia need prompt antidysrhythmic therapy in this setting. Continuous monitoring is the most effective way to detect these dysrhythmias.

Intravenous (IV) access should also be obtained early in any patient with chest pain when myocardial ischemia is suspected or IV therapy is anticipated. IV access is needed to treat dysrhythmias and to administer IV nitrates, thrombolytics, anticoagulants, or analgesics. A second line is often needed to avoid mixing incompatible drugs and to maintain more than one continuous drug infusion. In patients with presumed pulmonary embolism, IV anticoagulants, fluids, or pressor agents are often administered. In patients with presumed aortic dissection, IV antihypertensives such as nitroprusside are indicated early and before the CT scan, echocardiogram, or angiography. In any patient with hemodynamic instability or potential hemodynamic instability, IV access is needed to administer fluids, pressor agents, or antidysrythmics. IV access is much easier to establish before cardiovascular collapse than afterward.

▌▌▌▌▌▌▌KEY CONSIDERATIONS

WHAT IS THE LIFE THREAT?

Myocardial infarction, pulmonary embolism, aortic dissection, and unstable angina are life-threatening conditions that appear with chest pain.

Other potentially life-threatening conditions include pneumothorax and ruptured esophagus.

DOES THE PATIENT NEED ADMISSION?

Admit the patient to a monitored bed for myocardial infarction and unstable angina. Admit patients with pulmonary embolism for anticoagulation. Obtain a surgical consultation for aortic dissection.

WHAT IS THE MOST SERIOUS DIAGNOSIS?

Myocardial infarction, pulmonary embolism, aortic dissection, and unstable angina are the most serious diagnoses.

HAVE I PERFORMED A THOROUGH WORK-UP?

Obtain a thorough history of the pain, including a description of its character, location and radiation, onset, timing, intensity, aggravating factors, relieving factors, and associated symptoms (e.g., syncope, diaphoresis, hemoptysis, nausea, vomiting, or shortness of breath).

Obtain a history of cardiac risk factors, including smoking, family history, diabetes, elevated blood lipids, hypertension, cocaine use, and previous coronary disease.

Obtain a history of risk factors for pulmonary embolism, aortic dissection, and pneumothorax.

Obtain cardiac enzymes if unstable angina or myocardial infarction is suspected.

Obtain arterial blood gases and a ventilation/perfusion scan for suspected pulmonary embolism.

Recommended Reading

American College of Emergency Physicians: Clinical policy for management of adult patients presenting with a chief complaint of chest pain, with no history of trauma, Dallas, 1990, ACEP.

Gibler WB et al: Acute myocardial infarction in chest pain patients with nondiagnostic ECGs: serial CK-MB sampling in the emergency department, *Ann Emerg Med* 21:504-512, 1992.

Kelley MA et al: Diagnosing pulmonary embolism: new facts and strategies, *Ann Intern Med* 114:300-306, 1990.

The PIOPED Investigators: Value of the ventilation/perfusion scan in acute pulmonary embolism, *JAMA* 263:2753-2759, 1990.

Pozen MW et al: A predictive instrument to improve coronary care unit admission practices in acute ischemic heart disease, *New Engl J Med* 310:1273-1278, 1984.

Chapter *Twelve*
ABDOMINAL PAIN

ALEXANDER TROTT

Although abdominal pain is a common problem and accounts for 5% of all emergency department visits, it is one of the most challenging symptoms to confront the emergency physician. Distinguishing between the various causes of acute abdominal pain is difficult because a wide variety of factors complicate the evaluation process. The subjective nature of pain, its complex neuroanatomic pathways, and the fact that it is a common symptom that can arise from a large and diverse group of diseases makes abdominal pain hard to define and diagnose. In fact, even after extensive emergency department and inpatient evaluations, almost 50% of all patients with abdominal pain remain undiagnosed (nonspecific abdominal pain). Table 12-1 displays the range of the most common causes of abdominal pain in adults that are likely to be seen in the emergency department.

Extremes of age significantly modify the diagnostic possibilities. In children under the age of 2, the most common causes of abdominal discomfort are colic, gastroenteritis, viral illness, and constipation. Appendicitis is uncommon but assumes a much greater importance over the age of 2. In addition to appendicitis, the most common causes of abdominal pain in children and adolescents are functional disorders, constipation, and gastroenteritis.

Elderly patients over the age of 70 are much more likely to have a surgical cause of pain. Acute cholecystitis, malignant disease, and bowel obstruction account for approximately 50% of all cases, whereas nonspecific pain accounts for only 10%. Despite the seriousness of these disorders, elderly patients are more likely to have vague histories, diminished physical findings, and unhelpful laboratory values.

NEUROANATOMY AND PERCEPTION OF PAIN

Probably the most important factor affecting the clinician's ability to assess and diagnose accurately the cause of abdominal pain is the complex and imprecise manner in which pain is generated and transmitted from the abdomen to the central nervous system. Understanding pain generation is crucial to the physician's ability to recognize diagnostic limitations yet manage the patient safely and effectively. Two major pain pathways are activated to produce the patient's subjective symptoms and objective signs: the visceral and the somatic pathways. Referred pain, a result of the varying activation of either pathway, falls into recognizable patterns that can aid the physician in diagnosis.

Visceral Pain

Visceral pain is mediated through nerve fibers that are located in the walls of hollow organs

Table 12-1

COMMON CAUSES AND FREQUENCY OF ABDOMINAL PAIN IN THE EMERGENCY DEPARTMENT

Cause	Frequency (%)	Cause	Frequency (%)
Abdominal pain of unknown cause	40-50	Acute cholecystitis	2-4
Gastroenteritis	7-10	Intestinal obstruction	2-4
Pelvic inflammatory disease	7-10	Constipation	2-4
Urinary tract infection	4-6	Duodenal ulcer	1-2
Ureteral stone	3-5	Other causes	15-25
Appendicitis	3-5		

and in the capsules of solid organs. The most common mechanism by which visceral pain is generated is through abdominal stretching or distension of a wall or capsule. Ischemia and inflammation of an abdominal organ can also cause visceral pain. Each abdominal organ is innervated by visceral afferent fibers from both sides of the spinal cord, which explains why visceral pain is most often felt in the midline despite the fact that most organs are located in a lateral position in the abdomen.

Visceral pain is often the earliest symptom of an organ disorder. Visceral pain tends to be vague, poorly localized, and is often described as "cramping," "dull," and "gaseous." The pain can be either intermittent, such as from early bowel obstruction, or continuous, such as with biliary colic. This type of pain is accompanied by autonomic responses that lead to nausea, vomiting, pallor, and diaphoresis. Although visceral pain cannot be localized to a specific organ, the general location of the discomfort suggests various organ groups. Visceral pain from the liver, stomach, gallbladder, and duodenum is felt in the epigastrium. The periumbilical, or midabdominal, area is the cutaneous site for sensation from the small intestine, appendix, and cecum. Pain from the colon, kidneys, ureters, bladder, and pelvic organs manifests itself below the umbilicus.

Somatic Pain

The parietal peritoneum, the root of the mesentery, and the anterior abdominal wall are all invested with pain receptors and fibers. These receptors and fibers return to the spinal cord via specific unilateral dermatomes that correspond to the anatomic site from which the pain arises. Somatic pain is often initiated by chemical or bacterial inflammation and is described by patients as sharp and more specifically localized than visceral pain. Once the peritoneum becomes irritated, objective tenderness can be elicited. Involuntary guarding and rebound tenderness develop as the peritoneum becomes increasingly involved. Somatic, localized tenderness on physical examination provides the best direct evidence that a specific organ is responsible for the pain.

Referred Pain

Any pain felt at a site distant from a diseased organ is commonly known as referred pain. The embryologic origin of the organ in question and the cutaneous referral site are often similar. For example, the diaphragm originates from the fourth cervical segment and "migrates" to its more caudal position in the adult. For this reason, diaphragmatic irritation causes shoulder pain (Kehr sign). Other classic referral sites include the testes and groin for kidney pain (ureteral colic), the lower back area for pelvic disorders, the mid-back for pancreatitis, and the epigastrium for acute myocardial infarction.

Appendicitis provides a good example of how pain originates and evolves in the abdomen. Early in the course of this condition, symptoms are generated by obstruction of the lumen of the organ, usually by an appendicolith. As the appendix continues to secrete from its mucosa, the wall becomes distended and gives rise to vague, crampy pain that is diffusely or centrally referred. Examination of the abdomen may reveal either no tenderness or mild diffuse tenderness without peritoneal findings. As the secretion and distension continue, the vasculature becomes compromised, which leads to invasion by lumenal bacteria. Inflammation follows, and the pain "moves" to the right lower quadrant. At this point, somatic pain fibers localize the pain and give rise to peritoneal signs. Recognition of this and other pain patterns may prevent a premature assessment of the patient as having a nonsurgical condition.

INITIAL PATIENT MANAGEMENT

During the initial evaluation of the patient with abdominal pain, the emergency physician must assume that a serious life threat could be the cause of the pain. Certain diagnoses that are always kept in mind include abdominal aortic aneurysm, perforated viscus, mesenteric ischemia, myocardial infarction, and pulmonary embolism.

In addition, characteristic clinical risk factors and presentations point to the potentially unstable patient. These risk factors include extremes of age, immunosuppression, history of ulcer disease, alcoholism, cardiac risk factors, severe pain of acute onset, abnormal vital signs, pallor, diaphoresis, signs of dehydration, hematemesis, and hematochezia.

INITIAL PATIENT MANAGEMENT

Acquire vital signs
Unless patient is in shock, complete the
  following:
    Perform postural vital signs
    Disrobe patient completely
    Acquire full history
    Perform physical examination
Never omit the rectal or pelvic examinations

Once the patient arrives by rescue squad or once triage has been accomplished, the following initial management steps are performed (see the box above). The nurse confirms the patient's history, paying special attention to medical problems, medications, hospitalizations, and allergies. Vital signs are taken. Orthostatic measurements are obtained in patients with syncope, lightheadedness, significant vomiting, diarrhea, signs of dehydration, or a history of gastrointestinal or vaginal bleeding.

A rapid overview is performed while the patient is being completely undressed. Attention is given to the patient's level of consciousness and general appearance, including skin color and signs of dehydration. Breath sounds are assessed. A rapid assessment of the abdomen is carried out, including palpation for localized tenderness and degree of discomfort.

If the patient is short of breath (a respiratory rate of more than 20 breaths/minute), shows signs of peripheral or central cyanosis, or has a history that is compatible with myocardial infarction, supplemental oxygen is continued or administered. If myocardial ischemia is suspected or if there is a possibility of any serious illness, the patient is placed on a cardiac monitor and observed for dysrhythmias.

Establishment of intravenous (IV) access and drawing of initial blood are carried out simultaneously (see the box on p. 134). IV hydration is

---

IF THE PATIENT IS IN DISTRESS OR SHOCK

Start IV line and draw blood samples
Give 1 L normal saline wide open
Give fluids to follow at 50 ml/kg
    In child give initial bolus of 20 ml/kg
Place a nasogastric tube to low intermittent
    suction
Place an indwelling urinary catheter
Obtain early surgical consultation

---

indicated for patients who demonstrate orthostatic changes in vital signs, have dry mucous membranes, or have a history consistent with significant vomiting or diarrhea. The usual choice of IV solution is an isotonic crystalloid—either lactated Ringer's solution or normal saline. The rate of volume repletion is determined by the degree of hypovolemia, the cardiovascular status of the patient, and the response of the vital signs to initial therapy. A second large-bore IV is started for the more unstable patient in whom significant vomiting, diarrhea, bleeding, signs of severe dehydration, hypotension, or abnormal orthostatic vital signs are present. Boluses of 200 to 500 ml (for children, 20 ml/kg bolus, repeated if necessary) are initially given to assess the patient's response.

Depending on the severity of the illness, a nasogastric tube is placed as part of the early care. The tube has the therapeutic potential to relieve distension and to serve as a conduit for gastric lavage. A urinary catheter may be therapeutic in relieving bladder obstruction, but it is more often a diagnostic aid and is used to obtain urine for analysis and to monitor the patient's response to fluid therapy.

Despite the patient's major complaint of pain, analgesics have traditionally not been given by this time. A caring manner and a brief explanation of the hazards of analgesics in covering important pain symptoms can usually help gain the patient's cooperation for a short time. However, a growing number of physicians believe that analgesia or sedation does not mask the signs of true intraabdominal pathology. In fact, small doses of analgesics may well make the diagnosis easier because the patient becomes more comfortable and is better able to cooperate with the interview, physical examination, and adjunctive evaluations. Early and clear communication with surgical consultants must be maintained if analgesics or sedatives are to be administered.

In general, antiemetics are used for any patient with abdominal pain and vomiting. Antiemetics can also be useful in patients with gastroenteritis, gastritis, and renal colic.

For critically ill patients with a suspected abdominal infection, antibiotics should be administered in the emergency department. Antibiotics are chosen to cover the likely infecting bacteria, which most commonly include the various enteric bacteria, including anaerobes. Choices of antibiotics include ampicillin, sulbactam, cefoxitin, or clindamycin with an aminoglycoside.

CLINICAL ASSESSMENT

History

Once the patient has been briefly assessed and stabilized, a complete history and physical are performed. The main objective of the history is to characterize the quality, onset, and location of the patient's chief symptom, pain. The secondary objective is to elicit information about contributory symptoms and the patient's pertinent, recent, and past medical history.

Pain that begins abruptly and is severe often indicates a serious disorder such as a vascular catastrophe, perforation of a viscus, or renal colic. Inflammatory causes of pain, such as cholecystitis, appendicitis, and diverticulitis, tend to develop more slowly over hours or days and tend to be less severe at onset. Pain that clearly precedes the onset of nausea and vomiting is more often observed with surgical causes of abdominal pain than with nonsurgical disorders. Diffuse or poorly localized pain, especially early in the course of the patient's disease, may represent the "visceral" phase of the pain. In these cases, some time must pass before the localization takes place and specific somatic tenderness develops.

Age is a significant modifier of pain perception. When specifically studied for pain response, people over the age of 65 are found to have a significantly higher pain threshold than patients between 20 and 30 years of age. Therefore these older patients tend to significantly underestimate their distress.

Any noxious stimulus that affects the intraabdominal organs, peritoneum, or mesentery can cause anorexia, nausea, and vomiting by stimulating the vagus and sympathetic afferent nerves that return to the "vomiting" centers in the medulla. This triad of symptoms is so common that it has limited value in the differential diagnosis of disorders causing acute abdominal pain.

Although classically indicative of a urinary tract infection, genitourinary symptoms can occur as a result of irritation of the bladder or ureters from an inflamed appendix or another pelvic organ. Therefore distinguishing between a true urinary tract infection and other causes of urinary symptoms becomes important. A properly collected and interpreted urine specimen is crucial for making such a distinction.

Essential in the abdominal pain work-up is thorough questioning concerning cardiopulmonary symptoms. Pulmonary infection and embolism, and acute myocardial infarction are diseases in which abdominal pain may be the primary symptom.

Past and concurrent medical disorders can significantly influence the assessment of the patient with abdominal pain. Knowledge of prior surgeries is important, because as many as 70% of all patients with small bowel obstructions have had previous abdominal surgery. A complete detailing of medication and substance use is also important. Alcohol, salicylates, or corticosteroids can be either the source of abdominal pain or significantly exacerbate or complicate the underlying disorder. Medical disorders such as diabetes, heart disease, and chronic pulmonary disorders can complicate the evaluation and stabilization of patients with abdominal pain. Patients over the age of 70 years with acute abdominal disease can be expected to have at least one complicating medical illness in 65% of all cases. It is noteworthy that 84% of all patients with chronic abdominal pain have a concomitant psychiatric disorder.

With women, a complete menstrual and gynecologic history is especially important to help distinguish among various causes of abdominal pain. Acute salpingitis is one of the disorders most commonly confused with appendicitis. One of the main goals in taking a menstrual history is to determine if the woman is pregnant. A tubal pregnancy can mimic appendicitis. Advanced intrauterine pregnancy can make the diagnosis of appendicitis more difficult. The location of the appendix changes during the third trimester, which causes pain and tenderness to shift more toward the right upper quadrant. The clinical findings in pregnant women tend to be nonspecific or absent more often than in women who are not pregnant.

Physical Examination

For the physical examination, the general appearance of the patient is an important clinical observation. As a rule, patients with pallor, a quiet but distressed manner, and little or no body movement are more acutely and seriously ill. Perforated ulcers, vascular catastrophes, and pancreatitis can cause such a presentation. Patients with an inflamed peritoneum also tend to stay still to minimize their discomfort.

Hypotension combined with abdominal pain requires rapid assessment and stabilization. The pulse rate is a more subtle but equally important sign of serious physiologic distress. Tachycardia often indicates occult blood loss or volume contraction as a result of vomiting. Postural changes of pulse (an increase of 20 beats/minute) or blood pressure (a systolic decrease of 20 mm Hg) help to confirm the presence of hypovolemia.

Of all the vital signs, it is the temperature reading to which physicians most often look as a clue to the source and severity of a patient's abdominal pain. Unfortunately, fever is a nonspecific parameter that does not differentiate between acute abdominal disorders. In acute, uncomplicated appendicitis, temperature values lower than 37.8° C (100.2° F) can occur in as many as 50% of all patients. Patients who have temperatures higher than 38.5° C (102° F) often have a bacterial infection as a source of their pain, such as pneumonia, acute pyelonephritis, or acute salpingitis.

Inspection, auscultation, percussion, and palpation have traditionally formed the essential tetrad of the physical examination. Although inspection, auscultation, and percussion are necessary components of the physical examination, the information they provide is often not helpful.

Inevitably, the physician spends the most time with and pays the most attention to palpation. Localizing the area of maximal tenderness considerably narrows the diagnostic possibilities. To maximize the chances of making such a discovery, it is essential to have the patient's cooperation. A large component of that cooperation includes the patient's clear understanding of the difference between a subjective feeling of pain and the objective elicitation of tenderness by the physician. If this distinction is not clarified in advance with the patient, he or she might give an inappropriate response when the physician asks, "Does that hurt?"

Rebound tenderness has long been regarded as a hallmark of peritoneal inflammation. This sign must be interpreted with great care because it is not always accurate or specific for an inflamed peritoneum. False positive results occur in 25% of all patients and, conversely, false negative results occur in 14% of all patients.

The abdomen is divided into areas that roughly correspond to quadrants. The actual method of palpation should be a systematic, gentle search for an area of maximal tenderness. To make the patient calm and to gain his or her confidence, it is useful to place your hand on the patient's abdomen toward the end of the history. Ideally the history will have provided a clue about the possible cause and location of the patient's pain. The examination begins as far away from the suspected area as possible, proceeds in a gentle and thorough manner, and includes all the quadrants. Returning to previously examined quadrants in a back-and-forth manner can help both the patient and physician decide which area is most tender. When a point of maximal tenderness can be reliably determined, the diagnostic possibilities are significantly narrowed.

Although the rectal examination is a necessary part of the complete work-up of the patient with abdominal pain, it is not specific. It has been reported to be informative in as many as 60% of all patients with acute abdominal pain as a result of conditions other than appendicitis. In addition to the rectal examination, the pelvic examination is essential in women who have abdominal pain. No survey of the abdomen is complete without an examination of the heart, lungs, flanks, and external genitalia.

LABORATORY ANALYSIS

An abnormal elevation of the white blood cell count (WBC) helps confirm the presence of significant disease when historical and physical findings point toward an organic cause of the abdominal pain. The WBC is useful as an adjunctive test but should never be relied on as the sole factor in making a surgical, therapeutic, or disposition decision. For most causes of abdominal pain, this test lacks acceptable sensitivity and specificity. Because of the retroperitoneal location of the pancreas, its lack of a well-defined capsule, and the variability of clinical findings, pancreatitis is a difficult diagnosis to make. Therefore the serum amylase level is often used to confirm the presence or absence of this disorder. However, amylase is not elevated in all cases of pancreatitis; normal or only slightly elevated levels are found in as many as 20% to 36% of all patients proven to have this disorder through other clinical studies. Despite the shortcomings of the serum amylase value, it remains a key diagnostic test.

Interpretation of urinalysis results requires caution in patients with abdominal pain. It is occasionally tempting to ascribe vague abdominal pain and nonspecific clinical findings to a urinary tract infection if pyuria is present. Patients with proven appendicitis have been reported to have pyuria (a WBC of 5 or greater) in 20% of all cases. Therefore proper collection of the urine specimen and adherence to strict criteria for the diagnosis of a urinary tract infection are very important.

A pregnancy test for women of childbearing age is recommended whenever there is a possibility of pregnancy or a pregnancy-related disorder.

For the seriously ill or elderly patient with acute abdominal pain, several other tests are considered to better define the extent of the physiologic derangement. An ECG is obtained for any patient suspected of having myocardial ischemia or an underlying cardiac condition that might affect the patient's outcome. Arterial blood gases are obtained to measure oxygenation and acid-base balance in a patient with suspected pulmonary complications, severe hypovolemia, or pancreatitis. Electrolyte determination or blood urea nitrogen (BUN) are particularly important tests for a patient with protracted dehydration. Liver function tests are not routinely ordered for a patient with acute

---

SUGGESTED LABORATORY TESTS
Complete blood count Urinalysis Type and crossmatch for two units Electrolytes BUN and creatinine Glucose and amylase Special studies as individual patients warrant

abdominal pain but can reveal anicteric hepatitis as a cause of anorexia and vague, poorly localized abdominal comfort (see the box above).

IMAGING

Abdominal x-ray studies are often ordered for patients with acute abdominal pain. However, positive findings are relatively uncommon and vary between 10% and 40% of all cases. Abnormalities that actually lead to a change in patient management occur in only 10% to 15% of all cases. There are no strict guidelines for ordering x-ray studies in the clinical setting of abdominal pain. However, certain clinical findings are more likely to increase the yield of these studies. These findings include high-pitched bowel sounds, abdominal distension, a history of abdominal surgery, or the clinical possibility of ureteral calculi.

Ultrasonography is the primary modality for evaluating abdominal pain that is localized in the right upper quadrant. Cholecystitis, duct obstruction, and hepatic structures are well visualized by ultrasonography. Ultrasonography can also rapidly and effectively diagnose the presence and size of an abdominal aortic aneurysm. Evaluation of a urinary obstruction or abscess, especially in iodine-sensitive patients, is easily achieved through ultrasonography. Transvaginal ultrasonography provides much useful information in the female patient with acute abdominal pain of pelvic origin. Compared with standard transabdominal ultrasonography, all features of an intrauterine pregnancy are seen earlier and more distinctly with the transvaginal approach. Transvaginal ultrasonography is reported to be particularly advantageous for the diagnosis of an ectopic pregnancy, both because of improved

visualization and because of the ability to exclude a normal intrauterine pregnancy. In experienced hands, the use of graded-compression ultrasonography can be useful in the diagnosis of acute appendicitis. Sensitivity has been reported to range from 88% to a specificity that approaches 100%. The proper use of this tool can reduce the negative laparotomy rate.

A CT scan provides excellent visualization of

DIFFERENTIAL DIAGNOSIS OF ACUTE ABDOMINAL PAIN

Right upper quadrant pain

Perforated duodenal ulcer
Acute cholecystitis and biliary colic
Myocardial ischemia
Acute pancreatitis (bilateral pain)
Retrocecal appendicitis
Acute hepatitis
Pulmonary embolus
Hepatomegaly resulting from congestive failure
Herpes zoster
Right lower lobe pneumonia

Left upper quadrant pain

Acute pancreatitis
Myocardial ischemia
Gastritis
Splenic enlargement, rupture, infarction, or aneurysm
Herpes zoster
Left lower lobe pneumonia
Pulmonary embolus

Diffuse pain

Dissecting or leaking aneurysm
Mesenteric thrombosis
Peritonitis
Acute pancreatitis
Sickle cell crisis
Early appendicitis
Gastroenteritis
Intestinal obstruction
Diabetes mellitus

Right lower quadrant pain

Leaking aneurysm
Ectopic pregnancy
Appendicitis
Regional enteritis
Meckel diverticulum
Cecal diverticulitis
Twisted ovarian cyst
Pelvic inflammatory disease
Ureteral calculi

Left lower quadrant pain

Leaking aneurysm
Ectopic pregnancy
Sigmoid diverticulitis
Mittelschmerz
Twisted ovarian cyst
Pelvic inflammatory disease
Ureteral calculi
Incarcerated, strangulated groin hernia

the solid viscera and retroperitoneal organs. It is most useful in the diagnosis of abdominal aortic aneurysms in hemodynamically stable patients. Other tests that can be ordered from the emergency department include an IV pyelogram, a barium enema, and angiography.

DIFFERENTIAL DIAGNOSIS

Once the clinical, laboratory, and radiographic data have been collected, the emergency physician must try to construct a reasonable differential diagnosis on the basis of the available information. The pain history and pattern, as well as the site of maximal tenderness, are findings most likely to yield a workable group of diagnoses. It is useful to think anatomically when trying to arrive at a differential diagnosis (see the box on p. 138). For example, in the right lower quadrant, common or life-threatening diseases such as appendicitis and ectopic pregnancy reside at the top of the list, whereas uncommon disorders such as regional enteritis fall lower on the list.

The differential diagnosis changes somewhat when only diffuse or generalized tenderness can

---

GUIDELINES FOR SURGICAL CONSULTATION IN PATIENTS WITH ABDOMINAL PAIN

A rigid, silent, tender abdomen
Abdominal tenderness with peritoneal signs
Localized, reproducible tenderness
Tenderness with accompanying fever
Tenderness with mass
Pain or tenderness with a pulsatile mass
Tenderness with uncontrolled vomiting
Gastrointestinal bleeding
Suspected bowel obstruction
Suspected pancreatitis
Suspected mesenteric ischemia
Extremes of age (<2 years old, >65 years old)

---

be identified. Many early or atypical presentations of intraabdominal diseases may result in generalized pain. The reason for poor localization can be partially explained by the complex neuroanatomic pathways previously discussed. Poorly localized pain may also be caused by biochemical abnormalities, such as diabetes, or toxins, such as lead. Referred pain from extraabdominal sources (chest, back, genitalia) may mimic an acute abdominal syndrome. As mentioned previously, psychiatric causes must also be kept in mind when evaluating atypical abdominal pain.

CONSULTATION

Of all the decisions that an emergency physician must make when evaluating a patient with abdominal pain, probably the most difficult and important concern is when to obtain a consultation and when to discharge a patient. The decision is easy when the diagnosis is clearly evident or when the patient has symptoms and signs of surgical disease (see the box at left).

If the diagnosis is not immediately apparent and if the patient does not appear ill, the following is a suggested course of action to be considered: Patients with abdominal pain of unclear etiology, with or without mild tenderness and no associated peritoneal findings, can be observed in the emergency department. The patient should be evaluated for consistency of physical findings and for any changes in laboratory values. For example, a WBC can be repeated to detect a rise in the count. Depending on the clinical situation, observation for 4 to 6 hours with repeated examination is an acceptable option when the diagnosis is unclear and the situation does not appear to require urgent surgical intervention. If the patient's condition stays the same or worsens, a surgical consultation is recommended. Patients who improve considerably can be discharged with provisions made for follow-up care.

DISPOSITION

If consultation and admission to the hospital are considered unnecessary, the decision to send the patient home must be done with a clear understanding that the symptoms could worsen. In fact, the patient must be instructed to return immediately to the emergency department if the pain worsens or if other symptoms develop that indicate a serious or surgical disorder. As a precaution, most patients should be sent home with instructions for a clear liquid diet for 24 hours. This diet not only decreases the stimulus for vomiting and provides for hydration but also prevents dangerous gastric feeding should a surgical problem arise and the patient require a general anesthetic. Oral narcotic pain medications are discouraged. Most patients should be reexamined within a 24-hour period. The patient can be instructed to return to the emergency department; direct verbal communication should be made with a referral physician, and follow-up arrangements should be made before the patient is discharged from the emergency department.

KEY CONSIDERATIONS

WHAT IS THE LIFE THREAT?

Leaking aortic aneurysm, myocardial ischemia, perforated stomach or bowel, mesenteric thrombosis, peritonitis, severe pancreatitis, ectopic pregnancy, appendicitis, torsion of ovarian cyst, volvulus, and massive gastrointestinal hemorrhage constitute life threats.

DOES THE PATIENT NEED ADMISSION?

Patients with a life-threatening cause of abdominal pain or a "surgical" acute abdomen with peritoneal signs (rigid, tender, silent) require surgical consultation and admission.

Patients with pain of uncertain etiology with or without mild tenderness and no peritoneal findings can be observed in the emergency department for 4 to 6 hours or until the pain subsides. Surgical consultation should be obtained if the pain worsens, increased tenderness is noted, or the WBC rises.

WHAT IS THE MOST SERIOUS DIAGNOSIS?

Leaking abdominal aneurysm, perforated viscus, volvulus, mesenteric thrombosis, ectopic pregnancy, myocardial infarction, pulmonary embolus, and bowel obstruction are the most serious diagnoses.

HAVE I PERFORMED A THOROUGH WORK-UP?

In cases of severe abdominal pain in which a life-threatening or serious cause is considered, do the following:

Consider "nonabdominal," life-threatening causes of abdominal pain such as myocardial infarction, pneumonia, or pulmonary embolism.

Perform a history and physical examination, including an abdominal assessment that involves inspection, auscultation, and palpation of all quadrants.

Examine for rebound tenderness.

Perform a rectal examination.

Perform a pelvic examination.

Obtain a urinalysis, complete blood count, and serum amylase.

Consider liver function tests: BUN, creatinine, glucose, calcium, magnesium electrolytes.

Consider imaging studies, including abdominal and chest x-ray studies (supine and upright abdomen, upright chest), ultrasonography, and abdominal CT scans.

Recommended Reading

Brewer RJ: Abdominal pain: an analysis of 1000 cases presenting to the emergency room, *Am J Surg* 131:219, 1976.

Lukens TW, Emerman C, Effron D: The natural history and clinical findings in undifferentiated abdominal pain, *Ann Emerg Med* 22(4):690-696, 1993.

Reynolds SL, Jaffe DM: Diagnosing pediatric abdominal pain in the emergency department, *Pediatr Emerg Care* 8:126, 1992.

Rusnak RA, Borer JM, Fastow JS: Misdiagnosis of acute appendicitis: common features discovered in cases after litigation, *Am J Emerg Med* 12(4):397-402, 1994.

Silen W: *Cope's early diagnosis of the acute abdomen,* ed 17, New York, 1987, McGraw-Hill.

Temple CL, Hutchcroft SA, Temple CJ: The natural history of appendicitis in adults: a prospective study, *Ann Surg* 221(3):278-281, 1995.

Trott AT, Greenberg R: Acute abdominal pain. In Rosen P et al, editors: *Emergency medicine: concepts and clinical practice,* ed 3, St Louis, 1992, Mosby.

Way LW: Abdominal pain. In Sleisenger MH, Fordtran JS, editors: *Gastrointestinal disease,* ed 3, Philadelphia, 1983, WB Saunders.

Chapter Thirteen

GASTROINTESTINAL BLEEDING

PHILIP L. HENNEMAN

Gastrointestinal (GI) bleeding is a common problem encountered in emergency medicine that may manifest itself subtly or in dramatic fashion. The mortality rate is approximately 10% and has not changed in the past four decades. Diagnostic modalities have improved much more than therapeutic ones. Aggressive resuscitation and prompt consultation are the keys to appropriate management.

Patients who come to the emergency department with symptoms and signs of GI bleeding are often frightened. They are afraid of the possibility of painful procedures and of the real or perceived risk of death. It is important to approach these patients with understanding and compassion. GI bleeding may represent a significant life threat to the patient; therefore it is important to aggressively manage the patient to minimize the risk of significant complications. Remember to warn the patient about any painful or uncomfortable procedures before you perform them (e.g., intravenous line placement, nasogastric tube placement).

GI bleeding comprises upper and lower GI bleeding. Upper gastrointestinal bleeding (UGIB) is bleeding proximal to the ligament of Treitz (the duodenal suspensory ligament that at-

taches at the junction of the duodenum and jejunum). Each year, UGIB affects 50 to 150 persons per every 100,000 persons and results in 250,000 hospital admissions at an annual cost of almost 1 billion dollars. Lower gastrointestinal bleeding (LGIB) occurs distal to the ligament of Treitz and results in significantly fewer hospitalizations than UGIB.

GI bleeding can occur in individuals of any age but most commonly affects individuals who are between the fifth and eighth decades of life (mean age 59 years). Elderly patients are less able than younger patients to tolerate acute blood loss. Most of the deaths that occur from GI bleeding involve patients over the age of 60 years. A UGIB is twice as common in adult men than in women, and LGIB is more common in elderly women. Upper and lower GI bleeding stops spontaneously in at least 80% of all admitted patients.

ETIOLOGY

Upper Gastrointestinal Bleeding

The most common causes of UGIB in children and adults are listed in Table 13-1. Peptic ulcer

Table*13-1*

CAUSES OF SIGNIFICANT GASTROINTESTINAL BLEEDING*

Upper Gastrointestinal Bleeding	*Lower Gastrointestinal Bleeding*
Peptic ulcer disease	Diverticulosis
Gastric erosions	Angiodysplasia
Varices	Undiagnosed
Mallory-Weiss syndrome	Cancer/polyps
Esophagitis	Rectal disease
Duodenitis	Inflammatory bowel

*Listed in order of decreasing frequency.

disease, gastric erosions, and varices account for approximately three fourths of all patients with UGIB.

Peptic ulcer disease

Peptic ulcer disease is the most common cause of UGIB in children and adults and accounts for approximately 50% of all cases. Gastric or duodenal ulcer bleeding usually manifests itself with melena (black, tarry stools) or hematemesis (vomiting of blood). Hematochezia (red rectal bleeding) may occur if bleeding is brisk. Bleeding may be the initial presentation of an ulcer. Bleeding from duodenal or gastric ulcers accounts for approximately half of the deaths from UGIB.

Gastric erosions

Gastric erosions (small circumscribed mucosal defects) and gastritis (inflammation of the gastric mucosa) account for approximately one fourth of all cases of UGIB. Bleeding is usually less significant than that seen in peptic ulcer disease or varices; patients rarely die from bleeding as a result of gastritis or gastric erosions.

Varices

Bleeding from esophageal or gastric varices is a manifestation of portal hypertension. Portal hypertension and variceal bleeding is predomi-

nately a disease of adults but can occur in children. In the United States, most cases of portal hypertension are a result of alcoholic cirrhosis. A history of alcohol use and the findings of jaundice or ascites on physical examination often direct attention to the presence of liver disease and portal hypertension. Although bleeding in patients with cirrhosis is most commonly a result of varices, hematemesis and melena often arise from other sources, such as peptic ulcers and gastric erosions. Endoscopy is the most precise modality to diagnose the presence of varices, and it is often possible to acutely stop variceal bleeding with ligation or sclerotherapy. Bleeding from varices accounts for approximately 10% of all cases of UGIB, and such patients often rebleed. Variceal bleeding is responsible for one third of all deaths from UGIB.

Mallory-Weiss syndrome

Mallory-Weiss syndrome (bleeding resulting from small lacerations in the gastric mucosa in the area of the esophagogastric junction) accounts for fewer than 10% of all significant UGIBs. They occur predominately in adults following vomiting. Patients commonly report multiple episodes of vomiting followed by hematemesis. Bleeding is usually mild to moderate and stops spontaneously. People rarely die from Mallory-Weiss tears.

Esophagitis and duodenitis

Although it is a common disorder, esophagitis is a relatively uncommon cause of UGIB. Careful questioning of the patient often reveals a history of esophageal reflux. Esophagitis is the most common cause of UGIB during pregnancy. Duodenitis is also a relatively uncommon cause of UGIB and is often associated with aspirin use. In both esophagitis and duodenitis, bleeding is usually mild and self-limited.

Drug ingestion

Approximately one half of all patients with peptic ulcer disease and UGIB report a recent use of aspirin. Aspirin ingestion is associated with the development of gastric ulcers, gastric erosions, and gastritis. Alcohol and aspirin have a synergistic effect in precipitating UGIB. Nonsteroidal antiinflammatories are also associated with GI bleeding but to a lesser extent.

Lower Gastrointestinal Bleeding

The causes of LGIB vary with the age of the patient (see Table 13-1 for a list of the most common causes). Significant LGIB in the elderly is most commonly a result of diverticulosis or angiodysplasia. In young adults, massive LGIB is most often a result of ulcerative colitis. *Campylobacter jejuni* can also cause bloody diarrhea. Significant LGIB in children is most often a result of a Meckel diverticulum or intussusception. In all ages, minor LGIB is usually related to a rectal abnormality.

Diverticulosis

Diverticulosis occurs in one half of all patients over the age of 60 years but results in serious bleeding in fewer than 5%. In the past, most cases of LGIB in the elderly were attributed to diverticular disease because no other lesions were noted on the barium enema. Diverticulosis occurs throughout the colon, but bleeding from diverticula predominately occurs in the ascending and proximal transverse colon; diverticular bleeding is arterial. Patients bleed massively and acutely and may complain of mild, crampy abdominal pain. Patients can have red rectal bleeding or black, tarry stools. Severe bleeding may produce signs and symptoms of shock. Elderly patients are often less able than younger patients to tolerate significant blood loss. Approximately one third of patients with diverticular bleeding rebleed. One fourth of patients with diverticular bleeding require surgery.

Angiodysplasia

Angiodysplasia (arteriovenous malformation) is an acquired disorder of unknown cause. It is most often found in the cecum and ascending colon but can occur anywhere in the GI tract. Arteriovenous malformations are found in one fourth of all patients over the age of 60 years. Many authorities believe that LGIB is caused by angiodysplasia at least as often as diverticulosis. Patients bleeding from an arteriovenous malformation may have black, tarry stools but more commonly have red rectal bleeding. These lesions are not seen on a barium enema but can sometimes be visualized through colonoscopy. The best way to demonstrate these lesions is with mesenteric angiography. Most patients have recurrent bleeding. Coagulation biopsy through a colonoscope is often successful, but massive bleeding is best treated with a hemicolectomy after localizing the bleeding site.

Carcinoma

Carcinoma rarely causes major LGIB but should be considered in elderly patients with occult bleeding or iron deficiency anemia. Polyps are a relatively common cause of mild-to-moderate LGIB in children and adults.

Meckel diverticulum

Meckel diverticulum is the most common cause of *significant* LGIB in children. Symptoms can occur at any age but most commonly are seen in the first 2 years of life. Painless rectal bleeding is the usual presentation.

Intussusception

Intussusception is the most common cause of intestinal obstruction in children between the ages of 2 months and 6 years. Typically infants have a sudden onset of crampy abdominal pain that recurs at regular intervals. Most children pass stool containing blood and mucus (currant jelly stool). The diagnosis of intussusception is made through the history, physical examination, and radiographic confirmation with a barium enema.

Rectal disease

Rectal disease is a common cause of mild LGIB. Anal fissures and hemorrhoids are the most common causes of rectal bleeding in children and adults, respectively; the bleeding is usually minor. Patients complain of bright red blood with, or after, the passage of stool. Anal fissures can be seen by spreading the perineal skin to evert the anal canal. Anoscopy may demonstrate hemorrhoidal bleeding. LGIB should not be attributed to anal fissures or hemorrhoids until objective evidence confirms their presence and more serious causes have been excluded.

Factitious causes

With factitious causes of GI bleeding the site of bleeding may be obvious or subtle. Common sites include the nose, mouth, and throat. Swallowed blood may result in hematemesis or melena. Black stools will result from 50 ml of swallowed blood, and 100 to 200 ml of swallowed blood will result in melena. Examination of the nares, mouth, and pharynx should help establish the diagnosis. A chest x-ray examination may reveal a pulmonary source of swallowed blood.

However, not everything that is red or black in the vomitus or stool is blood. Multiple items such as red wine, spaghetti sauce, and cherry gelatin (Jell-O), will result in red vomitus. Certain substances, including iron, charcoal, and bismuth preparations, cause black stools.

CLINICAL PRESENTATION

The presentation of patients with GI bleeding is often straightforward. Most patients with GI bleeding have hematemesis, melena, or hematochezia. They may also have more subtle signs of hypovolemia, such as weakness, dizziness, or syncope. Patients may also experience such signs as shortness of breath, ischemic chest pain, or myocardial infarction. They may deny or be unaware of having blood in their vomitus or stool. It is important to consider GI bleeding in patients who have any of these similar complaints.

Bleeding from the esophagus, stomach, or proximal small bowel usually results in hematemesis or melena. The color of vomitus can not be used to differentiate arterial from venous bleeding. Blood from the duodenum or jejunum must be retained in the intestinal tract for 8 hours before it turns black. Bleeding that occurs anywhere from the distal small bowel to the rectum usually results in melena or hematochezia. Hematochezia usually occurs when bleeding originates in the colon, but if transit time is delayed, colonic bleeding results in black stool. Red rectal bleeding may result from brisk UGIB and a short transit time.

In a study of 2225 patients with UGIB, 71% had melena, 56% hematemesis, 21% maroon stool, 43% presyncope, and 14% syncope. In studies of patients with LGIB, as many as 40% have black, tarry stools, and 60% have red stools.

EVALUATION

Patients who are hemodynamically unstable should undergo prompt fluid resuscitation at the same time that a brief history and physical examination are being obtained. Once a patient has been initially stabilized, a further history can be obtained.

History

When obtaining the patient history, specific questions should address the duration and quantity of bleeding, any previous history of bleeding and treatment, medications, allergies, alcohol or aspirin ingestion, associated medical illnesses, treatment by prehospital personnel, and the patient's response to the prehospital treatment. Patients with a documented GI lesion will be bleeding from that site only 60% of the time. A history of hematemesis is useful in indicating an upper GI source of bleeding. The amount of blood loss can be estimated by the duration, frequency, color, and volume of the vomitus or stool and by the presence or absence of symptoms of hypovolemia (e.g., dizziness, diaphoresis, dyspnea, pallor, confusion, syncope, and angina).

Vital Signs

Vital signs and postural changes in vital signs are essential in assessing the amount of blood loss that a patient has sustained. All patients with hypotension, tachycardia, or postural changes in vital signs, as well as a suggestive history, should be assumed to have significant bleeding. Previously healthy adult patients who arrive in the emergency department in profound hemorrhagic shock have lost at least 40% of their blood volume (>2 L blood in a 70 kg man).

However, vital signs and postural changes are not always reliable. Young adults with a 15% blood loss typically do not have changes in their supine vital signs but will have postural changes in their systolic blood pressure (a decrease >20 mm Hg) or heart rate (an increase >20 beats/minutes). In addition, postural changes in vital signs are not reliable when the blood loss is less than 10 ml/kg. Pediatric and elderly patients may also show postural changes in their vital signs in the absence of blood loss. Frequent reassessment of patients is important because their status may change quickly.

GI bleeding is not associated with an elevated temperature. Patients with hypotension, tachycardia, and fever are probably in septic shock. However they may also have GI bleeding.

Physical Examination

With an unstable patient, the physical examination should be performed while the history is being obtained. Careful attention should be given to the patient's mental status, skin signs (color, warmth, moisture, capillary filling time, and lesions such as telangiectasia, bruises, and petechiae), pulmonary and cardiac findings, and the abdominal, rectal, and stool examination. The presence of occult hemoglobin in stool is confirmed by such tests as guaiac (Hemoccult) or *o*-toluidine (Hematest).

Laboratory Tests

Blood should be drawn on the patient's arrival for determination of baseline hematocrit and hemoglobin, prothrombin time (PT), platelet count, and type and crossmatching. Hematocrit and hemoglobin are useful tests in the evaluation of patients with bleeding as long as its limitations are appreciated. Changes in hematocrit may lag significantly behind actual blood loss. Equilibration of hematocrit after untreated acute blood loss takes as long as 72 hours; 70% of equilibration occurs in the first 24 hours. Nonbleeding patients who are given 20 to 30 ml/kg of normal saline sustain drops in their hematocrit of 4% to 6%. With acute blood loss, bolus infusion of crystalloid causes rapid equilibration of hematocrit. Hematocrit changes of greater than 4% to 6% after bolus crystalloid infusion should be considered as evidence of hemorrhage. Hematocrit, like vital signs, should be repeated periodically to reassess the patient.

The PT is important to determine if a patient has a preexisting coagulopathy and to guide therapy with fresh frozen plasma. Serial platelet counts are used to determine the need for platelet transfusion (i.e., <50,000/mm^3 for major bleeding). Determinations of electrolytes, blood urea nitrogen, and calcium levels are rarely useful. Persistent elevation of blood urea nitrogen after 24 hours implies inadequate fluid resuscitation rather than blood in the GI tract. Patients with alcoholic liver disease may have hypoglycemia and should be evaluated for this condition at the bedside at arrival, especially if they have altered mental status.

An ECG should be obtained for elderly patients, those with coronary artery disease, and middle-aged patients with significant anemia. Upright portable chest radiography is indicated as soon as the patient can sit up to exclude a diagnosis of free peritoneal air (evidence of a perforated viscus, such as may occur in peptic ulcer disease), aspiration pneumonia, or congestive heart failure (high output failure secondary to anemia or iatrogenic fluid overload). GI bleeding alone is not an indication for abdominal x-ray studies.

Nasogastric Tube and Gastric Lavage

After initial resuscitation, it is important to localize the GI bleed as either upper or lower. This localization is accomplished by sampling the gastric contents. If the patient is vomiting in the emergency department, the vomitus can be evaluated; otherwise a nasogastric or orogastric tube should be placed. Gastric tubes can be placed for suspected varices or Mallory-Weiss syndrome without the risk of aggravating the bleeding. Care must be exercised when placing gastric tubes because pharyngeal and esophageal perforation or tracheal intubation can occur. The presence or absence of blood in the gastric contents is best determined by visual inspection. Nasal trauma from nasogastric tube insertion is the most common cause of false-positive results. A clear aspirate does not exclude bleeding from the duodenum, because

edema or spasm may prevent a reflux of blood into the stomach. However, the presence of bile in an otherwise clear aspirate does make the likelihood of bleeding above the ligament of Treitz unlikely.

Gastric lavage is unnecessary unless the patient is about to undergo endoscopy. Lavage is best performed with a large-bore Ewald tube that is placed orally with the patient in the left lateral decubitus position and with the bed in the Trendelenburg position. Additional holes may be cut in the distal portion of the Ewald tube to improve aspiration of blood and clots.

It is important to evaluate the gastric contents of patients with hematochezia, because as many as 20% of all patients with UGIB have maroon stools. An anoscopy and proctosigmoidoscopy should be performed if the gastric contents are negative for blood in patients with hematochezia.

Anoscopy and Proctosigmoidoscopy

Patients with mild rectal bleeding should undergo an anoscopy. A proctosigmoidoscopy should be performed if actively bleeding hemorrhoids are not visualized. During a proctosigmoidoscopy, it is important to determine if the stool above the rectum contains blood. The absence of blood above the proctoscope implies that the rectum is the source of the bleeding.

TREATMENT

After arrival to the emergency department, the patient should be transferred to a bed, undressed, placed on a cardiac and oxygen saturation monitor, given supplemental oxygen, and quickly assessed with respect to the airway, breathing, and circulation (ABCs). Airway is rarely a problem in patients with GI bleeding unless they are in shock. Altered mental status and vomiting is an indication for prompt intubation. Universal blood and secretion precautions should be observed in the emergency department.

Intravenous Lines and Fluid Management

One or two large-bore (14 or 16 gauge), peripheral intravenous lines should be placed if they were not placed in the field. Normal saline boluses (5 to 15 ml/kg and up to a maximum of 30 ml/kg) should be given to stabilize the patient. Patients who demonstrate signs of hemodynamic instability after 30 ml/kg of normal saline should have additional large-bore, peripheral intravenous lines placed and be transfused with blood. Venous cutdowns should be reserved for patients with persistent hypotension or shock that is unresponsive to initial resuscitation; these patients may also benefit from central venous line placement to monitor right atrial pressure.

Blood Products

Patients with impending cardiac arrest or persistent shock after 30 ml/kg bolus of crystalloid should be treated with O-negative red blood cells (usually 2 units). This type of blood should be immediately available. Uncrossmatched type-specific blood is usually available 15 minutes after the blood bank receives a sample of the patient's blood. Typed and screened whole blood takes 30 minutes, and crossmatched blood takes up to 1 hour to be available. Patients who are persistently unstable and require continuous transfusions can progress from O-negative to uncrossmatched type-specific blood, to typed and screened whole blood, and finally crossmatched blood. To decrease the viscosity of packed red blood cells and to increase the flow rate through the intravenous line, 100 ml of normal saline solution can be placed directly into the bag and mixed with the blood.

Serial platelet counts should be followed on all patients who are receiving massive transfusions because dilutional and consumptive thrombocytopenia may need to be treated (platelet count <50,000/mm^3). Fresh frozen plasma should be given when the patient has a documented coagulopathy (PT >15 seconds) and persistent bleeding.

Antacids and Histamine H$_2$ Antagonists

Antacids should not be given in the emergency department to patients with UGIB. Blood is an excellent buffer, and antacids may obscure the endoscopist's view. Histamine H$_2$ antagonists are indicated in patients with UGIB. Metaanlysis of randomized, clinical trials suggests that treatment of UGIB patients with H$_2$ blockers may reduce the rates of bleeding or the risk of rebleeding, surgery, and death. The benefit of this therapy may be limited to patients with gastric ulcers, but these patients cannot be identified in advance by the emergency physician. Therefore it is reasonable to treat all UGIB patients with histamine H$_2$ antagonists (e.g., cimetidine 300 mg).

Further Diagnostic Evaluation and Treatment

UGIB and LGIB usually stop spontaneously. In most patients, diagnostic testing to determine the source of bleeding can be delayed for 12 to 24 hours to allow them to stabilize. Endoscopy can be performed on patients with UGIB to identify the cause of the bleeding. Patients with LGIB who require less than 3 units of blood in the first 48 hours can undergo colonoscopy.

UGIB that is unresponsive to initial resuscitation or is recurrent requires emergency endoscopy or angiography because further therapy (sclerotherapy, ligation, electrocoagulation, or surgery) is often decided by identifying the cause of bleeding. When LGIB is profuse and persistent, angiography should be performed to determine the site of surgical resection.

Endoscopy

Endoscopy is the most accurate diagnostic tool available in the evaluation of patients with

UGIB. Endoscopy identifies a lesion in most patients if performed within 12 to 24 hours of their hemorrhage. Earlier endoscopy is indicated if the patient does not respond to initial resuscitation efforts. In the setting of variceal bleeding, sclerotherapy or ligation (banding) have proven effective in controlling acute hemorrhage. With nonvariceal bleeding, electrocoagulation, heater probe, and injection therapy are possible through the endoscope.

Angiography

With the advent of endoscopy, the use of angiography has diminished dramatically in patients with UGIB (now less than 1% of all patients with UGIB). Angiography is used primarily for patients with massive LGIB. It rarely diagnoses the cause of bleeding in such patients, but it does identify the site of bleeding in approximately two thirds of those patients who require surgical intervention. An angiography must be performed during active bleeding (>0.5 ml/minute). If the site of the bleeding is identified, the surgeon will resect a smaller portion of the bowel.

Vasopressin

Intravenous vasopressin may be used in select patients with UGIB and is most commonly used in patients with variceal bleeding. Unfortunately, no clinical trials have shown a positive effect on overall mortality. Vasopressin is associated with serious complications, and therefore its use should be limited. Vasopressin is most often recommended after a failure to stop bleeding through the endoscope. However, in the patient who is exsanguinating and who has suspected variceal bleeding a trial of vasopressin (0.2 to 0.6 U/minute) is certainly reasonable.

Sengstaken-Blakemore tube

The Sengstaken-Blakemore tube stops hemorrhage in most patients who are bleeding as a result of esophageal hemorrhages. The Linton tube is superior to the Sengstaken-Blakemore tube in patients with bleeding gastric varices. In general these tubes should not be used without endoscopic documentation of the source of bleeding because complications are frequent and significant; 14% of those complications are major, and 3% are fatal.

Radionuclide imaging and colonoscopy

Radionuclide imaging and colonoscopy are performed after the patient has left the emergency department. Radionuclide imaging is used primarily in stable patients with persistent or recurrent LGIB. It can grossly identify the approximate site of the hemorrhage in more than three fourths of all patients undergoing surgery. Colonoscopy is rarely used in the acute assessment of patients with LGIB. It is usually performed 48 to 72 hours after the bleeding episode (and after cleaning of the bowel).

Surgery

Surgery is indicated in all hemodynamically unstable patients with active bleeding who do not respond to appropriate intravascular volume replacement and correction of a coagulopathy. Approximately 25% of all patients who undergo emergency surgery for GI bleeding die. Most authorities recommend emergency surgery when blood replacement exceeds 5 units within the first 4 to 6 hours or when 2 or more units of blood are needed every 4 hours after replacing the initial losses.

Consultation with a surgeon should be obtained if it appears that more than 2 units of blood will be required in the initial emergency department resuscitation. A consultation is especially needed for patients over the age of 65 who have a history of peptic ulcer disease. Patients with aortic grafts who enter the emergency department with GI bleeding should receive prompt vascular surgical consultation for the possibility of aortoenteric fistula.

To identify the bleeding lesion, to exclude lesions treatable through the endoscope, and to guide surgical therapy, endoscopy is indicated in all patients who are being considered for surgical management of UGIB. Patients with massive LGIB should have an angiography to identify the site of bleeding; the angiography is followed by intraarterial infusion of angiospastic agents. This procedure works for more than three quarters of all patients; when this procedure is unsuccessful, a subtotal colectomy should be performed.

potension, or postural changes and who have only a mild anemia and no evidence of continued bleeding can be considered for admission to the ward. Patients with a history of GI bleeding but a normal examination or only trace hemepositive stool or gastric aspirate can be considered for outpatient management with follow-up the next day.

ADMISSION CRITERIA

Patients with significant GI bleeding should be admitted to the hospital. Patients who are unstable on presentation, have persistent bleeding, are elderly, or have significant complications should be admitted to an intensive care unit, and the appropriate emergency procedures should be performed (Table 13-2). Stable patients with a single episode of melena or hematemesis who never had tachycardia, hy-

SUMMARY

Recommended guidelines should be followed for the management of patients with GI bleeding (Figure 13-1). Initial resuscitation begins with the assessment and management of the ABCs. Large-bore, peripheral intravenous lines should be placed, and crystalloid resuscitation should be begun. Blood should be obtained for initial hematocrit, hemoglobin, coagulation studies, and type and crossmatching. Patients

Table 13-2

INDICATIONS FOR EMERGENCY PROCEDURES

Procedure	Indications
Endoscopy	Persistent UGIB that is unresponsive to initial resuscitation; uncontrolled bleeding that requires surgery; endoscopy before surgery to clarify site of bleeding and possible therapeutic interventions
Angiography	Persistent GI bleeding (lower > upper) to localize the site of bleeding before surgery; trial of embolization (upper) or selective vasopressin (upper and lower)
Vasopressin	Patient who is exsanguinating with probable variceal bleeding; endoscopy unavailable or unsuccessful
Sengstaken-Blakemore tube	Patient who is exsanguinating with probable variceal bleeding; endoscopy unavailable or unsuccessful and no response to vasopressin
Surgery	Unstable patient unresponsive to resuscitation; more than 5 U blood in initial 6 hours; more than 2 U blood every 4 hours required after the initial 6 hours

Modified from Henneman PL: Gastrointestinal bleeding. In Rosen P et al, editors: *Emergency medicine: concepts and clinical practice*, ed 3, St Louis, 1992, Mosby.

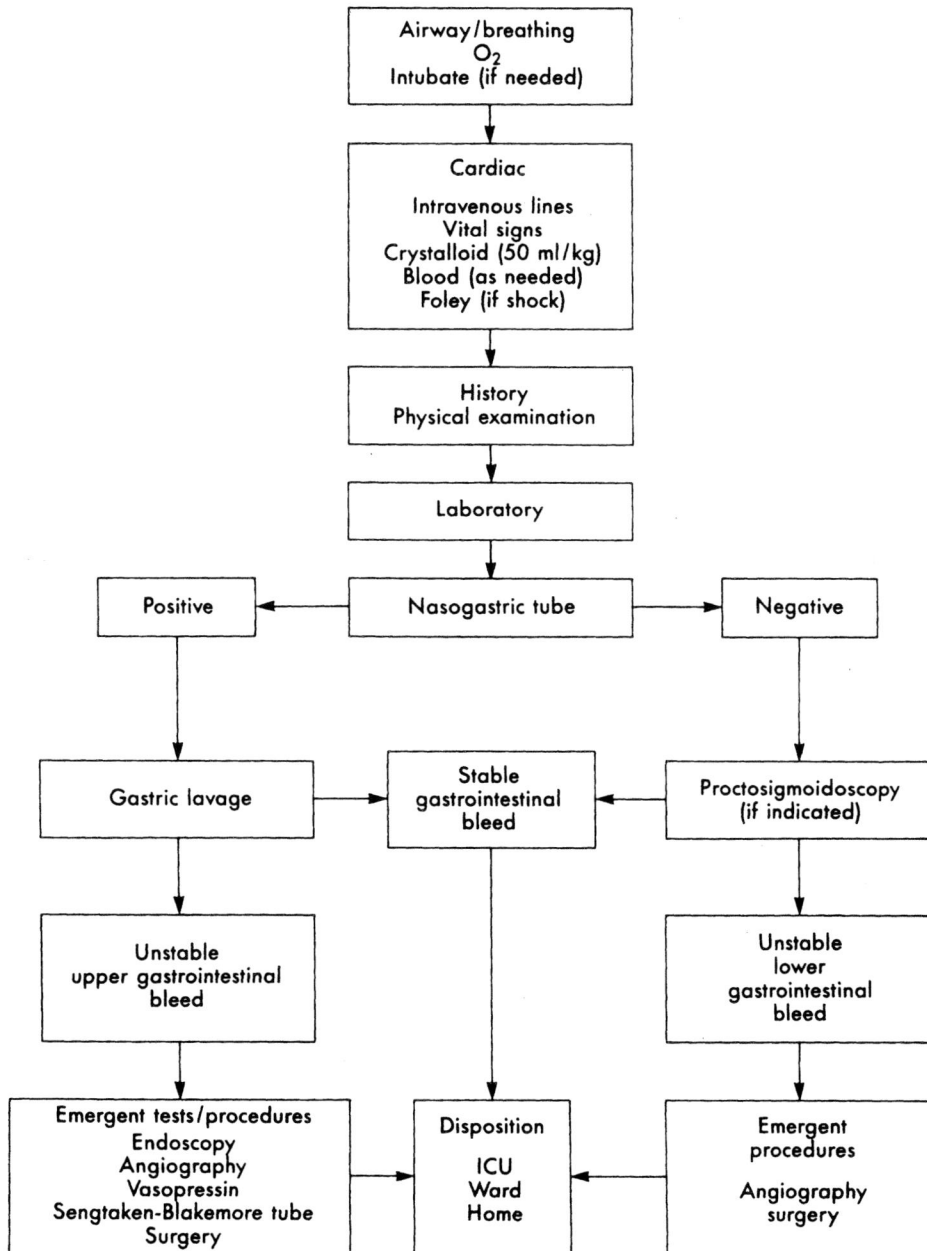

Fig.13-1   Management guidelines for gastrointestinal bleeding in the emergency department. (From Henneman PL: Gastrointestinal bleeding. In Rosen P et al, editors: *Emergency medicine: concepts and clinical practice,* ed 3, St Louis, 1992, Mosby.)

who do not respond to 30 ml/kg of intravenous normal saline solution should have more intravenous lines placed and be given blood. A nasogastric tube should be placed, and gastric aspirate should be inspected. Patients with hematochezia and a clear gastric aspirate should undergo anoscopy and proctosigmoidoscopy.

Stabilized patients should be admitted. Immediate consultation should be sought for all unstable patients requiring the emergency procedures listed in Table 8-2. Consultation with a gastroenterologist is appropriate for those who may need early endoscopy. Surgical consultation should be considered for patients requiring more than 2 units of blood during the emergency department resuscitation, especially if they are over age 65. Emergency endoscopy is appropriate for patients with persistent and profuse UGIB. Emergency angiography is appropriate for patients with massive LGIB.

KEY CONSIDERATIONS

WHAT IS THE LIFE THREAT?

Massive GI bleeding, if untreated, can lead to shock, exsanguination, and death.

DOES THE PATIENT NEED ADMISSION?

Patients with significant GI bleeding should be admitted to the hospital. Patients who are unstable on presentation, have persistent bleeding, are elderly, or have significant complications should be admitted to an intensive care unit. Stable patients with a single episode of melena or hematemesis who never had tachycardia or hypotension (including orthostatic hypotension) and who have only a mild anemia and no evidence of continued bleeding should be considered for ward admission. Patients with a history suggestive of GI bleeding who have a normal examination or only trace heme-positive stool or gastric aspirate can be considered for outpatient management with follow-up the next day.

WHAT IS THE MOST SERIOUS DIAGNOSIS?

Bleeding from esophageal varices, gastritis, gastric erosion, peptic ulcer, duodenal ulcer, diverticulosis, angiodysplasia, and carcinoma constitute the most serious diagnoses in adults. Bleeding from a Meckel diverticulum or intussusception constitute the most serious cases in children.

HAVE I PERFORMED A THOROUGH WORK-UP?

Assess the history of bleeding, and assess hemodynamic stability. Perform a rectal examination and nasogastric aspiration for UGIB. Assess coagulation status. Type and screen blood. Consider consultation for endoscopy, angiography, or surgery.

Recommended Reading

Barkin RM: Gastrointestinal hemorrhage: hematemesis and rectal bleeding. In Barkin RM, Rosen P, editors: *Emergency pediatrics: a guide to ambulatory care*, ed 3, St Louis, 1990, Mosby.

Brewer TG: Treatment of acute gastroesophageal variceal hemorrhage, *Med Clin North Am* 77:993, 1993.

DeMarkles MP, Murphy JR: Acute lower gastrointestinal bleeding, *Med Clin North Am* 77:1085, 1993.

Gupta PK, Fleisher DE: Nonvariceal upper gastrointestinal bleeding, *Med Clin North Am* 77:973, 1993.

Henneman PL: Gastrointestinal hemorrhage. In Rosen P et al, editors: *Emergency medicine: concepts and clinical practice*, ed 4 St Louis, 1996, Mosby.

Chapter Fourteen
VOMITING

GARY L. SWART

Vomiting represents the body's primary defense system against preingested, ingested, or absorbed toxins and signals a malfunction of the gastrointestinal tract. Nausea, retching, and emesis are protective responses caused by certain stimuli. Sight, smell, and taste, as well as complex sensations such as motion sickness and vertigo, commonly induce these responses. Anticipatory vomiting can occur when an individual experiences sensations previously associated with vomiting.

Afferents from the gastrointestinal tract include vagal, and to a lesser extent, sympathetic fibers. These fibers induce vomiting in response to gastrointestinal mucosal irritation or stretch from a variety of toxins, infectious agents, or mechanical abnormalities. Stimuli such as pregnancy, irradiation, or chemotherapy induce vomiting via unknown afferent mechanisms, although both nerve and humoral (i.e., bloodborne) inputs have been considered. Absorbed or injected drugs and toxins and other undefined peptides or hormones also act as humoral afferents to induce vomiting.

VOMITING SYSTEM

Chemoreceptor Trigger Zone

Two brainstem areas are the input centers for the vomiting system. The first of these, the chemoreceptor trigger zone (CTZ), lies in the floor of the fourth ventricle in the area postrema. This area remains outside of the blood-brain barrier and is therefore exposed to bloodborne toxins. In laboratory experiments, vomiting can be induced by electrical stimulation of the CTZ, and vomiting that is induced by bloodborne toxins can be blocked by ablation of the CTZ. However, vomiting that is induced by stimulation of vagal afferents from the gut is not affected by CTZ ablation. Therefore the CTZ is responsible for initiating vomiting that is related to bloodborne drugs and toxins but does not seem to be responsible for controlling the act of vomiting.

Vomiting Center

The second input area for the vomiting system has been referred to as the "vomiting center" and is responsible for motor control of the vomiting act. However, the name *vomiting center* is misleading because no such anatomically defined "center" actually exists. Many complex physiologic actions such as chewing, swallowing, and breathing are believed to be under the control of multiple brainstem nuclei and neurons that are referred to as "central pattern generators." Current theory suggests that vomiting is controlled by a central pattern generator in the nucleus tractus solitarii, which coordinates pharyngeal, gastrointestinal, and respiratory actions during retching and emesis. The central pattern generator for vomiting receives input from both vagal afferents and the CTZ; however, how it controls the act of vomiting remains unknown.

MECHANISM

The act of vomiting comprises three subactions: nausea, retching, and emesis. Nausea refers to the remarkably unpleasant epigastric sensation that occurs before emesis. It is often associated with other nonspecific autonomic signs such as tachycardia, tachypnea, salivation, diaphoresis, and mydriasis. Nausea may occur episodically and chronically without proceeding to retching or emesis. Interestingly, there is no definable neurologic pathway and no gastrointestinal motor activity that explains this very unpleasant subjective sensation.

Unlike nausea, which may not progress to emesis, retching and emesis usually do occur in series. Each retch is associated with a phase of esophageal dilatation, an emptying of the gastric contents into the esophagus, a return of the gastric contents to the stomach, and esophageal collapse. Motor activity of the stomach is relatively silent during retching and emesis. Emesis usually occurs after a series of retches in which reverse peristalsis of the small bowel and positive intrathoracic and intraabdominal pressure result in the expulsion of gastrointestinal contents from the mouth. Neurologically, retching and emesis require the coordinated activity of the gastrointestinal tract, respiratory muscles, diaphragm, abdominal muscles, and oropharyngeal structures.

ETIOLOGY AND ASSESSMENT

Vomiting is a physical sign, not a disease entity; however, it may be the most obvious physical sign that is present in the simplest or the most devastating illness. Therefore an in-depth history and examination followed by a carefully considered diagnostic work-up related to the vomiting itself is invaluable to determine the cause of the vomiting.

History

The historical aspects of vomiting that should be considered include timing, character/quality, associated symptoms, and aggravating/alleviating factors.

Timing

Both the time of day and timing after oral intake must be considered. Early morning vomiting before eating is associated with pregnancy, uremia, alcoholic gastritis, sinusitis with postnasal drip, and increased intracranial pressure. Immediate postprandial vomiting, within minutes of eating, is usually a result of psychogenic vomiting; however, psychogenic vomiting must remain a diagnosis of exclusion because gastric outlet obstruction as a result of a pyloric channel ulcer may also cause immediate postprandial vomiting. Peptic ulcer disease that occurs in locations other than the pyloric channel usually causes vomiting 30 minutes to several hours after a meal. Vomiting several hours after a meal may also suggest gastric retention caused by a motility disorder. Gastroparesis, literally a loss of peristalsis of the stomach, most commonly occurs in patients with diabetes but may also be seen in postvagotomy patients. It must be remembered that patients with diabetes vomit for reasons other than gastroparesis and that gastroparesis does not always cause vomiting. Therefore the term *gastroparesis* should be a diagnosis reserved for those in whom gastric atony and retention has been documented.

Character/Quality

The appearance of stomach contents at various states of digestion may give clues to the cause of vomiting. Most importantly, nondigested food that is vomited several hours after ingestion should suggest a gastric outlet obstruction or gastroparesis. Feculent vomitus suggest either bacteria overgrowth of the stomach or small bowel. Bacterial overgrowth may occur with long-standing atony, gastric outlet obstruction, distal intestinal obstruction, or ileus. Rare gastrointestinal catastrophes such as bowel ischemia or gastrocolic fistula may also result in feculent vomiting.

Bilious vomiting implies the presence of an open pylorus and therefore is not seen in gastric outlet obstruction. Bilious vomiting is otherwise a nonspecific sign. Blood in the vomit, or hematemesis, suggest upper gastrointestinal bleeding. Either fresh blood or a "coffee-ground" emesis may be secondary to bleeding in the esophagus (e.g., Mallory-Weiss tear, varices), stomach, or small bowel (e.g., peptic ulcer, tumor erosion into a blood vessel).

Some differentiation of vomiting can also be made on the basis of its forcefulness. Regurgitation is a low-force expulsion of stomach contents, but the mechanism is different from true vomiting. In the infant, regurgitation is a benign condition and is often confused with vomiting. In the adult, gastroesophageal reflux may result in the regurgitation of acidic stomach contents that taste like brackish water. *Projectile vomiting* is the term used for particularly forceful vomiting that occurs without prior nausea or retching. Projectile vomiting is characteristically associated with increased intracranial pressure, but its presence is neither unique to nor ubiquitous in this condition.

Associated symptoms

The presence and timing of pain associated with vomiting provides an important diagnostic clue. Abdominal pain is generally of two pathophysiologic types: obstructive and inflammatory. Obstruction of any peristalsing hollow viscus results in colicky, cramping pain. Conversely, peritoneal irritation resulting from inflammation, or peritonitis, results in constant localized or radiating pain with guarding, rigidity, and rebound tenderness of the abdomen. Obstructive pain and vomiting that occur close together suggest complete and proximal obstruction of the bowel or obstruction of a ureter. The onset of obstructive pain with a slower onset of vomiting may indicate a more distal obstruction. Peritonitis with vomiting close in onset suggests acute rupture of a hollow viscus (such as a duodenal ulcer), ischemia of the bowel, or torsion of an ovary or testicle. The peritoneal irritation that precedes the vomiting associated with appendicitis, diverticulitis, cholelithiasis, cholecystitis, pyelonephritis, and pelvic inflammatory disease is characteristic of an indolent inflammatory process.

Location and radiation of the pain associated with vomiting is of obvious importance because it may suggest the organ of origin. For example, obstructive pain in the flank that radiates to the groin is characteristic of ureteral obstruction. Right upper quadrant pain that radiates to the back may be crampy and obstructive with cholelithiasis or constant and inflammatory with cholecystitis. Peritonitis with vomiting and radiation of pain to the shoulders suggests peritoneal diaphragmatic irritation. This condition may be a result of a rupture of a hollow viscus with free intraperitoneal fluid or of inflammation localized near the diaphragm in splenic and hepatic disease.

Vomiting that is accompanied by an anatomically related symptom complex can also help achieve diagnostic certainty. Vomiting with chest pain, diaphoresis, or shortness of breath is associated with inferior myocardial infarction. Tinnitus or vertigo with vomiting suggests a cause of labyrinthine or cerebellar origin. Vomiting in association with constitutional symptoms such as fever, rigors, myalgias, arthralgias, cough, headache, and altered mental status may suggest viral or bacterial sepsis, gastroenteritis, pneumonia, meningitis, or a plethora of other infectious diseases.

Aggravating and alleviating factors

Additional diagnostic clues may be gained from having the patient describe what makes the vomiting better or worse. For example, vomiting in peptic ulcer disease is often made worse by eating, whereas for gastritis, eating often makes the vomiting better. Large or fatty meals in the patient with cholelithiasis may cause pain and vomiting. The vomiting in labrynthitis and benign positional vertigo is made worse by movement of the head. Finally, maneuvers that increase intracranial pressure, such as bending over or squatting, may induce projectile vomiting when some inciting cause of elevated intracranial pressure is already present.

Physical Examination

The ABCs

The potential for encountering severe illness in the emergency department setting makes it advantageous to begin each patient encounter with a brief consideration of airway, breathing, and circulation (the ABCs). For this initial assessment, the patient's general appearance and vital signs should be considered. Patients with vomiting and an altered level of consciousness must be assessed for the ability to protect the airway from aspiration. Unresponsiveness, sonorous respirations, or loss of a gag reflex suggests the need for airway protection, usually by endotracheal intubation. A brief assessment of circulation that considers abnormalities in mentation, pulse rate and blood pressure, or delayed capillary refill in children may provide evidence of shock.

Shock, by definition, is a state in which there is inadequate perfusion to meet the metabolic demands of the tissues. Shock may be related to hypovolemia, circulatory failure, sepsis, anaphylaxis, or neurogenic compromise. With dehydration and hypovolemia, shock may occur as a direct effect of vomiting. However, vomiting may also occur with sepsis, anaphylaxis, and circulatory failure. A prime example is the patient with an inferior myocardial infarction with chest pain, diaphoresis, dyspnea, and vomiting. Hypotension, tachycardia, and altered mentation in this patient are a result of circulatory failure, not hypovolemia.

Vital signs and general appearance

A postural, or orthostatic, increase in pulse and a decrease in blood pressure may be used to assess the degree of dehydration in the vomiting patient. However, other signs such as a resting tachycardia, subjective orthostatic dizziness, dry mucous membranes, lack of tear formation with crying, decreased urine output, sunken eyes or fontanelle, poor skin turgor, delayed capillary refill (>3 seconds), and an alteration in normal behavior or mental status are equally "vital" signs of dehydration in children and adults.

Fever can denote an infectious cause of illness in the vomiting patient. An increased respiratory rate with vomiting may represent a response to fever or respiratory compensation for metabolic acidosis. A deep and accelerated respiratory pattern called Kussmaul respirations is seen in patients with diabetic ketoacidosis, alcoholic ketoacidosis, or uremia as well as a result of intoxications with drugs that cause metabolic acidosis, such as aspirin, methanol, ethylene glycol, isoniazid, or paraldehyde.

Abdominal examination

Following a general assessment and vital signs, the abdominal examination provides much needed information in the vomiting patient. The abdominal examination is performed by inspection, auscultation, percussion, and palpation and centers around two important potential findings: obstruction and peritonitis.

Inspection. Gross inspection of the abdomen reveals distension when a bowel obstruction or ileus is present. Gastrointestinal ileus (literally "too roll up") can be caused by peritoneal irritation and by metabolic disturbances. Other extraabdominal causes of ileus include spinal fractures, pneumonia, and myocardial infarction. Vomiting occurs in both ileus and obstruction but occurs earlier and more intensely in proximal small bowel obstruction.

Auscultation. Auscultation of the abdomen normally reveals low-pitched, occasional peristaltic sounds. Very frequent or continuous sounds of normal pitch may represent bowel hyperactivity associated with intraluminal irritation such as gastroenteritis or the presence of blood in the gastrointestinal tract. High-pitched rushes and tinkling sounds of any frequency are typically a result of gastrointestinal obstruction. Absent sounds suggest bowel inactivity such as occurs in late obstruction or ileus.

Percussion. Percussion of the abdomen is performed to elicit sound and rebound tenderness. A hollow, tympanic sound generally implies a gas-filled bowel consistent with ileus or obstruction. A splashing sound over the stomach, the so-called "succussion splash," may be present as a result of incomplete emptying of the stomach with gastric outlet obstruction. Liver enlargement in hepatitis may reveal dullness to percussion in the right upper quadrant. Shifting dullness to percussion may be elicited if free fluid, particularly ascites, is present.

Rebound tenderness refers to abdominal pain that increases with sudden movement of the abdominal wall. Although its presence is variable, rebound tenderness is classically associated with peritoneal irritation. The presence of vomiting with peritonitis is also variable, but the presence of both rebound tenderness and vomiting suggests a surgical emergency. General causes of peritoneal irritation include (1) gastrointestinal rupture with leakage of contents, such as in a perforated gastric ulcer or necrotic gallbladder, or (2) any inflamed intraabdominal structure in contact with the peritoneal wall, such as in appendicitis, cholecystitis, cholangitis, pancreatitis, or pyelonephritis.

Palpation. Palpation of the abdomen is performed to identify the general state of abdominal tenderness as well as the presence of rigidity, masses, or organomegaly. The presence of severe abdominal pain with rebound tenderness, rigidity, and muscular guarding suggests the presence of peritonitis—a surgical emergency. The presence of a pulsatile mass in the abdomen with abdominal pain should raise the ominous suspicion of an abdominal aortic aneurysm. Such patients may experience vomiting, which can lead the physician into the false belief that the patient is experiencing some less morbid gastrointestinal illness. Patients with this disease progress rapidly into hypovolemic shock if the aneurysm is leaking or ruptures. Therefore immediate diagnostic studies and a surgical consultation should be obtained if such a diagnosis is considered.

Differential Diagnosis

It is clear that the differential diagnoses of vomiting are protean. In many cases, there are multiple levels of both gross mechanical and cellular physiologic processes between the true etiology and the physical sign of vomiting. Because of the enormity of the task, it seems most effective to consider the differential diagnosis of vomiting in a tabular formate from two etiologic perspectives: anatomy and stimulus. Broad categories rather than specifically named entities are presented for the less common diagnoses, which should facilitate the development of a mechanism-oriented differential diagnosis rather than a simple memorization of an extensive list of possibilities (see the box on pp. 158 and 159).

Pediatric Differential Diagnosis

In the pediatric population, the differential diagnosis of vomiting can be classified by age of occurrence as well as by anatomy and stimulus. The neonate (birth to 4 weeks of age) may exhibit the expulsion of gastric contents along a continuum of severity from simple "spitting up" through gastroesophageal reflux to true vomiting. Spitting up is of little concern as long as the birth history is without incident and the

DIFFERENTIAL DIAGNOSIS OF VOMITING BY ANATOMY AND STIMULUS

Cerebral

Elevated intracranial pressure
   Structural abnormality with hydrocephalus
   Mass effect with edema or hydrocephalus
      Benign or malignant tumor
      Hemorrhage
         Epidural hematoma
         Subdural hematoma
         Subarachnoid hemorrhage
         Intracerebral, intracerebellar, or
           brainstem hemorrhage
      Septic abcess
   Edema secondary to brain injury
      Contusion
      Diffuse axonal injury (concussion)

Ocular

Increased intraocular pressure

Auditory/labyrinthine

Meniere disease
Labyrinthitis
Benign positional vertigo
Seventh and eighth cranial nerve tumors
Motion sickness

Gastrointestinal

Pharyngeal gag reflex
Esophagus (often regurgitation rather than
  vomiting)
  Achalasia
  Zenker diverticulum
  Inflammation
    Barrett esophagus secondary to reflux
    Infectious
      Candidiasis
      Herpes
Stomach
  Inflammation
    Gastric ulcer
    Zollinger-Ellison syndrome
    Gastritis
      Alcoholic
      Stress-related
      Campylobacter jejuni infection

Gastrointestinal, cont'd

Stomach, cont'd
  Gastric outlet obstruction
    Pyloric channel ulcer
    Gastric carcinoma
  Gastroparesis
    Diabetic
    Postvagotomy
    Drug-induced
    Idiopathic
Liver, biliary tree, pancreas
  Inflammation
    Hepatitis, acute or chronic
      Infectious
      Alcoholic
    Cholecystitis
    Cholangitis
    Pancreatitis, acute or chronic
  Hepatic failure
  Hepatorenal syndrome
  Biliary obstruction
    Choledocolithiasis
    Primary biliary cirrhosis
    Carcinomatous
    Congenital anomalies
  Pancreatic carcinoma
Intestines and colon
  Infection
    Viral gastroenteritis, numerous agents
    Bacteria (more commonly bloody diarrhea)
      Direct invasion
      Endotoxin mediated
         Salmonella organisms
         Staphylococcal food poisoning
    Protozoa
  Inflammation
    Duodenal ulcer
    Crohn disease
    Ulcerative colitis
    Meckel diverticulum
    Appendicitis
    Diverticulitis, diverticulosis
    Mesenteric ischemia

Gastrointestinal, cont'd

Intestines and colon, cont'd
  Irritable bowel syndrome
  Chronic intestinal pseudo-obstruction
  Obstruction
    Superior mesenteric artery syndrome
    Volvulus
    Intussusception
    Stricture/adhesion
      Carcinomatous
      Postoperative
  Illeus
    Postoperative
      General anesthetic
      Direct handling of bowel
    Secondary to peritonitis, intraabdominal or
      retroperitoneal inflammation
    Pneumonia
    Myocardial infarction
    Spine fracture or surgery
    Institutional bowel

Renal and Urinary

Infection
  Pyelonephritis
  Perinephric abcess
Ureterolithiasis
Uremia secondary to renal failure, acute or
  chronic

Genital

Ovarian cyst
Ovarian torsion
Pelvic inflammatory disease
  Salpingitis
  Endometritis
  Tubo-ovarian abcess

Genital, cont'd

Pregnancy
  Morning sickness
  Hyperemesis gravidarum
  Molar pregnancy
Endometriosis
Testicular trauma
Testicular torsion
Epididymitis
Orchitis

Metabolic and Nutritional

Addison Disease
Ketacidosis
  Diabetic
  Alcoholic
  Starvation
Starvation ketosis
Hyperthyroid crisis
Hypoparathyroidism/hyperparathyroidism
Hypervitaminosis/avitaminosis
Congenital errors of metabolism

Psychologic

Bulimia
Psychogenic vomiting
Rumination

Common toxins in therapeutic dose and overdose

Digatalis glycosides
Erythromycin
Chemotherapeutic agents
Opiates
Aminophylline, theophylline
Estrogens
Iron preparations
Aspirin
Mushrooms

neonate appears well and gains weight appropriately. Gastroesophageal reflux, however, can be a more complex problem. Neonates with severe reflux may fail to gain weight and are subject to pulmonary complications of recurrent aspiration. A diagnosis of gastroesophageal reflux requires documentation of reflux, either by esophageal pH monitoring or by scintigram.

True vomiting in the neonate may be related to a congenital anomaly of the gastrointestinal tract, a systemic infection, a congenital error of metabolism, hydrocephalus, or a renal dysfunction. Congenital anomalies of the gastrointestinal tract often occur with vomiting in the first few days of life. These anomalies may include intestinal atresia or stenosis, malrotation, volvulus, meconium ileus or obstruction, Hirschsprung disease, and an imperforate anus.

Infants age 1 month to 2 years may have two age-specific causes of vomiting: pyloric stenosis and intussusception. Infants with pyloric stenosis are usually in the 4- to 6-week age range, with progressively increasing frequency of forceful vomiting and a failure to gain weight. Because of the level of obstruction, the vomitus in pyloric stenosis is not bilious as it may be in other more distal bowel obstructions. The hypertrophic pylorus, which is described as a "palpable olive" in the epigastrium, is a classically described but unreliable physical examination sign of pyloric stenosis.

Intussusception is the obstructive prolapsing of a proximal portion of bowel within a distal segment of bowel. It most commonly occurs in the 3-month to 1-year age range but may also occur well into childhood. Stools that contain mucus and are the color of "currant jelly" are touted as the essential diagnostic indicator of intussusception; however, this symptom tends to occur late in the disease and after the involved segments of bowel experience edema and bleeding. The intussusceptum may be palpable in the upper abdomen as a sausage-shaped mass, but like a "palpable olive," a "palpable sausage" is also an unreliable sign.

Other causes of childhood vomiting are not age-specific. By far the most common cause of vomiting in any pediatric age group is viral gastroenteritis. However, new-onset diabetes that appears as vomiting and acidosis; toxic ingestion; duodenal hematoma or traumatic pancreatitis related to blunt abdominal trauma (classically a bicycle handlebar injury); Reye's syndrome, intercranial masses or trauma; and psychologic causes such as stress, anorexia, or bulimia must also be considered.

DIAGNOSTIC WORK-UP

Because vomiting is a physical sign rather than a disease entity, much of the diagnostic work-up in the vomiting patient is directed toward identifying the cause of vomiting. However, potential complications of vomiting may be present regardless of the underlying cause. These complications include dehydration, electrolyte abnormalities, and acid-base status changes. The following discussion focuses on the identification and treatment of these complications.

Dehydration occurs with vomiting as a result of the loss of sodium and water in the vomitus, which cannot be replaced orally. The response to volume depletion is controlled by the renin-angiotensin-aldosterone system, which promotes reabsorption of sodium in the kidney. However, hydrogen chloride is also lost in the vomitus, which results in metabolic alkalosis. Metabolic alkalosis induces further sodium loss in the kidney in the form of sodium bicarbonate. In an attempt to recover the lost sodium, the kidney exchanges potassium for sodium during reabsorption. Loss of potassium results in hypokalemia and further exacerbates the alkalosis as hydrogen ions shift intracellularly in exchange for the potassium moving into the extracellular space. The result of these ion fluxes is a hypokalemic, hypochloremic metabolic alkalosis.

Not all vomiting patients require a laboratory

or radiologic evaluation. Patients who give a history consistent with a benign cause for vomiting and who appear mildly dehydrated on the basis of appearance, vital signs, and physical examination may be best served by a limited work-up. However, in some situations a more complete approach is prudent. Patients at the extremes of age who give a limited history, who have a complex medical history, who have a severe underlying disease process, who return to the emergency department for continued symptoms, or who simply look ill should have a work-up to determine the cause and severity of complications related to vomiting.

Laboratory Evaluation

The metabolic complications of vomiting can be best determined by obtaining serum electrolytes, blood urea nitrogen (BUN), and creatinine. Other helpful adjuncts to these tests are urinalysis and arterial blood gases. The patient who is vomiting and dehydrated may exhibit some degree of hyponatremia, hypochloremia, hypokalemia, or alkalosis. Furthermore, the decrease in glomerular filtration rate with volume depletion causes the BUN: creatinine ratio to exceed its normal 10:1 value. A concentrated urine with an elevated specific gravity is expected on urinalysis, and arterial blood gases may reveal a partially compensated metabolic alkalosis with elevated or compensated pH and normal or elevated PCO_2.

In most cases, measurement of serum electrolytes is sufficient to determine the extent of metabolic derangement resulting from vomiting. However, at times the underlying cause of the vomiting may affect these measurements. For example, when vomiting occurs with ketoacidosis, lactic acidosis, or aspirin toxicity, the result is a mixed acid-base disorder. The measurement of serum bicarbonate in these states must be supplemented with arterial blood gases to determine the extent of the acid-base abnormality. Prolonged vomiting can also result in

varying degrees of starvation ketosis. In these situations, the urinalysis may provide added information with the presence of urine ketones.

Radiologic Evaluation

Vomiting patients in whom the examination is suggestive of peritonitis or bowel obstruction should undergo abdominal radiography. This evaluation is often performed as a three-view series, including a chest film and upright and supine abdominal films. The chest x-ray study provides visualization of the lungs and diaphragms, which is important to rule out intrathoracic diaphragmatic irritation and to examine for free intraperitoneal air that may be trapped beneath the diaphragm. Abdominal films reveal the patterns of gas and fluid and degree of bowel distension. Paucity of gas in an area of the abdomen may suggest a mass, such as an appendiceal or diverticular abscess. A localized area of distended bowel may signify local irritation such as in the "sentinel loop" of pancreatitis. In bowel obstruction, the level of obstruction may be determined by the location at which the air/fluid levels are no longer seen. A large, distended stomach is expected in gastric outlet obstruction, whereas a hugely distended bowel emanating from the right or left lower quadrant suggests cecal or sigmoid volvulus, respectively.

MANAGEMENT
ABCs

Patients with a diminished level of consciousness as a result of head injury, shock, metabolic derangement, or intoxication are at risk for aspirating the gastric contents into the lungs if they vomit. Therefore such patients should be maintained in a lateral decubitus position so that the vomitus is expelled from the oropharynx. Endotracheal intubation must be considered if the patient is at risk for loss of a patent airway or is unable to be turned because of cervical immobilization.

An evaluation of the vomiting patient's circulatory status using general appearance, orthostatic vital signs, and capillary refill time may be normal or may reveal hypovolemic shock. However, for all of these patients the key issue is maintenance or replacement of hydration in a graded approach depending on their symptomatology and the suspected cause.

Intravenous Rehydration

Patients who have been vomiting for several days and who are experiencing subjective or objective orthostasis benefit from intravenous (IV) fluid therapy. IV fluid is given in the form of normal saline to the dehydrated patient because both sodium and chloride are required by the body. The amount and rate of IV rehydration can be determined according to several clinical criteria. In the patient with normally functioning heart and kidneys, several liters of fluid can be given rapidly at a "wide-open" rate because the patient will not suffer from excess hydration. Endpoints in these patients include the ability to tolerate oral fluid, the production of a dilute urine, and the resolution of measured orthostasis.

Patients with a history of renal dysfunction or congestive heart failure should be hydrated gently because excess sodium and water may exacerbate pulmonary congestion. Fluid should be given slowly as 250 to 500 ml boluses to avoid overshooting the required amount of fluid. Sometimes in such patients it is best to opt for hospital admission to provide the time for slow and observed rehydration.

Rehydration in the pediatric patient is based on the extent of dehydration. Mildly dehydrated children who tolerate oral intake may be rehydrated with clear liquids. However, an infant's inability to tolerate normal formula for more than 24 to 48 hours should prompt reevaluation because of electrolyte and nutritional requirements that are not met by clear liquids. Further-more, infants should be orally rehydrated with a balanced electrolyte solution to avoid hyponatremia from excessive free water. Infants and children who are moderately to severely dehydrated must be given IV fluid. Rehydration should be initiated with a 20 ml/kg bolus of 5% dextrose in normal saline over 30 minutes and may be repeated as a 10 to 20 ml/kg bolus over 30 minutes. Often this treatment is enough to allow the child to begin tolerating oral fluid. However, continued vomiting or severe initial dehydration should prompt hospital admission with a formal calculation of fluid deficit and replacement.

Other Management Issues

Patients who have laboratory evidence of hypokalemia also need potassium supplementation. However, it should be remembered that patients can be eukalemic by laboratory examination and still have a total body depletion of potassium if their vomiting persists for a period of days. Patients with evidence of starvation ketosis or alcoholic ketoacidosis require IV glucose to halt the production of ketones. This treatment can be given at 5% dextrose in normal saline as long as the measured serum glucose level is within the normal range. Patients with hypoglycemia require larger boluses of 50% dextrose, whereas patients with diabetic ketoacidosis should not be given the added glucose until insulin and fluid therapy has reduced their serum glucose to <300 mg/dl.

Antiemetic Medications

Medications to alleviate or prevent nausea and emesis are available if the cause cannot be treated readily (Table 14-1).

Both the antihistamines and the anticholinergics are thought to decrease excitability of the vestibular nuclei and to have central dopamine receptor blocking action. The antihistamines dimenhydrinate (Dramamine), diphenhydramine

Table*14-1*

COMMON ANTIEMETIC USES, ROUTES OF ADMINISTRATION, AND DOSAGE

Generic Name	Trade Name	Uses	Route	Adult Dosage
Dimenhydrinate	Dramamine	Motion sickness Vestibular disorders	PO, IM, IV	50-100 mg q 4-6 hrs
Diphenhydramine	Benadryl	Same as above	PO, IM, IV	25-50 mg q 4-6 hrs
Hydroxyzine	Vistaril	Same as above	IM	25-100 mg
Trimethobenzamide	Tigan	General use	PO PR, IM	250 mg q 6-8 hrs 200 mg q 6-8 hrs
Meclizine	Antivert, Bonine	Motion sickness Vestibular disorders	PO	25-50 mg q day 25-100 mg q day, divided
Prochlorperazine	Compazine	General use except motion sickness and vestibular disorders	PO PR IM IV	5-10 mg q 6-8 hrs 25 mg q 12 hrs 5-10 mg q 3-4 hrs 2.5-10 mg q 3-4 hrs
Promethazine	Phenergan	General use Postoperative	PO, IM, IV	12.5-25 mg q 4 hrs
Metoclopramide	Reglan	Gastroparesis Gastroesophagel reflux Chemotherapy	PO, IM, IV IV	10 mg 30 min qAC and HS 2 mg/kg before chemotherapy and 2× q 2 hrs
Cisapride	Propulsid	Gastroparesis Gastroesophageal reflux	PO	10 mg 30 min qAC and HS
Ondansetron	Zofran	Chemotherapy	IV PO	32 mg IV before chemotherapy 8 mg q 8 hrs

Data from *Physicians Desk Reference '94, AHFS Drug Information '92*, and Propulsid product insert.

(Benadryl), hydroxyzine (Vistaril, Atarax), trimeth-obenzamide (Tigan), and meclizine (Antivert, Bo-nine) are particularly effective for alleviating nausea and emesis resulting from motion sick-ness, labyrinthitis, and Meniere disease. The primary side effect of the antihistamines is drowsiness. The anticholinergic scopolamine is also effective as a prophylactic antiemetic for mo-tion sickness, particularly when used as a trans-dermal patch. Anticholinergic side effects include a dry mouth, blurred vision, and drowsiness.

The phenothiazine and derivative antipsy-chotics also have antiemetic properties. They are thought to be effective in reducing afferent sig-nals from the gut to the vomiting center and also in decreasing dopaminergic transmission in the CTZ. For this reason, these medications are ef-fective for vomiting secondary to toxins and drugs such as opiates, anesthetics, and chemo-therapeutic agents, as well as radiation sickness and gastroenteritis. They are less effective for vestibular causes of vomiting. Drugs in this class include prochlorperazine (Compazine), chlor-promazine (Thorazine), droperidol (Inapsine), and promethazine (Phenergan). The side effects of these drugs include drowsiness, parkinson-ism, and extrapyramidal dystonia.

Metoclopramide (Reglan) is a dopamine an-tagonist that crosses the blood-brain barrier only minimally at therapeutic doses but still exerts antidopaminergic effects in the CTZ. It is also a powerful cholinergic agonist peripherally and therefore speeds gut motility and gastric empty-ing. It is an effective antiemetic except in vestibular causes of vomiting and is particularly useful as a prokinetic agent in gastroparesis of any cause. Side effects related to central dopamine blockade do occur with metoclo-pramide and include drowsiness, parkinsonism, extrapyramidal dystonia, anxiety, insomnia, and confusion.

Cisapride (Propulsid) is a prokinetic agent that has few, if any, central side effects. It func-tions peripherally as a procholinergic agent. Cisapride is effective in gastroparesis, gastro-esophageal reflux, small bowel dysmotility, and pseudoobstruction.

Finally, ondansetron (Zofran) is a serotonin antagonist that is effective in reducing vomiting that is related to chemotherapeutic agents and is unresponsive to other antiemetics. It has min-imal side effects such as headache, constipation or diarrhea, and transient elevation of liver enzymes.

Recommended Reading

Brizzee KR: *Mechanics of vomiting: a mini-review, Can J Physiol Pharmacol* 68:221-229, 1990.
Barsan WG, Wolf LR: Disorders of the upper gastrointesti-nal tract. In Rosen Pet al, editors: *Emergency medi-cine: concepts and clinical practice*, ed 3, St Louis, 1994, Mosby.
Carpenter DO: Neural mechanisms of vomiting, *Can J Physiol Pharmacol* 68:230-236, 1990.

Friedman LS, Isselbacher K: Anorexia, nausea, vomiting, and indigestion. In Isselbacher K et al, editors: *Harri-son's principles of internal medicine*, ed 13, New York, 1994, McGraw-Hill.
Fuchs S, Jaffe D: Vomiting, *Pediatr Emerg Care* 6(2): 164-170, 1990.
Silen W: *Cope's early diagnosis of the acute abdomen*, ed 15, New York, 1979, Oxford University Press.

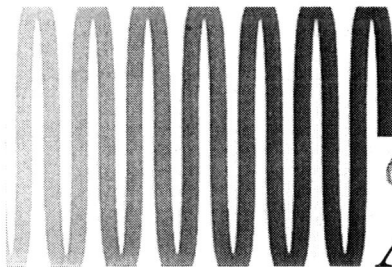

Chapter *Fifteen*
ACUTE INFECTIOUS DIARRHEAL DISEASE

ROBERT A. BITTERMAN

Acute infectious diarrheal disease represents a common entity in the emergency department and is associated with significant morbidity. It represents a common cause of dehydration that may require aggressive fluid resuscitation.

PATHOPHYSIOLOGY

As much as 9 liters of fluid enter the proximal bowel each day from diet and endogenous secretions. Normally 90% of this fluid is absorbed in the small bowel; the large bowel has additional reserve capacity. Water passively follows the osmotic gradients of electrolytes and other active substances such as sugars and amino acids. A bidirectional flux of electrolytes across the mucosa exists; the net water content of stool reflects osmotically active absorption and secretion of solutes. Glucose and certain amino acids are absorbed by active, carrier-mediated transport coupled to the sodium exchange.

Acute diarrheal disease may result from several mechanisms:

1. *Osmotic diarrhea.* Osmotically active substances create a gradient that leads to the movement of water and electrolytes into the lumen; hypertonic luminal fluid develops. Injury to the microvilli uncouple the sodium pump, decrease glucose absorption, and reduce the absorptive surface.

   Congenital or acquired carbohydrate transport deficits and the ingestion of nonabsorbable materials may be a cause of osmotic diarrhea.

   Stools are moderate in volume, have a reducing substance present (Clinitest positive, stool pH <6) and contain osmotically active, nonelectrolyte compounds. Improvement is noted with dietary restriction.

2. *Secretory diarrhea.* Pathologic activation of adenyl cyclase produces excessive luminal electrolytes. Sodium, chloride, and bicarbonate have diminished absorption.

   Vibrio cholerae, Escherichia coli enterotoxins, *Shigella* organisms, *Salmonella* organisms, *Clostridium difficile* organisms, and viral agents may be a cause of secretory diarrhea. Noninfectious causes include malabsorbed bile acids, prostaglandins found in chronic inflammatory disease or postinfection, and gastrointestinal hormones (calcitonin, vasoactive intestinal peptides).

   Large volume stools and a high electrolyte content are common. Diarrhea continues despite discontinuing oral intake.

3. *Motility excess.* Disrupted intestinal motility causes diarrhea. Increased motility may be

caused by osmotic or secretory diarrhea, exo-toxins, or drugs, whereas hypomotility allows for bacterial overgrowth, deconjugation of bile acids, and the short-circuiting of enterohepatic circulation resulting from neuromuscular disease, infection, or a shortened bowel.

Stool patterns and responses to dietary restrictions are variable.

ACUTE DIARRHEA: DIAGNOSTIC CONSIDERATIONS

Infection

Acute gastroenteritis
    Viral
    Bacterial
    Parasitic
Postinfectious malabsorption
Acute appendicitis/peritonitis
Extragastrointestinal
    Respiratory tract
    Urinary tract

Autoimmune

Ulcerative colitis
Regional enteritis (Crohn disease)
Gluten sensitivity (celiac)
Milk/food allergy

Intoxication

Anxiety/stress

Irritable bowel syndrome

Endocrine

Multiple endocrine adenoma
Hyperthyroidism

Neoplasm

Congenital

Hirschsprung disease
Intussusception
Cystic fibrosis

ETIOLOGIC AGENTS

Diarrheal disease is caused by a wide range of viral, bacterial, and parasitic agents, each with unique epidemiologic and clinical characteristics. Beyond infectious conditions, other considerations are required for the patient who has diarrhea or vomiting (see the boxes below).

Viral Agents

Viruses represent a leading cause of diarrheal illness in the United States. A number of agents have been incriminated. Parvovirus-like agents such as the Norwalk virus are primarily responsible for diarrheal disease in adults, whereas a human reovirus-like agent (or rotavirus) accounts for 10% to 80% of pediatric diarrheal disease during the winter and 20% during the summer.

ACUTE VOMITING AND DIARRHEA: DIAGNOSTIC EVALUATION

Chemistry
Electrolytes, blood urea nitrogen, glucose
Liver functions

Urinalysis

Complete blood count, platelets

Stool
Blood
Polymorphonuclear leukocytes
Culture
Ova and parasites

Vomitus
Blood
Bile
Undigested material

Manifestations

Following an incubation period of 2 to 3 days, patients develop an abrupt onset of watery diarrhea (which potentially leads to dehydration), vomiting, a low-grade fever, and minimal or no abdominal pain. Vomiting may be prominent, and diarrhea may persist for 4 to 7 days.

Management

Treatment for viral diarrheal disease involves fluid support and stabilization.

Bacterial Agents

A variety of agents cause an invasive pattern of gastroenteritis, which is accompanied by systemic illness and evidence of mucosal involve-

ment as noted by stool polymorphonuclear (PMN) cells on Gram stain and a mucousy, bloody appearance (Table 15-1). Enterotoxin-producing organisms can also be causative. The stool culture is diagnostic. Treatment is supportive, and antibiotic therapy is indicated as discussed later in this chapter.

Shigella organisms

Shigella flexneri is a common pathogen and partially reflects poor hygiene or sanitation problems. Person-to-person contact is common, but contaminated food may also be involved. Only a small inoculum is required.

Manifestations. A rapid onset of high fever, crampy abdominal pain, and diarrhea, are common after an incubation period of 24 to 72 hours. Vomiting is rare. Some cases progress to

Table *15-1*

EPIDEMIOLOGIC ASPECTS OF INVASIVE BACTERIAL GASTROENTERITIS

Organism	Source	Incubation Period	Features	Duration
Shigella	Person-to-person, fecal-oral	24-48 hours	Confined populations; poor personal hygiene and sanitation	4-7 days
Salmonella	Poultry, eggs, water, and domestic pets	8-24 hours	Family and cafeteria-type outbreaks common	2-5 days
Campylobacter fetus	Poultry, wild birds, water	2-5 days	High relapse rate; summer months; cases sporadic	5-14 days
Yersinia enterocolitica	Food or drink and person-to-person	12-48 hours (?)	Appendicitis; mesenteric adenitis-like syndromes; winter months	10-14 days
Vibrio parahaemolyticus	Seafood, especially shellfish	8-24 hours	High attack rates; summer months	24-48 hours

dysentery, with crampy lower abdominal pain, urgency, and tenesmus. Stool is profuse and often contains blood, mucus, and PMN leukocytes. Meningismus, respiratory symptoms, and significant fluid losses may occur. Febrile seizures (see Chapter 66) may occur early in children and often precede the onset of diarrhea. A carrier is unusual.

Cultures are usually diagnostic. The peripheral white blood cell count is variable and is usually accompanied by a shift to the left.

Management. Although the illness is self-limiting and lasts 3 to 7 days, treatment rapidly shortens the illness and reduces relapses and shedding. Oral ciprofloxacin in patients over 12 years old or trimethoprim-sulfamethoxazole (TMP-SMX) are effective medications. *Shigella* organisms are commonly resistant to ampicillin or amoxicillin.

Salmonella organisms

Person-to-person contamination and exposure to infected vehicles are common sources of salmonella transmission. Cattle, domestic animals, poultry, rodents, and egg products have been incriminated. Large turkeys cooked for holiday dinners are a common source of Salmonella infections. A large inoculum is required.

Manifestations. Fever, vomiting, and diarrhea develop 24 to 48 hours after exposure. Crampy abdominal pain, tenesmus, and urgency may also be present. Stools vary from mildly abnormal to profuse, green, slimy, and foul smelling. Stool PMN leukocytes are present. Meningitis, osteomyelitis, arthritis, pneumonia, and pyelonephritis have been reported. Septicemia may occur in children under 1 year of age and in those with sickle cell disease, hemoglobinopathies, and immunodeficiencies. A carrier state is common.

Salmonella typhi causes severe disease with high fever, diarrhea, malaise, headache, myalgia, hepatosplenomegaly, and rose spots (maculopapular erythematous 2 mm lesions on the upper abdomen).

Stool cultures are positive. The peripheral white blood cell count is elevated with a shift to the left.

Management. Patients who are ill when the diagnosis is made should be treated with antibiotics. Ciprofloxacin 500 mg bid × 5 to 7 days is the drug of choice for those over 12 years of age, but it cannot be used in children and during pregnancy. Trimethoprim-sulfamethoxizole (TMP-SMX 160mg/800mg) bid is a good alternate choice.

Campylobacter fetus

Campylobacter fetus is a gram-negative bacteria and has a primary reservoir in chickens, wild birds such as pigeons and sparrows, and domestic animals such as dogs; it can also be found in waterborne sources. Young children have a higher incidence, with an increased occurrence in summer months. The incubation period is 2 to 5 days.

Manifestations. With *Campylobacter fetus*, a rapid onset of fever, crampy abdominal pain, and diarrhea occur. Constitutional symptoms of anorexia, malaise, and arthralgia may precede the onset of diarrhea by 24 to 48 hours. Stools are typically loose and bile colored and often progress to being watery, grossly bloody, or melenic. Diarrhea may persist beyond a week. One fourth of all untreated patients suffer a relapse.

Stools demonstrate PMN cells and erythrocytes on microscopic examination and may be cultured on selective antibiotic-containing media.

Management. Supportive fluid management is essential. Erythromycin produces a rapid clinical and bacteriologic cure at a dosage of 250 mg four times daily by mouth for adults or 12.5 mg/kg every 6 hours by mouth for children (maximum of 250 mg qid). Ciprofloxacin 500 mg bid × 5 to 7 days is also effective for adults.

Yersinia enterocolitica

Increasingly recognized as a human pathogen, *Yersinia enterocolitica* may be transmitted person-to-person or through contaminated food.

Manifestations. Fever, colicky abdominal pain, and constitutional symptoms are common manifestations of *Yersinia enterocolitica.* Stools are usually watery, green, and bloody. A terminal ileitis or mesenteric adenitis that mimics appendicitis or Crohn disease may develop.

Stool examination reveals fecal leukocytes and blood. Cultures are positive but require special techniques and prolonged growth times.

Management. For infection with *Yersinia enterocolitica,* no specific treatment beyond support is indicated.

Enterotoxin-induced

Acute diarrheal disease is commonly associated with the introduction of toxins through ingestion of contaminated food. There is usually a rapid onset of explosive symptoms. A somewhat

Table **15-2**

EPIDEMIOLOGIC ASPECTS OF BACTERIAL TOXIN–INDUCED GASTROENTERITIS

Preformed Toxins				
Staphylococcal	Food-handler–related; potato salad, ham, eggs, mayonnaise, confectionaries	1-6 hours	Very high attack rates; large outbreaks	6-10 hours
Bacillus cereus				
Emetic toxin	Fried rice	2-4 hours	High attack rate; almost always fried rice	<10 hours
Diarrheal toxin	Meats, vegetables, especially gravies	6-14 hours	Food reheated or sitting out for long periods	24-36 hours
Scombroid	Tuna, mackerel, dolphin fish	5-60 minutes	Peppery or bitter taste; histamine intoxication; high attack rate	<6 hours
Toxins Produced After Colonization				
Clostridium perfringens	Meat, poultry, gravies, "steam table" meats	6-24 hours	Food reheated or sitting out for long periods	<24 hours
Vibrio organisms	Seafood, especially raw shellfish	24-48 hours	Summer months; dehydration common	6-8 days
Escherichia coli	Usually unsanitary drinking water	24-72 hours	Travelers; dehydration common in children	1-7 days
Clostridium difficile	Overgrowth of normal flora	Unknown	Antibiotic therapy; invasive colitis	Variable

more prolonged incubation period is associated with those toxins that are produced after introducing the organism into the gut (Table 15-2). Symptomatic support is indicated.

Enterohemorrhagic Escherichia coli 0157:H7

E. coli serotype 0157:H7 is an important and common cause of bloody diarrhea. Children, particularly those in day-care-centers, and the elderly, particularly those in nursing homes, are most often affected. The organism is transmitted through undercooked beef, especially hamburger, raw milk, apple cider, contaminated water, and via person-to-person contact.

Manifestations. After an incubation period of approximately 4 to 9 days, the patient experiences watery diarrhea followed by bloody diarrhea in the vast majority of cases. The diarrhea is typically accompanied by severe abdominal cramps, pain, and tenderness. In the elderly, this condition is often misdiagnosed as ischemic colitis. Hemolytic-uremic syndrome, primarily in children, and thrombotic thrombocytopenic purpura are two serious complications of *E. coli* 0157:H7. The mortality rate in elderly patients is as high as 30%.

Management. Diagnosis of *E. coli* infection requires culturing the stool on special growth media. The laboratory must be told to specifically look for the 0157:H7 organism. Treatment is supportive; antibiotics have not yet been proven effective. The public health department should be informed of the infection to prevent large outbreaks from occurring by the food-borne route.

Protozoan Agents

Giardia lamblia

A flagellated protozoan, *Giardia lamblia* is transmitted by the fecal-oral route and is a common cause of waterborne outbreaks of diarrhea. It is common for the patient to have a history of camping, travel, exposure to stream or well water, or poor hygiene. Giardiasis should be considered in homosexuals with diarrhea or in children with diarrhea who attend day-care centers. Incubation periods are noted to be 1 to 3 weeks.

Manifestations. Diffuse abdominal pain is associated with distension, colic, and flatulence. Explosive, foul-smelling pale stools are common. Symptoms may persist, which produces a malabsorption syndrome.

Cysts may be identified in the feces, or trophozoites may be found in the duodenal secretions, stool, or on jejunal biopsy.

Management. Metronidazole (Flagyl), 250 mg every 8 hours for 5 to 7 days is curative (children: 5 mg/kg tid for 5 to 7 days). Furazolidone is available as a suspension and is also curative in a dosage of 100 mg qid × 5 to 7 days (children: 1.5 mg/kg qid for 7 to 10 days). Patient contacts should be examined.

Cryptosporidium organisms

The *Cryptosporidium* organism is an intestinal protozoan parasite and is most often seen in persons who handle animals, in children in day-care centers, in healthy male homosexuals, and in immunocompromised patients. It is also occasionally a cause of large waterborne diarrheal outbreaks. Cryptosporidiosis is the most common cause of diarrhea in persons with AIDS.

Manifestations. After approximately a 1 week incubation period, profuse watery diarrhea develops and may persist for 1 to 2 weeks. In immunocompromised patients, especially patients with AIDS, the diarrhea may persist indefinitely.

Management. Treatment is supportive. No effective antibiotic treatment is available.

Other Agents

A host of other agents, including *Entamoeba histolytica* should also be considered. For more information, read Bitterman (1992).

ASSESSMENT

After quickly assessing the airway and breathing in the patient who has acute infectious diarrhea and vomiting, stabilize the patient's hemodynamic status. Orthostatic vital signs are helpful in the patient who is not already showing signs of volume depletion. Dehydration is common and requires rapid initiation of support and parenteral fluid administration to correct the deficits.

History

The history should focus on the nature of the acute onset of gastrointestinal signs and symptoms and on any previous similar episode. Determine the onset, progression, and response to alterations in diet. Check for associated abdominal pain, bloating, and tenesmus. Clarify the patient's stool pattern with respect to frequency, appearance (mucus, blood, water loss) and consistency. If vomiting is present, aspects that need focus include color, composition, appearance (blood, bile, digested/undigested food), odor, relationship to eating and position, and whether it is projectile. Explore any previous episodes of diarrhea and vomiting in great detail. Identify exposure, drug ingestion, travel, family incidence, sexual history, and trauma. Discuss previous episodes in detail with the patient. Look for associated findings such as dizziness, weakness, and evidence of hemodynamic instability. Note associated headaches, arthritis/arthralgia, fever, changes in mentation, and seizures.

Physical Examination

The physical examination should obviously define hemodynamic instability, which includes obtaining orthostatic vital signs. Carefully examine the abdomen for tenderness, masses, guarding, rebound, and other abnormalities. Perform a rectal examination to determine the presence of blood, tenderness, fissures, and perianal findings. Consider other contributing conditions, including neurologic disease and respiratory or urinary tract infections (see the box on p. 171).

Diagnostic Work-up

The diagnostic work-up may include initial evaluation of hydration by assessment of blood urea nitrogen (BUN), electrolytes, and glucose. Mild or moderate cases can be safely managed without obtaining any laboratory data. In the patient with normal renal function, the urinalysis, and especially urine specific gravity, may be a useful parameter. A complete blood count (CBC) reflects potential infectious origins.

Specifically examine the stool to determine the presence of stool PMN leukocytes, rotavirus, and ova and parasites; obtain a stool specimen for culture in patients with clinically infectious diarrhea (Fig. 15-1). The presence of multiple PMN leukocytes is associated with shigella or salmonella infections. Examination of vomitus for blood, bile, and undigested material is appropriate. Perform additional studies for liver function, ketones, and specific underlying conditions as indicated.

MANAGEMENT

Treatment should primarily focus on support and rehydration, as discussed in Chapters 5 and 66. After initial stabilization, correction of fluid deficits is imperative. Often the patient with even minimal or no orthostatic changes will benefit from intravenous infusion of a fluid bolus before undertaking oral intake. Patients who do not require circulatory support benefit from either a period of restriction of oral intake or from a significant dietary alteration. Patients often respond rapidly to bowel rest and then may be slowly advanced. Patients with diarrhea should have clear liquid dietary restrictions, whereas those with vomiting should have small sips of clear liquids. Further additions should reflect the initial response.

Empiric antibiotic treatment is indicated in patients who have diarrhea that appears to be infectious in origin; patients with fever, significant abdominal pain and tenderness, or constitutional symptoms; or those who appear toxic. A fecal smear wet mount that is stained with methylene blue and contains numerous PMNs helps confirm the need for such empiric treatment. The empiric drug of choice for adults is ciprofloxacin 500 mg bid or norfloxacin 400 mg bid, generally for 3 to 7 days. TMP-SMX 160mg/800mg bid is another choice. Ampicillin or the cephalosporins are poor choices because of the high frequency of resistance found in the usual enteric pathogens. Antibiotics are *not* indicated empirically in the management of patients with diarrhea that appears viral or toxigenic in origin or in patients with watery diarrhea and no fever, chills, significant pain, or systemic symptoms.

Antidiarrheal agents such as loperamide (Imodium) or diphenoxylate with atropine (Lomotil) should generally not be used in patients with infectious diarrhea. Such agents may increase the incidence of bacteremia, prolong the illness, or prolong a carrier state. The judicious use of antidiarrheals in patients with viral or toxigenic-appearing diarrhea is usually beneficial.

Education and strict adherence to diet are essential. Secondary spread can be reduced by good handwashing and by identifying the source of the infection.

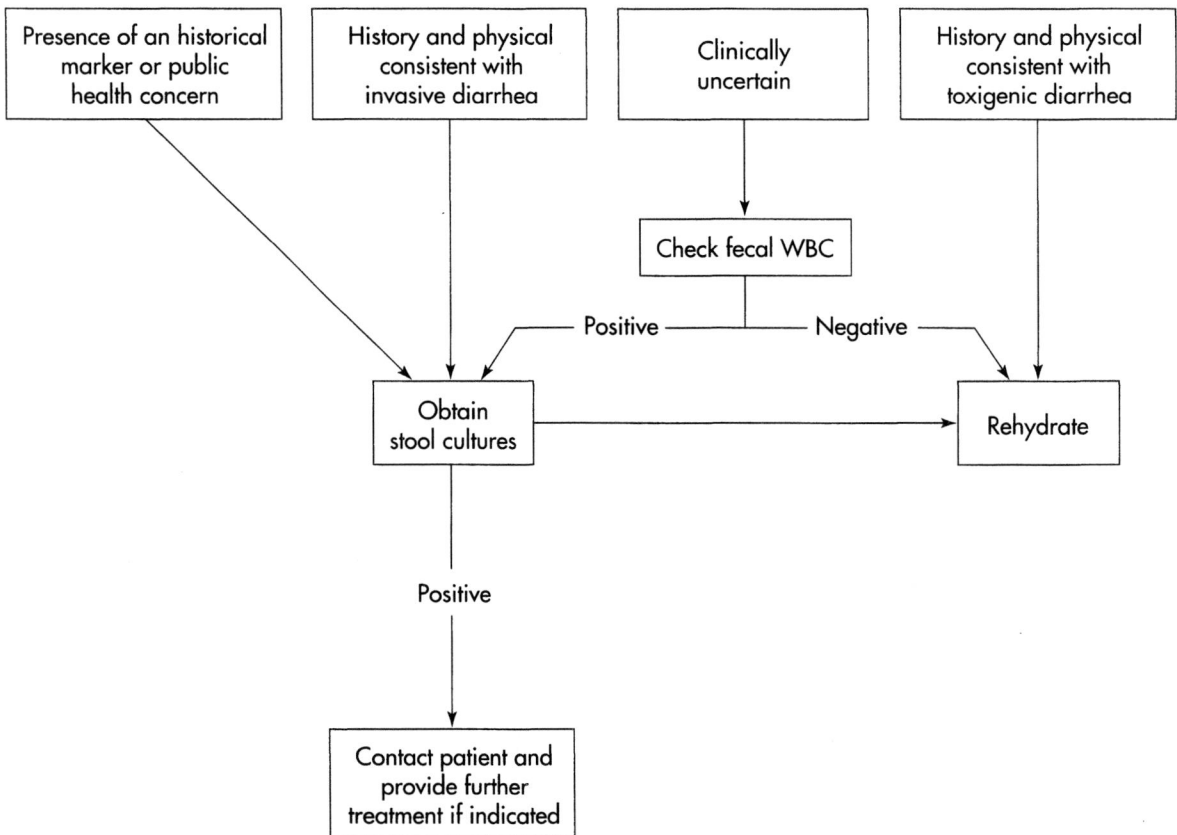

Fig. 15-1. Approach to use of fecal WBC test and stool culture to evaluate acute diarrhea. (From Bitterman RA: Acute gastroenteritis and constipation. In Rosen P et al, editors: *Emergency medicine: concepts and clinical practice,* ed 3, St Louis, 1992, Mosby.)

Recommended Reading

Bitterman RA: Approach to the patient with acute diarrhea, food poisoning, the patient with AIDS and diarrhea, and constipation. In Rosen P et al, editors: *Emergency medicine: concepts and clinical practice,* ed 3, St Louis, 1992, Mosby.

Foremark CE: AIDS and the gastrointestinal tract, *Postgrad Med* 93:143, 1993.

Giannella RA: Acute infectious diarrhea, *Gastroenterol Clin North Am* 22(3):483, 1993.

Guerrant RL, Bobak DA: Bacterial and protozoal gastroenteritis, *New Engl J Med* 325:327, 1991.

MacDonald KL, Osterholm MT: The emergence of *Escherichial coli* 0157:H7 infection in the US: the changing epidemiology of foodborne disease (editorial), *JAMA* 269:2264, 1993.

Taylor MB: *Gastrointestinal emergencies,* Baltimore, 1992, Williams & Wilkins.

Chapter *Sixteen*
PELVIC PAIN, VAGINAL BLEEDING, AND GENITAL INFECTION

GARY P. YOUNG

PELVIC PAIN

Pelvic pain has many causes. Some of the more common causes are listed in the box on p. 175. *Poorly localized visceral pain* may be caused by distension of a hollow viscus (e.g., the fallopian tube), distension of the capsule of a solid organ, or stretching of pelvic ligaments or adhesions. Irritation of the parietal peritoneum by an inflamed organ, blood, or purulent fluid may cause *well-localized pain,* but *more generalized pain* may be produced by the presence of large amounts of blood (such as is caused by the rupture of an ectopic pregnancy). The *sudden onset of pain* may be caused by acute ischemia (as produced by adnexal torsion) or by acute hemorrhage with peritoneal irritation. A more *gradual onset of pain* suggests evolving inflammation.

Genital Infection

A genital infection is the most common cause of pelvic pain encountered in emergency practice. Types of genital infection are discussed later in this chapter.

Adnexal Torsion

Torsion of a fallopian tube or ovary around its vascular pedicle almost always involves an adnexal (i.e., ovarian or fallopian tube) abnormality. Both *intrinsic* processes (e.g., ovarian cyst or tumor, pyosalpinx, hydrosalpinx, hematosalpinx, or tubal pregnancy) and *extrinsic* processes (e.g., pelvic adhesions, previous tubal ligation, masses, trauma) are precursors to torsion. Classically, the onset is a sudden, sharp, unilateral pain, but it may also be a dull ache with sharp exacerbations. The pain usually becomes increasingly severe but may subside by the time of presentation. Patients may give a past history of similar episodes, which indicates spontaneous detorsion. The occurrence of other signs or symptoms, including nausea and vomiting, urinary tract symptoms, and abnormal vaginal bleeding or amenorrhea, may confuse the clinical picture. The patient is usually afebrile, but a low-grade fever may be present. Tachycardia is commonly out of proportion to the degree of temperature elevation. Physical findings vary from slight unilateral lower abdominal tenderness to those reflecting frank peritonitis. Most

COMMON CAUSES OF PELVIC PAIN

Adhesions
Adnexal torsion
Dysmenorrhea
Endometriosis
Gastrointestinal-related
Genital infections
Ovarian cyst
Pregnancy-related
    Abortion
    Abruption
    Ectopic pregnancy
    Placenta
    Preeclampsia
    Premature labor
Sexual abuse
Tumors or masses
Urinary tract–related
Uterine leiomyoma
Uterine perforation
Vaginal foreign body
Vulvovaginitis

patients exhibit cervical motion and unilateral adnexal tenderness. In some patients the adnexal tenderness is bilateral. The emergency physician may find a tender, movable adnexal mass, but the ability to palpate such a mass is often hindered by abdominal guarding or patient discomfort.

Ultrasonography should reveal evidence of torsion and may reveal the predisposing pathologic condition. A culdocentesis is usually negative but may yield serosanguinous fluid. A diagnostic laparoscopy will establish the diagnosis, and a laparotomy is necessary if torsion exists. The consequences of a missed or late diagnosis may include scarring of the fallopian tube, necrosis of the ovary, peritonitis, and shock.

Ovarian Cyst

Enlargement of an ovarian cyst or neoplasm may produce pelvic pain by stretching supporting ligaments or by compressing contiguous pelvic organs. Functional ovarian cysts are nearly always asymptomatic until complicated by torsion, rupture, hemorrhage, or infection. Two types of such cysts occur with each menstrual cycle: follicular during the first 2 weeks and corpus luteum during the last 2 weeks. The corpus luteum of pregnancy persists to secrete progesterone for the first month of pregnancy. Ovarian cysts may also represent endometriosis, a benign dermoid cyst, or a malignant tumor.

The *rupture of an ovarian cyst* is often associated with exercise or sexual intercourse, and the patient usually experiences sudden, sharp, well-defined, unilateral pelvic pain. The duration and severity of the pain depend on the contents of the cyst. The pain usually resolves spontaneously when a functional serous cyst ruptures. However, when an endometrioma or dermoid cyst ruptures, severe prolonged pelvic pain occurs as a result of chemical peritonitis (see the section on endometriosis). Therefore the patient with a ruptured functional cyst usually requires only observation and reassurance unless significant ovarian hemorrhage occurs, but a ruptured endometrioma or a dermoid cyst requires a laparotomy for peritoneal cleansing.

The rupture of a *follicular cyst* with extrusion of the ovum occurs in midcycle and may be accompanied by slight bleeding from the ovarian surface. Up to one fourth of all ovulating women experience the resulting unilateral pain, which is known as mittelschmerz. Although there is usually no vaginal bleeding, some spotting may occur. The patient with a rupture of a *corpus luteum cyst* exhibits the same clinical picture except that the rupture occurs *just before* the menses. The physician may need to differentiate between a ruptured *corpus luteum cyst* of pregnancy and a ruptured ectopic pregnancy, both of which may require emergent laparotomy to prevent or treat hemorrhagic shock.

An *ovarian hemorrhage* can be either intra-ovarian or extraovarian. Hemorrhage into a cyst distends the ovarian capsule and causes sudden, sharp, and usually unilateral pelvic pain. Bleeding subsequent to rupture of the ovarian capsule causes hemoperitoneum and produces irritation of the peritoneum as evidenced by abdominal tenderness and guarding, which may be localized or diffuse. Hemorrhagic shock may develop depending on the size of the ovarian vessel torn during rupture.

Ultrasonography is the diagnostic study of choice in stable patients, either in the emergency department or in follow-up. In unstable patients, culdocentesis is more appropriate in diagnosing an intraperitoneal hemorrhage. A gynecologist may choose to perform a laparoscopy or immediate laparotomy to achieve hemorrhage control.

The overwhelming majority of small (less than 5 cm) ovarian masses that enlarge before ovulation or menstruation are benign. However, refer any woman with an adnexal mass that is thought to be a cyst to a gynecologist for reassessment at the end of menstruation, when hormonal stimulation is at a minimum. Because the ovaries are not normally palpable in premenarchal girls or in postmenopausal women, refer such patients with a palpable adnexal mass to a gynecologist for evaluation of a possible malignancy.

Endometriosis

Endometriosis is a syndrome produced by the growth of endometrial tissue outside the uterus. Such tissue is thought to arise from embryonic cell-rests or to be the result of retrograde regurgitation of endometrial fragments through the fallopian tubes. Implants (termed *endometriomas* or *chocolate cysts*) usually occur on the ovaries, in the posterior cul-de-sac, or on the uterosacral ligaments. In more advanced disease, the fallopian tubes, round ligaments, bladder, and intestines may also be involved.

Ectopic endometrial tissue responds to hormonal stimulation. During the latter half of the menstrual cycle, progressive pelvic aching may occur as the endometrial tissue proliferates; however, most patients complain of symptoms coinciding with menstrual flow. The pain is usually deep, constant, and bilateral. Patients may also experience dyspareunia, tenesmus, dysuria, or hematuria. Endometriomas can rupture early in pregnancy, and the clinical picture may resemble a ruptured ectopic pregnancy.

Sensitive nodules that are palpable in the cul-de-sac or adnexal areas suggest the diagnosis. However, many patients have nonspecific findings on pelvic examination. Diagnosis requires direct visualization and biopsy of ectopic endometrium during laparoscopy.

Uterine Leiomyoma

Uterine leiomyomata (*fibroids*) are the most common gynecologic neoplasms. These benign tumors are especially common in black women over the age of 30. High estrogen levels during the latter half of pregnancy and the postpartum period stimulate fibroid growth. Fibroids rarely undergo malignant transformation.

Fibroids may be asymptomatic or may cause dysmenorrhea, altered menstrual bleeding, pain, and pressure discomfort. They may be associated with menorrhagia but cause little change in menstrual timing. Ischemic necrosis can occur if fibroids outgrow their blood supply or if pedunculated fibroids twist on their vascular stalks; both conditions can cause severe lower abdominal cramps. A submucous fibroid or fibroid polyp may prolapse or even abort. Finally, large fibroids may produce urinary frequency, constipation, or neuropathy as a consequence of pressure applied to nerve roots or abdominal organs.

Pelvic examination reveals a large, sometimes tender uterus with distinct, firm nodules that disrupt the normal uterine contour. A negative pregnancy test should be followed up by an outpatient ultrasonography. Dilatation and curettage is necessary to rule out endometrial carcinoma.

Dysmenorrhea

Dysmenorrhea occurs at some time in nearly all women. Primary or idiopathic dysmenorrhea is defined by the absence of pelvic pathology. Secondary or acquired dysmenorrhea is the result of an underlying pelvic pathology. The patient usually describes a lower abdominal cramp or ache that may radiate to the back or thighs. The pain is often most intense on the first menstrual day and lasts from hours to days. Dysmenorrhea is often accompanied by increased menstrual flow or clotting. Associated symptoms may include nausea, vomiting, diarrhea, headache, fatigue, irritability, dizziness, or syncope. The physical examination is unremarkable if there is no underlying cause such as pelvic adhesions, endometriosis, inflammatory or infectious processes, intrauterine devices, congenital anomalies, ovarian cysts, fibroids, or other tumors or masses.

Treat moderate to severe dysmenorrhea with nonsteroidal antiinflammatory agents, such as ibuprofen, 600 to 800 mg po tid/qid, or naproxen, 550 mg at the start of menses followed by 275 mg po qid as needed.

Prepubertal Pelvic Pain

Sexual abuse and *vaginal foreign bodies* are the two most common causes of pelvic pain in the prepubertal girl. Although it varies with jurisdiction, the contact agency for sexual abuse is usually the police or child protective services.

A vaginal foreign body may cause pain accompanied by persistent malodorous or bloody discharge. The pain may occur primarily or exclusively with urination or defecation.

Other local disorders that cause pelvic pain in premenarchal girls include vulvovaginitis, cystitis, perineal and vulvar dermatitis, vaginal outlet obstruction, urethral prolapse, polyps, and neoplasms.

Pelvic Pain During Pregnancy

Pelvic pain during pregnancy may result from several causes. An *ectopic pregnancy* is the most important differential diagnosis to consider (see Chapter 45). Rupture of a corpus luteum cyst during early pregnancy can mimic the rupture of an ectopic pregnancy. Common causes of pelvic pain during pregnancy include the compression of intraabdominal structures and traction on the pelvic ligaments by the enlarging uterus.

Pelvic inflammatory disease is extremely unusual during pregnancy and therefore is not high on the differential list for the pregnant patient with pelvic pain. The emergency physician should consider appendicitis and pyelonephritis, which are both common during pregnancy, as nongenital causes of abdominal pain (see Chapter 45 for other complications of pregnancy).

Postmenopausal Pelvic Pain

Painful vaginal conditions are common in postmenopausal women. Decreased levels of circulating estrogens cause *atrophic vaginitis*, which results in dyspareunia and pruritus vulvae. Topical estrogen cream or vaginal suppositories and improved local hygiene are the initial treatments for these symptoms. Chronic hormonal replacement may also be indicated. Other common benign conditions that cause pelvic pain and postmenopausal bleeding are cervical polyps, uterine fibroids, and endometrial hyperplasia.

Pelvic examination of elderly patients with pain should include having the patient perform a Valsalva maneuver to observe for vaginal or uterine prolapse, cystourethrocele, and rectocele. A bimanual examination may be useful for detecting an endometrial or ovarian malignancy.

VAGINAL BLEEDING

The most common cause of vaginal bleeding is menstruation, which is a normal physiologic function. The physician should suspect as abnormal any vaginal bleeding that differs in interval or flow from that which is typical for the patient. The significance of abnormal vaginal bleeding varies according to the age of the patient. Functional bleeding is more common in younger women, whereas the physician should suspect malignancy in older women. During the reproductive years, the possibility of pregnancy and pregnancy-related disorders is always foremost.

Normal Menstrual Bleeding

The *cyclic* interval between menstrual periods varies between individuals but is fairly consistent for each individual. A cycle length of 18 to 40 days is within the normal range, with variations of as many as 5 days from the patient's normal pattern considered as normal.

The *duration* of menstrual flow ranges from 3 to 7 days and is fairly consistent for each woman. The amount of blood lost with each menstrual period varies widely among women and usually ranges from 25 to 60 ml. The average tampon or pad absorbs as much as 20 to 30 ml of blood when fully soaked. Therefore the number of tampons or pads used can help estimate the amount of blood lost. However, because habits of tampon or pad use vary widely among women, such comparisons may not be accurate.

Menstrual blood usually does not clot. *Clotting* typically occurs only with heavy uterine bleeding in which the blood does not remain in the uterine cavity long enough to undergo fibrinolysis. The presence of clotted menstrual discharge suggests brisk bleeding.

Cramping during menses is a phenomenon that occurs in nearly all women. The extent of discomfort varies widely among women but is relatively consistent for each individual. Signifi-

cant deviations from the norm may indicate a pathologic process.

Abnormal Vaginal Bleeding

Assessment

The patient with abnormal vaginal bleeding should be assessed like a patient with abnormal bleeding from any source. Abnormal vital signs, profuse bleeding, or other signs of hypovolemia indicate the need for resuscitation following the guidelines in Chapter 5.

In addition to a general physical examination (with special attention to the medical conditions that may produce abnormal bleeding), the patient with abnormal vaginal bleeding needs a thorough pelvic examination and a rectovaginal examination. Patients with bleeding in late pregnancy are an exception and should not undergo a bimanual examination. The external genitalia, vagina, and cervix should be inspected; the uterus and adnexa, including both ovaries, should be palpated.

Diagnostic aids

A stat hemoglobin and hematocrit are essential if bleeding is heavy and routine if serving only as a baseline. A serum quantitative or a qualitative urinary pregnancy test should also be obtained before the patient's discharge from the emergency department.

Pelvic ultrasonography has assumed a preeminent role in gynecologic diagnosis. It is useful in the diagnosis of ectopic pregnancy and in the delineation of pelvic masses (see Chapter 45). *Culdocentesis* may establish the presence of hemoperitoneum caused by an ectopic pregnancy or the rupture of an ovarian cyst.

Bleeding associated with organic pelvic disease

Tumors of the genital tract, including uterine leiomyomata, are a common cause of abnormal vaginal bleeding. The most common primary tumors are those of the cervix, uterus, and ovary.

Cervical polyps. Cervical polyps may cause vaginal bleeding that is characteristically light and intermenstrual (*metrorrhagia*). Coitus may provoke bleeding from cervical polyps. Polyps are generally small, red, pedunculated tumors that protrude from the cervical canal. These lesions rarely become malignant. Polyps are diagnosed by direct visualization during the speculum examination. The patient should be referred to a gynecologist for follow-up care.

Cervical carcinoma. Cervical carcinoma is a significant cause of abnormal vaginal bleeding by virtue of its frequency. Early treatment has the best chance for cure. It may be difficult to distinguish cervical carcinoma from infectious, erosive lesions of the cervix. All women of reproductive age should be reminded about the need for Pap smears. Patients suspected of having cervical carcinoma need a follow-up gynecologic evaluation for colposcopy.

Uterine carcinoma. Endometrial carcinoma occurs most often in the perimenopausal patient, but approximately one fourth of all cases develop during the reproductive years. All patients who have postmenopausal bleeding should be suspected of having endometrial carcinoma. These patients need urgent referral to a gynecologist.

Ovarian causes of vaginal bleeding. Ovarian lesions are common causes of menstrual abnormalities because of abnormal endocrine activity. Hormonal secretion may result in endometrial hyperplasia or anovulatory cycles that produce irregular (*metrorrhagia*) or increased (*menorrhagia*) vaginal bleeding. Associated symptoms may include pelvic pain or pressure sensation (see the section on pelvic pain). Ovarian tumors or cysts are also at risk for torsion (see the section on pelvic pain).

Trauma

Abnormal vaginal bleeding caused by trauma is less common than the nontraumatic causes. A common mechanism of perineal trauma is a straddle injury. The patient may also sustain injury from coital activity and sexual assault. The highest incidence of genital trauma occurs in the mother during childbirth.

Genital infection

Certain genital infections (see the section on genital infections later in this chapter) may be a cause of abnormal vaginal bleeding.

Dysfunctional uterine bleeding

Dysfunctional uterine bleeding (DUB) is a common form of abnormal vaginal bleeding. It generally results from hormonal imbalance.

The most common cause of abnormal vaginal bleeding not related to pregnancy relates to the use of *oral contraceptives*. Breakthrough bleeding often results from endometrial hyperplasia or from withdrawal bleeding, which is the consequence of noncompliant usage. For those patients with breakthrough bleeding, doubling the normal daily contraceptive dosage on a short-term basis sometimes is helpful. A pregnancy test should be performed before initiating such therapy. Patients should consult a gynecologist for long-term regulation therapy. They also need to be reminded that noncompliance with contraception places them at risk of pregnancy.

DUB not caused by oral contraceptives is related to abnormal endogenous hormone production and can be classified as either ovulatory or anovulatory. *Ovulatory* DUB is related to abnormal levels of circulating progesterone or estrogen or to a poor secretory response of the endometrium to normal circulating hormonal levels.

The most common cause of true DUB is an *anovulatory* cycle. Continued stimulation of the endometrium by unopposed estrogen following a failure to ovulate produces endometrial hyperplasia. The patient typically has several months of amenorrhea followed by frequent episodes of bleeding or a single bout of profuse bleeding.

The management of DUB consists of reducing the bleeding and treating the underlying cause. If the patient is stable and the hematocrit is within normal limits, 100 mg progesterone in oil can be administered IM. The progesterone stabilizes the endometrium and produces a cessation of bleeding. Withdrawal bleeding ensues several days later. Another therapeutic option is to place the patient on double- or triple-dose contraceptive therapy for 1 week. The estrogen builds up the endometrium, the progesterone stabilizes the endometrium, and withdrawal bleeding ensues. These patients require follow-up. If the patient is significantly anemic or hemodynamically unstable, intravenous fluids should be administered with blood transfusion as necessary. Conjugated estrogen 20 mg IV causes vasospasm of the uterine arterial vasculature and initiates coagulation-related functions. These patients should be hospitalized for dilatation and curettage and tissue specimen analysis.

Medical illness

Numerous medical diseases have been implicated as causes of abnormal vaginal bleeding, including coagulopathies, thrombocytopenia, cirrhosis, and anticoagulant therapy.

GENITAL INFECTION

Herpes Simplex Infection

A primary herpes simplex virus (HSV) infection produces painful, pruritic, vesicular, or ulcerated genital lesions. Urethral or cervical involvement may result in a mucopurulent discharge. The patient may have fever, chills, abdominal pain, myalgias, headache, malaise, lymphadenopathy, and photophobia. Tender grouped vesicles on an erythematous base are characteristic. Periodic recurrence of HSV infection is the rule, but recurrent episodes tend to be less severe than the primary infection.

The diagnosis is often obvious, but if doubt exists, a Tzanck test is positive in about half of all cases. Vesicular contents are stained with methylene blue or a Wright stain to reveal the characteristic multinucleated giant cells. A viral culture is also available.

Recommended therapy for initial HSV infection is acyclovir (Zovirax), 400 mg PO tid × 7 to 10 days; the alternative is 200 mg five times a day × 7 to 10 days. This treatment reduces the duration of viral shedding, accelerates healing, and decreases symptom duration. The best results are obtained when treatment is initiated within the first week of symptom onset. Only severe, recurrent episodes should be treated. It is recommended that acyclovir be started within 2 days of onset and that only 5 days of therapy be prescribed. Intravenous therapy is reserved for disseminated herpes or for immunocompromised hosts.

The major concern with HSV infection is that of possible transmission to the neonate by the pregnant patient. Beginning at 32 weeks of pregnancy, women with a history of HSV infection or of contact with sexual partners with genital HSV should be referred for screening for viral cultures. A cesarean section is the recommended delivery procedure for women who shed the virus near term. The use of condoms may help prevent transmission. Patients with herpetic lesions are at an increased risk of HIV transmission.

Bartholin Abscess

A Bartholin abscess is an infection of a Bartholin gland or duct cyst. These glands normally secrete fluid into a duct that exits at the mucosal surface of the labia, and they are not normally palpable or visible unless inflamed. Such infections may be caused by a number of organisms, including *Neisseria gonorrhoeae, Chlamydia trachomatis, Escherichia coli,* and *Proteus mirabilis.* Mixed infections are common.

The patient complains of unilateral pain and swelling at the lower introitus. Examination reveals an extremely tender fluctuant ovoid or spherical mass, often with surrounding erythema and edema of the labia majora. Like any closed-space infection, treatment of a Bartholin abscess requires incision and drainage. Make the incision on the mucosal surface of the vestibule just lateral to the hymenal ring. Insert a drain or a small balloon catheter (Word cathether) and leave it in place for 24 to 48 hours. Sitz baths are also recommended.

Vaginal Discharge

Patients who complain of abnormal vaginal discharge may note an increased amount of discharge or a change in color or odor. Associated symptoms may be perineal itching or swelling, dyspareunia, pelvic pain, or dysuria. Often such symptoms indicate the presence of cervicitis or vaginitis. Because discharge is often caused by venereal infections, screening for sexually transmitted diseases, especially gonorrhea and chlamydia infections, is necessary. Other causative organisms include *Trichomonas, Mycoplasma, Herpes viridae, Gardnerella,* and others. Concurrent venereal infections at different sites (e.g., pharyngeal or anorectal) or accompanied by early or incubating syphilis should be considered.

Gonorrhea cervicitis

N. gonorrhoeae is responsible for three patterns of involvement in women: pelvic inflammatory disease, (which is discussed later in this chapter); cervicitis; and asymptomatic carriers. Patients with cervicitis develop symptoms of increased vaginal discharge, dysuria, and abnormal bleeding 3 to 45 days after exposure. The cervix appears friable, erythematous, and congested. There is a purulent or mucopurulent discharge from the os externum uteri. However, Gram stain of the exudate is too insensitive to exclude the gonococcus as the causative agent. The enzyme immunoassay Gonozyme or the DNA ELISA Genprobe tests are useful. Culture is the standard diagnostic method.

Treatment should follow the Centers for Disease Control and Prevention recommendations for both gonorrhea and chlamydia (see the next section). For uncomplicated gonococcal cervicitis, ceftriaxone 125 mg IM or cefixime 400 mg PO is recommended. Alternative treatment options (e.g., in patients who are allergic to penicillin) include single doses of spectinomycin 2 g IM, ofloxacin 400 mg PO, or ciprofloxacin 500 mg PO. Follow-up is recommended to ensure compliance and a cure. Sexual partners also need treatment.

Chlamydial cervicitis

In addition to causing lymphogranuloma venereum, acute urethral syndrome, and pelvic inflammatory disease, *C. trachomatis* causes mucopurulent cervicitis that is difficult to distinguish clinically from that caused by *N. gonorrhoeae.* Symptoms are similar to those of gonococcal cervicitis. Physical findings include vaginal discharge, cervical edema, erythema, and friability. Yellow mucopurulent endocervical discharge and the presence of polymorphonuclear leukocytes on a Gram stain are characteristic of chlamydial cervicitis. The absence of intracellular gram-negative diplococci further supports the diagnosis.

First-line therapies for chlamydial cervicitis are doxycycline 100 mg PO bid for 7 days or azithromycin 1 g PO one time (i.e., during pregnancy). Alternatives include erythromycin 500 mg PO qid × 7 days or 250 mg PO qid × 14 days; ofloxacin 300 mg PO bid × 7 days; amoxicillin 500 mg PO tid × 10 days; or sulfisoxazole 500 mg PO qid × 10 days. Sexual partners also need treatment. Because of the strong likelihood of concurrent infection, one-dose therapy for *N. gonorrhoea* (see the previous section) should also be administered.

Trichomonas vaginitis

Trichomonas vaginalis is a common cause of vaginal discharge. Patients typically complain of a malodorous, itchy, profuse, frothy discharge that can be white, green, or gray. The discharge has a pH of 5 to 7. The vaginal mucosa and the

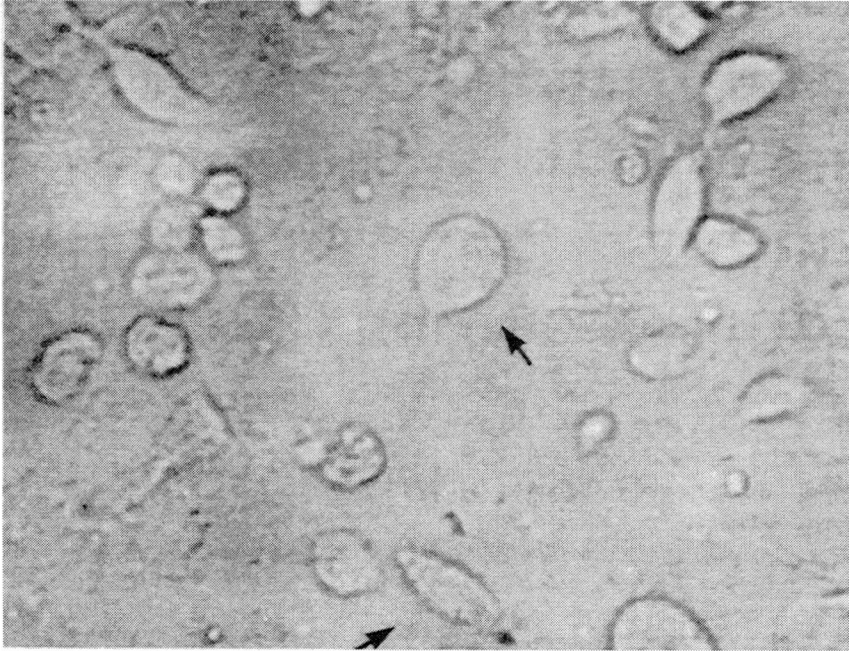

Fig. 16-1   *Trichomonas vaginalis.* (From Kaufman RH: Hosp Med. August 1981, p 15. Reproduced by permission.)

cervix may have a stippled or punctate "strawberry" appearance. A diagnosis is made by visualizing the motile trichomonad on a wet mount, but this technique may only be 60% sensitive. The organism is slightly larger than a leukocyte and is pear-shaped with three to five flagella at one end (Fig. 16-1). Trichomoniasis is best treated with metronidazole (Flagyl), either as a single dose of 2 g PO or 500 mg PO bid × 7 days. Because of the risk of an Antabuse-type reaction, alcohol must be avoided. Recurrences may require 500 mg PO tid × 7 days or 2 g PO qd × 3 to 5 days. Sexual partners must also receive treatment. Women in the first trimester of pregnancy should *not* receive metronidazole. Administering clotrimazole vaginal suppositories 100 mg bid × 14 days is a palliative alternative, with a 20% cure rate and symptomatic improvement in others. After the first trimester, metronidazole

2 g PO once or 250 mg PO tid × 1 week can be used if palliative treatments do not alleviate symptoms.

Bacterial vaginosis

In bacterial vaginosis, normal bacterial flora are replaced by *Gardnerella vaginalis*, *Mycoplasma hominis*, *Mobiluncus* organisms, or other organisms and anaerobes. One fourth of these organisms are associated with other pelvic infections, including pelvic inflammatory disease. Patients complain of a malodorous discharge that is gray or white with a pH above 4.5. The discharge has a fishy odor that becomes stronger after the addition of a drop of 10% potassium hydroxide to a sample (the "whiff" test). The presence of "clue cells" (vaginal epithelial cells to which the bacteria have become attached) establishes the diagnosis. A Gram stain that demonstrates curved gram-negative rods that are consistent with *Mobiluncus* organisms may be the most sensitive bedside test. First-line therapies are metronidazole vaginal gel 0.75%, 5 g bid × 5 days, or clindamycin vaginal cream 2%, 5 g qhs × 7 days. Alternatives include metronidazole 500 mg PO bid × 7 days or clindamycin 300 mg PO bid × 7 days.

Candida vaginitis

Candida albicans is probably the most common cause of vaginitis. Predisposing factors to *C. albicans* vaginal infection include a recent use of antibiotics, corticosteroids, and oral contraceptives; pregnancy; diabetes mellitus; and an immune compromise. Patients often complain of intense itching. Examination reveals a thick nonodorous discharge with a white "cottage cheese" texture and an inflamed mucosa.

Confirmation of *C. albicans* is obtained by identifying the budding spores and pseudohyphae with a wet mount using 10% potassium hydroxide. There are many recommended topical therapies, which are usually prescribed as an intravaginal applicator or suppository every night for 3 days to 1 week. These topical therapies include miconazole, clotrimazole, butoconazole, terconazole, and tioconazole. Recurrence is common. A single 150 mg PO dose of fluconazole is as effective as 3 days of intravaginal clotrimazole.

Pelvic inflammatory disease

Pelvic inflammatory disease (PID) is an infection that can involve the cervix, uterus, and adnexa. In the majority of cases, the responsible organisms are *N. gonorrhoeae* and *C. trachomatis.* Anaerobic bacteria (*Peptococcus, Peptostreptococcus,* and *Bacteroides* organisms) are associated with chronic, recurrent PID. Gram-negative bacteria can also cause PID. Risk factors include multiple sexual partners and the presence of an intrauterine device. Although rarely fatal, PID is a significant cause of ectopic pregnancy, infertility, and chronic pelvic pain.

The severity of the presentation does not correlate with the risk of chronic sequelae.

Acute PID is typically manifested by fever, increased vaginal discharge, pelvic pain, dyspareunia, and dysuria; it usually begins during the week following menstruation. These symptoms progress over a period of hours to days. Atypical presentations are common. Laparoscopic studies have revealed that the clinical diagnosis of PID is accurate in only approximately two thirds of all cases. Patients often have a history of antecedent irregular bleeding. Although PID can be seen during the first trimester of pregnancy, such an occurrence is rare.

On examination, tenderness is present with palpation of the lower abdomen. The hallmark finding is cervical motion tenderness. Salpingitis causes adnexal tenderness; adnexal fullness suggests that a tuboovarian abscess may also be present. Right upper quadrant pain and tenderness suggest the Fitz-Hugh-Curtis syndrome. Peritonitis may develop if the patient is left untreated.

The white blood cell count is often elevated with a shift to the left. The erythrocyte sedimentation rate is also elevated in the majority of patients. A Gram stain of cervical drainage may reveal leukocytes and gram-negative intracellular diplococci (if the infection is caused by *N. gonorrhoeae*).

Whereas exacerbations of acute PID are common, the clinical picture of chronic PID is often confusing and vague. Patients complain of constant aching pelvic pain that is exacerbated by sexual intercourse or menses. This pain is usually a result of pelvic adhesions. Abnormal uterine bleeding is also a common complaint. On examination, palpation often causes only nonspecific mild tenderness. Usually patients with chronic PID are afebrile and without signs of vaginitis, cervicitis, or urethritis.

Patients with the *intermediate PID* syndrome have a clinical picture between that of acute and chronic PID. Intermediate PID is most often caused by *C. trachomatis* or a secondary infection. Symptoms may be those of vaginitis, cervicitis, or urethritis. Pain is steady and aching rather than sharp and increases with sexual intercourse and menses. Unilateral or bilateral adnexal tenderness and signs of cervicitis are the pertinent findings during examination. Signs of peritonitis are generally absent.

The white blood cell count and sedimentation rate are usually normal in chronic and intermediate PID. The differential diagnosis of PID includes acute appendicitis, endometriosis, corpus luteum bleeding, ectopic pregnancy, and ovarian tumors.

Indications for hospitalization depend somewhat on local practice. Suggested guidelines for admission include the following: (1) a first episode of PID, especially in a young woman or one who is nulliparous; (2) an inability to tolerate oral medications; (3) treatment failure; (4) the presence of peritonitis; (5) sepsis; (6) the probability of pelvic or tuboovarian abscess; or (7) uncertainty about the diagnosis; (8) a history of diabetes or drug or alcohol abuse; (9) an immunocompromised state; or (10) a poor previous compliance.

Outpatient antibiotic therapy is similar to the management of gonorrhea and chlamydial cervicitis, but in this case, double the dosage of ceftriaxone to 250 mg IM, or administer cefoxitin 2 g IM with probenecid 1 g PO once. Then add doxycycline 100 mg PO bid × 14 days (during pregnancy, erythromycin 500 mg PO qid × 14 days). An alternative is ofloxacin 400 mg PO bid × 2 weeks plus either clindamycin 450 mg PO qid × 14 days or metronidazole 500 mg PO bid × 14 days.

Inpatient antibiotic therapy involves one of two regimens. The first consists of doxycycline 100 mg IV q12h, plus cefoxitin 2 g IV q6h or cefotetan 2 g IV q12h for at least 4 days or until improved. This dosage is followed by doxycycline 100 mg PO bid to complete 14 days of total therapy. An alternate regimen involves IV clindamycin 600 mg q6h or 900 mg IV q8h plus either gentamicin or tobramycin 2 mg/kg IV, fol-

lowed by 1.5 mg/kg IV q8h for at least 4 days or until improved in patients with normal renal function. This regimen should be followed by a course of doxycycline 100 mg PO bid or clindamycin 450 mg PO qid to complete a course of 14 days of treatment.

Condyloma accuminatum

Venereal warts are associated with exposure to the human papillomavirus, which places women at a higher risk for cervical cancer. Filiform to fungating fleshy growths appear on the vulva, cervix, vagina, and anus and are associated with pruritis or discharge. Atypical, pigmented, or persistent warts should be biopsied. Small, extravaginal lesions (not on mucous membranes) should be treated with podophyllum resin 10% with benzoin tincture applied only to warts and washed off in 1 to 4 hours, earlier if burning occurs. Surrounding skin should be protected by first applying petroleum jelly. Single lesions 1 to 5 mm in size may respond to gauze that has been saturated with 5% acetic acid (white distilled vinegar). Patients should abstain from sexual intercourse until treatment is complete and then use condoms. Patients should be told to keep long-term follow-up for their increased risk of cervical or anorectal carcinoma.

Granuloma inguinale

Granuloma inguinale is caused by *Calymmatobacterium granulomatis* (Donovan bodies). A painless, elevated "beefy red" zone of friable granulation tissue may extend to the inguinal nodes and cause intradermal and subcutaneous swelling or suppuration (Donovanosis). This condition is infrequent in the United States. A punch biopsy may be necessary. Treatment with doxycycline 100 mg PO bid or trimethoprim-sulfamethoxazole one double-strength PO bid may take as long as 4 weeks until all lesions are healed, but a treatment response is usually seen within 1 week. Treatment failures and recurrences are seen with doxycycline.

Lymphogranuloma venereum

Lymphogranuloma venereum is caused by *C. trachomatis*. A shallow, nonpainful herpetiform vesicle or ulcer lasts a few days but often heals without patient awareness. After 3 to 21 days of incubation, adenopathy (usually bilateral) appears, usually with a positive groove sign as the adenopathy is cleaved by the inelastic inguinal ligament. The nodes may coalesce to form caseous lesions that erode and form sinus tracts that may drain thick yellow pus. Complications include rectal stricture, hemorrhagic proctitis, proctocolitis, and elephantiasis of the vulva, scrotum, or perineum. A diagnosis is made on the basis of serology; a biopsy is contraindicated. Treatment is either doxycycline 100 mg PO bid × 21 days or erythromycin 500 mg PO qid × 3 weeks.

Chancroid

Chancroid is caused by *Haemophilus ducreyi*. Patients have deep, tender, nonindurated ulcers with irregular borders on a purulent base. Women may have multiple lesions. The incubation period ranges from 3 to 10 days. Half of the lesions are associated with painful, usually unilateral adenopathy, more commonly in men. The lesion may appear initially as a pustule. Nodes may be fluctuant with overlying red skin (bubo) that may suggest an abscess, but incision and drainage can result in a chronic draining fistula. As many as 10% of all patients with chancroid are coinfected with syphilis or herpes. There are many treatment options. Erythromycin 500 mg PO qid × 7 days is usually recommended. Other recommendations include ceftriaxone 250 mg IM, azithromycin 1 gm PO, or ciprofloxacin 500 mg PO bid × 3 days. Second-line alternatives include trimethoprim-sulfamethoxazole one double-strength PO bid × 1 week, or amoxicillin-clavulanate 500 mg PO tid × 1 week.

KEY CONSIDERATIONS

WHAT IS THE LIFE THREAT?

A ruptured ectopic pregnancy and ovarian torsion can constitute life threats.

A severe intraabdominal event such as an intestinal perforation, abscess, or ruptured blood vessel that causes pelvic pain can constitute a life threat.

Placental abruption can present a life threat to the fetus and mother.

DOES THE PATIENT NEED ADMISSION?

Admit patients with a ruptured ectopic pregnancy, ovarian torsion, incomplete spontaneous abortion, or severe vaginal bleeding, including placenta previa.

Indications for hospitalization for salpingitis include an inability to tolerate oral medications, treatment failure, the presence of peritonitis, sepsis, tuboovarian abscess, or uncertainty of the diagnosis in an ill or toxic-appearing patient.

WHAT IS THE MOST SERIOUS DIAGNOSIS?

A ruptured ectopic pregnancy, ovarian torsion, and uterine carcinoma are the most serious diagnoses.

HAVE I PERFORMED A THOROUGH WORK-UP?

Assess the pregnancy status in female patients with pelvic or abdominal pain or abnormal vaginal bleeding.

Consider appendicitis and pyelonephritis in the assessment of pelvic pain during pregnancy.

Obtain an ultrasonography of the pelvis for a suspected ovarian torsion, possible tubal pregnancy, pelvic masses, severe pelvic pain associated with pregnancy, or late trimester bleeding.

Recommended Reading

Bowie WR: Antibiotics and sexually transmitted diseases, *Infect Dis Clin North Am* 8:841, 1994.

Hochbaum SR: Vaginal bleeding. In Rosen P et al, editors: *Emergency medicine: concepts and clinical practice*, ed 3, St Louis, 1992, Mosby.

Pointer JE: Genital infections. In Rosen P et al, editors: *Emergency medicine: concepts and clinical practice*, ed 3, St Louis, 1992, Mosby.

Shapiro AG: Emergency treatment of menstrual disorders in a nonpregnant woman, *Emerg Med Clin North Am* 5:559, 1987.

Young, GP: Pelvic pain. In Rosen P et al, editors: *Emergency medicine: concepts and clinical practice*, ed 3, St Louis, 1992, Mosby.

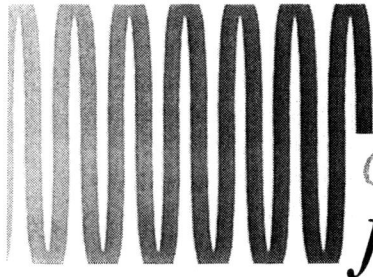

Chapter Seventeen
JOINT AND BACK PAIN

DAVID CHUNGSANG LEE

JOINT PAIN

Nontraumatic joint pain is a very common presentation in the emergency department. Although this type of pain rarely represents an acute life or limb-threatening condition, the emergency physician must be able to approach the evaluation and treatment properly and exclude those conditions that are life or limb threatening.

Pathophysiology

Diseases that affect the joints often interfere with the function of the joint by destroying the "lubricating" properties of the joint. Inflammation of the joint is characterized by an exudation of polymorphonuclear cells in the synovial cavity. These cells release lysosomal enzymes that degrade the various structures of the joint (Fig. 17-1).

Assessment

History

A joint-focused history should be obtained, and the following questions should be considered:

1. *Is the pain in the joint (articular) or around the joint (periarticular?)* The articular pain of arthritis is described as being generalized, with accompanying warmth and swelling. The periarticular pain of bursitis, tendinitis, and cellulitis is described as focal, with swelling and warmth localized to specific areas of the joint. Pain is often reproduced only with certain movements or positions.

2. *Does the pain involve one joint (monarticular) or several joints (polyarticular)?* Monarticular involvement often represents a local inflammatory condition (e.g., osteoarthritis, septic arthritis, gout, pseudogout, bursitis, tendinitis). Polyarticular involvement often represents a more systemic condition (e.g., rheumatoid arthritis, systemic lupus erythematosus, rheumatic fever, lyme disease).

3. *What is the distribution of the joint or joints involved?* Certain diseases have a predilection for specific joints. Gout predominantly affects the first metatarsophalangeal joint. Gonococcal arthritis often affects the knee or wrist. Rheumatoid arthritis often affects the metacarpophalangeal joints, but osteoarthritis affects the distal interphalangeal joints.

4. *What is the time pattern of the pain?* Does the pain occur suddenly, like gout or pseudogout? Does the pain appear gradually as in rheumatoid arthritis? Does the pain migrate from one joint to another as in acute rheu-

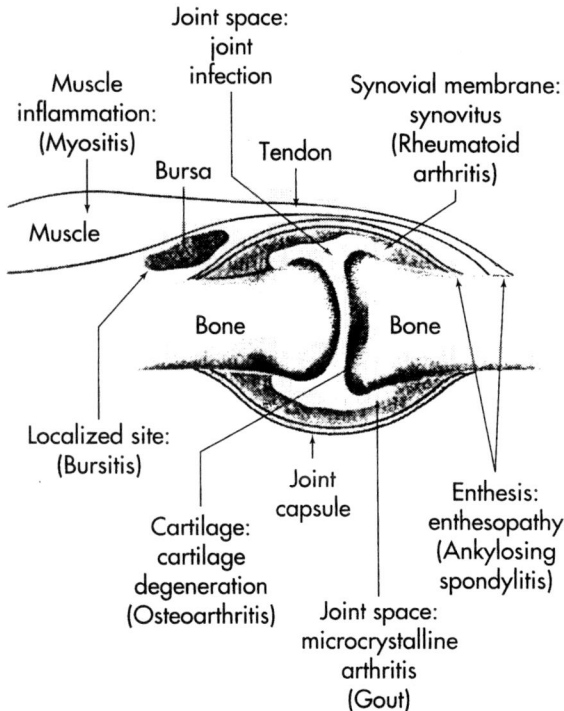

Fig.17-1 Sites and types of rheumatic disease. (From Wyngaarden JB, Smith LH, editors: *Cecil textbook of medicine*, ed 18, Philadelphia, 1988, WB Saunders.)

matic fever? Does the pain occur mainly in the morning as in osteoarthritis?
5. *Are there other associated symptoms?* Is there a high-grade fever to suggest septic arthritis? Is there a rash to suggest lupus, psoriasis, rubella, Lyme disease, or gonococcal arthritis?

Joint examination

Similar to other aspects of the physical examination, a joint examination should be approached in a systematic manner:
1. Inspect the overlying skin and the position of the rested joint.
2. Palpate the joint and surrounding structures, including the regional lymph nodes.

3. Evaluate joint function by having the patient go through a range of motion independently (active range of motion) and then by physically manipulating the joint without any effort from the patient (passive range of motion).

A joint examination should document the location of swelling; the location of maximum tenderness; the presence of crepitus, warmth, erythema, effusion or any obvious deformity; the limits of the range of active and passive motion; and the neurovascular status of the extremity or area of the body.

Radiographic and laboratory evaluation

Radiographic and blood studies (such as a complete blood count and erythrocyte sedimentation rate) have limited value in the evaluation of the patient in the emergency department who is complaining of nontraumatic joint pain. A single study usually does not confirm or exclude a diagnosis but may suggest a certain diagnosis. More sophisticated studies such as magnetic resonance imaging, serum antinuclear antibody levels, and complement levels are usually unavailable in the emergency department.

The most valuable laboratory test is the examination of the synovial fluid. In a healthy joint, synovial fluid is secreted by cells that line the synovial membrane; however, the amount of fluid and the chemical and cellular composition of the fluid changes with various disease processes. The most common reason to examine the synovial fluid is to differentiate between a septic joint and a crystalline-induced arthritic joint (Table 17-1). The most common causes of accumulating synovial fluid leading to an effusion are trauma and degenerative joint disease; other causes are listed in Table 17-2.

Observe the appearance and color of the synovial fluid. Fluid from a healthy joint should be thick and viscous, whereas fluid from an inflamed joint is often thin and watery. The fluid should be examined under the microscope to help confirm the diagnosis of gout or pseudo-

Table *17-1*

CLASSIFICATION OF SYNOVIAL FLUID

Group	Class	Appearance	Viscosity	Mucin Clot	White Blood Cell Count (/mm³)
I	Normal	Clear	High	Good	2000
II	Inflammatory	Turbid	Moderate	Medium	2000-100,000
III	Septic	Opaque	Low	Poor	Over 50,000
IV	Hemorrhagic	Bloody	Varies	—	—

gout. Gout is associated with uric acid crystals, which appear thin and needlelike. Pseudogout is associated with calcium pyrophosphate crystals, which appear rectangular or rhomboid (Fig. 17-2). These differences can be visualized better with a polarizing microscope.

The synovial fluid should be sent to the laboratory for the evaluation of glucose, protein, and a complete blood count with a differential. If infection is suspected, a Gram stain and a culture should also be obtained.

COMMON CHARACTERISTICS OF DISEASES THAT INVOLVE JOINTS

Monarticular Arthritis

Gout

Gout occurs when there is an accumulation and precipitation of uric acid crystals in the joint. Hypertension, diabetes, obesity, renal failure, certain medications (most notably thiazide diuretics) all predispose an individual to gout. Gout tends to occur in middle-aged men and postmenopausal women.

Patients with gout often complain of a recurring, severely painful swollen joint. The joint involved usually is the first metatarsophalangeal joint, but sometimes the ankle, foot, or knee (Fig. 17-3). A fever may be present. Consider the possibility of a septic joint in such cases. The ex-

amination may also reveal gouty deposits in the form of tophi that is located in the elbows, tendon sheaths, or the ear. A diagnosis is made by examining the joint aspirate under a polarized light with a first-order red compensator in the optic system; negative birefringent crystals will be seen.

The mainstay of treatment for acute painful gouty attacks is the use of nonsteroidal antiinflammatory drugs (NSAIDs). The most commonly prescribed drug is a tapering dose of indomethacin 75 to 200 mg/day titrated to symptoms. Other effective medications include colchicine, which can be given orally (0.6 mg orally every hour until pain is relieved or until the onset of nausea and vomiting; ten doses is the maximum recommended) or intravenously (1 to 2 mg diluted in 50 ml saline and administered over 10 minutes). The ease of administration of intravenous colchicine makes this method more suitable than the oral form in the emergency department. Patients with severe attacks can also benefit from a corticosteroid. A tapering dose of oral prednisone can be prescribed for several days (starting at 50 mg/day).

Pseudogout

Pseudogout occurs when calcium pyrophosphate dihydrate accumulates in the synovial fluid. The joint most commonly affected is the knee, but the disease also commonly occurs in

Table 17-2

JOINT FLUID GROUP DIFFERENTIAL DIAGNOSIS

Noninflammatory	*Inflammatory*	*Septic*	*Hemorrhagic*
Degenerative joint disease	Rheumatoid arthritis	Bacterial infection	Trauma
Trauma	Gout		Hemophilia
Neuropathic arthritis	Pseudogout		Bleeding diathesis
	Reiter syndrome		Synovioma
	Psoriatic arthritis		

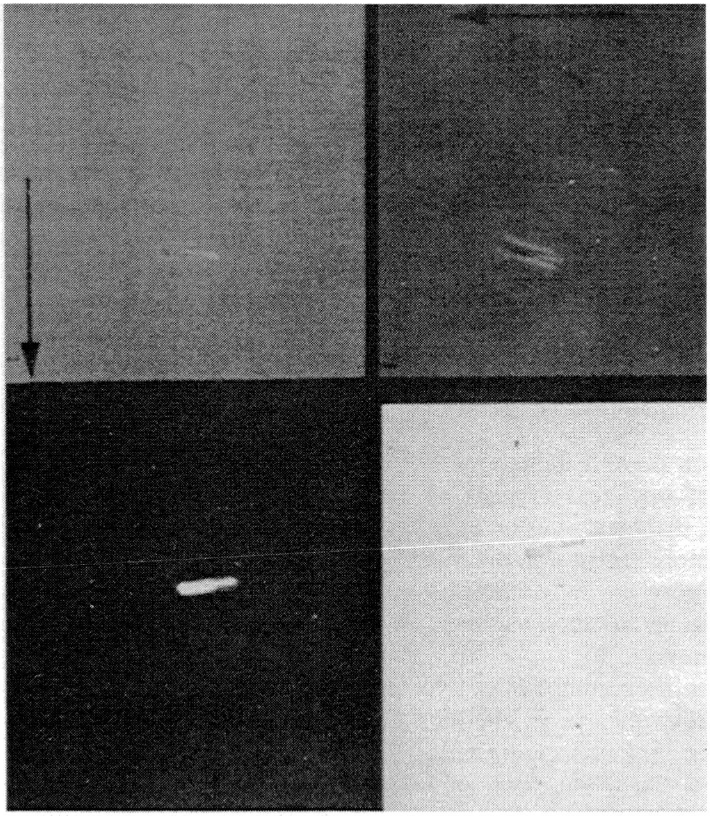

Fig. 17-2   Calcium pyrophosphate crystals.

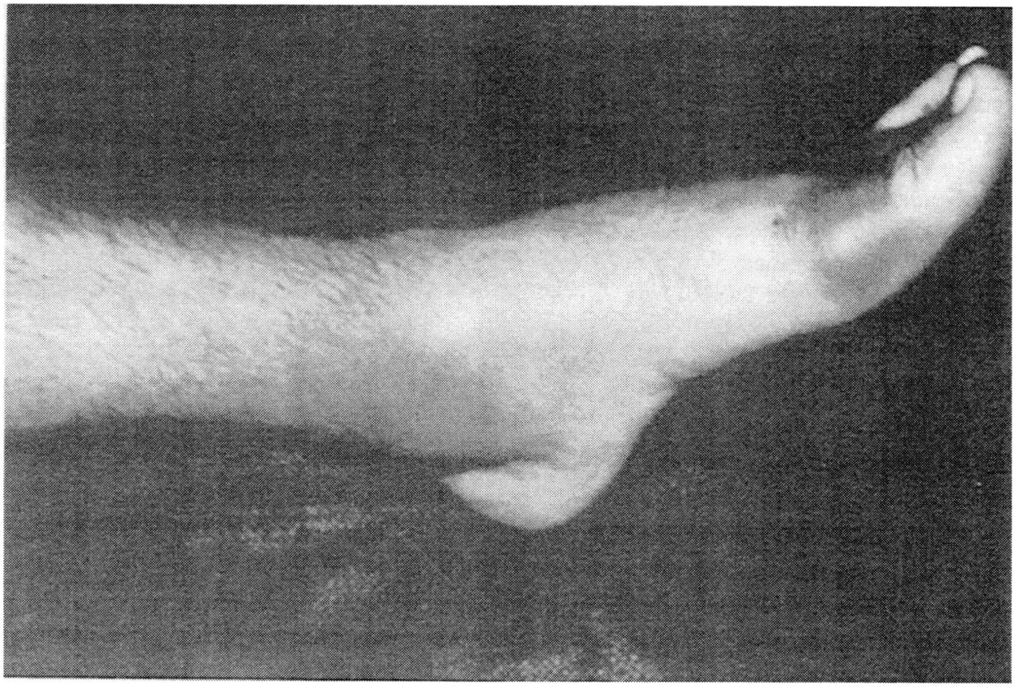

Fig. 17-3   Gouty arthritis of first metatarsal (podagra). (From the Clinical Slide Collection on the Rheumatic Diseases produced by the Arthritis Foundation. Copyright 1972. Reprinted by permission.)

the wrist, ankle, and elbow. Like gout, pseudogout usually occurs in those who are middle aged or older, but unlike gout, pseudogout has an equal gender distribution.

Patients with pseudogout often complain of recurring inflammation in one or more joints. Like gout, the diagnosis is made by examining the joint aspirate under a microscope using a first-order red compensator in the optic system. Weakly positive birefringent rhomboid crystals can be seen. Sometimes these crystals can be seen with a standard microscope. The treatment for pseudogout is similar to gout (see p. 189).

Septic arthritis

Bacteria can invade a joint by three mechanisms: (1) direct implantation into the joint such as a can occur with a puncture wound or during open surgery; (2) spread from infected local tissue as in osteomyelitis; and (3) by hematogenous spread from a septic site. Several common scenarios include the spread of gonorrhea to the knee from a venereal infection, the spread of *Haemophilus influenza* from an upper respiratory infection in children, and staphylococci from a distant skin infection. In all cases, the offending bacteria begins a cascade that leads to the release of synovial fluid and enzymes and causes joint destruction.

Patients complain of an acute onset (hours to days) of a painful monarticular joint with accompanying fever and possibly chills. The patient often has an underlying disorder that predisposes him or her to infection (e.g., positive HIV status, immunosuppressive medications, intravenous drug abuse, sickle cell disease). Examination of the joint reveals an erythematous, warm, painful joint accompanied by a fever. *All patients with monarticular joint pain and a fever must be considered to have septic arthritis until proven otherwise.* Radiographic studies are not particularly useful. Joint aspiration and examination of joint fluid is the key to a diagnosis (see Table 17-1). A complete blood count, erythrocyte sedimentation rate (ESR), and blood cultures are all indicated laboratory tests.

Patients who have a diagnosis of septic arthritis require inpatient treatment and orthopedic consultation for open drainage. The type of antibiotic should be customized to the underlying disorders and the route of infection.

Bursitis/tendinitis

Pain referred to a joint may actually be a result of the inflammation of structures surrounding a joint. This type of pain includes bursitis and tendinitis, the most common causes of which are trauma and chronic repetitive use. It is often very difficult to differentiate between articular joint pain and periarticular pain.

Patients with bursitis and tendinitis often complain of joint pain but may localize it to an area specific to a bursa or tendon. X-ray studies are usually not helpful but may show an area of focal calcification, which indicates chronic calcific tendinitis.

The mainstay of treatment includes rest, immobilization, and NSAID therapy. Local injection of steroids and the use of a topical anesthetic are also useful treatments.

Polyarticular Arthritis

Osteoarthritis

Osteoarthritis, or degenerative joint disease, is a chronic disorder that produces destructive changes of the joint and subchondral bone as a result of the loss of articular cartilage.

Patients with osteoarthritis often complain of chronic pain and deformity in one or more joints. Patients are usually more than 60 years of age. Osteophyte spurs in the proximal interphalangeal and distal interphalangeal joint can often be palpated (the Bouchard and Heberden nodes, respectively). Atrophy of local muscles often accompanies severe cases. X-ray studies often reveal a joint with an uneven, narrowed joint space and osteophyte formation at the margins.

The mainstay of treatment is pain control through the judicious use of NSAIDs, including salicylates. Physical therapy is often helpful in maintaining joint function.

Rheumatoid arthritis

In rheumatoid arthritis, immune complexes form in the joint and cause polymorphonuclear leukocytes to release destructive enzymes and proteins. This release leads to pain, inflammation, and scar formation. Rheumatoid arthritis appears to be familial and affects women much more often than men, often before or during middle age.

Patients initially complain of a prodromal period of various constitutional symptoms such as fever, fatigue, weakness, and muscular pain followed by joint pain and swelling. Examination shows warm and tender joints, often in a symmetric pattern. Patients with longstanding disease have multiple deformities of the hands and fingers, including bony changes of the metacarpal phalangeal and proximal interphalangeal joints (e.g., ulnar deviation, swan neck, and boutonniere deformities.) In severe disease, extraarticular manifestations in the skin, lung, and nervous system are present. To establish the diagnosis, an arthrocentesis should be performed and serum should be analyzed for rheumatoid factor. Anemia and an elevated ESR are common findings.

In mild disease, NSAIDs are the mainstay of treatment. Long-term care may include steroids, gold, penicillamine, azathioprine, and methotrexate.

Reiter syndrome

Reiter syndrome is a disease that is classified as a seronegative (rheumatoid-factor negative) spondyloarthropathy. This group includes ankylosing spondylitis, psoriatic arthritis, and arthritis associated with colitis. Patients with these diseases have a genetic predisposition that can be indirectly tested (HLA-B27 genetic marker.) It is believed that the combination of a genetic predisposition and an "environmental trigger" causes the disease. The classic triad of Reiter syndrome includes arthritis, urethritis, and conjunctivitis; however, the diagnostic criteria have been changing. Presently the diagnosis is suggested by arthritis that follows an infection, typically urethritis, cervicitis, or dysentery. Such infections cause a reactive inflammatory process in the synovial membrane. Patients are usually young, healthy men.

Patients complain of polyarticular, asymmetric joint pains usually of the weight-bearing joints of the lower extremities. Pain can be chronic and recurrent. One third of all patients also complain of lower back pain. There may be painful lesions in the mucosal areas of the eye or nasopharyngeal area. There may be a prior episode of diarrhea, dysuria, or vaginal discharge. Examination may reveal swelling of fingers and toes ("sausage-shaped" digits). Eye findings include conjunctivitis, uveitis, iritis, and corneal ulcerations. Skin findings include scaling, erythematous lesions on the palms and soles (keratodermia blennorrhagicum), and painless superficial ulcers on the glans penis. A diagnosis is usually made clinically. With the exception of the HLA-B27 marker, laboratory tests are not helpful. X-ray studies may show a fluffy periostitis characteristics of the bone.

NSAIDs are the treatment of choice. Antibiotics have not been shown to be effective in changing the course of the disease.

Gonococcal arthritis

Gonococcal arthritis is probably the most common type of bacterial-induced arthritis that occurs in otherwise healthy adults. It often is migratory and accompanied by a tenosynovitis. Such reactions are thought to be caused by an immune-mediated response. This condition occurs twice as often in women than in men.

Patients often complain of fever, chills, and migratory joint aches. Pain tends to localize in the knee, ankle, and wrist. Examination often reveals a mildly inflamed joint. Hemorrhagic necrotic pustules are also seen, especially over the distal extremities (Fig. 17-4). It is essential to obtain urethral, cervical, pharyngeal and rectal cultures in the appropriate medium because blood cultures reveal *Neisseria gonorrhoeae* only 20% of the time, and joint aspirate cultures are positive only 50% of the time.

Patients with a diagnosis of gonococcal arthritis are optimally treated as inpatients. The mainstay of treatment is either ceftriaxone, cefotaxime, or ceftizoxime. Spectinomycin or ciprofloxacin can be used if the patient is allergic to penicillin.

Lyme disease

Lyme disease is caused by the spirochete *Borrelia burgdorferi*. This infection is transmitted by the bite of the deer tick of the genus *Ixodes*. The arthritis that accompanies Lyme disease occurs late in the illness and is probably immune mediated.

Patients also may develop Bell palsy, meningitis, encephalitis, and atrioventricular block. Patients sometimes demonstrate a characteristic rash, called erythema chronicum migrans. This type of rash is a single red macule that spreads to form a large annular lesion; the lesion has a erythematous border but a partial central clear area. Several weeks to several months after developing the rash, patients often complain of painful joints, most commonly the knees. These joint pains may be recurring or chronic. Examination often reveals a painful joint with little or no effusion. Serum should be obtained for immunofluorescent antibody assays to confirm the diagnosis.

In early stages of suspected Lyme disease, an-

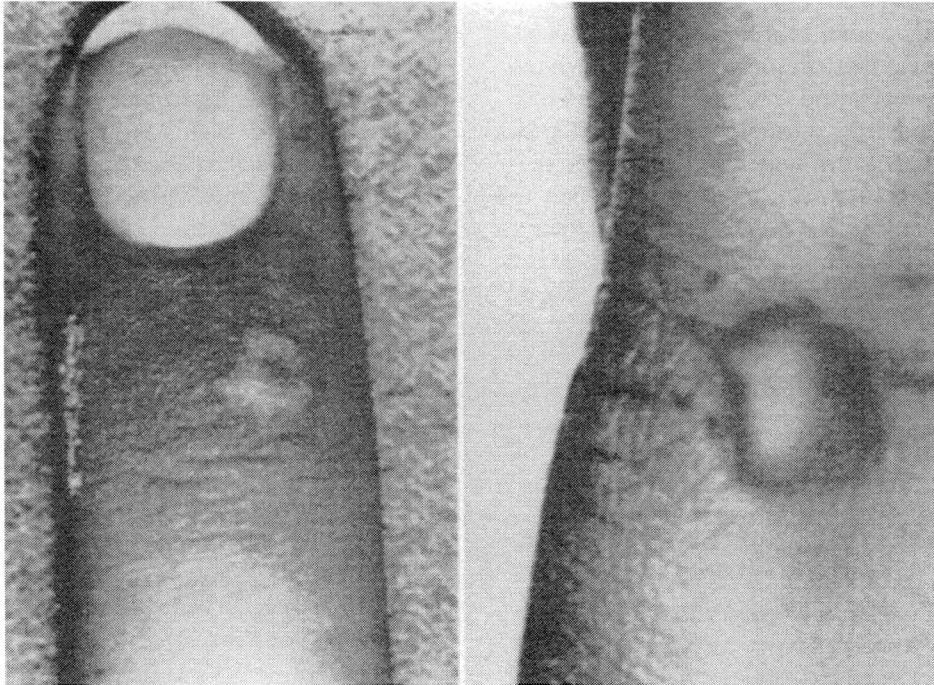

Fig.17-4   Gonococcemia: skin lesions. (From the Clinical Slide Collection on the Rheumatic Diseases produced by the Arthritis Foundation. Copyright 1972. Reprinted by permission.)

tibiotics can shorten the duration and severity of the disease (doxycycline 100 mg bid. for 10 to 21 days or amoxicillin 500 mg tid. for 10 to 21 days.) Patients with arthritis and suspected Lyme disease should be managed with NSAIDs and a long-term course of antibiotic treatment (doxycycline 100 mg bid for 30 days). Patients with a severe disease that manifests itself as persistent severe arthritis, myocarditis, or meningitis may require an inpatient course of ceftriaxone or a high-dose penicillin regimen.

Acute rheumatic fever

Acute rheumatic fever occurs as a result of Group A ß-hemolytic streptococcus. This type of bacteria causes immune complexes to form and deposit in various body tissues, including the joints. Arthritis is the most common finding, but myocarditis and chorea also occur.

Patients with acute rheumatic fever often complain of symmetric, migratory joint pain in various joints, especially the larger joints of the lower extremities. Sometimes a history of a sore throat can be elicited. Look for evidence of congestive failure secondary to carditis. Erythema marginatum, erythema nodosum, and subcutaneous nodules may also be present. The workup for acute rheumatic fever includes a documentation of streptococcal infection and includes a pharyngeal culture, anti-DNase, and the streptozyme test. Other helpful laboratory tests include ESR, antibody to streptolysin O, and C-reactive protein. An ECG is indicated.

Antibiotics are the mainstay of treatment

(penicillin V 2 g/day orally for 10 days or 1.2 million units of benzathine penicillin IM or erythromycin 2 g/day orally for 10 days). Arthritis responds well to salicylates.

Viral arthritis

Certain viruses cause a deposition of immune complexes in the joint, which leads to an inflammatory response. The most common offending viruses are those causing rubella and hepatitis B.

Most patients with virus-induced arthritis complain of a migratory asymmetric arthritis involving the hands and knees. Patients also have various constitutional complaints. In patients with rubella, the arthritis is accompanied by a characteristic rash. Rubella can also be isolated in the joint aspirate. In patients with hepatitis B, arthritis often heralds liver dysfunction.

Table 17-3 is an overview of monoarticular and polyarticular arthritis.

NONTRAUMATIC LUMBOSACRAL PAIN

Lower back pain is a very common problem. There are three groups of patients with this type of pain: the previously healthy patient with an acute episode, the chronically afflicted patient with an undetermined diagnosis, and the patient with chronic back pain with a defined pathologic state. The majority of patients fall into the first group.

History

Appropriate questions to pose during the history are the following: *o*nset, *p*osition, *q*uality, *r*adiation, associated *s*ymptoms, and *t*emporal relationships. Determine that the symptoms are not referred pain (see the box above). Differentiate between the pain arising from a musculoskeletal source and that of compression of a nerve root. Several questions that should be answered include the following: Is there urinary or fecal incontinence or retention? Are paresthesias present? Are there any changes in leg size?

DIFFERENTIAL DIAGNOSIS OF LOWER BACK PAIN

Renal
Pyelonephritis
Nephrolithiasis

Vascular
Aortic anuerysm

Gastrointestinal
Pancreatitis
Posterior penetrating peptic ulcer
Pilonidal cyst

Genitourinary
Pelvic inflammatory disease
Ectopic pregnancy
Ovarian cyst

Infectious
Epidural abcess
Musculi psoas abcess
Osteomyelitis
Meningitis
Shingles

Oncology
Malignancy with metastases to the lower spine, particularly the prostate

Physical Examination

The evaluation of a patient who is complaining of lower back pain includes careful abdominal, genitourinary, and rectal examinations. Note the patient's position. Most patients with severe musculoskeletal back pain lie flat and still. Observe how the patient moves. Check feet and toe walking strength. Document any obvious deformities, muscular atrophy, or signs of

Table 17-3

MONOARTICULAR AND POLYARTICULAR ARTHRITIS OVERVIEW

Diagnosis	Patient Type	Examination	Laboratory	Radiology	Treatment
Gout	Middle-aged patients; 9:1 male-to-female distribution	Occurs usually in first MTP joint; gouty tophi	Negative birefringent crystals	Assymetric bone destruction with overhanging edge	NSAIDs; IV colchicine; steroids
Pseudogout	Middle-aged patients; equal sex distribution	Most commonly affects knee, wrist, ankle, elbow	Positive birefringent crystals	Linear cartilage calcification	NSAIDs; IV colchicine; steroids
Septic arthritis	All age groups; immunocompromised	Fever accompanied with erythematous; warm, painful joint	Prurulent joint aspirate	Minimal changes in early stage; bone destruction in late stage	Antibiotics
Bursitis/tendinitis	More prevalent in older patients	Focal area of pain with distinct radiation	Nondiagnostic	Tendon calcification	NSAIDs; local steroids
Osteoarthritis	More prevalent in older patients	Joint deformities; Bouchard and Heberden nodes	Nondiagnostic	Uneven, narrowed joint spaces with osteophyte formation	NSAIDs

Rheumatoid Arthritis	Familial predominance; middle-aged women	Joint deformities; symmetric pattern	Rheumatoid factor; anemia; elevated ESR	Symmetric joint space narrowing; marginal erosions	NSAIDs; steroids, methotrexate; gold; azathioprine; penicillamine
Reiter syndrome	May be a familial predominance; adult men	Asymmetric conjunctivitis; urethritis; diarrhea	HLA-B27	Fluffy periostitis	NSAIDs
Gonococcocal arthritis	2:1 female-to-male distribution	Migratory arthritis; hemorrhagic, necrotic pustules	Blood, pharyngeal, urethral, cervical, pustule cultures	Nondiagnostic	NSAIDs; penicillin; possible steroids
Lyme disease	All age groups	Erythema chronicum migrans; neurologic/cardiac abnormalities	Lyme titers	Nondiagnostic	NSAIDs; antibiotics
Acute rheumatic fever	All age groups	Erythema chronicum migrans; subcutaneous nodules	Pharyngeal cultures; ASO; streptozyme, anti-DNase, C-proteins	Nondiagnostic	NSAIDs; antibiotics
Viral arthritis	All age groups	Migratory; assymetric	Varied	Nondiagnostic	NSAIDs

Table *17-4*

EXAMINATION FOR NERVE ROOT COMPRESSION

Site of Disk Herniation	Nerve Root Involved	Reflex Changes	Motor Changes	Pain Distribution and Sensory Changes	Comment
L3-L4	L4	Decreased knee jerk	Weakness of quadriceps	Anterolateral thigh, across knee, and down anteromedial leg	Uncommon site for disk herniation
L4-L5	L5	Usually not associated with reflex changes; occasionally knee jerk is decreased	Weakness of anterior tibial, peroneal, and extensor hallucis longus muscles (weak dorsal flexion of foot and big toe)	Posterolateral thigh, anterolateral leg, medial and dorsal foot, and big toe; occassionally numbness of heel and bottom of foot	Trouble with heel walking
L5-S1	S1	Decreased/absent ankle jerk	Weakness of gastrocnemius and soleus muscles (weakness of plantar flexion)	Posterior thigh, posterior leg, and lateral foot (fourth and fifth toes)	Trouble with toe walking or standing on tiptoes
Cauda equina syndrome	S2, S3, S4, S5; possibly lower lumbar roots	Decreased rectal tone; loss of bulbocarvernosus reflex and anal work	Diffuse motor weakness in lower extremities may progress to paraplegia	Perineal or "saddle anesthesia"	Bowel and bladder problems, especially urinary retention—may appear with bilateral sciatica

From Roberts JR: In focus: low back pain, sciatica, and disc disease, *Emergency Medicine and Ambulatory Care News*, p. 10, May 1989.

trauma. Palpate the spine and lower back, and look for tenderness or muscular spasms. Test straight-leg raising, because increased radiation of pain on the side opposite the straight-leg raising has been associated with a herniated lumbar disk. Palpate the lower extremities. Check the strength of the various muscle groups and the range of motion of the various joints. Document any change in sensation of the lower extremities and the perirectal area (diminished sensation in the perirectal area is seen with the cauda equina syndrome). Check the reflexes of the lower extremities: knee jerk (L3, L4) and ankle jerk (S1); check motor strength: first-toe dorsiflexion (L5) and plantar flexion of the foot (S1).

Radiology

Radiographic studies should be obtained in patients with the following characteristics: extremes of age (younger than 18 years and older than 50 years), chronic persistent back pain, the possibility of metastatic cancer, or osteomyelitis.

Computed tomography (CT scan), magnetic resonance imaging (MRI), and radionuclide imaging are other modalities that have proven helpful in evaluating lower back pain. The CT scan is probably the most common study used to evaluate disk lesions and bony abnormalities. In conjunction with myelography, the CT scan has been used to evaluate canal stenosis, but an MRI is more accurate and less invasive. A MRI can study multiple levels of spine in a sagittal orientation. Radionuclide imaging is the modality of choice for localizing metastatic or infectious causes of bone destruction.

Management

Musculoskeletal lumbosacral strain is the most common cause of lower back pain. The patient commonly relates a history of strenuous activity several hours before presentation. The pain is often exacerbated by hip flexion. Other than tenderness, the physical examination is normal.

Treatment includes strict bed rest for 2 days and NSAIDs. Muscle relaxants often help (e.g., cyclobenzaprine [flexeril] 10 mg tid). All patients benefit from weight loss, strengthening exercises, and using the correct position for lifting (i.e., bending and lifting with knee and hip flexion with a nonflexed spine).

Lumbar disk disease causes a degeneration of the annulus pulposus, which predisposes the disk to rupturing and herniation. Pain results from a physical compression or impingement on the nerve roots. The patient is often in severe distress, and minor motion often causes intense pain. The L4-L5 and L5-S1 levels are the most common area of disk disease (Table 17-4).

All patients with an acute neurologic deficit should have a neurosurgical consultation. A CT scan and MRI are useful to determine the need for emergent surgical decompression. Treatment also includes bed rest and analgesics.

Vertebral compression fractures usually are caused by a fall or acute flexion of the spine. The conditions of osteoporosis, metastatic malignancy, and metabolic bone disease predispose patients to these fractures. Pain occurs immediately, and point tenderness can be elicited on physical examination. Intestinal ileus can be a complication of vertebral fracture.

Although diagnosis is made by plain x-ray studies, the extent of spinal cord impingement is best determined with a CT scan or an MRI. Neurosurgical consultation is indicated when neurologic deficits are present. Management includes bed rest, analgesics, and physical therapy.

Recommended Reading

Campono, BA: Soft tissue spine injuries and back pain. In Rosen P et al, editors: *Emergency medicine: concepts and clinical practice,* ed 3, St Louis, 1992, Mosby.

Ezell SL, Kobernick ME, Benjamin GC: Arthrocentesis. In Roberts JR, Hedges JR, editors: *Clinical procedures in emergency medicine,* ed 2, Philadelphia, 1991, WB Saunders.

Jenkins J, Brown CG: Rheumatologic emergencies. In Harwood-Nuss A et al, editors: *Clinical practice of emergency medicine,* Philadelphia, 1991, JB Lippincott.

Resnick D, Niwayama G, editors: *Diagnosis of bone and joint disorders,* 4 vols, ed 2, Philadelphia, 1988, WB Saunders.

Roberts JR: In focus: low back pain, sciatica, and disc disease, *Emergency Medicine and Ambulatory Care News,* March, April, May, 1989.

Talbot-Stern JK: Arthritis, tendinitis, bursitis. In Rosen P et al, editors: *Emergency medicine: concepts and clinical practice,* ed 3, St Louis, 1992, Mosby.

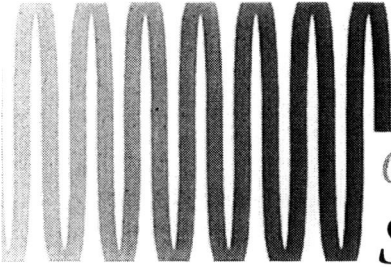

Chapter Eighteen

SEIZURE

MICHAEL CHARLES TOMLANOVICH

An epileptiform seizure represents the clinical expression of a paroxysmal and excessively disordered discharge of cerebral neurons and can be a sign of various neurologic and systemic disorders. Depending on the location of these hyperexcitable neurons, the seizure can be manifested as any combination of altered consciousness and disturbances in motor, sensory, or autonomic functions. The term *seizure* is generic, and other specific descriptions may be applicable according to the characteristics observed. Seizures may be isolated or repetitive. Seizures that spontaneously recur over a span of years are termed *epilepsy*. Generalized motor seizures are also called convulsions. Status epilepticus is a prolonged continuous seizure or a series of repetitive seizures without interictal consciousness.

ETIOLOGY

The causes of seizures are numerous, and the pathophysiologic categorization can be used as a guide in organizing the various etiologies (Table 18-1).

Almost any type of cerebral insult and many systemic disorders can evoke seizures. Etiologically, seizures are usually divided into primary, or idiopathic, and secondary, or acquired, types. The cause of primary seizures either cannot be determined or is attributed to a genetic predisposition. With the advancement of medical knowledge and the introduction of new diagnostic modalities, seizures are increasingly classified in the secondary category. The known cause of secondary seizures may be static (e.g., posttraumatic scars), dynamic (e.g., degenerative disease), or acutely transient (e.g., hypoglycemia). In addition to the underlying cause, various precipitating factors exist that are usually not themselves epileptogenic but that can activate a preexisting seizure focus. These precipitants include emotional stress, fatigue, sleep deprivation, hyperventilation, menstruation, photic stimulation, drug withdrawal, and alcohol abuse and other intoxications. Many experts support the probability that alcohol abuse can be an independent, dose-related causal factor for seizures in individuals who are otherwise normal. The search for the specific cause of a seizure is of prime importance, because identification of the cause helps determine the prognosis for seizure recurrence and guides therapeutic decision making.

CLASSIFICATION

Classification systems of seizures facilitate the recognition, management, and clinical investigation of seizures. The International Classification

Table **18-1**

CAUSES OF SEIZURES

Type	Cause	Type	Cause
Primary	Genetic	Neoplastic	Primary and metastatic CNS tumors
	Idiopathic	Perinatal	Infection
Secondary			Metabolic disorders
Degenerative	Hereditary myoclonus		Prematurity
	Multiple sclerosis		Trauma
	Myoclonic cerebellar dyssynergia	Toxic	Drug intoxication or withdrawal
	Presenile dementia		Heavy metal poisoning
	Sturge-Weber syndrome		Plant toxins
	Tuberous sclerosis	Traumatic	Cerebral contusion or laceration
Infectious	Cerebral abscess		Epidural or subdural hematoma
	Encephalitis	Vascular	Arteriosclerosis
	Jakob-Creutzfeldt disease		Arteriovenous malformation
	Meningitis		Cerebral infarction
	Neurosyphilis		Subarachnoid or intracerebral hemorrhage
	Parasitic infections		Vasospasm (migraine)
Metabolic	Addison disease	**Miscellaneous**	Burn encephalopathy
	Fluid and electrolyte disorders		Eclampsia
	Hepatic failure		Fever
	Hypercapnia		Hypertensive encephalopathy
	Hyperosmolar states		Menstruation
	Hypoglycemia		
	Hypothyroidism		
	Hypoxemia		
	Inborn errors of metabolism		
	Porphyria		
	Pyridoxine deficiency		
	Respiratory alkalosis		
	Thyrotoxicosis		
	Uremia		

of Epileptic Seizures is a useful conceptual framework (see the box on p. 203).

Generalized Seizures

Generalized seizures are characterized by the absence of signs and symptoms related to a focal anatomic or functional part of a single hemisphere. These seizures are also referred to as centrencephalic, and the EEG recordings demonstrate that symmetric and grossly synchronous discharges occur over both hemispheres from the onset. For this reason, there is no associated preictal aura. The common clinical features of generalized seizures include both an initial impairment of consciousness and ex-

INTERNATIONAL CLASSIFICATION OF EPILEPTIC SEIZURES

Generalized seizures (bilaterally symmetric and without local onset)

Absences (petit mal)
Bilateral massive epileptic myoclonus
Infantile spasms
Clonic seizures
Tonic seizures
Tonic-clonic seizures (grand mal)
Atonic seizures
Akinetic seizures

Partial seizures (seizures that begin locally)

With elementary symptomatology and generally without impairment of consciousness
    With motor symptoms (includes jacksonian epilepsy)
    With special sensory or somatosensory symptoms
    With autonomic symptoms
    Compound forms
With complex symptomatology and generally with impairment of consciousness
    With impairment of consciousness only
    With cognitive symptomatology
    With affective symptomatology
    With psychosensory symptomatology
    With psychomotor symptomatology (automatisms)
    Compound forms
Secondarily generalized

Unilateral seizures (or predominantly unilateral seizures)

Unclassified epileptic seizures (incomplete data)

---

tensive autonomic changes that are often accompanied by bilaterally symmetric motor changes. These motor signs can be manifested as either muscular contractions or atony.

Generalized seizures can be broadly classified as convulsive (e.g., tonic-clonic) or nonconvulsive (e.g., akinetic) and are reported to account for more than two thirds of all seizure episodes. However, this statistic may be excessively high because many partial seizures terminate with secondary generalization. The detection of an initial partial seizure largely depends on its duration and the presence of observable clinical manifestations. Retrograde amnesia can obscure initial partial sensory seizures.

Convulsive generalized seizures

The tonic-clonic seizure is the most prevalent type of generalized convulsion. Grand mal epilepsy is a chronic idiopathic tonic-clonic seizure disorder and has been extensively studied and described. It occurs equally in both sexes, and more than two thirds of all patients with this type of seizure are affected by the time they reach puberty. Seizure episodes can be provoked by drug withdrawal, photic stimulation, menstruation, fatigue, alcohol or other intoxications, and falling asleep or awakening.

One type of secondary tonic-clonic convulsion is the alcohol withdrawal seizure, which is a common emergency problem. The occurrence of a withdrawal seizure reflects physiologic dependence, which can develop after a few weeks of daily heavy alcohol exposure. These seizures occur in patients who have a continued long-standing problem with alcohol abuse, but they can also occur in spree or periodic drinkers and have been reported to occur after sprees as short as 5 days. Alcohol withdrawal seizures are a distinct and characteristic clinical syndrome. The seizures start in adult life and begin 6 to 48 hours after the cessation of a period of sustained heavy alcohol consumption. The entire convulsive disorder consists of one to five brief and spontaneously abating, generalized tonic-clonic seizures that occur over a period of usually less than 6 hours. The seizures can begin several days after the cessation of drinking and can be repetitive over several days, but these are rare occurrences. Alcohol withdrawal seizure is not a chronic epileptic disorder but is self-limited to the immediate abstinence period, with normal EEG recordings before and after the ictal episode. The acute abuse or cessation of alcohol can precipitate convulsions in patients with chronic idiopathic and secondary epilepsies such as posttraumatic seizures. Such patients are distinguished by a history of prior nonabstinence seizures, interictal EEG abnormalities, or focal convulsions.

Generalized clonic seizures are the prevalent pattern of febrile convulsions, which constitute the most common childhood neurologic problem and affect approximately 2% to 5% of all individuals under age 5 years. Various ictal characteristics are important in classifying febrile convulsions as either simple or complex. Together with other preictal and postictal features, these characteristics have a significant bearing on recurrence rates, long-term therapeutic considerations, and the prognosis for the

development of a chronic epileptic disorder. In general, a febrile convulsion can be defined as a seizure in a child younger than 6 years of age accompanied by a fever in excess of 38° C without evidence of intracranial infection or intoxication. Patients between the ages of 6 months and 5 years have 95% of all febrile convulsions, with peak incidence occurring during the second year of life. Most convulsions are generalized and subside within 20 minutes. They are usually seen within 2 to 6 hours after the onset of fever (almost always within 24 hours) and are usually associated with upper respiratory tract infections, primarily pharyngitis, and otitis media. Additionally, a high reported incidence of febrile convulsions is associated with both roseola infantum and Shigella gastroenteritis. Positive family histories of febrile convulsions have been reported in more than 50% of all such patients, and the inherited tendency to exhibit seizures seems to be greater with febrile convulsions than with other afebrile epileptic disorders. Simple febrile convulsions are characterized by an initial onset between the age of 9 to 18 months (rarely before 6 months). These convulsions tend not to occur in series, have no focal features, last less than 15 minutes, appear soon after a sudden rise in temperature, and have a high familial incidence. Febrile seizures that are long in duration, focal, or occur in a series are designated as complex. Complex febrile convulsions may indicate an underlying organic disorder or epilepsy precipitated by fever.

Nonconvulsive generalized seizures

Atonic, akinetic, simple absence, and complex absence seizures can be grouped as nonconvulsive generalized seizures. The EEG recordings are nonfocal, and the predominant clinical manifestations involve a loss of consciousness of varying degrees and one or more autonomic changes. Gestural and ambulatory automatisms can be observed along with motor activity that is usually minor and restricted to the head and neck. Loss of motor tone occurs in atonic seizures, and motor immobility occurs in akinetic seizures.

Simple absence (petit mal) seizures have an incidence of less than 5% among individuals with childhood epilepsy. The onset of these seizures almost always occurs in patients between ages 3 and 15 years, and the EEG findings are classic and pathognomonic of petit mal epilepsy. Petit mal epilepsy is a primary disorder with a rarely discoverable organic cause. The seizure is characterized by a complete suppression of all cognitive mental functions, which is manifested by sudden immobility and a blank stare. Associated simple automatisms and minor facial clonic movements may occur, particularly with the eyelids. The episodes are brief and last less than 30 seconds, with an abrupt onset and termination and no preictal or postictal elements. Amnesia for the ictal events is common; the patient usually continues with preictal activities but may have a subjective sense of lost time.

Partial Seizures

Partial seizures are distinguished by their initial manifestations and arise from epileptogenic discharges that are localized in a limited anatomic or functional part of a single hemisphere. The EEG recordings can be variable but at least initially are restricted to the affected region. Preictal auras can occur in patients in this group and have characteristics related to the ictal focus. There are many forms of partial seizures with simple or complex symptomatology, and they can be described in terms of the symptoms produced (e.g., somatomotor) or the involved anatomic site (e.g., frontal lobe).

Simple partial seizures

Simple partial seizures include sensory, autonomic, or motor manifestations. They are usually brief, begin and end abruptly, and involve little or no alteration of consciousness. Somatosensory seizures are characterized by various exteroceptive peripheral and afferent cranial nerve sensations (e.g., paresthetic, visual, olfactory) that occur without appropriate stimuli. Gastrointestinal, circulatory, respiratory, and genitourinary changes occur during autonomic seizures. Somatomotor seizures are usually clonic and show a predilection for the face, hands, and feet. These partial motor seizures may be static or dynamic. Jacksonian epilepsy demonstrates progressive motor involvement as the discharge spreads along the motor cortex. The sequence of motor propagation can follow the somatotopic arrangement of the precentral gyrus.

Complex partial seizures

Complex partial seizures involve extensive cortical regions; patients manifest mental and psychic symptoms that consist of affect changes, automatisms, confusion, disturbed ideations, hallucinations, and memory deficits. These seizures are usually longer in duration than simple partial seizures, have a more gradual onset and termination, and involve an associated impairment of consciousness. Most patients with partial seizures occasionally experience a progression of the local attack into a generalized convulsion. If this secondary generalization occurs rapidly, the focal phenomena may go unobserved.

The specific nature of a partial seizure is useful in localizing the area of epileptogenic focus, but neither the type or severity of the seizure nor the localization necessarily aids in identifying the underlying brain lesion. The most common causes of complex partial tumors include tumors, birth injuries, trauma, and postinflammatory scarring. Psychomotor or temporal lobe epilepsy is the most common type of partial seizure disorder and is classified in the group with complex symptomatology. The typical age of the patient at the initial seizure extends from late childhood into early adulthood. In many instances, psychomotor attacks are terminated by a generalized motor seizure. If the focal temporal lobe elements are brief or of an inconspicuous character, the seizure episode can be easily misinterpreted as a generalized convulsion rather than partial epilepsy with secondary generalization. Such misinterpretations may account for the wide variations in the reported prevalence of complex partial seizures and the apparent paucity or their appearances in the emergency department setting.

Temporal lobe seizures typically have a sequence of components that begin with the aura, are followed by various autonomic changes and automatisms (motor activity without voluntary control), and finally abate in any of several different ways. The nature of these attacks remains similar in an individual patient, but a broad diversity of manifestations occurs among patients who have psychomotor epilepsy.

Status Epilepticus

Status epilepticus is seizure activity that persists for more than 1 hour or involves repeated seizures that produce a fixed and enduring epileptic condition for more than 1 hour. Status epilepticus can be classified as two general types: convulsive and nonconvulsive. Convulsive status epilepticus may be generalized or focal and is distinguished by the presence of muscular contractions. Petit mal and psychomotor status are types of nonconvulsive status epilepticus and include mild-to-severe alterations in the level of consciousness and confusion with or without automatisms.

The incidence of status epilepticus among patients with epilepsy has been reported to be 1.3% to 10%. The difference between idiopathic and secondary epilepsy is remarkable. Convulsive status epilepticus occurs approximately six times more often in patients with secondary epilepsy and is probably related to the proposed major pathogenetic factors. On the other hand, nonconvulsive status epilepticus almost always occurs in patients with primary epilepsy or chronic epilepsy of unknown cause. Status epilepticus can occur in patients of any age, and although the causes are similar, the prevalence of each cause varies with the patient's age.

The list of underlying causes of status epilepticus is quite extensive; the most common causes are trauma, tumors, cerebrovascular disease, CNS system infections, and metabolic disorders. Individuals with idiopathic seizure disorders can experience status epilepticus, and these have been reported to constitute as much as one third of all cases. However, status epilepticus is rarely the initial manifestation of idiopathic epilepsy and generally appears many years after the onset of seizures. Status epilepticus is not considered to be an expected event in the course of a seizure disorder, and its occurrence requires specific explanation. Several underlying conditions are thought to give rise to the pathogenesis of status epilepticus, including gross brain damage, extensive cerebral dysfunction, involvement of the subcortical white matter, diffuse cerebral edema, or focal lesions involving the frontal lobes. When such conditions exist, various precipitating factors can trigger an episode of status epilepticus. Progressive cerebral disease, infection, acute trauma, anticonvulsant withdrawal, alcohol, and irradiation are some of the factors that play such a role.

DIAGNOSIS

The occurrence of a suspected or verified seizure warrants a comprehensive evaluation in an effort to identify a treatable illness or correctable focal cerebral lesion.

History

An assessment of the patient's history is usually the most revealing aspect of the diagnostic work-up. If appropriately detailed, the history can facilitate a more proficient course of investigative intervention, therapeutic decision making, and ultimate disposition. Interviews with relatives (or other observers when available) are at times necessary to obtain a detailed history. Individuals with established epileptic disorders are generally seen in the emergency department when the seizure episodes increase in frequency or duration or when they occur in an unfamiliar environment. It is useful to ascertain the patient's age at onset, prior adequate evaluation, ongoing care, anticonvulsant medication, and the degree of control of seizures. The cause of the seizure should be determined whenever possible. It should be noted that complete medical control of the seizure disorder cannot be achieved for a significant number of patients with epilepsy. The common precipitating factors should be reviewed, and in many instances poor medication compliance or alcohol abuse is discovered. A history of loss of consciousness or loss of awareness associated with abnormal movements or confusion is a strong suggestion for this diagnosis. The direct observation of a seizure by the physician is the best way of making the diagnosis, but a reasonable alternative is a reliable and thorough account of the witnessed ictal and postictal features, with particular attention given to any element that suggests localization. If possible, the patient should be questioned with regard to a possible precipitating event, the occurrence of a localizing aura, any acute illness, current medications, exposure to toxins or substance abuse, any past head injury or past cerebral infection, and any known chronic diseases, especially hepatic, renal, cardiovascular, neurologic, metabolic, or neoplastic disorders. With children, additional information needs to be elicited concerning the mother's history of any pregnancy or perinatal problems, developmental abnormalities or immunization reactions in the child, and the family history of febrile and afebrile seizures or any other genetically predisposing cerebral disorder.

Physical Examination

Although the findings are often normal, a careful general physical examination should be performed and occasionally provides clues to a possible underlying cause. Special emphasis should be placed on the neurologic evaluation in a search for mental status, cranial nerve, or peripheral motor, sensory, or reflex abnormalities. A transient focal paresis (Todd paralysis) in the postictal period is highly suggestive of a local brain lesion. A protracted confusional state can represent nonconvulsive status epilepticus.

The head and neck should be examined for papilledema, cranial bruits, fontanelle fullness, abnormal facies, gingival lead lines, focal infection, and nuchal rigidity. The presence of a pulmonary neoplasm or infection and cardiac murmurs or dysrhythmias may indicate a cerebral metastasis, abscess, or embolism. An examination of the skin can reveal peripheral hypopigmented macules and facial sebaceous adenomas associated with tuberous sclerosis (an inherited disorder manifested by a triad of seizures, mental deficiency, and adenoma sebaceum), cutaneous neurofibroma and cafe au lait spots associated with intracranial gliomas and neurofibromas (von Recklinghausen disease), and vascular nevi associated with cerebral hemangiomas. In patients with fever, an attempt should be made to determine the source. The evidence of acute intraoral injury and urinary incontinence also lend support to the diagnosis of a seizure.

Laboratory Tests

Laboratory procedures performed in the emergency setting are best guided by the historic and physical findings. An individual with a previously evaluated chronic seizure disorder who is otherwise normal may require only a determination of the serum anticonvulsant level or no studies at all. On the other hand, patients with new-onset seizures should have various baseline levels determined at least initially. Periodic repeat evaluations may also be beneficial to patients with partial seizures of undetermined cause.

Although not consistently abnormal in patients with chronic epilepsy, EEG recordings provide a definitive diagnosis. Such an evaluation is generally not available in the emergency department but should be planned for future follow-up when appropriate. Other routine studies can reveal indirect but useful data. An ECG, complete blood count, urinalysis, and determinations of the levels of serum electrolytes, blood glucose, blood urea nitrogen, serum calcium, and arterial blood gases (at least 1 hour after the seizure) furnish information about infection, blood dyscrasias, and metabolic and cardiac disturbances. Appropriate cultures should be obtained in the presence of fever or a suspected infection. Chest x-ray studies aid in assessing the cardiac status and pulmonary infections and neoplasms. In the absence of signs of high intracranial pressure or after a normal CT scan of the head, a lumbar puncture should be performed whenever the possibility of an intracranial infection exists. Cerebrospinal fluid examination should also be considered for all patients under the age of 18 months who have had either a first or a recurrent febrile convulsion because the clinical signs of meningitis are notoriously unreliable in these patients. In patients with normal cell counts, an elevated level of total protein favors the possibility of a tumor. An emergency CT scan is advantageous in patients with seizures that are attributable to perinatal complications or associated with acute head trauma or suspected intracranial bleeding.

TREATMENT

The vast majority of seizure episodes are relatively benign and short, with spontaneous termination and prompt recovery. The diagnostic evaluation prospectively guides therapeutic direction by differentiating those individuals who can be definitively treated for acutely reversible causes from those at risk for chronic recurrence who may require long-term prophylactic therapy or surgical intervention. The priority of therapy is to stabilize the airway, ventilation,

and circulation; correct the underlying disease, if possible; and control the seizures if necessary. Seizures are an immediate problem in the emergency department, and the priority of care is related to the stability of the patient's vital signs and state of consciousness. The patient should be placed in an area that facilitates ready observation for any further seizure activity. If a convulsion occurs, general supportive measures are usually all that is required. Tight clothing and dentures should be removed if possible. The patient should be placed in a lateral decubitus position to avoid aspiration and should be protected against injury by padding hard surfaces, particularly around the head. No attempt should be made to hold the convulsing extremities in a fixed position because doing so may result in bony fractures. A soft object such as a plastic airway tube may be placed in the mouth to prevent intraoral injury, but the benefits of this technique are debatable. Hard or wooden objects should not be used, and the closed tonic jaw should not be forced open because such maneuvers can produce dental or soft tissue injuries and possible tooth aspiration.

Anticonvulsant Therapy

Because most seizures spontaneously abate, there is no need for immediate anticonvulsant drug intervention, which could add certain risks and prolong the postictal period. However, a peripheral intravenous line is placed if possible in preparation for potential parenteral therapy as needed. If a convulsive generalized seizure continues for longer than 5 minutes, the use of a rapid-acting medication of short duration should be considered. Many benzodiazepines have significant anticonvulsant effects, which are mediated in the CNS by inhibiting seizure spread. Intravenous diazepam enters the brain in less than 10 seconds and achieves peak concentration in approximately 8 minutes. Because of rapid, extensive redistribution of diazepam from the central compartment to peripheral fat stores, the pharmacokinetics of its lipid solubility, protein binding, volume of distribution of free drug, and distribution half-life produce a duration of clinical effectiveness of 20 to 30 minutes. Diazepam is administered at intravenous rates of 0.2 to 0.5 mg/minute in infants, 1.0 mg/minute in children over age 5 years, and 2.0 mg/minute in adults up to a total acute dose of 0.15 to 0.25 mg/kg. Lorazepam has an anticonvulsant efficacy similar to diazepam but can take up to 3 minutes to enter the brain and approximately 23 minutes to reach peak concentrations. On the other hand, different pharmacokinetic properties of lorazepam in relation to protein binding and volume of distribution result in slower redistribution and produce a clinical effectiveness for several hours. Lorazepam is administered at intravenous rates similar to diazepam up to a total acute dose of 0.1 mg/kg.

The patient should be closely monitored for signs of respiratory depression and hypotension. The total quantity of a benzodiazepine given acutely is the smallest amount needed to stop the seizure. No specific loading dose is indicated because the use of a benzodiazepine is only a temporizing measure to provide seizure control until underlying reversible factors are corrected or until a loading dose of a long-acting anticonvulsant is administered. Benzodiazepines should not be used intramuscularly in this situation because their onset of action is too slow—they require approximately 1 hour to reach peak serum levels. Patients experiencing nonconvulsive generalized seizures or partial seizures do not usually require such acute drug intervention and can be observed for longer periods in anticipation of spontaneous termination. When the seizure is terminated, the decision to provide additional anticonvulsant therapy depends on the nature of the known or suspected underlying cause. Transient pathophysiologic processes such as hypoglycemia can be otherwise definitively corrected by glucose replacement. Some acute but reversible diseases such as meningitis may require short-term anticonvul-

sant therapy until the infection is adequately controlled.

Established chronic seizures

Individuals with established chronic seizure disorders who convulse because of poor medication compliance require the reinstitution or supplementation of their anticonvulsant medication to restore a therapeutic serum concentration. In such instances it is beneficial to prescribe a full or partial loading dose in the first 24 to 48 hours as indicated by the history and the type of anticonvulsant involved. If serum drug levels are available, the dose can be estimated by the following formula: the loading dose (in mg/kg) equals the volume of the body distribution (in L/kg) times the remainder of the desired serum concentration minus the observed serum concentration (in mg/L):

$$LD = V_D (DL\,[2] - DL\,[1]), \text{ in which}$$
$$LD = \text{loading dose,}$$
$$V_D = \text{volume distribution,}$$
$$DL\,(2) = \text{desired serum concentration and}$$
$$DL\,(1) = \text{observed serum concentration.}$$

Alcohol withdrawal seizures

Patients with alcohol withdrawal seizures and no other known epileptic disorder do not require long-term anticonvulsant therapy. These seizures, even if repetitive, are short with spontaneous termination and usually occur over less than 6 hours. Conservative management with a period of appropriate observation in the emergency department is an acceptable approach. If the patient demonstrates other elements of minor withdrawal such as tremulousness, a benzodiazepine can be used.

Febrile convulsions

In patients with febrile convulsions, the acute treatment is directed at lowering the body temperature with tepid water sponging and appropriate doses of acetaminophen. Patients with acutely prolonged and recurrent seizures should be treated with diazepam. Antibiotic medications are initiated as indicated. The potential need for chronic anticonvulsant therapy depends on the nature of the febrile convulsion, other interictal patient characteristics, and related long-term implications. Chronic prophylaxis for simple febrile convulsions is not recommended because of the magnitude of the population affected, the risks of medication side effects, and the benign nature of febrile convulsions. The ultimate decision to institute chronic treatment is best made in consultation with the physician responsible for the patient's long-term care.

New-onset seizures

Because of the susceptibility for recurrence, the initiation of anticonvulsant therapy should be considered for patients with new-onset seizures and no reversible, clearly defined, or identifiable causes. The institution of such treatment is appropriate in the emergency department when the patient to be admitted has had or is at risk for acute recurrence or when the patient is to be discharged for outpatient follow-up. The benefit of early prophylactic intervention is based on several factors. The patient with an untreated seizure disorder and multiple convulsions is subsequently more difficult to control medically. Each seizure also involves the risk of severe physical injury and potential socioeconomic handicap. Because anticonvulsant medical therapy has long-term implications, it should be begun with the patient's full knowledge and consent. The choice of a specific drug depends on the clinical type of seizure pattern, which is usually ascertained by the history or by observation. Some drugs are more effective with certain types of seizures but may aggravate others. Convulsive generalized seizures are usually the most controllable, and the drugs used also suppress partial seizures—a situation that may reflect a secondary origin of most generalized convulsions. An initial single-drug therapy is generally considered superior and is easier to assess and adjust in the event of an inadequate

response or adverse reaction. Although somewhat variable among individuals and age groups, the therapeutic ranges, toxic levels, half-life values, and volumes of distribution of these drugs provide useful information in determining the maximally effective treatment. Because different anticonvulsants have varied extents of tissue distribution, the achievement of a steady-state therapeutic serum concentration may take days to weeks when therapy is initiated with the usual maintenance dose. In these circumstances, the time interval can be calculated as approximately five to six times the half-life of the drug. However, in crucial situations such as cases of acute repetitive seizures or status epilepticus, a stable therapeutic level can be attained in considerably less time by delivering a loading dose. The rate and route of administration are determined by the life-threatening nature of the seizure activity. In patients with status epilepticus, intravenous routes are used, usually with continuous infusion at rates limited only by predictable serious side effects if too rapid. Under less serious conditions, the loading dose can be given in multiple increments over several hours. In most other instances, it is beneficial to achieve a timely steady-state therapeutic concentration by administering a loading dose orally over the first 24 to 48 hours, unless the dose is hindered by side effects. This strategy is particularly applicable to drugs with a long half-life, such as hydantoins and barbiturates. On the other hand, drugs with a short half-life reach stable therapeutic levels in a few days when the patient is started on only maintenance doses. In any event, the loading dose (in mg/kg) can be calculated as the product of the desired serum concentration (in mg/L) times the volume of body distribution (in L/kg):

$$LD = DL\ (2) \times V_D$$

Long-term Measures

As previously noted, the selection of a chronic maintenance anticonvulsant is related to the seizure pattern (Table 18-2). The drugs typically used in the treatment of convulsive generalized seizures include phenobarbital, phenytoin, mephenytoin, primidone, carbamazepine, and valproic acid. Phenobarbital is generally started first in patients with infrequent seizures and in children under 6 years of age. In instances of frequent seizures, phenytoin is the preferred initial drug. However, in young children, phenytoin may exacerbate seizure activity because of cerebral immaturity and may have adverse effects on developing connective tissue. When a single drug is ineffective, combination therapy can be instituted. Patients with simple partial seizures and those with complex partial seizures (psychomotor) usually respond well to the same drugs used for generalized convulsions. On the other hand, these anticonvulsants are relatively ineffective against nonconvulsive generalized seizures. Patients with these types of seizures are treated with valproic acid, ethosuximide, methsuximide, trimethadione, paramethadione, or clonazepam.

Status Epilepticus

Status epilepticus is a potentially life-threatening event that requires aggressive emergency care. Diagnostic and therapeutic measures should be instituted simultaneously. Blood specimens are obtained to assess the anticonvulsant level when appropriate and to detect possible underlying metabolic abnormalities. If indicated by the history and physical examination, additional microbiologic and toxicologic studies can be requested. General supportive measures are carried out, and an intravenous line is established. The choice of the intravenous fluid should include glucose to supply the metabolic substrate for increased cerebral energy requirements. It is also efficacious to give an appropriate bolus of 50% glucose immediately to reverse potential underlying hypoglycemia. If dextrose is administered, it should be accompanied by thiamine in patients with suspected nutritional deficiencies. Caution should be exercised with fluid ad-

ministration because excess hydration can worsen the cerebral edema secondary to prolonged seizure activity. The specific pharmacologic intervention depends on the type of status epilepticus involved.

The outcome of therapy often depends more on the underlying disease causing the status than on the drugs administered. Some of the conditions resistant to antiepileptic drugs include hypertensive encephalopathy, intracerebral hemorrhage, hypoxemic injury, and meningoencephalitis. Convulsive generalized status epilepticus is the most critical type of seizure because of the stress on the cardiovascular system; respiratory impairment; rhabdomyolysis with renal failure; hyperthermia; and acid-base, electrolyte, and glucose disturbances. The patient's cardiorespiratory and metabolic state should be closely monitored and supported as needed. Appropriate doses of calcium, glucose, and magnesium can be given on empiric grounds or as indicated by laboratory results, if available. It is recommended that neonates also receive pyridoxine. Patients with status epilepticus usually respond to appropriately administered antiepileptic drugs.

If anticonvulsant drug withdrawal is the suspected cause of status epilepticus, the withdrawn medication or its parenterally supplied equivalent should be replaced in doses guided by the serum anticonvulsant level. Otherwise phenytoin is the drug of choice for convulsive generalized status epilepticus because it is effective in more than 80% of these patients, is useful in neonates and infants, causes no respiratory or CNS depression, and is the preferred drug for long-term therapy of convulsive generalized seizure disorders. Phenytoin should be used with great caution when bradycardia, cardiac conduction block, or cardiac failure is present. Phenytoin is administered intravenously in doses of 15 to 18 mg/kg at a rate not to exceed 0.75 mg/kg/minute; this dosage provides a rapid, high therapeutic serum concentration that persists for 18 hours or more. In certain patients, 20 to 30 mg/kg of phenytoin may be necessary to stop status epilepticus. The patient

Table *18-2*

ANTICONVULSANT MEDICATIONS

Drug Group (Generic/Trade)	Therapeutic Use*	Loading Dose (mg/kg)*	Maintenance Dose (mg/kg)
Hydantoins			
Phenytoin (Dilantin)	CGS, SPS, CPS	10-20	4-8
Mephenytoin (Mesantoin)	CGS, SPS, CPS	8-20	3-10
Barbiturates			
Phenobarbital (Luminal)	CGS, SPS, CPS, A, F	8-20	2-5
Mephobarbital (Mebaral)	CGS, SPS, CPS, A, F, M	5-20	2.5-10
Deoxybarbiturates			
Primidone (Mysoline)	CGS, SPS, CPS, A	NIA	10-25
Iminostilbenes			
Carbamazepine (Tegretol)	CGS, SPS, CPS	NIA	10-20
Carboxylic Acids			
Valproic acid (Depakene)	CGS, M, A	NIA	15-30
Oxazolidinediones			
Trimethadione (Tridione)	A	NIA	10-25
Paramethadione (Paradione)	A	NIA	10-25
Succinimides			
Ethosuximide (Zarontin)	A	NIA	20-30
Methsuximide (Celontin)	A, CPS	NIA	5-10
Phensuximide (Milontin)	A	NIA	10-20
Acetylureas			
Phenacemide (Phenurone)	CPS	NIA	15-50
Sulfonamides			
Acetazolamide (Diamox)	A, CGS, SPS	NIA	5-15
Benzodiazepines			
Diazepam (Valium)	M	NIA	0.15-2.0
Clonazepam (Klonopin)	A, M, SPS, CPS	NIA	1-12 mg/day

Modified by J.V. Anandan, Pharm. D.

*CGS, Convulsive generalized seizure; CPS, complex partial seizure; M, myoclonic seizures; SPS, simple partial seizure; A, absence (petit mal); F, febrile seizures; NIA, no information available.

Therapeutic Serum Concentration (mg/L)	Plasma Half-life (hours)	Volume Distribution (L/kg)	Toxicity
10-20	12-80	0.5-0.8	Gastrointestinal distress, ataxia, sedation, gingival hypertrophy, rash, fever
15-40	34, 72-144 (metabolite)	NIA	
10-30	48-96 (↓ in children)	0.88 ± 0.33	Sedation, hyperactivity in children, ataxia, confusion, rash, anemia
10-30	24-25, 48-144 (metabolite)	NIA	
5-10	8.0 ± 4.8 (metabolite)	0.59 ± 0.47	Sedation, vertigo, dizziness, gastrointestinal distress, ataxia, diplopia, nystagmus, rash, anemia, thrombocytopenia
5-10	36 ± 15 (initial) 15 ± 5 (chronic)	1.4 ± 0.2	Diplopia, blurred vision, sedation, dizziness, gastrointestinal distress, leukopenia, jaundice, interstitial pneumonia
55-100	16 ± 3	0.15 ± 0.04	Gastrointestinal distress, sedation, ataxia, hepatitis, thrombocytopenia
>700	12-24, 144-312 (metabolite)	NIA	Sedation, blurred vision, rash, leukopenia, anemia, gastrointestinal distress, hepatitis
NIA	144-312 (metabolite)	NIA	
40-100	30 (child) 60 (adult)	0.72 ± 0.07	Gastrointestinal distress, sedation, dizziness, headache, blood dyscrasias
10-40 (metabolite)	2.6, 36-45 (metabolite)	NIA	
NIA	4	NIA	
NIA	NIA	NIA	Rash, anemia, hepatitis, leukopenia, psychic changes
10-14	4-10	NIA	Acidosis, sedation, hypasthesia, rash, anorexia
0.7	20-90	1.1 ± 0.3	Sedation, ataxia, behavioral changes, hypotension, respiratory depression
0.005-0.05	39 ± 12	3.2 ± 1.1	

must be closely observed for hypotension and bradycardia, which generally result from a rate of infusion that is too rapid. In such patients, the administration should be temporarily stopped and reinstituted at a slower rate. Direct intravenous injection is recommended to minimize precipitation, but phenytoin can be given as a controlled drip infusion using an on-line microfilter with concentrations not to exceed 7 mg/ml in a normal saline solution. Intramuscular phenytoin should not be used because of its extremely slow absorption; it requires 24 hours to reach the peak serum concentration after a single injection. Because phenytoin requires 15 to 20 minutes for safe infusion and may take 20 to 30 minutes to reach peak brain levels, a benzodiazepine can be administered concurrently. Diazepam 0.15 to 0.25 mg/kg or lorazepam 0.1 mg/kg are recommended and are intravenously administered at rates not to exceed 2 mg/minute.

Phenobarbital is the alternate choice to phenytoin in those individuals previously treated successfully with barbiturates, those with severe cardiac conduction disturbances, and those who are allergic to phenytoin. Phenobarbital should be used with caution in patients with myasthenia gravis and cardiorespiratory, hepatic, or renal disease. Phenobarbital can cause hypotension and respiratory depression, especially in patients who have previously received a benzodiazepine. The intravenous loading dose is 8 to 20 mg/kg, and the infusion rate should not exceed 0.75 mg/kg/minute. Phenobarbital may also be given by intramuscular administration. Continued failure to terminate the seizure may result from acute cerebral edema, untreated precipitating factors, a large underlying cerebral lesion, or inadequate anticonvulsant serum concentrations. Efforts directed toward the discovery of an acutely correctable cause need to be vigorously pursued. Particular attention should be given to continued maintenance of adequate ventilation, blood pressure support, euthermia, and metabolic homeostasis.

The use of a neuromuscular blocking agent should be strongly considered when continued status epilepticus produces severe physiologic dysfunction as evidenced by significant hypotension, hyperthermia, hypoxemia, hypercapnia, or acidosis. Neuromuscular blockade facilitates endotracheal intubation, airway protection, ventilation, oxygenation, and control of hyperthermia and rhabdomyolysis. A depolarizing blocking agent such as pancuronium bromide is preferable because of the potential to reverse it with an acetylcholinesterase inhibitor (e.g., neostigmine). The intravenous dose of pancuronium is 0.03 to 0.1 mg/kg, which produces gradual paralysis over several minutes without fasciculation. Although the neuromuscular blockade inhibits peripheral convulsive activity, cerebral electrical dysfunction persists, and the patient continues to be at risk for brain damage. Because the clinical manifestations are suppressed, the further assessment of the patient's ongoing convulsive activity requires EEG monitoring. If this is not feasible, the patient should be considered for transfer to a more appropriate facility where such monitoring capabilities are available or to the operating room for a general anesthetic.

Lidocaine has been used in patients with resistant status epilepticus and may be useful in those with acute CNS lesions. On the other hand, lidocaine may paradoxically enhance status epilepticus in patients with chronic epilepsy. Lidocaine is administered in a single intravenous dose of 2 to 3 mg/kg and is continuously infused at a rate of 3 to 10 mg/kg/hr in the event of recurrence. Finally, a general anesthetic may be used in the treatment of patients with severe generalized status who do not respond to intravenous anticonvulsant agents; halothane is the agent usually recommended.

It should be noted that the hazards of polypharmacy may outweigh the risks of ongoing seizure activity and that drug toxicity may be difficult to distinguish in the patient who is having a seizure. The decision to institute further drug therapy in the emergency department should be carefully evaluated and should reflect an ability to monitor closely and to support vital functions.

DISPOSITION

Although absolute dicta regarding disposition cannot be applied to all individuals with seizures, some general guidelines are useful. The final determination is facilitated by considerations that include the patient's present status and projected course, the appropriate setting for further diagnostic and therapeutic interventions, the potential for patient compliance, and the home environment. Patients with symptomatic seizures resulting from critical underlying disease entities such as meningitis and those experiencing status epilepticus or poorly controlled acute repetitive seizures require hospital admission. The disposition of individuals with new-onset seizures can be determined by the appropriate emergency department evaluation. Patients with a normal physical examination and normal emergency screening tests as previously described can be considered potentially acceptable for further outpatient evaluation and care. Additionally, patients who experience benign isolated seizure episodes but who are otherwise normal can also be safely discharged. These ictal episodes include alcohol withdrawal seizures, simple febrile convulsions, recurrent seizures in patients with chronic epilepsy, and isolated seizures secondary to acute reversible causes such as hypoglycemia. In these instances, proper patient instruction and appropriate, planned follow-up are essential.

PROGNOSIS

The long-term prognosis for patients with seizures is as varied as the underlying causes. The acute morbidity and mortality are related to the circumstances, character, and cause of the ictal episode and occur with the greatest incidence in patients with status epilepticus. Modern treatment has improved the overall course of patients with chronic epilepsy; 30% to 60% of all such patients are seizure free and another 25% are greatly improved after the initiation of therapy. However, a significant subgroup of approximately 20% of the epileptic population does poorly in both medical and social terms. With seizures of uncertain cause, the prognosis for medical control and life expectancy is related to several factors. Idiopathic epilepsy involves a more favorable outlook than seizures of known origin, especially those involving the temporal lobe. The type of seizure pattern has a distinct bearing on medical control, with single types responding better than mixed types. Patients with pure grand mal seizures have the best prognosis, followed by those with pure petit mal seizures, nontemporal lobe partial seizures, petit mal seizures complicated by convulsive generalized seizures, and psychomotor seizures. Associated neurologic deficits; the time interval before the institution of therapy; and the duration, frequency, and severity of the seizure episodes are of predictive value. Along with delayed treatment, multiple repetitive seizures or status epilepticus as the initial expression of epilepsy indicates a poor prognosis for the continuation of seizures. The patient's age at the time of onset is also significant, and initial seizures in individuals over age 45 are usually more easily controlled. However, the onset of seizure disorder in neonates is sometimes associated with subsequent deficient mental development.

Finally, the overall risk of death among epileptic patients ranges from that of the general population to a rate 200% greater and is significantly higher in the poorly controlled epileptic patient. Various factors contribute to an increased risk to the life and health of an epileptic patient, including ictal brain injury, medication side effects, trauma during seizure episodes, and an increased rate of suicide.

KEY CONSIDERATIONS

WHAT IS THE LIFE THREAT?

A seizure can be a manifestation of a life-threatening process such as intracranial hemorrhage, hypoglycemia, hypoxemia, meningitis, hyponatremia, drug overdose, eclampsia, or pediatric infection (febrile seizures).

An uncontrollable seizure (status epilepticus) can result in loss of airway as a result of aspiration of secretions.

DOES THE PATIENT NEED ADMISSION?

The new onset of seizures requires a diagnostic evaluation, including a head CT scan and a neurologic assessment. Seizures resulting from a chronic seizure disorder are usually associated with a subtherapeutic level of anticonvulsant. Such patients can usually be treated with an anticonvulsant regimen to sufficiently restore therapeutic levels of anticonvulsant and be discharged.

WHAT IS THE MOST SERIOUS DIAGNOSIS?

Intracranial hemorrhage or tumor, meningitis, drug overdose, hypoxemia, or eclampsia are the most serious diagnoses.

HAVE I PERFORMED A THOROUGH WORK-UP?

Obtain the history of seizures in the past and perform a physical examination, including a neurologic examination, and search for trauma. Evaluate the patient's oxygenation, glucose level, and CT scan in new-onset seizures.

Recommended Reading

Devinsky O: Epilepsy: diagnosis and treatment, *Neurol Clin* 11:737-990, 1993.

Engel J: *Seizures and epilepsy*, Philadelphia, 1989, FA Davis.

Levy R et al: *Antiepileptic drugs*, ed 3, New York, 1989, Raven Press.

Niedermeyer E: *The epilepsies: diagnosis and management*, Munich, West Germany, 1990, Urban & Schwarzenberg.

Porter R et al: *Alcohol and seizures*, Philadelphia, 1990, FA Davis.

Tomlanovich MC, Yee AS: Seizures. In Rosen P et al, editors: *Emergency medicine: concepts and clinical practice*, ed 3, St Louis, 1992, Mosby.

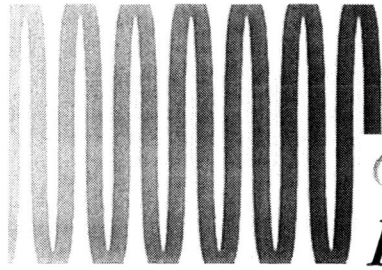

Chapter *Nineteen*
HEAD TRAUMA

PETER PONS

One of the principal causes of morbidity and mortality after multiple- or single-organ trauma is injury to the brain. Although the ultimate outcome often depends on the magnitude of the original insult, survival can be optimized with appropriate management of these grave injuries. Moreover, only a small percentage of head injuries encountered in the emergency department are critical. Nevertheless, it is for those few critical injuries that aggressive and compulsive care has the most to provide, and for those serious but subtle injuries for which timely intervention will preserve life or brain function.

PATHOPHYSIOLOGY

An almost infinite variety of mechanisms produce head injury. It is often hard to determine the exact mechanism of injury because of the amnesia that follows the original blow and because head injuries often occur in the context of alcohol consumption. One of the major challenges of emergency medicine is to distinguish between the coma of alcohol and the coma of head injury, which will be discussed later in this chapter.

Although the vast majority of head injuries are caused by blunt trauma, the brain is also subject to injury from penetrating trauma. Sometimes the penetration is hard to perceive, such

as with stab wounds of the head. However, the skull is not of uniform thickness, so cranial penetration must be sought aggressively. Less subtle are the penetrating injuries of gunshot wounds. Because not all of these injuries are lethal, aggressive and diligent care can preserve brain function and life itself.

Blunt injury of the brain may result from direct trauma to the head or indirectly from acceleration or deceleration forces. Several factors may be in action to produce brain injury. Fractures of the skull may disrupt arteries or veins, which leads to hematoma formation within the cranium. As it expands, the hematoma compresses the brain and may result in herniation. Blunt injury can also produce internal penetration via the mechanism of depressed skull fracture, with a spicule of bone being driven into the brain itself. Depressed skull fractures occur when great pressure is applied over a small area by devices such as high-heeled shoes or ball peen hammers. Finally, the brain can be injured without a direct blow to the head as when there is marked deceleration against a seat belt and the brain continues its forward motion within the skull. This continued motion may result in direct destruction of tissue as the brain strikes interior structures of the skull or dural shelves, shearing of brain tissue, or hemorrhage from torn blood vessels.

Common to all mechanisms of brain injury is that the brain is confined within a fixed space.

This fact is true even in the child whose sutures have not yet closed. The brain responds to injury of any type by retaining fluid and swelling. Therefore as the brain increases its volume, it does so against the fixed volume of the skull. Ultimately this progressive swelling produces the development of a variety of herniation syndromes. Often the pressure on the midbrain caused by the herniation effort leads to focal findings and the subsequent death of the patient.

Compounding the natural swelling in response to injury is the impairment of respiration that occurs with cerebral injury. As carbon dioxide is retained, blood flow within the cerebral vault increases and in turn increases brain volume at a time when the brain can least afford it. Because intracranial pressure is closely related to both hypoxemia and hypercapnia, the brain is ultimately compressed from both internal and external causes. Again these changes will be reflected by the development of focal neurologic findings as the brain attempts to escape the cranial vault.

As intracranial pressure increases, cerebral blood flow diminishes or ceases, which further compounds the vicious cycle that is occurring. By the time the changes known as the Cushing reflex—hypertension and bradycardia—are seen, cerebral function has been destroyed and the patient is essentially brain dead. It is therefore incumbent on the emergency physician to attempt to prevent intracranial hypertension and to reverse coning syndromes before they are fully developed. To await the development of focal findings or the Cushing reflex before aggressively treating the head injury is to ensure brain death.

ASSESSMENT

Many aspects of the patient's history, as well as an understanding of the injury mechanism are important in the assessment of a head injury.

> ### NEUROLOGIC EXAMINATION OF THE PATIENT WITH A HEAD INJURY
>
> Is the patient awake or unconscious?
> Are the eyes open, or will they open with pain?
> What are the reflexes, and are they equal?
> Can and does the patient move all limbs?
> What is the Glasgow Coma Scale score?
> Is there blood or spinal fluid in the nose or ear?
> What does the rectal examination reveal?

The physical examination of the patient should be performed rapidly and repeated at frequent intervals. It must not, however, be allowed to interfere with more urgent tasks such as intubation of the patient. It is always useful to have a baseline neurologic assessment before taking away the ability to assess the patient because of chemical paralysis. A suggested neurologic examination is shown in the box above.

It must always be considered that other organs may be injured besides the brain. Unfortunately the coma of severe head injury demands so much attention that the emergency physician often forgets to seek other pathologic conditions. Important clues include the mechanism of injury, if known, and the presence of shock because head injury almost never causes hypotension even in the child. Any patient from an automobile accident should be considered to harbor multiple organ trauma even if the head injury appears to predominate. Similarly, falls and batterings may injure much more than the head. Any patient with a severe head injury must be presumed to have a spinal injury, and immobilization precautions should be instigated while the head injury is being investigated.

Patient History

Loss of consciousness is hard to determine historically. There are well-documented cases of patients who were never observed to lose consciousness at the time of injury and yet have significant head injury and amnesia for the traumatic event. It also seems to be a common human response to report losing consciousness after any blow to the head. A more meaningful method of determining neurologic function immediately following injury is to ask the patient the last thing remembered before the injury and the first thing remembered after the injury. Any period of amnesia can be accepted as defining a loss of neurologic function. This concept of loss of function is more important to determine than "the loss of consciousness."

Witnesses should be questioned about the level of function even if the patient appears to be conscious. Repetitive questioning, irritable and high-pitched crying in the child, and an inability to focus intellectually are more common than loss of motor function or sensation and are significant in defining a functional neurologic injury.

It should also be determined whether consciousness was lost before injury to find a problem that may have caused the accident. For example, coma following an accident may be from syncope caused by an acute myocardial infarction. Any prior illness can contribute to, if not cause, the coma being observed. Reversible causes of coma should always be sought by the appropriate administration of naloxone (Narcan) and 50% dextrose.

Seizures can cause accidents or can be caused by the accident. Although quite common after childhood head injuries, posttraumatic seizures do occur in adults as well. They often complicate care because it is hard to immobilize a patient who is seizing.

Neurologic and Physical Examination

While performing the primary assessment of the multiple trauma (or any head-injured patient), quickly determine the Glasgow Coma Scale (GCS) score (Table 19-1). This scale was initially developed as a prognostic indicator rather than as a parameter of monitoring but nevertheless provides a good baseline for comparative observations. What is important about GCS is not any single absolute value but rather the rate and trend of the change. Immediately after a significant blow to the head, a GCS of 3 can often be observed, but if consciousness is quickly regained by the time the patient appears in the

Table *19-1*

GLASGOW COMA SCALE

Eye Opening	Talking	Motor	Score
Does not open eyes	Makes no noise	No motor response to pain	1
Opens eyes with pain	Moans, makes unintelligible sounds	Extensor response (decerebrate)	2
Opens eyes with loud verbal command	Talks, but nonsensical	Flexor response (decorticate)	3
Opens eyes on own	Seems confused, disoriented	Moves part of body but does not remove noxious stimulus	4
	Carries on conversation	Pushes away noxious stimulus	5
	Alert and oriented	Follows simple motor commands	6

emergency department, normal function and a GCS score of 15 is recorded. This information is useful because no single value can be determined in the field to predict outcome. It is ominous if the patient has a score lower than 8 in the field and continues at that level or actually decreases in function in the emergency department. The patient who starts out with a high score and deteriorates also has a poor prognosis. A quick rule is that the GCS score cannot be any higher than 5 or 6 if the patient is unconscious and only responds with motor movement to painful stimuli.

A common concern is the sedation of combative patients. There is no way to protect the spinal integrity if combative behavior is allowed, but sedating the combative patient removes the ability to perform serial neurologic assessments. In fact, once sedated, the patient may be more able to cooperate and demonstrate neurologic status. If not, the patient's pathologic condition will need to be defined with a CT scan rather than with clinical observations.

It can be difficult to determine the presence of *cerebrospinal fluid* in the ear or the nose. It is often mixed with blood, and the wrong conclusions can be drawn—either that the patient has a persistent epistaxis or that blood has run into the ear. In fact, if there is blood in the ear or persistent bloody ooze from the nostril, it should be concluded that there has been a basilar skull fracture and that one is looking at cerebrospinal fluid otorrhea or rhinorrhea.

The importance of an early *rectal examination* cannot be emphasized enough. It is easy to overlook a lack of motor movement of the limbs or to have a patient so intoxicated that there is no limb motion. However, rectal sphincter tone is a good clue that the spinal cord is intact. Moreover, in the male patient it gives useful information about the location of the prostate gland, which may help detect a urethral tear associated with a pelvic fracture.

The status of the patient's *cervical spine* must also be determined. The spine should be palpated, with the examiner checking for any obvious defect and for tenderness elicited during the examination. Until it can be proven otherwise, patients who are unconscious or under the influence of an intoxicant such as alcohol should be presumed to have a cervical spine injury if the mechanism of injury is compatible with the production of such an injury.

Radiologic Evaluation

The principal diagnostic modality for the patient with a head injury is the CT scan. Much controversy exists over whether conventional skull x-ray studies or CT scans should be used. The argument in favor of the skull films is that they are cheaper, show bony pathologic conditions better than the CT scan, and are more readily available. Much concern has been expressed about the cost of unnecessary diagnostic studies, and certainly skull films are overused. There is still a role for conventional skull films; they may be ordered for those patients in whom such films will alter the decisions concerning management. Those patients who have a potentially depressed skull fracture or a potential penetrating injury should be studied. The skull x-ray study also helps in the management decisions for the patient who has a known penetrating injury; for example, does the bullet cross the midline in a gunshot wound of the head?

For the patient with neurologic dysfunction, it is preferable to perform a CT scan. The neurologic dysfunction may range from a persistent headache and inability to concentrate to dizziness or prolonged unconsciousness. Seizures or a worsening of the GCS score also mandate a CT scan. In addition to these symptoms, patients with persistent vomiting (more than two times in an adult and more than three times in a child), weakness, retrograde or antegrade amnesia, or a documented loss of consciousness for longer than 10 minutes should be scanned. Finally, anyone who is to be discharged to an inad-

CRITERIA FOR CT SCANS
Loss of consciousness for > 10 minutes Persistent neurologic dysfunction Persistent vomiting GCS < 8 or deteriorating Retrograde or antegrade amnesia Inadequate social circumstances

CRITERIA FOR CONVENTIONAL SKULL X-RAY STUDIES
Potential for depressed skull fracture Potential for penetrating injury Missile penetration of the skull Potential for management alteration

equate social environment (the patient lives alone or a long distance from the hospital but is refusing admission) and cannot be observed in the hospital should be scanned. The criteria for conventional skull x-ray studies and CT scans are summarized in the boxes above. Less stringent criteria are often applied to children following head trauma.

If patients are unable to cooperate for the study, they will require sedation. If there is any question of neurologic deterioration, they must have active airway management before undergoing the study.

Although it is often desirable to know the results of the head CT scan before treatment, the patient's condition may preclude this knowledge. For example, if the patient is unstable and in hypovolemic shock from a torn spleen, it is wise to perform the laparotomy first and then acquire the CT scan postoperatively rather than have the patient exsanguinate in the CT scan gantry. When the patient develops a coning syndrome, it may be necessary at times to evacuate the mass that is producing the hematoma without the luxury of accurate diagnosis. Fortunately, with rapid new scanners it is possible to obtain quick information and perform a more leisurely detailed study after the patient has been stabilized.

For a suspected hemorrhage, the patient does not need to have contrast enhancement because acute bleeds should be hyperdense compared to surrounding brain tissue for as long as 1 week. Some patients have a normal CT scan when it is initially performed; if their condition worsens, it may be necessary to repeat the study. Many patients are victims of earlier traumas, especially the alcoholic population, and their problems may represent the worsening of a lesion that was already present.

MANAGEMENT

Airway Management

Once the initial assessment has been completed, protection and control of the airway is the first priority in the management of the patient with head injury. If the patient has a GCS score greater than 8, airway management may consist merely of supplemental oxygen unless there are other reasons that mandate active airway control (see the box on p. 224). If the airway needs active control, determine whether there is a cervical spine injury. If the GCS score is 8 or less, the rapid sequence intubation (RSI) (see Chapter 3) is the best route of intubation.

Hyperextension, hyperflexion, or hyperdistraction must be avoided; the neck can be safely stabilized by an assistant while oral intubation is performed. Because of the need to avoid intracranial hypertension, it is preferable not to nasally intubate a patient with a head injury. However, in the field or even with RSI, it may be the only route available. Traditional teaching has

---

MANDATORY AIRWAY MANAGEMENT

Massive facial injuries
Head injury with Glasgow Coma Scale < 8
Penetrating injury to the cranial vault
Missile penetrating injury to the neck
Blunt injury to the neck with expanding
   hematoma or alteration of the voice
Bilateral missile penetrating injuries of the
   thorax
Multisystem trauma with persistent shock

---

been that a cricothyrotomy should be performed. However, recent evidence suggests that the risk of oral intubation in the patient with a suspected neck injury but no evidence of spinal cord damage is less than originally thought and that oral intubation with in-line cervical immobilization is acceptable when the airway must be actively managed.

Once the patient has been actively intubated, it is important to *hyperventilate to a Pco$_2$ of approximately 25 mm Hg.* Below this level there is too little blood flow to the brain, which increases swelling. Above this level there is too much blood flow, which increases swelling. Hyperventilation is the fastest way to treat cerebral edema and an increased intracranial pressure. The patient must not be allowed to buck on the tube, and the tube must not be allowed to become kinked because this will result in a severe and rapid increase in intracranial pressure. For this reason it is often necessary to continue paralysis of the patient with pancuronium (Pavulon) or other longer acting paralytic agents. Although many seriously injured patients appear to have a spontaneous central hyperventilation they are rarely found to be down to the desired Pco$_2$ if the blood gases are measured. Moreover, such patients are unable to protect their airways and therefore are still at risk of aspiration.

Fluid Management

Intravenous fluids are controversial in the patient with a severe head injury. Although one does not want to increase cerebral edema, one does want to maintain perfusion. If the patient is hypotensive, assume that hypovolemia is the cause. A source must be aggressively sought and treated. In the meantime, it is important to give fluids as for other hypovolemic patients without head injuries. Early use of blood and increased attention to fluid quantities are necessary steps to prevent overhydration.

Another controversy is whether to treat the patient with *diuretics.* There appears to be no consensus on when to start osmotic agents. Osmotic agents require a lag time before affecting intracranial pressure and require continuous infusion once started to prevent rebound. Some trauma surgeons prefer not to use these agents while the patient is still hypovolemic, whereas others think that the protection they give the brain is worth the risk of compounding the fluid losses. Some neurosurgeons prefer furosemide (Lasix) to an osmotic agent with the reasoning that it more directly plays a role in keeping the brain cells from swelling; however, there is little clinical evidence that it makes much difference which is used. For the adult a dose of 10 mg of furosemide can be used, and a 1 to 2 g/kg dose of mannitol of a 20% solution can be used if an osmotic agent is desired. For the child, a 1 to 2 mg/kg dose of furosemide and 0.25 to 0.5 g/kg dose of mannitol can be given. It is agreed that the osmotic agents should be used in the presence of a coning syndrome, but in addition to, not instead of, intubation and hyperventilation.

Pharmacologic Management

There is absolutely no evidence that *steroids* are beneficial in the treatment of traumatic cerebral edema. Although they had been used for many years, some evidence is accumulating that suggests they may in fact be harmful.

There is no question that seizures should be

treated once present, but there is still debate regarding the value of *prophylactic anticonvulsant therapy.* Prophylactic anticonvulsant therapy may or may not prevent posttraumatic epilepsy, but it does prevent the acute seizures that often complicate a rising intracranial pressure. Any adult with a GCS score less than 8 and a brain injury demonstrated on a CT scan should be given 1 g phenytoin (Dilantin); children should be given 15 mg/kg. Seizures can be treated with diazepam (Valium) at a dose of 10 to 20 mg in the adult and 0.2 and 0.3 mg/kg in the child. If this dose does not stop the seizures, it may be necessary to add phenobarbital at a dose of 15 mg/kg. Patients in status epilepticus should be paralyzed early in their course, but it must be remembered that this action will stop only the motor manifestations of the seizures, not the seizure activity in the brain.

There is also controversy about the use of *prophylactic antibiotics* for basilar skull fractures. No evidence exists regarding their benefit, but most neurosurgeons still prefer to use them. There may be a difference in risk between rhinorrhea and otorrhea, but the consultant service can choose the therapy because they will be admitting and assuming responsibility for these patients.

The box below summarizes the management for the patient with a GCS score of less than 8.

SEVERE HEAD INJURY—GCS SCORE < 8

Immediate management

Active control of the airway
Hyperventilate to PCO_2 of 25 mm Hg
Paralyze with succinylcholine prn
Maintain paralysis with pancuronium
Phenytoin load

Optional

Prophylactic antibiotics
Osmotic diuretics

SPECIFIC INJURIES

Scalp Laceration

A scalp laceration is probably the most common injury to the head. The scalp is extraordinarily vascular, and it is common to underestimate the magnitude of blood loss from a large scalp laceration. This situation is one in which a head injury can produce hypovolemic shock. If the patient is too unstable for immediate repair of the bleeding scalp, control the bleeding with Raney clips. It is virtually impossible to put a compressive dressing on the head that is tight enough to stop bleeding, and large head dressings serve only as hiding places for large quantities of lost blood. It is easy to confuse a lacerated galea with a skull fracture. If there is uncertainty about the presence of a skull fracture, it may be necessary to order skull x-ray studies.

Concussion

It is hard to find an all-purpose definition of concussion that dictates appropriate management. Rather than limit the definition to the classic description of a brief loss of consciousness, *concussion* is defined as any transient neurologic abnormality with a return to normal function. Although in most instances the return to normalcy is rapid, it may take much longer than is routinely observed. Sophisticated psychologic testing might well demonstrate that what are thought to be minor head injuries are much more dysfunctional than they appear. As suggested previously, if there is an observed or historical loss of consciousness for more than 10 minutes or if there is a persistent loss of or diminished neurologic dysfunction, a CT scan should be performed. It is usually safe to discharge patients who have sustained mild concussions if they have full restoration of normal function, no skull fracture, have undergone a period of observation in the emergency department for at least 2 hours, and have someone available to observe them closely at home. The emergency physician might want to perform a CT scan to be more comfortable about the decision to discharge a patient who lives far from the hospital.

If the patient is to be discharged, narcotic analgesics should not be used. For most mild concussions, the patient experiences relief with aspirin or acetaminophen or a nonsteroidal anti-inflammatory agent. The reality of any discharge is that observation will not be as sophisticated or as thorough as in the hospital. If the person who is to do the observing feels uncomfortable and if it will not be easy for the patient and family to get back into the system, it is preferable to observe the patient for at least 8 hours at the hospital. This role is ideal for an emergency department observation unit.

Discharge instructions are written to ensure nonprofessional recognition of deteriorating neurologic status (see the box below). Even though it is often recommended to wake the patient every 2 hours, this task is hardly ever accomplished, especially with small children. If there is concern that this task will not be done, the patient should be kept at the hospital. If a patient has been discharged and the family calls the hospital for advice, it is safest and wisest to have them immediately return to the hospital. Even if the complaints sound trivial, they often represent true deterioration.

Virtually all other specific consequences of head injury require admission and in-hospital observation and management.

Skull Fracture

For some years it was thought that a skull fracture per se was not a mandate for admission. However, the presence of a skull fracture does represent a significant force applied to the head. Even if much of the force has dissipated by fracturing the skull, there must have been a transmission of force to the brain below. Some studies of complicated head injuries show that patients with skull fractures have many more complications and a poorer prognosis than patients without a fracture. It is much safer to admit all patients with skull fractures and, in most instances, acquire an immediate CT scan study.

Contusion

A cerebral contusion has been defined as a bruise of the brain, which suggests a less serious injury than in fact is present. This condition should be defined more properly as one or more areas of intracerebral hemorrhage, which implies that severe neuronal dysfunction may ensue. In fact, most cases of severe head injury have areas of contusion. When a patient is rendered unconscious from an initial blunt trauma and stays at the same poor GCS score, it is likely that the CT scan will demonstrate multiple areas of contusion accompanied by diffuse cerebral edema.

Any patient with a cerebral contusion should be admitted. In most instances, this is a moot point because these patients have initial GCS scores of 8 or less and should receive the imme-

---

DISCHARGE INSTRUCTIONS FOR MILD HEAD INJURY

Call or return immediately for the following:
Increasing or persistent headache not relieved by Tylenol or aspirin
Persistent vomiting
Inability to concentrate; dizziness; problems with walking, talking, chewing, or swallowing
Seizures
Incontinence
Change in personality or behavior
Increasing drowsiness or inability to be aroused

diate therapy outlined previously for such patients. Patients with cerebral contusion benefit most from intracranial pressure monitors and perhaps pharmacologic control of the intracranial pressure.

Intracranial Hemorrhage

The conditions that most puzzle the emergency physicians are those with subtle presentations. Foremost among these are the extracerebral collections of blood. Common to both epidural and subdural hematomas is a clinical course of initial depressed neurologic function, acute deterioration and, if not recognized and managed successfully, progression into a mass that leads to death or vegetation. Unfortunately, not every such patient runs a predictable or recognizable course. There are wide variations in the initial presentation, and recognizable physical patterns commonly represent the serious deterioration of a coning syndrome. It is for this reason that indications for performing CT scans and for observing the patients whose neurologic status is hard to define (e.g., the intoxicated alcoholic) should be liberal.

Subdural hematoma

A subdural hematoma, usually caused by a tear in bridging dural veins, has been classified in three groups: acute, subacute, and chronic. Perhaps a better classification is now available on the basis of the CT scan appearance: hyperdense, isodense, or hypodense. During the acute phase of a bleed, the blood appears as a hyperdense, crescent-shaped clot. Thus most acute diagnostic CT scans can be performed without an infusion of radiodense contrast material. After 1 to 3 weeks, as blood is reabsorbed from the hematoma, the density of the extracerebral fluid becomes isodense. At this point the subdural hematoma may be invisible on the CT scan without additional contrast material. After approximately 1 month, the extracerebral fluid becomes hypodense and approaches the density of cerebrospinal fluid. A contrast-enhanced study shows the lesions better and often shows a fascicular capsule around the hematoma.

An *acute subdural hematoma* carries the most dismal prognosis. Unless there is a significant collection of blood and unless there is a mass effect, immediate surgical drainage is probably of little benefit. This lesion is often found in a patient with a head injury from a major automobile accident. Most often there is an immediate onset of coma and a low GCS score. Even with aggressive field and emergency department management, there is often no improvement. An early coning syndrome in these patients usually represents massive cerebral edema rather than a hemorrhage. With appropriate pharmacologic and surgical management, the patient can sometimes survive the edema phase with return of good function.

The *subacute subdural hematoma* probably has the best prognosis. It can have a subtle presentation, probably because it is often found in alcoholics who cannot remember the original mechanism of injury as a result of a combination of chemical intoxication and blunt concussion-induced amnesia. The patient may return to fully normal neurologic function but often has a depressed sensorium that is written off as the "hangover" effects of the drinking episode. When an alcoholic or an alcohol-intoxicated patient is "found down," it is hard to distinguish between the alcohol effect and any potential head injury. Given the number of alcoholics with altered sensorium that are seen on any weekend shift, it is often impossible to do skull x-ray studies or CT scans on every alcoholic. Instead attempt to assess the acute blood alcohol level. A low blood alcohol level is an indication for an immediate CT scan. A high blood alcohol level suggests how long the coma caused by alcohol can be expected to continue. If the patient does not begin to awaken appropriately within the predicted time frame, this again indicates the need for a CT scan.

Other clues for further assessment are the

presence of seizures in a patient with a high blood alcohol level and, of course, any focal findings. In this context, the pupils become important. There is too much emphasis on anisocoria; it is almost unheard of as a sign of a mass effect from a coning syndrome in an awake patient. However, in the patient who is unconscious, even a tiny degree of anisocoria must be presumed to be evidence of herniation and vigorous diagnostic and therapeutic actions must be taken. These patients should be treated as any patient with a GCS score of 8 or less, and the treatment should commence before the CT scan. Because the hemorrhage is caused by venous bleed, these patients do well unless they deteriorate into massive herniation and edema.

A *chronic subdural hematoma* is also associated with a poor prognosis and is most often seen in an elderly patient with no history of trauma. It is not known whether this condition results from a trauma that was never observed or whether the bleeding was spontaneous or in response to hypertension. Whatever the case, the patient often has an acute organic brain syndrome or deteriorating cerebral function. All too often the patient is written off as being senile or as possessing "Alzheimer's disease." Order a CT scan on any patient with acute organic brain syndrome or for any elderly patient who has been observed to change in mental capacity. The actual surgical survival from a chronic subdural hematoma is good, but the prognosis for a return to normal brain function is much poorer. For unknown reasons the brain often does not properly expand after the hematoma is drained, and the patient often remains in a vegetative state.

A *subdural hematoma in an infant* has special considerations. First, it is almost always the result of child abuse. Second, the hematoma can sometimes be drained via a subdural tap performed through the anterior fontanelle. Third, the retina often shows hemorrhage—a sign that is almost never found in the adult. Fourth, the first manifestation may be a seizure

with a prolonged postictal state. Many of these children also have other injuries that should be sought as in any child with chid abuse.

Epidural hematoma

An epidural hematoma appears to occur in two forms. One form is a rapid deterioration of cerebral function within 8 hours of the initial trauma, which may have been minor. The patient often has a skull fracture, but sometimes that is hard to see on conventional or even CT scan studies. Bleeding is arterial, usually from a torn middle meningeal artery; there may also be significant brain injury from the initial trauma. The prognosis is poor, with death or vegetation being common. Patients sometimes complain of ear or jaw pain but not of neurologic dysfunction until they acutely lose consciousness, seize, and develop a coning syndrome. Even with rapid surgery, these patients tend to have a poor result.

The second form of epidural hematoma has a more insidious onset; the bleeding is a combination of both venous and arterial sources. The patient may have no fracture. There is little or no brain injury at the time of the original insult. The patient may have an acute concussive picture, with a return to a normal or almost normal level of consciousness. Following the gradual bleeding that occurs, the patient has a headache and usually a deterioration in neurologic function. If the condition is diagnosed before a coning syndrome develops, the patient usually has a good outcome.

With epidural hematomas, recommendations for skull x-ray studies or CT scans are liberal in hopes of defining the first group of patients before they crash. For the second group, the period of observation, careful discharge instructions, and ease of returning to the emergency department become most important.

Whichever clinical course is observed, the epidural hematoma is virtually always visible as a bean-shaped collection of blood outside the brain. Contrast enhancement is usually not necessary.

Intracerebral hemorrhage

For some patients, the blood accumulates within the cerebral substance, not outside the brain. This condition probably represents arterial bleeding and is often seen following the deceleration injuries described earlier. Although the patient often has an acute onset of coma, more desultory presentations are possible. The patient may appear to have a brain tumor, and the identity of the lesion is revealed only with the CT scan. Treatment should be the same as recommended previously for the patient with a GCS score of 8 or less, and surgery is defined by the neurosurgical consultant.

Penetrating Cranial Injury

A penetrating brain injury requires special considerations. A penetrating injury can be subtle and may be overlooked until the patient develops a septic complication. Even with missile penetration from low-velocity weapons and misfired ammunition, the patient may enter the emergency department awake and alert. Although the patient may be awake and alert, it is critical that treatment be as aggressive as for the patient with a GCS score of 8 or less. Waiting for the development of coma leads to so much cerebral swelling that much more brain is destroyed than that attributable to the path of the bullet alone. High-velocity missiles produce such a blast effect as they pass through tissue that the victims almost never survive and are almost always comatose from the moment of injury. Surgery for a penetrating injury is usually not urgent because it is not performed to correct a mass effect but rather to debride dead tissue and remove contaminated bone fragments.

If the missile passes the midline, especially at the level of the brainstem, survival is almost impossible. There will be difficult decisions about when and where to withdraw life support. In these cases early skull x-ray studies may reveal the hopelessness of the situation, and an end can be defined before too much life support is given to someone who is by all definitions brain dead. If there is any doubt about the extent of injury, it is preferable to admit the patient to the neurosurgical service and withdraw life support after the family has been appropriately counseled and prepared.

POSTTRAUMATIC SYNDROMES

A number of posttraumatic syndromes are often encountered in the emergency department. The most common of these is persistent headache and inability to concentrate. At times it is necessary to perform a CT scan to ensure that the patient is not developing a neurosurgically correctable lesion. Sometimes a short course of adequate analgesia and sedation is beneficial, but care must be taken to avoid producing an addictive situation. Some neurosurgeons have reported occasional success with treatment with anticonvulsant medications. Often only time clears these problems.

In general, long-term management does not fall to the emergency physician. Unfortunately many of these patients reappear in the emergency department, where there is often no information about their prior work-up. There is often no choice but to repeat the work-up and not assume that once negative, always negative.

Posttraumatic epilepsy is another common problem. There has been some suggestion that prophylactic anticonvulsant therapy prevents the appearance of a permanent seizure disorder, but there are no data as yet on how long this therapy must be maintained. Begging this question, it is important to load all patients with major head injuries with phenytoin during their acute management as described previously.

SUMMARY

Head injuries are a major responsibility of the emergency physician. Although many injuries result in death or a vegetative state from the moment of impact, many others benefit from aggressive, compulsive, and thoughtful diagnosis and management.

⫿⫿⫿⫿⫿⫿KEY CONSIDERATIONS

WHAT IS THE LIFE THREAT?

Intracerebral hemorrhage and extensive cerebral contusion with edema are life threats. Swelling of the brain in the confined space of the skull eventually causes cerebral ischemia, hypoxemia, herniation syndromes, and death.

DOES THE PATIENT NEED ADMISSION?

Patients with major head injuries require admission. A CT scan is required for patients whose injury resulted in prolonged loss of consciousness (longer than 5 to 10 minutes), persistent neurologic dysfunction, persistent vomiting, a GCS score less than 8, or deterioration, as well as for patients with inadequate social circumstances.

WHAT IS THE MOST SERIOUS DIAGNOSIS?

Epidural hematoma, massive subdural hematoma, and massive intracerebral bleeding are the most serious diagnoses.

HAVE I PERFORMED A THOROUGH WORK-UP?

Ensure that the airway is patent, and evaluate ventilation. Establish intravenous access.

Perform a neurologic examination.

Be alert for concomitant cervical spine injury; determine the status of the cervical spine by palpation and a cervical spine x-ray study before cervical immobilization is removed.

Obtain a CT scan for a major head injury.

Recommended Reading

Baxt WG: Head trauma. In Baxt WG, editor: *Trauma: the first hour,* Norwalk, Conn, 1985, Appleton & Lange.

Bowers SA, Marshall LF: Outcome of 200 consecutive cases of severe head injury treated in San Diego County: a prospective analysis, *Neurosurgery* 6:237, 1980.

Chestnut RM, et al: The role of secondary brain injury in determining outcome from severe head injury, *J Trauma* 34:216, 1993.

Lahaye PA, Gade GF, Becker DP: Injury to the cranium. In Mattox KL, Moore EE, Feliciano DV, editors: *Trauma*. Norwalk, Conn, 1988, Appleton & Lange.

Pons PT: Head trauma. In Rosen P et al, editors: *Emergency medicine: concepts and clinical practice*, ed 3, St Louis, 1992, Mosby.

Schackford SR, et al: The clinical utility of computed tomographic scanning and neurologic examination in the management of patients with minor head injuries, *J Trauma* 33:385, 1992.

Chapter *Twenty*
FACIAL AND ORAL TRAUMA

DOUGLAS A. RUND

GENERAL CONSIDERATIONS

In the presence of any injuries involving the face and its contents, the emergency physician must assess the status of the cervical spine. The worst facial injuries occur with direct forces transmitted to the face. Because there is no element of torque, the spinal column and the spinal cord are usually not affected; however, an accompanying head injury can occur.

Because the face has great capacity to swell, massive deformities of the facial structures are often hidden behind traumatic edema. Therefore the emergency physician should attempt to carry out a thorough facial examination early in the course of a resuscitation and before swelling occurs. Facial injuries can compromise the airway. Increased secretions, fragments of teeth, or other foreign bodies can obstruct the upper airway, and swelling can distort normally recognizable anatomic landmarks.

The supine position is often poorly tolerated by the patient with a facial injury. If it has been clinically or radiographically determined that the cervical spine is uninjured, the patient can be sat upright and encouraged to lean forward. Suction can be used to continuously clear the oral cavity. An alert patient who has no other complicated or critical injuries can often clear the airway by spitting into an emesis basin using a suction catheter. If the patient is not alert enough to clear the airway or if other factors preclude the upright position, the patient can be placed prone or in a lateral position to help keep the airway unobstructed.

If active airway management is indicated (see Chapter 3), it must be accomplished before the anatomy is massively distorted by the swelling process. In the conscious patient, an airway in jeopardy should be secured by oral intubation after rapid sequence induction and intubation while the head and cervical spine are manually stabilized as discussed in Chapter 3. In such cases, the emergency physician must be prepared to establish a surgical airway via cricothyroidotomy if oral intubation is unsuccessful. Nasal intubation is not recommended in patients with facial trauma because of the possibility of cribriform plate or laryngeal injury.

In some facial injuries, especially those involving the posterior pharynx or tongue, a hemorrhage can be exsanguinating and can obstruct the airway. More common is a persistent ooze from facial or scalp lacerations that over time can accumulate to produce a serious loss of blood.

If the patient's condition permits, assess the contours of the face. Determine if the patient has normal dental occlusion and normal function of the mandible. Place your fifth fingers in the patient's ears and ask the patient to bite down; movement of the mandibular condyles can normally be felt. An absence of movement on either side suggests a fracture of the mandibular condyle.

Assess function of the major nerves controlling facial musculature and sensation. The loss of seventh-nerve function can be partial and hard to assess but may be the only clue to a transverse temporal bone basilar skull fracture. If not detected and repaired early, a permanent loss of function is possible. Sensation around the orbit is often lost as facial edema increases but may also represent a blow-out or other orbital fracture.

Craniofacial separation can be detected with an assessment of maxillary integrity, which is best accomplished by attempting to rock the maxilla. Inspect the mouth first to be sure that the teeth or a local maxillary fracture are not responsible for the unusual degree of motion.

Assessing whether teeth have been lost in facial trauma can be difficult. Patients may have broken and even aspirated teeth without being aware of the injury. Careful inspection of the gums and dental sockets is necessary. At times, a chest x-ray study may be the only way to reveal a tooth aspiration.

SPECIFIC FACIAL INJURIES

Maxillary Fractures

Maxillary fractures may be hard to define, and plain x-ray studies often do not reveal the fracture line. Indirect evidence of a fracture is observed by seeing air fluid levels in the maxillary sinuses. CT scans have been helpful in delineating the full extent of injuries. In addition to searching for midface mobility, rhinorrhea and dental malocclusion should be assessed.

Le Fort described a series of facial-bone fractures that involve the maxilla. A Le Fort I fracture involves the maxilla to the level of the nasal fossa. A Le Fort II fracture involves the nasal bones and medial orbits and is generally pyramid shaped. A Le Fort III fracture represents craniofacial dissociation involving all the bones of the face (Fig. 20-1). Different combinations of fractures may be present in one patient. For example, the patient may have a Le Fort I injury on the right side of the face and a Le Fort II injury on the left side. The exact configuration of the fractures is of less importance to the emergency management of the patient than are correct airway management and the recognition of rhinorrhea.

At times, the patient with maxillary fractures has significant and major epistaxis. Normally this condition responds to anterior or posterior packing, but occasionally surgical arrangements may need to be made for control of epistaxis and repair of the fractures as needed.

Patients with maxillary fractures usually require hospital admission. They often have much discomfort; even when pain is relieved with adequate analgesics, pain with mastication interferes with eating. With more profound degrees of facial destruction, an accompanying head injury often requires inpatient evaluation and management.

Zygomatic Fractures

The zygoma is typically fractured from a direct blow with a blunt object. The zygoma conveys the angular appearance to the face, and when it is fractured, the cheek on the involved side appears flattened. A zygomatic fracture may be hard to detect after the traumatic edema has formed. The clue to diagnosis may then lie in an inability to chew. At times, the patient may experience such a fracture as trismus rather than painful mastication. The trismus is caused by impaction of the coronoid process of the mandible with spasm of the masseter muscle on the involved side. When the zygoma is fractured through the malar eminence, the patient may experience anesthesia of the cheek as a result of impaction of the fracture on the infraorbital nerve. At times, the patient may also have diplopia or entrapment of the inferior rectus

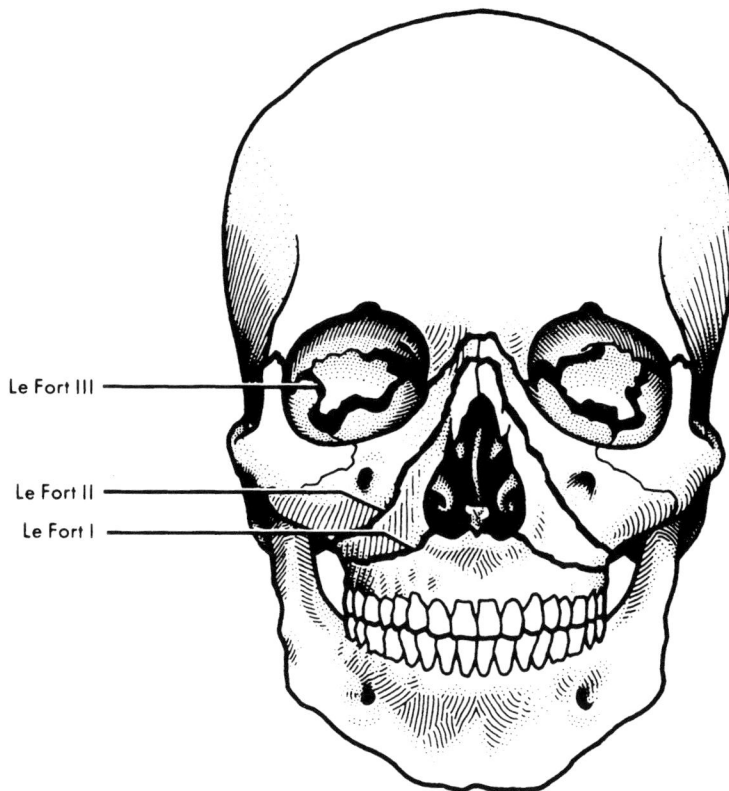

Fig.20-1 Le Fort classification of facial fractures. Le Fort I: palate facial dysjunction. Le Fort II: pyramidal dysjunction. Le Fort III: craniofacial dysjunction.

muscle or may develop a palpable stepoff at the level of the cheek bone. To demonstrate the fractures radiologically requires a combination of a Water position and a submental vertex view to show the angle of the zygoma.

When these fractures are isolated injuries, the patient can often be managed at home. However, if there is marked impaction of the zygomatic arch with trismus or impairment of mastication, inpatient management is best until the patient undergoes surgical elevation and repair of the fracture.

Orbital Fractures

The orbit may be fractured indirectly as in the malar fracture of the zygoma or by a direct blow to the orbit itself. When the blow is caused by an object that has a radius of 5 cm or less, the intraorbital pressures exceed the resistance of the orbital bone. The bone is especially weak on the inferomedial side. With an orbital bone fracture, the orbital contents may herniate into the maxillary sinus, which is known as a blow-out fracture. The physical findings may include enophthalmos, entrapment of the inferior rectus muscle, and hypesthesia in the distribution of the inferior orbital nerve. A useful clinical clue to the presence of an orbital fracture is the presence of a subscleral hemorrhage that extends to the orbital wall laterally or medially. If white sclera cannot be visualized when the patient gazes laterally or medially, it should be assumed that an orbital fracture is present, even if this diagnosis cannot be confirmed with plain x-ray studies. A CT scan is often helpful in delineating such fractures. Swelling is often profound and may prevent an accurate assessment of the orbit until the swelling subsides.

Other clues to an orbital fracture are the presence of subcutaneous emphysema in the orbital soft tissues or the inflation of the tissues around the eye when the patient blows the nose. These signs may be caused by a fracture into the ethmoid sinus rather than the antrum, and it may be difficult to detect any fracture line with an x-ray study. Also look for an air fluid level in the antrum on facial x-ray studies. Eye entrapment may not require surgical release; most surgeons who manage this problem prefer to await the relief of edema before making a final decision about surgical repair.

The patient may complain of diplopia, particularly while attempting to look upward. This condition usually subsides with relief of the edema but is another indication for surgical repair if it persists. Patients with an isolated blowout fracture rarely require hospital admission. Emergency department management consists of analgesics, an antiinflammatory drug such as piroxicam (Feldene) 20 mg PO daily, ice, and bed rest with the head up.

Mandibular Fractures

The mandible is a hemicircle of bone. Like the pelvis, it rarely breaks in a single location. Moreover, it is often fractured at a site distant from the point of impact. The most common clue to the presence of a mandibular fracture is maloc-

clusion. Because malocclusion is often hard to determine by inspection, asking the patient if he or she notes an abnormality of bite is most useful. If the patient is too intoxicated to cooperate or cannot respond because of the extent of the injury, ecchymosis in the floor of the pharynx sometimes provides a clue to the presence of the fracture.

The diagnosis of mandibular fractures is typically not easy with a conventional x-ray study. A panoramic view often shows the details of the mandible more accurately (Fig. 20-2). The condyles are better seen with a conventional view or with a CT scan.

The mandible is also subject to dislocation at the temporomandibular joint. There is no need to worry about a concomitant fracture if this dislocation occurs spontaneously after yawning or after minor trauma. However, after a more significant mechanism of trauma, it should be determined whether an accompanying fracture exists. In this case, a general anesthetic probably best accomplishes major muscle relaxation, and the fracture can be simultaneously fixated. When no fracture is present, the dislocation is usually easily reducible, often with no sedation. This technique involves standing behind the patient and pushing down and outward on the mandible. Gloves should be worn, and a tongue blade or bite block should be in place because an inadvertent occlusion of the mandible sometimes occurs with great risk to the physician's fingers. If the reduction cannot easily be accomplished, some sedation is required. A small dose of midazolam (Versed) should provide enough relaxation. If not, it must be determined whether a condylar or coronoid fracture exists.

Most patients with mandibular fractures require hospital admission. If no other injuries exist, some of these patients can be managed as outpatients with a soft or liquid diet and adequate analgesics until the mandible can be fixed. Treatment of open fractures requires penicillin and a staphylocidal antibiotic.

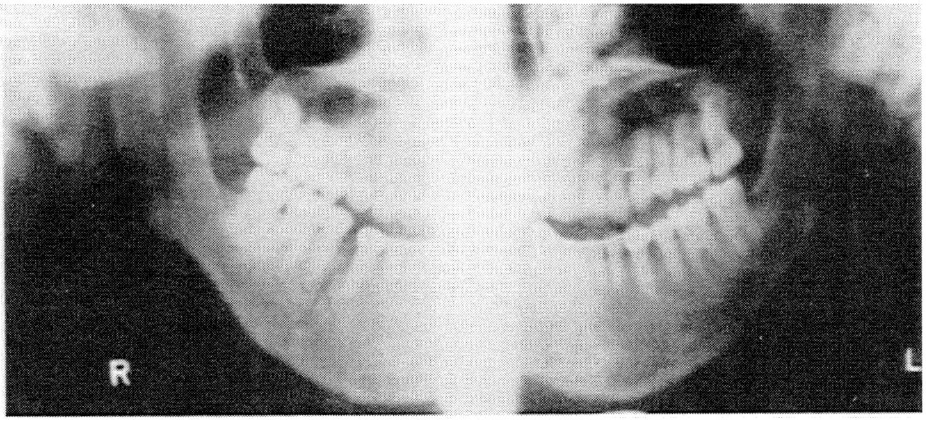

Fig. 20-2   Panoramic x-ray film of mandible. Note fractures in area of left angle and right body. (Dental retainer appliance is in place on lower incisors.)

Soft-Tissue Injuries

There should be no excessive pessimism about the cosmetic prognosis of facial injuries, even if there are extensive lacerations. With meticulous repair, cosmetic results are often remarkable. The face has an abundant blood supply, much elasticity, and considerable excess tissue. As a result, the surgeon can move tissue and cover large defects except in certain critical areas such as around the philtrum (Cupid's bow) of the upper lip, or around the nose and the eyebrows. Localized infections following facial lacerations are relatively infrequent for the following reasons: abundant blood supply, lack of weight bearing of the facial skin, the paucity of motion at the site of most lacerations, and the openness and dryness of the environment. Nevertheless, because the appearance of the subsequent scar is of major psychologic importance to the patient, the repair of facial lacerations should be carried out carefully.

The best results can be obtained by careful debridement of macerated tissue edges and meticulous approximation of the dermis. Anesthetize the wound, carefully irrigate it, and close it in layers. Use fine-diameter sutures, with 5-0 polyglactin 910 (Vicryl) for muscle fascia, 5-0 to 6-0 Vicryl for a dermal closure, and 5-0 to 6-0 monofilament nylon for the epidermis (see Chapter 25).

Close the dermis with interrupted buried vertical mattress sutures. Place enough sutures so that all tension is removed from the epidermis. Close the epidermis with running plain or locked sutures if the wound is straight or with interrupted simple sutures if the wound is jagged. If the edges of the wound tend to invert, evert them with several vertical mattress sutures.

Debridement should be performed carefully around the eyebrows, eyelids, and the corners of the mouth. If the philtrum or mouth corner angle is involved or if portions of the eyebrow are lost, refer the patient to a plastic surgeon. It is not always true that eyebrows fail to regrow after being shaved; they are not shaved because they provide an important landmark for repair to prevent stepoff in the final line of the eyebrow.

Close the lips with concern for the approximation of the edges of the vermilion border.

Even a small stepoff here produces a cosmetic deformity that is noticeable at a conversational distance. Mark the vermilion border with a small dab of methylene blue, or use a 28-gauge needle to inject an intradermal bead of lidocaine anesthetic at the border before injecting the lidocaine anesthetic. Alternatively, in a cooperative patient, place a stitch without an anesthetic to line up the vermilion border.

For through-and-through lip lacerations, always perform the repair in layers serially, and start with the inside of the mouth. Close the oral mucosa with interrupted 4-0 Vicryl, and test the closure with a syringe and No. 19 needle to be sure that a watertight closure exists. Close the muscle and subcutaneous layers with a few interrupted 4-0 Vicryl sutures, and finally close the dermis and epidermis as previously described. The risk of wound infection appears to depend on the adequacy of the mucosal closure.

Flaps of facial tissue formed by trauma are common. If the base of the flap is less than approximately one half of the height, the tip of the flap likely will necrose. Remove the flap and advance the skin edges to close the defect. This procedure invariably produces a dog-ear deformity at one or both corners of the advanced skin.

With the advent of modern safety glass in automobile windshields, the emergency physician does not see the extensive facial lacerations resulting from auto accidents that previously were common. However, what is common now is an abraded wound with multiple punctate lacerations, many of which harbor small slivers of glass. Finding and removing all of these slivers can be very difficult. An x-ray study obtained before and after the repair helps in the attempt to remove all fragments. Inject a field of damaged tissue with a local anesthetic agent before beginning the search. It is often impossible, and usually unnecessary, to place epidermal sutures in the hundreds of small lacerations. Remove road rash dirt particles, or they will form an unsightly permanent tattoo. With the appropriate anesthetic, scrubbing the area with a toothbrush is often effective in removing such particles.

Lacerations near the parotid gland are dangerous (Fig. 20-3). Not only can such lacerations damage the facial nerve, but they may also produce a significant and exsanguinating hemorrhage from the external facial artery or vein. In addition, there is always a risk of damage to the parotid duct. Check for this risk by inspecting the duct orifice at its exit into the mouth by the upper first molar. Refer the patient for repair of the Stenson duct if blood appears at the orifice of the duct spontaneously or after milking the duct through the face. If the parotid gland has been lacerated, refer the patient for plastic repair. If an immediate referral is not possible, drain the wound and admit the patient to the hospital.

In general, repair facial wounds of the face while using a local anesthetic. With small children who cannot cooperate, consider using a ketamine anesthetic. Give 6 mg/kg IM 10 minutes after giving 0.01 mg/kg of atropine IM. Also give diazepam 0.1 mg/kg IM before the child wakes up to try to eliminate the nightmares caused by ketamine. This regimen is especially useful for repairs that require meticulous sewing, such as around the eyes or lips, or for repairs inside the mouth, especially those that involve the tongue. The anesthesia lasts for 30 to 60 minutes; observe the child until responsiveness returns.

Most lacerations can be safely repaired, probably up until 24 hours after injury. If there is any question of contamination, simply clean the wound, dress it, and bring the patient back for inspection. When the wound is clean, do a delayed primary closure.

Remove epidermal sutures on the face in 3 to 5 days, and support the laceration edges with Steri-strips. Mucosal sutures are generally not removed if placed with an absorbable material such as Vicryl.

It is almost impossible to bandage most facial wounds. Cover the wounds with a thin layer of

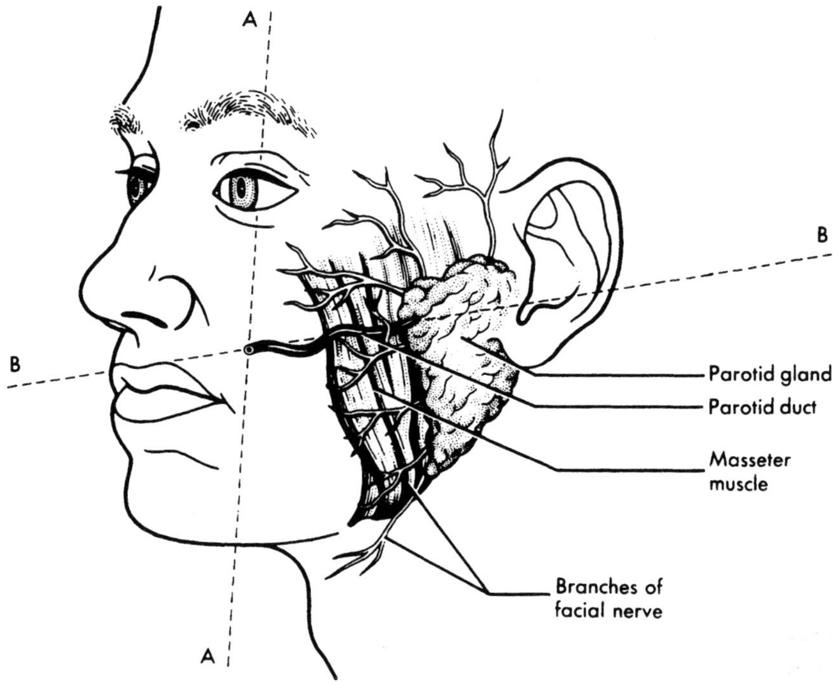

Fig.20-3 Parotid gland and parotid duct with nearby branches of facial nerve. Line *B* demonstrates approximate course of parotid duct from parotid gland, which enters mouth at junction of lines *A* and *B*.

Polysporin ointment. This treatment is used not to prevent infection but to keep the wound moist and to minimize the scab formation. Advise patients to clean the wound daily with hydrogen peroxide and saline and to reapply the ointment. Many complex facial lacerations ooze after repair, but a pressure dressing is not necessary. In the region of the temporal artery and when necessary, extend the laceration, identify the injured vessel, and ligate it to prevent massive hematoma formation.

OPHTHALMIC INJURIES

Fortunately, globe penetration rarely occurs with blunt trauma and most of the lacerations around the eye involve the skin of the eyelid but not the globe. Injury to the globe is easy to miss in a patient who is intoxicated or unconscious; search for it where its potential exists. Periorbital swelling often obscures the globe, and adequate examination may require the use of lid retractors from the operating room.

Assess visual acuity if the patient's condition permits. If the patient has too much discomfort to permit such testing, instill two drops of a topical anesthetic agent such as proparacaine (Ophthaine) into the involved eye. This procedure may lower visual acuity to some degree, but the change will be slight. If the patient does not have his or her own spectacles, estimate visual acuity with a pinhole.

As with all trauma, a history of the mechanism of injury is important. Any patient who may have had something fly into the eye, such as after hammering on metal, should undergo a search for foreign body penetration of the globe. The foreign body may be seen on a conventional x-ray study but at times a CT scan is necessary to find it.

Lid lacerations are common. If any fat is showing in the wound, assume that the lid has been penetrated and make a careful search for globe penetration. If the margin of the lid is involved or if there is close proximity to the lacrimal ducts, attempt to see if the patient has blood in the nostril or if it appears after milking the duct. If either the lid margin or the duct is involved, the patient should undergo repair by an ophthalmologist.

Traumatic iritis is not often seen in the emergency department but may have its onset within 24 hours of the initial trauma. With this condition, the patient has marked photophobia, tearing of the eye, a cloudy anterior chamber, and decreased visual acuity. The pain can be intense, and the eye resembles one that is affected by acute glaucoma. These patients require immediate attention from an ophthalmologist. If there is a question of narrow-angle glaucoma induced by the dilating solution, measure pressure in the eye and establish glaucoma treatment (see Chapter 68).

Following trauma, some patients develop an acute swelling of the retina with involvement of the optic nerve. This *Berlin edema* can be difficult to detect if the emergency physician has never seen a case. The only clue to its presence is an acute change in visual acuity. Therefore the visual acuity must be measured as soon as possible after an eye injury and the ophthalmologist must be involved as soon as any change in acuity appears.

Globe penetration should not be repaired in the emergency department. The emergency physician's responsibility is to recognize the injury, patch the involved eye with a metal patch and the uninvolved eye with a soft patch, and obtain an immediate consultation from an ophthalmologist.

OTOLARYNGOLOGIC TRAUMA

Nasal Fractures

The bony lesion in a nasal fracture is usually of little significance, but deformation of the cartilage and submucosal hemorrhage is important. Septal deformity from nasal injury is generally apparent with inspection of the nasal passages. Most otolaryngologists prefer to wait for edema to subside before reducing nasal deformities.

Determine whether a septal hematoma is present. An expanding hematoma can cause ischemic necrosis and a subsequent collapse of the septum. Such a hematoma should be drained acutely, usually by an otolaryngologist.

In cases of open fracture, a definitive setting of the septum and nasal bones can be left to the otolaryngologist. However, the emergency physician should repair the laceration overlying the nose. Silk sutures, rather than monofilament nylon, are preferable on the tip of the nose and around the lateral nares. The skin of the nose is oily, and monofilament sutures are uncomfortable to the patient and tend to pull through the skin. Antibiotics are not necessary because these wounds rarely become infected.

Although it may be impressive initially, traumatic epistaxis is usually of short duration. It is almost always an anterior bleed and rarely requires cauterization or nasal packing. With maxillary fractures, epistaxis can be more extensive and can require both anterior and posterior packing.

Otic Injuries

The ears are easily lacerated or contused. A subchondral hematoma is important to recognize in the ear because, as in the nasal septum, an enlarging hematoma can lead to necrosis of the ear cartilage. This type of injury is also very deforming. Bandaging the ear to achieve any pressure is difficult, and physicians have described a variety of techniques for sewing stents onto the area of hemorrhage. The wisest course is to refer these injuries immediately to a specialty consultant who can follow the patient. These patients should be admitted to the hospital unless extremely careful outpatient follow-up can be arranged.

Lacerations through the ear cartilage are common and can be safely repaired in the emergency department. Place several fine Vicryl sutures through the cartilage if necessary to line it up properly. Close the epidermis with interrupted 5-0 or 6-0 Ethilon. If the ear has been bitten off in a fight or has been partially detached, carry out the repair in the emergency department, but admit these patients to the hospital for careful management because the prognosis for survival of the tissue is poor.

Injuries to the inner ear are less common, and blood inside the ear canal commonly represents a basilar skull fracture or otorrhea. Avoid the common error of assuming that the blood is from a facial laceration and ran into the ear.

Mouth Injuries

Oral lesions become more dangerous and harder to manage as they become more posterior. Lacerations of the hard palate commonly occur, and although infection is always a modest risk, they rarely produce hemorrhage or airway obstruction. Lesions of the soft palate are most worrisome; they can produce a massive hemorrhage because the carotid artery is in close proximity. A rare but important injury is blunt trauma to the carotid artery. The earliest warning is persistent and increasing but hard-to-describe pain. Most oral lesions are uncomfortable, especially during swallowing. Pain during rest suggests ischemic pain; if the patient has a posterior pharyngeal injury, this type of pain may well represent an indication for admission and angiography.

The most common complications of an oral injury are hemorrhage and respiratory obstruction. The hemorrhage can be subtle. Blood may be swallowed by the patient, who may not be aware of the hemorrhage until a coffee-ground emesis occurs. Swelling in the retropharynx can produce upper airway obstruction, and the patient may not be aware of the impending catastrophe either because of alcohol ingestion or because he or she is asleep.

Most oral lesions do not require admission and are reparable in the emergency department either with a local anesthetic or with ketamine. Lean toward admitting patients with lesions that are posterior to the hard palate or that have a lot of bleeding or swelling, as well as patients who will have difficulty in communicating increasing symptoms or whose social circumstances preclude safe outpatient management.

Tongue injuries are common, especially in children. Base the decision for repair on the size of the wound, how much gaping exists, and how much bleeding is present. The tongue is almost impossible to repair easily without a general anesthetic, but ketamine offers a satisfactory alternative. Admit the patient for observation if much hemorrhage exists or if the tongue continues to swell after the repair is complete.

Frenulum injuries usually require no repair. In the absence of an underlying clotting dysfunction, these injuries usually have small, insignificant, and self-limiting amounts of bleeding. Bleeding is usually controllable with a single absorbable suture.

The uvula is occasionally injured by a penetrating object. It can bleed vigorously but usually does not. The uvula requires repair only to prevent the formation of a permanent window. In a small child, the repair requires ketamine or a general anesthetic. Swelling of the uvula is common and can be massive. If there is any airway obstruction, the patient requires intubation until the period of edema has passed. Consultation with an otolaryngologist is advisable.

Laryngeal Injuries

The larynx is unlikely to be injured from above but is subject to blunt trauma from blows to the anterior neck. Clinical signs of injury are changes in the voice and ecchymosis and swelling of the neck.

The mechanism of the injury provides the most useful clues to laryngeal injuries. Suspect injury to the larynx in patients who have received a blow to the neck. Perform a direct laryngoscopy if objective physical signs exist, such as contusions over the soft tissues of the neck or hoarse speech. Soft tissue x-ray studies of the neck, which are viewed best in a cross-table lateral study, sometimes reveal fractures of the laryngeal cartilages but more commonly show only soft tissue swelling or air in an abnormal location.

DENTAL INJURIES

Gingival lacerations are common but usually do not bleed extensively. They are often difficult to repair because of the close proximity to the tooth or mandibular or maxillary socket. If a dentist or oral surgeon is unavailable to assist in the management, repair the tissue either with small filament absorbable sutures (4-0 or 5-0 Vicryl) or fine silk, and refer the patient to the dentist or oral surgeon the following day.

The teeth are commonly injured, especially in athletic sports such as football when a mouth protector is not worn. Whenever a tooth is fractured, make a careful search for all fragments, because aspiration of broken teeth is unfortunately common. If the missing part cannot be found, obtain a chest x-ray study to search for an aspiration. If a broken tooth has been aspirated, consult a thoracic surgeon to arrange for a bronchoscopy and removal of the fragment.

Tooth fractures are generally managed according to the level of fracture, age of the patient, general condition of the tooth and

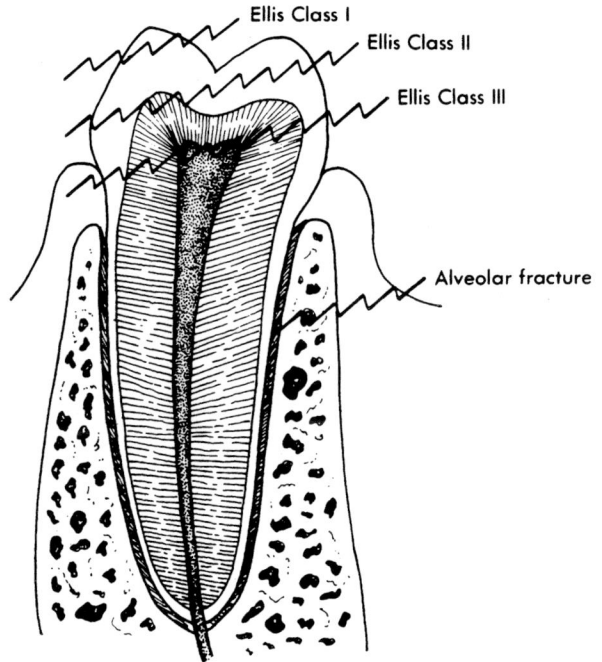

Fig. 20-4 Ellis classification for fractures of anterior teeth. From Tintinalli JE et al: *Emergency medicine a comprehensive study guide,* ed 4, by Amsterdam JT, New York, 1996, McGraw-Hill.

periodontal tissue, and accompanying injuries. The oral mucosa or tongue may be lacerated at the same time that the fracture occurs, and sometimes a subtle through-and-through laceration of the cheek or lip is missed because of attention to the broken tooth.

A commonly used dental fracture classification is that of Ellis (Fig. 20-4). An Ellis I fracture is minor and causes problems because of the rough edge that it produces in the enamel portion of the tooth. Either file the edge smooth, cover it with a temporary enamel bonding material, or leave it until the earliest opportunity to see a dentist.

An Ellis II fracture penetrates the dentin and exposes the pulp of the tooth to bacterial penetration, especially in children because their dentin is narrow. These injuries are painful, especially when exposed to air. The wisest course is to have a dentist see the patient as soon as feasible. In the meantime, the fracture can be covered with a calcium hydroxide paste. A temporary cap is advisable if available.

Ellis III fractures involve the full thickness of the teeth and include the pulp, the enamel, and the dentin. To distinguish Ellis III from Ellis II fractures, look for pink tissue or blood in the fracture. Teeth with an Ellis III fracture likely require root-canal work and are the most painful. If there is no immediate access to a dentist, place a long-acting bupivacaine (Marcaine) dental block, cover the tooth, and refer the patient to a dentist as soon as possible.

If the tooth is subluxed from its socket, a dentist or an oral surgeon must stabilize it. Have the patient bite on a gauze 4 × 4 until stabilization can be achieved.

A completely avulsed tooth should be replaced unless it is a deciduous tooth. For a deciduous, or "baby" tooth, avulsion, irrigate the socket and control bleeding if necessary. As already mentioned, search for the avulsed tooth because it may have been aspirated or may be totally hidden within a buccal wound.

The earlier that a permanent tooth avulsion can be replaced within the socket, the greater the chance of successful reimplantation. Most dentists feel that a reimplantation within 2 hours will be successful, but thereafter the success rate is low. Replacement is worth trying. Rinse the tooth with saline but do not wipe or scrub it. Replace the tooth in the socket and maintain manual pressure to set the tooth in place. The patient can bite gently on gauze to hold the tooth in place. It is helpful to have a dentist or oral surgeon see the patient at this point to secure the tooth in place.

Alveolar bone fractures are difficult to manage when other injuries preclude immediate attention. Because a loss of the alveolar plate is cosmetically deforming and because the patient can easily aspirate loose fragments of alveolar bone, the oral surgeon must be involved early in these injuries.

KEY CONSIDERATIONS

WHAT IS THE LIFE THREAT?

Airway compromise from facial trauma can occur from a number of sources, including the following: swelling in the neck and pharynx; distortion of the mandible following a fracture; hemorrhage in the mouth, nose, and pharynx; or the presence of foreign bodies such as loose teeth or dentures. If the mandibular symphysis is fractured in two places, the tongue can dislodge posteriorly and occlude the pharynx.

Some facial and oral injuries can bleed copiously and cause significant blood loss and shock.

Facial injuries can be associated with concomitant and life-threatening intracranial or cervical injuries.

Laryngeal injuries can compromise the airway.

DOES THE PATIENT NEED ADMISSION?

Extensive facial lacerations (especially those associated with an underlying fracture) may require the consultation of a plastic surgeon. An ophthalmic surgeon is usually consulted for through-and-through lacerations of the lid, for orbital fractures, or for lacerations of the globe.

Hospitalize patients whose airway has been compromised by swelling or bleeding.

WHAT IS THE MOST SERIOUS DIAGNOSIS?

Injuries that compromise or potentially compromise the airway are the most life threatening.

Evaluate the patient for an underlying intracranial and cervical spine injury.

HAVE I PERFORMED A THOROUGH WORK-UP?

Evaluate patients with facial injuries for a coexisting head and spine injury. Assess also for a soft tissue injury of the neck, including the airway.

Despite the dramatic nature of the facial injury, look for trauma to the head, neck, chest, abdomen, and pelvis.

Assess cranial nerves (especially the facial nerve) in cases of facial trauma and oculomotor nerve damage.

Evaluate for blow-out fracture of the orbit, including infraorbital facial sensation. Abnormal movement of the palate and maxilla suggests a loss of maxillary integrity as a result of fracture.

Evaluate the mouth and gums for missing teeth that may be aspirated; obtain x-ray studies of the chest and abdomen if aspiration is suspected.

Recommended Reading

Amsterdam JT: Dental disorders. In Rosen P et al, editors: *Emergency medicine: concepts and clinical practice,* ed 3, St Louis, 1992, Mosby.

Campbell WH, Cantrill SV: Neck injuries. In Rosen P et al, editors: *Emergency medicine: concepts and clinical practice,* ed 3, St Louis, 1992, Mosby.

Cantrill SV, McGill J, Kulig K: Facial trauma. In Rosen P et al, editors: *Emergency medicine: concepts and clinical practice,* ed 3, St Louis, 1992, Mosby.

Chapter Twenty-one
SPINAL INJURY

ROBERT S. HOCKBERGER

Spinal injuries are common, preventable, costly to society, and devastating to the victims and their families. Over 200,000 patients with spinal injuries now live in the United States, and that number increases by almost 10,000 each year. Most injuries occur in young men as a result of motor vehicle accidents, falls, and sports-related injuries. The annual cost to society from this disorder exceeds $5 billion, and the emotional and psychologic damage to patients and their families is incalculable.

Potential spinal injury victims are anxiety provoking for the emergency physician for two reasons. First, inadvertent movement of an injured spinal column may cause or worsen a spinal cord injury. Unfortunately, many patients with spinal injuries are uncooperative or combative as a result of alterations in their mental status from drug or alcohol intoxication, a head injury, or hypotension caused by other injuries. Secondly, almost every spinal injury case results in a lawsuit because of the patient's and family's anger and frustration, the psychologic need to assign someone with blame for the terrible event, and fear of huge costs associated with chronic care in light of lost income. Therefore patients with a potential spinal injury need to be evaluated systematically and completely; detailed documentation in the medical record should note the patient's neurologic status at presentation and should chronicle the course of their evaluation and treatment in the emergency department.

GENERAL APPROACH

The potential for a spinal injury should be suspected in all trauma victims with the following conditions: (1) impaired consciousness; (2) complaints of neck, back, or limb pain; (3) evidence of significant head or facial trauma; (4) localized spinal tenderness or paravertebral muscle spasm; (5) signs of neurologic deficit; (6) multiple painful injuries; or (7) unexplained hypotension.

The approach to evaluating and treating patients with a suspected spinal injury is depicted in Fig. 2-1. Although many of the steps outlined actually take place simultaneously and often by several members of a trauma resuscitation team, the order of prioritization is as follows: (1) immobilization of the spine to prevent the possible worsening of spinal injury, (2) airway management, (3) treatment of shock, (4) assessment of other potentially life-threatening injuries, (5) neurologic examination, (6) radiographic evaluation, and (7) treatment and disposition.

SPINAL IMMOBILIZATION

Most trauma victims have spinal immobilization, which is often termed *spinal precautions,* initiated in the field by paramedical personnel. Spinal immobilization is usually done by placing the patient supine on a backboard, anchoring the patient's torso to the backboard with straps, and immobilizing the head and neck with a plas-

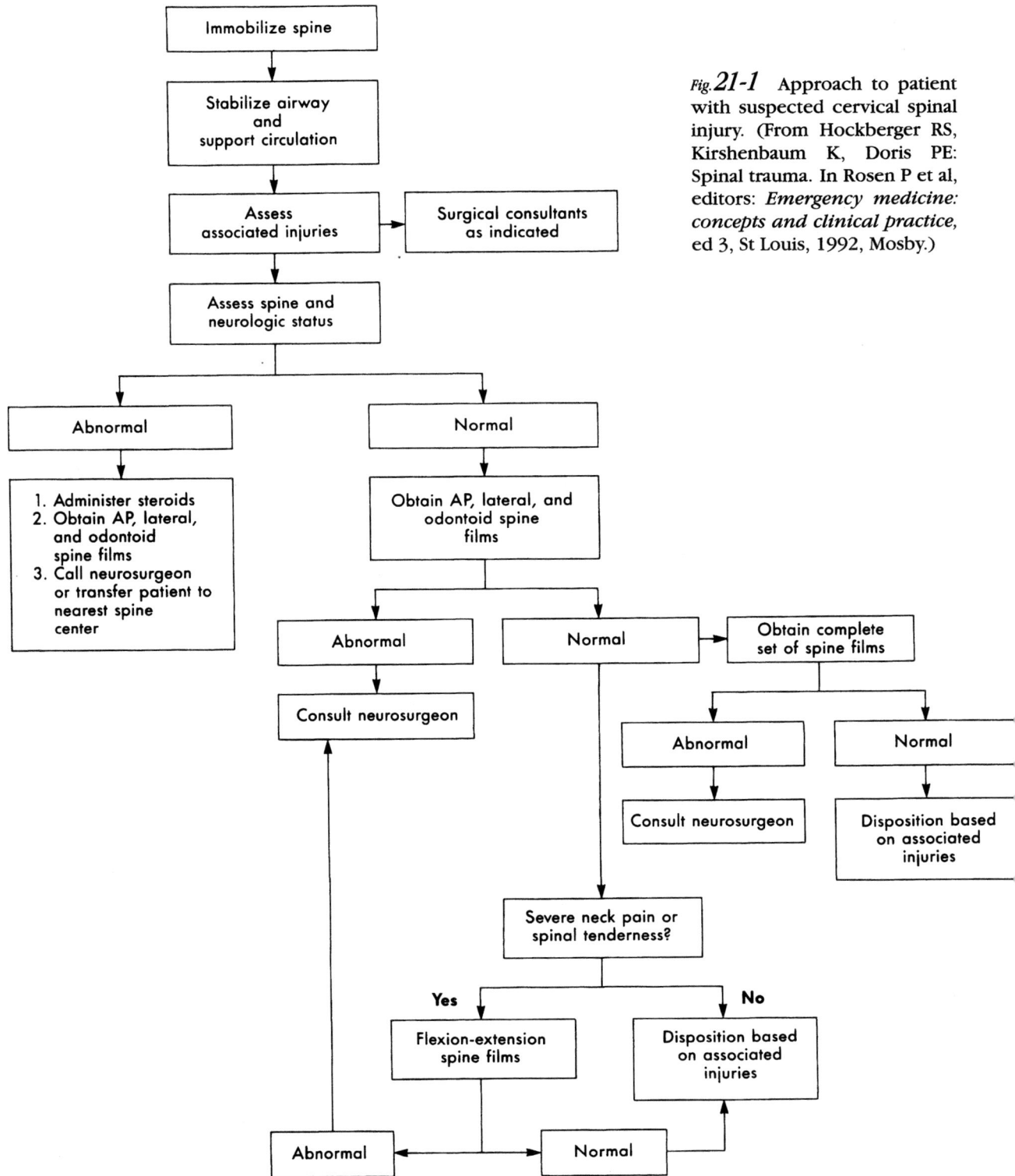

Fig. 21-1 Approach to patient with suspected cervical spinal injury. (From Hockberger RS, Kirshenbaum K, Doris PE: Spinal trauma. In Rosen P et al, editors: *Emergency medicine: concepts and clinical practice*, ed 3, St Louis, 1992, Mosby.)

tic cervical collar and sandbags placed on either side of the head and accompanied by the use of tape that extends across the patient's forehead and from one side of the backboard to the other. Spinal precautions should be maintained in the emergency department until the presence of a spinal injury is excluded through radiographic or clinical assessment.

Patients who have a normal mental status, no spinal pain or tenderness, and no other painful (and therefore potentially distracting) injuries are unlikely to have suffered a spinal injury and can be taken out of spinal precautions and assessed clinically. Patients who are conscious and cooperative but who are suspected of having a spinal injury should be cautioned against attempted movements until their assessment is completed. Uncooperative patients are best immobilized by an individual whose only assignment is to hold the patient's head in alignment with the longitudinal axis of the body. Most commercially available immobilization aids are ineffective with uncooperative patients, and placing these aids is difficult without further manipulation of the spine. Patients who are combative and therefore at risk for injury if they have an unstable spinal injury often require sedation, either alone or in conjunction with intubation and paralysis.

AIRWAY MANAGEMENT

Special attention must be paid to airway and ventilatory management in patients with a suspected spinal injury. Trauma patients may initially experience airway obstruction from displaced dentures, maxillofacial injuries, intraoral bleeding, or vomitus. Patients with spinal injuries may later develop acute pulmonary edema or respiratory paralysis, which is caused by lower cervical cord injury and results in delayed phrenic nerve paralysis from ascending spinal cord edema. Finally, trauma victims often have associated head or chest injuries that require airway control or respiratory support.

Patients suffering from traumatic cardiopulmonary arrest should undergo orotracheal intubation with in-line spinal immobilization. In-line spinal immobilization should not involve placing traction on the head or neck because such a procedure has been shown to cause both distraction and subluxation of unstable cervical spine injuries. Trauma victims who are unconscious, breathing, and in need of airway control or ventilatory support are best managed by careful orotracheal intubation, nasotracheal intubation, or cricothyrotomy. Although all airway management techniques result in some movement of the cervical spine, all three of these techniques appear to be safe when performed by experienced personnel. Combative patients should be orotracheally intubated following sedation and paralysis with neuromuscular blocking agents. Patients with significant maxillofacial injuries should have a cricothyrotomy performed or, if a cricothyrotomy is not possible, should be intubated orotracheally. Although there are reports of cases managed successfully with both a cricothyrotomy and orotracheal intubation, patients with a suspected laryngeal injury should ideally receive a tracheostomy. Following initial airway management, the patient's ventilatory status should be carefully monitored for the possibility of delayed respiratory deterioration.

CIRCULATORY SUPPORT

The term *spinal shock* refers to a clinical syndrome that is characterized by the loss of neurologic function and accompanying autonomic tone below the level of an acute spinal cord injury. Patients with spinal shock usually exhibit flaccid paralysis with a loss of all modes of sensory input, motor activity, deep tendon reflexes, and urinary bladder tone. Such patients also experience bradycardia, hypotension, hypothermia, and intestinal ileus from a loss of autonomic tone. Spinal shock usually lasts only a few days.

Neurogenic hypotension secondary to spinal shock should always be a diagnosis of exclusion in the trauma patient. A spinal injury should not be considered as the cause of hypotension unless (1) the patient is flaccid and areflexic, (2) there is an absence of the reflex tachycardia and peripheral vasoconstriction usually seen in patients with shock and, most importantly, (3) the possibility of coexisting hemorrhagic shock, cardiac tamponade, or tension pneumothorax has been eliminated. Because of the lack of sympathetic tone necessary to induce reflex vasoconstriction, pallor, and tachycardia, the signs of hypovolemic shock may not appear in a patient with spinal shock that is accompanied by injuries causing internal bleeding. Fortunately, neurogenic hypotension accompanying spinal shock is usually mild and readily treated with the Trendelenburg position and crystalloid fluid infusion. Other causes of shock should be considered if hypotension is severe, accompanied by tachycardia, or unresponsive to initial fluid resuscitation.

ASSOCIATED INJURIES

Injuries of the head, chest, abdomen, and pelvis are more commonly life threatening than a spinal injury and may be more difficult to diagnose in the presence of a spinal injury. Patients with suspected neurogenic hypotension should receive hematocrit determinations at frequent intervals because vital signs may not accurately reflect the patient's volume status. The abdominal examination is unreliable if a neurologic impairment is present and, as a result, the threshold for performing a peritoneal lavage or obtaining a CT scan of the abdomen should be low in a patient with a spinal injury. Trauma surgery or a general surgery consultation should be obtained for any neurologically impaired

trauma patient so that the patient can be followed closely for the possible progression of initially occult injuries.

NEUROLOGIC EVALUATION

Neurologic Examination

The initial neurologic examination of a patient with a suspected spinal injury should begin with simple *observation*. Careful inspection of the patient's entire body beginning with the head and proceeding downward may reveal indirect signs of spinal injury such as head and facial trauma or seat belt abrasions of the chest or abdomen. The patient's breathing pattern may provide an important clue to a cervical injury. The diaphragm is innervated by the phrenic nerve, which originates from the midcervical spinal cord, whereas the intercostal muscles of the rib cage are supplied by nerves that originate in the thoracic spine. Therefore abdominal breathing in the absence of chest-wall movement indicates a lower cervical injury. The presence of Horner syndrome (unilateral ptosis, miosis, and facial anhydrosis) may result from disruption of the cervical sympathetic nerves that run in close proximity to the lower cervical and upper thoracic spinal cord.

Motor activity should be assessed by testing for the presence and strength of those motions outlined in Table 21-1. For patients who exhibit an apparent total loss of function, every effort should be made to elicit even the most minimal of motor responses. Intact rectal sphincter tone or the presence of a slight toe flicker in an otherwise paralyzed individual is evidence of "sacral sparing" and indicates that the patient may ultimately have a substantial return of neurologic function. Along with the remainder of the neurologic examination, the motor examination should be repeated at frequent intervals in patients who exhibit an initial deficit, because cephalad progression of neurologic dysfunction

Table *21-1*

THE MOTOR EXAMINATION

Level of Lesion	Resulting Loss of Function
C4	Spontaneous breathing
C5	Shrugging of shoulders
C6	Flexion at elbow
C7	Extension at elbow
C8-T1	Flexion of fingers
T1-T12	Intercostal and abdominal muscles*
L1-L2	Flexion at hip
L3	Adduction at hip
L4	Abduction at hip
L5	Dorsiflexion of foot
S1-S2	Plantar flexion of foot
S2-S4	Rectal sphincter tone

From Hockberger RS, Kirshenbaum K, Doris PE: Spinal Trauma. In Rosen P et al, editors: *Emergency medicine: concepts and clinical practice,* ed 3, St Louis, 1992, Mosby.
*Localization of lesions in this area is best accomplished with the sensory examination.

Table *21-2*

REFLEX EXAMINATION

Level of Lesion (at or above)	Resulting Loss of Reflex
C6	Biceps
C7	Triceps
L4	Patellar
S1	Achilles

From Hockberger RS, Kirshenbaum K, Doris PE: Spinal Trauma. In Rosen P et al, editors: *Emergency medicine: concepts and clinical practice,* ed 3, St Louis, 1992, Mosby.

Table *21-3*

SENSORY EXAMINATION

Level of Lesion	Resulting Level of Loss of Sensation
C2	Occiput
C3	Thyroid cartilage
C4	Suprasternal notch
C5	Below clavicle
C6	Thumb
C7	Index finger
C8	Small fingers
T4	Nipple line
T10	Umbilicus
L1	Femoral pulse
L2-L3	Medial thigh
L4	Knee
L5	Lateral calf
S1	Lateral foot
S2-S4	Perianal region

From Hockberger RS, Kirshenbaum K, Doris PE: Spinal Trauma. In Rosen P et al, editors: *Emergency medicine: concepts and clinical practice,* ed 3, St Louis, 1992, Mosby.

secondary to proximal spinal cord edema is not uncommon.

Testing for the presence of *deep tendon reflexes* is a helpful localizing and diagnostic aid (Table 21-2). In the acute setting, muscle paralysis associated with intact deep tendon reflexes usually indicates an upper motor neuron (spinal cord) lesion, whereas muscle paralysis associated with absent deep tendon reflexes indicates a lower motor neuron (nerve) injury. This differentiation is important because the latter condition is often caused by a surgically correctable lesion.

Sensory function can be quickly evaluated by using a structured approach (Table 21-3) or by referring to a graphic representation of sensory nerve distribution for comparison (Fig. 21-2). After locating an area of hypesthesia, carefully delineate the area by slowly moving the

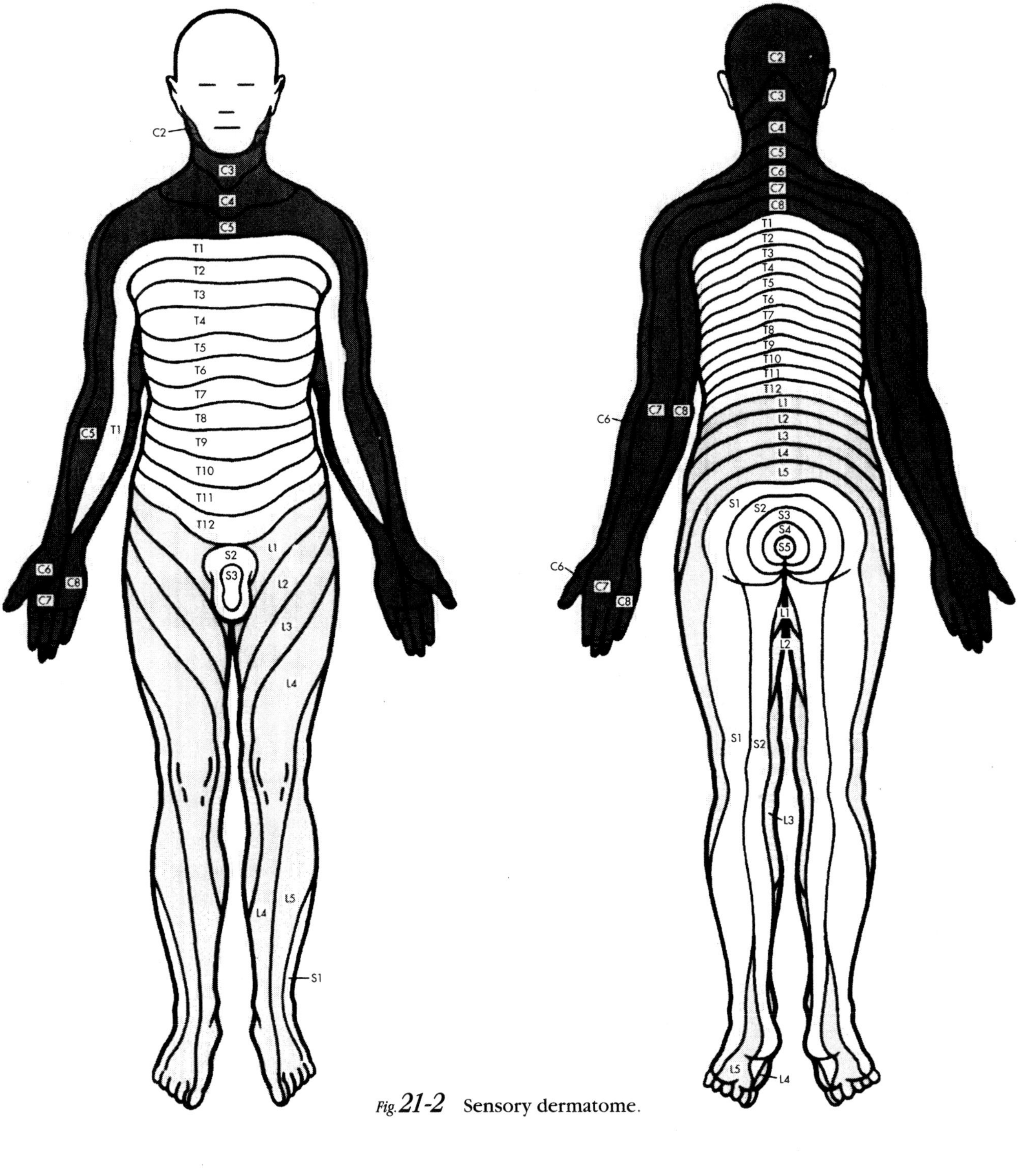

Fig. 21-2   Sensory dermatome.

stimulus from areas of decreased sensation outward rather than the reverse, because people are much more sensitive to the appearance of sensation than to its disappearance. Performing this test with a cotton wisp to assess sensitivity to light touch will assess posterior spinal column function. Repeating the test with a pin to assess pain sensation will assess anterior cord function (Fig. 21-3).

Complete Versus Incomplete Spinal Cord Lesions

A complete spinal cord lesion is defined as total loss of motor power and sensation distal to the level of a spinal cord injury. Patients with a complete spinal cord injury do not undergo functional recovery. However, two points should be considered before attempting to make this diagnosis. First, any evidence of minimal cord function, such as sacral sparing, excludes the patient from this group. Signs of sacral sparing include persistent perianal sensation, normal rectal sphincter tone, or slight flexor toe movement. The presence of any of these signs indicates a partial lesion, and the patient may have marked functional recovery, including bowel and bladder control and eventual ambulation.

A complete spinal cord lesion can also be perfectly mimicked by spinal shock. The end of spinal shock is heralded by the return of the bulbocavernosus reflex. This reflex is elicited by placing a gloved finger into the patient's rectum and squeezing the glans penis or tugging gently on the Foley catheter. An intact reflex results in a distinct rectal sphincter contraction. An absence of this reflex indicates the presence of spinal shock, and no accurate estimates of a patient's prognosis can be made until this reflex has returned. A complete spinal cord lesion remains unchanged following the cessation of spinal shock.

Most incomplete spinal cord lesions can be classified into one of three clinical syndromes: the central cord syndrome, the anterior cord syndrome, and the Brown-Séquard syndrome (see Fig. 21-3). The *central cord syndrome* is seen most often in older patients with degenerative arthritis whose necks are subjected to forced hyperextension, which causes a concussion or contusion of the central portion of the spinal cord. Patients have greater neurologic impairment in the upper extremities than in the lower extremities because the nerves supplying the lower extremities are found in the peripheral portion of the spinal cord. With more severe injuries, patients may appear to be almost completely quadriplegic and have only minimal evidence of sacral sparing. The prognosis for patients with this syndrome is directly related to how rapidly the clinical recovery progresses.

The *anterior cord syndrome* may result from cervical flexion injuries causing cord contusion, from the protrusion of bony fracture fragments or herniated intervertebral disks into the spinal cord, or by laceration or thrombosis of the anterior spinal artery. This syndrome is characterized by paralysis and hypalgesia below the level of injury, with preservation of posterior column functions (touch, position, and vibratory sensations). These patients require immediate evaluation with a CT scan or magnetic resonance imaging (MRI) to exclude compressive lesions that require surgical intervention.

The *Brown-Séquard syndrome*, or hemisection of the spinal cord, usually results from a penetrating lesion such as a bullet or knife wound but may occasionally be seen following certain cervical spine fractures. Patients with this type of lesion have ipsilateral motor paralysis and contralateral sensory hypesthesia distal to the level of injury. These patients rarely undergo surgery and do well functionally following rehabilitation.

RADIOGRAPHIC EVALUATION

Spinal x-ray studies are not indicated for every person who has experienced a motor vehicle

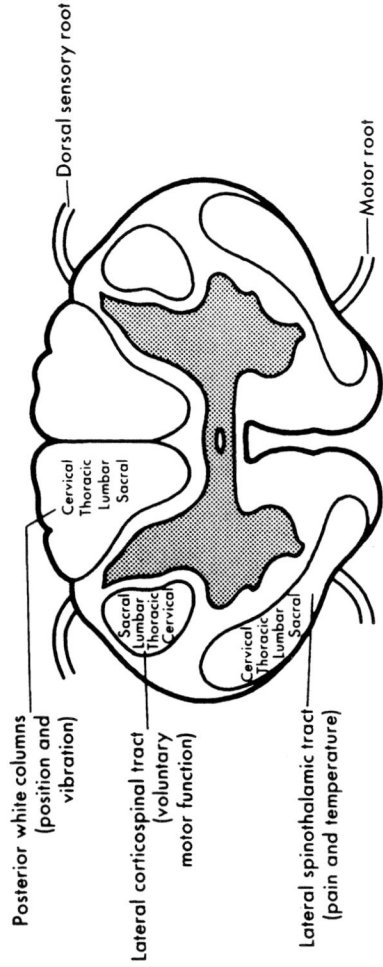

CROSS SECTION OF CERVICAL SPINAL CORD

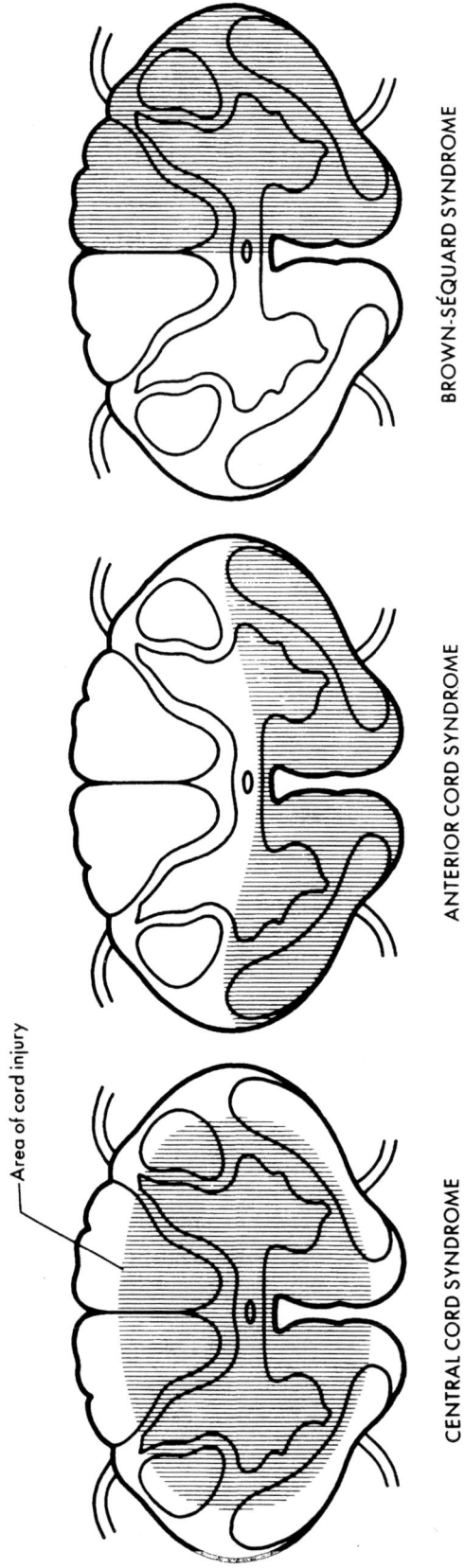

Dorsal sensory root

Motor root

Cervical
Thoracic
Lumbar
Sacral

Sacral
Lumbar
Thoracic
Cervical

Cervical
Thoracic
Lumbar
Sacral

Posterior white columns
(position and
vibration)

Lateral corticospinal tract
(voluntary
motor function)

Lateral spinothalamic tract
(pain and temperature)

BROWN-SÉQUARD SYNDROME

ANTERIOR CORD SYNDROME

CENTRAL CORD SYNDROME

Area of cord injury

Fig. 21-3 Incomplete spinal cord syndromes.

accident, fall, or sports-related injury; however, such persons are often brought to the emergency department in spinal precautions by paramedical personnel. The following questions should always be asked: Is the patient's mental status altered in any way? Is the patient under the influence of drugs or alcohol? Does the patient have other painful (potentially distracting) injuries? Does the patient exhibit spinal tenderness? Is the patient's neurologic examination abnormal? Does the patient experience more than mild discomfort with normal movement? Spinal x-ray studies are only indicated when the answers to one or more of these questions are positive. X-ray studies should not be obtained simply for medicolegal reasons.

When a spinal injury is suspected, the first x-ray study obtained is the lateral view. This single x-ray study diagnoses 70% to 90% of all spinal injuries. Adequate visualization of the junction of the lower cervical and upper thoracic (C7-T1) spine may require having someone pull downward on the patient's arms during the study or, alternatively, obtaining additional x-ray studies such as the transaxillary (swimmer's) view or a supine oblique view.

Because the lateral spine x-ray study does not diagnose all spinal injuries, an additional (anteroposterior) view is required for all spinal segments (cervical, thoracic, and lumbosacral), and a third (odontoid) view is required to adequately assess the cervical spine. The combination of these views diagnoses 90% to 98% of all spinal injuries.

Because the standard "trauma series" described above does not diagnose 100% of all spinal injuries, clinical judgment must be used to determine which patients require further radiographic assessment and which technique to use. The amount of force causing the injury, the level of patient discomfort, and the degree of tenderness on physical examination must be used to estimate the risk of injury. If the risk is high even in the presence of a normal trauma series, a CT scan of the spine (directed at the area of maximal pain or tenderness) or a flexion-extension x-ray study (to diagnose ligamentous injury in the absence of bony involvement) is indicated. A CT scan of the spine is also helpful to further evaluate questionable abnormalities on any of the trauma series x-ray studies. An MRI scan is occasionally used to better define soft tissue injuries of the spine.

TREATMENT AND DISPOSITION

Spinal Cord Injury

A patient may suffer *primary spinal injury* as the result of a contusion or laceration of the spinal cord, impingement on the spinal cord (from a fracture fragment, herniated intervertebral disk, or epidural hematoma), or from disruption of the vascular supply of the spinal cord. With the exception of surgery to relieve spinal cord impingement, there is no effective treatment for primary cord injury. During the posttraumatic period, particularly the first 4 to 6 hours, a complex series of molecular events results in progressive inflammation, edema, and tissue destruction within the injured spinal cord; this condition is termed *secondary spinal injury.* Much research has been done in an attempt to improve patient outcome by minimizing the effects of secondary spinal injury. Methylprednisolone is the only drug that currently shows promise. Beginning as soon as possible after the injury, spinal injured patients with evidence of neurologic impairment should receive a 30 mg/kg intravenous bolus of methylprednisolone followed by an infusion of 5.4 mg/kg/hr for 23 hours.

The role of surgery in the management of acute spinal injuries has been increasingly restricted and is today limited to relieving impingement on the spinal cord caused by foreign bodies, herniated disks, bony fracture fragments, or an epidural hematoma. Occasionally surgery is needed to reduce cervical spine dislocations. With these exceptions, patients with spinal injuries are best managed by early referral to a regional spine injury center, where rehabilitation directed by a team of spinal injury specialists can be initiated.

Musculoskeletal Injuries

Following clinical and radiographic assessment, the vast majority of patients evaluated for a possible spinal injury are given the nonspecific diagnosis of "musculoskeletal injury." These patients require reassurance, symptomatic treatment, and appropriate follow-up.

Minor musculoskeletal injuries are commonly associated with ongoing inflammation, soft tissue swelling, and muscle spasm that may cause symptoms to worsen during the first few days following injury. Patients should be apprised of this and told that ice packs for injured ligaments and hot baths for muscle aches are sometimes beneficial. Patients should receive a prescription for anal-

gesics appropriate to their degree of distress (usually nonsteroidal antiinflammatory agents), and muscle relaxants should be considered when significant muscle tenderness is present.

Providing patients with options for follow-up care is important. Underlying injuries can occasionally be missed at the time of initial evaluation, symptoms may worsen despite appropriate diagnosis and treatment, prescribed medications may prove ineffective or cause side effects, and litigation or worker's compensation issues may require ongoing medical evaluation. Therefore although specific follow-up appointments need not be scheduled for every injury victim seen in the emergency department, follow-up options should be offered to all patients. In addition, a patient should be told to return to the emergency department for evaluation if further or worsening symptoms develop or if it is not possible to obtain timely follow-up elsewhere.

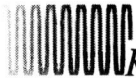

KEY CONSIDERATIONS

WHAT IS THE LIFE THREAT?

Spinal injury at the level of C4 and above interrupts neural input to the muscles of respiration and leads to death if airway and ventilatory support are not instituted. A cervical spine injury can eventually lead to respiratory paralysis because of phrenic nerve paralysis caused by ascending spinal cord edema.

Trauma to the cervical spine is often accompanied by serious injury to the head, chest, or abdomen, which should not be overlooked during the patient's evaluation.

Spinal shock resulting from spinal cord injury usually is mild and responds to intravenous fluids.

DOES THE PATIENT NEED ADMISSION?

The patient with a spinal cord injury needs neurosurgical consultation and admission.

WHAT IS THE MOST SERIOUS DIAGNOSIS?

Severe injury to the spinal cord resulting in paralysis, paresis, or death from respiratory failure are the most serious diagnoses.

HAVE I PERFORMED A THOROUGH WORK-UP?

In cases of spinal fracture or dislocation, the neurologic examination includes testing anal sphincter tone with a rectal examination.

The cervical spine series must adequately show the C7-T1 area and the rest of the cervical spine, including the ondontoid. Flexion-extension x-ray views are helpful if cervical instability is suspected. A CT scan or magnetic resonance imaging of the spine may be indicated if the patient has severe cervical pain, joint tenderness, and an injury mechanism that could have damaged the cervical spine.

Recommended Reading

Anderson DK, Hall ED: Pathophysiology of spinal cord trauma, *Ann Emerg Med* 22(6):987-992, 1993.

Bracken MB et al: Methylprednisolone or naloxone treatment after acute spinal cord injury: one year follow-up data, *J Neurosurg* 76:23-31, 1993.

Hockberger RS, Kirshenbaum K, Doris PE: Spinal trauma. In Rosen P et al, editors: *Emergency medicine: concepts and clinical practice,* ed 3, St Louis, 1992, Mosby.

Hoffman JR et al: Low-risk criteria for cervical-spine radiography in blunt trauma: a prospective study, *Ann Emerg Med* 21(12):1454-1460, 1992.

Scannell G et al: Orotracheal intubation in trauma patients with cervical fractures, *Arch Surg* 128:903-906, 1993.

Woodring JH, Lee C: Limitation of cervical radiography and the evaluation of acute cervical trauma, *J Trauma* 34(1):32-39, 1993.

Chapter Twenty-two

CHEST TRAUMA

DAVID J. VUKICH

Injuries of the chest may be trivial or life threatening, and because of this range of severity it is often difficult to discern one from the other. Regardless of the nature of the trauma and to avoid missing a serious injury, the emergency physician must focus on the basics: the adequacy and maintenance of respiration, ventilation, and circulation. This focus implies a primary survey for immediately correctable and life-threatening problems followed by a secondary, more detailed survey that includes a complete physical examination, laboratory studies, and x-ray studies. Occasionally this strategy may necessitate treatment before a complete diagnosis or before the underlying injury is diagnosed. Oxygen, large-bore IV lines (16 or 18 gauge), cardiac monitoring, and pulse oximetry should be applied immediately in all cases of significant chest trauma.

Once all basic functions have been ensured and the patient is stable, chest x-ray studies, ECGs, arterial blood gases, and other laboratory tests can be safely considered. As with all trauma patients, hypoxemia from chest trauma may masquerade as intoxication or head injury and must be considered immediately. Do not allow other dramatic but less life-threatening injuries (e.g., a bleeding scalp wound or an open fracture) to obscure a potentially lethal but more subtle chest injury such as a flail chest or cardiac tamponade.

Most salvageable patients with significant chest injuries can be successfully treated in the emergency department with basic resuscitation methods, a tube thoracostomy (if necessary), and airway control. Rarely is an emergency department thoracotomy indicated, and even more rarely does it result in survival. Obviously many patients need a surgeon, a formal operation, or admission to the hospital, and therefore the surgeon or trauma team should be involved as soon as possible in the patient's diagnosis and treatment. However, do not delay treatment nor postpone diagnostic maneuvers while waiting for members of the "team."

INITIAL ASSESSMENT AND MANAGEMENT

The earliest information concerning the chest injury usually comes from the prehospital care report before the patient arrives. The nature of the injury, vital signs, and level of consciousness help determine what interventions may be needed immediately. For example, the report of a penetrating chest injury and loss of breath sounds in the field should indicate the need to prepare for a thoracostomy. At the patient's arrival, the primary survey and initial monitoring should be performed at once. The depth and frequency of respirations, coordinated movement of the chest wall, color of the skin, and even the patient's voice provide clues about the adequacy of ventilation.

Look carefully at respiratory effort and the chest wall, and examine for flail segments, intercostal retractions, penetrating injuries, and subcutaneous air. If breath sounds are absent on the side of injury and the patient is in extremis, perform a needle or tube thoracostomy without waiting for a chest x-ray study. If the patient seems to be tolerating the injury and if the pulse oximetry indicates adequate oxygenation, it may be wiser to wait for the x-ray studies.

Injuries to the chest may produce hypotension as a result of bleeding from large or small vessels, direct cardiac injury or tamponade, tension pneumothorax, or direct pulmonary or chest wall injury with hypoxemia. After the primary survey, a more detailed examination should be performed. A secondary survey includes a "head-to-toe" examination of the patient, including an examination of the scalp, face, neck, trachea, jugular veins, heart sounds, back, abdomen, pelvis, and extremities, as well as a brief neurologic assessment. The chest is more closely observed by assessing the chest wall carefully.

To diagnose a subtle flail chest, it is often necessary to examine the chest wall in tangential light to see the segment moving paradoxically. Send laboratory studies, including a test to type and screen the patient's blood. An anteroposterior (AP) chest x-ray study should be taken in the upright position if the patient's condition allows it. With blunt trauma, look carefully at the x-ray study for two commonly missed findings: mediastinal widening and diaphragmatic rupture. If a pneumothorax is suspected but the diagnosis cannot be made on the initial chest x-ray study, order an expiratory view to increase the contrast between lung parenchyma and intrapleural air. Perform an ECG and pursue other modalities such as a CT scan or echocardiography when considering a mediastinal injury, cardiac contusion, or cardiac tamponade.

Hypotension and shock must be treated aggressively, but remember that injured lungs do not tolerate large volumes of crystalloid. A balance must be struck between adequate circulating blood volume and pulmonary function, which is analogous to a head injury situation. Therefore it may be wise to follow fluid therapy with central venous pressure or Swan-Ganz monitoring. Underlying lung diseases may also jeopardize treatment and recovery. The pulmonary reserve of the patient with asthma or chronic obstructive lung disease may be diminished, which may cause consideration of early intubation and ventilatory support, particularly with pulmonary contusion or flail segments. Control of pain in the patient with a chest injury can be difficult because most analgesics also reduce respiratory function. Narcotics should be used sparingly, and the use of intercostal blocks with bupivacaine should be used whenever possible.

BLUNT CHEST TRAUMA

Rib Fracture

The greatest concern with a rib fracture is not for the bony injury itself but for the potential damage to the underlying structures of the pleura, lungs, and mediastinal organs. Other than the pain of the injury, most undisplaced solitary rib fractures in an otherwise healthy individual are of little concern. Rib fractures are diagnosed clinically because they are not always visible on an AP chest x-ray study or rib series; however, they are easily treated with mild narcotics. Binders should not be used because they potentiate atelectasis and subsequent pneumonia, particularly in older individuals. Multiple rib fractures are a greater challenge for pain control, and intercostal blocks with 0.5% bupivacaine are often extremely effective. The short duration of the analgesia does make bupivacaine cumbersome for outpatient use, but it is effective and does not decrease respiratory excursion. A fracture of more than two ribs should prompt consideration of admission to

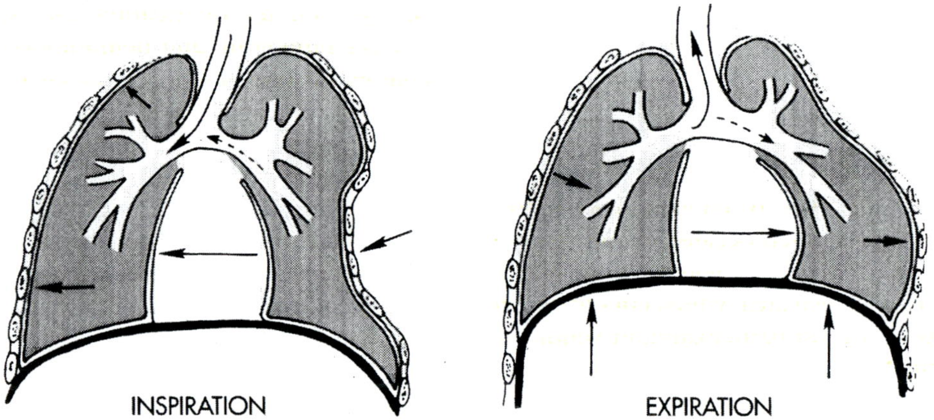

INSPIRATION   **EXPIRATION**

Fig.22-1   On inspiration, flail section sinks in as chest expands, impairing ability to produce negative intrapleural pressure to draw in air. Mediastinum shifts to uninjured side.
On expiration, flail segment bulges outward, impairing ability to exhale. Mediastinum
shifts to injured side. Air may shift uselessly from side to side in severe flail chest (*broken
lines*).

the hospital for pain control and pulmonary hygiene, particularly for the older patient. In any
age group, the risk of puncturing the pleura and
producing a pneumothorax increases with
more fractures.

The location of the rib fractures is also important. Fractures over the first and second ribs are
more commonly associated with potentially
lethal injuries to mediastinal structures. The increased force needed to break these relatively
protected ribs also indicates the possibility of
aortic or cardiac injury. A fracture of the last
three ribs, which are relatively mobile but prox-
imate to the liver and spleen, should increase
the search for injury of these organs.

Rib fractures can produce significant bleeding
from intercostal vessels or the internal mammary
artery. Despite their small caliber, intercostal vessels can cause a hemorrhage great enough to
threaten the patient's life. Ligating these small
vessels is technically very difficult, at least from
the exterior of the thorax. Ligation often requires
a formal thoracotomy to gain access and control.

Flail Chest and Pulmonary Contusion

The fracture of two or more ribs in two or more
places causes that portion of the chest wall to
be unstable. This instability allows the chest
wall to be pulled inward with inspiration and
forced outward with expiration; these movements are the opposite of normal chest wall dynamics (Fig. 22-1). This unstable portion of the
chest wall is called a flail segment; when multiple ribs are involved this flail segment is usually
apparent because it moves paradoxically to the
remainder of the chest. At one time this paradoxical movement was thought to be the most
important problem, and great efforts were made
to reduce this motion and to stabilize the chest
wall. Elaborate devices using towel hooks and
traction kept tension on the segment, and more
recently patients were intubated and ventilated
to "splint the chest from the inside." However,
for many years it has been recognized that the
most important issue is the condition of the underlying lung. A pulmonary contusion is often

produced by the trauma that was necessary to fracture these ribs; this situation is the true significance of flail chest injury.

The term *pulmonary contusion* belies the significance of this injury. As with a cerebral contusion, the effect can be dramatic and life threatening. The area of contusion, or hemorrhage, is not ventilated because of the blood in the tissues. Furthermore, blood flow is shunted around the damaged area, which effectively prevents this area from participating in ventilation or respiration. Several areas of the lung are often involved, and the respiratory embarrassment can be greater than predicted.

The chest x-ray study is not a good indicator of the degree of injury. Pulmonary contusion appears as an area of fluffy infiltrate, usually in continuity with the injured chest wall. These radiographic findings can be present early in the course or may be delayed 6 to 12 hours after injury. The extent of infiltrate on the chest x-ray study has little relationship to the degree of pulmonary injury. Patients with large infiltrates may have near normal function, whereas those with minimal radiographic findings can be severely affected and hypoxemic. Therefore patients with pulmonary contusions require careful observation and assessment of blood gases or pulse oximetry. A rising respiratory rate is also an indicator of a failing ventilatory status.

Patients with normal arterial blood gases, a stable respiratory rate, and adequate pain relief with analgesics do not require aggressive therapy or chest wall stabilization. When the pulmonary contusion is severe enough to cause respiratory distress or failure, the patient should be intubated and ventilated with positive pressure, which will allow more normal chest wall dynamics, overcome hypoxemia, and treat the contusion directly. Caution must be exercised because these patients are subject to barotrauma and possible tension pneumothorax. The material needed to perform a tube thoracostomy should be immediately available at the bedside. Further management should emphasize preventing or treating the sepsis, pulmonary embolism, and hemothorax that often complicate a pulmonary contusion.

Aortic Transection

Trauma that involves the delivery of massive energy to the chest, such as high-speed deceleration or overwhelming crush injuries, can transect the aorta within the thorax. Typical examples are high-speed auto accidents, falls from significant heights, and industrial crush injuries. The aorta has segments that are suspended and immobile and other portions that are relatively mobile, which allows tearing or transection to occur at these points. Most patients who sustain a complete tear die immediately in the field, but those with partial tears can survive 8 to 12 hours. During this latent period, it is possible to diagnose and operate successfully on these patients.

Although the plain chest x-ray study is one of the most helpful modalities for chest trauma, it is only modestly successful at diagnosing an aortic injury. Several findings are suggestive of aortic transection: pleural capping, elevation of the left main stem bronchus, a widened mediastinum, deviation of the nasogastric tube to the right or left, blurring of the aortic knob, and widening of the paravertebral stripe. Nevertheless, all of these signs may be absent in the presence of aortic injury. These findings are probably the result of bleeding from smaller mediastinal vessels and not from the aorta itself. A CT scan of the chest has not proven very useful. Aortic angiography is still the diagnostic gold standard for aortic transection, but this test may not be immediately available in many hospitals.

Because there are few reliable signs and symptoms of aortic transection, much debate exists over who should receive an angiography, particularly because this study is invasive and difficult to obtain. One of the most common protocols is to study anyone with an unexplained alteration of vital signs and a plausible mechanism of injury or anyone with a suggestive plain chest x-ray study. A few other clues to consider include the presence of paraplegia (present in 10% of those patients with aortic transection and resulting from spinal artery disruption) and hypertension (present in 25% of those with a transected aorta). Immediate surgery is the only lifesaving maneuver possible.

Myocardial Contusion

Blunt trauma to the anterior part of the chest may produce a myocardial contusion. Caught between the sternum and the vertebral column, the heart is suspended as it is concussed or compressed. Usually there are no signs or symptoms of myocardial contusion, but there may be bruising of the chest wall. There are also no physical findings or conclusive laboratory tests to positively diagnose a myocardial contusion, but the presence of a central flail chest injury or a fractured sternum is suggestive of this type of injury. The ECG and echocardiogram are somewhat useful in diagnosis and occasionally show ischemia or wall-motion abnormality, but radionuclide scanning may be slightly more sensitive and specific. Cardiac enzymes may also reveal the injury.

The most serious complication of myocardial contusion is acute dysrhythmia. Sudden cardiac death in this setting is probably caused by ventricular fibrillation or tachycardia and is labeled a myocardial contusion when this occurs. At times even minor chest trauma can produce dysrhythmias, even cardiac standstill. The most notable examples are in young children who have been struck in the middle of the chest while playing baseball and suffer sudden cardiac death. This effect is probably an electrical phenomenon rather than the contusion observed in adults.

The vast majority of patients with myocardial contusions survive the initial injury, probably without being diagnosed, and go on without complication or event. A few develop an area of electrical irritability that may be the source of a variety of dysrhythmias. Premature ventricular contractions often occur in the bruised myocardium and should be treated according to the same guidelines used for primary cardiac disease. Although sinus tachycardia is said to be the most frequent finding, it is so universal with trauma patients that it is useless as a diagnosis. A small percentage of patients with a myocardial contusion develop chest pain 5 to 7 days after the event; this pain is similar to ischemic cardiac pain. Most of these patients have normal coronary vessels, but rarely an individual has traumatic coronary artery occlusion. Only a coronary angiography can determine this type of injury, but currently there is little experience with thrombolytics and this condition is treated conservatively. The group without disease can be safely observed and treated for pain and dysrhythmia.

Adult patients with chest wall injury and associated hypotension, tachycardia, or other dysrhythmias, as well as patients with elevated CPK-MB and chest wall injury should be admitted for 48 hours of monitoring, bed rest, and treatment of any dysrhythmias. Serial cardiac enzymes, ECGs, and radionuclide scanning are the best methods for making the diagnosis, but in most patients the myocardial contusion resolves without complication.

Pneumothorax

A *collapsed lung* is the lay term for pneumothorax and is actually very descriptive of the pathophysiology of this type of injury. Normally the visceral and parietal pleura absorb any gas or fluid in the pleural space, which maintains a relative vacuum of -10 to -12 mm Hg. This vacuum keeps the otherwise elastic lung tissue expanded in the chest cavity and obliterates the pleural space. When an injury allows air to intrude between the pleural surfaces, the vacuum is lost and the lung "collapses." Both blunt and penetrating injuries can produce pneumothorax, but it is most common with a penetrating trauma.

The diagnosis of pneumothorax is made most often on a chest x-ray study, but the findings of intrapleural air can be subtle depending on the degree of collapse. The size of the pneumothorax may increase over time, but early in the course the findings may be minimal. The diagnosis can often be made by finding subcutaneous air in the chest wall, even though a pneumothorax is not directly visualized. With a penetrating injury it is tempting to attribute the subcutaneous air to the bullet or knife wound "dragging" air into the wound, but this air almost always originates from inside the chest and leaks into the chest wall through the pleural injury.

Physical examination may show decreased or absent breath sounds on the injured side and, occasionally, subcutaneous crepitus. The patient may be in extreme respiratory distress or may be minimally affected depending on the degree of collapse, the ability to compensate, and other injuries.

Three types of pneumothorax are recognized according to their anatomic description, but the treatment is similar for each.

Simple pneumothorax

A simple pneumothorax is the accumulation of air in the pleural space that is not under pressure and does not communicate freely with outside air. It is usually diagnosed by physical examination and a chest x-ray study but occasionally is not obvious on standard views. This is particularly true for a small or anteriorly located pneumothorax. An expiratory view often enhances a small pneumothorax, and the CT scan, usually performed for other reasons, has been shown to be extremely sensitive for the "invisible" anterior pneumothorax.

The treatment for a traumatic simple pneumothorax is tube thoracostomy. Oxygen should be administered and ECG and pulse oximeter monitoring should be applied. The preferred thoracostomy technique is to insert a size 32 to 40 French thoracostomy tube at the anterior ax-

illary line in the fifth intercostal space, direct the tube toward the apex, and connect the tube to an underwater seal with a 20 cm H_2O vacuum.

Tension pneumothorax

When air in the pleural space becomes trapped under pressure, it compresses the other thoracic structures and produces a tension pneumothorax. In this condition, the pleural injury acts like a ball valve, trapping air under pressure within the pleural space. This trapping of air in turn compresses the heart, great vessels, and contralateral lung and markedly embarrasses respiration and circulation; this condition may be rapidly fatal. Death is imminent unless the tension is immediately relieved.

One of the most frequent scenarios for tension pneumothorax is in the intubated patient who is being treated with a bag-valve-mask or ventilated with positive pressure. A simple but unrecognized pneumothorax can easily be converted to a tension pneumothorax under these circumstances. During the physical examination the patient is extremely anxious, in severe respiratory distress, and cyanotic. If a bag-valve-mask is being used, the lung compliance will decrease rapidly. The neck veins may be distended, and the trachea may be deviated to the side opposite the pneumothorax. There are absent breath sounds on the affected side. A cardiac monitor shows sinus tachycardia initially and begins to slow as cardiac arrest becomes imminent.

The only course of action with a tension pneumothorax is immediate relief of the pressure. Do not delay treatment for a chest x-ray study or any other diagnostic procedure. If a tube thoracostomy cannot be inserted immediately, a needle thoracostomy may work long enough to complete the formal procedure and is accomplished by inserting a large-bore IV catheter into the fifth intercostal space laterally.

Open pneumothorax

An open pneumothorax is not common in civilian practice because it occurs with massive wounds that remove large amounts of tissue from the chest wall. These types of wounds allow air to move freely into and out of the thoracic cavity, which greatly compromises respiration even if the lung itself is minimally injured. These wounds are obvious and are treated primarily by covering the defect and attempting to restore the integrity of the thorax. An occlusive dressing should be applied, and airway and circulation problems should be addressed aggressively. Once the occlusive dressing is in place, a tube thoracostomy must be placed to expand the lung. Do not be tempted to place the thoracostomy tube through the wound and into the chest. Placing the tube through an area of contaminated and devitalized tissue only complicates the course of treatment.

Hemothorax

A hemothorax is the accumulation of blood in the pleural space as a result of either a blunt or a penetrating injury. A hemothorax can cause hypovolemic shock and respiratory compromise by reducing vital capacity. The most common bleeding sites are the intercostal vessels and the internal mammary artery and less commonly the hilar vessels or the lung itself. An upright chest x-ray study will not demonstrate a hemothorax until at least 250 ml of blood has accumulated at the costophrenic angle. Many patients are not stable enough for an upright x-ray study, and the diagnosis is even more difficult with supine views.

Treatment consists of large-bore tube thoracostomy (36 to 40 French) with the tube directed posteriorly. Autotransfusion may be useful if the hemothorax is large and bleeding persists. Approximately 80% of all peripheral lung wounds respond to thoracostomy and volume replacement and do not need a thoracotomy. However, there are times when a thoracotomy is advisable, as is indicated in the box below.

Diaphragmatic Injury

Although a traumatic diaphragmatic rupture can often have immediate consequences, a diaphragmatic injury can also be silent for years until some intraabdominal organ is strangulated. Acutely it can cause severe respiratory compromise and can be catastrophic if a hollow viscus is entrapped or ruptures into the chest.

The left hemidiaphragm is more often ruptured by blunt trauma than the right hemidiaphragm. The classic chest x-ray study of a left hemidiaphragm rupture shows the air-fluid level of the stomach in the left side of the chest or shows an elevated diaphragm. This change can be very subtle because the normal location of the stomach shadow is not far away. Many of these injuries are missed because of the paucity of findings and because there may be no other signs of the herniation into the chest. If a nasogastric tube has been inserted, it may appear coiled in the lower left side of the chest on an x-ray study or may not pass easily.

Care should be taken when inserting a tube thoracostomy into a patient with blunt trauma. The area of the chest wall just inside the incision should always be swept with a gloved finger to ensure that the stomach or liver has not herniated into the chest.

INDICATIONS FOR THORACOTOMY

- Initial thoracostomy tube drainage is greater than 1500 ml of blood
- Persistent bleeding at a rate greater than 500 ml/hr
- Increasing hemothorax seen on chest x-ray studies
- Patient remains hypotensive despite adequate blood replacement, and other sites of blood loss have been ruled out
- Resumption of shock after successful initial resuscitation

If a diagnostic peritoneal lavage is performed, the level of red blood cells considered positive for a diaphragm injury should be lowered to 5000/ml rather than the standard 100,000/ml.

PENETRATING CHEST INJURY

Cardiac tamponade and esophageal injuries are almost exclusively a result of a penetrating injury. Although it may not ultimately be the most serious problem, penetration of the pleura is usually the first consideration with a penetrating injury of the chest. If a pneumothorax has occurred, all of the normal pressure relationships of the lungs are altered, respiration is severely compromised, and the patient is endangered. A tube thoracostomy must be placed immediately and at times before obtaining a chest x-ray study. This concept of stabilization before diagnosis may seem unnatural, but there is often no time to obtain diagnostic information.

The physical examination is not always completely informative and must be considered in context with the nature of the injury and the appearance of the patient. An elderly individual with underlying chronic obstructive pulmonary disease may normally have decreased breath sounds, whereas such sounds are more indicative of a hemothorax in a young person. Consider a gunshot wound to be more capable of causing significant harm than a knife. When primary survey and x-ray studies do not show a pneumothorax from either a bullet or a knife wound, it is standard to observe the patient for 4 to 6 hours and repeat the study. A pneumothorax should occur within this time, and assuming that there are no other injuries, the patient can usually be discharged for outpatient follow-up.

Regardless of the mechanism, most peripheral chest injuries do well with thoracostomy, oxygen, and volume replacement. Conversely, the center of the chest contains the mediastinal box (heart, great vessels, tracheobronchial tree,

and esophagus), and wounds to this area are not nearly so benign. If the patient is stable enough, an angiography, bronchoscopy, esophagoscopy, and esophagogram may be needed to determine if surgery is needed. Injuries to the low-pressure right side of the heart usually respond to conservative measures of thoracostomy and volume replacement. Injuries to the high-pressure left side of the heart require surgery and carry a much worse prognosis.

Cardiac Tamponade

Although it can occur with blunt trauma, cardiac tamponade is most often seen with penetrating injuries to the chest. Anterior wounds in the mediastinal box are most often associated with cardiac tamponade, but cardiac injury is possible from any thoracic penetration. A description of the wounding implement is somewhat helpful, but the history of a "small knife" or a "small caliber bullet" means nothing in this setting. Cardiac tamponade is much more common with knife wounds than with gunshot wounds because of the limited nature of the tissue destruction. A bullet usually destroys enough tissue to allow the pericardium to drain itself, but a stab wound will essentially seal off the wound track, which allows blood to collect under pressure within the pericardium.

With cardiac tamponade, the classical physical findings of muffled heart sounds, elevated jugular venous pressure, and pulsus paradoxus are often not present. The only clues for tamponade may be the penetrating injury to the chest and a deteriorating condition. The normal response to tamponade is an increase in heart rate to overcome a falling blood pressure. Some patients develop an intermittent tamponade that self-decompresses as pressure builds. This release of pressure is probably what allows these patients to survive more than a few minutes. When approximately 200 ml of blood accumulates in the pericardium, the ability of the pericardium to compensate is overcome, and intracardiac pressures rise rapidly.

If a cardiac injury is suspected, monitoring central venous pressure can be critical. Even in the absence of distended neck veins, the central venous pressure may be elevated, even with concomitant hypovolemia. With a penetrating injury, a rising central venous pressure in the face of falling blood pressure has few explanations other than cardiac tamponade or tension pneumothorax. Because it may be difficult to distinguish these two problems, a tension pneumothorax should be ruled out first before treating the patient for cardiac tamponade.

Treatment for cardiac tamponade is immediate decompression by one of three methods. If the patient is awake or at least responsive, a needle pericardiocentesis should be performed because it is the most rapid and least invasive technique. However, tamponade does tend to recur after needle drainage; therefore needle drainage should be considered a temporizing step until the either the patient is stable or a more definitive procedure is performed. If the patient has lost vital signs, an immediate thoracotomy should be performed, and the pericardium should be incised and drained. Some debate exists over the approach, but most physicians would enter laterally in the left side of the chest through the fifth intercostal space. The pericardium should be grasped with pickups and incised without damaging the phrenic nerve. A pericardial window is the third option for relieving tamponade, but this procedure is rarely performed in the emergency department.

Many patients with cardiac tamponade require intubation before any procedure because of the serious nature of the injuries; the omi-nous sign of worsening bradycardia should warn of immediate cardiovascular collapse. If a tension pneumothorax has been excluded, proceed directly to a thoracotomy in this premorbid setting. Although some patients can be completely treated with decompression in the emergency department, it is more likely that they will require a formal thoracotomy in the operating room.

Esophageal Injuries

The esophagus is rarely injured with blunt trauma, but a penetrating injury is capable of reaching this structure. Unfortunately, esophageal injuries are the most rapidly lethal injuries of the gastrointestinal tract and rapidly progress to fulminant infection. Because of its central location, the esophagus is usually injured along with other structures, most often the trachea. It can also be damaged iatrogenically during attempts to remove foreign bodies, intubation, or lavage.

X-ray studies of the neck and chest that may show air in the soft tissues may be the only early sign of a penetrating injury. A Hamman sign (a pericardial friction rub) is a late sign and suggests considerable involvement of the mediastinum as a result of a perforation. Injuries that penetrate the chest in the area of the esophagus should be studied with a combination of esophagoscopy and the esophagogram if the patient is stable. Once diagnosed, the emergency department treatment of an esophageal perforation should include nasogastric tube drainage, broad spectrum antibiotics, and an immediate surgical consultation.

KEY CONSIDERATIONS

WHAT IS THE LIFE THREAT?

Life-threatening injuries include airway obstruction, a ruptured bronchus, tension pneumothorax, massive hemothorax, penetrating injury to the heart, ruptured aorta, and cardiac tamponade.

DOES THE PATIENT NEED ADMISSION?

Patients with severe chest trauma require admission. Those with chest trauma and unstable vital signs require surgical consultation. Imaging techniques include a chest CT scan and angiography.

Depending on the nature of the injury, the patient will require surgery or admission to the intensive care unit. Those with a widening mediastinum need a chest CT scan or aortogram.

Patients with a fractured first rib have a high likelihood of more severe intrathoracic injury and deserve careful evaluation, including admission for observation.

WHAT IS THE MOST SERIOUS DIAGNOSIS?

A ruptured aorta, other ruptured intrathoracic blood vessels, penetrating injury to the heart, cardiac tamponade, and tension pneumothorax are the most serious diagnoses.

HAVE I PERFORMED A THOROUGH WORK-UP?

Assess vital signs repeatedly. Measure oxygenation or arterial blood gases. Obtain a CT scan if needed. Perform a tube thoracostomy for a pneumothorax or hemothorax. Check upper and lower extremity pulses and look for signs of a dissecting injury to or a rupture of the aorta.

Recommended Reading

French RS: Cardiac injuries. In Harwood-Nuss AL et al, editors: *The clinical practice of emergency medicine,* Philadelphia, 1991, JB Lippincott.

Hurst JM, Davis K, Branson RD: The thorax. In Moore et al, editors: *Early care of the injured patient,* ed 4, Toronto, 1990, BC Decker.

Kanowitz A, Markovchik V: Esophageal and diaphragmatic injuries. In Rosen P et al, editors: *Emergency medicine: concepts and clinical practice,* ed 3, St Louis, 1992, Mosby.

Markovchick V, Duffens KR: Cardiovascular trauma. In Rosen P et al, editors: *Emergency medicine: concepts and clinical practice,* ed 3, St Louis, 1992, Mosby.

Vukich DJ, Markovchick V: Thoracic trauma. In Rosen P et al, editors: *Emergency medicine: concepts and clinical practice,* ed 3, St Louis, 1992, Mosby.

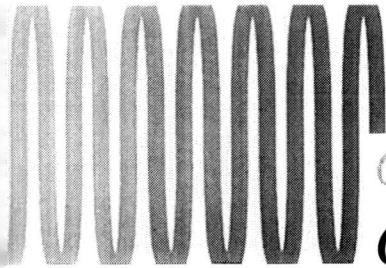

Chapter Twenty-three
CARDIOVASCULAR TRAUMA

VINCENT J. MARKOVCHICK

Trauma to the chest presents unique diagnostic and therapeutic challenges. Falls and high-speed automobile and motorcycle trauma result in acceleration/deceleration injuries to the chest with a subsequent risk for trauma to the cardiovascular system. Penetrating trauma from gunshots and stab wounds is the major cause of acute pericardial tamponade and has the potential for significant trauma to the aorta and other major vessels within the thoracic cavity. This chapter discusses blunt and penetrating trauma to the heart, aorta, and major blood vessels within the thoracic cavity.

MYOCARDIAL CONTUSION

The true incidence of trauma to the myocardium is unknown because there is no gold standard in detecting this type of injury. The estimated incidence of myocardial injury varies from 3% to 75% in the reported series of blunt, closed-chest trauma.

Blunt cardiac trauma may be viewed as part of a continuous spectrum that ranges from myocardial concussion to myocardial rupture. *Myocardial concussion* results from blunt trauma to the chest, which produces a "stunned" response in the myocardium. This response results in an acute dysrhythmia that results in a transient loss of consciousness if the dysrhythmia spontaneously re-

verses to a viable rhythm. This response also is thought to explain those instances in which blunt trauma to the precordium results in cardiac arrest and death of an individual whose postmortem examination reveals no demonstrable trauma to the myocardium. Cellular injury resulting from direct myocardial trauma is called a *myocardial contusion;* its natural history is to heal with no permanent sequelae. Because permanent myocardial damage is rare, it is thought that many cases of myocardial contusion go unrecognized. Blunt trauma to the myocardium may also result in a traumatic *myocardial infarction* secondary to occlusion of a traumatized coronary artery. The most common artery involved is the right coronary artery. The most severe form of cardiac trauma is *myocardial rupture,* which in rare instances manifests itself as acute pericardial tamponade but most of the time results in immediate exsanguinating hemorrhage.

Etiology

Trauma to the myocardium is usually the result of high-speed deceleration accidents, with auto accidents being the most common cause of myocardial injury. With a direct blow to the chest, energy is transmitted through the chest wall to the heart. A large force applied over the chest wall over a longer period causes the sternum to be displaced posteriorly, which compresses the heart between the sternum and the vertebrae or an elevated diaphragm and results in cardiac injury. In addition, the heart has relatively free movement in an anterioroposterior direction within the chest, and in cases of sudden deceleration of the chest wall, the heart continues to move forward because of its momentum when striking the sternum with considerable force.

Clinical Findings

Even though the diagnosis of myocardial contusion is easy to make at autopsy, it is impossible to make such a diagnosis clinically with 100% certainty. The history of significant blunt anterior chest trauma should lead to a consideration of this diagnosis, and the presence of any of the following should lead to the presumptive diagnosis of myocardial contusion: any new changes on an ECG, cardiogenic shock, or ischemic chest pain. The most common ECG changes include transient right bundle branch block, premature ventricular contractions, and persistent tachycardia, but other causes of tachycardia should be treated or ruled out first. If a large area of myocardium is involved, the patient may demonstrate a clinical picture of cardiogenic shock.

Treatment

Dysrhythmias and cardiogenic shock should be treated with standard pharmacologic therapy. Because a portion of the myocardium is dysfunctional, there is a decreased tolerance to fluid overload and care should be taken to avoid overzealous administration of crystalloid solutions. If signs of cardiogenic shock are present, Swan-Ganz catheterization and monitoring should be performed. Ultrasonography should be obtained for any patient who is exhibiting signs of cardiogenic shock to rule out pericardial tamponade and to assess wall motion.

If ECG findings are compatible with acute myocardial infarction, an immediate cardiology consultation should be obtained to determine if emergent coronary artery angioplasty is indicated because thrombolytic therapy is contraindicated in an acutely traumatized patient. If any of the preceding clinical signs are present in conjunction with moderate-to-severe trauma to the anterior chest, consideration should be given to admission and continuous cardiac monitoring for 24 hours.

MYOCARDIAL RUPTURE

Blunt trauma to the heart results in a variety of lesions; a myocardial rupture is the most serious and devastating heart lesion. A myocardial rupture results from violent trauma to the anterior chest and precordium and is nearly always fatal. The only real chance of survival occurs in those few cases in which the hemorrhage is limited by the pericardium and the patient survives to undergo a thoracotomy. In these rare instances, patients usually have pericardial tamponade, which is usually secondary to the rupture of an atrium.

Pathophysiology

Rupture of the myocardium occurs when there is closure of the outflow tract with violent ventricular compression of the blood-filled chamber; this mechanism is the most likely cause of ventricular rupture. The ventricles are the most commonly involved chambers in cardiac rupture; ruptures of the atria are less common, and the right side exceeds that of the left. Multiple chamber involvement occurs in approximately 30% of all patients. The vast majority of these patients experience cardiac arrest following blunt trauma; once this situation ensues, there is essentially no chance for survival, even with ideal care. The chances for survival are much improved if the hemorrhage is confined by the pericardium, if the patient comes to the emergency department with vital signs, and if there are no concomitant life-threatening injuries. Patients who have an intermittently decompressing pericardial tamponade secondary to a small laceration in the pericardium have the greatest chance of survival.

Isolated traumatic rupture of the pericardium from blunt chest trauma is rarely found in the absence of cardiac rupture. A principal complication of this lesion is the potential for cardiac or visceral herniation through the defect in the pericardium.

Treatment

The only chance of survival in patients with myocardial rupture is early emergency thoracotomy to gain direct access to the myocardium, control the hemorrhage, and relieve acute pericardial tamponade.

ACUTE PERICARDIAL TAMPONADE

Pericardial tamponade occurs in 2% of all patients with penetrating trauma to the chest or lower abdomen. It is rarely seen following blunt chest trauma. Pericardial tamponade is a surgical emergency because these patients can deteriorate in minutes. However, many can be saved if rapid and aggressive diagnostic and therapeutic interventions are implemented.

Etiology

Pericardial tamponade should be suspected in any patient who has sustained a penetrating wound or blunt trauma to the thorax, upper abdomen, or supraclavicular area. There is never any certainty regarding the trajectory of the bullet or the length and direction of the knife thrust. Obviously wounds directly over the precordium and epigastrium are most likely to produce a cardiac injury than those in the posterior or lateral thorax or superclavicular area.

Iatrogenic causes of tamponade include pacemaker insertion, cardiac catheterization, placement of central venous lines, intercardiac injections of medication, or attempts at pericardiocentesis.

Pathophysiology

The pericardium has very little capacity to distend in response to an acute increase in intrapericardiac pressure and volume. As a result, the volume of pericardial fluid encroaches on the capacity of the atria and ventricles to fill adequately, which results in a decreasing stroke volume. This phenomenon results in a decreased cardiac output and ultimately a diminished arterial systolic blood pressure and decreased pulse pressure. Concomitantly the central venous pressure rises because of the mechanical backup of blood into the vena cava. Next, several compensatory mechanisms occur. The heart rate and total peripheral resistance rise in an attempt to maintain an adequate cardiac output ($CO = SV \times HR$)* and blood pressure ($BP = CO \times TPR$).* A less effective compensatory response that results in an even greater rise in central venous pressure (CVP) is an increase in venomotor tone of the vena cava.

In a normotensive patient the earliest response to pericardial tamponade is a progressive rise in the CVP to a level greater than 15 cm of H_2O. A rising CVP in a hypotensive patient indicates that normal compensatory responses are unable to maintain an adequate cardiac output. Bradycardia or a simultaneous fall in both the CVP and blood pressure can occur precipitously and signals decompensation and imminent cardiac arrest.

Diagnosis

The most reliable clinical signs of pericardial tamponade are a CVP elevated to ≥15 cm of H_2O in association with hypotension and tachy-

---

*CO = cardiac output, SV = stroke volume, BP = blood pressure, TPR = total peripheral resistance.

cardia. The presence of acute pericardial tamponade must be considered when this triad is present either before or after volume replacement and the exclusion of a diagnosis of tension pneumothorax. For patients in hypovolemic shock, the elevation in CVP is not manifest until after adequate volume resuscitation. Additional physical findings include the presence of a pulsus paradoxus that may be detected by a palpable diminution or by the absence of the peripheral pulse during inspiration.

The only pathognomonic ECG sign of pericardial tamponade is complete electrical alternans. This sign is rarely if ever seen in acute pericardial tamponade and is most common in patients with chronic pericardial effusion. Electrical alternans is thought to be secondary to the "swinging heart" phenomenon. With large pericardial effusions it is thought that the heart may swing back and forth within the pericardial fluid, thus alternating its position and electrical axis.

A plain chest x-ray study is not helpful in diagnosing acute pericardial tamponade because changes in the cardiac silhouette do not occur in the acute situation. However, a chest x-ray film is useful in detecting the presence of concomitant pulmonary, bony, or mediastinal trauma.

The most rapid, highly sensitive, specific, and noninvasive study for making the diagnosis of fluid in the pericardial space is cardiac ultrasonography. If available, this study should be performed in the emergency department on all patients with suspected pericardial tamponade. Acute pericardial tamponade is defined by ultrasonography as a collapse of the right ventricle during diastole, although the presence of pericardial fluid is sufficient to warrant a pericardial window.

Treatment

Prehospital

In the field and in the emergency department, aggressive initial fluid resuscitation with crystalloid supports the initial compensatory mechanisms present in acute pericardial tamponade. A tension pneumothorax may mimic the clinical signs of acute pericardial tamponade and must be emergently treated if present. Patients with this suspected injury should be transported directly to a hospital that is capable of immediate operating suite thoracotomy. Prolonged transport times or deteriorating vital signs are two of the few indications for pericardiocentesis in the field.

Emergency department

In the emergency department, the standard ABCs of trauma resuscitation should be followed. In addition, early insertion of a CVP catheter is helpful for monitoring CVP changes and is often the earliest indicator of the development of acute pericardial tamponade. Cardiac ultrasonography should be obtained very early in the patient's course if available because it often reveals the presence of an acute pericardial effusion before the patient exhibits the classic clinical findings of this entity. If the ultrasonography is positive for fluid in the pericardial space or is not immediately available and the patient has developed the classic signs of acute pericardial tamponade (i.e., hypotension, tachycardia, and an elevated CVP), a pericardiocentesis should be performed as a temporizing measure while the surgeon and operating room team are prepared. Decompression of the pericardial sac may need to be performed several times while preparing the operating suite and mobilizing the surgical team for definitive care. Inserting a catheter into the pericardial space usually eliminates the need for recurrent needle pericardiocentesis.

Acute patient deterioration (e.g., bradycardia or profound hypotension) in the emergency department and unsuccessful pericardiocentesis compose the one clear indication for emergency department thoracotomy. A left lateral thoracotomy should be performed and exposure to the heart obtained. A vertical incision into the pericardium will immediately relieve the tamponade. The penetrating wound of the heart should be located and immediately tamponaded with digital pressure. If definitive surgical care is unavailable or is going to be delayed substantially, such wounds can be closed with horizontal mattress sutures over pledgets.

Prognosis

The vast majority of patients who sustain a penetrating trauma to the pericardium and have vital signs on arrival to the emergency department survive with no sequelae. Acute pericardial tamponade secondary to gunshot wounds and blunt trauma has a much poorer prognosis than that resulting from stab wounds. An aggressive approach to patients who have a systolic blood pressure greater than 50 mm Hg on arrival to the emergency department has resulted in survival rates as high as 95% in some series.

AORTIC TRAUMA

Aortic Rupture

Aortic rupture is one of the leading causes of death from automobile trauma, with an estimated 7500 deaths annually. Of those who sustain this type of injury 80% to 90% exsanguinate immediately as a result of free rupture into the thoracic cavity. The remaining 10% to 20% who survive at least temporarily do so because of the tamponade of aortic blood by the intact adventitia. The natural history of traumatic aortic bleeding that is confined by the adventitia reveals that the majority of these patients ultimately die from free rupture and exsanguination if this condition is not diagnosed and surgically repaired in a timely fashion. Fortunately, because few patients in this latter group sustain free rupture within the first 6 hours, more immediate life threats such as intraperitoneal or intracerebral hemorrhage can be treated before repair of the aorta.

Etiology

Automobile acceleration/deceleration injuries with transverse forces across the chest are the most common cause of an aortic tear. The ruptured sites of the tear occur 85% of the time at the isthmus, 9% at the origin of the ascending aorta, and 3% at the diaphragm. Tears of the ascending aorta have a high incidence of associated cardiac injuries. The mechanism for ascending aortic tears includes passenger ejection, pedestrian impact, falls from significant heights, and crush injuries.

Pathophysiology

Several theories about the mechanism of aortic rupture have predominated in the literature. The descending aorta is relatively fixed. Therefore with sudden deceleration, the more mobile aortic arch swings forward and produces a shearing force on the aorta at the isthmus. This shearing force results in a tear at the classic location in the descending aorta just distal to the ligamentum arteriosum. Ninety percent of all aortic tears occur in this area. The ascending aorta may also be involved, particularly in vertical acceleration/deceleration such as falls from significant heights. If it occurs within the reflections of the pericardium, a tear in the ascending aorta may appear as acute pericardial tamponade or a myocardial infarction if flow to the coronary arteries is compromised.

Clinical findings

The possibility of aortic rupture must be considered in every patient who sustains a severe deceleration injury to the chest. This consideration is especially important for high-speed auto accidents, in patients who were not wearing proper restraints, or in patients who were ejected. In contrast to pericardial tamponade, there are very few clinical signs of traumatic aortic tear and dissection, partly because most of these patients have significant associated multiple injuries that often mask the signs and symptoms of aortic injury. The most common symptom that is present in a minority of patients is retrosternal or interscapular pain.

A classic clinical sign, if present, is generalized hypertension secondary to stimulation of the sympathetic afferent nerve fibers located in the area of the aortic isthmus; stimulation of these nerve fibers causes a reflex hypertension in response to a stretching stimulus. A less common clinical finding is upper extremity hypertension along with absent or diminished femoral pulses, which is known as the pseudocoarctation syndrome. More often these patients initially show signs of hypovolemic shock or respiratory distress secondary to hemorrhagic or concomitant pulmonary trauma.

The lack of external physical trauma to the chest wall has been reported in approximately one third to one half of the patients who have had documented aortic injury. Therefore the lack of or minimal external signs of thoracic injury should not preclude the diagnosis if there is a concerning mechanism of injury. Younger patients are less likely to have associated fractures because of the increased compliance of the chest wall.

Diagnostic studies

An upright standard posteroanterior (PA) chest x-ray film remains a good screening study in patients whose condition permits such a study to be performed. A sensitive but nonspecific finding is increased mediastinal width. The condition of most major trauma patients requires that the initial screening chest study be performed in the supine position. A supine portable chest x-ray view often results in a falsely positive widened mediastinum; therefore an upright standard PA chest film should be obtained in the radiology suite if the patient's condition permits. There is a reported sensitivity of between 50% and 92%, with a very low specificity of approximately 10% because there are a myriad of causes of bleeding into the mediastinum other than an aortic dissection.

Additional clinical signs that have been de-

scribed on the plain chest x-ray film include an obscured aortic knob, a displaced nasogastric tube to the right, a widened peritracheal stripe, a widened right paraspinal interface, a left apical pleural cap, a depression of the left main stem bronchus below 40 degrees from the horizontal, a left hemothorax, a deviation of the trachea to the right, and fractures of the first or second ribs.

The predictive value of a negative or normal chest x-ray study is controversial. Some believe that it is 98% predictive of a normal arteriogram, but others state that in one series 6 out of 41 patients (15%) who had an acute traumatic rupture of the aorta had completely normal chest x-ray studies. A completely normal upright standard chest x-ray film associated with a mild-to-moderate mechanism of injury is probably a very reasonable screen to rule out the presence of an aortic tear. However, in those patients who have a major mechanism of injury, a normal chest x-ray film is not 100% reliable in ruling out this entity.

Aortography remains the gold standard for the diagnosis of an acute aortic injury, but recent studies have indicated that there are other noninvasive diagnostic studies that may reliably rule out the presence of an acute aortic tear: a dynamic CT scan of the chest and transesophageal echocardiography. In preliminary reports the absence of a mediastinal hemorrhage on a dynamic CT scan of the chest has an extremely high sensitivity but low specificity in regard to the presence of an acute aortic tear. In one preliminary series, 100% of the patients who had a negative dynamic CT scan of the chest had the absence of an acute aortic injury confirmed by a follow-up arteriography, which resulted in 100% sensitivity. However, an aortogram must be performed if a dynamic CT scan of the chest is positive for a mediastinal hemorrhage. In some instances, a dynamic CT scan of the chest has been shown to be diagnostic for an acute aortic injury if the intimal tear can be demonstrated on the CT scan. A transesophageal echocardiography to demonstrate the presence of a periaortic hemorrhage or intimal flaps has also shown great promise. The use of either a CT scan or transesophageal echocardiography in stable patients who have had a moderate-to-major mechanism of injury will probably reduce the number of aortograms necessary to rule out this life-threatening injury.

Aortography remains the initial procedure of choice and should be performed as soon as possible in unstable patients who have had a major mechanism of injury and who are exhibiting the classical signs of aortic rupture on a plain chest x-ray film. However, this study should not take precedence over the control and treatment of other acute life-threatening injuries such as intraperitoneal hemorrhage and acute subdural or epidural hematoma.

Treatment

Because the definitive care of the traumatic aortic tear requires timely aortography and surgical repair, any patient sustaining significant blunt chest trauma secondary to an acceleration/deceleration mechanism should be transported directly to a trauma center if possible. The repair of this lesion should be performed as soon as possible after the diagnosis is made because of the ever-present risk of free rupture and exsanguination. However, more immediate life threats such as significant intraperitoneal hemorrhage, acute epidural or subdural hematomas, or a significant retroperitoneal hemorrhage secondary to unstable pelvic fractures should take priority because they pose more immediate life threats.

If the patient develops hypertension, the blood pressure should be carefully regulated until definitive surgical repair can be obtained. The recommended agents for this condition are intravenous nitroprusside and intravenous beta blockers such as esmolol to minimize the shearing effect of hypertension on the intact adventitia of the aorta.

Most definitive surgical repairs of the descending aorta can be performed without a cardiopulmonary bypass. However, in type 1 or ascending aortic tears, a cardiopulmonary bypass is more often necessary. The surgical mortality from a descending aortic injury is as much as 30%, with a 5.7% reported incidence of postoperative paraplegia secondary to disruption of circulation to the spinal cord.

Associated Cardiovascular Injuries

Blunt injuries involving the major arterial branches of the aortic arch are uncommon but should be suspected when major forces have been applied to the upper chest, clavicles, or base of the neck. Symptoms and signs common to these injuries include decreased or absent upper extremity or carotid pulses, differential upper extremity blood pressures, bruits, large hematomas in the neck, an apical pleural cap on the chest radiograph, major intrathoracic hemorrhage, and neurologic deficits secondary to brachial plexus injuries or carotid artery injuries.

For patients who sustain penetrating injuries to zone 1 of the neck, to the area just above or below the clavicles, or high in the axilla, strong consideration should be given to early aortography, with studies assessing the integrity of the vessels exiting the proximal aorta. Angiography should be considered for patients sustaining gunshot wounds in proximity to major vessels to rule out intimal disruption, which can result in delayed sequelae such as thrombosis or stroke. Cardiovascular consultation should be obtained early in such patients because there is risk for an accelerated internal hemorrhage that may necessitate emergency operative control of the hemorrhage via the thoracotomy median sternotomy approach.

KEY CONSIDERATIONS

WHAT IS THE LIFE THREAT?

Myocardial rupture following blunt or penetrating trauma, acute pericardial tamponade, and aortic rupture are all life-threatening injuries.

DOES THE PATIENT NEED ADMISSION?

Patients with severe cardiovascular trauma require evaluation by a cardiac surgeon and admission to the operating room or intensive care unit.

Patients with a myocardial contusion may have associated dysrhythmias, dysfunctional myocardium, or traumatic coronary artery thrombosis. Patients with blunt injury to the chest who exhibit hypotension or ischemic chest pain or who exhibit ischemic change or dysrhythmia on the ECG should at least be hospitalized for observation and have a cardiology consultation.

WHAT IS THE MOST SERIOUS DIAGNOSIS?

Myocardial rupture, aortic rupture, or pericardial tamponade are the most serious diagnoses.

HAVE I PERFORMED A THOROUGH WORK-UP?

Obtain a good history of the mechanism of trauma if possible, including whether or not the steering wheel was damaged in auto accidents. Evaluate the chest carefully, noting seat-belt injury, rib tenderness or deformity, breath sounds, and heart sounds. Obtain a chest x-ray study, an ECG, and pulse oximetry. If necessary, evaluate with a dynamic CT scan, transesophageal ultrasonography, or aortography.

Evaluate the patient for myocardial contusion if the patient has a new change on an ECG, cardiogenic shock, or ischemic chest pain.

Recommended Reading

Agee CK et al: Computed tomographic evaluation to exclude traumatic aortic disruption, *J Trauma* 33(6): 876-881, 1992.

Baxter BT et al: Graded experimental myocardial contusion: impact on cardiac rhythm, coronary artery flow, ventricular function, and myocardial oxygen consumption, *J Trauma* 28:1411, 1988.

Brooks SW et al: The use of transesophageal echocardiography in the evaluation of chest trauma, *J Trauma* 32:761-768, 1992.

Kearney PA et al: Use of transesophageal echocardiography in the evaluation of traumatic aortic injury, *J Trauma* 34:696-703, 1994.

Kim FJ et al: Trauma surgeons can render definitive surgical care for major thoracic injuries, *J Trauma* 36(6):871, 1994.

Poole GV et al: Computed tomography in the management of blunt thoracic trauma, *J Trauma* 35(2): 296-302, 1993.

Rosenberg JM et al: Blunt injuries to the aortic arch vessels, *Ann Thorac Surg* 48:508, 1989.

Chapter Twenty-four

ABDOMINAL AND GENITOURINARY TRAUMA

JOHN MARX AND ROBERT E. SCHNEIDER

ABDOMINAL TRAUMA

BLUNT ABDOMINAL TRAUMA

The evaluation of blunt abdominal trauma has evolved considerably during the last three decades. Diagnostic peritoneal lavage (DPL) has provided a sensitive and rapid means of investigating the intraperitoneal cavity. However, it does have its shortcomings, including occasional oversensitivity, relative nonspecificity, an inability to coincidentally evaluate the retroperitoneum, and an acceptably low incidence of complications. A CT scan is a more specific method of delineating organ injury, but it lacks sensitivity for certain structures, and its ability to predict the need for operation is questionable. Ultrasonography is the latest addition to the diagnostic armamentarium, particularly for blunt trauma. It has undergone limited study in this country and is more widely used in parts of Europe and Asia.

Physical Examination

Even in the conscious and oriented patient, clinical manifestations of significant injury to intraperitoneal structures may be lacking following abdominal trauma. In addition, false positive signs of injury may be seen in the setting of abdominal wall contusions, thoracolumbar spine fractures, and preexisting disease. Most importantly, the majority of patients with significant multiple blunt trauma injuries have associated intoxication, a closed head injury, or distracting pain at extraabdominal sites. These and other factors combine to render the physical examination only 50% to 60% reliable in determining the presence of intraabdominal pathology that requires operation.

Clinical Indications for Laparotomy

It is occasionally appropriate following blunt trauma to pursue urgent laparotomy solely on the basis of clinical criteria and without the aid of other diagnostic measures. These indications include the following:

- *Unstable with suspected abdominal injury.* This indication is appropriate only when a patient presents with isolated injury to the thoracoabdominal region.
- *Peritoneal irritation.* This indication is generally unreliable early. It is more helpful in patients who present to the emergency department 12 or more hours following injury and in whom hollow viscus perforation is likely responsible.
- *Pneumoperitoneum.* This indication has high specificity in blunt trauma. However, it

is an insensitive finding in the presence of perforation and is relatively uncommon.

- *Evidence of diaphragmatic injury.* This indication mandates repair but may be undertaken in a nonurgent fashion. Both the physical and radiologic findings of diaphragmatic injury lack sensitivity and specificity.

Laboratory

Hematology

Baseline hematocrits reflect a premorbid state, endogenous plasma refill, and crystalloid administration. Serial hematocrits are more helpful but require integration with clinical findings to determine the need for transfusion.

Serum amylase, lipase, and pancreatic isoenzymes

Serum amylase, lipase, and pancreatic isoenzyme tests lack sensitivity and specificity and are not justified for routine use. Elevated levels rarely reflect the presence of pancreatic or proximal small bowel injury.

Liver functions

Elevated transaminases may increase the suspicion for hepatic injury, but given the widespread use of alcohol in trauma victims and the lack of prospective data, such tests are not routinely necessary.

Serum bicarbonate

A clinical history and physical examination is a less costly and more readily available method of determining the presence of shock.

Diagnostic Studies

Diagnostic peritoneal lavage

Advantages

- *Sensitivity.* DPL is exceptionally sensitive in the discovery of hemoperitoneum and has a false-negative rate of less than 2%. Therefore it is a superior triage instrument in the pa-

tient with hypotension and multiple blunt trauma.

- *Availability.* DPL can be performed in virtually any patient by individualizing the site and method.
- *Rapidity.* Less than 5 minutes is required to aspirate the peritoneum, and this is the more time-critical portion of the procedure.
- *Safety.* Although DPL is invasive, the complication rate is small in experienced hands.
- *Immediate triage.* In the patient with acute and multiple blunt trauma injuries, DPL allows for rapid recognition of hemoperitoneum. This recognition is decisive in determining whether a patient requires a laparotomy or if other urgent diagnostics can be pursued.

Disadvantages

- *Inaccuracies.* The retroperitoneal space is not sampled by DPL. False negatives are uncommon with DPL, but false positives can occur as a result of faulty performance of the procedure.
- *Sensitivity.* Strict reliance on findings of hemoperitoneum and absent consideration of the clinical scenario can result in a 6% to 12% unnecessary laparotomy rate. These unnecessary laparotomies usually result from minimal-to-moderate and self-limited injuries to the liver or spleen that at laparotomy are found to be nonbleeding and not requiring operative intervention.
- *Complications.* Less than 1%.

Interpretation

- *Bloody aspirate.* The presence of more than 10 ml of blood has a high association with the presence of intraperitoneal injury.
- *Red blood cells.* > 100,000: positive
            20,000 to 100,000: equivocal
            < 20,000: negative
- *White blood cells.* This test is insensitive for up to 3 to 5 hours postinjury and is thereafter a nonspecific test. This test should not be used in isolation as an indication to proceed to laparotomy.

- *Enzymes.* Lavage amylase (level ≥ 20 IU/L: positive; 10 to 19 IU/L: equivocal) can be an immediate marker of proximal small bowel injury. Lavage alkaline phosphatase (level ≥ 3 IU/L: equivocal) is suggestive but not as accurate as lavage amylase.

Computed tomography

Advantages

- *Specificity.* The CT scan is most accurate for liver and spleen pathology. It allows visualization and perhaps quantitation of variable amounts of hemoperitoneum.
- *Retroperitoneum.* A CT scan is able to evaluate simultaneously the intraperitoneal and retroperitoneal spaces.

Disadvantages

- *Inaccuracies.* A CT scan is generally excellent for solid visceral trauma but may be falsely negative for hollow injuries to the viscera and pancreas, as well as occasional moderate-to-large quantities of hemoperitoneum.
- *Logistical concerns.* The ability to perform a CT scan in a safe and moderate fashion, the time required for performance, and the ready availability of this procedure must be considered on an institutional basis.
- *Complications.* Complications include aspiration of oral contrast material and allergic reactions to intravenous contrast.

Ultrasonography

Two utilities have brought ultrasonography (US) to the forefront. First, this modality has been considered for use as a triage instrument similar to DPL for the detection of intraperitoneal hemorrhage. Second, US can determine injury to solid viscera such as the liver, spleen, and kidney. It is useful for late complications of pancreatic trauma, such as pseudocyst formation. Clinical experience suggests a sensitivity for detection of hemoperitoneum that ranges from 60% to 95%. When compared with DPL, US has been found to be less sensitive, with false-negative rates of 5% to 20%. Like a CT scan,

US is a more powerful tool with solid organs but the experiences reported are very uneven and dependent on the training and experience of the technician or interpreter.

Advantages

- *Safe.* No contrast agents or radiation.
- *Rapid.* US can be completed quickly if the emergency physician or trauma surgeon is able to perform.
- *Serial examinations.* US can be used to follow hemoperitoneum and specific organ injury.
- *Pregnancy.* No concerns.
- *Prior laparotomy.* A prior laparotomy is not a contraindication to the use of US, but compartmentalization of blood could theoretically lead to misinterpretation.

Disadvantages

- *Availability.* Clinicians or radiologists who are able to conduct US, as well as the necessary equipment, must be immediately available. Otherwise, US cannot serve in lieu of DPL as a rapid means of determining the need for laparotomy.
- *Accuracy.* The accuracy of US varies with equipment and with technical and reader expertise. Hollow visceral and acute pancreatic injuries are poorly visualized by this method.

Operative vs. Nonoperative Management

In the patient with acute blunt multisystem trauma, it is difficult to predict the need for an operation on clinical grounds alone. An exception to this rule is the patient who cannot be stabilized and who appears to have massive hemoperitoneum. Patients typically undergo one or more diagnostic procedures before laparotomy. Certain peritoneal injuries can be watched expectantly. Specifically, this technique has been effective with minimal-to-moderate and self-limited trauma to the liver or spleen; it is not appropriate for hollow viscus perforation.

The advantages of operative management of solid visceral intraperitoneal injury include the extra measure of safety of operative repair and the potential discovery of coincident injury, particularly to hollow viscera. Disadvantages of operative management are the hazards of the operation, including general anesthesia, intubation, and possibly an increased hospital stay and cost.

Expectant management potentially avoids laparotomy and its attendant risks. Its hazards include the possibility of increased transfusions, delayed laparotomy with attendant morbidity, and the greatest consequence of missed injuries. In particular, the patient with a closed head injury is very difficult to evaluate by serial clinical assessments.

PENETRATING TRAUMA

Stab Wounds

Peritoneal violation occurs in 50% to 70% of all stab wounds to the anterior abdomen. Approximately half of those injuries in which the stabbing implement violates the peritoneal cavity require a laparotomy. Thus only one fourth to one third of all patients who sustain stab wounds to the anterior abdomen ultimately require operative intervention. A mandatory laparotomy on the basis of mechanism was practiced before the mid-1960s and resulted in an enormously high number of unnecessary laparotomies. Subsequently, various strategies have been implemented to better define those patients who require operation. The combination of clinical criteria, local wound exploration (LWE), and DPL has wide support. Other modalities to discern the presence of worrisome injury have gained popularity in some camps. These modalities include serial clinical examinations, CT scans, and laparoscopy.

Diagnostic strategy

An algorithmic approach to a stab wound to the anterior abdomen can be broken down into three sequential steps (Fig. 24-1):
1. Is there a clinical need for a laparotomy?
   - *Unstable vital signs.* The presence of un-

stable vital signs is the most likely reason that a patient moves urgently to the operating room without preliminary diagnostic procedures. However, stab wounds, particularly to the epigastrium, may produce unstable vital signs as a consequence of intrathoracic hemorrhage or pericardial tamponade rather than intraperitoneal injury.
   - *Gastrointestinal hemorrhage.* A gastrointestinal hemorrhage may indicate violation of the stomach or duodenum but is an unusual occurrence.
   - *Evisceration.* Evisceration indicates coincident intraperitoneal injury in approximately two thirds of all cases. In certain institutions the physician reduces the evisceration in the emergency department and proceeds with other diagnostics to determine whether an operation is necessary.
   - *Diaphragmatic injury.* Penetrating trauma to the diaphragm produces small tears and evanescent clinical clues to their presence.
   - *Intraperitoneal air.* Intraperitoneal air may impute communication of the knife with the intraperitoneal space and not necessarily indicate hollow visceral perforation.
   - *Peritoneal signs.* Peritoneal signs are notoriously inaccurate, particularly in the early postinjury period. The high prevalence of alcohol and drug use among victims of penetrating trauma further undermines the reliability of a physical examination.
   - *Implement in situ.* The conservative and almost universally held maxim is to remove implements-in-situ of the torso in the operating room. However, if emergency resuscitation is impeded by the presence of the implement, the implement should be removed in the field or emergency department. For certain patients, in whom operative removal poses a prohibitive risk, other diagnostic studies (e.g., a CT scan) may be indicated.
2. Has the peritoneal cavity been violated?
   - *Free air*

1. Clinical mandate for OR?

No

Yes

2. Peritoneal entry?

(LWE)

Yes*

3. Injury?

No

(DPL†)

Yes‡

No

OR ◄─ ─ ─ ─ ─ ─ ─ ─ ─ ─ ─ ─ ─ ─ ─ Observe ─ ─ ─ ─ ─ ─► D/C

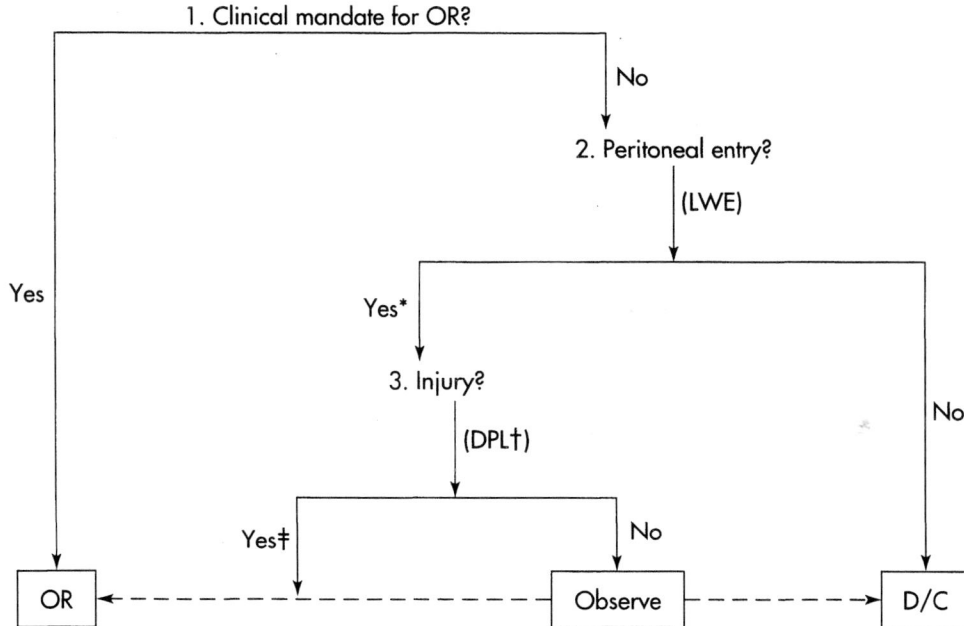

OR, Operation; *LWE*, local wound exploration; *DPL*, diagnostic peritoneal lavage; *D/C*, discharge.

*If LWE cannot be performed or results are equivocal, peritoneal entry should be presumed.
†Serial examinations, laparoscopy, or CT scan can complement or replace DPL.
‡Expectant management of injuries is infrequently attempted.

Fig. **24-1** Stab wound algorithm.

- *Evisceration*
- *Local wound exploration.* LWE is an effective and underused tool to determine the depth of a stab wound tract. Blind probing with digits and instruments is hazardous and inaccurate. LWE can be performed on the anterior abdomen, flank, and back. LWE is generally proscribed for stab wounds to the lower chest; however, slash-type wounds lend themselves to this type of evaluation as long as it is not taken beyond the anterior rib surface to prevent iatrogenic complications. A carefully per-

formed negative LWE that clearly delineates the end of a stab wound tract as anterior to the rectal fascia allows the patient to be discharged after appropriate wound care has been given.

3. Does an intraperitoneal injury exist, and does the injury warrant a laparotomy?

DPL has been the diagnostic standard to address this issue during the last 25 years. A CT scan is used in certain circumstances. Clinical examination alone has been advocated by some, and laparoscopy has received attention as an alternative diagnostic approach.

- *DPL.* DPL has a 90% to 95% accuracy for the discovery of intraperitoneal pathology: Gross blood. Generally accurate, but false positive studies can occur because blood from the abdominal wall stab site reaches the peritoneal cavity.

  Red blood cell (RBC) count. Cut-offs below 20,000/mm^3 produce an unacceptable incidence of unnecessary laparotomies. The RBC criterion for a stab wound of the lower chest should be lowered to 5000 RBC/ml to maximize sensitivity for isolated diaphragmatic injuries:

  Anterior Abdomen
  >100,000 RBC/mm^3: positive
  20 to 100,000 RBC/mm^3: equivocal
  Lower Chest
  5000 RBC/mm^3: positive
  Enzymes.
  Lavage amylase (LAM) $\geq$ 20 IU/L: positive; 10 to 19 IU/L: equivocal

- *Computed tomography.* A CT scan is excellent for the detection of a solid visceral injury following a penetrating mechanism but is less accurate for bowel and diaphragmatic injuries. Because these structures are far more commonly injured following a penetrating trauma, the application of a CT scan to a penetrating mechanism is limited. When a retroperitoneal injury, including a colorectal injury, is more likely a CT scan can serve as an important adjunctive diagnostic method.

- *Serial examinations.* Several reports suggest the reliability of serial clinical examinations for stab wounds of the anterior abdomen, flank, and back without the use of DPL or a CT scan. However, vigilant observation on a busy trauma service can be imposing.

- *Laparoscopy.* Experience with laparoscopy in trauma at certain institutions allows it to be used for direct inspection of the diaphragm and many intraperitoneal organs. It is especially useful for stab wounds of the lower chest, flank, and back.

Gunshot Wounds

There are few points of contention regarding gunshot wounds (GSWs) to the abdomen. An immediate laparotomy is indicated if patients are unstable or show clinical evidence that a missile has entered the peritoneal cavity. If a missile has entered this space, the risk of intraperitoneal injury requiring repair ranges from 89% to 98%. Therefore in these circumstances further diagnostics are unnecessary.

Diagnostic strategy

The approach to GSWs can also be separated into three steps (Fig. 24-2):

1. Is there a clinical indication for a laparotomy? These indications provide essentially the same value as for stab wounds:
   - *Unstable vital signs*
   - *Peritoneal signs*
   - *Gastrointestinal hemorrhage*
   - *Diaphragmatic injury*
   - *Evisceration*

2. Has there been peritoneal violation?

   Several methods determine whether a missile has entered or traversed the peritoneal cavity. However, the path of many GSWs is difficult to assess.
   - *Missile path.* Missile path is predicted on evaluation of entrance and exit wounds. Confusion may arise when missiles ricochet or when there are multiple injuries.
   - *Plain x-ray films.* An anteroposterior and lateral x-ray film can be used to estimate whether the missile lies within or has traversed the peritoneal cavity.
   - *Local wound exploration.* Because of greater depth to and more extensive tissue damage surrounding the missile tract, LWE is a less reliable tool for a GSW of the abdomen, flank, and back. LWE may be useful with low-velocity projectiles and suspected superficial entry.
   - *Laparoscopy.* Laparoscopy has been used to determine whether integrity of the peritoneal cavity has been broached.

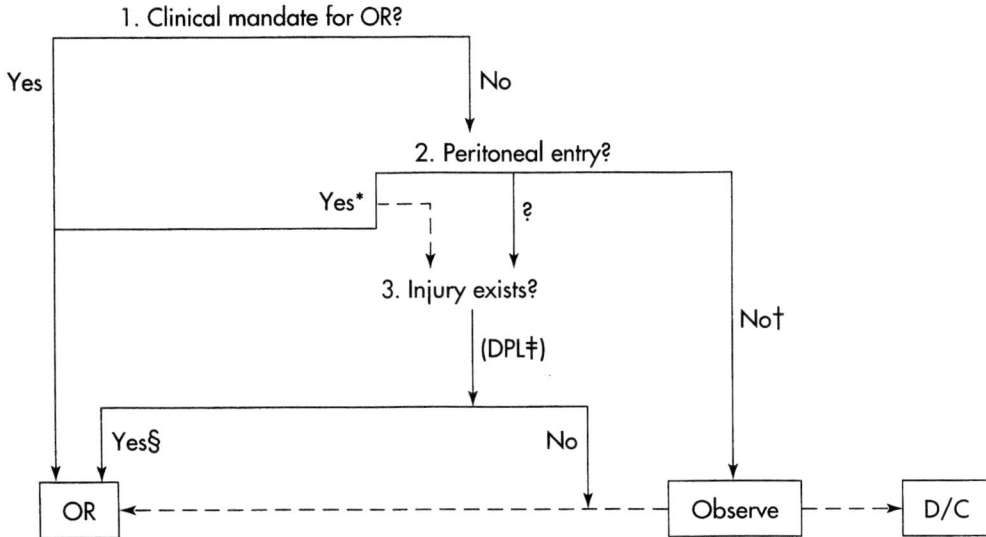

OR, Operation; *DPL*, diagnostic peritoneal lavage; *D/C*, discharge.

*Most centers proceed to laparotomy if peritoneal entry is suspected.
†Documented superficial low velocity injuries can be discharged; unknown depth or high-velocity injuries require further tests or observation.
‡Serial examinations, laparoscopy, or CT scan can complement or replace DPL.
§Expectant management of injuries caused by gunshot wounds is infrequently attempted.

Fig. 24-2 Gunshot wound algorithm.

3. Does injury exist? Does the injury warrant a laparotomy?

At most institutions, the algorithm ends with laparotomy after the second step. However, at selected centers, additional diagnostics may include DPL, serial physical examinations, CT scans, and a laparoscopy.

- *DPL.* DPL is reserved for patients in whom there is a question of intraperitoneal injury. If DPL is used, the RBC threshold should be lowered to 5000/mm^3 to maximize the sensitivity of the procedure.
- *Computed tomography.* There is a very limited need for a CT scan in the evaluation

of GSWs to the abdomen. A more precise location may be indicated, and contrast-enhanced enemas (CECTEs) have been used for colorectal injuries.

GENITOURINARY TRAUMA

GENITAL TRAUMA

Female

Trauma to the uterus, fallopian tubes, and ovaries is rare following blunt abdominal trauma, except with the gravid uterus. Genital trauma can follow seat belt injuries, especially when only the lap restraint is used. It may be seen with penetrating injuries, but even in these cases the lower abdomen is rarely the target. The most common source of penetration comes from the pelvic girdle after a major pelvic fracture.

Symptoms of genital trauma resemble those of most intraabdominal trauma, and the pathologic condition is often not defined until the laparotomy is performed. The physical examination is often nonspecific, and there may be no external bleeding source.

Blood at the vaginal introitus in a patient with a pelvic fracture is a hallmark for potential urethral or vaginal laceration or both. The vagina is more commonly injured by various combinations of blunt and penetrating trauma and may be the source of a severe exsanguinating hemorrhage. These patients require a general anesthetic and surgical repair. Control of the hemorrhage in the emergency department can be difficult, and at times the best option is to pack the vagina with laparotomy sponges and make no attempt at surgical control of the hemorrhage until the patient has been anesthetized.

Straddle injuries are common in young children, and although hymenal perforation can be bloody and is often of great concern to both the young patient and to the parents, the bleeding is never serious and does not require any operative repair. The potential for sexual abuse is ever present; if the mechanism of injury is questionable, the case should be reported to the appropriate authorities.

Male

The male genitalia are much more commonly injured, not only because they are more exposed but also because men are more commonly involved in fights and dangerous sporting events.

Blunt injury to a testicle is common, and a simple contusion is often difficult to differentiate from a torn testicle because scrotal hematoma is often minimal. Any patient with a history of testicular injury and an abnormal examination should undergo a testicular color Doppler ultrasonography examination; a urologic consultation is dependent on the results of this examination. A penetrating injury to the scrotum is less common, but the patient may require scrotal exploration if there is violation of the tunica vaginalis testis.

Degloving injuries of the penis and scrotum are relatively common and are best managed by the urologist or plastic surgeon.

Blunt injuries to the penis are most often sustained during vigorous intercourse, and although the patient experiences severe pain and a palpable hematoma, he is usually able to urinate. These patients should be evaluated by a urologist for possible surgical repair of the torn penile tunica albuginea.

Mutilating lacerations of the external genitalia may be self-inflicted but are also seen from external attacks. If the severed penis is recovered, wrap it in moist, saline-soaked gauze and refer the patient to a urologist or plastic surgeon. Reimplantation may be attempted if the injury is less than 8 hours old. Regardless of the time of injury, the patient requires operative intervention and benefits from early psychiatric consultation.

URINARY TRACT INJURIES

Upper Tract

Renal injuries are common events. Although most renal trauma is not serious, a full spectrum of injury is possible and occasionally can be life threatening. The kidneys are reasonably well protected from anterior trauma but are susceptible to lateral and posterior blunt forces. Even strenuous exertion, such as that experienced by jai alai players, can produce renal injury, and contact sports such as football are common causes of renal trauma.

Penetrating injuries may involve the ureter as well as the kidney. Although ureteral injury is uncommon following blunt trauma, it can be quite debilitating if missed.

Blunt trauma

The classification of a renal injury is important because it allows the physician to recognize which injuries require radiographic investigation and potential operative intervention. Renal contusion is the most common type of renal injury and is not serious. This type of injury is commonly experienced after blunt trauma, and symptoms can range from none to marked flank pain. The patient may experience microscopic hematuria, but gross hematuria is present with more severe contusions. Hematuria may alarm the patient and bring him or her to the attention of the emergency physician. Vital signs are often normal; abnormalities are most often a result of associated nonurologic causes.

All patients with any degree of gross or microhematuria used to receive a diagnostic workup with intravenous pyelography. However, guidelines are now much more selective and differ for adults and children.

Radiographic studies of the urinary tract are not recommended if the adult patient with blunt trauma has only microhematuria with no shock (systolic BP $\geq$ 90) in the field or emergency department and if the patient did not have a sudden deceleration mechanism of injury. If this patient is otherwise stable, he or she may be discharged from the emergency department with close urologic follow-up. In the presence of gross hematuria or any degree of microhematuria ($\geq$ 3 to 5 RBC/hpf) with a history of shock (systolic BP $\leq$ 90) in the field or emergency department, an intravenous (IV) contrast-enhanced CT scan of the kidneys is the diagnostic procedure of choice.

Children can have congenital abnormalities of the upper urinary tract, and they have less muscle mass and skeletal development to protect against blunt forces. In addition, they tolerate ongoing hemorrhage longer than adults before hypotension ensues. Therefore even if their vital signs have been stable, they must undergo an IV

contrast-enhanced CT scan of their kidneys for any history of blunt renal trauma and associated gross hematuria or microhematuria.

The remaining types of renal trauma involve some degree of urinary extravasation and perirenal hemorrhage. Investigation and staging of these remaining injuries is accomplished in the same fashion. Surgical intervention for these more serious injuries remains very controversial. Management of suspected renal pedicle injuries may be frustrating. An IV contrast-enhanced CT scan of the kidney is diagnostic. Further definition of a pedicle injury may require arteriography. It may not be possible to salvage the kidney because the injury is often not recognized within a time frame that permits ideal renal vascular repair. However, awareness of the injury may save a patient's life in very select cases and, on a larger scale, prevent the subsequent development of postinjury renovascular hypertension.

Penetrating trauma

In penetrating injuries, any degree of gross hematuria or microhematuria or proximity of

---

INDICATIONS FOR DIAGNOSTIC RENAL STAGING

Indications for bolus infusion intravenous pyelogram with nephrotomography

Isolated renal injury (rare)
No access to CT scan

Indications for IV contrast-enhanced CT scan of kidneys

Adult
   Gross hematuria
   Microhematuria ($\geq$ 3-5 RBC/hpf) with shock
     (systolic BP $\leq$ 90) in the field or
     emergency department)
Child
   Any degree of gross hematuria or
     microhematuria

the wound to the urinary tract dictates the need for an IV contrast-enhanced CT scan of the kidneys to determine the extent of upper tract injury. Immediate exploration may be necessary with penetrating trauma, especially GSWs. The CT scan is especially important in a penetrating trauma because approximately 1 out of every 2000 people are born with only one kidney; the operating surgeon must be aware of this situation when planning the operative approach to an injured kidney or ureter. In an unstable patient, an intraoperative bolus infusion intravenous pyelogram (IVP) should be done to define the upper tract injuries after life-threatening injuries have been addressed. The indications for an IV contrast-enhanced CT scan of the kidneys and bolus infusion IVP with nephrotomography are given in the box on p. 280.

Bladder

Most bladder injuries occur when blunt abdominal trauma is sustained while the bladder is full. Gross hematuria is common but can be confusing because it does not define the level of injury in the genitourinary tract and cannot be correlated with the amount of injury. Gross hematuria is definitely a marker for urinary tract injury, and most often the injured organ is in close proximity to the injury force (e.g., pelvic trauma and bladder injury, upper abdominal or chest trauma and renal injury).

A retrograde cystogram is needed to define a bladder perforation. This technique requires the retrograde instillation of contrast material through an indwelling Foley catheter to one of three endpoints: 100 ml and a kidney, ureter, and bladder (KUB) showing gross extravasation; 400 ml in an adult (50 ml/kg in a child to 400 ml maximum); or retrograde filling to the point of initiating a bladder contraction, then forcefully injecting an additional 50 ml more than the previous amount slowly but under pressure, clamping the catheter, and obtaining a filled bladder film. A postevacuation anteroposterior x-ray film is needed to evaluate posterior bladder perforation. Failure to follow the above guidelines may result in spurious examinations and missed perforations, especially in penetrating bladder trauma.

Urethra

In men, urethral injuries are caused by straddle falls and accompanying pelvic fractures. Although these types of injuries are less common in women, they do occur and can be missed. The patient often has blood at the urethral meatus or at the vaginal introitus. Physical examination findings suggestive of male urethral injury include blood at the urethral meatus; hematoma or ecchymosis of the penile shaft, scrotal skin, or perineum; and palpation of a boggy, ill-defined mass rather than a well-defined prostate during the rectal examination.

Any of these findings dictate the need for retrograde urethrography to define urethral integrity. Any evidence of urethral extravasation is consistent with urethral injury and requires a urologic consultation. A suprapubic catheter is often needed to decompress the bladder while the urethral injury is healing.

KEY CONSIDERATIONS

WHAT IS THE LIFE THREAT?

Hemorrhage from blunt or penetrating injuries to the abdomen occurs when the victim sustains a laceration of an intraabdominal blood vessel, aorta, vena cava, liver, or spleen. Gastrointestinal hemorrhage may also occur as a result of trauma. Massive intraabdominal or gastrointestinal hemorrhage can lead to shock, exsanguination, and death. If undetected, even a slower intraabdominal hemorrhage can pose a life threat.

Renal trauma can lead to laceration or rupture of the kidneys. This type of injury can constitute a life threat if bleeding is significant.

DOES THE PATIENT NEED ADMISSION?

Patients with gunshot wounds to the abdomen or knife wounds that violate the peritoneum require a laparotomy. With blunt injuries to the abdomen, indications for laparotomy include unstable vital signs, peritoneal irritation, pneumoperitoneum, and evidence of a diaphragmatic injury. Patients with a hemoperitoneum that has been diagnosed with diagnostic peritoneal lavage (DPL), ultrasonography, or an abdominal CT scan following trauma generally require a laparotomy.

Indications for laparotomy in penetrating trauma include unstable vital signs, evisceration, gastrointestinal hemorrhage, diaphragmatic injury, intraperitoneal air, peritoneal signs, and an implement in situ.

WHAT IS THE MOST SERIOUS DIAGNOSIS?

Vascular disruption as a result of trauma or a laceration to the spleen, liver, pancreas, or bowel is the most serious diagnosis.

HAVE I PERFORMED A THOROUGH WORK-UP?

Repeat assessment of the vital signs periodically and perform DPL, ultrasonography, or an abdominal CT scan in patients with suspected abdominal trauma and diminished consciousness as a result of head injury or intoxication.

Perform an IV contrast-enhanced CT scan of the kidneys for patients who undergo abdominal or flank trauma and have gross hematuria or a history of hypotension and microhematuria.

Perform a retrograde urethrography in patients with evidence of urethral injury, including blood at the urethral meatus, ecchymosis of the penile shaft or scrotum, or a boggy mass palpated around the prostate during the rectal examination.

Recommended Reading

Easter DW, Shackford SR, Mattrey RF: A prospective, randomized comparison of computer tomography with conventional diagnostic methods in the evaluation of penetrating injuries to the back and flank, *Arch Surg* 126:115-119, 1991.

Henneman PL, Marx JA, Moore EE: Diagnostic peritoneal lavage: accuracy in predicting necessary laparotomy following blunt and penetrating trauma, *J Trauma* 30:1345, 1990.

Ivatury I et al: Laparoscopy in the evaluation of the intrathoracic abdomen after penetrating injury, *J Trauma* 33:101-109, 1992.

Marx JA: Abdominal trauma. In Rosen P et al, editors: *Emergency medicine: concepts and clinical practice,* ed 3, St Louis, 1992, Mosby.

Mee SL et al: Radiographic assessment of renal trauma: a 10 year prospective study of patient selection, *J Urol* 141:1095-1098, 1989.

Moore EE, Marx JA: Penetrating abdominal wounds, *JAMA* 253:2705-2708, 1985.

Schneider RE: Genitourinary trauma, *Emerg Med Clin North Am* 11(1):137-145, 1993.

Chapter Twenty-five
SOFT-TISSUE INJURIES AND LACERATIONS

DANIEL R. MARTIN

Soft tissue injuries are among the most common reasons for emergency department visits. Although rarely life threatening, soft-tissue injuries require careful management to avoid infections, unsightly scars, and disability. The majority of subsequent serious problems in wound management are a result of retained foreign bodies and missed injuries such as tendon and nerve injuries.

Although their presentation is often dramatic, soft-tissue injuries should be approached methodically and carefully examined. During the primary or initial survey, attention should be given to controlling bleeding and removing obvious foreign bodies. The wounds should be covered with saline-moistened gauze, and attention should be directed to life- and limb-threatening injuries. Once these steps have been completed, the extent of soft-tissue injury can be determined and the neurovascular examination can begin.

HISTORY OF INJURY

Although the history can be easily overlooked when faced with a soft-tissue injury, the cause and mechanism of the injury may reveal important data that could drastically alter the patient's evaluation and management. The history may suggest neurovascular compromise or retained foreign bodies such as glass or gravel. The history can reveal important underlying conditions such as a seizure disorder, syncope, or child abuse. Host factors that put the patient at greater risk for infection should be assessed (e.g., heart valve replacement, immunocompromised state, prosthetic devices of any type, or inadequate tetanus immunizations).

WOUND ANATOMY AND PHYSIOLOGY

The most important tissue layers with regard to the repair of soft-tissue injuries or lacerations are the dermis and epidermis. Although the epidermis is the key layer from a cosmetic standpoint, the dermis is the crucial layer for tensile strength; therefore sutures need to be anchored in the dermis.

Wound healing is a complex physiologic process that depends on numerous factors. When a wound forms, serum, cells, and new proteins accumulate. The fibroblasts differentiate from the inflammatory cells and begin to form collagen as early as 1 to 2 days after the injury. Epithelialization occurs during the first 48 hours after the injury; dead tissue or infection impedes this process, and moisture (supplied by topical antibiotics or dressings) accelerates it. The rate of epithelialization depends on the absence of infection; the ability of the host to form new proteins; the presence of ascorbic acid; special proteins that come from leukocytes, platelets, and fibroblasts; and an absence of excessive motion at the wound site.

PHYSICIAN PREPARATION

The physician should routinely use universal precautions, which include eye protection and a mask. Even the most innocent-appearing wound can erupt blood from a vascular source without warning and contaminate the physician or other medical personal. Because the repair of extensive soft-tissue injuries can be time consuming, the physician should be comfortable and preferably seated with adequate lighting.

Despite the use of proper techniques in administering anaesthesis and analgesis, some degree of pain is unavoidable when manipulating the injury or when preparing to anesthetize the injury. Because patients respond to pain in various ways, the physician must always be prepared for the possibility of vasovagal syncope, which could lead to further injuries. For this reason, the patient should be on a cart and preferably in a suspine position, regardless of how minor the wound appears.

WOUND PREPARATION

Although several methods of wound preparation have been described, aggressive irrigation with sterile saline remains the most commonly recommended technique. Although povodone-iodine (Betadine) solution should be used on areas adjacent to the wound, highly concentrated solutions of any type, including Betadine and concentrated hydrogen peroxide used di-

rectly in the wound, cause cytotoxicity and can impair healing. Irrigation should be accomplished with a large (≥30 ml) syringe and several hundred milliliters of normal saline. A meticulous search for and removal of foreign materials such as dirt, gravel, and glass is an integral part of wound preparation. Unless the wound is very superficial, a radiographic evaluation to diagnose the presence of foreign material and a repeat x-ray film to verify its removal are needed. An ultrasonography evaluation to detect foreign material such as plastic or wood should be pursued if clinically indicated.

Nonviable tissue needs careful debridement. In general, hair should be clipped, not shaved, because shaving can interfere with landmarks and may cause infection. If the hair interferes with wound evaluation ·or closure, it can be plastered down with a topical antibiotic ointment.

Once the wound has been properly cleansed, it should be thoroughly explored, and the depth of the wound should be documented. Tendon, bone, joint, or cartilage involvement can be easily missed if the depth of the wound is not explored.

HEMORRHAGE CONTROL

Hemorrhage control is always best achieved by direct pressure rather than blind clamping inside the wound or compression of nearby arteries. Blind clamping inside the wound can injure vascular structures, tendons, or nerves; arterial compression can result in ischemic injury. Applying tourniquets to the extremities may result in increased venous pressure and continued blood loss and should be done with careful attention to the time elapsed.

Direct compression should be accomplished for at least 10 minutes. Compression or elastic bandages can be used successfully for scalp wounds, whereas direct pressure and elevation are best for the extremities.

WOUND CLOSURE

There is an incorrect tendency to close all wounds. The two goals of wound repair should be remembered:

1. Prevention of infection
2. Achievement of the best possible functional and cosmetic result

Ironically, although wounds are closed to prevent infection, the closure increases rather than diminishes the risk of abscess formation if the wound is dirty. Wound cosmetics are improved only if no infection is present. Wound closure can be delayed until there is a clear absence of infection (see the box below).

The nomenclature of wound repair must be understood. *Primary repair* is carried out before granulation tissue forms (it takes 5 to 7 days for a wound to produce granulation tissue). *Secondary repair* occurs after granulation tissue has formed. *Tertiary repair* (also known as repair by tertiary intent) occurs when a wound is allowed to close by granulation. Tertiary repair may be permitted on an extremity but tends to leave unsightly scarring on the face.

WOUNDS REQUIRING INITIAL OPEN MANAGEMENT

1. Any wound on the extremity that is more than 8 hours old
2. Any wound on the face that is more than 24 hours old
3. Any wound that is contaminated with bacteria-laden foreign particles
4. Any wound that requires excessive tension to approximate the edges
5. Gunshot wounds
6. Stab wounds of the extremities or those that puncture deeply into muscle
7. Animal (especially cat) and human bites in places other than the face
8. Puncture wounds

Materials Used for Wound Closure

Most emergency departments stock both absorbable and nonabsorbable sutures (Table 25-1). The common absorbable sutures include plain gut (sheep intestine mucosa), chromic gut (chromium trioxide–treated gut), polyglycolic acid (Dexon), and polyglactin (Vicryl). The nonabsorbable sutures usually include monofilament nylon or silk. Other materials, such as skin tapes or staples, can also be used.

Of those nonabsorbable sutures available in most emergency departments, monofilament nylon sutures are the least reactive and result in the least amount of scarring. Fine gauge, 6-0 monofilament nylon is recommended for the repair of facial lacerations. A heavy gauge, 5-0 nylon is usually recommended for other areas. In closing the scalp, a 4-0 gauge nylon on a medium-sized needle allows hemostat closure of the superficial layers. If the epithelial edges of the wound are well approximated when the patient is at rest, a single layer of ephithelial sutures may be used instead of several layers. Layered closure in facial wounds is important to provide tensile strength. Superficial sutures in facial lacerations should be removed in 3 to 5 days to prevent suture marks. Skin tapes can be used in partial-thickness or in some flap lacerations, and staples can be used with linear lacerations that require a single layer of sutures.

Minimizing the Pain of Wound Repair

A liberal amount of anesthetic should always be used when repairing lacerations. The two classes of anesthetic agents are amides and esters. Of the amides, lidocaine and bupivacaine are the most commonly used; procaine, tetracaine, benzocaine, and cocaine are used from the ester group. For patients who report an allergy to a specific anesthetic, crossreactivity between the amide and ester groups should not occur. However, preservatives such as methylparaben can cause allergic reactions. Therefore

Table 25-1

COMPARISON OF SUTURE MATERIALS

Type	Tensile Strength	Tissue Reactivity	Size	Metabolism by Body	Comments
Ideal	Infinite	Zero	Infinitely small	Yes; needs no removal	Does not collect bacteria; does not currently exist
Polyglycolic (Vicryl, Dexon)	Retained for up to 21 days	Occasionally rejected	3-0 to 6-0	Yes; does not require removal	May be rejected occasionally and cause abscess; recommended for internal use
Plain catgut	Broken down in 5 to 7 days	Inflammatory response can be excessive and appear like a wound infection	3-0 to 6-0	No; body rejects as foreign protein	Not recommended for internal use
Chromic catgut	Broken down in 7 to 10 days	Same as plain catgut	2-0 to 4-0	Same as plain catgut	Same as plain catgut
Wire	Very strong	Least of all sutures	3-0 to 5-0	No; must be removed with special cutters	Hard to use, uncomfortable for patient when used in skin or subcutaneous tissues; easily punctures surgeon's glove and skin and therefore not recommended because of AIDS risk

	Strength	Reaction	Size	Removable?	Comments
Monofilament plastic sutures (nylon, Dacron)	Very stiff	Almost as unreactive as wire	3-0 to 6-0	No; must be removed, but removal is quite easy if not tied too tightly	Easier to use than wire, but tends to slice through oily or macerated tissues; does not collect bacteria; is ideal epithelial suture; requires many extra throws in knots to prevent it from untying itself; although suture may be left in longer, it will not form suture hole scars if removed in 3 to 5 days
Silk and cotton	Strong	Form severe inflammatory reactions (but not as severe as with catgut) when left in too long	2-0 to 5-0	Rejected by body as foreign protein; must be removed	Limited use currently but useful in oily skin or on sensitive parts of the body such as the nipple; no longer used in mouth (replaced by polyglycolic sutures)
Paper tape	Weak	Minimal if any	NA	No	Used for superficial lacerations, especially in children; can help support a wound after epithelial sutures have been removed; should not be used in wounds that gape or those that ooze serum; works best on dry skin
Staples	Very strong	Minimal	4-0 to 5-0	No; removed with special devices	Quickly placed; work best on linear incisions and in wounds that do not require layered closure; in general, are uncomfortable for patient

patients reporting previous severe allergic reactions to an anesthetic should be given an anesthetic from the other group that does not contain preservatives or benadryl.

Several other methods to reduce pain have also been recommended, including injecting with a small needle (e.g., 27-gauge or smaller), injecting subdermally, injecting slowly and buffering the anesthetic with bicarbonate (1 ml of bicarbonate per 9 to 10 ml of lidocaine). Administering a small amount of topical anesthetic before a local or regional injection should also be considered. In addition, greater emphasis recently has been placed on regional anesthetics for areas such as the face, hand, and foot. Regional anesthetics with a long-acting agent such as bupivacaine provides longer anesthesia and causes less distortion of tissues.

PLACEMENT OF SUTURES AND DRESSINGS AND SUTURE REMOVAL

The correct placement of sutures should result in eversion of the wound edges, not inversion; inversions cause a shadow that accentuates the scar. The sutures should be placed equidistant from each other, and the intersuture distance should be roughly equal to the distance from the wound edge to the point at which the suture enters the skin. Vertical or horizontal mattress sutures may be used in deep or gaping wounds. Although subcutaneous absorbable sutures should be used for facial lacerations, their use in other areas, especially the distal extremities, increases the risk of infection and therefore should not be used on the hands and feet.

The use of barrier dressings (Band-aids) for at least the first 48 hours after wound repair aids wound healing by providing moisture and maximizing the environment for epithelialization. Applying topical antibiotics such as Neosporin twice a day has also been found to accelerate healing. Whenever possible, attempts should also be made to splint lacerations to prevent ex-

Table **25-2**

TIMING OF SUTURE REMOVAL

Location	Time of Removal (days)
Face	3-5
Scalp	7-10
Trunk	7-10
Arms/legs	10-14
Fingertip	10-12
Palms/soles	14
Joint extensor	14
Joint flexor	8-10

cessive movement of the laceration.

Suture removal varies according to the location of the wound (Table 25-2). Sutures should be removed from the face on Day 3 to Day 5, whereas sutures across joints should not be removed for at least 14 days. Because the tensile strength of wounds is minimal when sutures are removed, skin tapes should be applied for an additional 2 to 4 days after suture removal.

WOUND INFECTIONS AND INDICATIONS FOR PROPHYLACTIC ANTIBIOTICS

The incidence of wound infections varies from 2% to 10%. Factors that make infection more likely to occur include the presence of more than 10^5 bacteria/gram of tissue; the presence of wound contaminants such as feces, dirt, or saliva; and the location of wounds in areas of high flora counts (e.g., mucous membranes, perineum, or axilla) or decreased vascularity (e.g., distal extremities). Severely abraded or contused wounds and the use of epinephrine during wound repair have also been associated with a higher risk of wound infection.

Although controversy exists regarding the use of prophylactic antibiotics, several consensus indications have been described. These indications include lacerations associated with bone, cartilage, tendon, or joint injuries; most bite wounds (animal and human); a significant risk of subacute bacterial endocarditis (artificial valve); or the presence of other prosthetic devices (e.g., a total hip replacement). More controversial indications include contaminated wounds, oral lacerations, and wounds older than 8 to 12 hours.

The choice of antibiotics is usually a first-generation cephalosporin or a penicillinase-resistant penicillin. Erythromycin and ciprofloxacin have been recommended for patients allergic to penicillin. Because the goal of prophylactic antibiotic administration should be to deliver the antibiotic to the tissues as quickly as possible, the initial antibiotic dose should be given intramuscularly or intravenously.

SUTURING SPECIAL AREAS

Scalp

Scalp lacerations may be macerated and contused and can often harbor glass or dirt fragments. Even with direct palpation, it can be difficult to determine whether intact bone lies at the base of the wound, especially if the galea is torn. The galea can be so stiff that the edges may feel like fracture fragments. In most of these wounds, the laceration should be cleaned and irrigated, foreign bodies should be removed, and the wound edges should be repaired with interrupted 3-0 or 4-0 monofilament nylon sutures. The galea should be closed whenever possible with interrupted 3-0 absorbable sutures. Before repair, the scalp hair should be clipped, not shaved. If hair still obscures the view of the laceration, it can be plastered down with topical antibiotic ointment. Because the patient may become bald later in life, repair the wound with careful attention to cosmetics. Leave the sutures in place for 5 to 7 days. Most superficial scalp wounds do not require bandaging, but deeper wounds (i.e. those down to the skull) may need to be wrapped with an elastic bandage for 24 hours to prevent hematoma formation. Leave the ears outside the dressing unless they must be covered; in such a case, pad the posterior ear well to avoid creating a flexion crease on the ear. If hemostasis is a problem, control it by suturing the laceration carefully or by applying prolonged local pressure and subsequently expressing any hematoma from the wound before applying the dressing.

Nose and Ears

If the nasal cartilage is severed, approximate the edges with interrupted 5-0 absorbable sutures. Open nasal-bone fractures should be treated prophylactically with antibiotics. Careful attention should be given to rule out septal hematomas and cerebral spinal fluid rhinorrhea.

Field block anesthesia for the ear can be accomplished by anesthetizing the subcutaneous tissue or by raising a wheal around the ear by injecting anesthetic in the posterior auricular area and anterior to the tragus. If the ear is involved to the canal, suturing under an operating microscope may be needed in addition to an otolaryngology or plastic surgery consultation. Suture the cartilage with absorbable sutures. Partial and complete amputations of the ear are deforming injuries. Although surgical repair is not difficult, such patients are best referred to a plastic surgeon or oncologist and probably admitted to the hospital following repair. After repair of an ear laceration, the ear may need a compression dressing to prevent hematoma formation, which can be accomplished by placing a dressing between the skull and the ear and by wrapping the head with an elastic or Kerlix dressing for at least 24 hours.

Mouth and Lips

Facial lacerations need careful evaluation before repair. Particular attention should be given to ensure that the parotid duct is intact and that neither the recurrent labial nerve (below the corner of the mouth) nor the facial nerve (anterior to the ear) has been injured. This evaluation can be done by carefully examining the facial musculature while having the patient smile.

Through-and-through lacerations of the lips and cheeks are common and require careful, layered closure to achieve a low incidence of infection. Start inside the mouth and achieve a watertight seal of the muscosa with interrupted 4-0 or 5-0 absorbable (Vicryl or Chromic) sutures. Carefully inspect the wound for tooth fragments. After repairing the mucosa, repeat the irrigation from the external wound, and suture the fascia of the cheek musculature with interrupted absorbable sutures. Finally, close the dermis and epidermis. Many sources recommend prophylactic and antibiotics for such wounds.

Leave the tongue unrepaired if the laceration is small (less than 1 cm), if there is little hemorrhage, or if there is no persistent gape. For other lacerations, repair the tongue with interrupted 3-0 or 4-0 absorbable sutures. For a child, consider a general anesthetic, ketamine, or heavy sedation with fentanyl. The frenulum does not need to be repaired in most cases, nor does the uvula unless the bleeding is heavy or there will be a persistent opening.

The lips require special concern when the lacerations involve the vermilion border. If the border is not approximated to prevent more than 1 mm of step-off, a defect that is visible at conversational distance will remain. Mark the vermilion border with methylene blue, or use a 27-gauge needle and form a small intradermal bead at the border before distorting the anatomy with the infiltration of lidocaine. Anatomic distortion often can be avoided by administering a regional anesthetic whenever possible. Place the first suture through the marked borders; close the mucosa with interrupted 4-0 to 5-0 absorbable sutures and the skin with 6-0 monofilament nylon.

A plastic surgeon should repair lacerations that involve the philtrum or the corner of the mouth, as well as lacerations in which more than 1 inch of lip tissue is lost.

Neck

Neck wounds that penetrate the platysma need to be repaired by a surgeon in the operating room. Nonpenetrating wounds are generally long linear injuries that do not require layered closure. Although interrupted sutures are most commonly used, a continuous locked suture is equally effective. The principal responsibility in managing these wounds is the recognition of any penetration of the platysma so that the patient can be appropriately observed for deep injury. Avoid blind probing with a cotton swab in an attempt to define the limits of injury. If the platysma is penetrated, the extent of the wound is best determined by special diagnostic studies or by formal exploration in the operating room.

Upper Extremity

Wounds of the axilla are also sources of hidden danger. Not only is there a potential for injury to the axillary artery or vein, but also it is possible to penetrate the pleura or to involve the brachial plexus. Carefully examine the patient for all of these possibilities. Because of problems with serous fluid accumulation following the repair, some patients may need surgical consultation and possible admission for observation until it is clear that no infection has developed.

Lacerations are common over the bursa of the olecranon. Such wounds often become infected if closed primarily unless the bursa is excised. Leave these wounds open, use a splint with secondary closure, and arrange for follow-up by an orthopedic surgeon.

Hand

Injuries to the hand are common both in domestic and industrial settings. Hand dominance is important to ascertain; the dominant hand is commonly the one injured.

The skin on the hand is stiff, and sutures easily tear through it. Because of the tendons and neurovascular bundles present, close hand wounds in only one layer. In a hand wound, avoid clamping what appears to be a spurting vessel to achieve hemostasis because it is too easy to clamp structures such as nerves or tendons. Hemostasis can be achieved by direct pressure and elevation or, rarely, by tourniquet.

Before doing any repair, ascertain the mechanism of injury and the potential for foreign bodies to be present in the wound. As stated earlier, obtain an x-ray examination to find glass fragments if they may be present. If the patient was injured with a high-pressure injector, the skin wounds may appear very innocuous; however, all such wounds require exploration in the operating room to remove all foreign material.

Before any laceration is repaired, evaluate the degree of motor function that remains intact. Measure the natural grasping ability of the hand and the individual tendon functions. The location of the wound indicates whether damage is likely to involve the extensor or flexor mechanisms, but partial tendon injury does not reveal motor deficits. Therefore carefully inspect the wound visually and test it dynamically. Use an operating tourniquet for inspection and an adequate amount of anesthetic for the patient. Assess nerve function before anesthetizing the digit or hand. Achieve appropriate levels of anesthesia with digital, local, or regional blocks.

Test sensation both with pinprick and with fine touch; also determine two-point discrimination abilities. If the patient cannot cooperate because of age, pain, fear, or drugs or alcohol, the integrity of the digital nerves can be assessed by looking for wrinkling of the skin after immersion in hot water. If the digital sympathetic nerve is severed, the skin is not able to wrinkle. If wrinkling does occur, other digital nerve functions are also intact.

Partial extensor tendon injuries are common. Tendons less than 25% lacerated do not need surgical repair but can be treated by splinting the metacarpophalangeal joints in 10 to 20 degrees of flexion, the phalanges in full extension, and the wrist in 30 degrees or extension. Splint fingers other than the thumb in pairs—index or ring finger to the long finger, and the little finger to the ring finger.

Suture tendon lacerations that are complete or more than 25% lacerated with a buried mattress figure-of-eight suture of monofilament nylon; allow the knot to fall between the cut ends of the tendon. Do not repair the extensor tendon laceration (1) unless you have experience with the procedure and are prepared to follow the patient, (2) if the lacerated tendon is at the wrist or involves multiple tendons, (3) if the proximal tendon has retracted far from the site of injury or the wound is badly contaminated, or (4) if there is tendon missing. Few emergency departments are set up to do tendon repairs; for those that are not, it is wisest to involve the appropriate hand service. Do not repair flexor tendons in the emergency department because such repairs require very careful splinting, follow-up, and physical therapy.

Lacerations through the nail often involve the nail matrix. Remove part or all of the nail and suture the matrix with a fine-diameter absorbable suture. Some avulsions of the nail do not involve the germinal matrix, and the proximal portion of the nail can be reattached to provide a biologic dressing.

Contrary to previous beliefs, avulsions of the digit pad of the fingertip do not require grafting, even when more than a dime-sized piece of skin has been lost. Although a split-thickness graft can be taken from the forearm to provide coverage, the finger does epithelialize in approximately 21 days if the finger is kept dressed and clean. The dressing that is easiest for patient and physician is a layer of fine mesh petroleum- or vaseline-based nonadhering dressing on the wound and Tubegauz dressing for the involved digit. During the first 10 days, splint the digit with approximately 10 degrees of flexion at each joint. As described previously, the finger is best splinted to the adjacent finger.

Amputation of the digits is common with industrial accidents. Many hand services attempt to replant the digits with microsurgery when the amputation is proximal to the distal interphalangeal joint. Until the desires of the hand surgeon are known, handle the amputated digits as if they will be reimplanted. Wrap them in saline-moistened gauze, enclose them in a plastic bag, and place the bag in an ice cooler. Do not allow the digit to directly contact the ice. Although some hand surgeons like to tag vessels, nerves, and tendons, we prefer to control bleeding with direct pressure and elevation. Avoid using a tourniquet, and handle the tissues as little as possible before definitive repair is undertaken.

Thorax

Penetrating wounds of the chest from any cause can result in pleural penetration; therefore these patients usually need chest radiography and careful observation. It is usually impossible to ascertain the depth of the wound by probing it with a finger or cotton swab, and this step may produce pleural penetration and pneumothorax. If the wound was caused by a knife or bullet, do not close it primarily. A common error is to assign chest-wall bleeding to thoracic musculature or soft tissue when it is actually caused by intercostal vessels. If this fact is ignored, the patient may exsanguinate from an intrathoracic hemorrhage.

Abdomen

Abdominal wounds are often stab or bullet wounds. As with the chest, the significance of these wounds is their potential for damage to intraabdominal structures. With bullet wounds, assume that there has been intraperitoneal penetration and injury, and determine and repair these at laparotomy. Investigate stab wounds that have normal vital signs and no obvious penetration (e.g., herniated omentum or bowel). After the abdomen has been examined for peritoneal irritation, local wound exploration should be considered. The wound should be thoroughly prepared and anesthetized. The would may be extended with careful visualization of each successive layer of tissue. If the fascia of the rectus abdominis or external oblique muscle has been penetrated, a diagnostic peritoneal lavage to determine the extent of penetration into the peritoneal cavity may be indicated. Blind probing with cotton-tipped swabs, instruments, or fingers is inaccurate and may be harmful. If the fascia is intact, pack the wound open and treat it with delayed primary or secondary closure. Some trauma centers close the wound primarily after a thorough irrigation, but a prudent course with stab wounds is to suspect contamination and to treat the wound open.

Lower Extremity

The foot has many of the same characteristics as the hand, but because shoes are worn by most patients, the propensity for infection is higher. Repair lacerations as on the hand, using a single layer of skin sutures. Splinting the lacerations and crutch-assisted non–weight bearing are usually needed. Use a plaster posterior splint or a short-leg walking cast liberally.

Splint toes to adjacent toes as part of the bandaging technique. Search for foreign bodies using both an x-ray study and direct inspection. Both toothpicks and metallic foreign bodies (needles) are especially troublesome because toothpicks do not appear on conventional x-ray study techniques and because most emergency departments do not have access to xeroradiography. Needles are hard to locate even when seen on an x-ray study. They can sometimes be removed under fluoroscopic assistance in the radiology department, and the metallic objects can sometimes be removed with powerful magnets. Overall, however, these objects are hard to define, and at times the patient needs to go to the operating room for removal under an operating tourniquet.

CONCLUSIONS

When treating a wound, remember to include the following:
1. Explore and document the depth of all wounds.

2. Document the mechanism of injury, and perform a neurovascular examination distal to the laceration; be specific (i.e., **never** write "neurovascular examination is intact").
3. Irrigate all wounds; document the type and amount of solution used.
4. Consider asking the patient to return for a wound check in 48 to 72 hours unless the wound is extremely clean or the patient is extremely reliable.
5. Tape all facial wounds after removing the sutures.
6. Tell patients what to expect, and explain the signs of infection.

KEY CONSIDERATIONS

WHAT IS THE LIFE THREAT?

Although most soft-tissue injuries seen in the emergency department rarely pose a life threat, bleeding from wounds of the face and scalp or wounds that involve arterial bleeding can be extensive and lead to hypovolemia and shock from blood loss.

DOES THE PATIENT NEED ADMISSION?

Patients who require admission usually have accompanying head, chest, abdominal, or bone injuries that require hospital management. Extensive human-bite injuries of the hand may require admission for intravenous antibodies, particularly if a joint is involved.

WHAT IS THE MOST SERIOUS DIAGNOSIS?

Wounds that involve injury to blood vessels, nerves, tendon, and bone are generally the most serious. Extensive lacerations can create a significant blood loss that can lead to hypovolemia. Certain facial lacerations, such as through-and-through lacerations of eyelids, require specialized repair, usually by a plastic surgeon, maxillofacial surgeon, or ophthalmologist.

HAVE I PERFORMED A THOROUGH WORK-UP?

Evaluate tendon, muscle, nerve, and vascular function distal to an extremity laceration. Evaluate the trauma victim for other injuries. Such injuries may not be obvious in the unconscious or intoxicated patient.

Recommended Reading

Berk WA, Welch RD, Bock BF: Controversial issues in clinical management of the simple wound, *Ann Emerg Med* 21:72-80, 1992.

Cummings P, Del Beccaro MA: Antibiotics to prevent infection of simple wounds; a meta-analysis of randomized studies, *Am J Emerg Med* 13:396-400, 1995.

Henry GL: *Emergency medicine risk management: a comprehensive review*, Dallas, 1991, American College of Emergency Physicians.

Proceedings of the clinical advances track of the 1988 ACEP winter symposium, *Ann Emerg Med* 17:1264-1347, 1988.

Roberts JR, Hedges JR: *Clinical procedures in emergency medicine*, ed 2, Philadelphia, 1991, WB Saunders.

Rosen P et al: *Emergency medicine: concepts and clinical practice*, ed 3, St Louis, 1992, Mosby.

Trott A: *Wounds and lacerations: emergency care and closure*, ed 1, St Louis, 1991, Mosby.

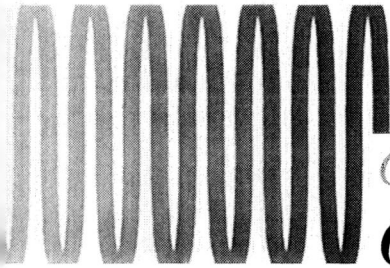

Chapter Twenty-six
ORTHOPEDIC INJURIES

JOEL GEIDERMAN

Skeletal injuries are among the most common reasons for visits to the emergency department. Some of these injuries are within the complete domain of the emergency physician, whereas many fractures and dislocations warrant definitive management by an orthopedic surgeon. It is the responsibility of the emergency physician to recognize these problems, stabilize the patient, and involve the orthopedic surgeon in a timely fashion, as appropriate.

GENERAL PRINCIPLES

Keep in mind the following guidelines for managing skeletal injuries:
- Most orthopedic injuries can be anticipated by knowing the age of the patient and the mechanism of injury.
- A careful history and physical examination will suggest x-ray findings; positive radiographs are corroborative.
- If x-ray studies are negative but a fracture is suspected clinically, treat the injury as a fracture.
- Be familiar with proper x-ray views; bad or incomplete films result in missed injuries.
- Take x-ray films of dislocations before and after reduction unless a delay would be injurious to the patient.

- Check and record neurovascular competence before and after all reductions.
- Circular casting is best left to the physician who is providing the ongoing care.
- Before they leave the emergency department, give the patients explicit follow-up instructions, including warning signs of neurovascular compromise.
- Check the patient's ability to ambulate safely before discharge from the emergency department.
- Although few orthopedic injuries are life threatening, some are limb threatening. Most orthopedic injuries should take a secondary role to the assessment and management of more life-threatening injuries to the head, chest, or abdomen. Exceptions include fractures or dislocations that can cause devascularization of the limb or those that are accompanied by tissue destruction and hemorrhage that will be fatal unless the limb is sacrificed.
- Dislocations of the hip and knee also require special attention. Aseptic necrosis of the femoral head can develop if the hip is not relocated in a timely fashion. With a knee dislocation, the popliteal vessels are at significant risk. Similarly, elbow dislocations may compromise the brachial artery.
- Finally, some fractures and dislocations

clearly compromise the vascularity of the limb. Although the general rule is to splint the limb in the position in which it is found, it is more prudent to relocate the dislocation when circulation is compromised.

COMMUNICATION AND DEFINITIONS

Fractures

Because many skeletal injuries are referred to another physician's care, it is most important to be able to provide an accurate and understandable description for that physician. The language of fractures is a shorthand communication that should be precise. The box below summarizes the terms used to describe a fracture.

The description of a fracture is important to the emergency physician and the following physician because it directs the initial and subsequent management decisions.

First, is the *fracture open or closed?* This terminology is preferred over *simple versus compound.* An open fracture needs antibiotics, a dressing, and usually an operative cleansing. Wounds that lie near a fracture may convert it from closed to open, and at times the area of skin

---

TERMS TO DESCRIBE A FRACTURE

Mandatory

Open versus closed
Exact anatomic location
Direction of fracture line
Position (displacement)

Additional modifiers

Complete versus incomplete
Avulsion
Impaction
  Depression
  Compression
Involvement of articular surface (%)

---

discontinuity may be small and easily missed when dealing with more significant injuries.

The *exact bone involved* and helpful anatomic landmarks or features should be mentioned; thus a "femoral neck fracture" means something entirely different than a "femoral shaft fracture," and either descriptions convey more information than simply a "femoral fracture." It is easy and common to confuse the sides of the body. Check the assessment of right versus left against an independent observer. If there is any discrepancy, the only recourse is to reexamine the patient. Mislabeled notes or x-ray studies should be corrected early.

The *direction and magnitude* of the fracture are also important. An oblique fracture of the humerus is more likely to involve the radial nerve than is a transverse fracture. Comminution (multiple fragments) also has an important significance.

Displacement describes the movement of the fracture fragments and is of great importance for management decisions. It is customary to describe the movement of the distal fragment relative to the proximal fragment.

A last designation that is important to communicate is whether a fracture extends into and involves an articular surface. Often the percentage of articular surface that is involved is estimated; in some cases the percentage that is involved dictates the need to perform a surgical repair. Involvement of the articular surface is important to note because it may change management from closed to surgical and because it worsens the prognosis when the joint surface is involved.

A *complete fracture* means that both cortices of bone are interrupted, but this need not include displacement. Incomplete fractures, which are often seen in pediatric injuries, involve only one cortex. *Avulsion* is the tearing away of a small fragment of bone, usually by extreme muscular contraction. *Impaction* is the collapse of one fragment on another; in the spine this collapse is often called *compression*. In the skull and tibial plateau, this collapse is called *depression* of the fracture fragment.

Subluxation is partial loss of continuity between two joint surfaces, whereas *dislocation* is a complete loss. Dislocations are described according to movement of the involved part relative to the normal skeleton; for example, a lateral dislocation of the patella or an anterior dislocation of the shoulder. The former means that the patella is outside its normal location at the knee and resting on the lateral side of the femur. The latter dislocation describes the humerus as being outside the glenoid fossa and anterior to the shoulder girdle. Dislocations can also occur in conjunction with fractures and are described according to the major involved joint, such as fracture-dislocation of the ankle (usually involving fractures of the medial and lateral malleoli with lateral displacement of the foot relative to the ankle).

A few other anatomic descriptors are important. In *valgus deformities* the distal segment lies away from the midline of the body, whereas *varus deformities* are those in which the distal segment lies toward the midline. In the hand, refer to the *radial* or *ulnar* side of any part, rather than the medial or lateral side. On the upper extremity, refer to *volar* and *dorsal* rather than anterior and posterior. When reference is made to fingers, it is confusing to talk about the first through the fifth finger because some people label the thumb as the first finger, whereas some label the index finger as the first finger. It is preferable to name each finger as follows: thumb, index, middle, ring, and little. Do the same with the toes: great (or hallux), index, middle, ring, and little toe.

Children's bones are necessarily soft and resilient, which predisposes them to a number of incomplete fractures. *Greenstick* fractures are incomplete, angulated fractures of long bones. The resultant bowing of the bone resembles a moist young branch that breaks when bent in a similar fashion. A *torus* fracture is another form of incomplete fracture and is characterized by a buckling or wrinkling of the cortex. It derives its name from Greek architecture, in which a torus is a bump at the base of a column.

In children, it is hard to remember all of the ossification centers and their dates of formation, as well as the dates of closure for various epiphyseal surfaces. If neither a radiologic table nor a pediatric radiologist is available, comparison views can be obtained for assistance in interpretation.

Epiphyseal injuries are usually classified by the Salter-Harris system (Table 26-1). Type I injuries are caused clinically by the same mechanism as those that cause fractures of closed epiphyses and sprains; the extremity has the same clinical deformity, but the x-ray study shows a slippage or widening of the epiphysis. A Type II injury shows an epiphyseal slip plus a fracture of the adjacent metaphysis. A Type III injury involves a fracture of the epiphysis as well as slippage. A Type IV injury has a fracture of both the epiphysis and metaphysis, as well as slippage. A Type V injury is caused by compression and may appear normal on an x-ray study. Magnetic resonance imaging (MRI) should be ordered to confirm or rule out this diagnosis in suspicious cases. The significance of a compressing injury to an epiphysis is that it can cause significant growth deformity in the patient.

Sprains and Strains

A soft tissue injury also has its own language. A *sprain* is the stretching, separation, or tear of a supporting ligament, whereas a *strain* is the separation or tear of a musculotendinous unit from a bone.

Sprains are graded by severity. A first-degree sprain has no joint instability because only a few fibers are torn. Swelling is minimal with minor discomfort. Hemorrhage is minimal, and often there is no ecchymosis. Second-degree sprains cause more disruption. The joint is still usually intact, but there is much more swelling and,

Table 26-1

SALTER-HARRIS CLASSIFICATION OF EPIPHYSEAL INJURIES

	Description	*Diagram*
Type I	Fracture extends through the epiphyseal plate, which results in displacement of the epiphysis (this displacement may appear merely as widening of the radiolucent area representing the growth plate)	
Type II	Same as above; in addition, a triangular segment of metaphysis is fractured	
Type III	Fracture line runs from the joint surface through the epiphyseal plate and epiphysis	
Type IV	Fracture line occurs as in type III but also passes through adjacent metaphysis	
Type V	This is a crush injury of the epiphysis; it may be difficult to determine by x-ray studies; an MRI may be necessary to confirm the diagnosis	

usually, visible ecchymosis. In a third-degree sprain, the ligaments are totally disrupted. If the joint is stressed, it will open. Although swelling may be visible and significant, it can be minimal with some total tears because the joint contents are no longer confined. A third-degree sprain of the knee is often accompanied by dislocation and spontaneous relocation. If the degree of tear is not appreciated, the danger to the popliteal vessels can go unrecognized until the limb loses its vascular supply.

Strains are also graded by severity. A first-degree strain is commonly referred to as a "pulled muscle." Overuse such as in unusual exertion of an unconditioned muscle may produce this type of injury; an example is the pain experienced in the rectus muscles after multiple sit-ups in an untrained individual. There is localized pain aggravated by movement or muscle tension. A second-degree strain involves more of the fibers of the muscle or musculotendinous unit but falls short of a complete disruption. There is a continuum of injury from first- to second-degree injury that is judged on clinical grounds. Swelling, ecchymosis, and loss of strength are greater than in first-degree strains.

In third-degree strains, the muscle or tendon is completely disrupted, with resultant separation of muscle from muscle, muscle from tendon, or tendon from bone. Disruption at the musculoskeletal junction may be accompanied by an avulsion fracture, which can be seen on an x-ray film. Third-degree strains often result from sudden, violent muscle contraction, particularly before warming-up and in middle-aged or older individuals. In some cases, a bulging or bunching of the muscle is present, and sometimes a palpable defect is appreciated. The gastrocnemius or soleus muscles or the Achilles tendon may be involved in the lower extremity. The biceps are most commonly involved in the upper extremity.

In addition to strains, tendons are subject to episodes of inflammation (tendinitis), which is probably caused by excessive use or repeated blows from the exertions of sport or industry.

The bursae that help cushion the tendinous insertions to bone can also become inflamed and result in bursitis. The bursae respond to this inflammation by producing more fluid and becoming swollen. Bursae can also become infected when there is any break in the overlying skin. It is sometimes difficult to distinguish between septic bursitis caused by infection, and inflammatory bursitis. Obtaining a history and a white blood cell count may be useful in distinguishing between the two entities; aspiration and examination of fluid is diagnostic. Lacerations in these areas (especially over the knee or elbow) are best left open for delayed primary or secondary closure.

METHODS OF FRACTURE TREATMENT

The major component of therapy has not changed for thousands of years: Achieve approximation of the fracture fragments, place the fracture site at rest to prevent motion at the pseudarthrosis caused by the fracture, and allow healing to occur.

Whether immobilization is achieved by splints or plaster, the principles are the same: The joints above and below the injury site must be placed at rest if the injury site is also to be at rest. In addition, if adjacent parts keep moving, the injury site will not be immobilized; therefore fingers and toes adjacent to the fracture must be splinted.

Upper Extremity

For *digit* splints, use foam-lined aluminum splints cut to the desired length. For digit extensor injuries, apply the splint on either the dorsal or palmar surface; most patients find the dorsal surface more comfortable and convenient.

The *wrist* can be splinted with either dorsal or volar plaster. Immobilization is better with a volar splint because the urge to keep using the hand with a dorsal splint is more than most patients can resist. The wrist should be neutral. The splint should extend to the level of the metacarpophalangeal joints if a dorsal splint is used and to the distal palmar crease if a volar splint is chosen. The splint need not extend past the elbow.

Splint the *elbow* from wrist to shoulder with the wrist pronated and the elbow flexed to 90 degrees. The arm can be supported with a sling, but the patient should be taught shoulder exercises and encouraged not to allow the shoulder to be immobile.

The *shoulder* is best splinted by placing the

arm against the torso; accomplish this by first placing the arm in a sling and then bandaging the arm to the thorax with the elbow at a right angle and the hand pronated. This position is also an effective splint for acromioclavicular separations or rotator cuff tears.

For *clavicle* problems, a figure-of-eight bandage or a commercial clavicle strap provides immobilization and a modicum of comfort.

Lower Extremity

Toes are harder to splint than fingers. An effective technique is to use plain roller gauze to bandage the toe to the adjacent uninjured toe, thus using the normal phalanx as a biologic splint (i.e., a "buddy" splint). Be sure to place cotton and apply baby powder between the toes to avoid maceration.

Immobilize the *ankle* with a posterior plaster splint that extends from midcalf to the toes. The splint can be made from either a rolled plaster bandage or plain linear splints, as well as padded plaster materials. Cover the skin with a layer of stockinette and bandage the splint with a layer of webril. When this type of splint is used, the patient must also use crutches to avoid weight bearing. Once the swelling diminishes, ankle immobilization can be achieved with a short-leg walking cast. Apply the protective heel of the cast at midfoot rather than over the calcaneum. The foot should be plantar flexed approximately 10 degrees at the ankle. The ankle is uncomfortable in the neutral (90 degree) position.

The *knee* can be splinted with plaster or with any of the commercially available knee immobilizers. If plaster is used, it need only extend from ankle to hip, but most patients are more comfortable if the ankle and foot are incorporated into the splint. The ankle should be at 10 degrees of extension, with the knee at 90 degrees of flexion. Instruct the patient in crutch walking.

Bed rest is required to immobilize the *hip*.

Whether a Buck traction or one of the long-leg femur splints such as a Thomas or Hare traction splint is used, the patient needs to be confined to bed with all its attendant problems.

Cast Complications

Although the emergency physician rarely applies a circular cast, he or she may be the first to see a patient who has a complication from such a cast that has been placed by the orthopedic surgeon. The first principle of cast management is that increasing pain or pain that persists after the first 8 hours following cast application must be interpreted as a sign of a complication. Pain that is induced with passive muscle stretching is a useful positive sign of increased compartment pressure. Pulses and capillary refill may remain normal even in the presence of an impending compartment syndrome. If ignored, these complications can lead to a Volkmann contracture or vascular insufficiency. The most prudent action when doubt exists is to split the cast; splitting should be done at two points, not on a single side, and the cast should be spread, not just split. It may also be necessary to split the stockinette and webril bandages that lie beneath the cast itself.

Other cast complications occur at pressure points. Pressure sores may form if bony protuberances are not well padded or if unexpected swelling occurs at or distal to the fracture site. If the patient complains of increasing pain over a bony prominence, it may be necessary to remove the cast to identify the problem. Even though it is undesirable to disturb the immobilization of a snug cast, this step is preferable to allowing a stasis ulcer to develop.

If the cast covers an open fracture, some drainage can be expected at the site of the open wound. It is wise to leave access to the wound to see if abscess formation is occurring. As with the suspicion of vascular compromise, often the most prudent action is to split the cast and inspect the wound directly.

FRACTURES AND DISLOCATIONS OF THE UPPER EXTREMITY

Hand

Phalanges

Fractures of the *distal phalanges* are significant in that they are usually open fractures. Treatment usually focuses on the soft-tissue injury, and the emergency physician may forget that this injury represents an open fracture and should be treated as such with thorough cleansing and antibiotics. These injuries can usually be treated in the emergency department rather than the operating room. Direct treatment of the bone is rarely necessary unless there is significant tissue loss of the distal phalanx with exposed bone. It may then be necessary to amputate a portion of the bone and perform a V-Y procedure on the digit.

As the fracture becomes more proximal, the joint tends to be involved. If more than 25% of the articular surface is involved, consult a hand surgeon to determine if a Kirschner wire should be placed for stabilization. These more proximal

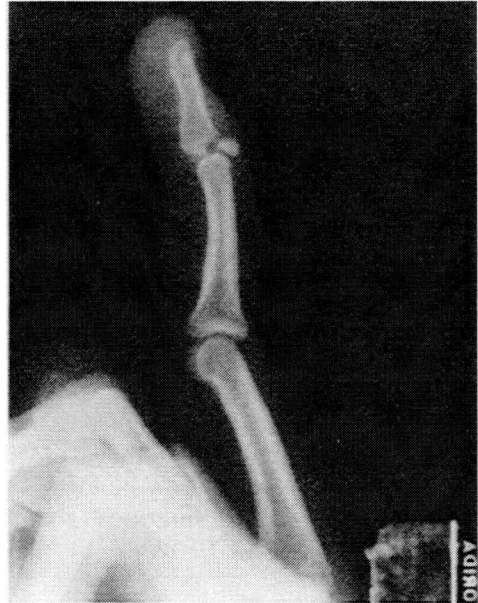

Fig.26-2 Mallet finger caused by avulsion fracture with subsequent disruption of extensor mechanism. Fracture fragment includes approximately 50% of joint surface and is optimally managed by percutaneous Kirschner-wire fixation.

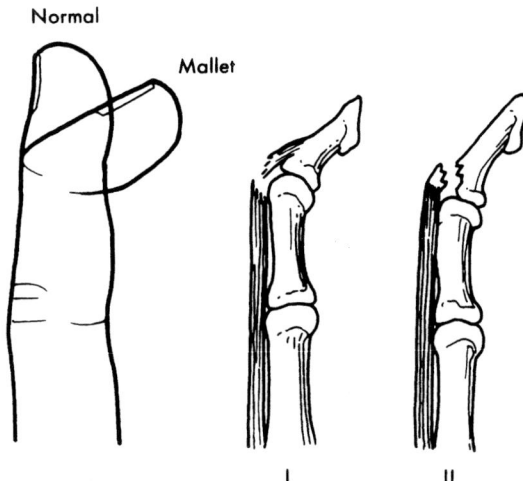

Fig.26-1 Mallet finger occurs with loss of extensor function to distal phalanx. This injury may be caused by a tear of tendon itself or by an avulsion fracture of dorsal base of distal phalanx.

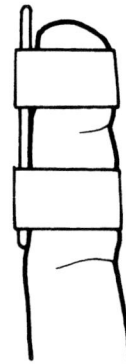

Fig.26-3 Paper clip wrapped in tape forms padded dorsal splint for mallet fingers. This splint should be tightened with daily retaping by patient.

injuries are usually caused by a blow to the end of the finger (as in miscatching a softball). In addition to the fracture, there is a more significant rupture of the extensor tendon insertion. The patient has a flexed distal digit and often has pain at the distal interphalangeal joint. Treat small fractures and minor articular involvement with a dorsal splint, with the distal interphalangeal joint in neutral or 5 degrees of hyperextension (Figs. 26-1 to 26-3).

Dislocations of the distal phalanx are common and often are reduced at the place of injury by coaches or trainers or by the patient. In light of such a history, the finger should be immobilized with approximately 5 degrees of flexion. If the finger could not be reduced in the field, it may require operative reduction. Make one or two gentle attempts after giving a digital block anesthetic, and if unsuccessful, refer the patient to a hand surgeon for operative reduction.

Fractures of the *middle phalanges* are less common and are usually caused by a twisting torque on the finger in which the patient has caught the finger during a vigorous motion of the hand (e.g., a football tackler who catches a finger on the opponent's face mask). Such injuries are serious because the fracture lines are usually spiral and can easily distort the normal alignment of the digit. Even though the fractures are easy to align, they are unstable and may require Kirschner wire fixation to achieve stability. If the fracture is stable, splint it to the adjacent finger. In the case of the ring finger, in-

corporate both the long and little fingers in the splint; use a short-arm cast with an extension for the fingers. The wrist should be extended in pronation to approximately 20 degrees. The metacarpophalangeal joints should be flexed to approximately 70 degrees, the proximal interphalangeal joints flexed to approximately 20 degrees, and the distal interphalangeal joints flexed to approximately 5 degrees. This "James position" is thought to be more physiologic than the "position of function" (as with a hand grasping a softball), because the collateral ligaments of the metacarpophalangeal joints are under more stretch in flexion than in extension as a result of a cam effect (Figs. 26-4 and 26-5).

A common problem with middle phalangeal fractures is the rupture of the central slip of the extensor tendon with tearing of the dorsal ligaments of the middle phalanx. The result is a "boutonniere" deformity, with flexion of the middle interphalangeal joint and extension at the distal interphalangeal joint (Figs. 26-6 and 26-7). If the rupture occurs to the ligament alone, splinting the proximal interphalangeal joint in extension is satisfactory; however, surgery is required when there is an accompanying avulsion fracture or a significant fracture of the middle phalanx.

Problems encountered with *proximal phalangeal fractures* are similar to those of the middle phalanges; however, distortion of alignment is even more common, and many of these fractures require surgical repair (Fig. 26-8).

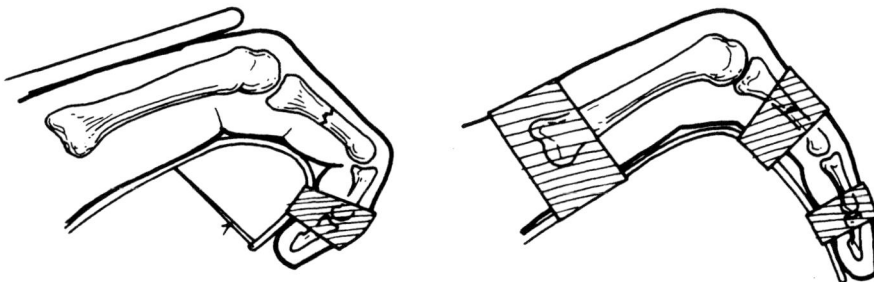

Fig. 26-4   James position with metal outrigger.

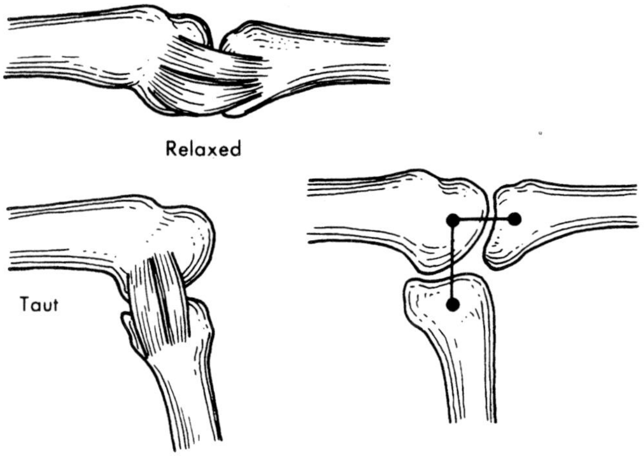

Fig. **26-5**   Collateral ligaments in stretch with meta-carpophalangeal joint flexed.

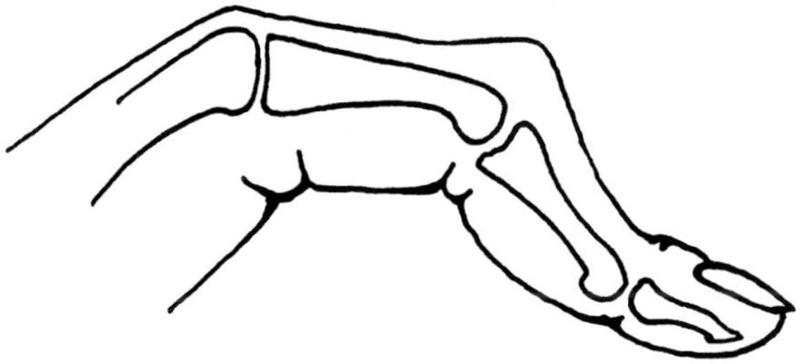

Fig. **26-6**   A boutonnière deformity resulting from disruption of the extensor tendon. (From Simon RR, Koenigsknecht SJ: *Emergency orthopedics: the extremities,* Norwalk, Conn, 1987, Appleton & Lange.)

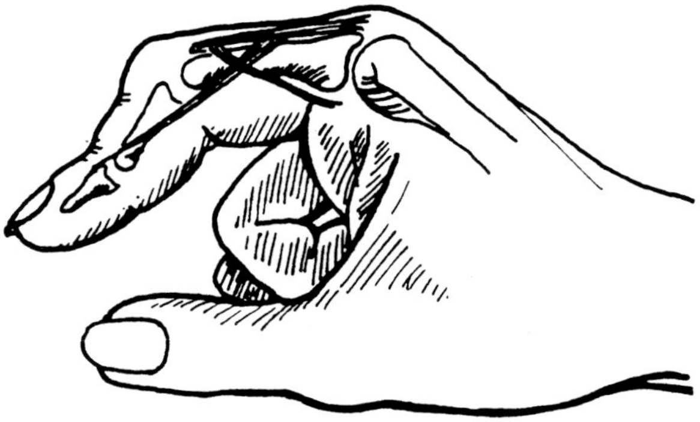

Fig. **26-7**   The boutonnière deformity. (From Simon RR, Koenigsknecht SJ: *Emergency orthopedics: the extremities,* Norwalk, Conn, 1987, Appleton & Lange.)

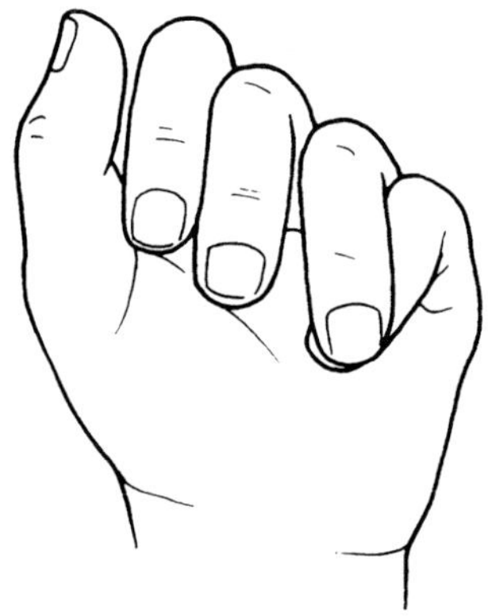

Fig. **26-8**   Rotational deformity through proximal phalanx.

Follow-up care for phalangeal fractures is important; do not assume that those injuries are trivial. Immobilization should not occur for more than 3 to 4 weeks because the finger will become stiff. The patient should be referred to an orthopedist or other hand surgeon if the emergency physician is not prepared to follow the patient and arrange for physical therapy if needed.

Metacarpals

Metacarpal fractures occur from blows to the hand, serious falls, or fisticuffs. In the context of fights, the *little finger* metacarpal is commonly injured, which results in a "boxer's fracture." It is imperative to note any break in the skin because such a break strongly suggests the teeth of another individual as the cause. Because the "fight bite" or clenched-fist injury has great potential for infection, many hand services prefer to wash the involved joint in the operating room and cover the patient with intravenous antibiotics.

The *index* and *middle finger* metacarpals must be aligned perfectly if the patient is to have a good outcome. Refer metacarpal fractures to a hand surgeon because many of these fractures cause angulation and are hard to align. A greater degree of angulation can be tolerated in the ring and little fingers, but it is still wise not to accept more than 10 to 20 degrees. Anesthesia for the reduction may be achieved with a Bier block. Use the James position for casting, which is a short-arm cast with a dual-finger extension for the two or three fingers adjacent to the fractured one.

Thumb metacarpal fractures require special attention; they tend to be proximal and are often spiral. They often require open reduction and internal fixation with a Kirschner wire; the only exception is the variation that is comminuted. Because the thumb is such an essential part of the grasping mechanism, refer all thumb metacarpal fractures to a hand surgeon.

Metacarpal dislocations may penetrate the extensor mechanism because virtually all of them are dorsal. Consider this possibility if the dislocation does not reduce easily. It will require an open reduction.

Wrist

Wrist injuries are often caused by falls on the outstretched hand or by direct blows. Because many *carpal bone* fractures are hard to visualize on the x-ray study, it is not unusual to pass off the injury as a sprain. The clinical presentation of localized pain must be respected. Even if no fracture is seen, splint the wrist and repeat the x-ray study if pain persists.

Navicular (scaphoid) fractures are often difficult to see on the x-ray study. Even a special coned-down view of the navicular bone may fail to reveal the acute fracture. If the patient has localized tenderness in the anatomic snuff-box despite a negative x-ray study, treat him or her as if the navicular were fractured. This treatment requires a short-arm cast with a thumb extension. The wrist should be in a neutral position with slight ulnar deviation. The hand should be pronated, and the thumb spica should extend to the interphalangeal joint. This cast should be left in place 1 to 4 weeks depending on the patient's symptoms and mechanism of injury. If the navicular fracture is still not apparent following a repeat x-ray study, remove the cast and have the patient begin mobilization of the hand. Even with careful care, the navicular fracture is subject to nonunion and may require bone graft surgery. Nonunion and avascular necrosis can result from unrecognized injuries, inadequate immobilization, or insufficient treatment periods.

Dislocations of the *lunate bone* or the bones surrounding the lunate (perilunate) are easy to miss in the anteroposterior (AP) x-ray view. It is much easier to detect such injuries on the lateral view. On the lateral view, the radius, lunate, and long finger metacarpal should form a straight line (Fig. 26-9), and the navicular should be at an angle of approximately 125 degrees. If these alignments are lost, there is probably a perilunate dislocation, and the patient should be referred to a hand surgeon. Lunate dislocations are easier to see because the lunate will be out of the line of the carpal bones.

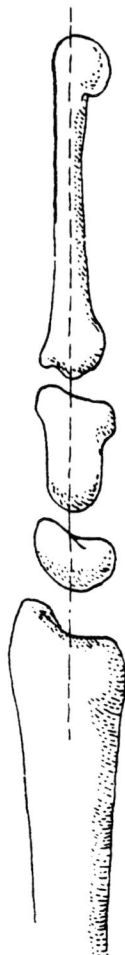

Fig. 26-9 Note that a line drawn through the midpoint of the radius and the capitate on the lateral view of the wrist traverses the midpoint of the lunate. If the lunate is dislocated or subluxated, the line will traverse only a fragment of the bone or miss it entirely. (From Simon RR, Koenigsknecht SJ: *Emergency orthopedics: the extremities,* Norwalk, Conn, 1987, Appleton & Lange.)

A Colles fracture is characterized by the classic "silver fork deformity" and is usually easily recognized (Fig. 26-10). It is the most common fracture in adults over the age of 50, is more common in women, and usually results from a fall on the outstretched hand. The term *Colles fracture* should not be used interchangeably with any fracture of the distal radius. The definition requires fracture of the distal radius with dorsal displacement and volar angulation, with or without an accompanying ulnar styloid fracture. Typically the radial fracture is approximately 2 cm from the distal end of the radius; the fracture rarely involves the articular surface. The ulnar styloid is involved approximately 60% of the time.

The goal of treatment for a Colles fracture is to restore the original length and volar tilt to the radius. If the normal volar tilt cannot be restored, the minimum goal is a neutral position (zero angulation) of the distal radial articular surface. Most Colles fractures are treated with closed reduction and cast immobilization.

Anesthesia can be achieved with a Bier block or with direct infiltration of the fracture site with 0.25% to 0.5% bupivacaine (Marcaine). Reduction can be difficult and usually requires longitudinal traction on the fingers while another person attempts to lengthen the radius by applying dorsal pressure at the fracture site. Traction may be applied by using hanging finger traps. Although a circular cast is ultimately required, it is not necessary initially. A volar splint from the distal palmar crease to the elbow will suffice until the swelling subsides. A long-arm cast is preferred in the young adult, whereas for an elderly patient it is preferable to retain mobility of the elbow. Also in the elderly patient, neutrality of the hand is preferable to ulnar deviation. If a circular cast has been applied, the patient must be seen within 24 hours and must be instructed about possible forearm compression syndromes. If a circular cast is applied, some physicians recommend immediate bivalving of the cast rather than awaiting the onset of vascular impairment.

The reverse of a Colles fracture is the *Smith fracture* (i.e., volar displacement of the fractured radius). This unusual injury generally occurs from a severe blow to the dorsum of the hand while the hand is flexed rather than from a fall on the outstretched, extended hand. This type of injury is more commonly seen after motorcycle accidents or automobile accidents. Unless attention is paid to the mechanism of injury and to the x-ray study appearance, it is tempting to treat these injuries as if they were Colles fractures. Reduce a Smith fracture with volar pressure on the distal fragment rather than dorsal pressure, with traction applied by finger traps. Although anatomic reduction may be achieved initially, many of these fractures are unstable and require surgical fixation. Because those fractures tend to cause even more swelling than do Colles fractures, any initial cast should be bivalved.

The *Barton fracture* involves the rim of the articular surface of the distal radius and may involve either the volar or dorsal aspect (Fig. 26-11). The dorsal rim injury is usually caused by an extreme flexed dorsiflexion of the wrist accompanied by a pronating force, although the mechanism of injury is variable. Because of volar ligament disruption, the carpus is subluxed dorsally and creates radiocarpal instability. Treatment is directed toward restoring the articular surface and reducing the carpal subluxation.

A *volar Barton fracture* results from a fall on

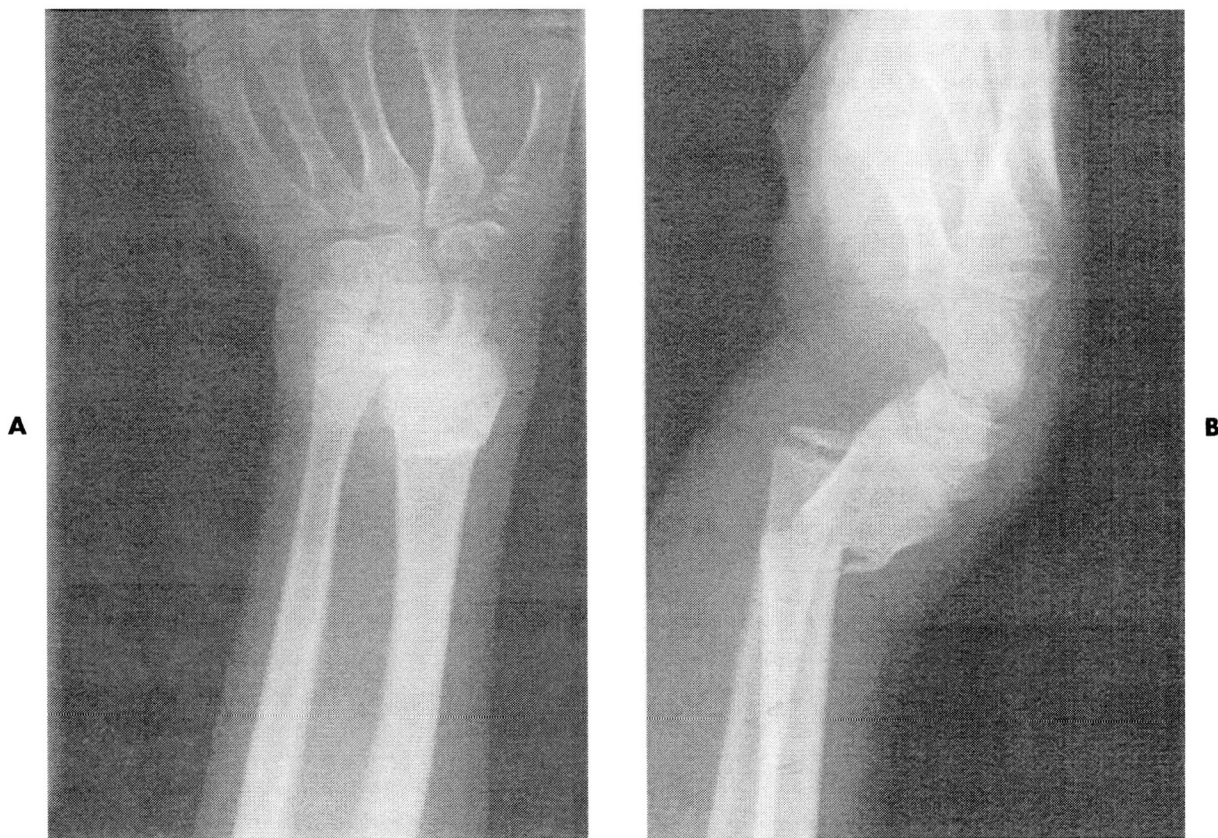

Fig. **26-10**   **A,** Colles fracture, AP view. **B,** Colles fracture, lateral view.

DORSAL BARTON'S

VOLAR BARTON'S

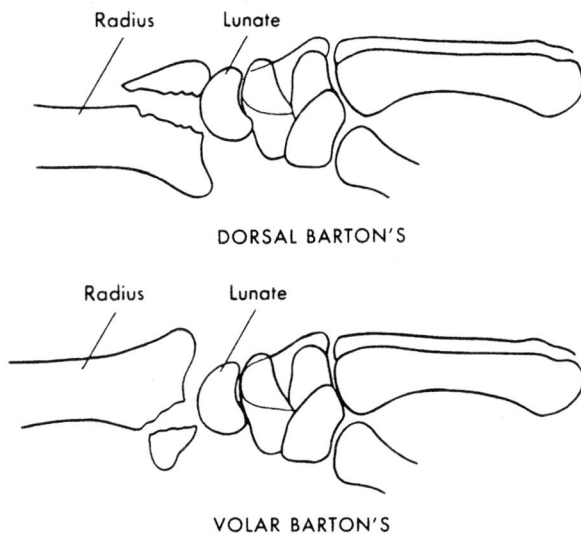

Fig.26-11 Barton fracture. (From Frykman GK, Kropp WE: Fractures and traumatic conditions of the wrist. In Hunter JM, Mackin EJ, Callahan AD, editors: *Rehabilitation of the hand: surgery and therapy,* St Louis, 1995, Mosby.)

an outstretched hand in supination. The injury is best demonstrated on the lateral x-ray study, which reveals a volar fragment of the distal radius and volar subluxation of the carpals. The goal of treatment is the same as for the dorsal rim injury. For either injury, fractures that involve less than 50% of the articular surface can usually be treated closed, whereas more extensive involvement may require open reduction and internal fixation.

Forearm

Fractures to either of the forearm bones are usually seen as paired injuries. Although separate, these bones work as a functional paired unit at both the wrist and the elbow. Thus it is especially necessary to get an x-ray study of the shafts of both the radius and ulna, as well as both joints. If there is angulation of a fracture of

either the radius or ulna, it is imperative to look at the wrist or elbow to ascertain whether the opposite bone is dislocated. For example, when the ulna is fractured in midshaft, a commonly missed injury is dislocation of the radial head at the elbow. If the radial injury is not diagnosed, the ulna will probably develop persistent angulation and nonunion; this injury is known as a *Monteggia fracture.* Similarly, if the radius is fractured and angulated, look at both the elbow and wrist; most often there will be a dislocation of the ulna at the wrist, which is known as a *Galeazzi fracture.*

Forearm fractures are notoriously unstable and often require operative intervention except in a child, who may sustain a torus fracture of both bones. If the fractures do not appear stable and are not displaced, comminuted, or angulated, treat them with a long-arm cast that extends from shoulder to hand. The hand should be pronated with the wrist neutral, and the cast should extend to the distal palmar crease. The elbow should be flexed to 90 degrees. The patient must be seen again within 24 hours and must have instructions concerning the possible development of a forearm compression syndrome. Any increase in pain or pain with finger movement should mandate the patient being seen again. The cast needs to be bivalved, otherwise the patient is at risk for developing a forearm compartment syndrome that will lead to a Volkmann contracture and a functionless, painful extremity.

Elbow

Fractures

Elbow fractures are commonly diagnosed with only indirect radiologic signs. A true lateral x-ray study is important for the detection and management of such fractures. On this view, if a posterior fat pad or a billowing of the anterior fat pad is seen, assume that there is a fracture of the radial head (Fig. 26-12). A visible posterior

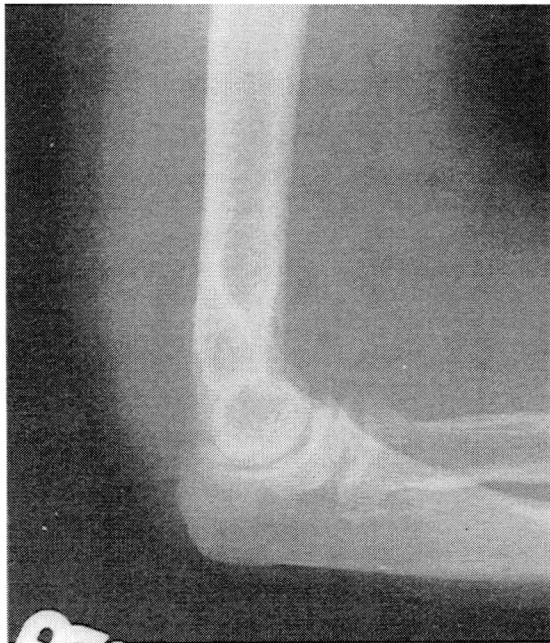

Fig.26-12 Examples of "fat pad sign" in lateral elbow x-ray film. **A,** Anterior fat pad. **B,** Posterior fat pad.

fat pad is always pathologic and is indicative of an effusion within the joint. Displacement or comminution of the radial head is much easier to see directly and may require excision of the radial head as part of the operative treatment. Often a tense hemarthrosis is associated with these fractures. Aspiration of the distended joint may provide great relief of the resultant pain. Treat the patient with a posterior splint that extends from wrist to shoulder and refer to an orthopedic surgeon for follow-up care.

Olecranon fractures are often seen following falls on or direct blows to the elbow. Displacement of the fracture fragments is often seen on x-ray study. If there are more than several millimeters of displacement, the patient needs an open reduction. Because the triceps inserts on the olecranon, interference in normal extension

of the elbow often exists, which also is an indication for surgical repair.

Dislocation or subluxation

All bones at the elbow are subject to dislocation. The patient with a dislocated elbow has a marked deformity of the elbow and usually considerable discomfort. The potential for neurovascular disturbance is great, especially with posterior dislocations that distort the brachial artery. Quickly evaluate the integrity of the brachial artery; if radial or ulnar pulses are diminished or absent, reduce the elbow as rapidly as possible. If there will be a delay in obtaining an orthopedic consultation or an operating room, reduce the dislocation in the emergency department. As the humerus is immobilized, apply traction distally at the wrist. Push the olecranon in the direction of the humerus, and gradually flex the elbow. As the dislocation reduces with an audible click, the elbow is flexed to approximately 120 degrees. It is important that the vascular function of the brachial artery be reassessed. If the hyperflexion causes loss or diminution of the pulses, reduce the angle of flexion. Apply a posterior plaster splint from shoulder to wrist and obtain a postreduction x-ray study. Because such limbs are at risk for compartment syndromes, observe the patient carefully for increasing pain, numbness of the fingers, pain on dorsiflexion of the fingers, or loss of forearm muscular function. Even if the pulses are still present, measure the compartment pressures for such signs. If pressure elevation occurs, a fasciectomy needs to be performed.

Lateral or medial dislocations of the *radius* or *ulna* can also occur. These dislocations require reduction in the emergency department only for relief of vascular compromise.

Massive swelling can occur following these dislocations and can interfere with testing the ligamentous stability of the elbow. Even if pulses are still present, an arteriogram may need to be performed to assess the integrity of the vascular system. Neurologic impairment is also common with these types of injuries, and the ulnar nerve is the most commonly injured nerve. Ulnar nerve injury may cause paresthesia along the hypothenar eminence or along the little finger and the ulnar half of the ring finger. There may be weakness of the lumbrical musculature with corresponding weakness while separating the fingers.

Subluxation of the radial head ("nursemaid's elbow") is a common problem in children. The child usually has been subjected to a longitudinal pull on the stretched arm, but spontaneous episodes have been reported in infants who rolled over in the crib. The child is usually under age 3 and often complains of arm pain. Sometimes the problem is noted because the child stops using the extremity; the arm is held in pronation. If the patient has a classic and reliable history, a gentle attempt at reduction may be attempted without an x-ray study.

In treating a subluxation of the radial head, the emergency physician should supinate the arm and gently press on the radial head. Often a click with relocation of the radial head is not felt, but the child will start to use the extremity within 5 to 10 minutes. If the child does not recover quickly, it is time to obtain an x-ray study. If the child does recover, a postreduction film is not needed.

Humerus

Proximal humeral fractures

The mechanism of injury for proximal humeral fractures is often a fall or a blow to the shoulder with the arm in abduction. Because this mechanism is the same one that produces a shoulder dislocation, the fracture may be accompanied by a dislocation. Fracture of the proximal humerus is primarily an injury of the elderly in whom osteoporosis weakens the bone. The overwhelming majority of such fractures are minimally displaced or impacted. Clinically, the presentation is usually characteristic:

the affected arm is held close to the body, and movement is restricted by pain. Tenderness, hematoma, deformity, or crepitus may be present over the fracture site.

X-ray evidence of the fracture is not difficult to detect if the shoulder is in alignment or if there is distraction of the fracture fragments. Impacted fractures occasionally go unnoticed on an x-ray film. It is often difficult to see an undisplaced fracture line in a shoulder that is also dislocated, which may lead to difficulties in reducing the humerus within the glenoid fossa. Moreover, the shaft but not the head of the humerus may reduce. Such a case requires an open reduction and fixation of the fracture. If there is a combination of fracture and dislocation, it is wise to involve an orthopedic surgeon in the patient's care. He or she may wish to reduce the fracture with an anesthetic and try to retain approximation of the fracture fragments as the shoulder dislocation is reduced. If an orthopedic consultation is not readily available, a gentle effort at reduction can be made. If the fracture fragments distract, the patient needs an open reduction, which would have been necessary anyway. In the meantime, the patient is usually much more comfortable. Immobilize the arm in a Velpeau bandage.

Minimally displaced or impacted fractures should be immobilized with a sling and swath, as well as prescribed ice packs and analgesics. To avoid a frozen shoulder, functional exercise should be initiated as soon as possible after union has been achieved.

Humeral shaft fracture

Humeral shaft fractures usually occur in the proximal part or middle third of the shaft as a result of direct blows or falls in which there was some delay in extending the arm to protect from the fall. This delay may explain why the fracture tends to occur in the elderly and in the inebriated patient. If the arm is extended early in the fall, navicular or Colles fractures are more likely to occur.

Fig. 26-13 "Sugar-tong" splint for humeral shaft fractures. **A,** Gentle traction is applied as splint is placed from over deltoid laterally, under elbow and up into axilla. **B,** Ace wrap holds splint in place. Axilla must be padded, and sling is used. (From Simon RR, Koenigsknecht SJ: *Emergency orthopedics: the extremities,* Norwalk, Conn, 1987, Appleton & Lange.)

Bony crepitus is usually felt over the fracture, and there is visible swelling and loss of function. The arm may be shortened or rotated depending on the displacement of the fracture fragments. Radiographically, the fracture is usually spiral. X-ray views should include the elbow and shoulder joints. Be sure to look for pathologic bone changes because the humerus is a common site for metastatic disease. Nondisplaced fractures are treated with a "sugar tong" splint and a sling and swath (Fig. 26-13). Displaced fractures should have a hanging cast applied by the orthopedic surgeon (Fig. 26-14).

In a humeral shaft fracture, there is a 15% to 20% incidence of involvement of the radial nerve as it spirals around the humerus; this involvement is often a benign neuropraxia and resolves in 80% of all patients. If there is a wrist drop, loss of sensation in a radial distribution of the hand, and no relief with fracture reduction, the nerve may be entrapped in the fracture fragments. Occasionally the neuropathy occurs

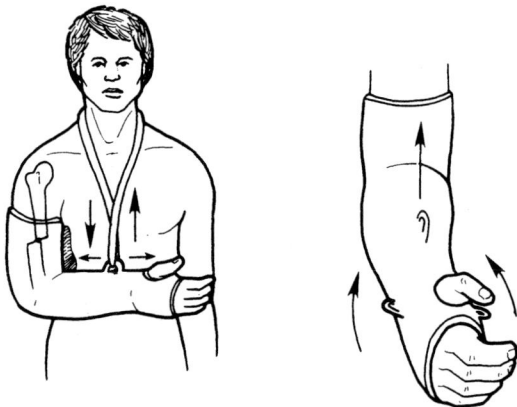

Fig. 26-14 Hanging cast technique. (From Magnusson AR: Humerous and elbow. In Rosen P et al, editors: *Emergency medicine: concepts and clinical practice,* ed 3, St Louis, 1992, Mosby.)

with reduction, which also suggests entrapment. Refer the patient to a neurosurgeon and orthopedic surgeon for surgical release of the trapped nerve.

Vascular damage to the brachial artery is also a possible complication of these types of fractures. If there is loss or diminution of the pulse in the brachial arteries or its branches, an angiogram or surgical exploration should be performed by an orthopedic surgeon.

Distal humeral fractures

Distal humeral fractures that are proximal to the humeral epicondyles are referred to as *supracondylar fractures.* Supracondylar fractures are especially common in children; 95% of these fractures result from falls on the outstretched arm with the elbow either fully extended or hyperextended.

The child with this type of injury holds the upper extremity immobile in extension to the side, with a typical S-shaped configuration and tenderness and swelling in the region of the elbow. Prominence of the olecranon attached to the posteriorly displaced distal fragment is similar to posterior dislocation of the elbow. When there is an incomplete supracondylar fracture, the diagnosis may be less obvious, with an elbow effusion as the only clinical sign. A careful neurovascular examination is essential. A lateral x-ray view is critical because 25% of these injuries are nondisplaced greenstick fractures, and a positive fat pad sign may be the only sign of fracture. Displaced fractures may be visible only after careful inspection of the AP and lateral views. Consider this type of injury when youngsters appear with trauma to this region.

Unrecognized, supracondylar fractures often lead to loss of the normal carrying angle of the arm, an inability to fully extend the elbow, osteoarthritis of the elbow joint, ulnar neuropathy, and loss of forearm strength. Although admission for observation is a prudent course with this type of injury, it is safe to discharge the patient if the fracture is undisplaced, if there is no vascular compromise when the elbow is flexed, if there is an adequate home environment with someone who can watch for compartment compromise, and if the child has been seen and recommended for discharge by the orthopedic surgeon. Displaced fractures often need to be reduced with the patient under general anesthesia, but conscious sedation may be a satisfactory substitute.

Dislocations

Shoulder dislocations are commonly seen following a fall or blow to the shoulder with the arm caught in abduction.

Anterior dislocations. Most shoulder dislocations are *anterior* (i.e., with the humerus outside the glenoid fossa anterior to the shoulder girdle). Usually the humeral head also lies inferior to the glenoid. The patient does not abduct the arm, and there is a loss of deltoid fullness to the shoulder. The head of the humerus can be palpated in the axilla. There is often compression of the axillary nerve, with loss of sensation over the deltoid muscle and lateral upper arm. It is impossible to test deltoid muscle strength while the shoulder is dislocated, and it is unwise to test it after reduction because such a test may cause the shoulder to dislocate again. Therefore sensory testing is the best method to determine axillary nerve involvement. Nerve compression or contusion is usually transient. Most patients recover function shortly after reduction of the shoulder, but some patients may require several days or even weeks before nerve function is recovered.

In most instances, it is important to have both prereduction and postreduction x-ray film studies to ascertain whether there is an associated fracture. In many instances, an undisplaced fracture fragment of the humerus is not detectable until after reduction.

Anterior dislocation is a painful injury while the bone is dislocated; the best way to relieve this pain is to reduce the dislocation. The earlier the reduction is attempted, the less muscle

spasm there is to overcome. It is also easier to accomplish reduction in children and elderly patients, who do not have the same muscle development as young athletic adults.

The key to reduction is gentleness: To overcome the muscle spasm, to lower the glenoid fossa, and to elevate the humeral head. In most instances it is not necessary to use large doses of opiates. If the patient is seen early after the injury is sustained and before much muscle spasm has ensued, the shoulder can sometimes be relocated with no supplementary medications and without much discomfort for the patient. Reduction can be made easier using a hypnotic dose of midazolam (Versed) or diazepam (Valium) because these medications provide muscle relaxation and some amnesia. These drugs need to be titrated until the desired effect is achieved. The dose for midazolam usually ranges from 1 to 10 mg intravenously, and for diazepam, 5 to 20 mg intravenously. Start an intravenous line and slowly inject the medication while talking to the patient. When the patient's speech becomes slurred and the eyelids begin to close, the hypnotic level has been achieved and it is possible to attempt the reduction.

Many different techniques of reduction have been described, but one should never use the "Hippocratic" method, in which the operator places a foot in the axilla and pulls longitudinally on the arm in the direction of the long axis of the humerus. The danger of this method is the high incidence of problems with the axillary nerve or brachial plexus, as well as the increased risk of fracturing the humerus.

In reducing anterior dislocated shoulder, any one of the following four methods can be used:

• *Method One:* If the patient's muscle spasm is minor or can be overcome with a hypnotic medication, place the patient in an upright seated position. Gradually elevate the arm, and ask the patient to place his or her hand on the occiput of his or her head. While someone applies gentle stabilization to the trunk of the patient, apply traction in the line of the long axis of the humerus. At the same time, gently push up on the humeral head with one hand. The humerus usually reduces with a popping sensation and relief of patient discomfort. The arm should be abducted to the thorax, and a postreduction x-ray film should be obtained.

If the shoulder has been dislocated for many hours (as in the intoxicated patient who is not aware of the dislocation until he or she becomes sober), this method will probably not work, even with maximum sedation and muscle relaxation. Method Two, Three, or Four can be attempted; if none of these methods work, the dislocation probably needs to be reduced with the patient under general anesthesia in the operating room.

- *Method Two:* The traction/countertraction technique to reduce anterior dislocations of the shoulder is usually safe and effective. Wrap a folded sheet under the axilla and around the chest, and securely grasp it in a direction 45 degrees caudad to the long axis of the body, not directly up into the axilla. After the patient has achieved adequate sedation and muscle relaxation, apply traction to the arm by grasping the lower third of the forearm and pulling backward. It may be desirable to loop another sheet around your waist and tie the ends of the same sheet around the patient's distal forearm. By leaning backward into the sling that has been created, the entire body weight can be applied to the traction force, which usually distracts the humeral head and results in reduction. Caution should be taken in individuals with thin skin, such as the elderly or those on steroids, to prevent tearing the skin where the sheet is attached at the distal forearm.
- *Method Three:* Place the patient prone on a gurney, with the involved arm hanging over the side of the stretcher. While gently pushing upward on the humeral head in the axilla, abduct the tip of the scapula toward the midline. The shoulder again reduces with a palpa-

ble pop; the arm is fixed to the thorax, and postreduction films are acquired. This method is most successful in the elderly patient who may have difficulty sitting up, especially after sedation; however, it is also worth trying in the younger patient before resorting to Method Four.

- *Method Four:* With the patient in the same position as for Method Three, ask him or her to grasp the handle of a water bucket. Tape the hand to the bucket and fill the bucket with enough water to place traction on the arm. Someone need not attend the patient unless he or she is groggy from the sedation. Within 10 to 15 minutes, the shoulder usually reduces spontaneously. The arm is fixed as in Method Three, and a postreduction x-ray study is obtained.

Refer all patients to an orthopedic surgeon for follow-up care. If this was a recurrent episode of dislocation, shoulder immobilization need be carried out only for 12 to 24 hours, after which the patient should begin exercising the shoulder to prevent stiffness. If this is a first episode, the shoulder should probably be immobilized for 4 to 6 weeks for younger patients, but this is controversial. Some authors prefer early resumption of activity to prevent the development of a chronic pain syndrome of a frozen shoulder; early resumption of activity is especially important in the elderly patient, and there is agreement that immobilization should be relatively brief. Patients with anterior shoulder dislocations also have an increased incidence of an accompanying rotator cuff injury; therefore early orthopedic referral is advised.

Posterior dislocations. *Posterior dislocations* are quite rare and are usually seen following unusual types of violent injury, such as electric shocks or after an epileptic seizure. The patient may not be aware of the injury because loss of consciousness occurred with the primary event. Because of altered consciousness afterward, the patient may not note pain until he or she attempts to use the shoulder.

With a posterior dislocation, there is often

not as much visible deformity of the lateral and anterior shoulder; however, it is often possible to palpate the head of the humerus as a posterior swelling. The x-ray study is much harder to interpret without a true lateral or a Y-view of the shoulder. It is possible to miss the dislocation because the humerus appears to lie within the glenoid fossa, but it is actually lying behind it.

Reduction of a posterior dislocation is often accomplished in the operating room with the patient under general anesthesia, but some of the anterior techniques also work, such as the traction with water bucket. After adequate sedation, one method that can be attempted is as follows: Place the patient in a prone position. With the patient's elbow flexed to 90 degrees and while gently pushing on the humeral head in the direction of the glenoid fossa, apply traction in the long axis of the humerus. When the shoulder reduces, a popping sensation should be felt similar to that of the anterior reduction. Immobilize the arm as with an anterior dislocation and obtain a postreduction x-ray study. Refer the patient to an orthopedic surgeon for follow-up care.

Shoulder and Clavicle

Clavicular fractures are common athletic and playground injuries and can occur from falls and from blows directed to the shoulder. At one time they were common football injuries, but the modern shoulder pad seems to protect against clavicular fractures.

Although a clavicular fracture is not normally serious, with proper force applied to the shoulder the bone fragment may be driven into the thorax with injury to the subclavian vessels. Such an injury may be suspected when larger amounts of swelling and ecchymosis than one expects to see from a simple clavicular fracture are found. Moreover, with this complication a pseudoaneurysm of the subclavian artery or an arteriovenous fistula between the artery and vein is often formed. The latter may produce a bruit over these vessels that stops abruptly at the heart. There may be no diminution of pulses. If this injury is suspected, it may be necessary to perform an angiogram for a definitive diagnosis.

Examine the patient for any signs of a *brachial plexus injury,* with appropriate referral to a neurosurgeon if this type of injury is found. Most of these fractures are in the middle third of the clavicle. In the toddler it is often a greenstick fracture.

Treatment of midshaft fractures traditionally requires a figure-of-eight bandage or a commercial clavicle strap applied when the patient is asked to "come to attention." This strap serves as a splint and provides some degree of pain relief. The axillae should be well padded, and the device should not be applied too tightly to avoid numbness. With proximal fractures, this strap may distract the fracture fragments, in which case a simple sling will suffice. Some physicians now treat all clavicle fractures with only a sling.

Acromioclavicular separations are common injuries, especially after skiing or horseback riding falls in which the patient lands directly on the point of the shoulder. Although all degrees of such injuries can be managed without surgery, complete separations are preferably managed surgically, both for speed of recovery and for cosmetic considerations.

Acromioclavicular separations are described in degrees as with sprains. A first-degree separation is a sprain of the acromioclavicular (AC) ligament. There is minor tearing of this ligament but not enough to produce subluxation. There is tenderness to palpation over the joint but x-ray studies, including stress views, are negative.

A second-degree separation is constituted by disruption of the AC ligament, with partial subluxation of the distal end of the clavicle from the acromion. Stress x-ray studies should be taken bilaterally and may be necessary to reveal the injury. With a second-degree injury, the coracoclavicular injury is not sufficient to completely disrupt the AC joint, and there is no increase in the distance between the coracoid process and the clavicle when compared to the normal shoulder.

A third-degree injury involves complete disruption of both the AC ligament and the coracoclavicular ligament. The coracoclavicular ligament, comprises the conoid and trapezoid ligaments and functions to anchor the distal clavicle to the coracoid process of the scapula. When all of these ligaments are disrupted, there is upward displacement of the clavicle, which may be appreciated clinically and confirmed by x-ray studies.

Treatment of first- and second-degree separations requires a sling or Velpeau bandage; the commercially available AC straps rarely work any better. When discomfort is gone, the patient should begin shoulder mobility exercises. With a third-degree separation, consult the orthopedic surgeon for a decision regarding the need for and timing of surgical intervention.

Rotator cuff tears are also common ski and football injuries. The mechanism can be an extra strong effort to serve in tennis or throw a baseball, especially when not warmed up; excessive weight lifting; or a fall with the arm abducted but not externally rotated. The patient has severe pain in the shoulder and cannot or will not elevate the arm above the waist. If the tear is partial, the failure to elevate is caused by pain. Distinguishing a partial from a complete tear can be done by injecting the shoulder with a combination of lidocaine and dexamethasone (Decadron). If the relief of discomfort does not enable function, the patient has a complete tear; with a partial tear, there is a resumption of function after the injection. At times an arthrogram or MRI needs to be performed to distinguish the two entities. If the former reveals extravasation, the tear is complete.

Treatment for partial tears is immobilization until the discomfort has abated followed by resumption of shoulder activities. Complete tears require surgery. For equivocal cases, it is acceptable to try a period of conservative management before embarking on surgical repair.

Scapular fractures are usually caused by direct blows to the back during high speed vehicular accidents, falls, or crush injuries. The patient complains of pain over the bone, but little swelling or deformity is observed. The real significance of the injury comes from the associated intrathoracic or extrathoracic injuries that the patient may have sustained. These injuries must be evaluated and dealt with before paying much attention to the scapula. A Velpeau bandage is satisfactory for immobilization. The patient should be encouraged to commence shoulder exercises as soon as tolerable.

NONFRACTURE PROBLEMS OF THE CERVICAL, THORACIC, AND LUMBOSACRAL SPINE

The most common mechanism for a nonfracture neck injury of the *cervical spine* is minor automobile trauma. The car is struck from the rear, and the patient's head is thrown backward and rebounds forward. Although most new cars have headrests, they must be elevated to have any effectiveness. The same mechanism can occur in reverse with front-end collisions, especially if the patient is restrained. The precise pathophysiology of the subsequent flexion-extension injury is hard to elucidate; it is not known if this injury is a true strain, sprain, or nerve compression. Occasionally a patient develops some prevertebral calcification, but in most patients, there are no true x-ray study findings. There may be loss of the normal lordotic curve, or there may be findings of chronic disease, such as osteoarthritis. There are few specific physical findings. Patients complain of tenderness along the paravertebral musculature and may complain of radiation of this tenderness onto the occiput of the skull. There may be spasm of the cervical muscles posteriorly.

It is prudent to search for bony injury if the patient complains about immediate onset of pain at the time of the accident or within the first hour afterward. However, if the pain and muscle spasm do not begin until some time afterward, it is not necessary to obtain a cervical x-ray study.

Treat a cervical spine injury with a nonsteroidal antiinflammatory agent combined with a muscle relaxing agent. Antiinflammatory agents are especially effective for patients who have developed prevertebral calcification.

It is common to treat this type of injury with a soft cervical collar. However, the longer the neck is immobilized, the greater the risk of atrophy of the paraspinous muscles. It is better to give adequate muscle relaxation and antiinflammatory agents and encourage early range-of-motion exercises of the neck. Because the use of diazepam (Valium) by outpatients is accompanied by the risk of substance abuse or dependency, some physicians prefer to use diazepam in the emergency department and to discharge the patient with methocarbamol (Robaxin). The dosage for methocarbamol should be 750 to 1500 mg four times a day. These patients require careful follow-up with their primary physicians and may benefit from early physical therapy.

The *thoracic spine* is rarely subjected to strains or sprains. Pain syndromes in the midspine are rare except in conjunction with compression fractures. Therefore when a patient complains of pain in this area of the back, one must aggressively pursue causes other than the benign. Serious causes include osteomyelitis of the spine or metastatic disease. If there are no obvious findings on the x-ray study, it may be necessary to perform a bone scan, a CT scan, or an MRI.

Lower back problems are experienced by virtually all humans, and the cause is not often identified. Back pain can occur in an acute incapacitating form after such benign forces as coughing, turning the torso, or sneezing. Lower back problems may also occur after lifting heavy objects, but flexion of the spine alone rarely causes the problem.

In general, x-ray studies are not needed because there rarely is any observable pathologic condition. A fall on the buttocks may produce a compression fracture, especially in the elderly; back pain in this setting or the presence of a calcaneal fracture after a fall from a height warrants an x-ray examination. Physical findings may include spasm of the lumbar paravertebral musculature. It is important to detect acute neurologic deficits because they indicate emergent diagnostic and therapeutic interventions to prevent permanent loss of function. Examine the patient for sensory loss in the extremities or in the saddle area of the perineum. In addition, ask the patient about fecal or urinary incontinence. Occasionally a patient has urinary retention. Test the deep tendon reflexes bilaterally, and test the anal sphincter for both sensation and tonus. If there is any abnormality that represents an acute neurologic change, the patient should be seen immediately by a neurosurgeon. A CT scan or MRI may be needed, and the patient may require an emergency laminectomy.

In the absence of any signs of neurologic involvement, treat the patient as for a cervical sprain. A combination of a muscle relaxant, an antiinflammatory agent, an analgesic, and ice in addition to a brief period of bed rest is the most beneficial treatment. Although most patients may be managed at home, some patients have such a poor home situation that they must be admitted to the hospital.

As soon as the patient regains some mobility, consider referring the patient for physical therapy to learn stretching and flexion exercises that help keep the back limber and free from recurrent problems. Weight control is also helpful, because obesity is one of the stresses on the spine that induces chronic pain syndromes.

An important cause of lower back pain does not have anything to do with the back or spine; this problem lies in the retroperitoneal space. A leaking abdominal aortic aneurysm, or a pelvic or retroperitoneal abscess can produce severe back pain. Patients with back pain and syncope should be evaluated immediately for an abdominal aortic aneurysm. Even if the pulses are normal and the blood pressure is not low, consider this diagnosis in patients who are considered at risk.

LOWER EXTREMITY

Pelvic Fractures

Before 1900, hypovolemic shock was almost a certain cause of death to patients with pelvic fractures. In 1890 the mortality rate from pelvic fractures was almost 90%.

Because a pelvic fracture is rarely an isolated injury, conflicting life-threatening injuries often occupy the trauma team's attention, and the pelvic injury is not recognized or treated aggressively. Therefore a routine AP pelvic view should be ordered for any multiple-trauma patient with a major mechanism of injury. The rectum and urethra should also be evaluated. Pelvic fractures are also commonly seen in the elderly after falls, but these injuries are often less serious.

Pelvic fractures are divided into those that are stable and those that are unstable. Stable fractures involve a single area of avulsion or an undisplaced break in the ring. Unstable fractures involve a double break in the ring, usually with marked displacement.

When an unstable fracture is defined, the emergency physician must search for an accompanying injury to the genitourinary tract, which usually involves the bladder or urethra. Moreover, he or she must be prepared for massive blood loss. These patients often maintain their vital signs until movement for other diagnostic studies; at that time a precipitous loss of stability can occur that can be hard or impossible to recover. Early detection, early aggressive volume replacement, and early efforts to stabilize the pelvis can help prevent this loss of stability. In the field and the emergency department, stabilization may be done with a military antishock trouser (MAST) suit. In the trauma unit, there may be continued use of the MAST suit or early application of an external fixation device. For cases in which there is no possibility of applying an external fixator, it may be necessary to control the hemorrhage with angiography and embolization of the bleeding pelvic vessels.

In addition to a urinary tract injury, the pelvic fracture may involve the vagina or uterus. In the press of resuscitation it is often forgotten to either acquire a history of present menstruation patterns or to perform a vaginal examination.

Sacral Fractures

Sacral fractures are unfortunately associated with neurologic deficits, but these deficits are often missed in the trauma room because it is difficult or impossible to test function of the sacral and gluteal musculature. It is also impossible to test gait before the amount of spinal and vascular integrity has been determined. Similarly, with sciatic nerve injuries the patient may be unaware of the characteristic motor and sensory deficits (see p. 317).

Patients with stable fractures need not be admitted to the hospital except for social reasons, such as an elderly patient who lives alone with no caretaker. Treatment for sacral fractures involves analgesics and antiinflammatory agents. Young athletes with avulsion injuries should rest from the sport that produced the injury.

Patients with unstable fractures require admission. Care of associated injuries often takes precedence over the care of the bony problem.

Acetabular Fractures

Acetabular fractures occur from medially directed blows against the greater trochanter, most often as a result of an automobile-pedestrian collision. The injury can also occur from striking the dashboard of an automobile with the knee. The fracture is often associated with fractures of the femur or femoral head and may also be seen with posterior dislocations.

This type of fracture may be hard to visualize on an x-ray study and may be detected only because of persistent pain and an inability to bear weight. A CT scan is very useful in defining the injury.

Admit patients with acetabular fractures for treatment. Treatment varies with associated injuries, the amount of displacement, and the age of the patient.

Sciatic Nerve Injury

The *sciatic nerve* is most commonly traumatized by posterior hip dislocations, deep penetrating wounds to the thigh or buttock, or inadvertent injections into the nerve. Sciatic nerve injuries may also be caused by femoral shaft fractures, as well as by intraneural or extraneural hemorrhages in patients who are taking anticoagulants. With posterior dislocation of the hip, sciatic nerve damage usually is partial with a predominantly peroneal distribution. The most sensitive clinical indicator of damage to the peroneal nerve is weakness of the extensor hallicus longus. Complete sciatic nerve neuropathy results in paralysis of the hamstring muscles and all of the muscles below the knee. Sensory loss involves the posterior thigh and most of the leg below the knee.

Traumatic injury of the sciatic nerve carries a poor prognosis, even under conditions of optimal repair.

Hip Fractures

A hip fracture is one of the more common injuries of the elderly patient and may occur from simple stress on the bone rather than from a fall. For example, some patients give a history of a sudden pain in the hip that caused them to fall rather than vice versa.

When the hip is fractured, the leg is typically shortened and externally rotated. However, intracapsular fractures that do not displace do not demonstrate this deformity. Efforts to ambulate or move the leg cause discomfort. Careful physical examination should reveal the possibility of the fracture.

Only a minor amount of blood loss is associated with femoral head and neck fractures because they are contained by the joint capsule. Conversely, intertrochanteric fractures, which

are extracapsular, may behave more like a fractured femoral shaft and be accompanied by significant hemorrhage. Femoral neck fractures are rarely seen in the young patient and, if found, should elicit a search for a pathologic cause of the fracture. Although usually found in elderly women with osteoporosis, femoral neck fractures can occur from falls. Such fractures can be impacted and cause only minor discomfort. Nevertheless, ambulation is not safe because the impaction may give way, with marked destabilization of the fracture.

Admit patients with hip fractures to the orthopedic service unless the fall was caused by multiple trauma or there is an underlying medical problem that needs attention.

A serious problem in the adolescent is the *slipped capital femoral epiphysis.* The patient is usually a pubescent male, often somewhat obese, and usually complains of a minor trauma sustained on the playground or at football practice. The physical examination may initially be normal except for some limping with weight bearing. An x-ray study of the hip may also be normal or show very subtle abnormalities. Comparison to the noninjured side is useful. When plain x-ray studies are normal but this injury is suspected, a CT scan or MRI may be useful in diagnosing the "preslipping" stage. Early recognition is important so orthopedic repair can be obtained for the injury before total slippage occurs. Total slippage appears clinically like a hip fracture, with shortening, external rotation, and abduction of the hip. Refer the patient immediately to an orthopedic surgeon to avoid aseptic necrosis of the femoral head.

Hip Dislocations

Hip dislocations are usually posterior and occur from blows to the knee when both knee and hip are flexed. The injury is very painful. The involved leg is shortened, abducted, internally rotated, and often there is a palpable mass posterior to the hip. The amount of time between injury and reduction is important, because the longer the hip is dislocated, the greater the risk of aseptic necrosis of the femoral head. Often the sciatic nerve is compressed by the dislocation. There may be an inability to flex the knee, loss of strength in the lateral leg musculature, and loss of sensation in the foot or great toe depending on which nerve bundles are dysfunctional.

Relocation of the hip is usually performed in the operating room with the patient under general anesthesia. If there will be a long delay before the patient can go into surgery, an attempt to reduce the hip should be made in the emergency department using adequate sedation and analgesia. Relocation should be done in conjunction with the orthopedic surgeon if immediately available; if not, the emergency physician should proceed. Pull in the line of the femur with the knee and hip flexed while an assistant holds the iliac crests in place by pushing posteriorly against the table on which the patient rests. A postreduction film is necessary.

Because reduction is often hard to sustain with an associated fracture, traction is also recommended to prevent recurrence, even in dislocations without fracture. Traction is easiest to arrange on the inpatient service.

Anterior dislocations occur much less commonly. Forced abduction and forces tearing the femoral head through the anterior capsule of the hip joint cause anterior hip dislocation. If the hip was in extension at the time of injury, either an iliac or pubic dislocation occurs. The head of the femur can be palpated anterior and lateral to the hip. If the hip was in flexion, an obturator dislocation occurs. The head of the femur is palpated in the thigh just lateral to the perineum. All of these dislocations cause the patient to lie with the extremity in abduction with external rotation. With an obturator dislocation, there is marked flexion of the hip.

As with posterior dislocations, time is important. These reductions are best performed in the operating room, but if there are unavoidable delays in scheduling operating time,

an attempt to reduce can be made in the emergency department with adequate sedation and analgesia.

Reduce an obturator dislocation by having an assistant stabilize the leg in abduction. With the knee flexed, pull in the direction of the femur, gradually flex and internally rotate the hip, and abduct the leg. For the other anterior dislocations, hyperextend the hip and pull downward in the line of the femur while gradually internally rotating the leg and while an assistant stabilizes the pelvis. A postreduction x-ray study and a period of traction are required for all of the previously mentioned relocations.

Until the orthopedic surgeon can arrange appropriate traction in the inpatient setting, a simple Buck traction or a long-leg splint (Hare or Thomas) can be used to stabilize the extremity.

Femoral Shaft Fractures

A major force is needed to fracture the femur. Femoral shaft fractures are commonly seen as the result of automobile accidents, and in children such an injury often results from being struck by a car in an automobile-pedestrian accident. In the infant, abuse is an unfortunate cause of this injury.

The fracture is almost never subtle because the powerful thigh muscles produce distraction of the fracture fragments. The patient has a shortened leg and has a midthigh mass. The leg is usually found in external rotation.

The potential for a life-threatening hemorrhage into the fracture site is often underestimated. It is important to immobilize these fractures in the field with a long-leg splint (such as a Thomas or Hare) to minimize the amount of hemorrhage. The patient must be typed and crossmatched but often does not require transfusion if immobilization is carried out early and effectively. In addition to minimizing volume depletion, immobilization also helps control pain by overcoming the muscle spasms produced by the competing flexion and extension forces at the fracture site.

There is always a potential for sciatic nerve injury with femoral shaft fractures; if such an injury is present, it is prudent not to apply traction to the long-leg traction device because doing so may further aggravate the nerve damage.

If the femur fracture is open, it is also preferable not to use traction on the long-leg device because reduction of contaminated bone increases the risk of infection. It is still wise to immobilize the extremity to avoid the hemorrhage potential of the injury.

Often the patient who has sustained a femoral shaft fracture has other injuries that may take precedence over management of the fracture. The patient can be left in the long-leg traction device while the other injuries are assessed and managed. The orthopedic surgeon can decide the optimal timing of definitive care in conjunction with the other necessary operative procedures.

Treatment of the fracture is either a period of bed rest with traction or operative repair with placement of an intramedullary rod. Although this is outside the province of the emergency physician, it is helpful to know what the orthopedic surgeons prefer within the institution; such knowledge allows for intelligent disposition of the patient and better communication with relatives.

Knee

Fractures of the patella are often seen after falls on the flexed knee and as a result of dashboard injuries. The patella takes the brunt of such trauma, but as noted previously, the same mechanisms produce hip dislocations and acetabular fractures. Because such injuries are much more likely to capture the attention of the emergency physician, it is important to check the patella whenever such mechanisms of injury are encountered. Sudden and violent contraction of the quadriceps muscles along with flexion of the knee may also produce a patellar fracture.

Loss of the extensor mechanism with a patellar fracture is an indication for operative intervention. It is also common to have a break in the skin overlying the patellar fracture, which is another indication for operative intervention. In this case, start the patient on broad-spectrum antibiotics, as with any open fracture.

The patellar ligament can rupture without a patellar fracture from a mechanism similar to that which produces a patellar fracture. If the extensor mechanism is affected and the patient is unable to extend the leg, the injury requires early referral to the orthopedic surgeon for operative repair.

The same mechanism of injury—strenuous contraction of the quadriceps—can cause the quadriceps tendon to rupture or the patellar ligament to avulse a bone fragment from the tibial tubercle (Fig. 26-15). Disruption of the infrapatellar portion of the patella may produce a "high riding" patella, which can be seen clinically or radiographically.

Another common injury is *patellar dislocation.* The patella always dislocates laterally. The leg is held in flexion and the patella is palpated lateral to its normal location. It is often desirable to reduce this dislocation in the field to enable extrication of patients from difficult environments (such as a squash court in which the door does not permit entrance of an ambulance stretcher). Relocation can often be achieved without sedation or anesthesia. While applying medial pressure to the patella, slowly bring the leg into extension at the knee. A postreduction film is necessary to rule out any associated patellar fracture. Further treatment involves a knee immobilizer, minimal weight bearing, and a referral to the orthopedic surgeon for consideration of operative management. If dislocation is a repeated problem, immobilization is not needed after the knee is no longer uncomfortable.

Sprains of the knee are common athletic injuries and arc especially prevalent in football and skiing. The sooner the knee stability is tested, the more accurate the assessment of the ligamentous integrity will be. Often the patient is not seen until hours or days after the injury, and in such cases joint effusion prevents an ac-

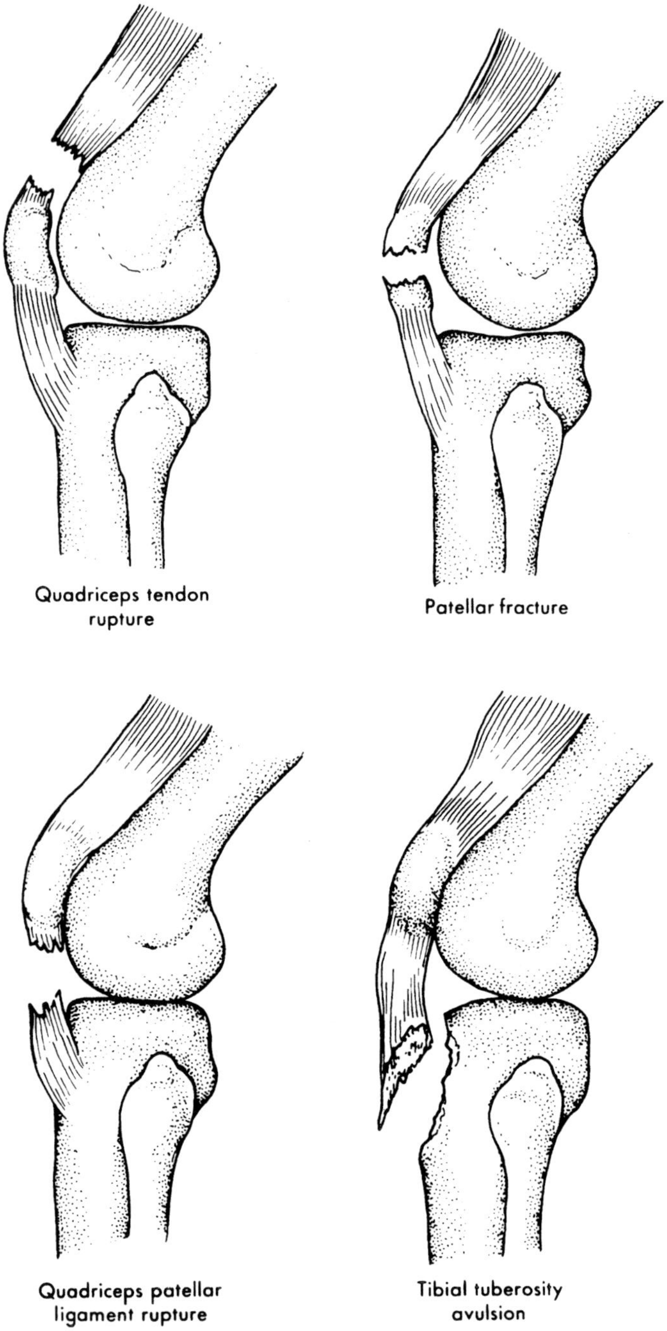

Quadriceps tendon
rupture

Patellar fracture

Quadriceps patellar
ligament rupture

Tibial tuberosity
avulsion

Fig. 26-15 Quadriceps apparatus may rupture in any one of four locations.

curate assessment. The anatomy of the knee joint is complex (Figs. 26-16 to 26-18), and any combination of ligamentous tears may be encountered.

A first-degree sprain of the medial collateral ligament is the most common knee sprain. This type of sprain is most likely because the outside of the knee is most exposed to contact forces that stress the medial joint line.

Test the leg using varus and valgus forces medially and laterally. If the knee opens up on lateral stress, the lateral collateral ligament is torn; if it opens medially with valgus stress, the medial collateral ligament is torn. While holding the foot, and with the knee in flexion, move the leg anteriorly and assess abnormal laxity. Abnormal excursion is referred to as a *positive drawer sign*. If present, the anterior cruciate ligament is torn.

Aspirate tense effusions to provide some diagnostic information and to provide comfort for the patient. If the effusion is bloody, there is likely to be a meniscal tear in addition to a ligamentous injury.

Third-degree sprains and anterior cruciate tears should be referred immediately to an orthopedic surgeon to be evaluated for surgery. Lesser sprains can be treated with ice, elevation, knee immobilization, non–weight bearing, antiinflammatory agents, analgesics, and a referral to the orthopedic surgeon.

If the mechanism of injury was trivial and the patient heard or felt a click or pop, the patient has probably sustained a meniscal tear. To test for this, extend the hip, partially flex the knee, and twist the knee by rotating the foot. Palpate over the medial joint line while *externally* rotating the foot to test the medial meniscus, and palpate over the lateral joint line while *internally* rotating the foot to test the lateral meniscus. If a grinding or internal popping sensation can be felt over the joint line and if the patient experiences pain, there is a probable tear of the meniscus. The presence of this finding is referred to as a positive *McMurry sign*. Because these injuries

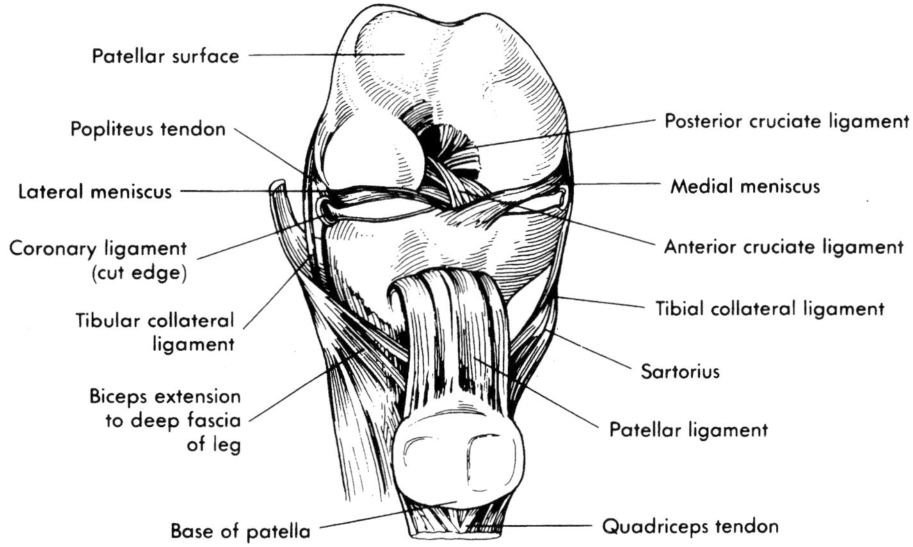

Fig. 26-16 Ligaments of the knee. (Redrawn from Anderson JE: *Grant's atlas of anatomy,* ed 8, Baltimore, 1983, Williams & Wilkins.)

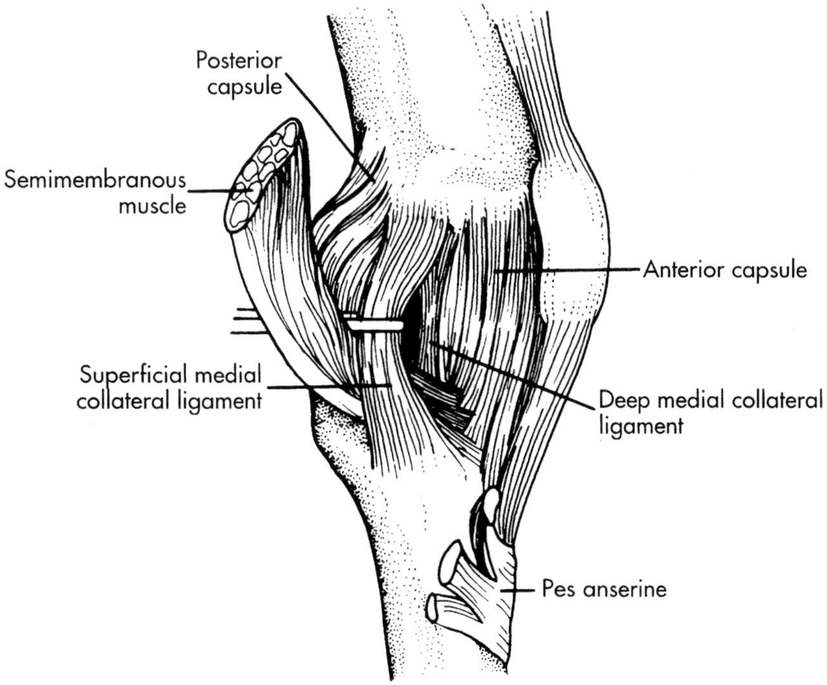

Fig. 26-17 Medial aspect of capsule of knee and its supporting ligaments. Note superficial and deep portions of medial collateral ligament. Semimembranous muscle interdigitates with capsule in its posterior and medial aspects.

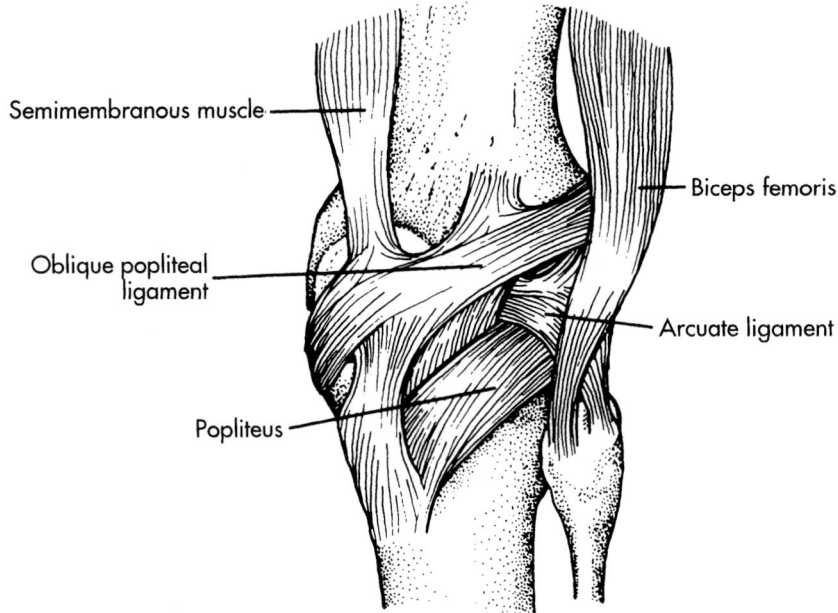

Fig. 26-18 Posterior aspect of knee. Multiple tendinous attachments of semimembranous muscle are shown. Note oblique popliteal ligament.

are usually not repaired acutely, the patient can be treated as previously described for sprains and referred to an orthopedic surgeon for a possible MRI or arthroscopy.

Knee dislocations are serious injuries sustained after major falls such as from bicycles, motorcycles, and water skiing. The injury usually involves all of the knee-establishing ligaments and may spontaneously reduce. As mentioned earlier in the chapter, the proximity of the popliteal vessels is the source of the most significant complication. The popliteal artery is injured in 30% to 40% of all knee dislocations, and usually in the anterior type. All of these injuries should be seen by a vascular surgeon as well as an orthopedic surgeon, even if the distal pulsations are adequate. An angiogram is necessary to rule out injury to the popliteal vessels in all anterior and posterior dislocations.

Leg Fractures

Tibial condyle and *tibial plateau fractures* are serious because they often extend into the knee joint. Fractures that extend into the joint produce a characteristic "fat-fluid level" on a cross-table lateral x-ray study of the knee. A fracture of the proximal third of the fibula has great potential for disturbing the trifurcation of the popliteal artery. Vascular repair is especially difficult in this location, so amputation is a common outcome when the arterial injury occurs. Angiography should be used aggressively.

The peroneal nerve may also be injured with fractures in this location. Tibial plateau fractures are usually the result of a varus or valgus stress. The combination of axial compression and an abduction force may cause major ligamentous damage or meniscal injury in addition to the fracture. Minimally displaced fractures without associated injuries may be treated conservatively. A residual step-off of greater than 5 mm in the weight-bearing area is universally associated with an unsatisfactory result. An early orthopedic consultation is advisable.

Proximal fibula fractures may be encountered after minor blows to the leg. This type of fracture is significant because of the proximity of the peroneal nerve and because of the potential for compartment compression. Assess the patient for foot drop, lateral leg weakness, and for signs of a compartment syndrome as evidenced by paresthesias, increasing pain, pain at rest, or pain on dorsiflexion of the toes. Arrange to measure the compartment pressures, if any of these are present. If the compartment pressures are elevated, the patient requires a fasciotomy.

Tibial shaft fractures occur from falls on ice, skiing, contact athletic sports, and automobile accidents. Because of the paucity of soft tissue surrounding the anterior tibia, open fractures are common. Open tibial shaft fractures should be splinted without reduction and treated with broad-spectrum antibiotics. Because the incidence of osteomyelitis is high with these open fractures, it is important to have the leg cleaned in the operating room as soon as possible. The patient often has other serious injuries when an automobile accident has caused the fracture, whereas the fracture is often an isolated injury if caused during sports or falls.

Closed shaft injuries are often treated with a long-leg cast. These fractures are especially slow healing when they are spiral or oblique and should be referred to an orthopedic surgeon.

Ankle

Fractures

The bones forming the ankle mortise are among the most commonly injured bones of the body, exceeded only by the distal radius. Most ankle injuries are produced by forces that are directed perpendicular to the normal motion of the joint. The only pure motion of the joint is plantar flexion and dorsiflexion. Several classifications of ankle fractures have been developed and take into account the presumed position of the ankle and foot at the time of injury and the direction of the force causing the fracture. In general, the following motions of the foot/ankle produce fractures that should be considered: inversion (adduction, supination), eversion (abduction, pronation), internal rotation, and external rotation. In addition, vertical compression may produce serious fractures. Routine x-ray views of the ankle should include AP, lateral, and mortise views. (The latter is an AP view with 20 degrees of internal rotation.) Although fractures are usually easily visualized, a search for abnormalities of the mortise must be performed. The clear zone around the talus should be uniform all the way around; ligamentous rupture may result in widening on the medial side.

The most common mechanism of injury involves inversion or supination of the foot with the ankle in some degree of plantar flexion. There is some inherent instability in this position because the talar dome is narrower posteriorly than it is anteriorly; therefore there is greater room for motion. The lateral malleolus is often fractured in this position. The typical x-ray appearance is that of an oblique fracture that begins at the joint line and extends upward. For this isolated injury, treatment involves a short-leg walking cast. When more force is applied (and if there is a lateral rotation force) the medial malleolus will fracture or the deltoid ligament will rupture in addition to the lateral malleolus fracture. Rupture of the deltoid ligament is signified by a widened mortise. Either of these medial injuries is considered equivalent, and both usually require surgery to stabilize.

With even more force, as the body carries the tibia forward and over the foot, the posterior margin of the tibia (posterior malleolus) also fractures. The combined injury is referred to as a *trimalleolar fracture* and often results in dislocation. If a dislocation is present and the skin is tented or there are signs of vascular compromise, the ankle should be reduced in the emergency department. A surgical consultation should be arranged. Even with aggressive and early therapy, the outcome of trimalleolar fractures is often poor.

At other times, the injury occurs with the foot in pronation (everted). In this instance the initial injury is either a rupture of the deltoid ligament or an avulsion fracture of the medial malleolus. With more force, the anterior inferior tibiofibular ligament ruptures, and then the fibula fractures. With severe torquing, the force sometimes is transmitted up the symdesmosis, which results in an accompanying *proximal* fibular fracture. This type of fracture is referred to as a Maissonneuve fracture. If an isolated medial malleolus fracture is seen on the x-ray film, always examine the proximal fibula for tenderness; obtain an x-ray study if tenderness is present.

Because the soft tissue coverage of the ankle is slim, open fracture dislocations are not uncommon. Immobilize and treat open fracture dislocations with broad-spectrum antibiotics and timely operative intervention. Because these injuries are often associated with injuries in other organ systems (especially when the mechanism is an automobile accident), the latter often takes precedence over early operative attention to the ankle.

Isolated ankle dislocations may occur. These types of dislocations are incapacitating injuries and often lead to permanent stiffness.

Sprains

Lateral sprains. The lateral aspect of the ankle is often injured in sports, dance, and everyday activities. Ankle injuries account for up to 10% of all emergency department visits, and 90% of the sprains in this location involve the lateral ligaments. Inversion of the foot is the basic motion that produces this injury. The ankle is usually plantar-flexed when the injury occurs, and there also may be external rotation of the leg relative to the ankle. The most commonly injured structure is the talofibular ligament. More serious injuries may also involve the calcaneofibular ligament and the posterior talofibular ligament.

With a lateral ankle injury, the patient experiences swelling and tenderness over the lateral malleolus in varying degrees depending on the force of injury; ecchymosis and an inability to bear weight are variable signs. Recurrent sprains are common. The severity of the injury and the need for thorough treatment is often underestimated, as is the length of time required to convalesce after a second-degree sprain.

An elastic (Ace) wrap is inadequate for more serious sprains. Emergency physicians should be aggressive in the use of plaster splints to immobilize these injuries. Even first-degree sprains can be incapacitating, and the patient is more prone to attempt ambulation too soon if the ankle is not splinted appropriately.

Immobilization in a gelocast or with an elastic anklet is effective for *first-degree sprains.* A combination of protected weight bearing until the discomfort is relieved, with ice packs applied for 15 minutes at a time 4 times/day, and antiinflammatory agents should lead to recovery in 3 to 7 days.

Second-degree sprains are the most underestimated of the sprain injuries. A significant degree of ligament disruption occurs, but the ligament and the ankle mortise are preserved, and the swelling is confined. The ankle is weakened because the ligaments are torn and because the lateral side of the ankle is naturally the weakest point. There is also a proprioceptive defect that is believed to predispose the patient to recurrences because of abnormal foot planting during exercise. The recovery period should not be rushed. The patient should expect to have a prolonged and possibly a future disability.

The severely sprained ankle should be completely immobilized. If the patient is seen early after injury, a plaster figure-of-eight or posterior splint is preferable. In addition, it is important for the patient to apply ice and elevate the ankle for the first 48 hours. If the edema has subsided, immobilize the ankle with a short-leg walking cast for 3 to 6 weeks. After removing the cast, have the patient wear a metal strutted ankle brace for another 2 to 4 weeks. Thereafter, the patient should support the ankle with an elastic anklet or tape whenever exercising and should be advised to wear high- or three-quarter–top sneakers for any sport that requires sudden turns. Crutch support is essential with the initial splint, but a walking heel can be used when the short-leg cast is applied.

Third-degree tears cause the ankle instability. The ankle may not be as swollen as with a second-degree tear because the bleeding is not confined in the ankle. The mortise may be widened on x-ray study, and the joint opens to stress testing. The decision to repair the ankle surgically or treat it as with the second-degree tear can be left to the orthopedic surgeon.

Second- and third-degree sprains have the potential for accompanying injuries. Always palpate the proximal fibula. Request an x-ray study if there is tenderness over this bone, because fracture of this bone is significant for neurologic impairment or compartment syndrome.

Medial sprains. The *medial deltoid ligaments* of the ankle are much stronger than the lateral ligaments and are less commonly injured. Deltoid ligament injuries account for approximately 10% of all ankle injuries. Significant injuries to this ligament result in widening of the ankle mortise on the medial side when a proper mortise-view x-ray study is obtained. When the ankle is subjected to an eversion stress, the ankle is often fractured because the deltoid ligament avulses the medial malleolus instead of tearing. The ankle often dislocates laterally, and the lateral malleolus is fractured.

Foot

Fractures of any of the bones of the foot can be encountered. Clinical symptoms should be correlated with x-ray study appearance. If there is any doubt, treat the patient as if the fracture is present (Figs. 26-19 to 26-21). Treatment usually involves a posterior splint and no weight bearing. Fractures that include dislocations should be managed by an orthopedic surgeon.

Calcaneal (os calcis) fractures are usually produced by falling or jumping from a significant height. Although they are usually not subtle, os calcis fractures are often associated with occult lumbar fractures. If the patient is conscious and not intoxicated, he or she can often report pain in the areas of involvement. However, if distracted by pain from other injuries or by drugs or alcohol, the patient may not be aware of the spinal injuries. Spinal injuries should be sought on a routine basis. Calcaneal fractures may also be associated with hip fractures and knee injuries.

If a calcaneal fracture is suspected, be sure to order AP, lateral, and axial (os calcis) views. Open reduction is recommended if the lateral view reveals significant loss of the Bohler angle (Fig. 26-22). Unfortunately, if there is significant comminution or compression, there is a high incidence of poor outcome regardless of the treatment.

The *Lisfranc fracture dislocation* refers to a dislocation or fracture dislocation at the tarsometatarsal (Lisfranc) joint. This joint is named for one of Napoleon's field surgeons, who described a midfoot amputation at this level. The mechanism of injury may be a direct blow such as from a horse stepping on the foot, or from an indirect injury, which commonly occurs when the plantar flexed foot is braced against the floorboard in a traffic accident. X-ray studies of this region may be difficult to interpret, and the injury is initially missed in 20% of all cases. Suspect this type of injury in patients who have significant pain and an appropriate mechanism of injury. The major complication of this injury is circulatory compromise. Immediate orthopedic consultation should be arranged.

Fractures of the *metatarsal shafts* commonly occur from direct blows; they are also a common site of stress fracture (a "march fracture"). Because stress fractures are often invisible or missed on an x-ray study, it is important to respect the patient's clinical complaints. A follow up x-ray study in 2 to 4 weeks reveals callus formation. If there is no distraction or midfoot dislocation, treat the fracture with a posterior splint and refer the patient to an orthopedic surgeon for follow-up. With distraction or dislocation, the patient needs to be seen immediately by an orthopedic surgeon.

A fracture of the *base of the fifth metatarsal*

is among the most common type of foot fracture. The usual mechanism of injury is an inversion stress on the forefoot, such as when stepping off a curb. This stress produces an avulsion fracture where the peroneus brevis tendon attaches to the base of the fifth metatarsal. The patient has tenderness, swelling, and often bruising over the injury, and x-ray studies reveal a characteristic transverse fracture. A longitudinal lucent line in this region represents an ununited apophysis rather than a fracture. The goal of treatment is to maintain

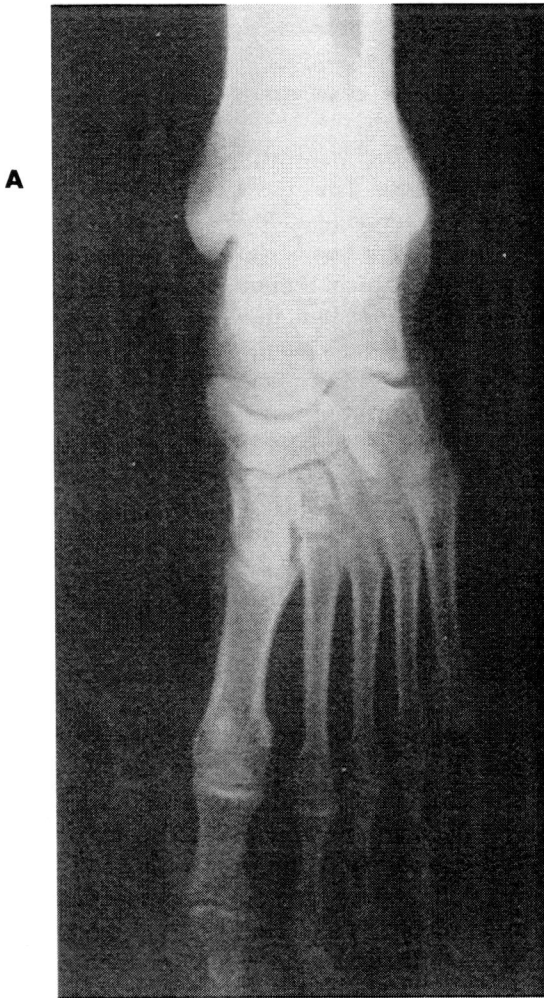

Fig. 26-19 **A,** Standard anteroposterior view of foot. **B,** Anatomic points of interest. (From Mann RA: *Surgery of the foot,* ed 5, St Louis, 1985, Mosby.)

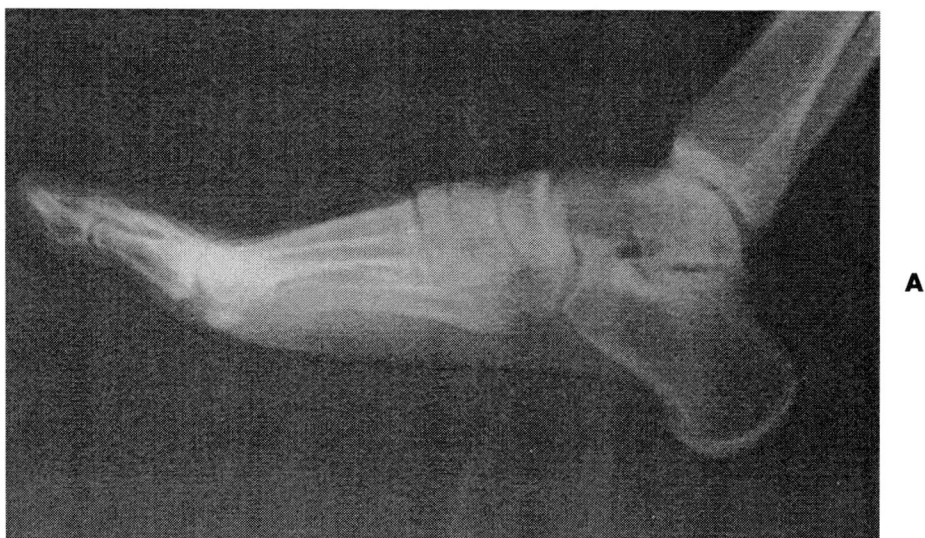

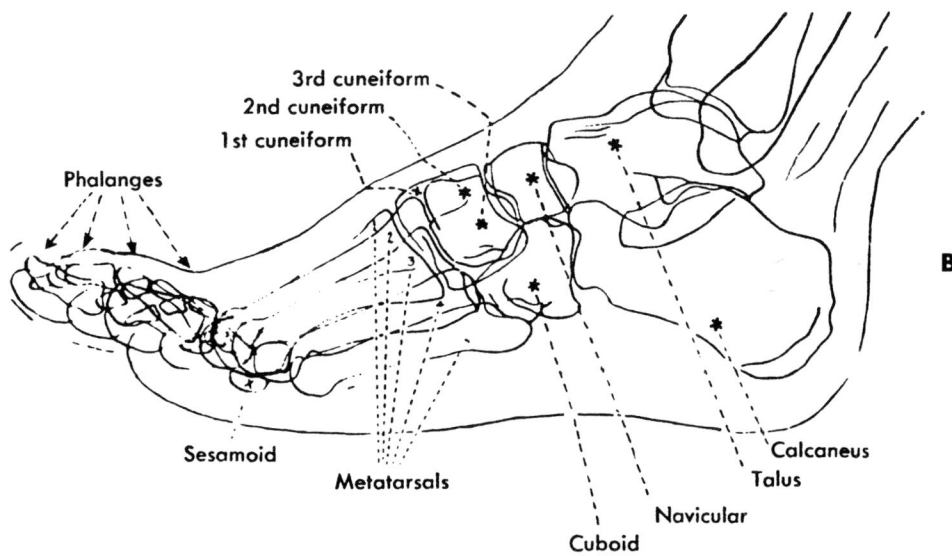

Fig. *26-20* **A,** Standard lateral view of foot. **B,** Anatomic points of interest. (From Mann RA: *Surgery of the foot,* ed 5, St Louis, 1985, Mosby.)

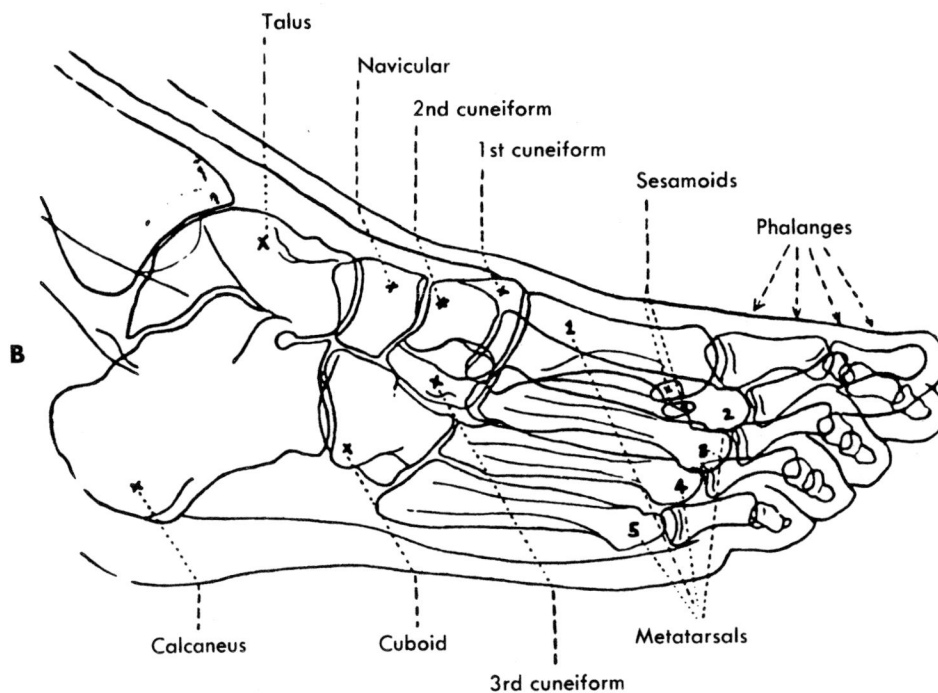

Fig. 26-21 **A,** Standard oblique view of foot. **B,** Anatomic points of interest. (From Mann RA: *Surgery of the foot,* ed 5, St Louis, 1985, Mosby.)

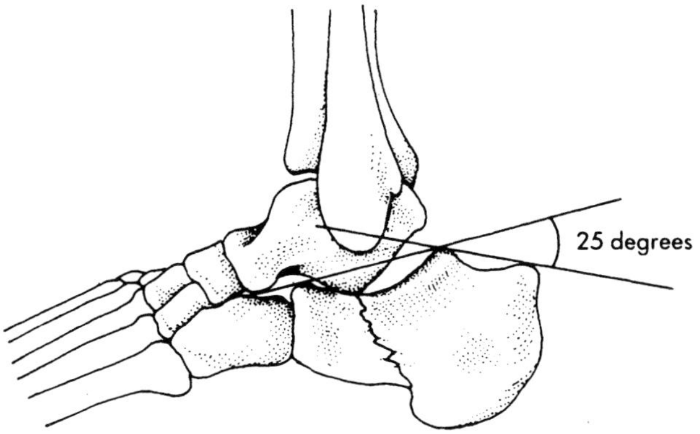

Fig. *26-22*   Bohler angle. (From Mayeda DV: Ankle and foot. In Rosen P et al, editors: *Emergency medicine: concepts and clinical practice,* ed 3, St Louis, 1992, Mosby.)

enough immobilization to provide comfort for 4 to 6 weeks as the fracture heals. Unna paste boots are often used for immobilization; casts are rarely necessary.

Avulsion fractures of the tuberosity must be distinguished from the more serious Jones fracture, which is a transverse fracture of the metatarsal shaft that occurs distal to the insertion of the peroneus brevis. This type of injury tends to occur in young athletes engaged in running and jumping sports. These fractures have a high incidence of delayed union or nonunion. Immobilization in a short leg cast is mandatory for at least 6 weeks.

Digit fractures are often caused by "stubbing" the toe on an immovable object. Unless open, the fracture is usually best treated by splinting or "buddy taping" the affected toe to an adjacent toe. If the fracture is markedly displaced, reduction is usually easily accomplished after digital block anesthesia. Fixation with a Kirschner wire may be required if the fracture involves greater than 25% of the articular surface of the hallux. If the fracture is open, treat it as other open fractures and consult a podiatric surgeon.

KEY CONSIDERATIONS

WHAT IS THE LIFE THREAT?

Few isolated orthopedic injuries are life threatening, but some can be limb threatening. An exception is inward dislocation of the claviculosternal joint, in which inward displacement of the clavicular head can compress the trachea and cause airway compromise.

Fractures and dislocations associated with laceration, thrombosis, or mechanical pressure on the artery that supplies the distal limb pose a threat to the survival of the limb.

DOES THE PATIENT NEED ADMISSION?

Patients with unstable pelvic fractures and, in most cases, vertebral fractures require admission. Patients whose fractures or lacerations are serious enough to require initial management in the operating room are usually admitted.

WHAT IS THE MOST SERIOUS DIAGNOSIS?

Compromised airway or ventilation from a bony injury, such as flail chest, constitutes a serious injury.

Vascular compromise that causes ischemia distal to the injury is limb threatening.

HAVE I PERFORMED A THOROUGH WORK-UP?

Evaluate distal neurologic and vascular function in soft tissue injuries and fractures; repeat the evaluation following reductions.

Check the patient's ability to ambulate safely before discharge from the emergency department.

Consider epiphyseal injuries (Salter-Harris classification I) in children with joint injury, joint tenderness, and a negative x-ray study.

In cases of rib fracture, evaluate the patient for underlying lung, liver, or spleen injury; evaluate for injury to pelvic blood vessels, the urinary system, the uterus, and the ovaries in cases of pelvic fracture.

Consider the possibility of a slipped capital femoral epiphysis in an adolescent who has a limp.

Recommended Reading

Campana BA: Cervical hyperextension injuries and low back pain. In Rosen P et al, editors: *Emergency medicine: concepts and clinical practice,* ed 3, St Louis, 1992, Mosby.

Cwinn AA: Pelvis and hip. In Rosen P et al, editors: *Emergency medicine: concepts and clinical practice,* ed 3, St Louis, 1992, Mosby.

Geiderman J: Orthopedic injuries. In Rosen P et al, editors: *Emergency medicine: concepts and clinical practice,* ed 3, St Louis, 1992, Mosby.

Gruber JE: Proximal femur and femoral shaft. In Rosen P et al, editors: *Emergency medicine: concepts and clinical practice,* ed 3, St Louis, 1992, Mosby.

Mayeda DV: Management principles. In Barkin RM, Rosen P, editors: *Emergency pediatrics,* ed 3, St Louis, 1990, Mosby.

Mayeda DV: Ankle and foot. In Rosen P et al, editors: *Emergency medicine: concepts and clinical practice,* ed 3, St Louis, 1992, Mosby.

Mayeda DV: Knee and lower leg. In Rosen P et al, editors: *Emergency medicine: concepts and clinical practice,* ed 3, St Louis, 1992, Mosby.

Orban DJ: Forearm and wrist. In Rosen P et al, editors: *Emergency medicine: concepts and clinical practice,* ed 3, St Louis, 1992, Mosby.

Orban DJ: Hand. In Rosen P et al, editors: *Emergency medicine: concepts and clinical practice,* ed 3, St Louis, 1992, Mosby.

Orban DJ: Humerus and elbow. In Rosen P et al, editors: *Emergency medicine: concepts and clinical practice,* ed 3, St Louis, 1992, Mosby.

Orban DJ: Shoulder. In Rosen P et al, editors: *Emergency medicine: concepts and clinical practice,* ed 3, St Louis, 1992, Mosby.

Rockwood CA, Jr, Green DP, Bucholz RW, editors: *Fractures,* ed 3, New York, 1991, JB Lippincott.

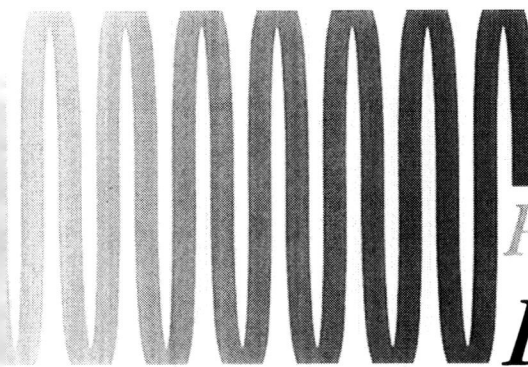

Part IV

ENVIRONMENTAL EMERGENCIES

Chapter Twenty-seven
THERMAL AND CHEMICAL INJURIES

RICHARD N. NELSON

GENERAL CONSIDERATIONS

Few injuries cause as much fear and even panic in patients and the medical team as do hot thermal injuries (burns). Even superficial burns can be a source of marked discomfort, incapacitation, and often visible cosmetic deformities that may not be surgically correctable. The long-term sequelae can be a continuous problem, and the patient with a serious deep burn has much to endure before being able to return to a functional existence. Severe burns, especially in the elderly, are among the rare injuries that can cause inevitable death and in which the patient should participate in the choice for comfort care only.

An estimated 2 million people are burned annually in the United States; 100,000 of those people require hospitalization. As many as 20,000 people die from the burn itself or die later from complications. Serious burns are particularly common in childhood and are the second leading cause of death in the 0 to 12-year age group. This chapter focuses on the emergency management of thermal burns, chemical burns, and smoke inhalation.

PATHOPHYSIOLOGY

The skin is the largest organ of the body and accounts for 15% of body weight. The skin functions as the body's chief barrier to infection and water loss and also regulates body temperature. All of these functions are potentially compromised when the skin is burned. In the early postburn period, fluid losses are substantial and can lead to hypovolemic shock. In addition, evaporative heat losses may result in hypothermia. Later in the course of the severe burn, sepsis and pulmonary injury are the most likely complications that can cause death.

Burns are classified as first, second, third, or fourth degree on the basis of depth of involvement to skin and subcutaneous structures. First-degree burns involve only the epidermis and do not cause tissue death. The skin surface is red and painful, but blistering does not occur and sensation is intact. A minor sunburn is an example of a first-degree burn.

Second-degree, or partial-thickness, burns are more serious because both the epidermis and deeper dermal structures are involved. Tissue death and permanent scarring can occur. Super-

333

ficial second-degree burns are red and painful, and blistering is almost always present. Sensation is preserved but may appear decreased as a result of edema and separation of the epidermis by the blister. Deep second-degree burns appear waxy and mottled and are nearly insensate. Portions of the dermis remain viable and may give rise to new skin if treated properly. Deep second-degree burns are often indistinguishable from third-degree burns in the initial postburn period, but management is virtually the same.

Third-degree, or full-thickness, burns result in the death of all skin layers, including sweat glands, hair follicles, and nerve endings. The skin appears waxy, leathery, and lifeless. Capillary refill is absent, and thrombosed skin veins may be visible. These burns are painless, and the skin is insensitive to touch. Charring may be present if there was exposure to flame.

Fourth-degree burns involve not only the epidermis and dermis but also subcutaneous tissue, muscle, and sometimes even bone. Charring is usually present.

Burn depth should always be determined in context with the mechanism of injury. For example, burns caused by flames or by direct contact with molten liquids such as grease, metals, or certain chemicals are more likely to produce full-thickness burns than are scald burns or exposures to a brief flash of flame. Electrical burns are also often deceptive because initially they may appear small and superficial but over time develop into a fourth-degree burn because of the vascular injury that often accompanies them.

MANAGEMENT OF THE BURN VICTIM

Airway

Patients exposed to large amounts of smoke and heat, particularly in an enclosed space, are likely to have an associated inhalation injury. Facial burns, singed nasal hairs, wheezing, respiratory distress, hoarseness, stridor, pharyngeal edema, and a cough that produces carbonaceous sputum should alert the physician to the need for early endotracheal intubation and ventilatory management.

Breathing

Administer 100% humidified oxygen to all patients who have significant burns or an inhalation injury. Frequent suctioning may be necessary with an inhalation injury. Third-degree burns around the chest and trunk may restrict ventilation and require an early escharotomy (see p. 336).

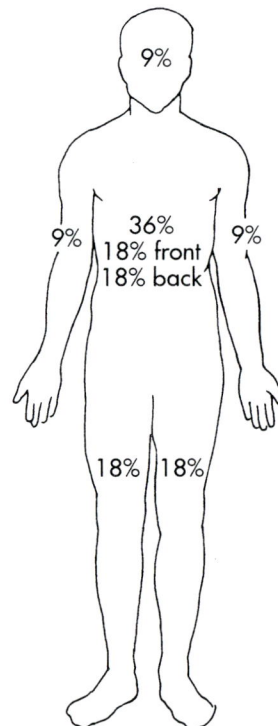

Fig. **27-1** Percentages used in determining extent of burn by "Rule of Nines." (From Miller RH: *Textbook of basic emergency medicine,* ed 2, St Louis, 1980, Mosby.)

Circulation

Aggressive fluid management in burn patients is essential to prevent or minimize renal failure. The fluid requirements of burn victims are often underestimated. Although it is well recognized that fluid loss is an early cause of death, there is still a tendency to be too slow in commencing fluid resuscitation. Once behind in fluid requirements, it is difficult to catch up.

Initial fluid requirements are based on the amount of body surface area burned. The amount of surface involved can be quickly estimated from two charts (Figs. 27-1 and 27-2). Although the "Rule of Nines" (i.e., dividing the body into regions equivalent to 9%) works reasonably well in the adult, children generally have larger head surfaces and smaller leg surfaces, especially during the first 2 years. For smaller burns, an area equal to the size of the patient's

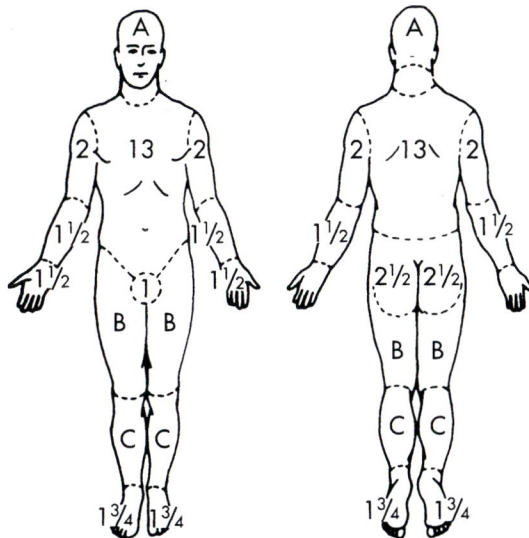

Relative percentages of areas affected by growth
(age in years)

	0	1	5	10	15	Adult
A: half of head	9½	8½	6½	5½	4½	3½
B: half of thigh	2¾	3¼	4	4¼	4½	4¾
C: half of leg	2½	2½	2¾	3	3¼	3½

Second degree _____ and Third degree _____ =
Total percent burned _____

Fig. 27-2 Classic Lund and Browder chart. The best method for determining percentage of body surface burn is to mark areas of injury on a chart and compute total percentage according to patient's age. (From Artz CP, Yarbrough DR III: Burns: including cold, chemical, and electrical injuries. In Sabiston DC, Jr., editor: *Textbook of surgery: the biological basis of modern surgical practice*, ed 11, Philadelphia, 1977, WB Saunders.)

palm is equivalent to a 1% body surface area.

Patients with second-degree or more severe burns that involve greater than 15% body surface area require intravenous fluid therapy. The most commonly recommended protocol for fluid resuscitation of the burn patient is the Parkland formula. Lactated Ringer's solution is infused at 4 ml/kg × percentage of body surface area burned. Half is given in the first 8 hours, and the other half is given in the next 16 hours. Patients with an inhalation injury or electrical burns may require more fluids.

Intravenous access in nonburn areas is often difficult in the burn patient. Do not hesitate to place a line through burned tissue. Because in deep burns the superficial veins may be destroyed or thrombosed, the only access may be via cutdown or central line placement. Intraosseous infusion may be necessary in children younger than 6 years old.

GENERAL MEASURES

Patients with severe burns should be approached with the utmost care to avoid further wound contamination. Emergency department personnel should wear surgical caps, gowns, masks, and gloves. Strict sterile technique when performing procedures is essential.

Remove the patient's clothing, and examine the patient carefully to determine the extent of burns and the presence of associated injuries. Remove all rings and other jewelry in anticipation of swelling. Apply cool, sterile saline compresses to relieve pain, but do not cover more than 10% of the body surface with cool compresses to avoid hypothermia. Never apply ice directly to a burned area. If chemical contamination is present, irrigate the involved areas with copious amounts of water.

Body heat is easily lost through burned skin, which not only increases the patient's metabolic demands but may also lead to hypothermia and subsequent cardiac dysrhythmias and refractory resuscitation. Use warmed intravenous fluids whenever possible, and keep the patient covered with sterile sheets and blankets as much as possible. The resuscitation room should be sufficiently warm, with heating lamps readily available.

Because the patient with a bad burn is often frightened and in pain, a combination of sedatives and analgesics is often necessary. Narcotics and benzodiazepines should be given intravenously to avoid the erratic absorption that occurs with intramuscular or subcutaneous administration. Give these drugs cautiously in patients who are not fully fluid resuscitated.

To counteract ileus and gastric distension, all patients with severe burns should have a nasogastric tube inserted and connected to low suction. An indwelling Foley catheter is also essential to monitor urine output. A urine output under 50 ml/hr in the adult or 1 ml/kg/hr in the child indicates the need for more aggressive fluid resuscitation. The presence of pink or red urine should alert the physician to possible hemolysis or myoglobinuria.

In patients with severe burns, central venous pressure monitoring, a Swan-Ganz catheter, and arterial lines are essential to accurately monitor hemodynamic parameters. These procedures should be performed in the emergency department if admission or transfer delays are encountered.

Circumferential full-thickness burns of the extremities or trunk may result in circulatory or mechanical compromise when edema builds up under the eschar. Such compromise is manifested by absent pulses in the involved extremities or, in the presence of deep burns to the chest, difficulty ventilating the lungs. An escharotomy should be performed when such compromise occurs. An escharotomy is done on an extremity by making bilateral incisions as if bivalving a cast. Escharotomies of the chest wall are made at the anterior axillary lines from the second to the twelfth ribs; the superior and inferior aspects of these incisions are connected with anterior incisions. The incisions are made through the eschar down to subcutaneous fat. A local anesthetic is not necessary because these full-thickness burns are insensate.

All burn patients should receive tetanus prophylaxis as needed, but prophylactic antibiotics are not indicated. Antacids and intravenous H_2 blockers are indicated to prevent burn-induced duodenal ulcerations (Curling ulcers) and may be initiated in the emergency department.

[handwritten margin note: Curling ulcers → late complication]

LABORATORY AND X-RAY STUDIES

Baseline laboratory studies should include arterial blood gas with carboxyhemoglobin levels, a complete blood count, coagulation studies, electrolytes, blood urea nitrogen, creatinine, and glucose. A type and crossmatch may be useful, but blood products are generally not needed during the first 24 hours. Urine should be checked for the presence of free hemoglobin (hemolysis) or myoglobin. Blood alcohol and toxicologic screens are obtained as indicated.

Obtain a chest x-ray study on all patients with severe burns to assess for infiltrates that are indicative of an inhalation injury or acute respiratory distress syndrome and to check for placement of the endotracheal tube.

OUTPATIENT MANAGEMENT OF THE BURN PATIENT

Most burns seen in the emergency department can be managed safely on an outpatient basis. Principles of care include cleaning the wound, debridement, correctly appreciating the depth of the burn, preventing infection, and achieving epithelialization.

Use a mild antiseptic soap or detergent to gently cleanse the wound after the initial pain has decreased. Repeated applications of cool, saline-soaked dressings are also useful. Small, intact burn blisters can be left in place, but remove and debride larger and ruptured blisters, particularly if present over joints.

Dress partial wounds with a layer of Adaptic or other nonadherent gauze; follow this layer with a layer of sterile absorbent gauze to produce a wick effect for weeping tissue. Finally, cover the wound with Kling or Kerlex to provide some protective bulk. Because the maximum amount of wound seepage occurs within the first 24 hours and because early wound infection needs to be aggressively treated, inspect the wounds and change the dressings the next day. If the wound is clean and does not show signs of infection, redress it in the same fashion as before. This dressing can be left in place for 2 to 4 days, depending on the preference of the emergency physician and the ability of the patient to keep the dressing clean.

After 5 to 7 days, the wound can be left open and allowed to scab. It must be kept clean and protected from extremes of temperature. The wound should epithelialize in approximately 3 weeks; however, epithelialization may not occur for 2 to 3 months if the wound is a deep second-degree burn in which the only skin remnants are the hair follicles or sweat glands.

Any partial-thickness burn will convert to a full-thickness burn if it becomes infected, especially with *Streptococcus* organisms. If the burn appears to be becoming infected, the patient must be admitted, treated with intravenous antibiotics, and given the topical wound care of a full-thickness burn.

Many dressings have been found to be effective, but those previously described are universally available, easy to apply, and inexpensive. Xenografts (pigskin) work well but are not readily available and are expensive. They are most useful for the immunocompromised patient because they minimize the risk of infection. Some of the new agents such as Biobrane also work very well but are expensive. These agents should be reserved for special situations.

Many physicians prefer to use topical antibiotic creams and ointments, including silver sulfadiazine, mafenide acetate, and silver nitrate solution. Silver sulfadiazine (Silvadene) is the most commonly used agent. Apply it in a thin layer with a tongue blade, and cover it with absorbent gauze. Silvadene dressings should be changed every 12 hours. The wound is cleansed with mild antiseptic soap and water before reapplying a new dressing.

Some burns require no dressings at all. First-degree burns should be left open to air. Second-degree burns of the face (e.g., flash burns from lightning, a furnace pilot, or a gas grill) may be treated with Bacitracin or Neosporin ointment applied directly to the burn with no overlying dressing.

ADMISSION TO BURN UNIT

Since the advent of specialized care units for burns, the mortality rate for severely burned patients has decreased dramatically. Decisions on whether to transfer a patient to a burn unit are based on several factors, including depth and location of burns, percentage of body surface area involved, age of the patient, type of burn, and associated medical or sociologic conditions (see the box at right).

All patients who are being transferred to burn units should be adequately stabilized before transport to prevent further deterioration enroute. If endotracheal intubation is indicated, it should be performed before the transfer. Fluid resuscitation should be well underway before the transfer. Do not waste time applying antibiotic dressings because they are removed immediately after arrival at the burn center; a sterile burn sheet is sufficient. Administer oxygen to all patients during transfer. Do not forget to send all laboratory results, x-ray films, treatment records, and historical data.

CHEMICAL BURNS

Few burns instill more fear in both patients and health care workers than those caused by chem-

---

CRITERIA FOR BURN CENTER ADMISSION*

1. Second- and third-degree burns greater than 10% total body surface area (TBSA) in patients less than 10 or more than 50 years of age
2. Second- and third-degree burns greater than 15% TBSA for other age groups
3. Second- and third-degree burns of the face, hands, feet, genitals, perineum, and major joints
4. Third-degree burns greater than 5% TBSA in any age group
5. Electrical burns
6. Chemical burns
7. Burns with an associated inhalation injury
8. Burns in patients with underlying medical disorders such as diabetes, peripheral vascular disease, immunosuppression, or cardiovascular disorders
9. Burns in patients with sociologic problems that may prevent adequate outpatient burn care or predispose them to further injury (e.g., substance abuse, suspected child abuse, mental incompetence, elderly abuse)

*These are recommendations only; local policies and protocols should take precedence.

---

icals. Care should be taken to ensure that not only does the patient receive proper care but also that health care workers, other patients, and health care facilities are protected.

Before arriving at the emergency department, most patients exposed to hazardous chemicals will have been decontaminated by local hazardous materials (HAZMAT) teams. Any patient who arrives without prior decontamination should be decontaminated during initial treatment. Ideally, such patients should be isolated from other patients in a decontamination station, which should be well ventilated and have available large volumes of water for irrigation. All water used for irrigation should be collected in plastic containers for later disposal. Medical personnel should wear protective gowns, masks, gloves, and eye protection. All emergency departments should have written protocols and practice drills to prepare for chemically contaminated patients.

Most chemical burns are treated with copious water irrigation to both dilute and remove the offending chemical. Exceptions are elemental sodium, potassium, and lithium, which react with water; and phenols, which should be irrigated only if large amounts of water are immediately available.

Acids and Alkalis

Acids and alkalis cause coagulation necrosis that will progress to full thickness depending on the concentration of the chemical. Alkalis generally penetrate more rapidly and thus cause damage more quickly. All such burns must be irrigated with copious amounts of water, sometimes for hours, particularly if sensitive areas such as the corneas are involved.

Hydrofluoric Acid

Hydrofluoric acid is a powerful acid that rapidly penetrates the skin and deeper to cause local and systemic toxicity. Pain is generally out of proportion to physical findings. Treatment should start with copious water irrigation for 15 to 30 minutes. If continued pain or an obvious burn is present, calcium gluconate therapy is indicated. This chemical binds with the fluoride ion and thus reduces its toxicity. Calcium gluconate may be applied topically as a dressing soaked with a 10% solution. Alternatively, 3.5 g of calcium gluconate may be mixed with 150 ml K-Y jelly to form a gel that is applied to the burn. For severe burns or continued pain, administer 10% calcium gluconate subcutaneously and slowly through a 27- to 30-gauge needle. Inject a maximum of 0.5 ml per cm^2 of burn to 0.5 cm beyond the margin of burned skin.

Phenol

Phenol (carbolic acid) and its derivatives, the cresols, are used as disinfectants, sanitizers, and deodorizers. Direct contact with skin causes severe coagulation necrosis with dense eschar that may trap the chemical underneath the skin. Systemic absorption causes CNS depression. The skin must be irrigated with water immediately and in copious amounts because dilute phenol penetrates skin more rapidly than concentrated phenol. The treatment of choice is a 5- to 10-minute application of a 2:1 solution of polyethylene glycol and methylated spirits. Alternative solutions are glycerol or isopropyl alcohol.

Lime

Lime (calcium oxide) is found in concrete mix. Lime reacts with moisture to form calcium hydroxide, which is an extremely caustic agent. Burns are often seen in construction workers who get lime on their boots or gloves. Treatment consists of copious water irrigation that is followed by burn care. Avoid using small amounts of water, because small amounts can increase the exothermic reaction. Always brush away any lime from the skin before irrigating it.

Phosphorous

Phosphorous is used in fertilizers, insecticides, rodenticides, and military munitions. Phosphorous causes thermal and chemical burns when exposed to air. Treatment consists of the immediate removal of visible particles and contaminated clothing. Irrigate burns with copious amounts of water or submerse them in water to prevent exposure to air. A brief (less than 30 minutes) rinse with 1% copper sulfate solution turns phosphorous particles black for easy identification and removal. After the copper sulfate rinse, irrigate the wound again to prevent systemic copper absorption.

Elemental Metals

Sodium, potassium, and lithium in elemental form produce an intense exothermic reaction when exposed to water. Therefore water irrigation is contraindicated in these exposures. Douse existing flames with sand or a class D fire extinguisher. Cover or immerse the burned area with mineral oil or cooking oil, and remove the metal fragments immediately.

SMOKE INHALATION

Respiratory complications are currently the leading cause of death among burn patients. These complications result from direct thermal injury to the upper airways and lungs, hypoxemia, chemical exposures (primarily carbon monoxide and cyanide), pulmonary edema and, later, pneumonia and sepsis.

Suspect an inhalation injury in any patient who was burned in a closed space. Other clues to a possible inhalation injury are hoarseness, stridor, sooty sputum, facial or pharyngeal burns, and burned nasal hairs.

Management

Airway and oxygen are the critical interventions in a patient with an inhalation injury. An unconscious patient or one with an altered mental status probably has hypoxemia and should be intubated early. Likewise, a patient who has other signs of inhalation injury as described above is at risk of losing the airway to edema and should also be intubated. Use a large-bore (#8) endotracheal tube for adults because these patients often require later bronchoscopy. Administer 100% humidified oxygen to a patient with an inhalation injury. Wheezing is a common finding and often responds to inhaled bronchodilators. Besides 100% humidified oxygen, all such patients should be placed on cardiac monitoring and continuous pulse oximetry. Maintain intravenous fluids at a rate sufficient to replace and keep up with fluid losses from burns; however, avoid overhydration because it may cause pulmonary edema.

Obtain arterial blood gas, carboxyhemoglobin level, and a chest x-ray film early in the treatment. Metabolic acidosis as a result of a combination of tissue hypoxemia and hypovolemia is a common finding. The chest x-ray study is often normal initially but later may show diffuse infiltrates consistent with noncardiogenic pulmonary edema.

High levels of carbon monoxide are extremely common in patients with smoke inhalation. Carbon monoxide toxicity is treated with 100% oxygen via an endotracheal tube or a nonrebreather mask. Patients with high blood levels of carbon monoxide (>25%) or those with findings consistent with carbon monoxide toxicity regardless of blood levels (e.g., loss of consciousness, altered mental status, ischemic chest pains, or ECG abnormalities) are candidates for hyperbaric oxygen therapy (see Chapter 65). Hyperbaric oxygen rapidly reduces the blood and tissue levels of carbon monoxide and dramatically improves signs and symptoms of toxicity. Consider transferring patients with high levels of carbon monoxide to a hospital that is equipped with a hyperbaric unit.

Another common type of poisoning associated with smoke inhalation is cyanide poisoning. This type of poisoning is particularly common with smoke produced from burning plastics and other synthetic materials such as furniture components. House trailer fires also produce large amounts of cyanide gas. Because cyanide levels are not readily available, many poison experts recommend empirically treating patients who have severe smoke inhalation and suspected cyanide exposure with a cyanide antidote. Use 25% sodium thiosulfate, which is found in the Lilly Cyanide Antidote kit; the dose is 50 ml for adults and 1.65 ml/kg for children. Do not use the sodium nitrite and amyl nitrite also found in the kit because these chemicals may worsen the tissue hypoxemia resulting from the carbon monoxide.

KEY CONSIDERATIONS

WHAT IS THE LIFE THREAT?

The mortality rate associated with thermal burns increases with the patient's age, severity of the burn, and the extent of the body surface involved. An immediate life threat is also posed by airway compromise and inhalation of carbon monoxide and other toxins. Third-degree burns around the thorax can restrict ventilation, and an early cause of death in the burned victim is from fluid loss with inadequate fluid replacement.

DOES THE PATIENT NEED ADMISSION?

Follow the recommendations in this chapter for guidelines about admitting patients to a burn unit. In general, admit patients with burns involving greater than 25% of total body surface area in adults, 10% in infants, and 20% in children up to age 10. Admit any patient with third-degree burns involving more than 5% body surface area. Admit patients with severe burns that involve the hands, feet, perineum, or face.

WHAT IS THE MOST SERIOUS DIAGNOSIS?

Airway compromise and fluid loss are the most serious diagnoses.

HAVE I PERFORMED A THOROUGH WORK-UP?

Estimate the total body surface area involved according to the "Rule of Nines" or a similar method. Determine the depth of burns according to appearance and sensation.

Evaluate the patient for evidence of thermal injury to the airway, for circumferential burns of the thorax that may restrict breathing, or for circumferential burns of the extremities that may impair circulation.

Estimate fluid loss and replace intravenous fluids according to the Parkland formula.

Remove chemicals that burn the skin on contact according to the recommendations in this chapter and those provided by the regional poison center.

Recommended Reading

Braen GR: Chemical injuries. In Rosen P et al, editors: *Emergency medicine: concepts and clinical practice,* ed 3, St Louis, 1993, Mosby.

Dimick AR: Burns and electrical injuries. In Tintinalli J, editor: *Emergency medicine: a comprehensive study guide,* ed 3, New York, 1992, McGraw-Hill.

Griglak MJ: Thermal injury, *Emerg Med Clin N Am* 10(2):369-383, 1992.

Martin ML, Harchelroad FP: Chemical burns. In Tintinalli J, editor: *Emergency medicine: a comprehensive study guide,* ed 3, New York, 1992, McGraw-Hill.

Ulin LS: Hazardous material accidents and toxic exposures. In Nelson R, editor: *Environmental emergencies,* Philadelphia, 1985, WB Saunders.

Chapter *Twenty-eight*

ELECTRICAL AND LIGHTNING INJURIES

MARY ANN COOPER

GENERAL CONSIDERATIONS

Electrical injuries may be conveniently divided into three groups on the basis of both their cause and their symptom presentation:
1. High voltage electrical injuries
2. Low voltage electrical injuries
3. Lightning injuries

Electrical energy, whether from manmade sources or from the heavens, may injure a person in three ways:
1. Thermal injury
2. Blunt injury
3. Electrochemical/cellular damage

Thermal injury can cause a variety of burns and thermal injuries depending on the amount of energy involved, the type of current source, and the duration of contact. Severe burns that result in amputations and major fluid resuscitation are most often associated with high voltage exposure, but lightning may on rare occasions cause severe thermal damage.

Blunt injury may occur because electrical contact causes a violent generalized muscle contraction that throws the person away from the source. It may also occur after an electrical explosion that throws the person or from falls associated with the injury (e.g., falling off a roof

or cliff). Blunt trauma protocols should be used in evaluating the patient.

Electrochemical damage was postulated as a mechanism of trauma early in this century but fell out of favor, probably because there was no real way to investigate it. The technology now exists, and electrochemical damage is again being turned to as an explanation for many of the signs and symptoms that cannot be explained by blunt or thermal injury. All cells and enzymes function on the basis of tiny changes in their electrical charges. Even if cells are exposed to electrical energy that is too low to cause thermal damage, injury and cell death may still result from irreversible changes in the protein configuration caused by charge changes in the enzymes and cell membrane structure. For example, if the sodium/potassium pump is damaged, the cell may not be able to maintain intracellular sodium and potassium concentrations. *Electroporation* is a term for the holes or "pores" that are opened on or inside a cell as the charges on the membranes are modified, which sometimes threatens cellular integrity. An exciting area for research is determining whether some acute treatment can be developed to plug or repair these holes and mitigate much of the injury experienced by victims of electrical injuries.

COMMON INJURIES

Although the precise dysrhythmias and complications may vary, cardiac arrest may occur with any of the three mechanisms of electrical injury. Asystole is more common for electrical injuries, and fibrillation is more common for lightning injuries. All of these injuries may be accompanied by hypoxemic brain damage in survivors, which complicates the recovery. Because lightning causes a longer respiratory arrest than cardiac arrest, respiratory support may need to be continued even after a life-sustaining heart rhythm resumes.

As suggested previously, a blunt trauma may injure the head, chest, abdomen, or musculoskeletal system, including fractures and dislocations. The patient should be treated as a general blunt trauma patient until such injuries have been ruled out by history, physical examination, or other means.

Central nervous system injuries may occur as a result of the electrical energy as well as the blunt trauma. These injuries run the gamut of intracerebral hemorrhage and contusion (with diagnostic evidence obtained from a CT scan and magnetic resonance imaging [MRI]) to no radiologic damage but significant long-term disability and neuropsychologic deficits similar to patients with a traumatic brain injury. There is good evidence for permanent sympathetic nervous system damage in some patients. Long-term dysethesias may be present in survivors. Other delayed neurologic sequelae have been reported with all forms of electrical injury.

Patients sustaining any of these three types of injury may have cataracts and many forms of eye injury, but more different types and more frequent cataracts are reported with lightning than with manmade electricity.

Because fetal damage is common with all three mechanisms, fetal monitoring and an immediate obstetrical consultation is indicated for pregnant patients.

The burns produced by electrical and lightning injuries are variable and depend on the mechanism of injury. High-voltage electrical injuries tend to have severe, deep burns that often result in limb amputation and significant myoglobin release. High-voltage electrical injuries act more like crush injuries than burns in many ways. Myoglobinuric renal failure may be prevented with proper alkalinization, generous fluid resuscitation, and furosemide or mannitol administration. Renal damage may also result from hypotension that accompanies severe injury and cardiac arrest. Fasciotomies, not just escharotomies, may be necessary for significant electrical burns that show evidence of compartment syndrome. In the days following a high-voltage injury, limbs and tissue that originally appear to be viable may suffer ischemia and necrosis as a result of progressive swelling and vascular damage, which necessitates frequent neurovascular checks.

Burns are usually much less severe with low-voltage (under 1000 volts) injuries, and deep burns are rare with lightning injuries. Fluid restriction may actually be preferable for patients with lightning injuries (if otherwise stable) to avoid further brain damage from edema. Care should be taken in obtaining the history of a low-voltage injury, because all things that are plugged into the wall are not necessarily sources of only 110 volts. With the expanding range of appliances that contain capacitors (e.g., microwave ovens, computer displays, televisions), large amounts of energy can be released.

Otologic damage is common with lightning injuries but relatively uncommon with other electrical injuries. Good experimental evidence shows that lightning uses the cranial orifices as portals of entry to the brain and cardiovascular system, which results in a number of eye, ear, brain, and cardiac problems.

MANAGEMENT CONSIDERATIONS

First, the patient must be released from the current source in a safe manner that does not place the rescuers at risk. This method should preferably involve turning off the current rather than rescuing the patient from the circuit.

The number of patients in lightning incidents may overwhelm the number of rescuers; in such cases, triage must be instituted but with preference given to those who appear to be in cardiac arrest. This protocol varies from the usual rules of disaster triage, in which those who are apparently dead are left for dead. It is unlikely for a lightning victim to die unless he or she has suffered an immediate cardiac arrest. Therefore those who are moderately affected have a good prognosis for survival and can be bypassed initially to care for those more severely injured.

Routine ABCs will need to be instituted, with generous fluid resuscitation particularly important for the patient with a high-voltage injury. Cardiac arrest is treated in the standard fashion, and all victims must be treated like trauma victims with spinal immobilization. Lightning victims may have a primary cardiorespiratory arrest, spontaneously recover cardiac function, and suffer a secondary arrest as they become hypoxemic from the much more prolonged respiratory arrest that accompanies such an injury. Cardiopulmonary resuscitation may indeed be a life-saving measure for such patients.

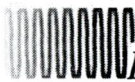

KEY CONSIDERATIONS

WHAT IS THE LIFE THREAT?

Cardiac arrest, respiratory arrest, and blunt injury to the head and chest pose an immediate life threat in victims of an electrical or lightning injury.

DOES THE PATIENT NEED ADMISSION?

The patient should be hospitalized for observation and intravenous hydration if myoglobinuria is present.

WHAT IS THE MOST SERIOUS DIAGNOSIS?

Cardiac arrest is the most serious diagnosis.

HAVE I PERFORMED A THOROUGH WORK-UP?

Examine the patient for evidence of burns and blunt injuries. Evaluate for evidence of myoglobinuria, and provide adequate intravenous fluid resuscitation to prevent renal failure as a result of myoglobinuria.

Recommended Readings

Andrews CJ, Darveniza M: Telephone-mediated lightning injury: an Australian survey, *J Trauma* 29:665, 1989.

Andrews CJ et al: *Lightning injuries: electrical, medical, and legal aspects,* St Louis, 1992, Mosby.

Andrews CJ et al: The pathology of electrical and lightning injuries. In Wecht CJ, editor: *Forensic science,* New York, 1995, Mathew Bender.

Cooper MA, Andrews CJ: Lightning injuries. In Auerbach P, editor: *Wilderness medicine: management of wilderness and environmental injuries,* St Louis, 1995, Mosby.

Cooper MA, Cherington M: *Seminars in neurology.* David Goldblatt, editor. Volumes 15(3) and 15(4), 1995.

Chapter Twenty-nine

NEAR-DROWNING

ROBERT KNOPP

Drowning accounts for more than 8000 deaths each year in the United States. The death rate is rising because of a greater number of swimming pools, population growth, and increased alcohol abuse.

Factors causing such accidents include an inability to swim, boating accidents, diving incidents, barotrauma, head or neck trauma, hypothermia, exhaustion, seizures, cardiac ischemia or dysrhythmia, suicide, hyperventilation with anxiety, intoxication (alcohol, sedatives, PCP, LSD), and child abuse.

The terminology associated with submersion accidents may be confusing:

- *Drowning:* suffocation from submersion in a liquid medium
- *Dry drowning:* death occurs from laryngospasm and hypoxemia without pulmonary aspiration in approximately 10% to 15% of all drownings.
- *Near-drowning:* recovery following submersion
- *Secondary drowning:* death occurring minutes to days after initial recovery; usually caused by pulmonary complications
- *Immersion syndrome:* sudden death after submersion in very cold water

Freshwater and saltwater drowning have distinct pathophysiologies leading to hypoxemia, but clinically the distinction is not usually important. Freshwater drowning disrupts surfactant, which causes atelectasis and, ultimately, pulmonary edema. Salt-water drowning causes fluid movement along an osmotic gradient, which floods the alveoli with protein-rich plasma; pulmonary edema again results. Electrolyte and erythrocyte abnormalities may develop; however, this phenomenon rarely occurs because large amounts of water are usually not aspirated.

Factors affecting outcome include low water temperature (usually provides a better outcome), duration and degree of hypothermia, age, water contamination, duration of cardiac arrest, and promptness and effectiveness of treatment. The box on p. 346 lists factors associated with a poor outcome.

CLINICAL PRESENTATION

The clinical presentation reflects pulmonary and cerebral hypoxemic injury. The spectrum of illness may range from minimal or negative findings initially, with a delayed onset of symptoms in 2 to 6 hours, to complete cardiac arrest.

Pulmonary findings may include cyanosis, pallor with pulmonary edema, or aspiration pneumonia, which is often associated with intrapulmonary shunting. Patients may develop

FACTORS ASSOCIATED WITH POOR
PROGNOSIS FOLLOWING NEAR-DROWNING

Under 3 years of age
Submersion longer than 5 minutes
Resuscitation not initiated for 5 minutes
Seizures with fixed or dilated pupils and
  posturing
Cardiopulmonary resuscitation required on
  admission
Arterial pH under 7

rales, frothy sputum, and rhonchi or wheezing
and progress to respiratory failure, adult or
childhood respiratory distress syndrome, or cardiac arrest from dysrhythmias.

Seizures, an altered mental status, and stupor
or coma may be present with or without focal
findings, which reflects hypoxemia and cerebral
edema. The patient may have drowned after a
seizure while swimming or bathing.

Evidence of trauma, particularly head and
neck injuries, should be sought. Other underlying precipitating factors should be considered.
In addition to pulmonary and central nervous
system injuries, the physician should assess the
patient's renal status. Acute tubular necrosis can
result from prolonged anoxia. Although infrequent, freshwater aspiration can produce hemolysis and hemoglobinuria, which may cause
acute renal failure.

ASSESSMENT

The initial assessment should focus on the ABCs,
vital signs, and protection of the cervical spine
(if indicated). Attempts to drain fluid from the
patient are unnecessary and inappropriate; if an
upper airway obstruction exists, the usual methods for relieving an obstruction should be used.
A rectal temperature is often necessary for accuracy because most electronic thermometers

cannot detect readings below 34° C. Once the
patient has been stabilized, determine the need
for laboratory and x-ray studies. The most important initial studies are a pulse oximeter measurement of the oxygen saturation, an arterial
blood gas, cardiac monitoring, and serial vital
signs. Other laboratory studies may be indicated
depending on the condition of the patient, including hemoglobin and hematocrit, electrolytes, blood sugar, creatinine, urinalysis for
hemoglobin, and ECG.

Radiographic studies should include a chest
x-ray examination on all patients and a cervical
spine x-ray examination if there was a history of
diving, if the patient is comatose, or if there are
other signs or symptoms of possible cervical injury.

MANAGEMENT

After first contact in the field or after arrival in
the emergency center, stabilize the airway,
breathing, and circulation while protecting the
cervical spine. Hypoxemia must be corrected.

All patients with a history of submersion
should be started initially on 100% oxygen. For
patients with hypoxemia, the most effective
method for reversing hypoxemia is continuous
positive airway pressure (CPAP). In the awake
and cooperative patient, CPAP may be administered using a tight-fitting mask. However, in
many situations, CPAP requires tracheal intubation and mechanical ventilation. The determination whether to apply CPAP during spontaneous
respiration or combine it with mechanical ventilation depends on the condition and response
of the patient.

The decision to intubate the patient in the
emergency department is based on the patient's
ability to protect the airway, respiratory distress,
pulmonary edema, and an arterial oxygen tension less than 60 mm Hg despite an FiO_2 of
100%.

No controlled studies have demonstrated the

effectiveness of steroids in the management of aspiration pneumonitis. Restrict antibiotics to those patients who demonstrate signs of infection or sepsis. Controversy still exists over the use of prophylactic antibiotics in patients who have aspirated grossly contaminated water such as sewer water.

The treatment for anoxic brain injury remains uncertain. In the 1980s, Conn and others reported improved outcomes after treatment with hypothermia, barbiturates, and other interventions. However, a comparison of patients treated with and without such treatment protocols reveals no improvement in outcomes. Because cerebral resuscitation protocols have not been demonstrated to be effective, emergency physicians should concentrate their efforts on treating hypoxemia. Metabolic acidosis may result from hypoxemia, but treatment with a bicarbonate is not usually necessary.

Cervical spine immobilization should continue until the integrity of the spine can be determined. If a spinal cord injury is detected, methylprednisolone (30 mg/kg) should be administered intravenously, with the remainder of the steroid protocol to follow (see Chapter 21).

The prognosis is poor for patients who arrive in the emergency department without spontaneous pulse or respirations. However, with extremely cold-water accidents, hypothermia may prolong the period that separates clinical from biologic death. Published reports document survival after prolonged cold-water submersion without neurologic impairment; one patient was successfully resuscitated and survived 66 minutes of submersion. Core rewarming is often necessary to reestablish spontaneous circulation in these patients. Deciding when to stop resuscitation is difficult. Unless the submersion occurred in extremely cold water, resuscitation is unlikely to be successful in patients who have no spontaneous pulse or respirations and have been submerged for longer than 20 to 30 minutes.

In alert patients with a history of submersion but no signs or symptoms of pulmonary problems, the emergency physician must decide whether to admit the patient or observe him or her in the emergency department for a given period of time. Outpatient management is a reasonable decision with reliable adults who remain asymptomatic after 8 hours of observation, including a normal chest x-ray examination and pulse oximetry readings. With toddlers and small children, overnight observation in the hospital is the prudent course.

Emotional support is imperative for family and friends, especially in young patients.

The most effective method for reducing the incidence of submersion accidents is prevention. Specific efforts include installing adequate fences around swimming pools, training children and adults in water safety, and recognizing the role of alcohol in water accidents.

||||||||||KEY CONSIDERATIONS

WHAT IS THE LIFE THREAT?

Hypoxemia and cerebral edema constitute major life threats in the postresuscitation period following a near-drowning episode.

DOES THE PATIENT NEED ADMISSION?

Patients who are resuscitated from a near-drowning episode should be hospitalized.

WHAT IS THE MOST SERIOUS DIAGNOSIS?

Hypoxemia and cerebral edema are the most serious diagnoses.

HAVE I PERFORMED A THOROUGH WORK-UP?

For cold-water drownings, continue resuscitation until hypothermia has resolved.

Evaluate oxygenation with pulse oximetry and arterial blood gases. Provide supplemental oxygen and continuous positive airway pressure, or perform a tracheal intubation and institute mechanical ventilation.

Measure electrolytes, calcium, magnesium, blood urea nitrogen, creatinine, hemoglobin, and glucose.

Evaluate the cervical spine.

Recommended Reading

Knopp RK: Near-drowning. In Rosen P et al, editors: *Emergency medicine: concepts and clinical practice,* ed 3, St Louis, 1992, Mosby.

Modell J: Drowning. *N Engl J Med* 328:253-256, 1993.

Orlowski JP: Drowning, near-drowning and ice-water submersion. *Pediatr Clin North Am* 34:75-93, 1987.

Orlowski JP: Drowning, near-drowning and ice-water drowning. *JAMA* 260:390-391, 1988.

Ornato JP: The resuscitation of near-drowning victims, *JAMA* 256:75, 1986.

Simmons CW, Neuman TS: Near-drowning: what to look for, how to treat, *J Resp Dis* 13:1084-1094, 1992.

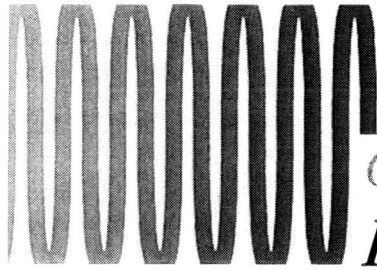

Chapter Thirty

HEAT- AND COLD-INDUCED INJURIES

DANIEL F. DANZL

HEAT ILLNESS

Healthy individuals are usually able to dissipate any environmental heat stress applied to the body. Because cellular metabolism also produces heat, the body temperature would rise at a rate of 1.1° C/hour without efficient cooling mechanisms. During strenuous exercise, this potential rate of rise could increase to 5° C/hour.

Heat loss mainly occurs through radiation, convection, and evaporation. High ambient temperatures and humidity interfere with normal heat loss. Most of the heat loss from diaphoresis results from the evaporation of sweat on the skin. Thermoregulation is maintained by these normal mechanisms of heat dissipation unless the environmental heat stress or endogenous heat production, such as fever or heavy muscle activity, exceeds heat dissipation.

Environmental and individual physiologic characteristics also influence the risk of developing heat illness (Fig. 30-1). Because all heat illnesses are readily preventable, education should focus on the importance of risk factors, acclimatization, and adequate hydration.

Clinical Presentation

Minor heat illness syndromes are not often seen by the emergency physician because they are vague or minor enough that patients may never seek treatment. Minor heat illness syndromes include the following:

1. *Heat edema.* Self-limited, mild swelling of the hands and feet that occurs in nonacclimated patients during the first few days of exposure
2. *Heat tetany.* Carpopedal spasms that may be associated with a variety of heat illnesses and with hyperventilation
3. *Heat syncope.* Occurs in unacclimatized subjects during the early phase of exposure; results from a decrease in vasomotor tone and peripheral venous pooling
4. *Prickly heat.* Results from blockage of sweat pores and a secondary staphylococcal infection; occurs primarily in hot, moist climates
5. *Anhidrotic heat exhaustion.* Accompanies prolonged prickly heat with symptoms of excessive fatigue from physical exertion; this syndrome parallels mild heat exhaustion.

Heat cramps are painful cramps that occur in the heavily exercised skeletal muscles, particularly the calves, during and after hard exercise. The cramping often accompanies profuse sweating in patients who replace fluid losses with water or other hypotonic, salt-poor solutions. The body temperature is almost normal. Usually

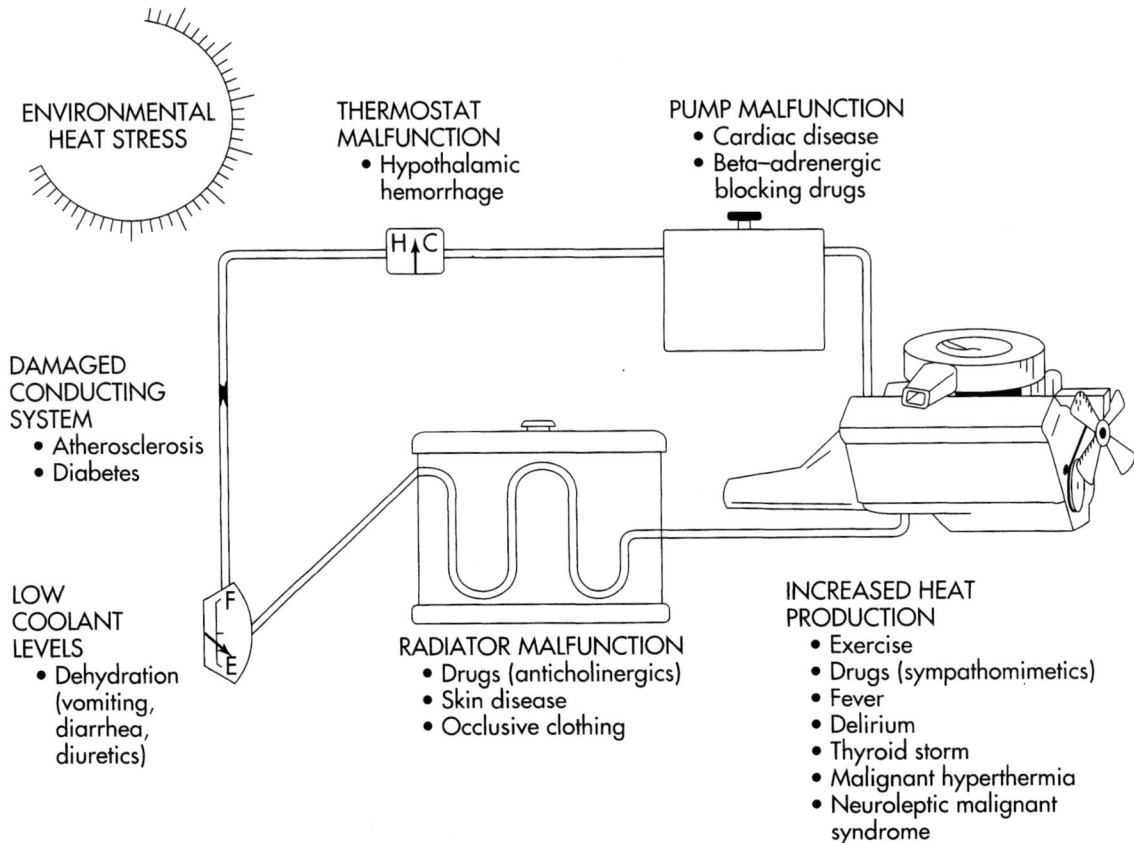

ENVIRONMENTAL
HEAT STRESS

THERMOSTAT
MALFUNCTION
• Hypothalamic
  hemorrhage

PUMP MALFUNCTION
• Cardiac disease
• Beta–adrenergic
  blocking drugs

DAMAGED
CONDUCTING
SYSTEM
• Atherosclerosis
• Diabetes

LOW
COOLANT
LEVELS
• Dehydration
  (vomiting,
  diarrhea,
  diuretics)

RADIATOR MALFUNCTION
• Drugs (anticholinergics)
• Skin disease
• Occlusive clothing

INCREASED HEAT
PRODUCTION
• Exercise
• Drugs (sympathomimetics)
• Fever
• Delirium
• Thyroid storm
• Malignant hyperthermia
• Neuroleptic malignant
  syndrome

Fig.30-1 Predisposing factors for heat illness: an automotive analogy. (From Jolly BT, Ghezzi KT: Accidental hypothermia, *Emerg Med Clin North Am* 10:311, 1992.)

oral electrolyte solution replacement coupled with rest is sufficient treatment.

Heat exhaustion results from volume and electrolyte depletion during a heat stress, which causes tissue hypoperfusion. The signs and symptoms of heat exhaustion often resemble a viral syndrome and can be very misleading. Unlike with heatstroke (see the discussion that follows), thermoregulatory control is still present. Heat exhaustion is a diagnosis of exclusion: first consider all potential infections (see the box on p. 351). Initial treatment is crystalloid rehydration, which is guided by the specific electrolyte

abnormalities that are identified. Many of these patients require hospitalization.

Heatstroke begins when a patient has lost all thermoregulatory control. After exposure to a heat stress, heatstroke is the combination of hyperpyrexia, classically over 40.5° C (105° F); and CNS impairment such as confusion, delirium, seizures, or coma. Heatstroke develops when all physiologic mechanisms to maintain heat loss have failed. The blood pressure can only be maintained by the development of peripheral vasoconstriction, which causes radiative heat loss to plummet.

HEAT EXHAUSTION DIAGNOSIS

Vague malaise, fatigue, headache, myalgias
Core temperature often normal or slightly
  elevated
Mental status intact
Tachycardia, orthostatic hypotension, clinical
  dehydration (may occur)
Other major illnesses have been ruled out
If in doubt, treat as heatstroke and cool
  rapidly

Classical heatstroke usually strikes the elderly, the chronically ill, and infants when access to fluids and a cool environment is restricted for several hot days. These patients are significantly dehydrated and may cease sweating. Exertional heatstroke is more common in fit, young individuals and in athletes who are not acclimatized (Table 30-1).

Initial symptoms of heatstroke are those of heat exhaustion that eventually progress to an elevated core temperature and CNS abnormalities. Sinus tachycardia and hyperventilation often precede the dysrhythmias and hypotension. Systemic involvement also is common; anticipate acute tubular necrosis, hepatic failure, rhabdomyolysis and myoglobinuria, and coagulopathies with disseminated intravascular coagulation and thrombocytopenia.

Management

Given the potential life-threatening nature of heatstroke, it is essential to aggressively cool the patient while administering oxygen. Airway protection is always necessary. Remember the aphorism: "It does not take long either to boil an egg or to cook neurons."

Heatstroke requires aggressive intravenous fluid support and additional close monitoring of the central venous pressure (or pulmonary capillary wedge pressure if appropriate). Maintain an adequate urinary output.

Initially stabilize the circulation by rapidly administering 20 to 40 ml/kg of normal saline. Remove clothing and facilitate evaporation by keeping the skin moist and using a fan. Get the core temperature below 39° C immediately. An ice-water bath is not ideal and is far less effective than evaporative cooling; icing the extremities often induces peripheral vasoconstriction and shivering. A practical alternative involves spraying the patient with lukewarm water and placing ice chips in the axillae and groin. An-

Table 30-1

HEATSTROKE GENERAL CLINICAL CHARACTERISTICS

Exertional	*Classical*
Younger, healthy adults	Older adults with predisposing health factors or medicines
Diaphoresis is common	Anhidrosis is common
Sporadic occurrences	Heat waves
Hypoglycemia and hypocalcemia are common	Hypoglycemia and hypocalcemia are uncommon
DIC, ARF, LA, and rhabdomyolysis are common	DIC, ARF, LA, and rhabdomyolysis are uncommon

DIC, Disseminated intravascular coagulation; *ARF,* acute renal failure; *LA,* lactic acidosis

FACTORS PREDISPOSING TO HYPOTHERMIA

Decreased heat production

Endocrinologic failure
  Hypopituitarism
  Hypoadrenalism
  Hypothyroidism
Insufficient fuel
  Hypoglycemia
  Malnutrition
  Marasmus
  Kwashiorkor
  Marathon exertion
Neuromuscular inefficiency
  Age extremes
  Impaired shivering
  Inactivity
  Lack of adaptation

Increased heat loss

Environmental
  Immersion
  Nonimmersion
Induced vasodilatation
  Pharmacologic
  Toxicologic
Erythrodermas
  Burns
  Psoriasis
  Ichthyosis
  Exfoliative dermatitis
Iatrogenic
  Emergent deliveries
  Cold infusions
  Heatstroke treatment

Impaired thermoregulation

Peripheral failure
  Neuropathies
  Acute spinal cord transection
  Diabetes
Central failure
  CNS trauma
  CVA
  Toxicologic
  Metabolic
  Subarachnoid hemorrhage
  Pharmacologic
  Hypothalamic dysfunction
  Parkinson disease
  Anorexia nervosa
  Cerebellar lesion
  Neoplasm
  Congenital intracranial anomalies
  Multiple sclerosis

Miscellaneous associated clinical states

Recurrent hypothermia
Episodic hypothermia
Sepsis
Pancreatitis
Carcinomatosis
Cardiopulmonary disease
Vascular insufficiency
Uremia
Paget disease
Giant cell arteritis
Sarcoidosis
Shaken baby syndrome

From Danzl DF: Accidental hypothermia. In Rosen P et al, editors: *Emergency medicine: concepts and clinical practice*, ed 3, St Louis, 1992, Mosby.

Table 30-2

PHYSIOLOGIC CHARACTERISTICS OF THE THREE STAGES OF HYPOTHERMIA

Stage	°C	°F	Characteristics
Mild	37.6	99.6 ± 1	Normal rectal temperature
	37	98.6 ± 1	Normal oral temperature
	36	96.8	Increase in metabolic rate
	35	95	Urine temperature 34.8° C; maximum shivering thermogenesis
	34	93.2	Amnesia and dysarthria develop; normal blood pressure; maximum respiratory stimulation
	33	91.4	Ataxia and apathy develop
Moderate	32	89.6	Stupor; 25% decrease in oxygen consumption
	31	87.8	Extinguished shivering thermogenesis
	30	86	Atrial fibrillation and other dysrhythmias; poikilothermy; pulse and cardiac output two-thirds normal; insulin ineffective
	29	85.2	Progressive decrease in level of consciousness, pulse, and respiration; pupils dilated
	28	82.4	Ventricular fibrillation susceptibility; 50% decrease in oxygen consumption and pulse
Severe	27	80.6	Losing reflexes and voluntary motion
	26	78.8	Major acid-base disturbances; no reflexes or response to pain
	25	77	Cerebral blood flow one-third normal; cardiac output 45% normal; pulmonary edema may develop
	24	75.2	Significant hypotension
	23	73.4	No corneal or oculocephalic reflexes
	22	71.6	Maximum risk of ventricular fibrillation; 75% decrease in oxygen consumption
	20	68	Lowest resumption of cardiac electromechanical activity; pulse 20% of normal
	19	66.2	Flat EEG
	18	64.4	Asystole develops
	16	60.8	Lowest accidental hypothermia survival in an adult
	15	59.2	Lowest accidental hypothermia survival in an infant
	10	50	92% decrease in oxygen consumption
	9	48.2	Lowest therapeutic hypothermia survival

From Danzl DF: Accidental hypothermia. In Rosen P et al, editors: *Emergency medicine: concepts and clinical practice*, ed 3, St Louis, 1992, Mosby.

tipyretics are not useful during cooling. Intense shivering may need to be controlled with benzodiazepines.

Early baseline laboratory parameters should include a complete blood count (CBC); electrolytes; hepatic, clotting, and renal studies; and arterial blood gases *un*corrected for temperature. Aggressively treat the common complications of heatstroke, including seizures, prolonged hypotension, and acute renal failure with hyperkalemia.

HYPOTHERMIA

Accidental hypothermia is an unintentionally induced decrease in the body's core temperature in the absence of preoptic anterior hypothalamic pathology. The normal compensatory responses to heat loss via conduction, convection, radiation, and evaporation may be overwhelmed by exposure. Conduction is the transfer of heat by direct contact across a temperature gradient (from a warm body to the cold environment). Heat loss may increase 5 times in wet clothing and up to 25 times in cold water. Convection is the transfer of heat by air movement such as occurs when the wind disrupts the layer of warm air surrounding the body. Radiation, evaporation, and respiration further contribute to heat loss.

The disruption of normal heat regulation may result from decreased heat production, increased heat loss, or impaired thermoregulation. Some of the predisposing factors to more severe hypothermia include injury, exposure, age, health, nutrition, medication, and intoxicants (see the box on p. 352).

Clinical Presentation

Historical circumstances often suggest the diagnosis when exposure is obvious. Multi-organ involvement is typical (Table 30-2). Below 32° C, an adynamic stage progresses with a general slowdown of metabolic function, which is accompanied by impaired inotropic and chronotropic cardiac function. Dysrhythmias are prevalent below 30° C, and the risk increases as the temperature decreases. The Osborn (J) wave appears as a slow, positive, "camel-humped" deflection during the QRS-ST junction (Fig. 30-2). Although the Osborn wave is not correlated with any specific lowering of temperature, it strongly suggests the diagnosis when present.

All atrial dysrhythmias are common but should have a slow ventricular response and be considered innocent. If there is a tachycardia that is disproportionate for the temperature, check for hypovolemia, hypoglycemia, or an overdose. A preexistent ventricular ectopy may

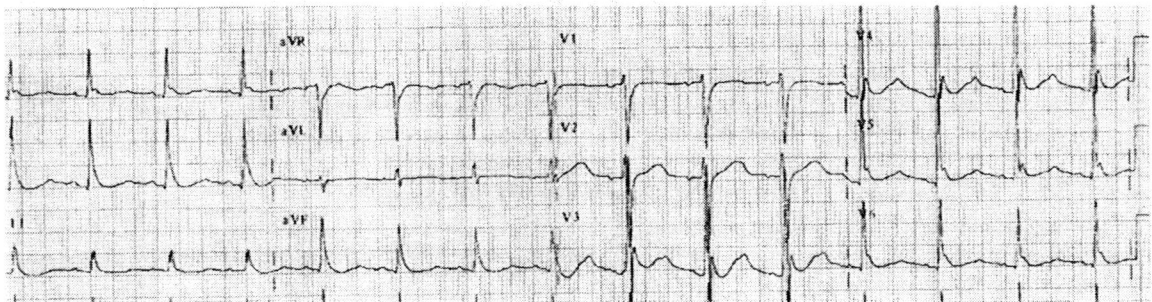

Fig.30-2 The J (Osborn) wave is present at the junction of the QRS complex and ST segment.

be suppressed by the cold and reappear during rewarming.

Similarly, carbon dioxide production drops with the temperature. Persistent hyperventilation should suggest an organic acidosis or a CNS pathology. If the level of consciousness is not consistent with the temperature, suspect an overdose or a CNS trauma or infection.

Management

Confirm hypothermia by measuring core temperature (e.g., rectal, esophageal, tympanic, bladder). Stabilization of the patient and treatment of any underlying conditions is mandatory (see the box on p. 352). Define the resuscitation goals (see the box below).

To avoid precipitating a fatal dysrhythmia, minimize rough handling. Preoxygenate the patient before performing any procedures. Hypothermia adversely affects tissue oxygenation.

RESUSCITATION REQUIREMENTS

Prevention of additional heat loss
    Conduction
    Convection
    Radiation
    Evaporation
    Respiration
Maintenance of tissue oxygenation
    Adequate circulation
    Adequate ventilation
Rewarming options
    Passive external rewarming
    Active external rewarming
    Active core rewarming
Other considerations
    Treat precipitating disease
    Treat underlying disease

From Danzl DF: Frostbite. In Rosen P, Barkin RM et al, editors: *Emergency medicine: concepts and clinical practice,* ed 3, St Louis, 1992, Mosby.

Administer warmed, humidified oxygen; glucose; and warmed IV solutions to correct hypoxemia and hypoglycemia. Generally, 250 to 500 ml of D_5NS should be administered empirically because of the relative dehydration and hemoconcentration that results from fluid shifts.

Routine hematologic evaluations should include arterial blood gases *un*corrected for temperature. An uncorrected pH of 7.4 and a PCO_2 of 40 mm Hg reflects acid-base balance at all temperatures. Laboratory assessment should also include a CBC, electrolytes, glucose, and renal and coagulation studies.

Uncontrolled trials have been unable to rigidly define the ideal management protocol for treating hypothermia. Several flexible approaches may be initiated in patients with temperatures below 32° C. Generally, passive external rewarming is adequate for patients with less severe hypothermia.

Passive external rewarming minimizes heat dissipation. Simply cover the patient with an insulating material, such as warmed blankets, in a warm and ambient temperature. This technique helps maintain peripheral vasoconstriction in the extremities. Spontaneous rewarming should occur at a rate between 0.5° C and 2° C/hour. This method is ideal for most mild cases in previously healthy patients.

Active external rewarming involves direct application of heat to the thorax using hot water immersion, warmed blankets, radiant heaters, or heated objects such as hot water bottles. Heat applied to the extremities may increase the cardiovascular load and lower the blood pressure. Ideally, truncal active external rewarming can be combined with various active core rewarming techniques.

Active core rewarming options include inhalation of heated humidified oxygen; heated intravenous (IV) fluids; irrigation of the thorax, peritoneum, or gastrointestinal tract; and extracorporeal rewarming.

All patients with a body temperature below 32° C benefit from airway rewarming; preoxy-

PREDISPOSING FACTORS TO PERIPHERAL COLD INJURIES

Physiologic

Genetic
Core temperature
Prior cold injury
± Acclimatization
Dehydration
Overexertion
Trauma: multisystem/extremity
Dermatologic diseases
Physical conditioning
Diaphoresis/hyperhidrosis
Hypoxemia

Cardiovascular

Hypotension
Atherosclerosis
Arteritis
Raynaud syndrome
Cold-induced vasodilatation
Anemia
Sickle cell disease
Diabetes
Hypovolemia; shock
Vasoconstrictors/vasodilators

Psychologic

Mental status
Fear/panic
Attitude
Peer pressure
Fatigue
Intense concentration on tasks
Hunger; malnutrition
Intoxicants

Environmental

Ambient temperature
Humidity
Duration of exposure
Wind chill factor
Altitude ± associated conditions
Quantity of exposed surface area
Heat loss: conductive, evaporative

Mechanical

Constricting/wet clothing
Tight boots
Vapor barrier/alveolite liners
Inadequate insulation
Immobility/cramped positioning

From Danzl DF: Frostbite. In Rosen P et al, editors: *Emergency medicine: concepts and clinical practice,* ed 3, St Louis, 1992, Mosby.

genation and gentle intubation helps prevent ventricular dysrhythmias. Heating IV fluids is not very efficient as an isolated rewarming technique but can be important during massive volume resuscitations, such as in trauma cases.

Both a peritoneal dialysate infused at 40° C to 45° C and a thoracostomy tube irrigation efficiently transfer heat. However, irrigating the gastrointestinal tract has very limited value. Extracorporeal rewarming should be considered for potentially salvageable patients who are in cardiac arrest or for those with completely frozen extremities or severe rhabdomyolysis.

Peripheral cold injuries include nonfreezing syndromes, as well as freezing injuries such as frostbite. A nonfreezing injury from dry cold is called chilblains (pernio). These are "cold sores" that are usually found on the face and dorsa of the hands and feet. Trench foot results from exposure to wet cold. Erythema, edema, and bullae often develop.

The severity of the cold injury reflects the temperature, duration of exposure, wind-chill factor, immobility, tightness of clothing, and dampness (see the box above). The presence of ice crystallization in the cells coupled with pe-

EMERGENCY DEPARTMENT REWARMING PROTOCOL

Prethaw

Protect part
Stabilize core temperature
Address medical/surgical conditions
Hydration
No friction massage

Thaw

Rapid rewarming in 38° C to 41° C circulating
   water until distal flush (thermometer
   monitoring)
Requires 10-30 minutes with active motion of
   part without friction massage
Parenteral analgesia

Postthaw

Clear vesicles—aspirate (if intact) vs. debride
Hemorrhagic vesicles—aspirate
Apply topical aloe vera (Dermaide) q6h
Ibuprofen 400 mg q12h
Tetanus prophylaxis
Streptococcal prophylaxis for 48-72 hours
Elevation

From Danzl DF: Frostbite. In Rosen P et al, editors: *Emergency medicine: concepts and clinical practice,* ed 3, St Louis, 1992, Mosby.

ripheral vasoconstriction markedly increases tissue damage. The most commonly affected areas are the digits, hands, feet, ears, and nose.

Frostbite was historically classified into degrees of injury, similar to burns. However, it seems more useful to simply consider frostbite "superficial" if it does not entail eventual heat loss, and "deep" if it does. Remember that the initial clinical presentation is often deceptively benign.

Consider the possibilities of life-threatening hypothermia and other medical conditions before initiating frostbite management. Initial treatment in the field must include careful handling; consider rewarming in severe cases only if there is *no* chance of a second refreezing during transport.

Deep frostbite requires a rapid rewarming—do not use hot air. Completely immerse and re-

warm the frozen part for approximately 20 minutes in warm water that is between 38° C and 41.4° C. Incomplete thawing is a common error because the reestablishment of perfusion is very painful. Protect the involved tissue from further damage by elevating the extremity (see the box above).

Amputation should be delayed until there is good demarcation of necrotic tissue, which may take months ("Frostbite in January—amputate in July"). Anticoagulants, low–molecular-weight dextran, and regional sympathectomy have not proved valuable. Recommendations regarding frostbite vesicle management vary. Large clean blisters can initially be left intact, aspirated, or debrided. Hemorrhagic blisters should be left intact to prevent desiccation. Topical thromboxane inhibition with aloe vera cream or systemic inhibition with ibuprofen may also be helpful.

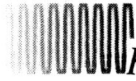

KEY CONSIDERATIONS

WHAT IS THE LIFE THREAT?

Heatstroke and accidental hypothermia are life-threatening conditions. With hypothermia, the degree of life threat increases as the body temperature drops.

DOES THE PATIENT NEED ADMISSION?

Patients with heatstroke and those with a core temperature less than 32° C require hospital admission. Patients with less severe hypothermia require admission if they have had a cardiac dysrhythmia or diminished consciousness, are elderly, or are taking medication that makes them susceptible to a recurrent episode.

WHAT IS THE MOST SERIOUS DIAGNOSIS?

Heatstroke and accidental hypothermia with a core temperature less than 30° C.

HAVE I PERFORMED A THOROUGH WORK-UP?

Protect the airway and administer oxygen. Provide aggressive intravenous fluid support. Cool the body using a water spray mist and fans to promote evaporation and ice packs to groin and axillae.

Recommended Reading

Costrini A: Emergency treatment of exertional heatstroke and comparison of whole body cooling techniques, *Med Sci Sports Exerc* 22:15, 1990.

Danzl DF: Accidental hypothermia. In Rosen P et al, editors: *Emergency medicine: concepts and clinical practice,* ed 3, St Louis, 1992, Mosby.

Danzl DF: Frostbite. In Rosen P et al, editors: *Emergency medicine: concepts and clinical practice,* ed 3, St Louis, 1992, Mosby.

Danzl DF, Pozos RS: Accidental hypothermia, *N Engl J Med* 331:1756-1760, 1994.

Jolly BT, Ghezzi KT: Accidental hypothermia, *Emerg Med Clin North Am* 10:311, 1992.

Yarbrough B: Heat illness. In Rosen P et al, editors: *Emergency medicine: concepts and clinical practice,* ed 3, St Louis, 1992, Mosby.

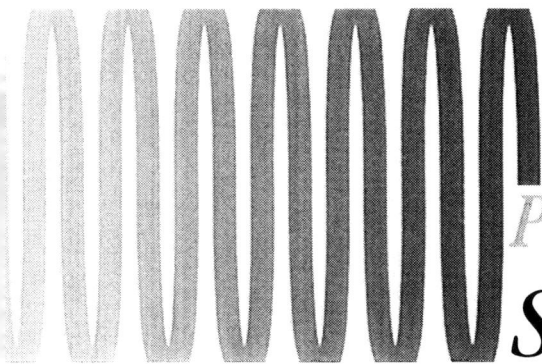

Part V

SYSTEMIC DISORDERS

Chapter Thirty-one
ACUTE RESPIRATORY TRACT INFECTION

JOHN J. KELLY

Acute disorders of the upper and lower respiratory tract are a common complaint for patients visiting the emergency department. Although the majority are viral and therefore self-limited, significant morbidity is associated with such infections, and they may occasionally progress to respiratory failure as a result of respiratory distress and hypoxemia.

UPPER RESPIRATORY TRACT

The upper respiratory tract comprises the nasopharynx and oropharynx, with intimate connections between the paranasal sinuses, middle ear, and larynx. Multiple organisms colonize the nasopharynx and oropharynx, whereas the paranasal sinuses and airway below the epiglottis are normally sterile.

Host defenses provide protection against infection. Mechanical protective mechanisms include sneezing, gagging, and coughing, whereas the localized expulsive ciliary action of the respiratory tract epithelium provides a complementary barrier. Systemic defenses include a rich blood supply, secretory IgA antibodies, and lymphoid tissue.

Pharyngitis

Acute pharyngitis is commonly associated with tonsillitis and soreness, fever, and minimal nasal involvement. Group A streptococcus accounts for 20% to 30% of all cases; other pathogens are commonly noted (Table 31-1). As many as 50% of all patients with pharyngitis have no definable bacteriologic or virologic pathogen.

Clinical presentation and assessment

Although no single finding can accurately separate streptococcal from nonstreptococcal pharyngitis, clinical observations of pharyngeal erythema, exudate, palatal petechiae, temperature more than 38.3° C, and anterior cervical adenitis are relatively sensitive. A scarlatiniform rash is diagnostic of a streptococcal infection.

Infants rarely have a sore throat, but streptococcal disease is more commonly associated with nasal discharge, excoriated nares, and diffuse cervical lymphadenopathy.

Exudative pharyngitis accompanies group A streptococcus, the Epstein-Barr virus (infectious mononucleosis), and adenovirus infection. Exudative pharyngitis is commonly caused by a virus in those under 3 years of age and by group A streptococcus in those over 6 years of age.

*Table*31-1

CAUSES AND CLINICAL CHARACTERISTICS OF COMMON TYPES OF PHARYNGITIS

Type	Clinical Characteristics	Type	Clinical Characteristics
Bacterial		**Viral**	
Group A streptococcus	Tonsillar exudate Fever greater than 101° F (38.3° C) Tender cervical adenopathy	Influenza virus	Associated with fever, myalgia, headache, malaise Pneumonia is common complication
Neisseria gonorrhoeae	Patient practices fellatio or cunnilingus, complains of "sore throat" May be no signs of pharyngitis Can be source of gonococcemia with dissemination	Rhinoviruses and coronaviruses	Common "cold," acute coryza, fever, chills, malaise
		Epstein-Barr virus	Mononucleosis syndrome; exudative pharyngitis; fever; cervical adenopathy, anterior and posterior Associated with splenomegaly, hepatitis, aseptic meningitis
Mycoplasma pneumoniae and *Chlamydia* organisms	Sore throat with non-productive cough, fever, alveolar infiltrate of lower lobes Crowded living conditions Bullous myringitis in 2% to 8% of all cases	**Noninfectious**	
		Trauma	Burns, physical injury, foreign body, mandibular or maxillary fractures
Haemophilus influenzae	Usually occurs in children Associated with otitis media, epiglottitis, meningitis	Inhaled irritants	Chemicals, smoke, gases
		Thyroiditis	Subacute form associated with chronic symptoms Acute form associated with severe symptoms, toxic patient
		Sinus drainage	Acute or chronic; irritative, often with cough
		Candida albicans	White plaque over shallow ulcer Common in infants and patients with immunodeficiency.

Soft palate petechiae are found with group A streptococcus and Epstein-Barr virus infection, vesicles or ulcers on the posterior tonsillar pillars with enterovirus infection, and ulcers on the anterior palate with adenopathy in herpes infections.

Adult epiglottitis commonly causes an extremely painful sore throat that may evolve with dysphagia and significant airway obstruction and worsen over several days. Common symptoms include fever, a muffled voice, poorly handled secretions, and stridor.

Throat culture remains the diagnostic tool of choice for group A streptococcus. However, total reliance on these cultures may create problems:

1. A negative culture does not exclude the diagnosis of group A streptococcus. A second swab culture can reduce the false-negative rate.
2. A positive culture (usually low colony count) does not substantiate an infection in the absence of an immune response. The strep-

tozyme test or the Aso test may be used to investigate the carrier state, which is usually associated with a low titer. The carrier rate in nonepidemic areas is 10% to 50%. These patients are not at risk for rheumatic fever or acute glomerulonephritis.

3. Rapid simple diagnostic tests are available to identify group A streptococcus and make immediate diagnosis a reality. In view of the high false-negative rate, it is essential to confirm negative tests with a routine culture.

Infants should have their nares rather than their throats cultured. Symptomatic family members should have cultures done, but routine cultures of all relatives are not cost effective.

Management

The patient can obtain symptomatic relief initially by gargling with warm water; sucking hard candy; and using aspirin, acetaminophen, or ibuprofen. Oral prednisone (1 mg/kg/day × 5 to 10 days) may help in reducing pharyngeal edema and pain in cases of extreme swelling.

Table *31-2*

TREATMENT ALTERNATIVES FOR GROUP A STREPTOCOCCAL PHARYNGITIS*

Drug	Dosage	
	Adults	Children
Penicillin V potassium	250-500 mg qid po × 10 days	25-50 mg/kg/24 hr qid po
Penicillin G benzathine	1.2 million units IM	900,000 units benzathine; 300,000 units procaine (Bicillin C-R†)
Erythromycin	250 mg tid po × 10 days	30-50 mg/kg/24 hr tid po

*Second- or third-generation oral cephalosporins provide adequate treatment but are often more expensive.
†Procaine Bicillin C-R is 75% benzathine and 25% procaine preparation:

Weight	Bicillin C-R
<30 lb	300,000:100,000
31-60 lb	600,000:200,000
61-90 lb	900,000:300,000

If the infection is streptococcal, prescribe antibiotic therapy for 10 days of therapy (unless given intramuscularly) (Table 31-2). Symptomatic improvement is noted following early therapy with antibiotics. Treatment also allows patients to return to work or school in 24 hours, thereby decreasing the associated social disruption. The risk of developing acute rheumatic fever and acute glomerulonephritis is not increased if antibiotics are started within 7 days of the onset of symptoms.

Specific treatment for *Candida* organisms, *N. gonorrhoeae,* and *Chlamydia trachomatis* may be considered, as indicated.

Deep Infections

Soft tissue infections in and around the pharynx may extend by contiguous spread through the lymphatic and venous system. The numerous fascial planes facilitate spread to deep structures, including the peritonsillar, retropharyngeal, parapharyngeal, and prevertebral spaces.

A *peritonsillar abscess* occurs with suppurative infection beyond the tonsillar capsule into surrounding tissues. Group A streptococcus is the most common pathogen, but *H. influenzae* and *S. pneumoniae* are also reported causes. Patients usually have toxicity accompanied by fever, severe sore throat, progressive trismus, drooling, alterations in speech ("hot potato voice"), and dysphagia. The involved tonsil is often displaced medially, with erythema and edema of the soft palate. The uvula deviates to the opposite side.

If there is any airway compromise, active intervention should be an immediate priority. Initiate ceftriaxone or clindamycin early, with the possible addition of nafcillin or a third-generation cephalosporin if resolution is slow. Incise and drain the abscess if it is fluctuant. A needle aspirate may initially be both diagnostic and therapeutic, with a definitive incision and drainage being completed in the operating room.

A *retropharyngeal abscess* may complicate otitis media or nasopharyngeal infections associated with suppurative adenitis of the small lymph nodes between the buccopharyngeal and prevertebral fascia. If untreated, this condition can lead to abscess formation, particularly in children less than 3 years of age. Group A streptococcus, *Staphylococcus aureus, H. influenzae,* and anaerobes are common. The infection may spread from otitis media, nasopharyngitis, vertebral osteomyelitis, or from wound infections following a penetrating injury of the posterior pharynx or palate.

Patients develop swallowing difficulties, drooling, and severe throat pain. Nuchal rigidity may result from irritation of the paravertebral ligaments. Potential respiratory obstruction may be associated with labored respirations and gurgling and hyperextension of the head. A definite unilateral posterior pharyngeal wall mass is present and often becomes fluctuant. Lateral cervical x-ray films demonstrate an increased soft tissue mass between the anterior wall of the cervical spine and the pharyngeal wall. The limits of normal soft tissue measurements in the neck are as follows:

1. At the level of C2-C3, the average distance from the anterior edge of C2-C3 to the posterior pharynx is 3.4 mm (range 1 to 7 mm)
2. At the level of C6, the average distance from the anterior edge of C6 to the posterior trachea is 14 mm (range 9 to 22 mm)
3. In children, the retropharyngeal soft tissue should not be more than 5 mm at the level of C3 or 40% of the anteroposterior (AP) diameter of the body at C4 at that level.

After ensuring adequacy of the airway, begin parenteral administration of a penicillinase-resistant penicillin or cephalosporin. In children, *H. influenzae* should also be covered if the child is not immunized against this type of bacteria.

Prevertebral space infections, which are located between the prevertebral fascia and cervical spine and are caused by osteomyelitis of the cervical spine, are diagnosed by lateral neck films demonstrating bony and soft tissue involvement. *S. aureus* is a common pathogen. Antibiotics and surgical intervention are usually indicated.

Parapharyngeal infections of the deep neck structures are rare and cause unilateral neck pain, tenderness, and swelling at the angle of the mandible. Airway compromise may occur and require urgent antibiotic and surgical intervention.

Ludwig's angina is a rapidly spreading cellulitis with brawny edema of the floor of the mouth; it involves the sublingual and submandibular spaces and often follows dental manipulation or pharyngeal trauma. A "bull neck" appearance is common. Mixed pathogens are usually causative, including a variety of anaerobic bacteria.

If evidence of obstruction is present airway stabilization is the highest priority. Prescribe antibiotics, including a penicillinase-resistant penicillin and aminoglycoside; substitute a third-generation cephalosporin in children.

Epiglottitis is seen more commonly in adults than in children (see Chapter 66). Clinically, patients complain of a severe sore throat of 2 to 4 days' duration, with accompanying fever and dysphagia. The throat pain is disproportionate to the objective signs of pharyngitis.

Treatment should commonly include third-generation cephalosporins. *S. aureus* has been reported as a pathogen in addition to the more common *H. influenzae*. Intubation may not be as necessary as in the child, but the adult must be admitted to an ICU for observation. In all of these deep infections, IV steroids (i.e., Decadron) may be used to reduce pharyngeal/airway edema, inflammation and pain.

Sinusitis

Swelling of the nasal mucosa and obstruction of the sinus ostea result in an acute inflammatory reaction within the sinuses. Allergic vasomotor changes, atmospheric pressure changes, chemi-cal irritants, mechanical obstructions, systemic disease, and viral infection can impair normal defenses and drainage.

Although the bacteriology is unclear, predominant infecting bacteria include *H. influenzae, S. pneumoniae, M. catarrhalis,* Group A streptococcus, and a variety of anaerobic and aerobic organisms. Viruses may also be important pathogens, whereas fungal infections are of concern in patients with diabetes and in immunocompromised individuals.

Clinical presentation and assessment

Rhinorrhea is present in 78% of patients, and 64% have a purulent discharge. A cough, often worse at night (50%); sinus pain or headache; and temperatures above 38.5° C are common. Concurrent upper respiratory tract infections and malodorous breath are common presentations. Only 8% of patients have tenderness over the frontal, ethmoid, or maxillary sinuses. Transillumination is commonly noted to be asymmetric. Sphenoid sinusitis is associated with occipital pain and potential toxicity. Chronic sinusitis may be asymptomatic or associated with purulent nasal discharge. Partial opacification or dullness to transillumination is nonspecific and may not correlate with bacteriologic verification of infection.

Associated complications may include periorbital cellulitis (especially ethmoid sinusitis); osteomyelitis of the sinus wall (frontal involvement appears as a Pott's puffy tumor, a midfrontal swelling); brain, subdural, or epidural abscesses; or meningitis.

Radiologic examination reveals clouding, mucosal thickening (>8 mm), or air-fluid levels within the sinuses; the latter is the most helpful in defining an acute infection. A CT scan may be required in difficult cases.

Management

The symptoms of bacterial sinusitis usually resolve in 48 to 72 hours. The use of decongestants remains controversial. Many physicians use sys-

Table 31-3

COMMONLY USED ANTIBIOTICS FOR BACTERIAL SINUSITIS

	Dosage	
Drug	**Adults**	**Children***
Amoxicillin	250-500 mg q6h po	50 mg/kg/24 hr q6h po
Amoxicillin/clavulanate (Augmentin)	250-500 mg q8h po	40 mg/kg/d divided q8h
Clarithromycin	500 mg q12h po	15 mg/kg/d divided q12h
Clindamycin	150-300 mg q6h po	8-16 mg/kg/24 hr q6h po
Erythromycin	250-500 mg q6h po	30-50 mg/kg/24 hr q6h po
Trimethoprim/sulfamethoxazole	One double-strength bid	—

*Second- or third-generation oral cephalosporins may also be used.

temic decongestants (pseudoephedrine or phenylpropanolamine) in combination with oxymetazoline spray (Afrin); the latter is usually used for 3 days or less. Guaifenesin is a mucolytic that liquifies secretions and helps clear the sinuses. Antihistamines should not be used. Use antibiotics in patients with an unresolving illness, patients with toxicity, and those with complications. Commonly used antibiotics are listed in Table 31-3. Failure to respond justifies otolaryngic consultation and a CT scan of the sinuses. Sphenoid sinusitis often requires parenteral therapy.

LOWER RESPIRATORY TRACT

Acute Bronchitis

Inflammation of the bronchi, trachea, and bronchioles is commonly referred to as bronchitis, tracheobronchitis, and bronchiolitis. Infection may be caused by viruses, *mycoplasma clamy-*

dia, or pertussis; bacterial superinfection is common with *S. pneumoniae, H. influenzae, S. aureus,* or *M. catarrhalis.* Coughing is constant and is usually found in afebrile patients with an upper respiratory tract infection. Concurrent chest pain and general malaise are also noted. Sputum production is generally minimal in viral disease, becoming purulent and productive with bacterial (purulent) bronchitis. Rarely, vigorous coughing may cause pneumothorax, pneumomediastinum, and headache. Radiographically, x-ray films generally contribute little, but increased bronchopulmonary markings may be noted.

Treatment may include cough suppressants. Antibiotic therapy may be efficacious in reducing sputum volume, particularly in chronic bronchitis. Suggested antibiotics may include erythromycin, amoxicillin, or a cephalosporin. Bronchodilator therapy using inhaled ß-agonists and oral steroids are indicated and effective in bronchospastic disease.

Text continued on p. 375.

Table*31-4*

HELPFUL CLINICAL CLUES TO DIAGNOSIS OF PNEUMONIA

Organism	Fever (°F)	Chills	Sputum	Chest X-ray Studies	Other Features
Bacteria					
Streptococcus pneumoniae	Sustained 101° to 106°	Shaking at onset	Productive in 75% Rusty, muco-purulent	May be normal despite clinical signs Usually lobar con-solidation Patchy lobar, more common in immuno-compromised individuals	Pleuritic chest pain, cyanosis, confusion Lobar consolida-tion Sepsis and other organ involve-ment, espe-cially in patients with hyposplenism
Staphylococcus aureus	Hectic 102° to 105°	Multiple	Productive	Sometimes lobar Usually multi-centric Pneumatoceles and pyopneu-mothorax	Especially fol-lowing influenza Pleuritic pain Debilitated host, IV drug abusers 10% of hospital-acquired pneumonia May be associ-ated with endocarditis Look for distant foci (abscesses)
Group A beta-hemolytic *Streptococcus pyogenes*	Hectic 104° to 106°	Multiple	Productive Purulent and bloody	Multilobar in ad-jacent lobes common Frequent pleural effusion and empyema Slow to clear	Pleuritic pain common High mortality Rapidly progres-sive

Continued.

Table *31-4*

HELPFUL CLINICAL CLUES TO DIAGNOSIS OF PNEUMONIA—cont'd

Organism	Fever (°F)	Chills	Sputum	Chest X-ray Studies	Other Features
Bacteria—cont'd					
Haemophilus influenzae (usually type B)	Variable	Not pronounced	Purulent	Bronchopneumonia often multilobar Lobar consolidation and pleural effusion may occur	Compromised host, especially alcoholics or patients with a chronic viral infection High mortality, especially patients with hyposplenism Wheezing and dyspnea common
Klebsiella pneumoniae	Variable, often remittent 102° to 104°	Multiple	Productive Purulent, tenacious, often bloody	Upper lobe common, especially with aspiration Abscess formation common "Bulging" of lobes from swelling and necrosis	Especially alcoholic men over 40 years old; also diabetics and patients with chronic lung disease Severe pleuritic pain
Francisella tularensis (Pasteurella tularensis)	Sustained 102° to 105°	Variable Prodromal	Scanty Cough variable	Bronchopneumonia with hilar adenopathy	Agitation and tachycardia Rodent and arthropod exposure (bite, inhaled, or ingested) Dermal site of entry with lymphadenopathy

Table **31-4**

HELPFUL CLINICAL CLUES TO DIAGNOSIS OF PNEUMONIA—cont'd

Organism	Fever (°F)	Chills	Sputum	Chest X-ray Studies	Other Features
Bacteria—cont'd					
Pasteurella (Yersinia) pestis	Sudden onset 103° to 106°	Common with myalgias	Cough may be delayed Late, frothy, bloody, and runny	Bronchopneumonia, may be diffuse Hilar adenopathy common	Vague chest pain, agitation Rodent and arthropod exposure (usually airborne) Chest examination may be normal Possible hematogenous spread from obscure dermal site of entry with proximal tender bubo Fulminant and often fatal
Legionella pneumophila	Consistent High and sustained 104° to 106° in 50%	Common Intermittent and repeated	Scant or absent	Patchy, often nodular areas of consolidation Cavitation may occur	Usually during summer months in outbreaks; also sporadic Smokers with lung or renal disease; immunosupressed middle to older age group
Chlamydia pneumoniae	May be minimal	Variable	Slow onset Cough and purulent sputum	Single or multiple infiltrates	10 days of sore throat/hoarseness Abnormal breath sounds Can range from subclinical to severe pneumonia

Continued.

Table *31-4*

HELPFUL CLINICAL CLUES TO DIAGNOSIS OF PNEUMONIA—cont'd

Organism	Fever (°F)	Chills	Sputum	Chest X-ray Studies	Other Features
Bacteria—cont'd					
Chlamydia psittaci (psittacosis, ornithosis)	Usual 101° to 105°	Shaking in 30%	Cough may be delayed Scant mucoid, some blood streaking	Scattered, although mostly perihilar infiltrates not coinciding with physical examination Progressive	Bird excrement exposure Influenza-like; often self-limited Headache prominent; malaise, axial severe myalgias, delirium Often fatal when progressive Sparse physical findings Malaise, headache, myalgia, diarrhea, confusion Physical examination shows few rales
Anaerobic bacteria (many)	Variable	Variable	Foul smelling	Variable pneumonitis pattern, often involving right middle lobe or lingula Abscess and empyema common	Usually aspiration; usually polymicrobial with aerobic bacteria as well in 50% Altered consciousness, dysphagia

Table *31-4*

HELPFUL CLINICAL CLUES TO DIAGNOSIS OF PNEUMONIA—cont'd

Organism	Fever (°F)	Chills	Sputum	Chest X-ray Studies	Other Features
Bacteria—cont'd					
Mycoplasma					
Mycoplasma pneumoniae	Variable 101° to 104°	Uncommon	Usually scant or nonproductive Mucoid when present	Mostly interstitial, multicentric, perihilar, but highly variable pleural effusions may occur	Intractable cough Headache frequent, with coryza, myalgias, sinusitis, pharyngitis, otitis, and bullous myringitis Up to 20% to 40% of community-acquired pneumonia; may be epidemic Usually self-limited, but symptoms persistent Chest pain uncommon but may occur
Virus					
Influenza A	Usual 104° to 105°	Rare without bacterial superinfection	Persistent hacking Scant, may be slightly bloody	Patchy, interstitial and alveolar infiltrates May progress rapidly	Marked dyspnea, tachypnea, cyanosis Bacterial superinfection common Susceptible host in epidemic
Rickettsiae					
Rickettsia burnetii (Q fever)	Abrupt onset Up to 105° Sustained and fluctuating	Common	Slight Cough late Scant sputum	Patchy, usually perihilar	Pleurisy common late Headache and myalgia prominent Sheep, cattle, and goat exposure

Table 31-5

LABORATORY AND DIAGNOSTIC FEATURES OF PNEUMONIA

Organism	Sputum Smear	Sputum Culture	Blood Culture	WBC Count*	Other
Bacteria					
Streptococcus pneumoniae	Gram-positive, lancet-shaped diplococci, often intra-cellular, encapsulated	Usually positive, but less reliable than blood cultures	Positive in 20% to 40%	Usually up (10,000 to 30,000) Leukopenia is bad sign	PCN-resistant strains common. Most common type of pneumonia. Serotyping helpful in epidemic situations. High-risk patients should be vaccinated
Staphylococcus aureus	Often helpful—gram-positive clumps of cocci	Usually positive	When positive, suggests extra-pulmonary focus or endo-carditis	Usually up (10,000 to 30,000) Leukopenia is bad sign	Early treatment to prevent further lung destruction
Group A beta-hemolytic streptococcus	Positive, but not diagnostic in expectorated sputum	Usually positive	Often positive	Usually very high (20,000 to 30,000)	Necrotizing and fulminant
Haemophilus influenzae	Small gram-negative bipolar rods or coccobacilli	Usually positive	Usually positive	Usually high (15,000 to 30,000)	Increasing ampicillin resistance
Klebsiella pneumoniae	Short, plump, gram-negative, encapsulated rods, often paired	Usually positive	Uncommonly positive	Usually very high (20,000 to 40,000) Leukopenia is bad sign	Cavitation empyema and necrosis may require surgical intervention
Francisella tularensis	Generally not helpful (scant sputum)	Positive when cultured on blood-cysteine agar (use caution in handling)	Usually negative	May be normal or markedly elevated (20,000 to 40,000)	Specific skin test and complement fixation titers

*Per mm^3.

Table *31-5*

LABORATORY AND DIAGNOSTIC FEATURES OF PNEUMONIA—cont'd

Organism	Sputum Smear	Sputum Culture	Blood Culture	WBC Count*	Other
Bacteria—cont'd					
Pasteurella (Yersinia) pestis	Careful examination of bubo or when sputum is available reveals small gram-negative bacilli	Usually positive on blood agar	Usually positive	Moderately high with neutrophilia	Serodiagnostic tests confirm diagnosis retrospectively Often must treat before diagnosis
Legionella pneumophila	Almost always negative except with special stains of tissue	Almost always negative	Negative	Moderately high with shift to the left	Elevated erythrocyte sedimentation rate, liver enzymes; hematuria and proteinuria Diarrhea common Often fatal Serodiagnostic tests being developed Immunofluorescent staining of tissue useful Biopsy often necessary for diagnosis
Chlamydia pneumoniae	Complement fixation and microimmunofluorescence	Monoclonal antibody testing	Usually negative	Often normal	Symptoms after treatment may necessitate repeat course of treatment Associated with adult-onset asthma

*Per mm³.

Continued.

Table 31-5

LABORATORY AND DIAGNOSTIC FEATURES OF PNEUMONIA—cont'd

Organism	Sputum Smear	Sputum Culture	Blood Culture	WBC Count*	Other
Bacteria—cont'd					
Anaerobic bacteria	Multiple organisms Specimen should be obtained anaerobically without oropharyngeal contamination	Anaerobic culture techniques usually reveal multiple organisms Anaerobes are not normal flora in chronic lung disease	Occasionally positive	Variable	Must often treat associated condition
Mycoplasma					
Mycoplasma pneumoniae	Negative	Positive in 5% to 80% if proper culture techniques followed	Usually negative	Usually less than 10,000 but may be elevated in 10% to 15% of patients	Common cold hemagglutinins, hemolytic anemia Rising hemagglutinin titer Definitive diagnosis by culture and immunofluorescent antibody titers
Virus					
Influenza	Positive only with bacterial superinfection	Negative except with special viral cultures	Negative except with special cultures	Moderate elevation common (10,000 to 20,000) with lymphocytosis	Cold agglutinins may be positive Throat swab may reveal virus for culture Serodiagnosis may be useful

*Per mm^3.

Pneumonia

Inflammation of the pulmonary parenchyma may result from bacterial, viral, fungal, mycoplasmal, rickettsial, or parasitic pathogens. Viral pneumonia is by far the most common, and *S. pneumoniae* remains a significant pathogen in bacterial pneumonia. The responsible pathogen is never defined in up to 50% of all cases.

Clinical presentation

Typically patients have fever, a nonproductive cough, and some respiratory discomfort. This mild viral-type illness often progresses with accompanying secondary infection; patients may have dyspnea, fever, tachypnea, pleuritic chest pain, shaking chills, and a cough productive of purulent or rusty sputum. On physical examination, patients are variably ill and toxic with elevated temperatures. Splinting on the affected side, dullness to percussion, increasing fremitus, egophony, coarse rales, and bronchial breath sounds may be noted on physical examination.

Factors contributing to severity of infection include the patient being over age 65; underlying conditions such as diabetes, chronic obstructive lung disease, chronic renal failure, and alcoholism; musculoskeletal abnormalities; suspected aspiration; and forms of immunosuppression such as a postsplenectomy state and AIDS.

Assessment

Clinical clues (Table 31-4) and laboratory evaluations (Table 31-5) provide parameters in determining suggested causes and treatment plans.

Expectorated sputum is inconsistently reliable because of the uneven distribution of pathogens, the overlooking of fastidious pathogens, deficiencies in the processing of specimens, and previous antibiotic therapy. Only bronchoscopic techniques and percutaneous transtracheal aspiration are reliable. Such invasive techniques may be indicated in immunocompromised patients, those failing to respond, and those with suspected aspiration or superinfection and hospital-acquired infections. Consider tuberculosis in all patients with pulmonary infiltrates.

Management

Treatment should focus on assessment and stabilization of respiratory distress. Focus on the adequacy of the airway and ventilation, followed by assurance that hydration status is normal. Use antibiotic therapy for most bacterial pneumonias, as well as rickettsial, mycobacterial, mycoplasmal, *Pneumocystis carnii,* and some fungal disease. Pneumococcal pneumonia remains the most common and treatable, but penicillin is no longer the drug of choice (see the boxes on pp. 376 and 377).

Other treatment modalities include tracheobronchial toilet (encouraging coughing, suction, postural drainage), drainage of abscess, supportive care, and monitoring of respiratory status. Admit patients who are over age 65, as well as those with respiratory distress or failure; toxicity; underlying conditions such as chronic obstructive pulmonary disease (COPD), multilobar infections, hypoxemia, or splenectomy; immunocompromise; and complicated disease.

OUTPATIENT PNEUMONIA WITHOUT COMORBIDITY AND 60 YEARS OF AGE OR YOUNGER[*†]

Organisms
  S. pneumoniae
  M. pneumoniae
  Respiratory viruses
    C. pneumoniae
    H. influenzae
  Miscellaneous
    Legionella organisms, *S. aureus,*
    M. tuberculosis, endemic fungi, aerobic
    gram-negative bacilli
Therapy
  Macrolide[‡]
  OR
  Tetracycline[§]

From ATS Board of Directors: American Thoracic Society
Statement, *Am Rev Respir Dis,* vol. 148, pp. 1418-1426, 1993.
[*]Excludes patients at risk for HIV.
[†]In roughly one third to one half of the cases no etiology
was identified.
[‡]Erythromycin. The newer macrolides, clarithromycin or
azithromycin, should be considered in those intolerant of
erythromycin, and in smokers (to treat *H. influenzae*).
[§]Many isolates of *S. pneumoniae* are resistant to
tetracycline, and it should be used only if the patient is
allergic to or intolerant of macrolides.

OUTPATIENT PNEUMONIA WITH COMORBIDITY AND/OR 60 YEARS OF AGE OR OLDER[*†]

Organisms
  S. pneumoniae
  Respiratory viruses
    H. influenzae
  Aerobic gram-negative bacilli
    S. aureus
  Miscellaneous
    Moraxella catarrhalis, Legionella
    organisms, *M. tuberculosis,* endemic
    fungi
Therapy
  Second-generation cephalosporin
  OR
  TMP/SMX
  OR
  Beta-lactam/beta-lactamase inhibitor
  ±
  Erythromycin or other macrolide[‡]

From ATS Board of Directors: American Thoracic Society
Statement, *Am Rev Respir Dis,* vol. 148, pp. 1418-1426, 1993.
[*]Excludes patients at risk for HIV.
[†]In roughly one third to one half of the cases no etiology
was identified.
[‡]If infection with *Legionella* organisms is a concern.

HOSPITALIZED PATIENTS WITH COMMUNITY-ACQUIRED PNEUMONIA[*][†]

Organisms
  S. pneumoniae
  H. influenzae
  Polymicrobial (including anaerobic
  bacteria)
  Aerobic gram-negative bacilli
  Legionella organisms
  S. aureus
  C. pneumoniae
  Respiratory viruses
  Miscellaneous
      M. pneumoniae, Moraxella catarrhalis,
      M. tuberculosis, endemic fungi
Therapy
  Second- or third-generation cephalosporin[‡]
  OR
  Beta-lactam/beta-lactamase inhibitor
  ±
  Macrolide[§]

From ATS Board of Directors: American Thoracic Society Statement, *Am Rev Respir Dis,* vol. 148, pp. 1418-1426, 1993.
[*]Excludes patients at risk for HIV.
[†]In roughly one third to one half of the cases no etiology was identified.
[‡]See comments about third-generation cephalosporins in text.
[§]Use a macrolide if infection with *Legionella* organisms is a concern; rifampin may be added if *Legionella* organism is documented.

SEVERE HOSPITALIZED COMMUNITY-ACQUIRED PNEUMONIA[*][†]

Organisms
  S. pneumoniae
  Legionella organisms
  Aerobic gram-negative bacilli
  M. pneumoniae
  Respiratory viruses
  Miscellaneous
      H. influenzae, M. tuberculosis
      Endemic fungi
Therapy
  Macrolide[‡]
                PLUS
  Third-generation cephalosporin with anti-*Pseudomonas* activity[§]
                OR
  Other antipseudomonal agents such as imipenem-cilastatin, ciprofloxacin

From ATS Board of Directors: American Thoracic Society Statement, *Am Rev Respir Dis,* vol. 148, pp. 1418-1426, 1993.
[*]Excludes patients at risk for HIV.
[†]In roughly one third to one half of the cases no etiology was identified.
[‡]Rifampin may be added if *Legionella* organism is documented.
[§]Although uncommon because of high mortality associated with *P. aeruginosa* pneumonia, an aminoglycoside should be added, at least for the first few days of treatment, whether one is using a third-generation cephalosporin, imipenem, or ciprofloxacin.

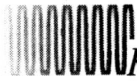

KEY CONSIDERATIONS

WHAT IS THE LIFE THREAT?

Epiglottitis, peritonsillar abscess, retropharyngeal abscess, parapharyngeal abscess, and infection of the floor of the mouth (Ludwig's angina) can cause airway compromise that is life threatening. Airway assessment and stabilization are key considerations in patients with such conditions. Pneumonia can be life threatening, especially in those who are immunocompromised. Patients with shortness of breath, cough, fever, or chest pain should be assessed for adequacy of oxygenation, including pulse oximetry; such patients should receive supplemental oxygen if necessary.

DOES THE PATIENT NEED ADMISSION?

Admission is usually required for treatment of pneumonia in the elderly, those who are immunocompromised, and those with diabetes, alcoholism, or severe COPD. Other patients with hypoxemia and pneumonia require admission. Patients with impending airway compromise require admission and intubation or close observation depending on the degree of compromise and the underlying condition.

WHAT IS THE MOST SERIOUS DIAGNOSIS?

Impending upper airway obstruction from infection or impaired ventilation and oxygenation from lung infection constitutes a life threat.

HAVE I PERFORMED A THOROUGH WORK-UP?

Obtain throat and sputum cultures as needed.

Consider a sputum Gram stain in the assessment of pneumonia.

Consider epiglottitis, peritonsillar abscess, retropharyngeal abscess, and peripharyngeal abscess in patients with a sore throat.

Recommended Reading

Brillman JC, Quenzer RW: *Infectious disease in emergency medicine,* Boston, 1992, Little, Brown, & Co.

Mabry RL: Therapeutic agents in the medical management of sinusitis. In Rice DH, editor: *Inflammatory diseases of the sinuses: the otolaryngologic clinics of North America,* Philadelphia, 1993, WB Saunders.

Niederman MS et al: Guidelines in the initial management of adults with community-acquired pneumonia: diagnosis, assessment of severity and initial antimicrobial therapy. *Am Rev Respir Dis* 148:1418-1426, 1993.

Vukmir RB: Adult and pediatric pharyngitis: a review, *J Emerg Med* 10:607-616, 1992.

Wallace RJ: Lower respiratory tract infections, *Infect Dis Clin North Am* 5:3, Philadelphia 1991, WB Saunders.

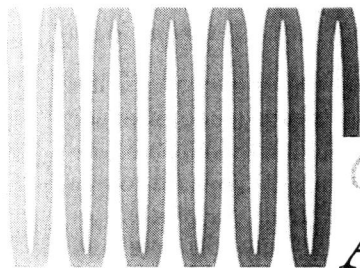

Chapter Thirty-two

ACUTE ADULT ASTHMA AND EXACERBATIONS OF CHRONIC OBSTRUCTIVE PULMONARY DISEASE

RICHARD M. NOWAK AND CHARLES L. EMERMAN

ACUTE ADULT ASTHMA

The most recent definition of asthma is that found in the National Asthma Education and Prevention Program's Guidelines for the Diagnosis and Management of Asthma. According to this source, asthma is a lung disease with the following characteristics: (1) airway obstruction (or airway narrowing) that is fully or incompletely reversible either spontaneously or with treatment, (2) airway inflammation, and (3) airway hyperresponsiveness to a variety of stimuli.

Asthma affects approximately 5% of the United States population, or approximately 10 to 15 million persons; its prevalence, mortality, and morbidity is increasing. In 1990 it was estimated that 1.8 million people with asthma visited emergency departments for treatment of acute exacerbations of the disease. The direct and indirect costs (e.g., loss of work days) related to asthma in 1990 have been estimated to be 6.2 billion dollars.

Pathophysiology of Exacerbations

Airflow obstruction is determined by the diameter of the airway lumen and can be affected by numerous factors, including airway smooth muscle contraction and hypertrophy, edema of the bronchial wall, and mucus production. The initiating events are thought to be inflammatory. An initial trigger may cause the release of inflammatory mediators from bronchial mast cells, macrophages, and epithelial cells. This release produces an inflammatory infiltrate composed of eosinophils and neutrophils with release of leukotrienes and results in epithelial injury, abnormalities in neural mechanisms, increases in airway smooth muscle responsiveness, and airflow obstruction.

Airway inflammation is an important factor that causes airway hyperresponsiveness (exaggerated bronchoconstrictor responses) to many physical, chemical, and pharmacologic agents (e.g., allergens, environmental irritants, viral respiratory infections, cold air, exercise).

Clinical Presentation

Most patients with acute exacerbations of asthma experience a constellation of symptoms that consist of coughing, dyspnea, and wheezing. Coughing often starts early in an attack and may be the major complaint in association with shortness of breath (cough-equivalent asthma). Dyspnea is present and may not correlate to the severity of the airway obstructions. Wheezing depends on air movement velocity and turbulence. With severe airway obstruction, wheezing vanishes because there is insufficient air movement velocity to produce turbulence.

Ascertaining a pertinent past history is important because patients tend to have similar acute courses. Therefore their past patterns help with decision making concerning therapy and admission.

Severely ill patients may have tachycardia, tachypnea, or diaphoresis; may be unable to lie supine; and may be using the accessory muscles

of respiration. However, the absence of such signs does not rule out the existence of major flow limitations. The current increases in morbidity and mortality are possibly related to the underestimation of the severity of symptoms of an acute exacerbation by both patients and physicians, which results in inadequate and delayed treatments.

Not all wheezing is necessarily asthma related. The wheezing patient requires a broad differential diagnosis as listed in the box at left.

Clinical Assessment

The severity of the current airflow obstruction and its response to therapy must be assessed. Many indices can be used to diagnose severe asthma (see the box below) but measurement

DIFFERENTIAL DIAGNOSIS OF WHEEZING

Acute exacerbations of COPD
Allergic or anaphylactic reactions
Carcinoid tumors
Cardiac asthma (congestive heart failure with wheezing as the predominant manifestation)
Chemical irritants, insecticides, and cholinergic drugs
Endobronchial disease
  Bronchial stenosis
  Foreign body inhalation
  Neoplasm
Eosinophilic pneumonias
Invasive worm infestation
Pulmonary embolus
Upper airway obstruction
  Foreign body inhalation
  Laryngeal edema
  Neoplasm

INDICES OF ACUTELY SEVERE ASTHMA IN ADULTS

Symptoms
Severe breathlessness and wheezing
Difficulty speaking
Syncope or near syncope

Physical findings
Pulsus paradoxus that does not change with therapy
Use of accessory muscles of respiration
Diaphoresis; inability to lie supine
Heart rate >120 beats/minute
Respiratory rate >30 breaths/minute

Expiratory flow
FEV_1 or PEFR <40% baseline (predicted or personal best)
Failure to improve expiratory flow by ≥10% after initial treatment

Arterial blood gases/oximetry
O_2 saturation <90%
PaO_2 ≤60 mm Hg or $PaCO_2$ ≥40 mm Hg

of expiratory flow using the peak expiratory flow rate (PEFR) or forced expiratory volume in 1 second (FEV_1) is the most useful test. Decisions to draw arterial blood gases or to use pulse oximetry can be guided by expiratory flow measurements. A patient will not be hypercarbic ($PaCO_2 > 42$ mm Hg) or markedly hypoxemic ($PaO_2 < 60$ mm Hg) unless such measurements are less than 25% to 30% of the predicted or the patient's personal best values.

Chest x-ray studies should be ordered if there are clinical signs of asthma complications such as pneumonia, pneumothorax, or pneumomediastinum. Patients who are sick enough to be admitted to the hospital may have clinically unrecognized infiltrate or atelectasis, which is detectable on an admission chest x-ray film. If a patient is on chronic theophylline therapy, a theophylline level needs to be obtained, and appropriate adjustments in dosage need to be made. Therapeutic levels are 5 to 15 µg/ml. A complete blood count is of no value in the overall assessment. However, given the increasing dosages of ß-agonists now used to treat exacerbations of this disease with their known side effect of inducing hypokalemia, it may be prudent to measure the serum potassium level.

Management of the Acute Attack

The principal goals of treating the acute attack are to abort the symptoms of the episode and to pre-

Table *32-1*

INITIAL ASSESSMENTS/TREATMENTS

Measurement/Therapy	Severe	Moderate	Mild
PEFR, FEV_1 % predicted or personal best	Unable or <40%	40%-60%	>60%
Supplemental O_2	Yes	As needed	As needed
ß-agonist therapy, wet nebulization of albuterol	2.5-5.0 mg every 20-30 minutes × 3, (continuous if necessary, especially in intubated patients)	2.5 mg every 20-30 minutes × 3	2.5 mg, may repeat another 2 times if necessary
Corticosteroids	Methylprednisolone 60-125 mg IV **or** Hydrocortisone 200-500 mg IV	Same as for severe asthma **or** Prednisone 60 mg po	Consider steroids in same dosages if not rapidly responding to ß-agonists or if already on oral steroids
Anticholinergic therapy, wet nebulization of ipratropium bromide	0.5 mg mixed with ß-agonist inhalation therapies	May be helpful in some cases	Not indicated
Magnesium sulfate 2-3 g IV at 1 g/minute rate	If not responding and continuing to deteriorate, consider in conjunction with aggressive ß-agonist therapy	Not indicated	Not indicated

vent progression to a more severe, life-threatening situation. For those with obvious respiratory failure and for those who are fatiguing, immediate intubation and mechanical ventilation should be instituted as soon as possible. Otherwise, the aggressiveness of the therapeutic approach depends on the severity of the exacerbation as reflected mainly by the expiratory flow parameters (Table 32-1). The inhalation of selective β_2-agonists is the cornerstone of therapy, and the dosages used continue to escalate with no set maximum yet determined. Medications delivered to patients from metered-dose inhalers using spacer devices often produce bronchodilatation that is equivalent to that produced by nebulization. The optimal way to deliver inhaled medications is under continued investigation; until further developments, wet nebulization is considered the treatment of choice in patients with severe exacerbations of asthma. Albuterol is the drug of choice for the majority of emergency physicians. Corticosteroids, either intravenously (IV) or by mouth, are given to the majority of patients to suppress airway inflammation, whereas anticholinergic therapy (Atrovent) is reserved for those with the most severe airway obstruction. With severe asthma, intravenous magnesium sulfate may cause a short period of bronchodilatation.

After the initial treatments, patients are graded into good, incomplete, or poor responses or respiratory failure, and treatments are continued as outlined in Table 32-2. Decisions to admit or discharge are driven mainly by the expiratory flow measurements.

Many drugs may decrease or increase theophylline clearance, which predisposes patients to toxic or subtherapeutic effects. Drugs that may in-

Table 32-2

CONTINUING THERAPY BASED ON RESPONSES TO INITIAL TREATMENTS

Response	Therapy
Good (PEFR, FEV$_1$ ≥ 70%)*	Observe 30-60 minutes. Discharge with close medical follow-up and on appropriate outpatient medications.
Incomplete (PEFR, FEV$_1$ >40 but <70%)	Continue inhaled ß-agonists hourly. Consider subcutaneous epinephrine (.3 mg 1/1000 s-cut) or terbutaline (.25 mg s-cut). Continue clinical and objective monitoring every 30-60 minutes. At 4 hours reassess; if now >70%, discharge home; if now >40% but <70%, make clinical decision to admit or discharge using historical and psychosocial information.
Poor (PEFR, FEV$_1$ <40%)	Continue as with incomplete response. At 4 hours reassess; if still <40%, admit to hospital; if now >40% but <70%, make clinical decision as with incomplete response; if >70%, discharge home as with good response.
Respiratory Failure (PEFR, FEV$_1$ <25%) and (Paco$_2$ ≥ 40 mm Hg)	Admit to Intensive Care Unit. Consider endotracheal intubation, ventilatory support, and sedation/muscle paralysis.

*All PEFR, FEV$_1$ % indicate predicted or personal best.

crease serum levels include allopurinol, cimetidine, thiabendazole, propranolol, and macrolide antibiotics (erythromycin, troleandomycin). Drugs that may decrease levels include carbamazepine, isoproterenol, phenobarbitol, phenytoin, rifampin, and marijuana (smoked). If the patient has been on chronic theophylline, guided therapy is used to optimize the measured serum level. Each milligram per kilogram of administered loading dose of aminophylline increases the serum theophylline level by approximately 2 µg/ml.

Management of the Intubated/Mechanically Ventilated Patient With Asthma

With the exception of apnea or coma, there are no absolute indications for intubation and immediate institution of ventilatory support. Relative indications include persistent hypercarbia or normal or elevating $PaCO_2$ levels in a patient with dyspnea, as well as exhaustion, depression of mental status, and continuing poor or decreasing pulmonary function values.

In preparation for endotracheal intubation, most emergency physicians choose to sedate and paralyze patients. Ketamine is a very useful agent

---

INSTRUCTIONS FOR METERED-DOSE INHALER (MDI) USE

1. Remove cap from the MDI container.
2. Assemble the MDI and hold it upright.
3. Shake the canister.
4. Place the mouthpiece loosely between the teeth (or hold it 3-4 cm in front of the open mouth).
5. Exhale fully (to functional residual capacity).
6. Actuate the inhaler at the beginning of a slow and full inhalation (as if "sipping hot soup") over 5-6 seconds.
7. Hold breath for at least 10 seconds.
8. Wait 1 minute before reuse.

---

because it has a bronchodilating effect. Once the endotracheal tube is in place, the strategy for ventilator management should be to maintain oxygenation while limiting peak inspiratory pressures (<50 cm H_2O), barotrauma, and the development of the auto–positive end-expiratory pressure phenomenon, even if this results in elevated $PaCO_2$ levels (permissive hypercapnia). Thus ventilator settings need to be at a long expiratory time (inspiration:expiration <1:2), a low tidal volume (<10 ml/kg), and a low ventilator rate (<10 cycles/minute). Today mortality rates for mechanically-ventilated patients with asthma should be low in spite of the obvious severity of the disease.

If at any time a patient with asthma has a *sudden* cardiac arrest, bilateral chest tubes should be placed while appropriate life-saving measures are being taken and without prior chest x-ray study because pneumothorax is a complication of asthma.

Discharge Planning

All discharged patients must continue inhaled ß-agonist regimens because ongoing inflammation and peripheral airway obstruction are going to be present for several days. Physicians should ascertain how patients are using their metered-dose inhalers (MDI) because ineffective usage results in inadequate medication delivery (see the box at left). If there is a persistent problem with "hand-lung coordination," the use of a self-actuated MDI should be considered. Currently in the United States there is only one such MDI available (pirbuterol [Maxair] 200 µg/puff).

Almost all patients, except those with mild and rapidly responsive asthma, should receive a tapered course of oral corticosteroids over several days. An example is 60 mg initial dose of prednisone that decreases over several days to none. If the patient has an overall symptom frequency of coughing and wheezing more than 1 to 2 times/week (lasting a few days, requiring occasional emergency care, and affecting sleep

Table 32-3

INHALED STEROID THERAPY OPTIONS

Drug	Dosage Options	
Beclomethasone dipropionate (Vanceril; Beclovent)	42 µg/puff, 8-20 puffs/day	qid dosing
Flunisolide (Aerobid)	250 µg/puff, 4-8 puffs/day	bid dosing
Triamcinolone acetonide (Azmacort)	100 µg/puff, 8-16 puffs/day	qid dosing

and general activity), he or she requires antiinflammatory therapy on a chronic basis. Inhaled corticosteroid therapy is optimal, and the options available are listed in Table 32-3. This type of patient might require additional chronic therapy such as a long-acting ß-agonist (salmeterol [Serevent]), an oral theophylline product, or an oral ß-agonist.

Patients with severe ongoing symptoms such as daily wheezing, frequent nocturnal awakening, and marked limitation of activity require oral steroids on a daily basis.

Discharged patients should have close (2 to 3 day) outpatient follow-up and should also be encouraged to obtain a peak flow meter, to create a daily peak flow rate diary, and to develop with their physician a home medication strategy on the basis of changes in peak flow measurements. These actions allow optimal patient care, which results in better overall asthma control and fewer visits to the emergency department.

Asthma and Pregnancy

Uncontrolled asthma during pregnancy has been associated with maternal complications (preeclampsia, gestational hypertension, hyperemesis, vaginal hemorrhage, eclampsia, induced and complicated labors) and fetal complications (increased risk of perinatal mortality, intrauterine growth retardation, preterm birth, low birth weight, neonatal hypoxemia). Goals of management involve controlling the disease and rapidly

correcting exacerbations. Oxygenation is thus maintained while preventing harm to the fetus.

Pregnant patients coming to the emergency department for acute exacerbations are to be aggressively treated in a similar manner to nonpregnant patients, with the following caveats:

1. The combination of hypoxemia and respiratory alkalosis commonly seen can have serious detrimental affects on the fetus. Therefore supplemental oxygen should be routinely delivered to maintain arterial oxygen saturations of ≥95%, especially during the last trimester when there is normally a physiologic decrease in arterial Po_2.

2. The Collaborative Perinatal Project showed a significant rise in the incidence of congenital malformations in mothers who received epinephrine; therefore it is prudent to avoid using this agent.

3. Immediate antepartum fetal assessment (continuous electronic fetal heart-rate monitoring) is indicated in asthma exacerbations with an incomplete or poor response to therapy or with significant maternal hypoxemia.

Because asthma creates a high-risk pregnancy, it is imperative for the mother to have close prenatal care.

CHRONIC OBSTRUCTIVE PULMONARY DISEASE

Chronic obstructive pulmonary disease (COPD) is a syndrome that includes patients with emphysema, chronic bronchitis, or chronic airflow limitation, either alone or in combination. Emphysema is manifested by destruction of the alveolar structure. Patients with emphysema have long thin chests with evidence of lung hyperexpansion. On physical examination, the lung is hyperresonant and the diaphragm is depressed. Chronic bronchitis is defined as sputum production for 2 years in a row for at least 3 months out of the year. Chronic airflow limitation is demonstrated by persistent abnormalities during pulmonary function testing. Most patients develop COPD as a consequence of cigarette smoking. Occasionally, patients may develop COPD as a result of genetic factors, environmental exposure, or occupational exposure.

Initial Evaluation

The initial evaluation of the patient with an acute exacerbation of COPD may be limited by the patient's respiratory distress. At some point during the evaluation, the patient should be questioned to determine potential precipitating causes for the exacerbation, baseline medications, results of prior therapy, and the presence of co-existing diseases. Exacerbations may be caused by a variety of causes, including pulmonary infection, pneumothorax, pulmonary embolism, or exposure to noxious substances. The patient should be questioned to determine the types and dosages of current medications; an assessment of the patient's compliance with medical therapy should also be made. Because many older patients have difficulty coordinating the use of metered-dose inhalers, the patient's method of using this type of inhaler should be reviewed. Additional questions should be directed at other medication use, including the history of steroid use. Finally, the patient should be questioned about frequency of emergency department visits, hospitalizations, and ICU admissions. Previous intubations may be an indication of a high-risk patient.

The clinical evaluation should be directed at assessing the severity of the patient's illness and

BACTERIAL CAUSES OF BRONCHITIS IN COPD
Haemophilus influenzae *Haemophilus parainfluenzae* *Streptococcus pneumoniae* *Branhamella catarrhalis* *Chlamydia* organisms

identifying precipitating co-existing factors such as bronchitis (see the box above) or inhalation of noxious stimuli. The presence of jugular vein distension, rales, and peripheral edema may indicate congestive heart failure or may be a consequence of cor pulmonale. The extremities should be inspected for evidence of deep venous thrombosis because pulmonary embolus may also be present with dyspnea. The lung examination should be directed at finding evidence of consolidation or pneumothorax.

Diagnostic Testing

Diagnostic testing is used to assess the severity of distress and to identify precipitating factors. Approximately 15% of all patients with an acute exacerbation of COPD have abnormalities on chest x-ray film. It is difficult to predict the presence of radiographic abnormalities; therefore most patients should receive an x-ray examination as part of the evaluation. Arterial blood gases are useful in guiding therapy and in identifying patients who are at risk for respiratory failure. Pulse oximetry is useful in identifying patients who are markedly desaturated, as well as in following the course of therapy. Physicians perform poorly in estimating the degree of airway obstruction. Spirometry or peak-flow measurements should be obtained initially, during therapy, and as part of the disposition decision. The advantage of measuring peak-flow rates is that the test is easier to perform in acutely ill pa-

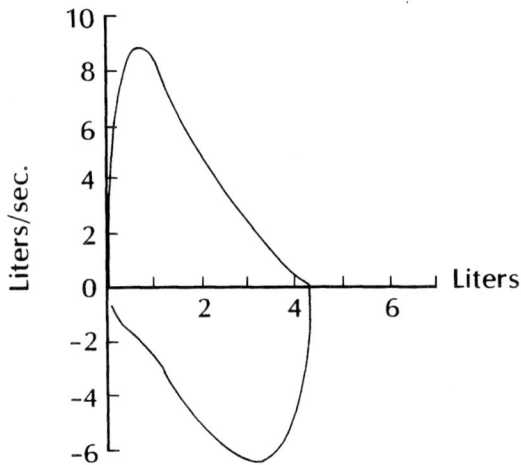

Fig.32-1 Normal flow volume loop demonstrating initial expiration and volume limited flow. The expiratory loop on the upper half of the graph has a sharp spike, which demonstrates good initial effort. A poor tracing might show a rounded upward curve with a jagged tracing caused by coughing or a sudden termination caused by an interrupted exhalation.

tients and is easy to teach to ancillary personnel; the devices used to measure peak flow are also inexpensive and portable. The disadvantage of peak-flow measurements is that the PEFR is highly effort dependent. Spirometry can be performed in the emergency department with computerized and relatively inexpensive equipment. The FEV_1 is the most commonly followed parameter and is more effort independent than is PEFR. Examination of the flow-volume loops can help differentiate between restrictive and obstructive lung disease (Figs. 32-1, 32-2, 32-3). The patient with obstructive lung disease has a concave-up appearance on the flow-volume curve in addition to a depressed FEV_1 and FEV_1/forced vital capacity (FVC) ratio. The patient with a primarily restrictive disease has a depressed FEV_1, but the FEV_1/FVC ratio is normal.

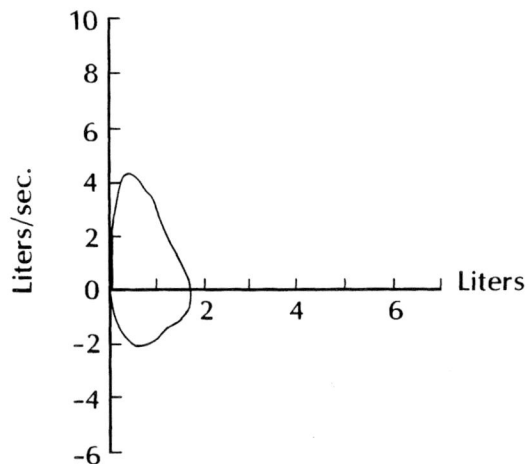

Fig.32-2 Flow volume loop showing obstructive pattern with concave-up appearance. The concave-up appearance reflects airway collapse during exhalation. With treatment, these changes may reverse.

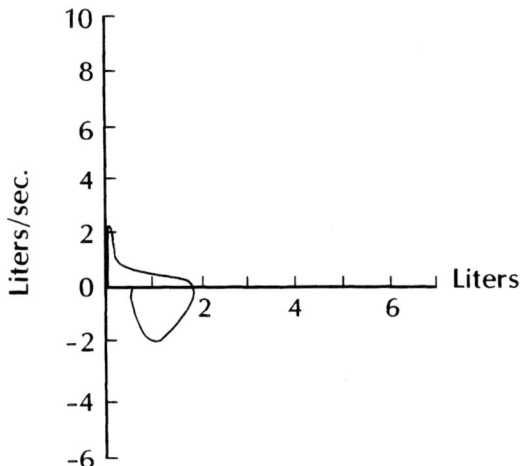

Fig.32-3 Flow volume loop demonstrating restrictive pattern with decreased flow and expired volume. Many patients with an acute exacerbation of COPD initially have this pattern because of chest wall pain from prolonged coughing. This pattern may also change with treatment if it is a result of these causes.

Treatment

Treatment of the patient with an acute exacerbation of COPD is initiated with aerosolized ß-adrenergic agents (see the box below). Albuterol is long lasting and $ß_2$ selective. Subcutaneous administration of terbutaline or epinephrine may be considered in patients who are severely obstructed, who are uncooperative, or who are unable to coordinate the use of the nebulizer. There is little evidence to support the routine use of other agents in managing patients with an acute exacerbation of COPD. In patients who fail to respond to ß-adrenergic therapy, consideration should be given to adding an anticholinergic agent. Ipratropium, atropine, and glycopyrrolate have all been studied for use in acute exacerbations of COPD. Aminophylline has not been shown to influence the course of emergency department therapy for a large number of patients; however, in patients with severe respiratory distress it may be reasonable to add this drug to the regimen. All patients with an acute exacerbation of COPD should receive oxygen therapy. Patients with chronic CO_2 retention may be susceptible to hypercarbia. For many years hypercarbia was thought to be a result of depression of the central respiratory center, but now it is recognized that a ventilation/perfusion mismatch may be an important cause of hypercarbia. In these patients, controlled oxygen therapy with a Venturi mask should be initiated with careful monitoring by pulse oximetry and arterial blood gases. The use of magnesium sulfate has not been studied in large numbers of patients with COPD, but again it should be reserved for patients in severe respiratory distress or respiratory failure. Steroids have not been found to influence the course of emergency department therapy in patients with COPD. There are studies that indicate that steroids may be useful over the course of 24 to 48 hours for hospitalized patients with an acute exacerbation of COPD.

EVALUATION AND MANAGEMENT OF ACUTE EXACERBATION OF COPD

Initial evaluation

Chest x-ray examination, arterial blood gases, spirometry, or peak flow measurement

Initial treatment

Oxygen therapy 2-3 L/minute by nasal cannula (note use 24% to 28% ventimask in patients with chronic CO_2 retention)
Aerosolized beta-agonist q 20-30 minutes
Albuterol 0.5% 0.5 ml in 2 ml normal saline
Give hourly after first three treatments

Additional therapy (if needed)

Epinephrine 0.3 ml and subcutaneously, may repeat twice q 30 minutes **or**
Terbutaline 0.25 ml subcutaneously, may repeat once in 30 minutes
Ipratroprium 500 µg by aerosol **or**
Glycopyrrolate 2 mg in 10 ml normal saline
Methylprednisolone 80-120 mg IV (most useful in patients being admitted)
Aminophylline 5.6 mg/kg if theophylline level is 0; otherwise loading dose is calculated as
    0.5 mg/kg × (10 − theophylline level)
Magnesium sulfate 1-2 g IV over 10 to 20 minutes (should be reserved for patients in respiratory failure)

Ventilatory Management

Occasionally patients may require intubation for drug-resistant respiratory failure. Intubation for these patients should be preceded by oxygenation using the bag-valve-mask technique. After intubation, therapy should be continued via ß-agonist agents administered through the endotracheal tube. A newer therapy that is currently being studied involves the use of nasal biphasic airway pressure (Bipap). This form of ventilation requires careful patient selection and education. The role of Bipap is not yet clear, but it may provide an alternative to intubation in selected patients.

Disposition

Patients may be discharged from the emergency department if they have demonstrated an im-

INDICATIONS FOR ADMISSIONS IN COPD
Continued dyspnea
Respiratory failure
PO_2 <50 mm Hg
PCO_2 >45 mm Hg with pH <7.36
Posttreatment FEV_1 or PEFR <40% predicted normal (some patients with chronic airflow limitation may be discharged with PFT <40% if they no longer have dyspnea)
Posttreatment FEV_1 or PEFR <65% of baseline
Pneumonia
Pneumothorax

Table 32-4

ANTIBIOTICS FOR BRONCHITIS

Drug	Dose	Frequency	Comments
Amoxicillin	250 mg	tid	May not cover beta-lactamase–producing *H influenzae*
Trimethoprim/ Sulfamethoxazole	Fixed dose	bid	Bacteriostatic
Erythromycin	250 mg	qid	High incidence of gastrointestinal effects; interferes with theophylline metabolism
Tetracycline	250 mg	qid	Bacteriostatic
Azithromycin	250 mg	2 tablets first dose; then 1/day	Broad coverage
Cefaclor	500 mg	tid	*B catarrhalis* commonly resistant
Cefuroxime	500 mg	bid	Slightly better coverage against *B. catarrhalis* and *H influenzae* over other second-generation cephalosporins such as cefprozil and loracarbef
Cefixime	400 mg	1/day	Effective against beta-lactamase–producing organisms
Ciprofloxacin	500 mg	bid	Good coverage against *H. influenzae* and *B catarrhalis*
Amoxicillin/ clavulanate	500 mg	tid	Good coverage against beta-lactamase-producing organisms

provement in their pulmonary function and relief of dyspnea (see the box on p. 388). Patients are generally safe for discharge if their FEV_1 is at least 40% of predicted normal or if they no longer have dyspnea. Alternatively, improvement in pulmonary function may be measured against the baseline FEV_1, using 65% of baseline as the target for discharge. Discharge planning should include a review of the patient's medication along with the patient's techniques for using metered-dose inhalers. Patients with purulent sputum production should receive broad-spectrum antibiotics (Table 32-4). There is little evidence to suggest that any one antibiotic leads to a better outcome than another. Inexpensive regimens such as trimethoprim sulfamethoxazole lack the extensive coverage of newer antibiotics such as azithromycin or cefixime, but there is little evidence to suggest a difference in clinical efficacy. Theophylline can be added to the patient's regimen if he or she has difficulty coordinating the use of the metered-dose inhaler or is otherwise on maximum therapy. Similarly, ipratropium may be beneficial for patients with COPD. Steroid therapy should be considered for selected patients who have a history of frequent relapses, have a combined diagnosis of asthma and COPD, or have been demonstrated in the past to be responsive to steroids.

KEY CONSIDERATIONS

WHAT IS THE LIFE THREAT?

A severe asthma attack can cause such a decreased airflow through the bronchi that the process is life threatening.

Severe chronic obstructive pulmonary disease (COPD) may result in death. Special attention should be devoted to causes of exacerbation of dyspnea in COPD, including pneumonia, pneumothorax, or pulmonary embolism.

DOES THE PATIENT NEED ADMISSION?

Admission of the patient with asthma depends on the response to treatment, including the measured peak expiratory flow rate (PEFR). Patients with a peak expiratory flow rate less than 25% of predicted despite treatment require admission to the ICU and possibly intubation. Patients with persistent PEFRs between 40% and 70% despite treatment should be considered for admission; the decision should be based on historical and psychosocial situations. The elderly, the immunocompromised, and those who have required intubation in the past deserve admission. Those living alone or without social supports should also be considered for hospitalization. Patients with a persistently low Po_2 or elevated Po_2 compared to baseline also require admission.

WHAT IS THE MOST SERIOUS DIAGNOSIS?

Serious diagnoses are severe hypoxemia resulting from severe asthma or severe COPD. Pneumonia can seriously exacerbate asthma and COPD. If the patient has dyspnea, consider other life-threatening processes such as myocardial infarction, pulmonary embolus, or pneumothorax.

HAVE I PERFORMED A THOROUGH WORK-UP?

Assess the patient's history of airway disease, and perform a physical examination. Measure PEFR and oxygen saturation by pulse oximetry. Obtain arterial blood gases as needed to assess severity; determine therapy and assess the need for admission.

Recommended Reading

American Thoracic Society: Standards for the Diagnosis and Care of Patients with Chronic Obstructive Pulmonary Disease (COPD) and Asthma, *Am Rev Respir Dis* 136:225-243, 1987.

Canadian Association of Emergency Physicians, Lung Association, and Thoracic Society: *Guidelines for the Emergency Management of Adult Asthma,* Emergency Department Poster.

Emerman CL, Cydulka RK: Evaluation of high yield criteria for chest radiography in acute exacerbation of COPD, *Ann Emerg Med* 22:680-684, 1993.

Emerman CL, Effron D, Lukens TW: Spirometric criteria for hospital admission of patients with acute exacerbation of COPD, *Chest* 99:595-599, 1994.

Ferguson GT, Cherniack RM: Management of chronic obstructive pulmonary disease, *N Engl J Med* 328:1017-1022, 1993.

Francis PB: Acute respiratory failure in obstructive lung disease, *Med Clin North Am* 67:657-667, 1983.

McFadden ER: Evaluating concepts in the pathogenesis and management of asthma, *Adv Intern Med* 39:357-394, 1994.

McFadden ER, Gilbert IA: Asthma, *N Engl J Med* 327:1928-1937, 1992.

National Asthma Education Program: *Guidelines for the diagnosis and management of asthma,* National Heart, Lung, and Blood Institute, Bethesda, Md, 1991; Publication No 91-3042.

National Asthma Education Program: *Management of asthma during pregnancy,* National Heart, Lung, and Blood Institute, Bethesda, Md, 1993; Publication No 93-3279.

Nowak RM, Tokarski GF: Adult acute asthma. In Rosen P et al, editors: *Emergency medicine: concepts and clinical practice,* ed 3, St Louis, 1992, Mosby.

Schmidt GA, Hall JB: Acute or chronic respiratory failure: assessment and management of patients with COPD in the emergency setting, *JAMA* 261:3444-3453, 1989.

Weiss KG, Gergen PJ, Hodgson TA: An economic evaluation of asthma in the United States, *N Engl J Med* 326:862-866, 1992.

Chapter Thirty-three
ASPIRATION AND FOREIGN BODIES

PETER PONS

Aspiration of foreign material produces inflammation of the lung parenchyma. The extent of injury is affected by the pH of the material aspirated, the volume of the aspirate, and the presence of particulate matter.

Fluid aspirated into the trachea quickly disperses in the alveoli and interstitial space, which produces immediate ventilation-perfusion mismatches with subsequent hypoxemia. *Nontoxic fluids* (water and saline) tend to produce short-lived effects. *Lipids* produce insidious and chronic changes: Oil in the airway may lead to a granulomatous reaction in the lungs. *Gastric juices* produce patchy atelectasis and pulmonary edema followed by intraalveolar hemorrhage and marked interstitial and peribronchial edema. Small foci of frank necrosis of the lung parenchyma, necrotizing bronchitis, and bronchiolitis are seen. The severity of the reaction reflects the volume aspirated and the acidity of the fluid. The greater the acidity of the aspirate, the more severe the reaction.

Dissolved food with particles produces a prolonged inflammatory process similar to acid aspiration. Extensive hemorrhagic pneumonitis is followed after 48 hours by a granulomatous reaction.

Pyogenic material is significant if the normal protective mechanisms of the upper airway are disrupted. Sterility is usually maintained by the reflexes that keep foreign bodies out of the airway in combination with pulmonary macrophages and the mucociliary membrane. Aspiration of a heavily infected inoculum produces a necrotizing pneumonia, lung abscess, or empyema if the defense system is overwhelmed. Gastric acid aspiration, by itself, does not primarily produce pulmonary infectious problems.

Particulate matter or foreign body aspiration of neutral material produces a response that reflects the size, location, and composition of the particles. The location of the object determines the clinical picture. Bronchial obstruction may be caused by a variety of mechanisms:

- *Check valve:* air is inhaled but not expelled, leading to emphysema.
- *Stop valve:* no inhaled air is allowed to pass, resulting in distal atelectasis
- *Ball valve:* the foreign body is dislodged during expiration, but reimpacts on inspiration, resulting in atelectasis
- *Bypass valve:* a partial obstruction to inflow and outflow with decreased aeration on the affected side.

Food and vegetable matter (nuts, seeds, grapes, raisins, candy, sausage-shaped meat such as hot dogs, or raw carrots) are most commonly aspirated by children. Objects are usually ≤32 mm, with round objects more likely to plug the airway completely.

High-risk patients are those who have lost reflex protection of the airway, or control or coordination of the muscles involved in swallowing or regurgitation, as well as those who have a structural defect in the gastrointestinal tract (see the box above).

CLINICAL PRESENTATION

Although a history of aspiration is useful, the absence of a positive history is not definitive. Silent regurgitation in a patient with an abnormal level of consciousness is more dangerous than actual emesis.

Over 90% of patients become symptomatic within 1 hour of the aspiration event; few may have a time lag as long as 6 hours. Immediately following the aspiration event, there is a sudden onset of coughing, choking, wheezing, and shortness of breath; one third of these patients develop apnea. Symptoms may progress to cyanosis and hypoxemia and, ultimately, impaired mentation and cardiopulmonary arrest.

The clinical presentation of an airway particulate foreign body reflects the acuteness and location of the obstruction. Laryngotracheal foreign bodies typically produce an acute obstruction, with an acute onset of respiratory distress and often stridor. Bronchial foreign bodies produce a more subacute course. Bronchial obstruction may result from material lodging in the bronchus, which causes relative or total obstruction.

Examination reveals fever, tachypnea, coughing, diffuse rales, and variable respiratory distress and failure.

ASSESSMENT

The approach to assessment and treatment reflects the degree of obstruction or respiratory failure. A number of diagnostic modalities may be useful.

Radiologic studies, which should be done immediately after the aspiration, often show no changes. Atelectasis may develop in the first hour followed in 6 to 12 hours by the development of infiltrates resembling pulmonary edema. These infiltrates progress over 24 to 36 hours and are most commonly seen in the right lower lobe. Radiographic changes may be unilateral (26%) or localized to one lobe (38%).

Inspiratory and expiratory x-ray films may be diagnostic of bronchial particulate foreign bodies. Tracheobronchial tree findings may indicate an obstruction (13%), a radiopaque foreign body (11%), and pneumonia (5%). Five percent of the x-ray films are normal.

Radiopacity is a relative quality rather than an absolute property. It is often important to distinguish a foreign body in the trachea from one in the esophagus. Foreign bodies lie in the plane of least resistance. Flat foreign bodies, such as coins in the esophagus, lie in the frontal plane and appear as a full circle on the posteroanterior (PA) view. Those in the trachea rest in the sagittal plane and appear end-on in the PA chest x-ray film and flat on a lateral view.

An *arterial blood gas study* should be obtained as a baseline from which to assess hypoxemia and ventilatory status.

Hemodynamic monitoring may be required if progression to adult respiratory distress syndrome (ARDS) occurs or if unresponsive pulmonary edema is present. Central venous or pulmonary wedge pressure monitoring may be required.

MANAGEMENT

Rapid Intervention

Rapid intervention is required. Initial stabilization must ensure attention to the airway and ventilation while managing shock, respiratory or cardiac arrest, complications of hypoxemia, and respiratory acidosis. Hypovolemia may develop because of extravasation of fluid across the pulmonary capillary membrane into the alveolar spaces.

Reduce Quantity Aspirated

Place the patient who has aspirated in a left lateral decubitus position with the head down. Vigorously suction the mouth and trachea.

Relieve Obstruction

In particulate foreign body aspirations, initiate efforts to clear the airway on first contact. This effort is followed by back blows and manual thrusts.

If the patient is less than 12 months of age, the rapid increase in pressure resulting from four back blows may expel or loosen a foreign body because many of these foreign bodies lodge high in the trachea or throat. If the material is not expelled by the patient, immediately perform manual chest thrusts to provide a more sustained increase in pressure and airflow. Repeat as indicated.

In older children and adults, a manual abdominal (Heimlich) thrust is the primary technique. Repeat as indicated.

The patient who is talking or coughing should be allowed to continue doing so. Blind probing of the airway is discouraged.

Bronchoscopy may be useful for removing particulate matter. Irrigation of the airways with neutral or alkaline solutions has no documented beneficial impact.

Reduce Hypoxemia

Monitor hypoxemia. Intubation and intermittent positive-pressure ventilation (IPPV) are useful in reversing hypoxemia. Positive end-expiratory pressure (PEEP) may be necessary if respiratory distress syndrome develops.

Other Measures

Steroids have not been proven to be efficacious in reducing sequelae.

Use antibiotics only for specific indications, including fever, an expanding infiltrate that appears more than 36 hours after aspiration, leukocytosis, culture-proven bacterial pathogen, and unexplained deterioration of the patient. Prophylactic administration of antibiotics is not indicated.

Bronchodilators such as albuterol or epinephrine may be administered for the relief of bronchospasm induced by the aspirated material.

Prevent Aspiration

Prevention is key to aspiration. Recognize high-risk patients and intervene before aspiration. Airway protection in high-risk patients, gastric acid reduction, and gastric emptying in patients with altered consciousness may be helpful. Prohibit the ingestion of particulate mater that may easily be aspirated, particularly in children between 1 and 2 years of age.

KEY CONSIDERATIONS

WHAT IS THE LIFE THREAT?

One-third of all patients with acute aspiration of gastric contents become apneic. If untreated, the aspiration of gastric juices and particulate food matter constitute an immediate life threat.

A foreign body that occludes the larynx is an immediate threat to life.

DOES THE PATIENT NEED ADMISSION?

Patients surviving significant aspiration require admission to the hospital and perhaps to the ICU for airway support and monitoring of ventilation, oxygenation, and hemodynamic status.

WHAT IS THE MOST SERIOUS DIAGNOSIS?

Laryngeal obstruction, tracheal or bronchial obstruction, and aspiration of gastric contents are most serious diagnoses.

HAVE I PERFORMED A THOROUGH WORK-UP?

Perform the Heimlich maneuver for an acute laryngeal obstruction, especially in settings outside the hospital.

Perform a laryngoscopy as needed to remove laryngeal obstructions dislodged by the Heimlich maneuver.

Obtain a chest x-ray examination, and make arrangements for a bronchoscopy and bronchial lavage for severe aspiration. Monitor oxygenation and ventilation.

Recommended Reading

American Heart Association: Guidelines for cardiopulmonary resuscitation (CPR) and emergency cardiac care (ECC), *JAMA* 268:2171, 1992.

Kosloske AM: Bronchoscopic extraction of aspirated foreign bodies in children, *Am J Dis Child* 136:924, 1982.

Lumpkin JR, Jayne HA: Aspiration. In Rosen P et al, editors: *Emergency medicine: concepts and clinical practice,* ed 3, St Louis, 1992, Mosby.

Pons PT: Foreign bodies. In Rosen P et al, editors: *Emergency medicine: concepts and clinical practice,* ed 3, St Louis, 1992, Mosby.

Schlass MD, Pham-Dang H, Rosales JK: Foreign bodies in the tracheo-bronchial tree: a retrospective study of 217 cases, *J Otolaryngol* 12:212, 1983.

Chapter Thirty-four

DEEP VENOUS THROMBOSIS AND PULMONARY EMBOLISM

CRAIG F. FEIED

Venous thromboembolic disease, the syndrome in which blood clots form in the deep veins and break loose to travel to the lungs, is a difficult and serious problem. A pulmonary embolism (PE) is a common complication of deep venous thrombosis (DVT). In 60% of all patients with DVT, fragments of loose venous thrombus float through the right side of the heart and lodge within the pulmonary circulation. Two thirds of these pulmonary emboli initially create no clinically apparent signs or symptoms, but they cannot be considered benign. Recurrent embolism is the rule, and pulmonary hypertension may cause chronic illness or sudden hemodynamic collapse and death.

The true incidence of venous thromboembolism is unknown. Published estimates suggest that between 1 million and 3 million cases of DVT occur yearly in the United States alone and result in between 650,000 and 2 million cases of PE. Prompt diagnosis and treatment can reduce the mortality of PE from 30% to 8% or less.

PATHOPHYSIOLOGY OF DEEP VENOUS THROMBOSIS

Flow stasis, altered coagulability, or extensive vessel wall injury may cause microthrombi to propagate, resulting in macroscopic thrombi.

Vessel wall endothelial damage is the most significant of these factors, because even a minor endothelial injury often results in an accumulation of macroscopic thrombus in the veins.

Hemostasis

The initiating event in venous thrombosis is platelet adhesion. Initial platelet adhesion and aggregation are stimulated by a component of endothelial cells, most likely a substance known as amorphous electron-dense substance (AEDS). The release of this substance is enhanced by activity of the intrinsic coagulation cascade and is inhibited by platelet antiaggregating agents, by thrombolytics, and by anticoagulants. Platelet activation causes the release of platelet proaggregants thromboxane A_2 and serotonin, resulting in the aggressive recruitment of additional platelets to form a "hemostatic plug." Thromboxane A_2 and serotonin also cause local vasoconstriction. Exposed platelet membrane phospholipids catalyse the activation of factor X and the local (endothelial) formation of thrombin, which is itself a powerful proaggregant. Thrombin-mediated platelet aggregation is unaffected by aspirin and nonsteroidals, but aggregation caused by platelet-derived thromboxane A_2 depends on platelet cyclooxygenase, which is reversibly inhibited by nonsteroidal antiinflammatory agents and is irreversibly inhibited by aspirin.

Coagulation

After a hemostatic plug has been well established, coagulation pathways are activated and thrombin is generated. Fibrin cross linking builds a true thrombus out of what was initially a loose aggregation of blood elements. If this series of events were unopposed, any small vascular endothelial injury would result in thrombus propagation throughout the venous system. However, three factors serve to retard and prevent propagation from becoming out of control: flow dilution, natural anticoagulants, and natural thrombolytics. If blood flow is reduced, activated coagulation factors accumulate rather than being carried away. If this happens, or if there is any defect in the production or function of the natural anticoagulants or thrombolytics, a thrombus forms more vigorously than appropriate for a given vascular injury. The patient will develop recurrent venous thrombosis and PE.

Anticoagulation

Protein C, protein S, and antithrombin III are the best understood of the natural circulating anticoagulants. Antithrombin III, which interferes with the action of serine proteases such as thrombin, is a general inhibitor of the intrinsic pathway. Protein C (with its cofactor, protein S) inhibits factor V and factor VIII, which are principal components of the common coagulation pathway. Paradoxically, a deficiency of the procoagulant factor V increases resistance to the anticoagulant effects of activated protein C; this deficiency is present in nearly half of all patients with venous thrombosis. Many other plasma proteins serve as activators, inhibitors, or cofactors in the coagulation cascade, and together these plasma proteins prevent minor endothelial injury from initiating an uncontrolled intravascular coagulation.

Fibrinolysis

Fibrinolysis is the organism's defense against the formation of thrombus. Fibrinolysis is initiated by tissue activators and circulating activators that transform the inactive precursor plasminogen into the active fibrinolytic agent plasmin. Plasmin attacks and degrades fibrin and, if present in excess, also attacks and degrades fibrinogen. Damaged endothelial cells release tissue-type plasminogen activators at the same time that they bind platelets and initiate the clotting process. This balancing process ensures that under normal conditions the formation of thrombus remains localized to the injured area in which it is needed. Any disturbance of this delicate balance leads either to increased bleeding or to increased propagation of thrombus.

CLINICAL PRESENTATION OF DEEP VENOUS THROMBOSIS

The classical signs and symptoms of DVT are those associated with obstruction of venous drainage: pain, tenderness, and unilateral leg swelling. Symptoms of DVT may be present or absent, unilateral or bilateral, and mild or severe. A thrombus that does not cause a net venous outflow obstruction is often asymptomatic. A nonobstructing thrombus may appear with localized pain as an isolated symptom. An obstructing thrombus that involves the iliac bifurcation, the pelvic veins, or the vena cava produces bilateral leg edema. Partial obstruction often produces mild bilateral edema that is mistaken for the dependent edema of right-sided heart failure, of fluid overload, or of hepatic or renal insufficiency.

Severe venous congestion produces a clinical appearance that is indistinguishable from cellulitis. All patients with a warm, swollen, tender leg must be evaluated for both cellulitis and DVT because patients with primary DVT often develop a secondary cellulitis, whereas patients with a primary cellulitis often develop a secondary DVT. In addition, superficial thrombophlebitis is often associated with clinically inapparent underlying DVT; thus a clinical diagnosis of superficial phlebitis warrants an investigative work-up to rule out deep vein involvement.

If a patient has suspected or documented PE, the absence of tenderness, erythema, edema, or a palpable cord on examination of the lower extremities does not rule out thrombophlebitis, nor does it imply a source other than a leg vein. More than two thirds of all patients with proven PE lack any clinically evident phlebitis. Nearly one third of all patients with proven PE have no identifiable source of DVT despite a thorough investigation. Autopsy studies suggest that even when the source is clinically inapparent, it is hidden within the deep venous system of the lower extremity and pelvis in 90% of all cases.

Deep Venous Thrombosis Below the Knee

Although it is widely believed that DVT below the knee is benign, this belief is untrue. Most cases of proximal DVT originate in the venous sinuses of the calf; propagation to the popliteal vein and the femoral vein occurs in 40% of all cases.

There are three principal pairs of deep veins in the lower leg: the anterior tibial (drains the dorsum of the foot), the posterior tibial (drains the sole of the foot), and the peroneal (drains the lateral aspect of the foot). DVT isolated to the anterior tibial vein results in PE in 30% of all cases. Other deep vein groups draining the lower leg include the gastrocnemius plexus and the soleal plexus. These plexi and the deep venous groups drain via the popliteal vein at the knee. Thrombosis of the popliteal vein results in PE in 66% of the cases—a frequency identical to that of DVT in the thigh.

Deep vein thrombophlebitis in the calf is an important cause of morbidity quite aside from any risk of propagation or of embolization. Isolated calf vein thrombophlebitis results in clinical postphlebitic syndrome in 20% to 40% of all cases. Postphlebitic syndrome is caused by re-

canalization of thrombosed deep veins, which leads to the destruction of the venous valves and thus to chronically elevated ambulatory venous pressure within the legs. Incompetence of the valves in the popliteal segments of the deep venous system leads to elevated ambulatory venous pressures that average 72 mm Hg. More than 60% of those patients with popliteal valve failure develop severe clinical signs of chronic venous insufficiency. This postphlebitic syndrome is responsible for chronic pain, edema, hyperpigmentation, and ulceration (Fig. 34-1) as well as many cases of recurrent DVT and PE.

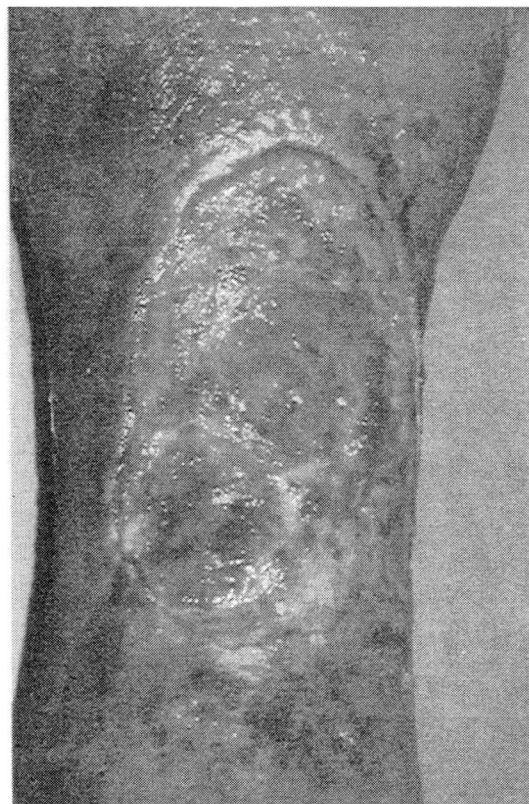

Fig. **34-1**   Postphlebitic changes at the ankle.

CLINICAL PRESENTATION OF PULMONARY THROMBOEMBOLISM

A PE is suspected when a patient complains of the sudden onset of pain, shortness of breath, anxiety, tachypnea, tachycardia, hypoxemia, or hypotension. Highly suggestive symptoms and severe clinical signs are helpful in the small subset of patients who have one of the three classic syndromes of PE, which are pulmonary infarction, massive embolization, and submassive embolization:

- *Pulmonary parenchymal infarction* occurs when small emboli lodge in the peripheral lung, where the flow through anastomotic bronchial arteries is insufficient to sustain the parenchyma. Inflammation of parietal pleura causes pleuritic chest pain. The pain often is associated with the chest wall in the distribution of the intercostal nerves. Radiation of pain to the shoulder or neck is typical. Patients may develop a cough and hemoptysis.
- *Massive embolism* presents as acute cor pulmonale, with a mixture of pulmonary and cardiac manifestations. The pain is described as retrosternal, dull, heavy, and aching, sometimes with a superimposed respirophasic component. Shortness of breath is profound, and patients often have hypoxemia and hypotension. Massive PE can appear with a pain picture very suggestive of myocardial ischemia, and such cases are commonly misdiagnosed as acute myocardial infarction or as septic or hypovolemic shock. Angina pectoris is the initial diagnosis in as many as 30% of the patients for whom a final diagnosis of PE is made.
- *Submassive proximal embolism* causes the sudden onset of painless or minimally painful acute and unexplained dyspnea, either on exertion or at rest. Such patients are often misdiagnosed as having asthma, hyperventilation syndrome, or panic attacks. If the chest x-ray study is abnormal, these patients may appear to have congestive heart failure or pneumonia.

Unfortunately, fewer than half of all patients with PE have the classical syndromes previously described. The majority of patients with symptomatic pulmonary emboli have only vague and nonspecific clinical findings. PE may appear with abdominal or back pain. It often causes pulmonary infiltrates and such confounding clinical findings as fever, cough, and leukocyto-

Table 34-1

SYMPTOMS IN HOSPITAL INPATIENTS WITH ANGIOGRAPHICALLY PROVEN PE

Symptom	Percentage
Dyspnea	84
Chest pain, pleuritic	74
Apprehension	59
Cough	53
Hemoptysis	30
Sweating	27
Chest pain, nonpleuritic	14
Syncope	13

Table 34-2

SIGNS IN HOSPITAL INPATIENTS WITH ANGIOGRAPHICALLY PROVEN PE

Sign	Percentage
Tachypnea >16/minute	92
Rales	58
Accentuated second sound	53
Tachycardia >100/minute	44
Fever >37.8° C	43
Diaphoresis	36
S_3 or S_4 gallop	34
Thrombophlebitis	32
Lower extremity edema	24
Cardiac murmur	23
Cyanosis	19

sis, whereas more "typical" findings of pain or shortness of breath are often absent.

PE can mimic pneumonia in every detail. 60% of patients with PE have a fever above 38° C over the first 3 days, and 10% remain febrile for a full week. A cough is present in 50% to 70% of patients with PE, and the white blood cell count is often above 11,000 and may be as high as 20,000. The infiltrates caused by PE are indistinguishable from those caused by infection. Pneumonia and PE may be clinically indistinguishable, but if the patient has no fever, lacks a leukocytosis, or has a chest x-ray study that is normal or shows an effusion, then pneumonia is much less likely and pulmonary thromboembolism is a more likely diagnosis (Tables 34-1 and 34-2).

THROMBOGENIC AND HYPERCOAGULABLE STATES

The clinical settings most commonly reported as risk factors for venous thrombosis are listed in the box below. The following list further explains some of these risk factors:

- *Cancer.* Malignancy is an important risk factor for DVT, and spontaneous DVT without an obvious cause is an important marker for a possible occult malignancy.
- *Cerebrovascular accidents and neurotrauma.* A DVT is common after a stroke or neurologic trauma.
- *Chemotherapy.* Many types of chemotherapy increase the risk of DVT and PE.

RISK FACTORS FOR VENOUS THROMBOSIS AND PULMONARY EMBOLISM

Acute myocardial infarction	Malignancy
AIDS (lupus anticoagulant)	Multiple trauma
Antithrombin III deficiency	Obesity
Behçet disease	Oral contraceptives
Blood type A	Phenothiazines
Burns	Polycythemia
Chemotherapy	Postvenography
Congestive heart failure	Postoperative (especially pelvic and orthopedic
Disorders of plasminogen activators	procedures)
Drug-induced lupus anticoagulant	Postpartum period
Dysfibrinogenemia	Pregnancy
Dysplasminogenemia	Previous history of DVT
Estrogen replacements	Protein C deficiency
Familial hyperlipidemias	Protein S deficiency
Fractures	Resistance to activated protein C
Hemolytic anemias	Significant varicosities
Heparin-induced thrombocytopenia	Systemic lupus erythematous (lupus)
Homocystinuria	Thrombocytosis
Immobilization	Ulcerative colitis
Increasing age	Venous pacemakers
Indwelling venous infusion catheters	Warfarin (first few days of therapy)
Intravenous drug abuse	

- *Coagulopathy.* Patients with a familial deficiency of protein C or protein S or with an inherited resistance to activated protein C often suffer multiple episodes of DVT or PE before age 35.
- *Fibrinolysis.* Impaired fibrinolysis occurs in several inherited syndromes but is most common in postoperative patients, those on synthetic estrogens of any type, and in pregnant or postpartum women.
- *Increasing age.* Increasing age leads to an increased risk of DVT and PE, but it is not known whether this factor is entirely independent of associated factors such as other underlying illnesses and immobility.
- *Inflammatory bowel disease.* Patients with ulcerative colitis and Crohn disease are at increased risk for DVT and PE.
- *Obesity.* Obesity, defined as a weight greater than 20% above ideal weight, has long been accepted as a risk factor for DVT and PE, but the evidence supporting this association has been questioned.
- *Oral estrogens.* Patients taking oral contraceptives have a 3 to 12 times higher risk for DVT and PE compared with those not taking them.
- *Polycythemia and thrombocytosis.* The risk of venous and arterial thrombosis increases linearly with increasing hematocrit. Approximately 40% of the deaths in patients with polycythemia vera are related to thrombosis, but only a third of these are a result of venous thrombosis.
- *Pregnancy and puerperium.* PE is the most common nontraumatic cause of maternal death in pregnancy, and the incidence is even higher in the postpartum period.
- *Prior DVT.* Prior DVT raises the risk of new postoperative DVT from 26% to 68%. A past history of clinically apparent PE raises the risk of new postoperative DVT to nearly 100%. In general, those with a prior history of DVT have a 500% increase in the risk of new DVT.
- *Postoperative state.* The most common and most important risk setting for DVT is the post-operative period. Abdominal and pelvic surgery entails a risk nearly as high as that of knee and hip surgery, in which 30% to 60% of patients develop DVT if not adequately anticoagulated.
- *Acute myocardial infarction.* 15% of patients who die during an admission for acute MI are found at autopsy to have died from unsuspected PE.

DIAGNOSIS OF DEEP VENOUS THROMBOSIS

The diagnostic tools most useful in assessing the deep venous system are plethysmography, continuous-wave Doppler ultrasonography, and B-mode ultrasonography. The invasive technique of contrast venography has long been the gold standard in the diagnosis of DVT, but venography may occasionally miss thrombus in certain areas where B-mode ultrasonography can be more sensitive. Magnetic resonance imaging (MRI) of the lower extremity has approximately the same sensitivity and specificity for DVT as venography and may be more helpful in suggesting an alternate diagnosis when DVT is not the cause of an acutely swollen leg.

The usefulness of plethysmography and of continuous-wave Doppler ultrasonography tests depends strongly on the skill and experience of the operator and on the patient population in which the tests are used. False-positive and false-negative results are quite common. Test sensitivity is lowest in patients who are at high risk for venous thromboembolism but who lack the symptoms of leg edema and pain that are caused by significant obstruction of a major venous outflow tract.

Detailed B-mode ultrasonography imaging is the most sensitive and specific of the noninvasive tests but is far from perfect, even when color-flow Doppler mapping is added to the image. Ultrasonography is poor at identifying patients with obstructing DVT at a location other than the thigh and is even less reliable in patients without leg pain and swelling.

Negative results from a noninvasive venous evaluation, including color-flow duplex imaging (B-mode ultrasonography), do not rule out an occult thrombus in patients without clinical evidence of DVT. In fact, when a patient has symptoms of PE, even a negative venogram cannot rule out an occult thrombus because an extensive work-up fails to reveal a source of thrombus in 30% of patients with proven PE. Such a negative result may occur if the entire thrombus has embolized to the pulmonary vascular bed (leaving no detectable thrombus at the original site), if the thrombus is smoothly applied to a quadrant of the vessel wall in a nonoccluding manner, or if a residual thrombus is located below the knee or above the groin, where diagnostic tests are insensitive. The critical thing to remember about tests for DVT is that if a patient has signs and symptoms of PE, a negative work-up for DVT does not markedly reduce the likelihood of PE.

DIAGNOSIS OF PULMONARY THROMBOEMBOLISM

The ECG and chest x-ray study cannot confirm the diagnosis of PE, but those tests may be suggestive. The diagnosis of PE virtually always rests on one of two tests: the nuclear pulmonary scintigram (often referred to as the ventilation/perfusion [V/Q] scan) or the pulmonary angiogram. Spiral CT scans of the chest are now being investigated to determine their sensitivity and specificity for PE, and it is possible that these will ultimately supplant or supplement either the V/Q scan or the angiogram.

The ECG may be normal or may show any abnormality whatsoever. Sinus tachycardia and nonspecific ST-T wave abnormalities are common. Atrial fibrillation or other dysrhythmias may be seen. It is rare to see classic "pulmonary strain" patterns such as a large "P-pulmonale" in lead II or the *S1-Q3-T3* pattern of a deep S-wave in lead I along with a deep Q-wave and an inverted T wave in lead III (Fig. 34-2).

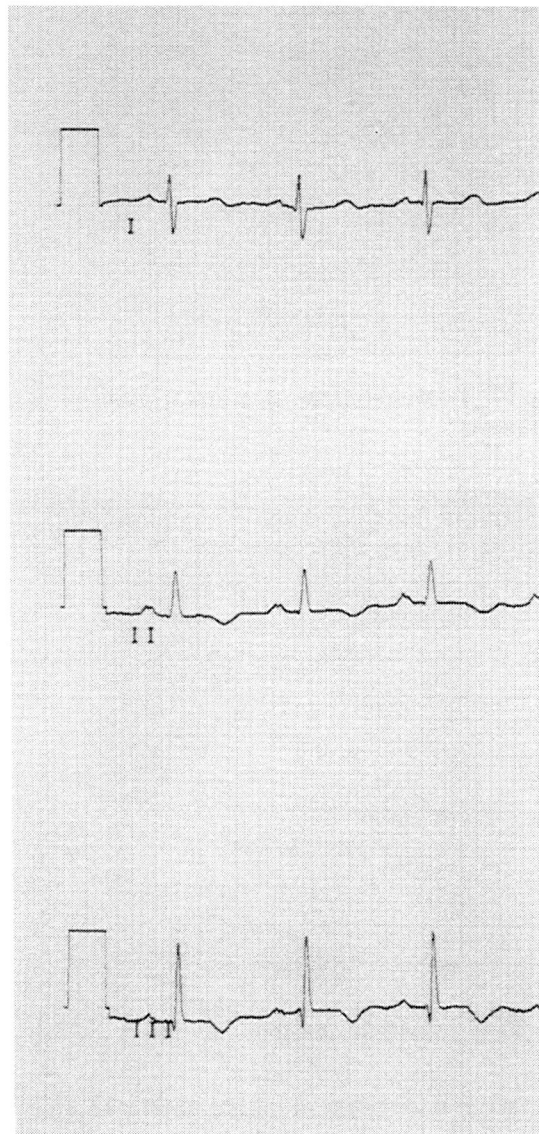

Fig. **34-2** Classical pattern in acute PE showing a deep S-wave in lead I and a Q-wave with an inverted T-wave in lead III, hence the name "S_1-Q_3-T_3." This pattern is rarely seen and is nonspecific.

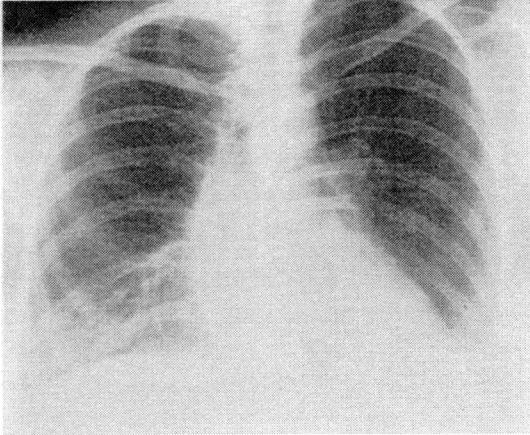

Fig. **34-3** Westermark's sign and a small pleural effusion.

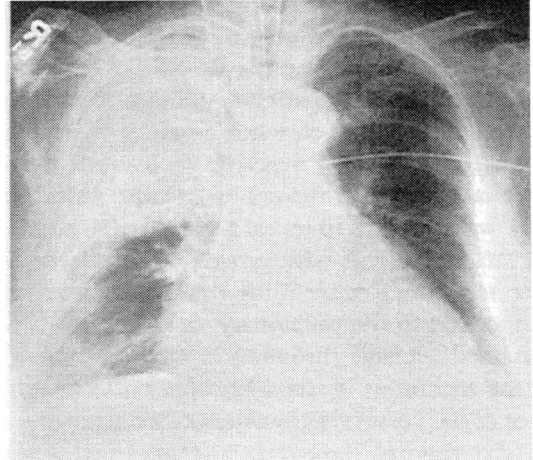

Fig. **34-5** Infiltrates from PE.

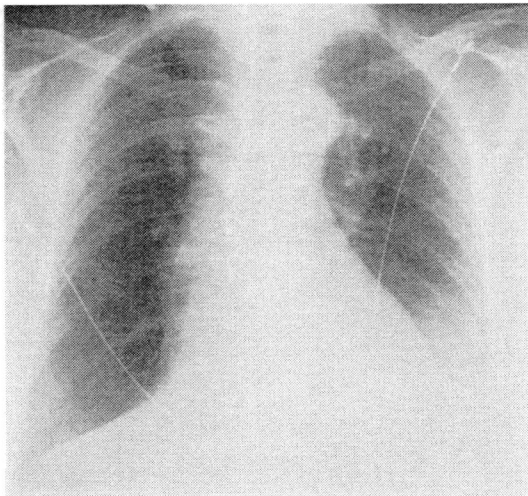

Fig. **34-4** Moderate effusion.

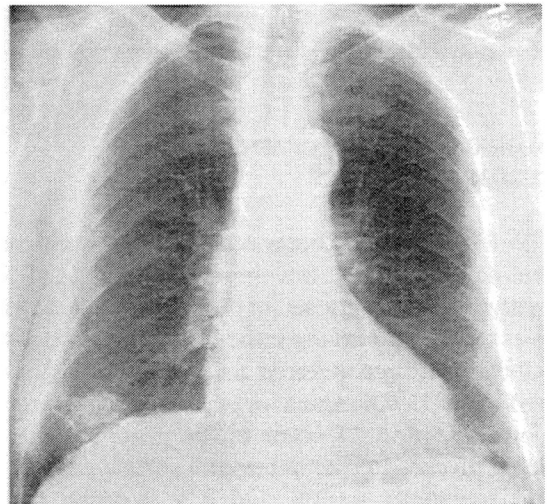

Fig. **34-6** Hampton's hump.

In the acute phase of PE, the chest x-ray study is virtually always normal and may remain so throughout the course of the disease. The only abnormal finding that can appear acutely is *Westermark's sign,* an abnormal increase in the density and size of pulmonary vessels in one area accompanied by an abnormal paucity of vessels in another area (Fig. 34-3). The most common chest x-ray abnormality in PE is a pleural effusion, which may be large (Fig. 34-4) but is often so small that it is missed (see Fig. 34-3). By the third day, many pulmonary emboli have produced infiltrates that are indistinguishable from those of pneumonia (Fig. 34-5). Over time, an area of pulmonary infarction near the diaphragm may produce a classic pulmonary scar pattern known as *Hampton's hump* (Fig. 34-6).

V/Q SCAN WORKSHEET Patient: Date:

Clinical Information

Chest x-ray:

V/Q Narrative:

Modified PIOPED Classification

Normal Scan

☐ No perfusion defects seen

- *At least 2 percent of patients with PE will have this pattern.*
- *96 percent of patients with this pattern do not have PE, and 4 percent do.*

High Probability

☐ Two or more segmental or larger perfusion defects with normal CXR and normal ventilation.

☐ Two or more segmental or larger perfusion defects where CXR abnormalities and ventilation defects are substantially smaller than the perfusion defects.

☐ Two or more subsegmental and one segmental perfusion defect with normal CXR and normal ventilation.

☐ Four or more subsegmental perfusion defects with normal CXR and normal ventilation.

- *41 percent of patients with PE will have this pattern.*
- *13 percent of patients with this pattern do not have PE, and 87 percent do.*

Nondiagnostic Scan

Formerly graded as low probability

☐ Small perfusion defects, regardless of number, ventilation findings, or CXR findings.

☐ Perfusion defects substantially smaller than CXR abnormality in the same area.

☐ Matching perfusion and ventilation defects in less than 75% of one lung zone or in less than 50% of one lung, with normal or 'nearly normal' CXR.

☐ Single segmental perfusion defect with normal CXR, regardless of ventilation match or mismatch.

☐ Nonsegmental perfusion defects.

- *16 percent of patients with PE will have this pattern.*
- *86 percent of patients with this pattern do not have PE, and 14 percent do.*

Formerly graded as intermediate probability

☐ Any V/Q abnormality not otherwise here classified as 'high' or 'low' probability.

- *41 percent of patients with PE will have this pattern.*
- *70 percent of patients with this pattern do not have PE, and 30 percent do.*

Fig.34-7 V/Q worksheet.

The least invasive test that has the potential to prove or disprove the diagnosis of PE is the nuclear ventilation/perfusion (V/Q) scan. The Q scan uses radiolabelled microaggregates of albumin to detect areas of the lung with reduced blood flow, and the V scan uses inhaled radioisotopes to detect areas of the lung with impaired ventilation. If the V/Q scan shows *normal perfusion,* the work-up need not proceed further. Only 5% of all patients with a normal perfusion scan ultimately prove to have PE.

If the scan is *high probability,* it will show two or more perfusion defects that correspond to anatomic pulmonary segments (or one segmental defect and two that correspond to pulmonary subsegments); at least one of the perfusion defects is in an area of normal lung on a chest x-ray study. This scan pattern means that the diagnosis of PE is overwhelmingly likely. Confirmatory angiography is needed only if the patient has strong contraindications to treatment.

All other V/Q patterns are *nondiagnostic* and are rarely of any clinical value. In particular, if perfusion defects are entirely limited to areas of the lung with a corresponding chest x-ray abnormality or ventilation scan abnormality, the V/Q scan is not diagnostic because it is equally possible that perfusion defects of this type may be primary (from a pulmonary embolism) or secondary (from air space disease).

Fig. 34-7 shows a worksheet that may assist in the clinical application of V/Q scan reports. This worksheet documents two very important points: First, that the majority of all V/Q scans are nondiagnostic, and second, that most patients who do have PE also have a nondiagnostic scan. Fig. 34-8 contains the same information and is formatted to fit on a 3″ × 5″ reference card.

When the V/Q scan is nondiagnostic, the deep venous system should be investigated to look for evidence of DVT. Duplex color-flow ultrasonographic imaging of the veins of the lower extremities has a high positive predictive value in patients with suspected PE but a very low negative predictive value. A positive duplex scan finding of DVT at any location essentially proves the diagnosis of PE, and the patient should be treated accordingly. Unfortunately, many patients with PE have both a nondiagnostic V/Q pattern and a negative deep vein work-up. A negative duplex scan is not a valid endpoint when working up a patient with suspected PE; if the duplex scan is negative or cannot be performed, the patient should have a pulmonary angiogram.

Modified PIOPED Classification of V/Q scans

Normal Scan

☐ No perfusion defects seen
At least 2 percent of patients with PE will have this pattern.
At least 4 percent of patients with this pattern DO have a PE.

High Probability

☐ Two or more segmental or larger perfusion defects with normal CXR and normal ventilation.
☐ Two or more segmental or larger perfusion defects where CXR abnormalities and ventilation defects are substantially smaller than the perfusion defects.
☐ Two or more subsegmental and one segmental perfusion defect with normal CXR and normal ventilation.
☐ Four or more subsegmental perfusion defects with normal CXR and normal ventilation.
41 percent of patients with PE will have this pattern.
87 percent of patients with this pattern DO have a PE.

Nondiagnostic Scan

Formerly graded as low probability

☐ Small perfusion defects, regardless of number, ventilation findings, or CXR findings.
☐ Perfusion defects substantially smaller than CXR abnormality in the same area.
☐ Matching perfusion and ventilation defects in less than 75% of one lung zone or in less than 50% of one lung, with normal or 'nearly normal' CXR.
☐ Single segmental perfusion defect with normal CXR, regardless of ventilation match or mismatch.
☐ Nonsegmental perfusion defects.
16 percent of patients with PE will have this pattern.
14 percent of patients with this pattern DO have a PE.

Formerly graded as intermediate probability

☐ Any V/Q abnormality not otherwise here classified as 'high' or 'low' probability.
41 percent of patients with PE will have this pattern.
30 percent of patients with this pattern DO have a PE.

Fig. 34-8 Modified PIOPED classification of V/Q scans (can be copied onto a 3″ × 5″ card for handy reference).

Pulmonary angiography is performed by placing a pigtail catheter through the right side of the heart and into the pulmonary artery, and then injecting contrast material into the right and left pulmonary arteries and their tributaries. It is a common practice to look first at the iliac veins and the vena cava, then at any area of x-ray study or V/Q scan abnormality, and finally at successive portions of the pulmonary circulation. The angiogram is complete when an abnormality has been found or when the entire pulmonary bed has been visualized bilaterally.

A pulmonary angiogram is not a perfect test. The pulmonary tree branches 26 times before reaching the end capillaries, but an angiogram can identify a thrombus only within the first three branches. Pulmonary emboli that were not detected angiographically are very often found at autopsy.

TREATMENT

When a diagnosis of DVT or PE is seriously suspected, anticoagulation should be instituted without delay. If the diagnosis is confirmed, modern treatment alternatives include anticoagulation, thrombolysis, and thrombectomy. A pair of 30 to 40 mm gradient compression stockings should always be placed, because they can increase the flow rate through the deep veins by a factor of five and can dramatically decrease the progression of thrombosis.

Heparin

All patients with DVT or PE should be started on full heparin anticoagulation, regardless of whether thrombolysis or thrombectomy are indicated. Heparin anticoagulation was introduced into clinical practice in the 1930s and reduced the mortality of PE from 30% to less than 10%. Heparin anticoagulation does not guarantee a successful outcome because a recurrence or extension of DVT and PE often occurs despite full

and effective heparin anticoagulation. Heparin does not dissolve an existing clot nor can it prevent thrombosis in the presence of sufficient venous endothelial injury, but it can prevent the normal process of thrombus organization, which in the absence of heparin is well established in 1 week. Heparin interferes with the coagulation cascade by activating antithrombin III to inhibit the action of thrombin and to slow or prevent the progression of DVT. A deficiency of antithrombin III renders heparin ineffective as an anticoagulant.

Heparin metabolism follows first-order kinetics, with a half-life of 90 minutes. An activated partial thromboplastin time (APTT) of at least 1.5 times the control value is necessary for a therapeutic heparin effect. A recurrence of DVT and PE is 15 times more frequent if the APTT is not immediately therapeutic. Unfortunately, clinical surveys have found that 60% of those patients given heparin are not adequately anticoagulated within the first 24 hours. To achieve and maintain effective anticoagulation, an initial intravenous bolus of unfractionated heparin should be 10,000 units, and the initial maintenance infusion should be approximately 20 units/kg/hour. The APTT values should be monitored 6 hours after each change in therapy, and any subtherapeutic APTT should be addressed with an immediate rebolus and an increased infusion rate. Extremely high APTT results should be met with only a brief (30 minute) interruption of the infusion and a small decrement in heparin dosage. The box on p. 406 provides a guide to monitoring heparin therapy. In some hospitals an assay for heparin may be followed in lieu of monitoring the APTT; anticoagulation is achieved with serum heparin levels of 0.3 to 0.5 units/ml.

Fractionated low–molecular-weight heparin (LMWH) has recently become available in the United States and has been shown to be at least as safe and effective as unfractionated heparin. Fractionated LMWH is given as a subcutaneous injection twice daily; there is no need to measure the activated partial thromboplastin time

HEPARIN DOSING

Recurrence or progression of venous thromboembolism is 15 times more common when a therapeutic APTT is not achieved within the first 48 hours. Most patients treated with heparin as a 5000 unit bolus and a drip of 1000 units/hour do not have a therapeutic APTT within the first 48 hours.

The following regimen achieves a therapeutic APTT rapidly in most patients and does not increase the likelihood of bleeding complications:

Initial Bolus

10,000 units of heparin IV push

Initial Maintenance Drip

Mix 20,000 units heparin in 500 ml D5W or normal saline
Start the maintenance drip as soon as possible
Begin the maintenance drip at 32 ml/hour (1280 units/hour)
Check the APTT 6 hours after the initial bolus

Dose Adjustment

Adjust the heparin maintenance drip according to the following schedule:

APTT (seconds)	Hold Drip (minutes)	Adjust Drip	Check APTT
<50	0	+3 ml/hour	6 hours later
50-59	0	+3 ml/hour	6 hours later
60-85	0	No change	Next morning
86-95	0	−2 ml/hour	Next morning
96-120	30	−2 ml/hour	6 hours later
>120	60	−4 ml/hour	6 hours later

(APTT) because the drug has an extremely wide therapeutic window and does not usually prolong the APTT.

Heparin is a safe and valuable drug, but it is not without risks. It is the most common cause of drug-related deaths in hospitalized patients and causes bleeding complications in 10% to 15% of all patients. A serious hemorrhage is more common when the APTT is prolonged more than 3 times the control values, and it is exacerbated by the concomitant use of aspirin or other platelet inhibitors. If necessary, the anticoagulant effect of heparin may be reversed by protamine sulphate (15 mg infused over 3 minutes). Fresh frozen plasma and platelet transfusions are ineffective when excessive bleeding is a result of heparin. In addition to bleeding complications, heparin may result in a syndrome of heparin-associated thrombocytopenia (HAT) that may be mild or severe. Paradoxically, HAT can trigger significant venous or arterial thrombosis. If HAT occurs, one may substitute porcine heparin for the usual bovine heparin, use a low-molecular weight fractionated heparin, or switch from heparin to an oral anticoagulant such as warfarin.

Heparin is not teratogenic and may be used in pregnancy; however, its use is associated with a 20% incidence of fetal demise and a 14% incidence of prematurity. It does not cross the placenta and is not secreted in breast milk.

Oral Anticoagulants

After effective anticoagulation has been achieved with intravenous heparin, most patients are switched to warfarin. Warfarin competitively inhibits the regeneration of the reduced active form of vitamin K; it therefore interferes with the action of the vitamin K–dependent clotting factors II, VII, IX, X, as well as with the action of the anticoagulant factors protein C and protein S. Anticoagulation is usually effective when the prothrombin time is approximately 1.5 times normal. The International Normalized Ratio (INR) accounts for variations in reagent strength and is gradually replacing prothrombin time as a measure of anticoagulation. An INR of 2 to 3 is consistent with effective "low-intensity" anticoagulation.

Warfarin should never be given for thromboembolic disease without prior heparinization and a therapeutically prolonged APTT. Protein C and factor VII have short half-lives compared to the other vitamin K–dependent proteins. Therefore the administration of warfarin without heparin anticoagulation results in an early reduction in anticoagulant protein C and protein S function before procoagulant activity is affected. This phenomenon has been proven to cause or worsen venous thrombosis and PE and is also responsible for the syndrome of warfarin skin necrosis, in which large areas of skin and sometimes portions of the distal extremities become gangrenous and may require amputation. To prevent this, heparin should be continued for 3 to 5 days after the initiation of warfarin.

Warfarin, like heparin, may cause significant hemorrhage. Hemorrhagic complications are controlled by the transfusion of fresh frozen plasma and by the administration of parenteral vitamin K (10 mg IV), which reverses the warfarin effect within a few hours. Warfarin is teratogenic and cannot be used in pregnancy. It is secreted in breast milk in small quantities but may nonetheless be used in nursing mothers. Pregnant patients with venous thromboembolism are generally kept heparinized for the entire duration of their therapy, and serious consideration should be given to the placement of a venous filter device.

A 3- to 6-month course of oral anticoagulation reduces the incidence of recurrent PE to below 8%. For most patients, more prolonged oral anticoagulation offers little further improvement in the incidence of DVT and PE.

Thrombolysis and Thrombectomy

Primary fibrinolytic therapy has become the standard of care for the patient with PE and hemodynamic instability or profound hypoxemia, and it is also indicated for selected patients with PE who are not hemodynamically unstable and do not have hypoxemia.

Thrombolysis and thrombectomy for DVT

Anticoagulant prevents thrombus extension but does not promote lysis of a preformed thrombus; therefore anticoagulation alone is not an optimal treatment for DVT. At least 65% of all patients treated with heparin and warfarin for DVT develop persistent deep vein valve incompetence and altered venous return. More than half of these patients suffer a lifelong postphlebitic syndrome of recurrent pain, swelling, stasis dermatitis, ulceration, and recurrent DVT. Of all patients with DVT, 50% to 80% develop a venous ulcer within 10 years. These sequelae are common both from isolated calf vein thrombosis and from proximal thrombosis.

Valve damage in a thrombosed vein is directly related to the duration of thrombosis. Three fourths of all thrombosed venous valves regain functionality if thrombolysis or thrombectomy occurs within 24 hours, but only 16% of the valves are competent when a thrombus remains in place for longer than 24 hours. Lytic therapy produces more rapid clot resolution, more complete clot resolution, a marked reduction in late symptoms, and a reduced likelihood of recurrent DVT. If peripheral systemic lytic therapy is ineffective, a partial catheter thrombectomy and direct catheter infusion of lytic agents into the remaining thrombus is effective for large DVT in a low-flow area.

Thrombolysis and thrombectomy for pulmonary thromboembolism

Immediate thrombolysis is the current treatment of choice for virtually all patients with any degree of hypotension or hypoxemia caused by a proven PE. Hypotension and hypoxemia are signs that the cardiovascular system has exhausted its reserves and has no further adaptive capacity. Even a small additional embolic episode is likely to be fatal in such a patient. Heparin slows the formation of new thrombus, but only thrombolysis can rapidly reverse right ventricular hypokinesis, ventricular dilatation, tricuspid regurgitation, and hemodynamic compromise in patients with PE. Full-dose heparin anticoagulation should be started along with any thrombolytic therapy, because thrombolytic agents do not prevent the accumulation of new thrombus.

Pulmonary thrombectomy, once the only alternative for patients with acute decompensated right-sided heart failure, is reserved today for patients who cannot receive thrombolysis (such as those who have just undergone intracranial, spinal, or ocular surgery) and for those whose condition continues to worsen despite thrombolysis. Because PE is a disease of frequent and early recurrences, it is generally accepted that thrombolysis should be performed for any patient who is unlikely to tolerate further embolization:

- Those whose condition is critical because of a severe underlying illness

- Those with massive PE (even without hypotension or hypoxemia)
- Those with severely reduced pulmonary reserves

Angiographic evidence of obstruction to pulmonary blood flow persists following therapy with anticoagulants alone, but thrombolytic therapy results in significant (50% or more) resolution of thrombus within 24 hours.

Risks and complications of thrombolysis

With thrombolysis, the incidence of systemic bleeding is the same for lytic agents and for heparin, but excess bleeding at angiography puncture and cutdown sites raises the overall incidence of hemorrhagic complications in patients treated with lytic agents to nearly twice that of patients who receive only heparin.

The management of life-threatening bleeding complications from lytic therapy requires that the infusion of the lytic agent be stopped. Fresh frozen plasma and cryoprecipitate will reverse the lytic state. Aminocaproic acid is an inhibitor of plasminogen activator that is effective when given as a 5 g IV load over 30 minutes followed by a drip of 1 g/hour as long as bleeding continues.

SUMMARY

Venous thromboembolic disease is a common cause of death and disability in the United States. Early diagnosis and treatment can significantly reduce the morbidity and mortality of DVT and PE. The current standard of care for venous thromboembolic disease is full anticoagulation for all patients with DVT and PE with the addition of thrombolytic therapy for patients with massive PE, any degree of hypotension or significant hypoxemia, and for selected patients who cannot tolerate recurrences of thromboembolism.

▌▌▌▌▌▌▌KEY CONSIDERATIONS

WHAT IS THE LIFE THREAT?

Massive PE constitutes an immediate threat to life. The degree of threat correlates roughly with the patient's underlying medical condition, the degree of obstruction to pulmonary blood flow, and the presence of a deep vein source of future impending embolization.

DOES THE PATIENT NEED ADMISSION?

The patient with PE should be hospitalized for treatment with heparin, evaluation for DVT, and consideration of thrombolytic therapy.

WHAT IS THE MOST SERIOUS DIAGNOSIS?

Assess the patient with dyspnea and chest pain for risk factors associated with thromboembolism, including the following: recent surgery, immobilization, cancer, immunodeficiency, coagulopathy (deficiency of protein C or protein S or a resistance to activated protein C), oral estrogens, obesity, and prior venous thrombosis. Examine for calf tenderness or enlargement. Perform a chest x-ray study. Initiate anticoagulation as soon as the diagnosis of PE is seriously suspected, without waiting for test results. Interpret results of the ventilation/perfusion scan with caution. A completely negative scan signifies a low probability of a pulmonary embolus (5% or less). A high probability scan means that the diagnosis of pulmonary embolus is extremely high. All other scans are nondiagnostic. Additional tests to order when the scan is nondiagnostic include a duplex color-flow imaging of the lower extremities. If this is negative, proceed to pulmonary angiography. Most patients with a high-probability scan will not require a pulmonary angiogram to confirm the diagnosis.

HAVE I PERFORMED A THOROUGH WORK-UP?

Consider PE in cases of chest pain, dyspnea, and syncope. Evaluate vital signs. Arterial blood gases may be helpful, but remember that the PO_2 and the O_2 saturation (as measured by pulse oximetry) are normal in the vast majority of patients with PE. Most important, do not abandon the work-up of a patient with suspected PE until a firm diagnosis has been made.

Recommended Reading

Feied CF: Pulmonary chest pain, cor pulmonale, and pulmonary thromboembolism. In Aufderheide T, Gibler B, editors: *Emergency cardiac care.* New York, 1994, Mosby.

PIOPED Investigators: Value of the ventilation/perfusion scan in acute pulmonary embolism, *JAMA* 263:2753, 1990.

PIOPED Investigators: Tissue plasminogen activator for the treatment of acute pulmonary embolism: a collaborative study by the PIOPED investigators, *Chest* 97:528-533, 1990.

Sharma GVRK, Folland ED, McIntyre KM: Long-term hemodynamic benefit of thrombolytic therapy in pulmonary embolic disease, *J Am Coll Cardiol* 15:65A, 1990.

Research Committee of the British Thoracic Society: Optimum duration of anticoagulation for deep-vein thrombosis and pulmonary embolism, *Lancet* 340:873-876, 1992.

Chapter Thirty-five
PERIPHERAL ARTERIOVASCULAR DISEASE

TOM P. AUFDERHEIDE

PATHOPHYSIOLOGY

The peripheral arterial vascular system can be considered as a single end-organ that manifests a wide variety of pathologic conditions. Eight basic pathophysiologic processes or conditions produce disease manifestations of this system: atherosclerosis, aneurysm, embolism, thrombosis, inflammation, trauma, vasospasm, and arteriovenous fistula.

VASCULAR HISTORY

Patients with peripheral arterial disease complain of pain, a change in skin sensation or appearance (swelling, discoloration, or temperature change), or tissue loss (ulceration or gangrene). Atherosclerosis and thrombosis account for the majority of peripheral arterial problems.

Atherosclerosis is the primary cause of peripheral arterial disease. Conditions that result from atherosclerosis and may constitute secondary evidence of its presence are cardiac disease, myocardial infarction, cardiac dysrhythmias (including atrial fibrillation), stroke, transient ischemic attacks, and renal disease. Risk factors for atherosclerosis are cigarette smoking, diabetes, hypercholesterolemia, and hypertension.

Historical factors important to the vascular history of but not related to atherosclerosis include prior injuries or operations, major illnesses, a history of phlebitis or pulmonary embolism, the presence of autoimmune disease or arthritis, and a history of prior coagulation abnormalities. Intravenous drug abuse can lead to arterial injury.

Acute Arterial Occlusion

Patients with acute arterial occlusion usually demonstrate some variation of the five "*P*s": pain, pallor, pulselessness, paresthesias, and paralysis. Paresthesias and paralysis indicate limb-threatening ischemia that requires emergency surgical intervention regardless of the cause. In patients with non–limb-threatening ischemia, patient management is determined by an accurate differentiation between embolism and in-situ thrombosis as the cause of acute arterial occlusion. Arterial embolism is best managed by emergency Fogarty catheter embolectomy. Non-limb-threatening ischemia from in-situ thrombosis is often aggravated by emergency surgical intervention and is therefore initially best managed nonoperatively, if possible (Fig. 35-1).

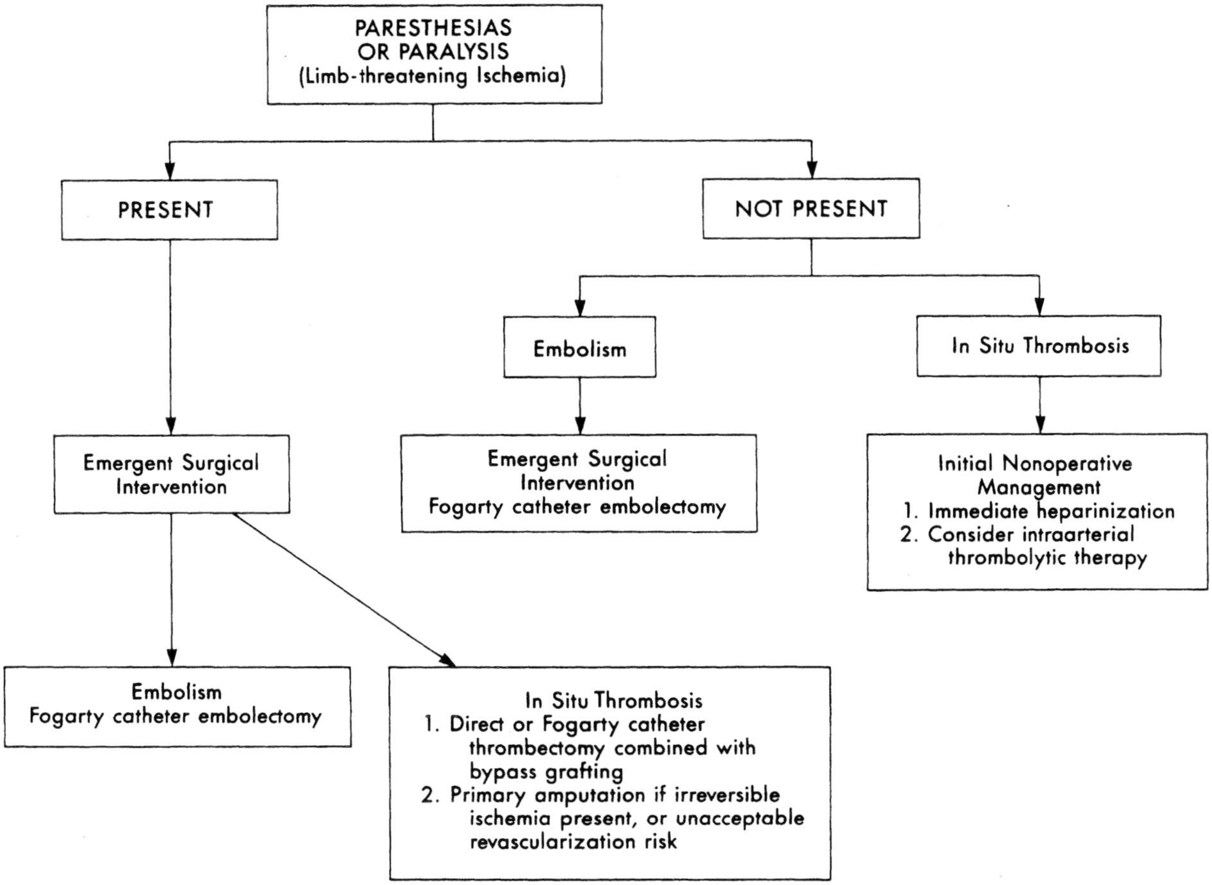

Fig.35-1 Clinical presentation and management of acute arterial occlusion. (From Aufderheide TP: Peripheral arteriovascular disease. In Rosen P et al, editors: *Emergency medicine: concepts and clinical practice,* ed 3, St Louis, 1992, Mosby.)

Acute arterial embolus

Acute arterial embolus usually occurs in patients without significant peripheral atherosclerosis and without well-developed collateral circulation. For these reasons, acute arterial embolus usually appears as a sudden, limb-threatening ischemia. Patients describe a sensation of the leg being suddenly "struck" by a severe shocking pain, which forces the patient to sit or fall to the ground during the event.

In-situ thrombosis

In-situ thrombosis is usually manifested in patients who have long-standing, significant peripheral atherosclerosis and well-developed collateral circulation. For these reasons, in-situ thrombosis often appears subacutely with non–limb-threatening ischemia. A prior history of claudication is common with in-situ thrombosis and rare in patients with arterial embolus.

Chronic Arterial Insufficiency

Intermittent claudication and ischemic rest pain are the two characteristic types of pain caused by chronic arterial insufficiency. The level of arterial occlusion is closely correlated with the location of intermittent claudication pain. Calf claudication is associated with femoral and popliteal occlusion. Patients complain of cramping pain, which is reliably reproduced by the same degree of exercise and completely relieved by several minutes of rest. Aortoiliac occlusive disease commonly causes claudication in the buttocks and hips in addition to the calves. Aortoiliac occlusive disease that is severe enough to produce bilateral claudication is almost always associated with impotence (Leriche syndrome).

Progression of chronic arterial insufficiency eventually results in ischemic pain at rest. Rest pain often begins in the foot distal to the metatarsals and awakens the patient from sleep. Ischemic rest pain is characterized as a severe, unrelenting pain that is aggravated by elevation and unrelieved by analgesics. Patients often sleep in a chair or with the leg dangling over the side of the bed, which improves perfusion pressure to distal tissues. Patients report a prompt relief of pain by assuming the standing position.

PHYSICAL EXAMINATION

A thorough and systematic evaluation of the peripheral vascular system is imperative. Palpation of the pairs of brachial, radial, femoral, posterior tibial, and dorsalis pedis arteries should be performed and documented on a 0-to-4 scale. Carotid arteries should be gently palpated independently and the findings documented.

The lower extremities should be examined for evidence of chronic and advanced ischemia, which is characterized by muscular atrophy, loss of hair growth over the dorsum of the toes and foot, and thickening of the toenails. The skin becomes shiny, scaly, and "skeletonized" from atrophy of the skin, subcutaneous tissue, and muscle as the ischemia becomes more advanced.

The physical examination can be helpful in differentiating arterial embolism from in-situ thrombosis in patients who have acute arterial occlusion. The absence of a previously present pulse is characteristic of arterial embolus. Chart review should be undertaken to objectively determine the prior pulse status of the limb. It is important to recognize that a bounding pulse may often be felt initially at the location of an embolism as the result of transmitted pulsations through a fresh clot. Patients with arterial embolus have few physical findings that suggest long-standing peripheral vascular disease with normal proximal and contralateral limb pulses. Tenderness to palpation may occasionally be noted at the site of an embolic occlusion.

Searching for the Source of a Suspected Embolus

The physical examination should be directed toward identifying the source of a suspected arterial embolus. Left ventricular mural thrombus secondary to a prior myocardial infarction and left atrial thrombus in a patient with mitral valve disease are the two most common sites. Coexistent atrial fibrillation is present in 60% to 75% of all cases.

The limb distal to an embolic occlusion is initially chalk white, and demarcation between ischemic and nonischemic tissue is sharp. Cyanosis may appear with the persistence of ischemia. Paresthesias or paralysis indicate limb-threatening ischemia. The presence of sensitivity to light touch is often the best guide to tissue viability. Complete anesthesia demands immediate surgical intervention. Paralysis represents severe skeletal muscle and neural ischemia that may be irreversible. Involuntary muscle contracture with woody hardness represents irreversible ischemia.

The physical findings of long-standing atherosclerotic occlusive disease are usually present in patients with in-situ thrombosis. Proximal or contralateral limb pulses are usually diminished or absent. An identifiable source for an embolus, such as mitral valve disease or atrial fibrillation, is usually not present. Demarcation of limb ischemia is less well defined because of well-established collateral circulation.

Auscultation of the carotid and femoral arteries should be undertaken to determine the presence or absence of bruits. The midabdomen should be similarly auscultated for evidence of abdominal aortic aneurysm or renal arterial bruits. If an occlusion of the upper extremity vessels is suspected, the subclavian artery should be evaluated by palpating for thrills and listening for bruits in the supraclavicular fossa.

A funduscopic examination allows direct visualization of retinal arterioles that may demonstrate evidence of arteriosclerosis or hypertension. Atheromatous emboli in the retinal arterioles, termed *Hollenhorst plaques,* may be detected. Roth spots (round or oval white spots seen near the optic disc) may be present in patients with infective endocarditis.

Inflammatory vascular disease manifests physical signs primarily by skin involvement. A palpable purpura is the typical lesion; however, other cutaneous manifestations of vasculitis, including macules, papules, vesicles, bullae, subcutaneous nodules, or ulcers, may occur. Skin lesions may be pruritic or even painful, with a burning or stinging sensation. Skin lesions more commonly occur in dependent areas—in the lower extremities in ambulatory patients or in the sacral area in bedridden patients. Hyperpigmentation often occurs in areas of recurrent or chronic lesions.

Emboli can cause diverse end-organ damage—hemiplegia from cerebral emboli, flank pain with hematuria from renal emboli, left upper quadrant abdominal pain from splenic infarcts, and pleuritic pain or hemoptysis from pulmonary emboli. Septic pulmonary emboli from right-sided endocarditis may be confused with pneumonia.

Lower Extremity Ulcers

The cause of lower extremity ulcers should be determined carefully. Approximately 5% of all lower extremity ulcerations are a result of arterial insufficiency. They are usually located distal to the ankle and typically at the terminal portion of the digits, around the nail beds, or between the toes as a result of friction of one toe on another. Arterial insufficiency ulcers are painful, but the pain is somewhat relieved when the extremity is in a dependent position. Arterial insufficiency ulcers are associated with evidence of coexisting chronic arterial insufficiency. Ulcers are initially small, shallow, and dry. The base is gray, yellow, or black, with minimal or no granulation tissue present. The rim of the ulcer is sharp and shows no signs of cellular proliferation or epithelialization.

Approximately 90% of all lower extremity ulcers are caused by chronic venous insufficiency. They are usually located proximal to or in the region of the ankle, particularly near the medial malleolus. Venous stasis ulcers are only mildly painful and improve with elevation of the extremity. Edema, prominent superficial veins, stasis dermatitis, and other evidence of long-standing chronic venous insufficiency are present. Ulcers are moderate in size with a weeping base and extensive granulation tissue. A rapidly developing ulcer is more suggestive of venous insufficiency.

Vasospastic Disorders

Vasospastic disorders are characterized by a sharp demarcation between ischemic and normal tissue. Intermittent attacks of triphasic skin color changes (pallor, cyanosis, and rubor) characterize Raynaud disease. Two other vasospastic disorders, livedo reticularis and acrocyanosis, have characteristic cutaneous manifestations. Livedo reticularis has a persistent cyanotic mottling of the skin with a "fishnet" appearance that typically involves the extremities and trunk. Acrocyanosis is the most uncommon of the vasospastic disorders and is characterized by persistent, painless, diffuse cyanosis of the fingers, hands, toes, and feet. The involved parts are nearly always cold, exhibit excessive perspiration, and have normal arterial pulsation.

Arteriovenous malformations and fistulae must be distinguished from vascular bruits or aneurysms. True aneurysms or arterial stenoses are associated with a systolic murmur. Pseudoaneurysms generally have a loud systolic and sometimes a separate faint diastolic murmur. Arteriovenous fistulae have a constant systolic and diastolic (to-and-fro) murmur, which is usually best heard directly over the lesion and often associated with a palpable thrill. Unless congenital, arteriovenous fistulae occur at prior operative or trauma sites. Large and long-standing arteriovenous fistulae produce high cardiac output and a widened pulse pressure. The tachycardia that may be observed in these patients may suddenly decrease when the artery leading to the fistula or fistula itself is occluded (Branham sign).

Bedside Testing

Any suspected area of ischemia can be tested by blanching with finger pressure. A delay in return of normal color on relieving the pressure (capillary refill) compared with that of the nonaffected extremity implies reduced perfusion.

Buerger sign

The *Buerger sign* provides reliable evidence of severe advanced ischemia. With the patient supine, the patient's feet are elevated more than 12 inches above the estimated level of the right atrium, and any change in the color of the feet is noted. If the color does not change, the patient dorsiflexes the feet five or six times. Latent color changes induced by exercise are noted.

With the patient sitting, the feet are next allowed to hang over the side of the stretcher, and the time of normal color return is recorded. Normal color should return within 10 seconds, and the veins should fill within 15 seconds. If the veins require more than 20 seconds to become distended, advanced ischemia is present. With severely restricted inflow and chronic dilatation of the peripheral vascular bed, the foot turns chalk white on elevation and intensely hyperemic after one minute of dependency. Localized pallor or cyanosis associated with poor capillary filling is usually a prelude to ischemic gangrene or ulceration.

Allen test

The *Allen test* is helpful in assessing the patency of the radial or ulnar artery distal to the wrist. The patient initially opens and closes the hand and clenches the fist to expel as much blood from the hand as possible. The examiner then compresses the radial and ulnar arteries. When the patient opens the fist, the hand is pale. The examiner then releases pressure from the radial artery but maintains it on the ulnar artery. If the radial artery distal to the wrist is patent, the hand rapidly becomes pink. If it is occluded, the hand remains pale. The maneuver is repeated by maintaining pressure on the radial artery while releasing the ulnar artery. A comparison can be made with the opposite hand.

Doppler ultrasonography

Doppler ultrasonography should be used in the emergency department in all patients with questionable or absent pulses. Doppler testing is more sensitive than palpation in detecting peripheral pulses. An estimate of the blood flow to the lower extremities can be made by measuring the systolic blood pressure at the level of the ankle and comparing it to the brachial systolic pressure. With patient supine, a blood pressure cuff is applied just proximal to the malleolus, inflated above brachial systolic pressure, and deflated slowly. Ankle systolic pressure can be accurately measured with a Doppler probe placed over the dorsalis pedis or posterior tibial arteries. This pressure is normally at least 90% of the brachial systolic pressure. With mild arterial insufficiency, it is between 70% and 90%; with moderate insufficiency, between 50% and 70%; and with severe insufficiency, below 50%.

Ancillary Evaluation

B-mode ultrasonic imaging

Real-time *B-mode ultrasonic imaging* uses differences in sound wave reflection from the interfaces between tissues with different acoustic impedances to provide anatomic detail of underlying structures. B-mode ultrasonography is noninvasive, painless, less expensive than some other modalities, such as arteriography, and widely available. The use of this technology by emergency physicians can lead to rapid diagnosis of immediate life-threatening conditions and can reduce the number of delayed or invasive diagnostic methods. B-mode ultrasonic imaging is the diagnostic procedure of choice for initially evaluating and determining the size of peripheral artery aneurysms.

Angiography

Angiography is the most definitive diagnostic test of abnormal peripheral artery anatomy but often gives inconclusive information about the physiologic condition of the tissues. Adverse effects of contrast media and catheter-related complications (complication rate averages 0.5%; mortality rate is 0.03%) must be weighed against the benefits of this procedure. An emergency angiography is commonly required in the following circumstances: (1) acute arterial embolus or thrombosis if the clinical diagnosis is uncertain (2) consideration of emergency vascular bypass grafting, and (3) for characterization of a vascular abnormality before emergency surgical correction. A decision to proceed with an angiography should be made in consultation with a vascular surgeon.

Other diagnostic modalities

Other diagnostic modalities are available to objectively assess the severity of arterial occlusive disease and are generally performed on an elective basis in a vascular surgery laboratory. Plethysmography, Doppler ultrasonography waveform analysis, duplex scanning, transcutaneous measurement of oxygen tension, radioisotope clearance, CT scans, and magnetic resonance imaging can be helpful in further characterizing reduced tissue perfusion or more accurately defining anatomic abnormalities.

CHRONIC ARTERIAL INSUFFICIENCY

Arteriosclerosis Obliterans

Arteriosclerosis obliterans most commonly affects the lower abdominal aorta, the iliac arteries, and the arteries supplying the lower extremities. Upper extremity manifestations are uncommon.

Exercise-induced claudication must be distinguished from the nocturnal muscle cramps that are commonly experienced by elderly patients during rest. The pain from osteoarthritis of the hip must be differentiated from aortoiliac occlusive disease. Osteoarthritis of the hip tends to vary from day to day, is not relieved completely with rest, and is not reliably reproduced by the same amount of exercise. The cauda equina syndrome is caused by a narrowing of the lumbar canal and may produce pseudoclaudication, but it is less closely related to exercise and rest than true claudication.

Buerger Disease (Thromboangiitis Obliterans)

Buerger disease is an idiopathic inflammatory occlusive disease that primarily involves the medium and small arteries of the hands and feet. Patients are usually men between the ages of 20 and 40 who use tobacco. The initial arterial inflammatory process progresses to affect the adjacent veins and nerves and often leads to venous thrombosis and progressive fibrous encasement of these structures. This process results in the hallmark finding termed phlebitis migrans, which is characterized by painful, tender, reddened, or dark nodules over a peripheral artery in which the pulse is either reduced or absent.

Virtually all patients with Buerger disease chew or smoke tobacco. Clinical criteria for the diagnosis of Buerger disease include the following: (1) a history of smoking, (2) onset before the age of 50, (3) infrapopliteal arterial occlusive lesions, (4) upper limb involvement or phlebitis migrans, and (5) absence of atherosclerotic risk factors other than smoking.

Infrapopliteal arterial occlusion results in the most characteristic symptom of Buerger disease, which is foot or instep claudication. Foot pulses may be absent in the presence of normal femoral and popliteal pulses. Hand involvement is often bilateral and symmetric and leads to hand claudication or fingertip ulcers. Phlebitis migrans occurs early in the disease. Approximately one half of all patients with Buerger disease experience a Raynaud-type triphasic color response to cold.

ACUTE ARTERIAL OCCLUSION

Arterial Embolism

Approximately 50% of all acute arterial occlusions are caused by arterial embolism; the other 50% are caused by in-situ thrombosis. The clinical differentiation of arterial embolism and thrombosis has already been reviewed (see Fig. 35-1).

Atheroembolism (Blue Toe Syndrome)

Atheroemboli are microscopic aggregates of cholesterol, calcium, and platelets that have dislodged from proximal complicated atherosclerotic plaques or aneurysms; atheroemboli result in multiple sites of acute arterial occlusion in the distal end arteries of the digits and toes.

Showers of atheroemboli result in the sudden onset of multiple small painful areas on the foot and toes, which are cyanotic and tender to touch. If involvement is bilateral, the distribution is not symmetrical. Because atheroemboli lodge in distal end arteries, the posterior tibial and dorsalis pedis pulses are present. The physical examination should be directed toward identifying a proximal source of atheroemboli, such as an atherosclerotic aneurysm of the aorta, iliac, femoral, or popliteal arteries.

Arterial Thrombosis

Acute arterial thrombosis is almost always caused by intense thrombogenesis of a complicated atherosclerotic plaque. Its subacute onset and lack of sharply demarcated ischemic borders in a patient with long-standing peripheral arteriovascular disease helps differentiate it from acute arterial embolism.

PERIPHERAL ARTERIAL ANEURYSMS

Peripheral arterial aneurysms rarely rupture but instead cause symptoms of distal acute arterial occlusion as a result of embolism or thrombosis.

Lower Extremity Aneurysms

The most common peripheral aneurysms are *popliteal aneurysms.* Sixty percent of all popliteal aneurysms are bilateral. There is an 80% incidence of a coexisting abdominal aortic aneurysm in patients with a bilateral popliteal aneurysm.

Femoral aneurysms are the second most common type of peripheral aneurysm. Patients with peripheral arterial aneurysms usually experience claudication, thromboembolic events, atheroembolic events, or gangrene. Aneurysmal dilatation can cause venous compression with associated deep venous thrombosis. Femoral or popliteal aneurysms can be diagnosed by palpation of a pulsatile mass with unilateral or bilateral calcified aneurysms demonstrated on bilateral plain x-ray studies.

Upper Extremity Aneurysms

Peripheral arterial aneurysms in the upper extremities are rare. Because atherosclerosis generally spares the upper extremities, localized trauma is the most common cause of an upper extremity aneurysm.

Subclavian artery aneurysms are primarily caused by thoracic outlet obstruction and trauma. With acute aneurysm expansion, patients may have chest, neck, or shoulder pain. Compression of the right recurrent laryngeal nerve can lead to a voice change. Compression of the trachea results in stridor or other respiratory complaints. A distal embolic phenomenon may produce acute limb ischemia.

Subclavian-axillary artery aneurysms are most common in women and in the dominant upper extremity and are caused by a complete cervical rib that articulates with the first rib to produce a poststenotic dilatation. *Axillary artery aneurysms* are most commonly caused by blunt trauma from an inappropriate and prolonged use of crutches. The rare syndrome of *ulnar artery aneurysms* is associated with occupational trauma in which the heel of the palm is used to hammer, push, or twist objects. This syndrome, alternately termed *hypothenar hammer syndrome,* is most often seen in industrial workers such as mechanics, carpenters, and machinists.

Infected Aneurysms

Currently the most common cause of an infected aneurysm is sepsis with hematogenous spread of bacteria to atherosclerotic arteries. Organisms associated with these infected aneurysms are *Salmonella* organisms, *Staphylococcus* organisms, and *Escherichia coli.* The incidence of infection in preexisting atherosclerotic aneurysms

has been estimated to be between 3% and 4%. Gram-positive organisms, especially *Staphylococcus* organisms, predominate (60%). *Posttraumatic infected aneurysms* result from invasive hemodynamic monitoring, angiography, and intravenous drug use. *Staphylococcus aureus* is associated in 30% to 70% of all cases. *Mycotic aneurysms* are infected aneurysms caused by septic emboli that results from bacterial endocarditis. Gram-positive cocci are most common.

Traumatic Aneurysms

A *traumatic aneurysm* refers to a perforation of the arterial wall with formation of a perivascular hematoma. Traumatic aneurysms may or may not be associated with an arteriovenous fistula. Synonyms for traumatic aneurysm include a pseudoaneurysm and false aneurysm.

The usual presentation of a traumatic aneurysm is a pulsatile mass found near the course of an extremity artery that has a past history of trauma (or surgery) more than 1 month earlier. A loud systolic and possibly a separate diastolic murmur are characteristic of a traumatic aneurysm.

VASOSPASTIC DISORDERS

An abnormal vasomotor response in the distal small arteries characterizes the vasospastic disorders; the cause of the heightened vasospastic response is unknown. True histologic changes within the vessel wall are absent.

Raynaud Disease

Raynaud disease is the most common vasospastic disorder and occurs at least five times as often in women as in men. By definition, Raynaud disease has no evidence of an underlying cause. The following criteria assist in diagnosis: (1) episodes are precipitated by cold or emotion, (2) symptoms are bilateral, (3) gangrene is absent or is minimal and confined to the skin, (4) the absence of any disease or condition that may cause a secondary Raynaud phenomenon, and (5) symptoms have been occurring for at least 2 years. The classic Raynaud attack is triphasic: the fingers become chalk white, then blue, and finally red. This phenomenon is produced initially by complete closure of the palmar and digital arteries, which produces cessation of capillary perfusion. When slight relaxation of arterial spasm occurs, a slight flow of blood returns to the dilated capillary bed, where it rapidly dissipates and produces cyanosis. When arterial flow returns to baseline, reactive hyperemia produces a red extremity.

Raynaud Phenomenon

Raynaud phenomenon is Raynaud disease that occurs secondary to an identifiable underlying disorder. Connective tissue disorders such as scleroderma, rheumatoid arthritis, and systemic lupus erythematosus are the most common underlying disorders.

Other Vasospastic Disorders

Benign *livedo reticularis* is caused by a spasm of the dermal arterioles in response to cold and is characterized by a persistent cyanotic mottling of the skin, which gives the skin a typical "fishnet" appearance. *Acrocyanosis* is the most uncommon of the vasospastic disorders. It occurs more often in women; is intensified by exposure to cold; and is characterized by bilateral, persistent, painless, symmetric cyanosis of the fingers, hands, and, less commonly, the feet. Excessive perspiration is a common accompanying feature. Primary *erythromelalgia* is a rare syndrome of paroxysmal vasodilatation with burning pain, increased skin temperature, and redness of the feet and, less often, the hands. Attacks are not triggered by cold.

No treatment is required for livedo reticularis. No consistently effective treatment has been found for acrocyanosis or erythromelalgia.

NECROTIZING VASCULITIDES

The necrotizing vasculitides are characterized by inflammation and necrosis of blood vessels and are thought to be induced by immune complexes. The clinical manifestations of different forms of vasculitis depend on the size and location of the vessels involved.

Temporal arteritis is a representative example of a vasculitis of medium and large arteries; it characteristically involves one or more branches of the carotid artery, particularly the temporal artery. It is most common in elderly women in the United States and Europe, with a prevalence of approximately 1 out of every 1000 patients age 50 and over. The classic presentation is that of fever, anemia, a high erythrocyte sedimentation rate (greater than 100 mm/hour), and headaches in an elderly patient. The temporal artery may be thickened, nodular, or tender to palpation. It is imperative to ask about visual symptoms such as diplopia or occasional ptosis. Retinal or optic nerve ischemia rapidly occurs following the initial visual symptoms, and the vision loss is usually irreversible. Patients with impending visual complications require hospitalization and treatment with high-dose intravenous steroids. The first dose should be administered in the emergency department. Jaw claudication from stenosis of the arteries that supply the muscles of mastication is a clinical hallmark of temporal arteritis.

THORACIC OUTLET SYNDROME

Thoracic outlet syndrome involves compression of the brachial plexus, subclavian vein, or subclavian artery at the superior aperture of the thorax. Compression of the brachial plexus causes the neurologic type of thoracic outlet syndrome and constitutes approximately 95% of all thoracic outlet syndrome cases. The onset of symptoms occurs between the ages of 20 and 50 years, with women predominating approximately three to one. Compression or thrombosis of the subclavian vein constitutes the venous type of thoracic outlet syndrome and is responsible for 4% of all cases. It occurs most commonly in men between the ages of 20 and 35 years. The arterial type of thoracic outlet syndrome is rare and occurs in approximately 1% of all cases. Men and women are affected equally in a bimodal age distribution of young adults and patients greater than 50 years of age.

The subclavian artery, subclavian vein, or brachial plexus can be compressed from a cervical rib, variations in the insertion of anterior scalene muscle, hypertrophy of the subclavius muscle, abnormalities of the first rib, or old clavicular fractures (Fig. 35-2).

Compression or irritation of the brachial plexus most commonly affects the two lower nerve roots, C8 and T1, which produces pain and paresthesias in the ulnar nerve distribution. The second most common anatomic pattern involves the upper three nerve roots of the brachial plexus—C5, C6, and C7—with symptoms referable to the neck, ear, upper chest, upper back, and outer arm in the radial nerve distribution. Venous compression eventually progresses to intimal damage and subclavian

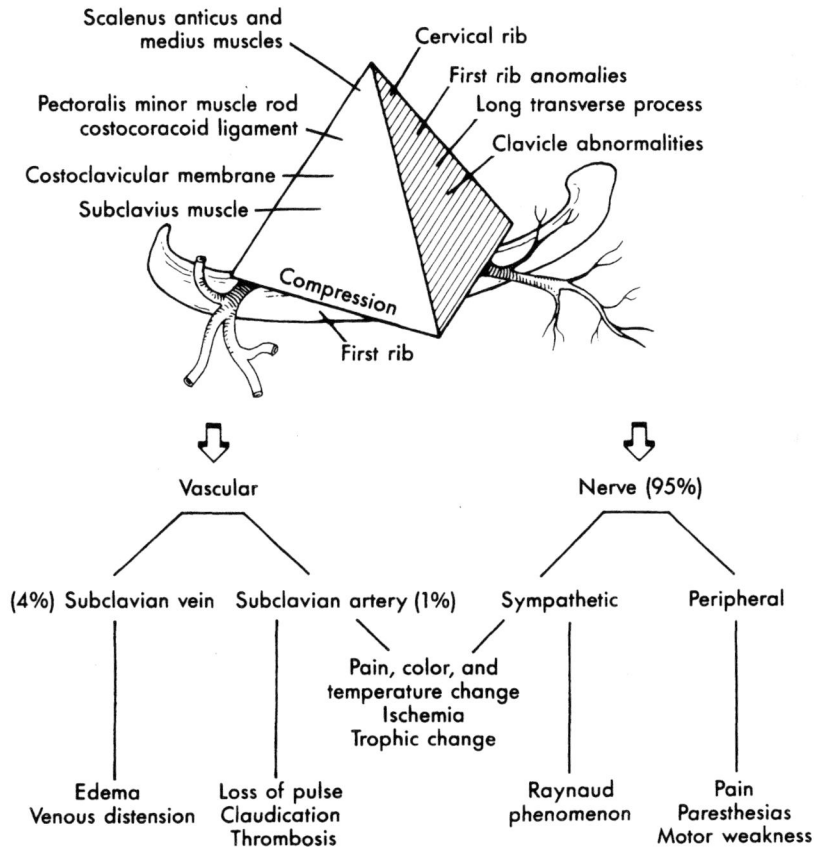

Fig.35-2 Schematic diagram showing relations of muscle, ligament, and bone abnormalities in thoracic outlet that may compress neurovascular structures. (From Urschel HC Jr, Razzuk MA: Thoracic outlet syndrome, *N Engl J Med* 286:1140, 1972.)

vein thrombosis, with venous engorgement and swelling of the affected extremity. Persistent subclavian artery compression eventually results in poststenotic aneurysm formation and its pathologic sequelae (see Fig. 35-2).

The Adson, costoclavicular, and hyperabduction maneuvers are unreliable as diagnostic tests for thoracic outlet syndrome. Only 1% of all patients with thoracic outlet syndrome have involvement of the subclavian artery. Furthermore, most (92%) asymptomatic patients have variation in the strength of the radial pulse during positional changes.

The most reliable test in screening for thoracic outlet syndrome is the elevated arm stress test (EAST). To perform this test, the patient sits with the arms abducted 90 degrees from the thorax and the elbows flexed 90 degrees and with the shoulders braced slightly behind the frontal plane. The patient is asked to open and close the fists slowly but steadily for 3 minutes and to describe any symptoms that develop. Normally, a patient can perform this test without any symptoms other than mild fatigue. A patient with thoracic outlet syndrome develops symptoms of early heaviness and fatigue of the involved limb, gradual onset of hand numbness, and progressive aching through the arm and top of the shoulder. Within 3 minutes of test initiation, the patient usually drops the hand to the lap for relief of the progressive distress that becomes intolerable. Patients with carpal tunnel syndrome may experience dysesthesias in the fingers but do not have shoulder or arm pain. Patients with cervical disk syndrome may have pain in the neck and shoulder but have no arm or hand symptoms.

The EAST evaluates all three types of thoracic outlet syndrome: neurologic, venous, and arterial. Radial pulses may be palpated by the examiner during the test. The presence of a radial pulse and a positive EAST result are strong indications that the basis of the symptoms is neurologic involvement of the brachial plexus.

The differential diagnosis of thoracic outlet syndrome is extensive and includes a herniated cervical disk, cervical spondylitis, a spinal cord tumor, ulnar nerve compression at the elbow, carpal tunnel syndrome, orthopedic shoulder problems, trauma, postural palsy, angina pectoris, and a variety of neuropathies.

PERIPHERAL ARTERIOVENOUS FISTULAE

Acquired peripheral arteriovenous fistulae are most commonly caused by trauma, including gunshot wounds, stab wounds, or surgery. The correct diagnosis may be made with a clinical examination alone. A constant systolic and diastolic (to-and-fro) murmur associated with a palpable thrill is characteristic of peripheral arteriovenous fistulae. Sixty percent of all arteriovenous fistulae are also associated with a coexisting false aneurysm.

Recommended Reading

Aufderheide TP: Peripheral arteriovascular disease. In Rosen P et al, editors: *Emergency medicine: concepts and clinical practice,* ed 3, St Louis, 1992, Mosby.

Connett MC, Murray DH Jr, Wenneker WW: Peripheral arterial emboli, *Am J Surg* 148:14, 1984.

Crawford ES: Aorto-iliac occlusive disease: factors influencing survival and function following reconstructive operations over a 25-year period, *Surgery* 90:1055, 1981.

Kumagai K: Increased intracardiovascular clotting in patients with chronic atrial fibrillation. *J Am Coll Cardiol* 16:377, 1990.

Roos DB: New concepts of thoracic outlet syndrome that explain etiology, symptoms, diagnosis, and treatment, *J Vasc Surg* 13:313, 1979.

Rutherford RB, editor: *Vascular Surgery,* ed 3, Philadelphia, 1989, WB Saunders.

Sicard GA: Thrombolytic therapy for acute arterial occlusion, *J Vasc Surg* 2:65, 1985.

Chapter Thirty-six
ISCHEMIC HEART DISEASE

EDWIN CARY PIGMAN

The physiologic basis of ischemic heart disease (IHD) is that the cellular myocardial oxygen demand exceeds the capacity of the coronary vasculature to deliver oxygen. This impaired capacity of the coronary arteries is a result of partial or complete obstructions. In stable angina, the myocardium receives sufficient supplies of oxygen except when there is significant exertion and the increased needs of the myocardium cannot be met. Unstable anginal syndromes and acute myocardial infarction (AMI) result from the abrupt blockage of a coronary artery by a thrombus, usually at the site of a fixed coronary artery narrowing and principally as a result of atheromas. Similar data support the "wave" concept of myocardial necrosis, in which cell death first occurs at the endocardial layer, gradually extends transmurally to the epicardium, and involves more at-risk myocardium like ripples in a pond.

This phenomenon has led to the "open infarct-related artery" theory, which states that the more rapidly the occluded artery is made patent, the greater the myocardial salvage. This greater myocardial salvage translates into better myocardial function and improved survival. This early intervention is the challenge to emergency medicine physicians.

ASSESSMENT

History

The patient's description of his or her symptoms is one of the two most critical evaluation components for the emergency medicine physician. The patient with pain resulting from myocardial ischemia will typically complain of a retrosternal chest discomfort that is pressure like, constricting, or squeezing. A classic description is of a weight on the chest. The pain may be burning or cramping in nature. Some patients may even hesitate to call it a "pain" but prefer to call it a "feeling" or "sensation in my chest." The pain may radiate into the neck, arm, or abdomen or be noted only in the epigastrum, shoulder, mandible, back, or arm.

The pain of myocardial ischemia is typically exertional in nature, requiring several seconds to minutes to crescendo with exertion and easing with rest. Often a careful history reveals a prior history of exertional-type symptoms. Associated symptoms typically are present, such as dyspnea, diaphoresis, nausea, emesis, near syncope, or syncope.

The presence of risk factors should be sought in the patient who is being evaluated for chest pain (or any symptom suggestive of IHD) and who does not already have a history of IHD. A history of prolonged smoking, uncontrolled or poorly controlled hypertension, hyperlipidemia, diabetes mellitus, or the presence of IHD in family relatives (especially in those younger than 50 years of age) increases the likelihood of IHD.

Physical Examination

IHD is responsible for few direct signs that are apparent on physical examination. Because IHD represents diseased coronary arteries, findings consistent with peripheral vascular disease (e.g., diminished peripheral pulses or skin ulcerations) support the possibility that the patient's chest pain or other symptom may represent IHD. Hereditary hyperlipidemias may be suggested by certain skin lesions such as xanthelasmas.

The typical signs present in IHD are those of myocardial dysfunction. The value of the physical examination is to assess the degree of congestive heart failure. The examination is important as a tool to guide therapy and assess prognosis. The patient in florid pulmonary edema is easy to identify, but the patient with subtle cardiac auscultatory findings is not. An S_3 or S_4 gallop may be present during myocardial ischemia. However, neither gallop is specific for IHD. Rales on chest auscultation may indicate pulmonary edema as a result of left ventricular dysfunction;

peripheral edema and ascites may indicate right ventricular dysfunction. A new murmur may indicate papillary muscle dysfunction or necrosis.

Another use for the physical examination is the identification of signs that suggest an alternative diagnosis in the patient at low risk for IHD. Point tenderness at the costrochondral junction in a young person suggests costrochondritis, a precordial rub suggests pericarditis, and in an older patient a typical vesicular eruption in a dermatomal distribution suggests herpes zoster.

Electrocardiogram

The ECG is the second most critical evaluation component for the emergency medicine physician. It is critical to understand that a normal ECG does not exclude a diagnosis of IHD. If the first ECG is not diagnostic and the suspicion of AMI is high, the emergency physician is often best served by one or two additional tracings in the emergency department. Having an older tracing for comparison can be very beneficial. Accurate interpretation of the ECG is critical because decisions regarding thrombolytic therapy are made on the basis of ST segment findings.

An early indicator of transmural myocardial infarction is the presence of prominent T waves

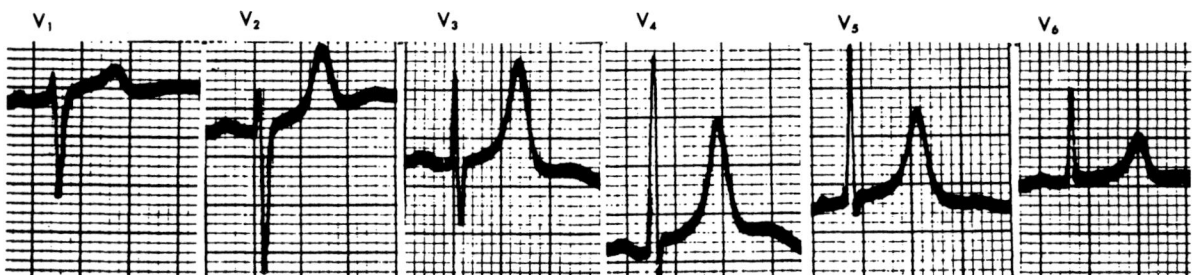

Fig.36-1 Precordial leads showing hyperacute T waves. Precordial T waves are abnormal, symmetric, and prominent (over 10 mm in leads V_3 and V_4). Normal T wave is assymmetric, with steeper descending than ascending limb. (From Schamroth L: *The electrocardiology of coronary artery disease*, Oxford, 1975, Blackwell Scientific Publications.)

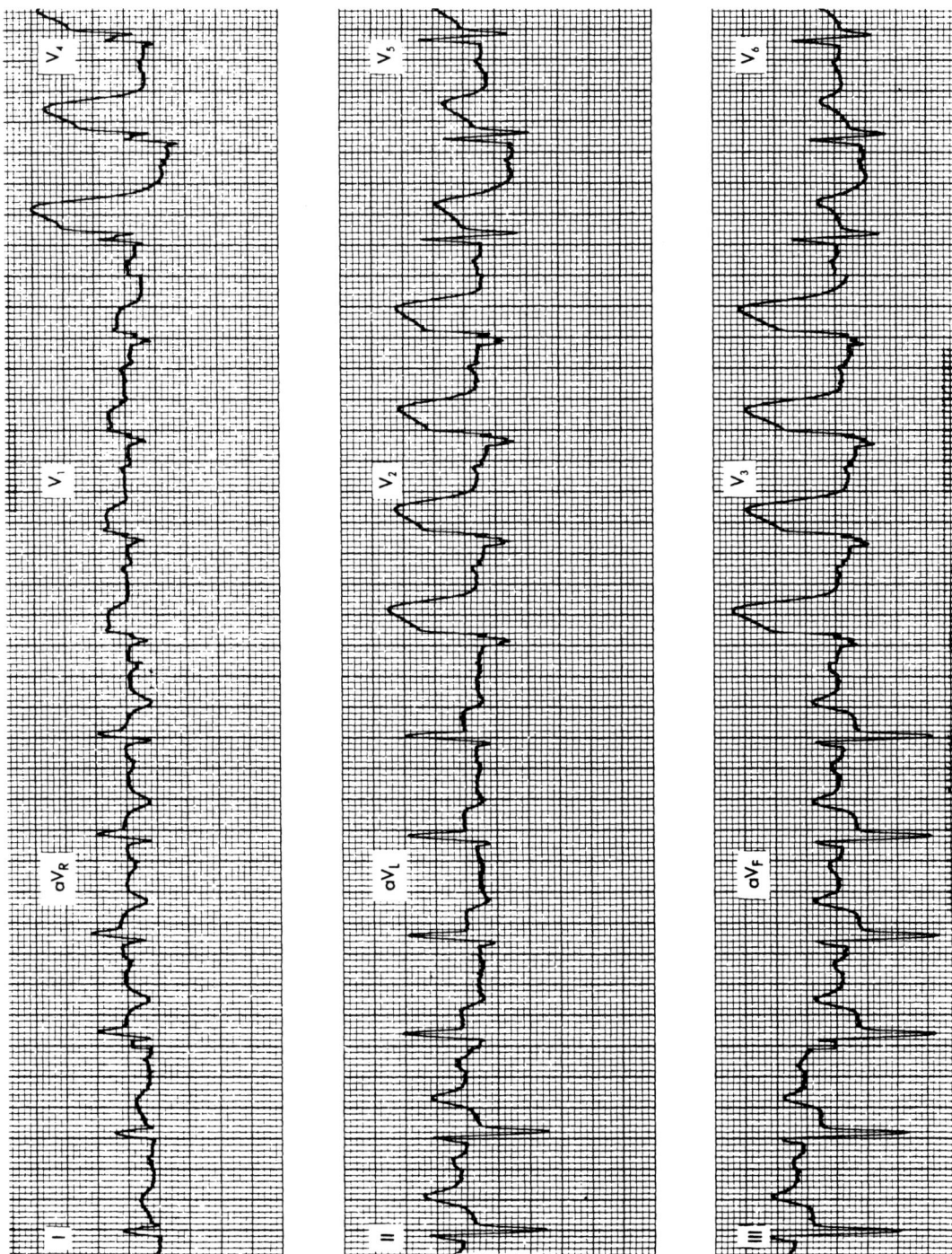

Fig 36-2   Acute anteroseptal myocardial infarction. Acute current of injury and hyperacute T waves are seen in leads I, aV$_L$, and V$_1$ to V$_5$. Elevated ST segments blend with prominent T waves. Pathologic Q waves are present in leads aV$_L$ and V$_1$ to V$_3$.

(Fig. 36-1). T waves are best seen in the precordial leads and are usually greater than 7 mm in height. They are peaked symmetrically and usually associated with ST-segment elevation. ST-segment elevation is a second early sign of severe ischemia (Fig. 36-2). This elevation may range from 1 to 10 mm. ST-segment depression is also associated with ischemia but is less specific.

Pathologic Q waves are initial negative QRS deflections of 0.04 seconds or longer in leads other than aV_R and V_1. They typically appear within 24 hours of a transmural infarction, but a

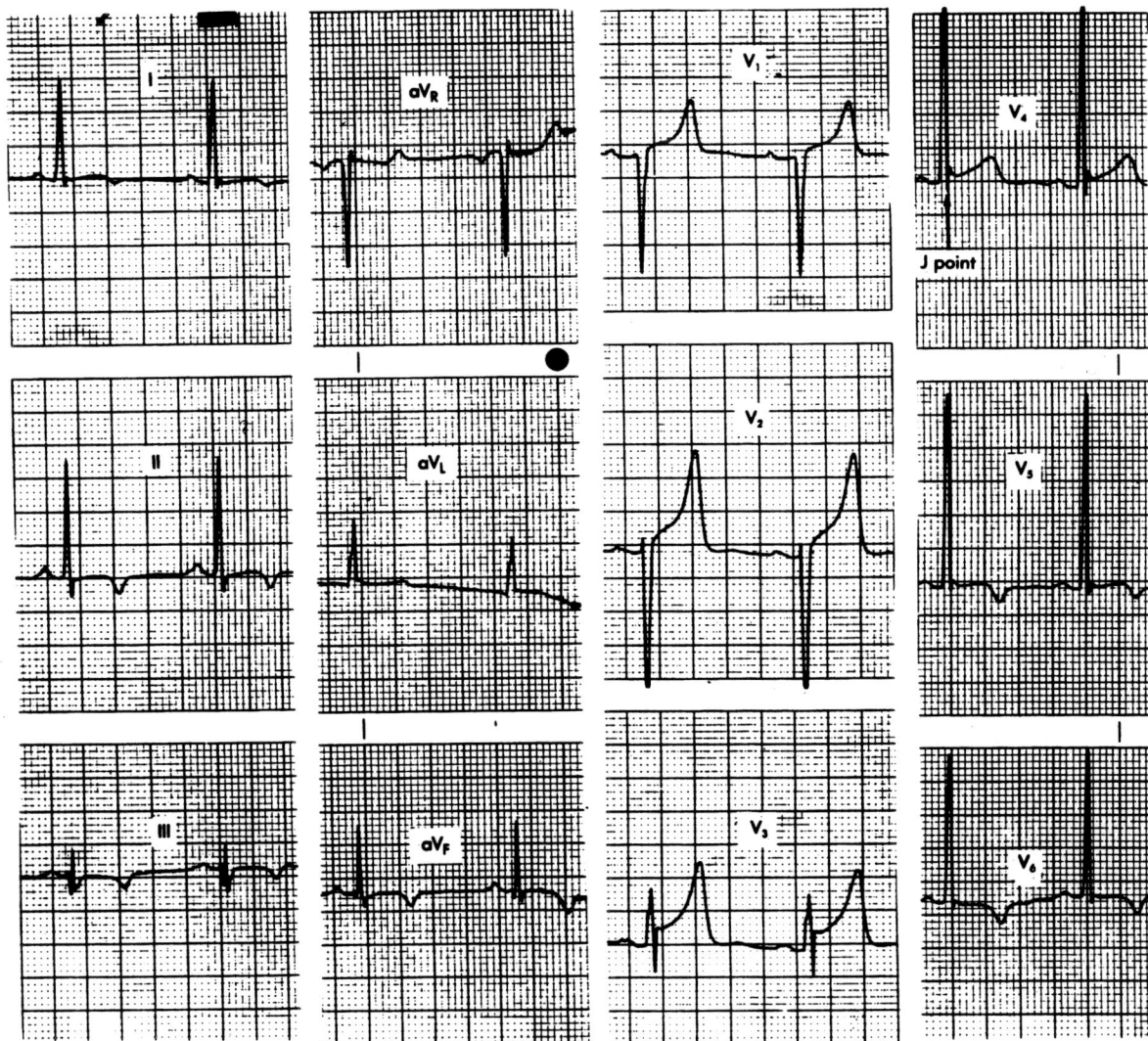

Fig.36-3 Benign early repolarization. Elevated ST segments with upward concavity are seen in leads V_1 to V_4. A notched J point, the hallmark of benign early repolarization, is evident in the left precordial leads.

significant number of AMIs never demonstrate Q-wave evolution.

Certain conditions may be electrocardiographically confused with myocardial ischemic patterns. Benign early repolarization (BER) is often found in healthy young adults and is characterized by ST-segment elevation and prominent T waves (Fig. 36-3). A notched J point (the junction of the ST segment and the QRS complex) is very suggestive of BER. Acute pericarditis may produce diffuse ST-segment elevations that are similar to those produced with myocardial ischemia (Fig. 36-4). They may be distinguished by their diffuse presence and are typically present in each bipolar limb lead (I, II, III) and all precordial leads. PR-segment depression is occasionally seen and is very suggestive of pericarditis. Hyperkalemia can also produce prominent T waves and elevated ST segments.

A bundle branch block (BBB) pattern obscures the changes of an AMI, especially a left bundle branch block (LBBB) (Fig. 36-5). Although bundle branch patterns may exist without any underlying coronary artery disease, cardiac ischemia is suggested by the new appearance of a BBB (especially an LBBB) associated with any symptom complex consistent with IHD.

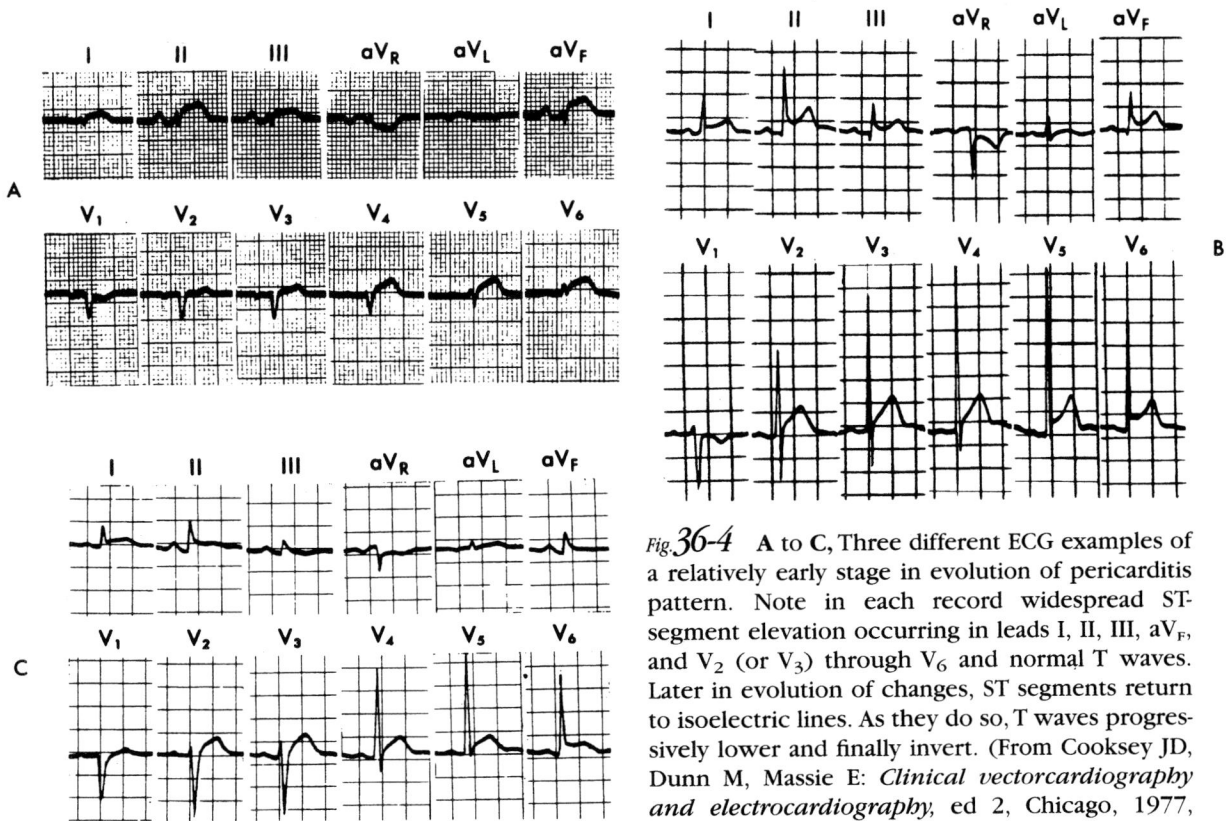

Fig.36-4 **A** to **C,** Three different ECG examples of a relatively early stage in evolution of pericarditis pattern. Note in each record widespread ST-segment elevation occurring in leads I, II, III, aV_F, and V_2 (or V_3) through V_6 and normal T waves. Later in evolution of changes, ST segments return to isoelectric lines. As they do so, T waves progressively lower and finally invert. (From Cooksey JD, Dunn M, Massie E: *Clinical vectorcardiography and electrocardiography,* ed 2, Chicago, 1977, Year Book Medical Publishers.)

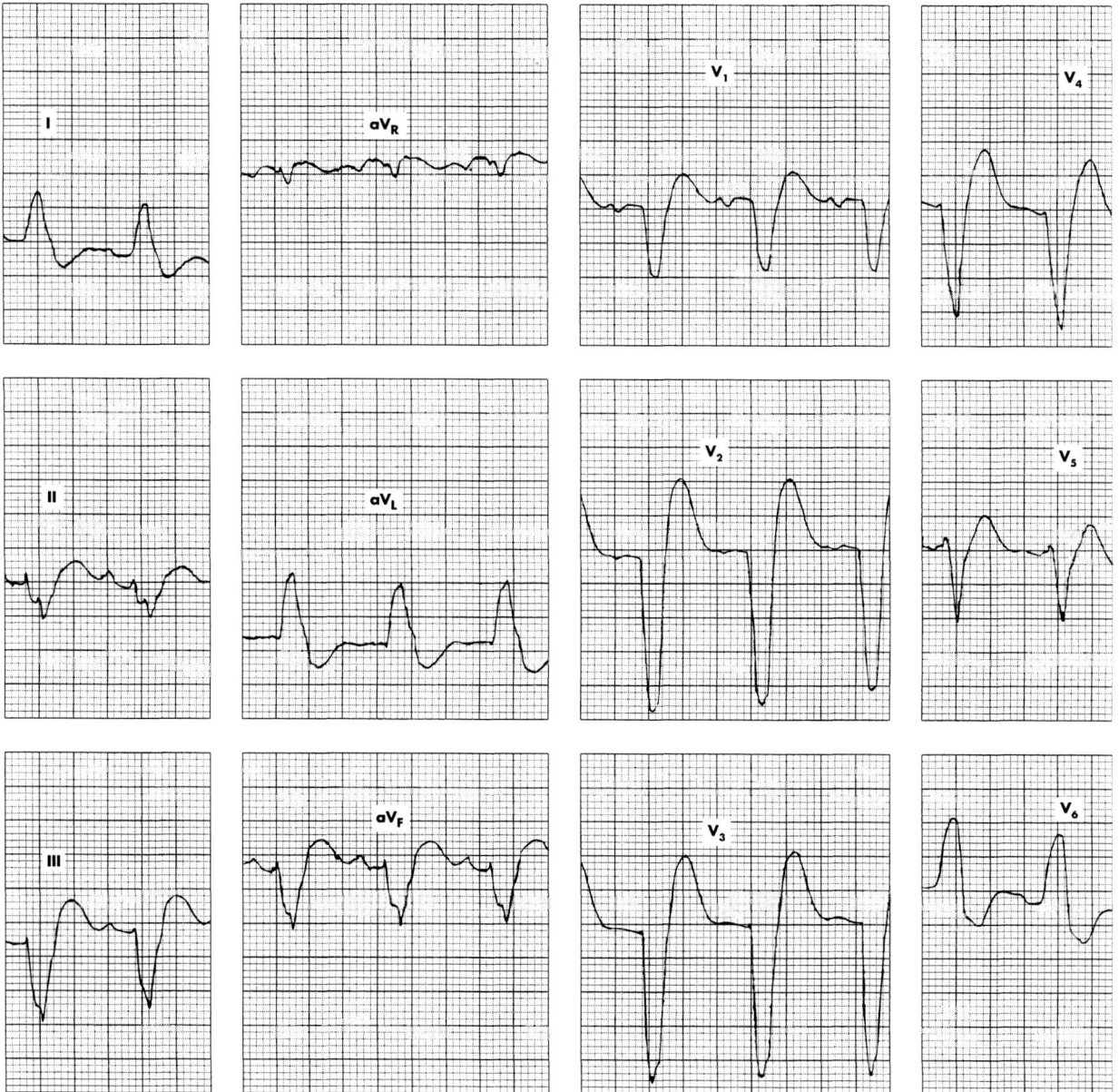

Fig. 36-5   Left bundle branch block with left axis deviation and concordant ST-T wave abnormalities.

Chest Radiography

A portable chest x-ray study may reveal evidence of cardiac decompensation not suggested by the physical examination. Cardiomegaly and pulmonary congestion may be demonstrated and may contribute to the emergency management of the patient with unstable angina or AMI.

Cardiac Enzymes

The detection of intracellular cardiac macromolecules in the peripheral circulation is the sine que non for the diagnosis of myocardial cellular damage.

Creatinine kinase (CK) rises within 4 to 6 hours of an AMI and peaks within 10 to 18 hours. Monoclonal antibody techniques allow rapid, bedside testing for CK. At least 95% of all myocardial infarctions are associated with an elevated total CK. A limitation of CK is that it is found in skeletal muscle and the brain; therefore any condition that damages these two systems also elevates CK. CK is composed of three isoenzymes: CK-BB (found in brain), CK-MM (found in skeletal and myocardial tissues), and CK-MB (found exclusively in myocardial tissue). Normal myocardial tissue contains 85% CK-MM and 15% CK-MB. Testing directed at determining the elevation of CK-MB not only increases the specificity by eliminating positive results from skeletal or brain injury, but it also increases the sensitivity by detecting small myocardial infarcts (especially small subendocardial AMIs) in which the amount of cellular damage is too small to raise the total CK but large enough to raise that portion of CK made up by the MB isoenzyme.

Several additional methodologies are under study to allow more rapid detection of AMI, which is an especially important determination for those patients without a diagnostic ECG. Isoforms of CK are being studied. The CK-MM$_3$, a tissue form of the MM isoenzyme that is rapidly broken down into MM$_2$ and MM$_1$ isoforms, may hold promise. An MM3:MM1 ratio that increases

above 0.8 (normal value is 0.5) may be detectable before total CK or CK-MB values increase. Myoglobin, a small intracellular oxygen transport molecule, rises within 1 to 2 hours and peaks within 4 hours of an AMI. Both of these new methods benefit from allowing earlier detection of myocardial damage, but they both have a reduced specificity as a result of the many noncardiac causes that can result in their release from an intracellular site. Serum cardiac troponin has also been studied as an early indicator of myocardial damage.

Cardiac Sonography

Cardiac sonography can be useful as a diagnostic aid to evaluate the presence of an acute manifestation of IHD in addition to providing information regarding cardiac wall thickening, the presence of ventricular thrombi, and valvular function. Wall motion abnormalities, which would be present during acute ischemia or with a transmural infarction, can be detected reliably with two-dimensional echocardiography. This technique may become part of the emergency physician's diagnostic armamentarum.

Differential Diagnosis

The differential diagnosis for the acute manifestations of IHD is large and includes practically all conditions related to the chest and abdomen. Major alternative diagnoses include thoracic aortic dissection, pulmonary embolism, pericarditis, pneumonia, pneumothorax, peptic ulcer disease, esophageal disorders, biliary colic, and chest wall conditions such as costrochondritis or herpes zoster.

CLINICAL PRESENTATIONS

Stable Angina

A patient with stable angina, in which the frequency and quality of chest pain has not changed recently, is unlikely to come to the emergency department because of the chest pain. However, this patient may have an unrelated complaint in which the review of systems reveals a history of stable IHD. The goal for the emergency physician is to determine that the new complaint is, in fact, unrelated.

Unstable Angina

Any change in chest pain frequency, intensity, quality, or initiating factor in the patient with IHD constitutes unstable angina. Pain occurring at rest is of particular concern for the patient with IHD. It is presumed that this type of patient is experiencing increasing coronary artery stenosis with intermittent occlusion; these patients are at high risk for subsequent complete occlusion, with AMI and death. They require admission to the hospital and to a coronary care unit or a telemetry-monitored unit depending on the ease of control of their symptoms. Therapeutic interventions include supplemental oxygen, nitroglycerin (sublingually, topically, or intravenously), aspirin, heparin, and opiates.

The patient with new onset angina must also be considered as having unstable angina. Often the diagnosis for this type of patient is unclear.

Acute Myocardial Infarction

The patient with AMI typically complains of severe and unrelenting chest pain with radiation into the neck or shoulder. The patient is often pale, dyspneic, diaphoretic, and appears to be in significant distress. This pain will have been constant for more than 15 minutes. However, a large number of patients have less clear complaints, and some patients suffer an AMI and never have chest pain. Other symptoms, such as dyspnea or abdominal pain, may represent an anginal equivalent and be the only complaint.

An inferior wall AMI manifests changes in leads II, III, and aV$_F$. Isolated right coronary artery or left circumflex artery disease is suggested when these are the only leads involved. More extensive disease of the left anterior descending branch of the left coronary artery is present when the infarct pattern also involves changes in V$_1$ to V$_4$. Inferior wall AMIs are associated with less myocardial impairment than anterior wall AMIs. Complete heart block may develop gradually, often progressing from first-degree and type I second-degree blocks. Usually this block is transient and does not require permanent pacing. Inferior wall AMIs tend to be associated with an increased vagal tone and have a high incidence of symptomatic bradycardia. Because of diaphragmatic irritation, these infarcts are often associated with gastrointestinal symptoms such as nausea, emesis, and epigastric discomfort.

An anterior wall AMI manifests changes in the precordial leads and limb leads I and aV$_L$. The diseased artery is the left anterior descending branch of the left coronary artery. An anterior wall AMI represents a more extensive amount of myocardial damage than an inferior wall AMI. These patients are at greater risk for abrupt and dramatic onset of complete heart block. Patients with anterior wall AMIs who have any evidence of intraventricular block should be paced in anticipation of complete heart block.

A true posterior wall infarct manifests only reciprocal changes. There may be tall R waves in V$_1$ to V$_3$. The T waves may be tall, symmetric, and upright with depressed, concave-up ST segments.

Some AMIs are characterized by a serum cardiac enzyme elevation (indicating myocardial damage) but also produce an ECG that never demonstrates a typical injury pattern of Q-wave formation. These AMIs have several names, such as subendocardial, nontransmural, or non–Q wave infarcts. The unifying concept is that these infarcts have not involved the entire thickness of the myocardium. Although the short-term mortality with this "partial" AMI is not great, it is associated with a high risk of subsequent larger, full-thickness AMIs. Because of this reinfarction risk, a 1-year mortality rate is greater with subendocardial AMIs than with full-thickness AMIs.

Sudden Death

Sudden death, which is defined as death that occurs within 1 hour of symptom onset, is a common presentation of AMI. It can result from papillary muscle rupture, cardiac wall rupture, or malignant dysrhythmia. However, myocardial death does not need to be present for sudden death. The successful early resuscitation of the victim of sudden death requires the prompt response by scene witnesses and emergency medical services.

MANAGEMENT

All patients with an acute manifestation of IHD should be placed on continuous electrocardiographic monitoring and should have intravenous access established. The emergency department team must be vigilant and prepared to respond to the complications common to unstable angina and AMI. Supplemental oxygen, at 2 to 6 L/minute by nasal cannula, should be administered to all patients; infarct size may be reduced with this supplemental oxygen. A lower flow rate of oxygen may be used in those with a history of chronic lung disease who retain CO_2.

Nitroglycerin

Nitroglycerin results in dilatation of the coronary circulation and results in improved collateral blood flow to areas of ischemia. It also causes venous dilatation of the mesenteric vessels, which results in reduced ventricular filling pressure and improves coronary microvascular perfusion by reducing the ventricular transmural pressure. These changes improve the balance of myocardial oxygen supply and demand.

Nitroglycerin can be administered as 0.2, 0.4, or 0.6 mg sublingual doses every 5 minutes and as a topical ointment of 1 to 2 inches. The most easily controlled route is constant intravenous infusion. The infusion is started at 10 µg/minute and titrated to relief of pain or reduction of the systolic pressure to less than 90 or 100 mm Hg.

Aspirin

Aspirin can reduce the mortality of AMIs by more than 20%. Only a low dose of aspirin is needed to block the cyclooxygenase-dependent pathway for platelet aggregation. Patients with unstable angina or AMI should receive 160 mg of aspirin in the emergency department unless they have a history of hypersensitivity.

Heparin

Heparin, which catalyzes antithrombin III and inhibits thrombin and factor Xa, is beneficial in unstable angina and AMI. The principle benefit is in preventing reocclusion of a coronary artery that has undergone spontaneous or pharmacologic thrombolysis. These diseased coronary arteries typically have ulcerated lesions with high concentrations of fibrinogen and are at great risk for rethrombosis. An additional benefit is in preventing ventricular mural thrombus (which may occur with large anterior wall AMIs) and therefore reducing the risk of a subsequent embolic cerebrovascular accident. Heparin is also effective in preventing deep vein thrombosis during the immediate post-AMI period.

For true efficacy, heparin must be administered intravenously. Some controversy exists concerning the appropriate dose of heparin. A bolus of 5000 to 10,000 units of heparin should be followed by a constant infusion of 1000 to 1250 units/hour. The rate of administration should be adjusted to achieve an activated partial thromboplastin time of 1.5 to 2 times the control.

Opiates

Morphine is an analgesic and anxiolytic. By producing arterial and venous dilatation and reducing myocardial afterload and preload, morphine also reduces cardiac work. It may be administered intravenously in doses of 2 to 5 mg every 5 minutes. Morphine also has vagomimetic properties, causes histamine release, and is a central nervous system depressant. The patient must be monitored for hypotension, bradycardia, and respiratory depression.

Lidocaine

The indications for lidocaine in the patient with AMI who has not had ventricular fibrillation or ventricular tachycardia include greater than six premature ventricular contractions/minute, multifocal or closely coupled premature ventricular contractions, and short runs of nonsustained ventricular tachycardia. Lidocaine is administered as a 1 mg/kg intravenous bolus followed by a 1 to 4 mg/minute constant infusion. A 0.5 mg/kg rebolus should occur 10 minutes after the initial bolus.

Lidocaine is associated with central nervous system toxicity and a higher incidence of asystole, an almost always fatal dysrhythmia. It is no longer recommended prophylactically for all patients with AMI. An exception would occur under circumstances in which immediate electrical defibrillation is not available.

Beta-Adrenergic Blocking Agents

Long-term administration of ß-adrenergic blocking agents is associated with a marked reduction in mortality, reinfarction, myocardial rupture, and sudden death. By reducing the heart rate and contractility, these agents reduce myocardial oxygen requirements in the initial postinfarction hours and may reduce the amount of damaged myocardium. Many contraindications to their use exist, including any hypotension, bradycardia, A-V conduction abnormalities, congestive heart failure, and a history of reactive airway disease. However, in the patient with an AMI who has no contraindications and is hemodynamically stable, the administration of metoprolol in the emergency department, three doses of 5 mg intravenously every 2 minutes, may have substantial benefit.

Thrombolytic Agents

The thrombolytic agents represent the most exciting development in the emergency-department care of AMI of the last several years. Two thrombolytic agents are widely available. Strep-

CONTRAINDICATIONS TO THROMBOLYTIC THERAPY

Absolute

Active bleeding
History of hemorrhagic CVA
Major trauma or surgery within 2 weeks
Suspected aortic dissection
Recent head trauma
CNS tumor or A-V malformation
Persistent hypertension (>200/120)
Bleeding disorder
CNS surgery within 2 months

Relative

Active peptic ulcer disease
History of CVA
Major trauma or surgery within 2 months
Subclavian or internal jugular venous cannulation
Current use of anticoagulants

Table *36-1*

DOSAGE SCHEDULES FOR THROMBOLYTIC THERAPY

Agent	Intravenous Schedule
Recombinant tissue plasminogen activator (rt-PA)	15 mg bolus 50 mg over 30 min 35 mg over next 60 min
Streptokinase (SK)	1.5 million units over 60 min

tokinase (SK), produced by ß-hemolytic strepto-cocci, forms a complex with plasminogen to pro-duce the fibrinolytic agent plasmin. SK can be associated with hypersensitivity reactions. Re-combinant tissue plasminogen activator (rt-PA) is produced by recombinant DNA technology. It is "clot specific" and activates fibrin-bound plas-minogen to produce plasmin far more effectively than freely circulating plasminogen. These two agents have been compared head-to-head in sev-eral large studies. The benefit of rt-PA over SK is in establishing faster coronary artery patency, which may be particularly important within the first hour of an AMI. However, rt-PA has not shown a consistent improvement in mortality or ventricular function over SK and may be associ-ated with a higher rate of reocclusion of the infarct-related artery and a higher rate of intra-cerebral hemorrhage.

Thrombolytic agents may be indicated in any patient who has 12 hours or less of chest pain or an anginal equivalent symptom and who has suitable ECG findings. These findings are ≥1 mm ST-segment elevation in two or more contiguous limb leads, ≥2 mm ST-segment elevation in two or more contiguous precordial leads, or a new BBB pattern. Contraindications to thrombolytic therapy are listed in the box on p. 430. Dosage schedules are listed in Table 36-1.

Coronary Angiography and Revascularization

Some early data have suggested that emergent coronary angiography with percutaneous angio-plasty or coronary artery bypass grafting may be better therapy than the emergent administration of thrombolytic agents. The lack of wide avail-ability of these complicated and resource-intense modalities suggests that more patients with AMI will benefit from thrombolytic agents. However, the patient who would benefit from thrombolysis on the basis of pain duration and ECG findings but who has a contraindication to the administration of thrombolytic agents should be promptly transported to a facility that has in-vasive cardiac capability. Additionally, the patient who has postinfarct angina, significant conges-tive heart failure, or malignant dysrhythmias may also benefit from early coronary angiography and revascularization procedures.

KEY CONSIDERATIONS

WHAT IS THE LIFE THREAT?

Acute coronary ischemia can result in lethal dysrhythmia or myocardial infarction that can lead to immediate death from cardiac arrest or acute pump failure.

DOES THE PATIENT NEED ADMISSION?

Patients with unstable angina or AMI require admission to a unit where they can be monitored for acute dysrhythmia.

Thrombolytic therapy is indicated for patients with AMI who meet the inclusion criteria outlined in the text.

WHAT IS THE MOST SERIOUS DIAGNOSIS?

AMI and unstable angina are the most serious diagnoses. Other serious causes of chest pain, such as pulmonary embolism and acute aortic dissection, should be considered.

HAVE I PERFORMED A THOROUGH WORK-UP?

Obtain a history of the chest pain and risk factors for coronary disease, including smoking, hypertension, lipid abnormality, family history of coronary disease, previous coronary disease, diabetes, and cocaine use.

Obtain an electrocardiogram (ECG), chest x-ray study, arterial oxygenation, and cardiac enzymes.

Obtain an ECG as early as possible to assess patient for the use of thrombolytic agents.

Recommended Reading

ACC/AHA Task Force Report: Guidelines for the early management of patients with acute myocardial infarctions, *J Am Coll Cardiol* 16:249, 1990.

The GUSTO Investigators: An international randomized trial comparing four thrombolytic strategies for acute myocardial infarction, *N Engl J Med* 329:673, 1993.

ISIS-3 (Third International Study of Infarct Survival) Collaborative Group: ISIS-3: a randomized comparison of streptokinase vs tissue plasminogen activator vs anistreplase and of aspirin plus heparin vs aspirin alone among 41,299 cases of suspected myocardial infarction, *Lancet* 339:753, 1992.

Marriott HJL: *Practical electrocardiography,* ed 8, Baltimore, 1988, Williams & Wilkins.

National Heart Attack Alert Program Coordinating Committee—60 Minutes to Treatment Working Group: *Emergency department: rapid identification and treatment of patients with acute myocardial infarction,* September 1993; Baltimore; NIH publication no 93-3278.

Scott JL et al: Ischemic heart disease. In Rosen P et al, editors: *Emergency medicine: concepts and clinical practice,* ed 3, St Louis, 1992, Mosby.

Chapter *Thirty-seven*
HYPERTENSION

JAMES MATHEWS

Hypertension is one of the major long-term health problems in the United States. Approximately 20 million people have some degree of elevated blood pressure. The prevalence of systolic hypertension rises steadily with age; there is a less dramatic increase in diastolic pressures after the fifth to sixth decades of life. Men have a higher incidence of hypertension than women, and hypertension is both more prevalent and more severe in blacks (both men and women) than in whites. A patient with hypertension is more likely to have a family history of elevated blood pressure.

Arbitrary values are used to define hypertension. A systolic blood pressure less than 140 mm Hg and a diastolic blood pressure less than 90 mm Hg are considered normal values. If the systolic pressure is between 140 and 159 mm Hg and the diastolic pressure is between 90 and 95 mm Hg, the term *borderline hypertension* is applied. A systolic blood pressure of 160 mm Hg or higher or a diastolic blood pressure higher than 95 mm Hg is considered hypertension.

A single elevated blood pressure reading does not warrant a diagnosis of hypertension. The measurement should be repeated after a period of time and should be obtained in both arms. Obese patients pose a special problem because the use of a standard size cuff may result in a false elevation of blood pressure.

Hypertension is not a disease in itself but rather the end result of a number of pathophysiologic processes and risk factors. By far the most common type of hypertension is *essential hypertension,* for which a specific cause has not been identified. However, there are a number of other specific causes (see the box on p. 434). All types of renal disease have been associated with hypertension.

Abnormalities of the large arteries can also produce hypertension. Although rare, coarctation of the aorta is an important cause of secondary hypertension. Upper extremity hypertension, a systolic murmur best heard over the back, and delayed femoral pulses together suggest coarctation. Loss of elasticity in the larger arteries because of aging may produce systolic hypertension. Fibromuscular disease of the renal arteries is a disease of young white women.

Excessive glucocorticoid levels are associated with hypertension. The most common cause of these excessive levels is steroid therapy. Endogenous overproduction is relatively uncommon but may result from excessive adrenocorticotropic hormone (ACTH) production by a pituitary tumor, ectopic ACTH production by a nonpituitary tumor, or ACTH production by tumors of the adrenal cortex. Patients affected in this way show other signs of hyperadrenalism. This type of hypertension is usually not severe

CAUSES OF HYPERTENSION

Systolic

Arteriosclerosis
Thyrotoxicosis
Anemia

Systolic and diastolic

Renal disease
   Pyelonephritis
   Glomerulonephritis
   Congenital renal lesions
   Renal vascular occlusion
Endocrine disease
   Aldosteronism
   Cushing syndrome
   Pheochromocytoma
Other
   Coarctation of the aorta
   Eclampsia
   Polycythemia
   Essential hypertension

COMMON CAUSES OF PEDIATRIC HYPERTENSION AT VARIOUS AGES

Neonates

Coarctation of the aorta
Renal artery thrombosis
Renal artery stenosis
Congenital renal malformations
Bronchopulmonary dysplasia
Intracranial hemorrhage

Children under 6 years

Coarctation of the aorta
Renal artery stenosis
Renal parenchymal disease
   Polycystic kidney
   Hydronephrosis
   Pyelonephritis
   Wilms tumor

Children 6-10 years

Renal artery stenosis
Renal parenchymal disease
Essential hypertension

Children older than 10 years

Essential hypertension
Renal parenchymal disease

Table 37-1

NORMAL BLOOD PRESSURE RANGES IN YOUNG CHILDREN

	Blood Pressure (Torr)	
Age	Systolic	Diastolic
Newborn (1-2 kg)	50 ± 10	28 ± 8
Newborn (2-3 kg)	60 ± 10	37 ± 8
1 month	80 ± 16	46 ± 16
6 months	89 ± 29	60 ± 10
1 year	96 ± 30	66 ± 25
2-3 years	99 ± 25	64 ± 25
4-5 years	99 ± 20	65 ± 20

Mean ± 2 SD.

and can be controlled by treating the underlying disease process.

Pheochromocytomas are responsible for fewer than 1% of all cases of hypertension. The characteristic features of pheochromocytoma are paroxysms of hypertension associated with palpitations, tachycardia, malaise, and sweating. A prodrome of apprehension and abdominal pain that progresses to headache, palpitations, and angina may also be seen.

The normal blood pressure ranges of children are found in Table 37-1. Hypertension in children under 12 years of age is usually associated with anatomic pathologic conditions, whereas elevated blood pressure in older children more commonly represents essential hypertension. Conditions that suggest an increased risk of hypertension in infants include the presence of an abdominal mass or bruit, coarctation of the aorta, congenital renal hyperplasia, neurofibromatosis, failure to thrive, and unexplained heart failure or renal disease. Common causes of hypertension in children of various ages are listed in the box on p. 434.

HYPERTENSIVE CRISIS

The term *hypertensive crisis* includes both hypertensive emergencies and hypertensive urgencies. Hypertensive emergencies require reduction of blood pressure within 1 hour to lower a real risk of morbidity and mortality. Hypertensive urgencies require a lowering of the blood pressure over the next 24 to 48 hours. The determining factors for this division are whether or not the patient appears "sick" and whether there is evidence of acute and progressive end-organ involvement. This determination requires an appropriate assessment of the patient within the emergency department and cannot be based on the level of blood pressure alone.

EMERGENCY DEPARTMENT ASSESSMENT OF THE PATIENT WITH HYPERTENSION

A difficult decision is whether or not to admit the patient with hypertension to the hospital. Admission is usually indicated if the diastolic pressure is greater than 135 mm Hg. Many patients with diastolic pressures between 120 and 135 mm Hg may also require admission for hypertension management. Below these levels, patients seldom require admission on the basis of blood pressure levels alone.

Patients with severe hypertension, which is defined as a diastolic pressure greater than 115

mm Hg, must be carefully evaluated. This evaluation includes a thorough history and physical examination that is oriented toward the organs commonly affected by hypertension, namely the heart, kidneys, and brain. A careful funduscopic examination must be performed. Laboratory testing should include electrolyte, blood urea nitrogen, and creatine levels; a urinalysis; and an ECG. A chest x-ray study is indicated if there is clinical evidence of heart failure. Unanticipated positive findings indicate a hypertensive emergency that requires intervention. (Specific therapeutic agents are discussed later in this chapter.) If this assessment is negative, the patient is not a hypertensive emergency and may be discharged for outpatient management. However, patients whose blood pressure is so high that prudency discourages discharge should be admitted as observation patients and have urgent reduction of blood pressure over the next 24 hours.

Patients with hypertension must be carefully followed. If the patient has been on a regimen of antihypertensive medications that has been unsuccessful in controlling the blood pressure or if the patient has altered the regimen without a physician's advice, that regimen should either be restarted or changed in communication with the patient's primary physician.

HYPERTENSIVE EMERGENCIES

Hypertension is a life-long condition, and complications are related to the duration and level of the elevated blood pressure. The most serious long-term complications involve an increased risk of atherosclerosis, cerebrovascular disease, renal disease, and myocardial infarction. These complications often produce medical emergencies, and their management is made more difficult by the presence of an elevated blood pressure. In addition, several syndromes occur as a direct result of severe hypertension.

Hypertensive Encephalopathy

Hypertensive encephalopathy occurs when there is an abrupt, sustained rise in blood pressure that exceeds cerebral autoregulation limits of the small resistance arteries of the brain. Above a mean arterial pressure of 150 to 200 mm Hg, cerebral autoregulation may be unable to control cerebral blood flow. The result is marked vasospasm with consequent ischemia, increasing vascular permeability, and cerebral edema.

The onset of hypertensive encephalopathy is acute. Patients have severe generalized headache, vomiting, drowsiness, and confusion. Seizures are commonly observed, and the patient may experience blindness, focal neurologic deficits, confusion, or coma. Other signs of severe hypertension may be present, including hematuria and elevated levels of creatinine and blood urea nitrogen.

Hypertensive encephalopathy constitutes a grave condition. Although the effects are potentially reversible, untreated patients develop a coma of increasing depth, and death may ensue within hours. Rapid reduction of blood pressure is mandatory. Several agents are widely used, including nitroprusside, diazoxide, intravenous (IV) labetalol, and nifedipine.

Management

Nitroprusside. When careful monitoring of blood pressure over the duration of therapy can be obtained, nitroprusside is the agent of choice for treatment of the majority of hypertensive emergencies. Nitroprusside is a potent vasodilator that directly affects the smooth muscle of both resistance and capacitance vessels. To date, no case of hypertension has been found to be resistant to this agent. The rate of onset of its effects is rapid, and the duration is very short. Cessation of administration returns blood pressure to pretreatment levels within 1 to 10 minutes. Nitroprusside does not produce increased angina, which has been associated with agents such as diazoxide and hydralazine.

Nitroprusside is given intravenously using an infusion pump, and the rate of infusion must be carefully monitored and controlled. The patient should be kept in the recumbent position because of the hazard of orthostatic hypotension. The degree of blood pressure drop is dose related. The starting dose should be between 0.25 and 1.0 µg/kg/minute. The average dose required for control of hypertension is 3 µg/kg/minute. Nitroprusside is unstable in ultraviolet light, and the solution should be wrapped in opaque material, such as metal foil. Elderly patients and those previously receiving antihypertensive medications are more sensitive to the effects of this agent. Patients treated with nitroprusside infusion should be admitted to an intensive care unit for close monitoring of their blood pressure by an arterial line. An arterial line is not mandated to initiate therapy with nitroprusside as long as blood pressures are recorded at frequent intervals, especially when the infusion rate is adjusted. An arterial line is required for prolonged administration of the agent.

The therapeutic goal of nitroprusside therapy in hypertensive encephalopathy is a 30% to 40% reduction of blood pressure from the pretreatment level. Side effects are directly related to excessive vasodilatation and resultant hypotension, and they can be avoided by carefully monitoring the patient's blood pressure and regulating the infusion rate. Extreme caution must be taken to avoid the extravasation of nitroprusside, because local necrosis can be severe. Nitroprusside is relatively contraindicated in pregnancy because of the potential accumulation of the cyanide ion in utero.

Nifedipine. Nifedipine, a calcium channel blocker, has replaced many of the other agents in the treatment of hypertensive emergencies. It may be administered by the sublingual, buccal, oral, or rectal routes; all routes produce approximately the same effect. Nifedipine can result in a profound lowering of the blood pressure, especially in dehydrated and elderly patients; it should be used with extreme caution in these circumstances. The usual dose is 10 mg either sublingually or orally. Blood pressure reduction occurs within 10 to 15 minutes of administration and reaches its maximum effect within 1 hour. The actions of this agent last 4 to 6 hours. Because of the ability to titrate the response and the short duration of action, nitroprusside remains the agent of choice when absolute control of blood pressure is mandated by the clinical circumstances or when there is an increased risk for profound reduction of blood pressure by nifedipine.

Labetalol. Labetalol is both an α_1- and nonselective ß-adrenergic receptor blocker. It produces vasodilatation without reflex tachycardia. Although oral administration of labetalol usually does not produce significant orthostatic changes, marked orthostatic hypotension may be observed after IV administration, and the patient should be kept in the supine position for several hours.

When labetalol is given intravenously, a significant fall in blood pressure generally occurs in 5 to 10 minutes, with a maximum effect in 30 minutes. Therapy is begun with 20 mg infused over 2 minutes. The blood pressure is checked every 5 minutes, and an additional dose may be given every 10 minutes to a total of 300 mg. Because labetalol is a nonselective beta blocker, it should not be given to patients with congestive heart failure, heart block, or asthma.

The effects of labetalol therapy cannot be so closely controlled nor so quickly reversed as those of nitroprusside; however, the use of labetalol does not require intensive care unit admission, and it is an excellent alternative when constant monitoring of blood pressure is not feasible. When used as previously described, it has not caused the profound drop in blood pressure associated with diazoxide. Furthermore, coronary artery disease is not exacerbated.

Malignant Hypertension

Malignant or accelerated hypertension is a phase of hypertension that can occur during the clinical course of any patient with a persistent blood pressure elevation. It may also be the initial presentation of a hypertensive patient. During the malignant phase of hypertension, serious damage may develop in various organ systems within the body, particularly the renal, cardiac, and cerebral systems.

Patients with malignant hypertension appear ill and may have complaints of severe headache, blurred vision, dyspnea, chest pain, or symptoms of uremia. Hypertensive encephalopathy may be associated with malignant hypertension, but this correlation is not universal. Although it is less critical than hypertensive encephalopathy, malignant hypertension is a medical emergency.

If left untreated, malignant hypertension may result in acute renal failure, cardiac decompensation, myocardial infarction, cerebral hemorrhage, or hypertensive encephalopathy. The level of diastolic blood pressure usually seen is higher than 130 mm Hg. Readings below this level are seldom associated with malignant hypertension or hypertensive encephalopathy, but both conditions have been reported with diastolic pressures as low as 110 mm Hg. Most patients with hypertension never develop either of these syndromes.

Assessment

Malignant hypertension cannot be diagnosed with blood pressure readings alone. The physical examination in most cases reveals an enlarged left ventricle and rales at the lung bases. Papilledema, linear hemorrhages, and cotton wool exudates may be present on funduscopic examination. Laboratory evaluation reveals evidence of diminished renal function, with hematuria, proteinuria, or elevated serum levels of creatinine and blood urea nitrogen. Red cell fragments may be visible on a blood smear, and fibrin degradation products may be elevated, which is a picture compatible with microangiopathic hemolytic anemia. Additional findings include left ventricular hypertrophy with strain

Table 37-2

COMMONLY USED ANTIHYPERTENSIVE MEDICATIONS

Drug	Common Brand Name	Dose (daily)	Major Action	Common Side Effects	Unique Problems
Thiazide diuretics	Diuril Hydrodiuril Esidrix Zaroxolyn	0.5-2 g 25-50 mg 25-100 mg 5-10 mg	Renal sodium and water increase by inhibition of Na^+ reabsorption in distal tubule	Hypokalemia, decreased glomerular filtration rate, increased uric acid	Further compromise of impaired renal or hepatic functions, severe hyperglycemia
Furosemide	Lasix	40-200 mg	Inhibits Na^+ reabsorption in ascending limb of Henle loop	Fluid and electrolyte imbalance, hyperuricemia	Eighth nerve damage (rare)
Propranolol	Inderal	80-160 mg (may be much higher)	ß-adrenergic blockade	Exacerbates congestive heart failure, exacerbates asthma, many central nervous system side effects (e.g., depression, hallucinations)	Masks signs and symptoms of hypoglycemia
Clonidine	Catapres	0.4-2 mg	Many actions both peripheral and central (most important); causes stimulation of central centers that inhibit sympathetics	Dry mouth, sedation	Hyperirritability, marked rebound of hypertension with acute withdrawal
Hydralazine	Apresoline	100-200 mg/day, rarely more than 400 mg/day	Direct relaxation of smooth muscle, arteries much more than veins	Numerous effects, including headaches, palpitations, dizziness, nasal congestion, flushing, peripheral neuropathy, myocardial ischemia	Acute rheumatoid states (10%), lupus-like syndrome
Spironolactone	Aldactone	100 mg	Competitive antagonist of aldosterone in renal tubules	Hyperkalemia with or without other diuretics	Gynecomastia, masculinization, gastrointestinal upset

Generic	Trade name	Dose	Mechanism	Side effects	
Triamterene	Dyrenium	200-300 mg	Direct action on tubular transport; not competitive antagonist of aldosterone	Hyperkalemia	Gastrointestinal symptoms, megaloblastic anemia (rare)
Prazosin	Minipress	3 mg to start, with first dose 1 mg only; may increase to 20 mg slowly	α-adrenergic blocking agent at postsynaptic receptors	Postural hypotension; syncope, especially in salt-depleted patient (first-dose phenomenon); palpitations; drowsiness; headache	Positive antinuclear factor (⅔ of patients)
Minoxidil	Loniten	10-40 mg	Vasodilatation by direct relaxation of arteriolar smooth muscle	Fluid retention, reflex activation of sympathetic nervous system	Pericardial effusion
Labetalol	Normodyne	600 mg	Vasodilatation by α_1-adrenoreceptor blockade; also ß-blockade	Fatigue, dizziness Postural hypotension (uncommon) Bradycardia (uncommon) Contraindications: Asthma Heart failure Heart block Severe tachycardia	Hypertensive crisis possible if used when pheochromocytoma is present
Captopril	Capoten	75-450 mg	Competitive inhibition of angiotensin 1–converting enzyme	Proteinuria Hypotension, especially when CHF is present Elevated BUN	Agranulocytosis
Nifedipine	Procardia	30-60 mg; should not exceed 180 mg/day	Vasodilatation by calcium-channel blockade in arterial smooth muscle	Excessive vasodilatation with edema and dizziness; 20% of patients, but most are benign and abate with time or by lowering dose	Myocardial ischemia from hypotension, tachycardia, profound hypotension (greatest risk in elderly and volume-depleted patients)

From Mathews J: Hypertension. In Rosen P et al, editors: *Emergency medicine: concepts and clinical practice*, ed 3, St Louis, 1992, Mosby.

evident on the ECG, as well as cardiomegaly as seen on the chest x-ray study.

Management

Treatment of malignant hypertension consists of judiciously lowering the blood pressure by 30% to 40% from pretreatment levels within the first hour and more gradually normalizing the blood pressure over several days. Nitroprusside remains the agent of choice for the initial phase of treatment, particularly if the patient is hyperacute, but nifedipine is an excellent alternative in many circumstances. In all cases the patient should be hospitalized. The patient should be switched to oral medications as soon as possible for long-term control.

Hypertension With Cerebrovascular Accident

Hypertension is commonly associated with stroke syndromes, and the emergency physician is often faced with the difficult decision of whether and how much to reduce blood pressure. Guidelines are presented in Chapter 50.

The majority of patients suffering from embolic or thrombotic strokes without an associated hemorrhage do not show a profound elevation of blood pressure. In these patients, the degree of hypertension is usually mild to moderate, and its presence has little acute effect on the clinical course. The blood pressure can be gradually controlled over several days in the hospital with a number of oral agents (Table 37-2).

If hypertension has been long-standing, the rapid reduction of blood pressure further reduces cerebral blood flow and causes increased ischemia. Therefore do not begin immediate antihypertensive therapy unless the diastolic pressure is greater than 140 mm Hg. In this instance, check the blood pressure at frequent intervals; if this level persists after the first hour, institute a 30% reduction with nitroprusside.

Patients suffering from intracranial hemorrhage commonly have a profound elevation of blood pressure. In the majority of such patients hypertension is transient and is caused by increased intracranial pressure and irritation of the autonomic nervous system. This type of hypertension often disappears rapidly and has little effect on the clinical picture of the patient. The exception is the patient in whom the hemorrhage results from hypertensive vascular disease. Small arteries can rupture when malignant hypertension is present, and in this circumstance control of the blood pressure is mandated by using nitroprusside. Because the exact cause of an intracranial bleed is not always clear, it is prudent to monitor the patient's blood pressure for approximately 1 hour and initiate nitroprusside therapy only if recordings remain markedly elevated.

Hypertension With Pulmonary Edema

Severe hypertension with pulmonary edema is a critical medical emergency. In the majority of patients with this combination of entities, the hypertension is caused by increased peripheral vascular resistance as a result of elevated catecholamine levels associated with the stress of pulmonary edema. With standard treatment of pulmonary edema, catecholamine levels fall and blood pressure rapidly returns to normal. Less commonly, pulmonary edema is caused by severe elevation of blood pressure and resultant acute left ventricular failure. In this situation, blood pressure must be lowered to reverse the process. Nitroprusside remains the preferred agent because it does not cause sodium retention, improves function of the failing heart, and can be carefully titrated and its effects rapidly reversed. Another agent that may be effective in this clinical situation, either alone or in conjunction with nitroprusside, is nitroglycerin by IV infusion.

Hypertension With Congestive Heart Failure and Angina

Most patients with congestive heart failure have some degree of increased peripheral resistance and resultant hypertension. The degree of elevation is moderate and does not represent a critical medical emergency. Long-standing hypertension produces myocardial hypertrophy, which continues until the increased myocardial mass can no longer overcome the elevated peripheral vascular resistance and the left ventricle begins to fail. A patient with a combination of moderate-to-severe hypertension and congestive heart failure without pulmonary edema requires admission and long-term control rather than the institution of immediate antihypertensive therapy.

Angina and hypertension are also commonly associated. Blood pressure must be lowered immediately if severe hypertension is present and angina is increasing. The preferred drug is nitroprusside, especially if the blood pressure is markedly elevated. In many patients, nitroglycerin may be used either alone or in combination with nitroprusside.

Hypertension With Renal Failure

The most important cardiovascular complication of chronic renal failure is hypertension. Hypertension may appear at any time during the course of chronic renal failure and eventually becomes a problem for most patients in advanced stages of renal failure. Uncontrolled hypertension accelerates the cardiovascular problems that commonly cause death in both dialysis and renal transplant patients; it also causes further damage to diseased kidneys.

The primary cause of hypertension in patients with chronic renal failure is an actual or relatively increased extracellular volume. The mainstay of treatment in a patient who has some remaining renal function is careful balance of sodium intake and augmentation of excretion with a diuretic such as furosemide. Antihypertensive agents should be added to the treatment regimen if this treatment fails. Unless hypertension is associated with severe congestive heart failure, aortic dissection is suspected, or other worrisome findings are noted, treatment of hypertension that occurs with renal failure should be initiated in the emergency department only if

the level of diastolic pressure is more than 140 mm Hg. Nitroprusside is also the preferred drug when malignant hypertension with renal failure is encountered. Nifedipine is another alternative therapy. Diazoxide is contraindicated in chronic renal failure because it enhances sodium retention.

Hypertensive Emergencies of Pregnancy

The standard definition of hypertension as a blood pressure over 140/90 mm Hg has no meaning in pregnancy. A blood pressure greater than 125/75 mm Hg before 32 weeks of gestation is associated with increased fetal risks. Elevation of the systolic pressure by 20 mm Hg or a rise of 10 mm Hg in the diastolic pressure during pregnancy should be considered abnormal.

Eclampsia of pregnancy is defined as the onset of hypertension, edema, and proteinuria after the twentieth week of gestation. Preeclampsia is eclampsia without seizures, whereas eclampsia is defined by the occurrence of hypertension, edema, and proteinuria during pregnancy, with seizures of no other apparent cause. Eclampsia occurs most commonly in young primiparous and older multiparous women, and the syndrome usually disappears after delivery. Although uncommon, eclampsia can occur after delivery, usually within the first 24 to 48 hours; however, it may be seen as late as 7 days after delivery.

Eclampsia usually occurs after 32 weeks of gestation but may occur earlier if there is a preexisting renal disease of hypertension. Eclampsia may also be associated with an hydatidiform mole during the first trimester. The onset of eclampsia is often silent, with gradual development of edema and hypertension occurring first. Proteinuria follows, but at times it is the first finding. Visual disturbances, headaches, anxiety, and epigastric pain gradually appear.

Assessment

The physical examination reveals edema of the face and hands and prominent diastolic hypertension. The systolic pressure is usually less than 160 mm Hg. Funduscopic examination may reveal segmented arteriolar narrowing with a glistening fundus suggestive of retinal edema. If convulsions have occurred, hemorrhages and exudates may be present. The excitability of the central nervous system is reflected by the presence of hyperactive deep tendon reflexes. The urinary sediment is usually only minimally abnormal and reveals only a few red blood cells. Proteinuria may be profound and range from 1 g/L to more than 30 g/L. Thrombocytopenia or the hemolytic-uremic syndrome may develop in patients with severe eclampsia. The most common cause of maternal death from eclampsia is a cerebral hemorrhage.

Management

The treatment of eclampsia is aimed at prevention and early detection through proper prenatal care. The onset of proteinuria during pregnancy is an ominous sign and is one indication for admission. If there have been no convulsions, blood pressures lower than 140/90 mm Hg do not necessarily require immediate therapy in the emergency department. Admission and management with bed rest in the left lateral recumbent position is indicated. Sodium restriction is not indicated, and some patients may benefit from careful volume expansion with normal saline.

In the United States, magnesium sulfate is usually given to prevent seizures, but there are not controlled studies to support this practice. A loading dose of 4 g is given intravenously over 5 minutes. Maintenance therapy involves 1 to 3 g/hour. The therapeutic range is a serum magnesium level of 4.8 to 8.6 mEq/L. The patient should be monitored carefully for signs of magnesium toxicity by patellar reflexes, renal function, and respiratory rate. Calcium channel blockers should not be used with magnesium therapy.

A diastolic pressure of more than 110 mm Hg during pregnancy is suggestive of a hypertensive emergency unless these levels were present before the pregnancy. The immediate reduction of blood pressure is required. The agent of choice remains IV hydralazine, if available within the institution. Administer hydralazine by IV bolus, starting with a 5-mg test dose and repeating 10-mg doses every 20 minutes until the diastolic pressure is below 100 mm Hg. The amount of hydralazine usually required to achieve this endpoint is 5 to 20 mg. Hydralazine may be given by continuous IV infusion. Labetalol has also been used widely and is safe except in those patients who have a contraindication to beta blockade. Nifedipine also appears to be safe to use but should not be used with magnesium sulfate. Finally, nitroprusside, although relatively contraindicated in pregnancy because of the potential accumulation of the cyanide ion in utero, may be used if other agents fail.

After blood pressure reduction and clinical stabilization, delivery of the fetus is indicated, especially if seizures have occurred. The onset of seizures indicates the presence of severe disease. Magnesium sulfate is the preferred drug to prevent both initial and recurrent seizures, but it is not effective in stopping an eclamptic seizure; use diazepam and phenobarbital for this purpose. This type of seizure may prove extremely difficult to control. In certain patients, seizures and blood pressure cannot be controlled; these patients require early delivery. It is essential that the obstetrician be made aware of these patients as soon as possible and have early involvement in their management.

Aortic Dissection

Aortic dissection is not necessarily a complication of hypertension, but a major component of the therapy for this condition is aimed at reducing blood pressure. Most patients with aortic dissection are hypertensive, middle-aged men, but other conditions (e.g., Marfan syndrome and various congenital connective tissue disorders) also predispose an individual to dissection.

Aortic dissection begins as a tear in the aortic

intima, with blood dissecting within the aorta and through the media. Approximately 50% of all dissections begin in the descending aorta; 30% begin in the arch; the remainder begin in the ascending aorta. The dissection may extend either proximally or distally; specific clinical signs depend on the vessels involved. The carotid arteries may be included in the dissection, which results in severe cerebral ischemia. If a proximal dissection occurs, the coronary arteries may be involved, which leads to myocardial infarction. Proximal dissection may also result in acute aortic insufficiency. Rarely, rupture of the dissection into the pericardium occurs and produces an acute cardiac tamponade.

Spinal arteries may be affected, which results in paraplegia or anesthesia below the level of the cord ischemia. If the renal vessels are involved, the resultant renal ischemia may aggravate hypertension. If the orifices of major arteries are involved, there may be asymmetric or absent pulses, but this occurs in only a small number of cases.

The majority of patients with an aortic dissection are men between the ages of 40 and 70. Most patients complain of severe pain that requires differentiation from that of myocardial infarction. Usually the pain of an aortic dissection radiates to the back or abdomen and is described as a "tearing" sensation.

Assessment

Aortic dissection is a diagnosis that is often not obvious on clinical grounds. Plain chest x-ray studies are often abnormal in patients with aortic dissection. Many radiographic signs of dissection exist, including dilatation of the ascending aorta, blurring of the aortic knob, displacement of the trachea by the aneurysm, mediastinal widening, and displacement of intimal calcium more than 6 mm from the outer edge of the aortic shadow. A normal x-ray study does not exclude the presence of aortic dissection. Unfortunately, many of the radiologic findings associated with aortic dissection are extremely subtle.

Aortography is the definitive diagnostic study. The CT scan, which is also useful in evaluating the aorta, has specific limitations. It is limited in its ability to evaluate the branches of the aorta, especially the abdominal and coronary branches. Both false-positive and false-negative studies can occur with a CT scan, but this process has become much more reliable with the advent of rapid infusion techniques. Ultrasonography can depict some complications of aortic dissection, such as pericardial effusion, but this procedure is imprecise in the diagnosis of dissection itself.

Management

In the emergency department, the patient's vital signs, cardiac rhythm, central venous pressure, and urinary output should be continuously monitored. Definitive treatment may be either medical or surgical. Initial therapy in all cases involves aggressively reducing blood pressure to a systolic level of 100 to 120 mm Hg. The preferred drug is nitroprusside (see the discussion earlier in this chapter).

In conjunction with blood pressure reduction, the systolic ejection force of the heart should be reduced. Propranolol 1 to 3 mg IV is used in combination with nitroprusside. The therapeutic goals are to reduce the cardiac rate and to lower the systolic ejection force, which further reduces the strain on the weakened aortic wall.

Whether definitive therapy is to be medical or surgical depends on multiple factors, including the portion of the aorta involved, end-organ compromise, and stability of the patient (see the Key Considerations). Medical therapy is often the sole treatment for dissections that are limited to the descending aorta. Surgical therapy is generally applied to the ascending aorta, especially if there is evidence of aortic valvular insufficiency. Additional indications for surgery in patients with descending aortic dissection include occlusion of a major branch of the aorta, aortic rupture, or an inability to control pain or blood pressure with medical management.

||||||||||KEY CONSIDERATIONS

WHAT IS THE LIFE THREAT?

A hypertensive crisis is associated with hypertensive encephalopathy, intracranial hemorrhage, and acute heart failure; therefore it is a life-threatening condition.

A hypertensive crisis or urgency occurs at much lower elevations of blood pressure for patients who are unaccustomed to hypertension, such as the pregnant patient with new-onset preeclampsia.

DOES THE PATIENT NEED ADMISSION?

If the diastolic pressure is greater than 135 mm Hg, admission is usually indicated. Patients with a diastolic pressure between 120 to 135 mm Hg require admission if their pressure cannot be lowered easily with an oral agent (e.g., nifedipine) or if there is evidence of acute end-organ impairment such as encephalopathy, CNS hemorrhage or ischemia, chest pain, heart failure, or renal injury. A preeclamptic patient or a patient with significant postpartum hypertension (compared to her baseline) should be admitted for evaluation and treatment.

WHAT IS THE MOST SERIOUS DIAGNOSIS?

A hypertensive emergency is the most serious diagnosis.

HAVE I PERFORMED A THOROUGH WORK-UP?

Evaluate the patient for acute end-organ damage, including retinal hemorrhage, diminished visual acuity, and other signs of retinopathy. Evaluate kidneys with BUN, creatinine, and urinalysis.

Evaluate the heart with an ECG and a chest x-ray study.

Evaluate serum electrolytes. Evaluate cerebral function with a neurologic examination and mental status assessment.

Recommended Reading

Gifford RW: Management of hypertensive crisis, *JAMA* 266:829, 1991.

Mathews J: Hypertension. In Rosen P et al, editors: *Emergency medicine: concepts and clinical practice*, ed 3, St Louis, 1992, Mosby.

Ram CVS: Management of hypertensive emergencies: changing therapeutic options, *Am Heart J* 122:357, 1991.

Svensson A: Hypertension in pregnancy, *Clin Exper Hyper* 15:1353, 1993.

Yong L et al: Longitudinal study of blood pressure: changes and determinates from adolescence to middle age. The Dormot High School follow-up study, 1957–1963 to 1989–1990, *Am J Epidemiol* 138:973, 1993.

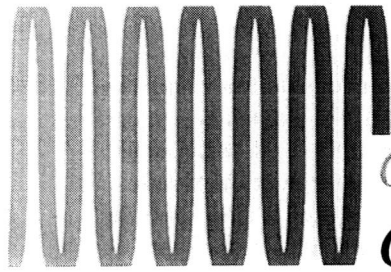

Chapter Thirty-eight
CONGESTIVE HEART FAILURE

STEPHEN R. HAYDEN

Congestive heart failure (CHF) affects approximately 2% of the U.S. population (4 million people) and has a higher mortality rate than many forms of cancer. The incidence of CHF increases twofold for each decade of life, and the presence of CHF increases the age-adjusted mortality rate eight times for men and five times for women. Approximately one half of all deaths in patients with CHF result from ventricular dysrhythmias. Nondysrhythmic causes of death include cardiogenic shock, pulseless electrical activity, and myocardial rupture. The most common causes of CHF are myocardial infarction resulting from coronary artery disease and longstanding hypertension.

CHF can be defined as a failure of the heart to pump oxygenated blood at a rate sufficient to satisfy organ demands. Additionally, in certain types of CHF, cardiac output may be normal, or even high, but is inadequate for metabolizing tissues. Furthermore, the elevated cardiac output is produced only by maintaining abnormally elevated ventricular filling pressures. Conditions that may lead to the development of CHF include decreased myocardial contractility (resulting from myocardial ischemia or infarction, primary cardiomyopathy, and decreased contractile efficiency from drug-related or metabolic conditions), pressure overload states (hypertension and valvular or congenital abnormalities), restricted cardiac output (constrictive pericardi-

tis, tamponade, and myocardial infiltrative diseases), and certain miscellaneous conditions (thyrotoxicosis and severe anemia). CHF should be distinguished from congested states resulting from abnormal salt and water retention; it should also be distinguished from iatrogenic administration, in which there is no abnormality in cardiac function.

FORMS OF HEART FAILURE

Heart failure may be described in many ways, such as high output vs. low output, acute vs. chronic, right sided vs. left sided, and systolic vs. diastolic. It is important to classify the type of heart failure and to identify precipitating causes. The treatment strategy may differ, and alleviation of an acute precipitant may be lifesaving.

Cardiac output in *low-output CHF* is decreased as a result of myocardial ischemia or infarction, cardiomyopathy, valvular or pericardial disease, and hypertension. In *high-output failure,* cardiac output is elevated. Conditions causing high-output failure include hyperthyroidism, severe anemia, pregnancy, beriberi, and Paget disease.

Acute heart failure often results from a precipitating event in a heart that lacks the reserve to compensate for an additional burden. Examples of such an event may include a large myocardial infarction, pulmonary embolus, severe infection, dysrhythmia, hypertensive crisis, severe environmental or emotional stress, discontinuation of CHF medications, or rupture of a cardiac valve. In contrast, *chronic heart failure* is typically observed in patients with slowly progressive ischemia, dilated cardiomyopathy, or prolonged hypertension. The clinical distinction between the two forms can sometimes be difficult in a patient with chronic heart failure that worsens acutely as a result of a sudden precipitating event.

Many of the clinical manifestations of heart failure result from the backup of fluid behind the involved cardiac chamber. When the abnormal hemodynamic load is placed primarily on the left ventricle, pulmonary congestion occurs; this is referred to as *left-sided failure*. *Right-sided failure* develops when the hemodynamic burden is placed primarily on the right ventricle. Right-sided failure occurs with pulmonary hypertension or pulmonary stenosis. Peripheral edema, hepatic congestion, and venous distension result. Right- and left-sided failure are not mutually exclusive conditions. In addition to pulmonary congestion, a long-standing burden on the left ventricle with chronic elevation in left ventricular end diastolic pressure and a subsequent rise in pulmonary capillary wedge pressure eventually results in elevated right-sided pressure and the manifestations associated with right-sided failure.

The term *systolic dysfunction* is applied if the principal cardiac abnormality is reduced myocardial efficiency and a decreased ability to pump sufficient blood. *Diastolic dysfunction* occurs when the ventricles' ability to relax and fill normally is impaired, which results in elevated ventricular filling pressures and increased myocardial workload. Recent studies have shown that as many as 30% to 40% of all patients with CHF have normal systolic function and primary diastolic dysfunction. The two primary causes of diastolic dysfunction are left ventricular hypertrophy and ischemic heart disease.

Patients with diastolic dysfunction and systolic dysfunction often have similar clinical presentations. Echocardiography and radionuclide angiography are two noninvasive methods of distinguishing between systolic and diastolic dysfunction. Therapy with diuretics, vasodilators, beta blockers, and phosphodiesterase inhibitors may be beneficial in both systolic and diastolic dysfunction. Because digitalis glycosides improve contractility, they would not be beneficial in diastolic dysfunction, in which contractility is normal. Calcium channel blockers, although potentially effective in diastolic dysfunction, reduce contractility and activate neurohumeral mechanisms that may make systolic function worse.

SYMPTOMS OF HEART FAILURE

Dyspnea, although not specific to CHF, is one of the most common and early symptoms of CHF. Initially, it may occur only with exertion and may be quantified by asking the number of stairs a patient can comfortably climb or the number of blocks a patient can walk. In more severe CHF, dyspnea occurs even with minimal activity or with rest. Cardiac dyspnea results from an elevation in pulmonary venous and capillary hydrostatic pressures.

Orthopnea is dyspnea in the recumbent position and occurs later in the progression of CHF than dyspnea on exertion. Orthopnea develops in part by elevation of the diaphragm and increased venous return from the lower extremities and abdomen when supine. These changes produce increased pulmonary capillary hydrostatic pressure, which results in interstitial and alveolar edema. Orthopnea can be quantified by the number of pillows a patient must use to sleep comfortably without shortness of breath.

Paroxysmal nocturnal dyspnea (PND) refers to an attack of severe breathlessness and coughing that occurs after a period of recumbency. Several factors may play a role in the development of PND. Reduced ventilation during sleep may induce low-grade hypoxemia, ventricular function may be impaired during sleep as a result of decreased adrenergic stimulation, and increased transudation of fluid through pulmonary capillaries occurs from increased pulmonary capillary hydrostatic pressure. Such factors result in interstitial and alveolar edema. Unlike orthopnea, PND may persist despite sitting upright and may progress to severe pulmonary edema.

Generalized symptoms such as fatigue and weakness are common in CHF and result from diminished skeletal muscle perfusion. Decreased appetite and nausea result from hepatic and portal congestion. Alterations in cognitive ability and a decreased level of consciousness result from diminution in cerebral perfusion.

SIGNS OF HEART FAILURE

The general appearance of a patient with CHF is often that of a patient who is chronically ill. The mental status may be characterized by anxiety, agitation, confusion, and even lethargy. Cyanosis of the lips and nailbeds may be present. Tachypnea and tachycardia are often observed.

The third and fourth heart sounds (S_3, S_4) are audible. An S_3 gallop results from rapid blood flow into a noncompliant ventricle in early diastole; an S_4, which may be heard in normal adults, is present late in diastole and synchronous with atrial contraction in pressure overload situations. The presence of both creates a summation gallop. *Pulsus alternans* is produced by alternating weak and strong cardiac contractions, and a retrosternal heave from right ventricular hypertrophy may be palpable.

Pulmonary findings are variable. In milder cases moist crepitant rales at the lung bases that do not clear with coughing are typical. In more advanced disease, coarse rales and even wheezing may be present diffusely, with dullness at the bases from pleural effusion.

Increased systemic venous pressure is manifested by an abnormally elevated external jugular venous pulsation that is measured when the patient is semireclined at approximately forty-five degrees. An increase in liver span from hepatic congestion may be noted, and the jugular venous pulsation may rise with sustained abdominal pressure (positive hepatojugular reflex).

Dependent edema (pedal, scrotal, or presacral) occurs when the increased systemic capillary hydrostatic pressure exceeds both the capillary oncotic pressure and the ability of the lymphatic system to remove interstitial fluid.

LABORATORY DATA

The chest x-ray study is most valuable in assessing CHF. The appearance of the x-ray study may be divided into three types of images depending on the phase of the CHF. The early phase is characterized by redistribution of the pulmonary blood flow in the upper position, with distension of upper lobe pulmonary veins, which is called *cephalization of vessels*. The next phase is characterized by interstitial pulmonary edema. Pulmonary vessels are indistinct because of perivascular fluid, and Kerley A and B lines may be seen; they represent interlobular septal edema and appear as 1 to 2 cm horizontal lines at the lung periphery. Interstitial fluid accumulating between lobes in the fissures may produce an oval, lens-shaped mass termed a *pseudotumor*. Bilateral pleural effusions commonly occur in CHF, and when unilateral are more common on the right side. In this stage, the classic butterfly-shaped interstitial infiltrate from the hila is an unmistakable finding of pulmonary edema. In the third phase, interstitial edema progresses to frank alveolar edema that may produce asymmetric, large patchy infiltrates that can be mistaken for bronchopneumonia and other pneumonic processes.

Cardiomegaly on a chest x-ray study is very common but relates more to the progression of the underlying disease process than to the severity of the clinical symptoms present. Occasionally pericardial effusion is present in CHF and may result in a large "water bottle" appearance of the heart.

Arterial blood gas analysis may be useful in patients with CHF but does not necessarily reflect clinical severity. Variable degrees of hypoxemia and an increased alveolar-arterial oxygen gradient (A-aO$_2$) may be present. An increased base deficit indicates progressively poor perfusion as hypoxemia at the tissue level forces a greater proportion of anaerobic metabolism. Hypercapnea is uncommon unless underlying lung disease coexists or the severity of the disease has progressed to a critical point.

TREATMENT

The treatment strategy for CHF is threefold. First, identify and correct the underlying cause, if possible; second, identify and remove any precipitants of CHF; and third, control the CHF condition. The third strategy can further be divided into several components, including reducing myocardial workload, optimizing both preload and afterload, controlling excessive fluid retention, and increasing myocardial contractility.

Reducing Cardiac Workload

Physical and emotional rest are important in reducing cardiac workload. Mean arterial pressure is lowered, adrenergic stimulation that increases myocardial oxygen demand is reduced, tissue metabolic requirements are lowered, and enhanced diuresis occurs from redistribution of body fluids. Absolute and prolonged bedrest are rarely required and should be discouraged because of the increased risk of thromboembolic disease.

Control of Excessive Fluid Retention

A number of the signs and symptoms of CHF are related to the expansion of interstitial fluid vol-

ume. Treatment is directed toward lowering total body sodium stores by restricting sodium intake but more importantly by increasing urinary excretion through the use of diuretics. Many diuretic agents are available (Table 38-1). Decreasing fluid volume also decreases preload and enhances myocardial performance.

The *thiazide diuretics* act mainly by inhibiting sodium reabsorption in the distal renal tubules. Their advantages include low cost, single daily dosing, good gastrointestinal absorption, and relatively few serious side effects. Disadvantages include hypokalemic alkalosis, hypercalcemia, hyperglycemia, and hyperuricemia. Thiazide diuretics are not effective in renal insufficiency, except for metolazone (Zaroxolyn). The prototype drug, hydrochlorothiazide (Dyazide, HydroDIURIL), has an onset of action in 2 to 4 hours and a duration of 12 to 18 hours. Numerous formulations combine hydrochlorothiazide with other diuretics and antihypertensive agents. Metolazone is a weak diuretic when used alone but is synergistic with the loop diuretics.

The *loop diuretics* are the most powerful diuretics available and produce diuresis by inhibiting sodium reabsorption in the ascending Henle loop; they are administered orally or parenterally. The dosage range is wide, and the response varies when these agents are initiated. Therefore in the urgent situation, keep the initial intravenous (IV) dose small and then, in subsequent doses, double the initial level every 1 to 2 hours. Patients with renal insufficiency often require extremely high doses to achieve effective diuresis.

Furosemide (Lasix) is the most widely used loop diuretic. In patients with normal renal function the usual oral starting dose is 20 to 40 mg once daily, which can be increased as necessary. Patients with renal failure generally need higher doses. In addition to its diuretic action, furosemide has a venodilating effect that quickly follows intravenous (IV) administration and makes the drug particularly useful in acute pulmonary edema. Bumetanide (Bumex) is approximately 40 times as potent as furosemide;

Table **38-1**

DIURETICS

Drug	Mechanism of Action	Physiologic Changes	Dosage
Thiazides			
Hydrochlorothiazide (HCTZ)	↑ reabsorption in distal tubule	Blood: ↓ K^+, Cl^-; ↑ HCO_3^-, uric acid, glucose	25-100 mg/day po
Chlorthalidone	Same	Urine: ↑ Na^+, K^+, Cl^- Blood: same as HCTZ	25-100 mg/day po
Metolazone	↓ reabsorption of Na^+ in proximal and distal tubules	Urine: ↑ Na^+, K^+, Cl^-	5-20 mg/day po
Loop Diuretics			
Furosemide	↓ reabsorption of Na^+ and Cl^- in ascending Henle loop	Same as Thiazides	20-320 mg/day po, IV
Bumetanide	Same	Same as Thiazides	0.5-2 mg/day po, IV
Potassium Sparing			
Spironolactone	Distal tubule aldosterone inhibition	Blood: ↑ K^+, H^+ Urine: ↓ K^+, H^+; ↑ HCO_3^-	50-200 mg/day po
Triamterene	Same	Same	100-300 mg/day po
Amiloride	Inhibition of Na^+-K^+ ATPase		5-10 mg/day po

diuresis begins quickly after oral administration and within minutes after IV administration. The half-life is 1 to 1.5 hours, and it has a similar side effect profile as furosemide except that it does not produce ototoxicity as often.

The side effects of the loop diuretics are similar to those of the thiazides. In addition, they may produce hypernatremia and hyponatremia. Ototoxicity may occur at high doses. Furosemide and metolazone have been found to be particularly synergistic.

The *potassium sparing diuretics* represent the third major group of diuretics. Because their action is relatively weak, these drugs are often combined with the thiazides or loop diuretics.

The potassium sparing agents act on the distal tubule to promote a mild saluresis and potassium reabsorption. They may produce life-threatening hyperkalemia in patients with renal insufficiency. Other side effects include drug rash, renal calculi (triamterene), and gynecomastia (spironolactone).

Spironolactone in doses of 100 to 200 mg daily has an onset of action in 2 to 4 hours and a duration of 8 to 12 hours. Use the same dosing schedule with triamterene (Dyrenium). Amiloride (Midamor) is used in a single daily dose and has an onset of action of 2 to 4 hours with a duration of 12 to 24 hours.

Optimizing Preload and Afterload

A complex interaction of neurohumeral influences in CHF patients results in peripheral vasoconstriction and increased afterload. Some of these influences include increased adrenergic activity, a rise in the level of circulating catecholamines, and activation of the renin-angiotensin system. Although these mechanisms are generally considered compensatory, the myocardium of heart failure patients is already operating on the flat portion of the Starling curve. Any additional increase in preload or afterload may significantly decrease stroke volume and cardiac output. Reduction of both preload and afterload by vasodilatation allows the ventricle to operate closer to the steep portion of the Starling curve and improve hemodynamic performance, decrease left ventricular end diastolic pressure, and improve subendocardial perfusion.

Vasodilator therapy has recently become one of the most important pharmacologic interventions in the treatment of CHF (Table 38-2), particularly the *angiotensin converting enzyme (ACE) inhibitors.* ACE inhibitors are considered balanced vasodilators because of their effect on both preload and afterload. In numerous recent trials, ACE inhibitors were the only drug class that reduced mortality and hospitalization without concomitant administration of another drug. One-year mortality can be decreased by as much as 30%, but there is no reduction in the incidence of sudden death. ACE inhibitors competitively inhibit the conversion of angiotensin I

Table 38-2

VASODILATORS

Drug	Mechanism of Action	Preload Effect	Afterload Effect	Dosage
Nitrates				
Nitroglycerin	Direct vasodilator (DV)	3+	1+	0.4 mg sublingual, ½-2 inches topically
				5-200 μg/min IV
Isosorbide	DV	3+	1+	20-60 mg q6h po
ACE Inhibitors				
Enalapril	ACE inhibitor	3+	2+	2.5-20 mg/day po
Lisinopril	ACE inhibitor	3+	2+	5-20 mg/day po
Captopril	ACE inhibitor	3+	2+	6.25-25 mg q6h po
Other				
Nitroprusside	DV	2+	3+	5-100 μg/kg/min IV
Hydralazine	DV	—	3+	10-50 mg q6h po
				5-10 mg q6h IV, IM
Minoxidil	DV	—	3+	10-40 mg/day po
Prazosin	α-adrenergic blocker	3+	1+	1-5 mg q8h po
Nifedipine	Calcium channel blocker	1+	2+	10-40 mg q6h po
Diltiazem	Calcium channel blocker	1+	2+	30-120 mg q8h po

to angiotensin II, thus promoting vasodilatation and, in addition, lower aldosterone production.

Currently, ACE inhibitor therapy for CHF is most commonly begun with enalapril (Vasotec), or lisinopril. The usual starting dose of enalapril is 2.5 mg once daily with a total dosage range of 2.5 to 20 mg. Peak concentrations occur approximately 1 hour after oral administration, and the half-life is approximately 12 hours. Lisinopril therapy is initiated at 5 mg once daily with a range of 5 to 20 mg; it also has a half-life of 12 hours. Both of these agents can produce hypotension in patients concurrently taking diuretics unless therapy is begun at the low-dose range. Angioedema has been reported in approximately 0.2% of those patients taking an ACE inhibitor. Captopril (Capoten) is now used less often because of its side effect of agranulocytosis.

Nitrates are principally venodilators and therefore reduce preload; moreover, they increase coronary artery blood flow. Their side effects include headache, dizziness, hypotension, and flushing. Sublingual nitroglycerin 0.4 to 1.2 mg, as well as intravenous nitroglycerin, can be used for rapid treatment of pulmonary edema. Nitroglycerin ointment, paste, and patches are widely used for treating angina and CHF. A variety of long-acting oral nitrates are available, of which isosorbide (Isordil) is the most common. Whereas nitrates have been shown to improve hemodynamics and exercise tolerance, they have not been demonstrated to reduce mortality in CHF patients.

Hydralazine (Apresoline) is a direct arteriolar dilator that was developed as an antihypertensive agent. Its side effects are numerous, including a lupus syndrome, peripheral neuropathy, blood dyscrasias, hypotension, reflex tachycardia, and tachyphylaxis. With IV dosing, the onset of action is 5 to 10 minutes, and the duration of action is 2 to 4 hours. Onset of action after oral dosing is 2 to 4 hours, and the duration is 8 to 12 hours.

Nifedipine (Procardia) and *diltiazem* (Cardizem) are calcium channel blockers that predominantly affect afterload reduction. Side effects of nifedipine include hypotension, negative inotropy, thrombocytopenia, edema, and headache. Diltiazem produces less hypotension. These agents do improve hemodynamics in patients with diastolic dysfunction, but they have not been shown to improve survival. In fact, they may be detrimental in patients with systolic dysfunction because of their tendency to produce negative inotropy and hypotension.

Increasing Myocardial Contractility

Digitalis has traditionally been the single most important drug used to increase myocardial contractility in CHF. Other inotropic agents (Table 38-3) may be used parenterally in the treatment of acute pulmonary edema. Although the development of vasodilators has surpassed the importance of digitalis in managing chronic CHF, it remains a commonly prescribed medication.

In CHF patients, digitalis increases cardiac output and causes a reflex decline in peripheral vascular resistance. Digitalis has a narrow therapeutic range, and toxicity is common. Digoxin is the most commonly used form of digitalis. After oral administration the onset of action is 2 to 3 hours, and the peak effect occurs at 4 to 6 hours. The usual dosage range is 0.125 to 0.375 mg daily. The dosage must be reduced in patients with impaired renal function, and digoxin levels must be monitored closely. IV digitalis is not effective in acute pulmonary edema unless it is associated with atrial fibrillation.

Intracellular acidosis and the accumulation of phosphate, as well as a deficiency of cyclic adenosine monophosphate (cAMP), has been suggested as a mechanism that may cause contractile failure in acute CHF resulting from myocardial ischemia. The *phosphodiesterase inhibitors,* such as amrinone and milrinone, are inotropic vasodilators that improve contractility and hemodynamic performance. However, no beneficial effects on survival have yet been demonstrated. Table 38-3 gives the dosage range.

Table 38-3

INOTROPIC AGENTS

Drug	Mechanism of Action	Heart Rate Effect	Oxygen Demand	Dosage
Digoxin	Inhibits Na^+-K^+ ATPase	Decreases	Increases	1 mg load over 24 hrs; 0.125-0.375 mg/day po
Dopamine	Enhances cAMP	Increases	Increases	5-20 µg/kg/min IV
Dobutamine	Enhances cAMP	No effect	Increases	5-20 µg/kg/min IV
Amrinone	Phosphodiesterase inhibitor	No change	Decreases	0.75 mg/kg IV load 5-10 µg/kg/min IV
Milrinone	Phosphodiesterase inhibitor	No change	Decreases	50 µg/kg IV load 0.5 µg/kg/min IV

In summary, the treatment of patients with symptomatic CHF should be initiated with a combination of diuretics, ACE inhibitors, and possibly digoxin for patients with systolic dysfunction. Patients who remain symptomatic may benefit from the addition of a direct-acting vasodilator like hydralazine, as well as a nitrate. The use of stronger inotropic agents and phosphodiesterase inhibitors may improve hemodynamics and exercise tolerance but have not been shown to improve survival. For patients refractory to conventional therapy, cardiac transplantation may offer new hope.

ACUTE PULMONARY EDEMA

Acute pulmonary edema is a life-threatening emergency consisting of the abrupt onset of left ventricular failure. It is often the result of an acute precipitating event, which should be sought and corrected if possible.

The patient with acute pulmonary edema is typically anxious, pale, clammy, acutely dyspneic and tachypneic, sometimes cyanotic, and often confused. Most individuals sit upright and resist efforts to force recumbency. Tachycardia

and hypertension are common. Hypotension is an ominous sign because it indicates that cardiac contractility is substantially reduced even under maximum adrenergic stimulation.

A cough with pink frothy sputum production is a classic sign but is often absent. Increased jugular venous pulsation, pedal edema, and congestive hepatomegaly may be present. Cool distal extremities from poor perfusion and catecholamine-induced vasoconstriction is common. Auscultation of the chest often reveals diffuse rales, wheezes, or both. A ventricular heave and an S_3 gallop rhythm can often be detected.

Management of pulmonary edema requires immediate, aggressive intervention. Administering high-flow oxygen, cardiac monitoring, maintaining the patient in the upright position, and establishing IV access are correct initial interventions. Achieve venodilatation to reduce preload (and to a lesser extent arteriolar dilatation) by administering rapid-acting nitrates 0.4 to 1.2 mg every 5 to 10 minutes as long as the systolic blood pressure remains above 100 mm Hg. Morphine sulfate to reduce adrenergic vasoconstrictor stimuli and to reduce emotional stress may be administered in increments of 2 to 4 mg IV, and furosemide 40 to 120 mg IV or bumetanide

(Bumex) 1 mg IV may be given to promote diuresis and increase venous capacitance.

If these measures do not result in significant and rapid improvement, nitroglycerin may be used intravenously beginning at 5 to 10 µg/minute; increase the dosage by 5 µg/min increments until the desired effect is achieved or until the systolic blood pressure drops below 100 mm Hg. Sodium nitroprusside is also an effective afterload reducer in the face of severe, persistent hypertension or increased systemic vascular resistance. Give an initial dose of 10 µg/minute, and titrate according to the effect on systemic blood pressure.

Provide ventilatory support as indicated. Several recent reports have suggested the efficacy of continuous positive airway pressure (CPAP) and nasal bi-PAP ventilation to acutely improve oxygenation and reduce pulmonary edema. This effect may be balanced by the increase in intrathoracic pressure and the subsequent effect on cardiac output. In severe pulmonary edema with impending respiratory failure, endotracheal intubation and ventilatory support may be necessary.

Initial laboratory tests include a chest x-ray examination, arterial blood gas analysis, a complete blood count, serum electrolytes, blood urea nitrogen, creatinine, glucose, creatine kinase isoenzyme levels, and a 12-lead ECG. A urinary catheter often is necessary to monitor the diuresis and determine subsequent doses of furosemide. The use of a pulmonary artery catheter can be useful in directly measuring hemodynamic parameters so that specific interventions can be guided more precisely.

Hypotension precludes the use of nitroglycerin, morphine, and other vasodilators. In this instance the use of parenteral inotropic agents (see Table 38-3) may be indicated. Dopamine is the most common inotropic agent recommended. Start the dose at 5 to 10 µg/kg/minute and monitor the blood pressure carefully. An intraarterial line is often required. The onset of action occurs within minutes of IV administration; the duration of action following cessation is similarly brief. Dobutamine is a catecholamine, and its actions in decreasing afterload are similar to those of dopamine. Dobutamine does not, however, increase renal blood flow or produce as significant a tachycardia. The dosage range is similar to dopamine. Consider adding dobutamine once the systolic blood pressure reaches 100 mm Hg by previous administration of dopamine.

Amrinone is a noncatecholamine phosphodiesterase inhibitor that acts as an inotropic agent to increase cardiac output and decrease left ventricular filling pressure. Administration of a 0.75 mg/kg loading dose followed by a 5 to 10 µg/kg/minute maintenance infusion may be needed if the patient is not responding to therapy.

In extremely refractory cases, patients may be considered for insertion of aortic balloon counterpulsation to augment diastolic function. Patients in renal failure who develop acute pulmonary edema are characteristically refractory to traditional treatment modalities and often require emergent dialysis.

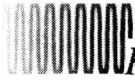

KEY CONSIDERATIONS

WHAT IS THE LIFE THREAT?

Acute congestive heart failure may be precipitated by an extensive myocardial infarction, pulmonary embolus, hypertensive crisis, severe infection, dysrhythmia, or rupture of a cardiac valve. Exacerbations are caused by discontinuing previously prescribed medications or severe environmental stress. Because the symptoms and signs of congestive heart failure reflect impairment of tissue perfusion and oxygenation, the condition is life threatening when severe.

DOES THE PATIENT NEED ADMISSION?

Patients with only minimal exacerbation of previously established congestive heart failure are sometimes treated in the emergency department with diuretics and released when asymptomatic. It is best to consult with the patient's physician and ensure good follow-up within a few days. Other patients, including those with new-onset failure, acute pulmonary edema, chest pain, a ruptured valve, and severe worsening of a preexisting condition, require consultation and admission.

WHAT IS THE MOST SERIOUS DIAGNOSIS?

Acute pulmonary edema, massive myocardial infarction, pulmonary embolism, and a ruptured cardiac valve are the most serious diagnoses.

HAVE I PERFORMED A THOROUGH WORK-UP?

Search for causes of acute heart failure that can be corrected. Such causes include a ruptured cardiac valve, dysrhythmia, pulmonary embolism, cardiac tamponade, severe anemia, thyrotoxicosis, or a severe underlying infection.

Recommended Reading

Armstrong PW, Moe CW: Medical advances in the treatment of congestive heart failure, *Circulation* 88:2941-2952, 1993.

Braunwald E: Heart failure. In Wilson JD et al, editors: *Harrison's principles of internal medicine,* ed 12, New York, 1991, McGraw-Hill.

Dei Cas L, Leier CV: Strategies for initial management of acute congestive heart failure, *J Crit Illness* 7(10):1612-1623, 1992.

Leier CU, Binkley PF, Cody RJ: Alpha-adrenergic component of the sympathetic nervous system in congestive heart failure, *Circulation* 82 (suppl 11):1168-1176, 1990.

Shesser R: Heart failure. In Rosen P et al, editors: *Emergency medicine: concepts and clinical practice,* ed 3, St Louis, 1992, Mosby.

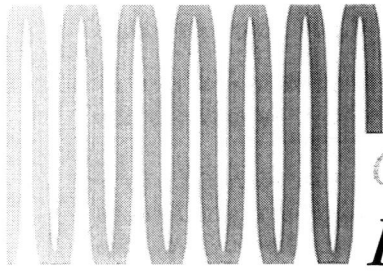

Chapter Thirty-nine
DYSRHYTHMIAS

J. STEPHEN STAPCZYNSKI

Evaluating disturbances in cardiac rhythm is an important skill for the emergency physician. This chapter reviews the management of commonly encountered dysrhythmias. Although the emphasis is often placed on diagnosis, precise identification is not always necessary for effective treatment.

GENERAL ASSESSMENT

Hemodynamic Stability

The most important issue during the assessment of dysrhythmias is hemodynamic stability: Is the cardiac output adequate for cerebral and myocardial perfusion? Hemodynamic instability is defined by the criteria noted in the box at right.

If the patient is hemodynamically unstable, the second issue is whether the instability is a result of an abnormal rhythm. A normal heart can tolerate ventricular rates between 40 and 160 beats/minute because physiologic adjustments are able to maintain an adequate cardiac output between these rates. However, adults with cardiac or arterial disease may develop ischemia in susceptible organs at rates below 50 or above 120 beats/minute. If the patient is hemodynamically unstable because of a dysrhythmia, immediate treatment is needed (Table 39-1).

The third issue is the potential for deterioration despite apparent hemodynamic stability. For example, ventricular tachycardia may appear stable but can suddenly deteriorate into ventricular fibrillation. Such dysrhythmias deserve urgent treatment despite the appearance of hemodynamic stability.

If the patient is stable, evaluation and treatment can be approached in an orderly manner. Specifically determine the following:
1. Is the ventricular rate fast or slow?
2. Are the QRS complexes narrow or wide?
3. Is the ventricular rhythm regular or irregular?
4. Are P waves present and associated with each QRS complex?

Tachycardias

If the patient is unstable with a rapid rhythm, the recommended treatment is direct current

---

SIGNS OF HEMODYNAMIC INSTABILITY

Hypotension: systolic blood pressure less than 90 mm Hg
Evidence of inadequate cerebral perfusion: confusion, coma
Pulmonary edema: dyspnea, rales
Evidence of myocardial ischemia: chest pain

Table 39-1

MANAGEMENT ON THE BASIS OF HEMODYNAMIC STABILITY

Hemodynamic State	Rhythm	Treatment
Unstable	Rapid	Direct current cardioversion
Stable	Rapid	Vagal maneuvers IV antidys- rhythmics
Unstable	Slow	IV atropine Transcutaneous pacemaker Transvenous pacemaker

electrical cardioversion. Two important steps before cardioversion are (1) to assess for an adequate airway (intubate if required), and (2) to assess for adequate ventilation (ventilate the patient with a bag if necessary). An intravenous (IV) access and sedative administration are desirable but should not delay cardioversion in an unstable patient.

If the patient is stable with a rapid rhythm, vagal stimulatory maneuvers such as carotid sinus massage or the Valsalva maneuver may be helpful in differentiating supraventricular from ventricular rhythms. These vagal maneuvers impair atrioventricular (AV) node conduction that may either slow the ventricular response to rapid atrial dysrhythmias or terminate the dysrhythmia if the AV node is a crucial part of a sustaining reentry circuit. Stable patients with rapid rhythms who require emergent treatment are usually given IV antidysrhythmics to either (1) slow the ventricular response, or (2) terminate the dysrhythmia and allow resumption of sinus rhythm. An example of the first approach is the use of digoxin or diltiazem to slow the ventricular response in atrial fibrillation; an example of

the second approach is to use adenosine or verapamil to abolish reentrant supraventricular tachycardia.

A regular tachycardia with wide QRS complexes (duration >120 msec) can pose a therapeutic dilemma. Wide-complex tachycardias may represent either ventricular tachycardia or supraventricular tachycardia with aberration. Adenosine and procainamide are generally safe, often effective, and thus recommended in cases of unknown wide-complex tachycardia. Lidocaine and verapamil are contraindicated.

Bradycardias

In the unstable patient with bradycardia, the therapeutic goal is to increase the ventricular rate. The initial treatment should be IV atropine, and if ineffective, start pacing with a transcutaneous pacemaker.

IRREGULAR BEATS

Irregular, extra beats originate from myocardium that undergoes spontaneous depolarization, manifests pacemaking activity, and temporarily usurps control of cardiac contraction. These ectopic beats commonly originate from either atrial or ventricular myocardium. Such ectopic beats are premature—occurring before the next expected normal beat—and are differentiated from escape beats, which occur after the time in which the next expected normal beat should have occurred.

Premature Atrial Contractions

Premature atrial contractions (PACs) originate in atrial myocardium other than the sinus node. PACs have several electrocardiographic characteristics: (1) the ectopic P′ wave is premature and appears sooner than the next expected sinus beat, and (2) the ectopic P′ wave has a different configuration or direction than the sinus

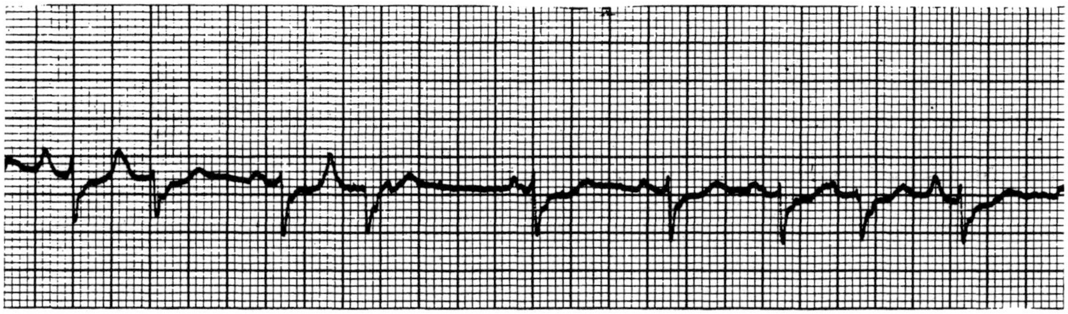

Fig.39-1 Premature atrial contractions.

P wave (Fig. 39-1). The PAC may encounter the AV node during the complete refractory period and not be conducted into the ventricle (no following QRS), may be conducted through the infranodal system aberrantly (wide QRS) or, most typically, may be normally conducted through the ventricles (normal QRS). The sinus node is often depolarized and "reset" by the PAC; therefore although the interval following a PAC is often slightly longer than the previous cycle length, the pause is less than fully compensatory.

PACs are common in all ages and are often seen in the absence of heart disease. Stress, fatigue, alcohol, tobacco, or coffee may precipitate PACs. Frequent PACs may occur in chronic lung disease, ischemic heart disease, atrial dilatation associated with congestive heart failure, or digitalis toxicity. A PAC may trigger atrial tachycardia, flutter, or fibrillation. Treatment is initiated by discontinuing any precipitating drugs or toxins and by treating underlying disorders. PACs that initiate sustained dysrhythmias may need to be suppressed with oral antidysrhythmics.

Premature Ventricular Contractions

Premature ventricular contractions (PVCs) are ectopic beats that originate in the ventricular myocardium. The impulse is conducted slowly from cell to cell rather than by the faster Purkinje network. PVCs have several electrocardiographic characteristics: (1) a premature and wide QRS complex, and (2) no preceding P wave (Fig. 39-2). With PVCs, the T wave is usually directed opposite the major deflection. With PVCs, the sinus node is usually not affected (not "reset"), and therefore there is a fully compensatory pause after the PVC (Fig. 39-3).

PVCs are very common and occur even in patients without heart disease. They also are seen in most patients with ischemic heart disease and are nearly universally present in patients with acute myocardial infarction. Other common causes of PVCs include digitalis toxicity, congestive heart failure, hypokalemia, alkalosis, hypoxemia, and sympathomimetic drugs.

There is no need to suppress PVCs in most clinical settings. However, with acute myocardial infarction, PVCs are believed to represent underlying electrical instability and the potential for sudden ventricular fibrillation. Many physicians do treat PVCs in this setting, especially if the PVCs are frequent, coupled, or multiform.

Lidocaine is the preferred drug of treatment: 75 mg (1.0 to 1.5 mg/kg) IV over 60 to 90 seconds followed by a constant infusion at 1 to 4 mg/minute (10 to 40 μg/kg/minute). A repeat dose of 25 to 50 mg (0.5 mg/kg) may be necessary during the first 20 minutes to prevent a sub-

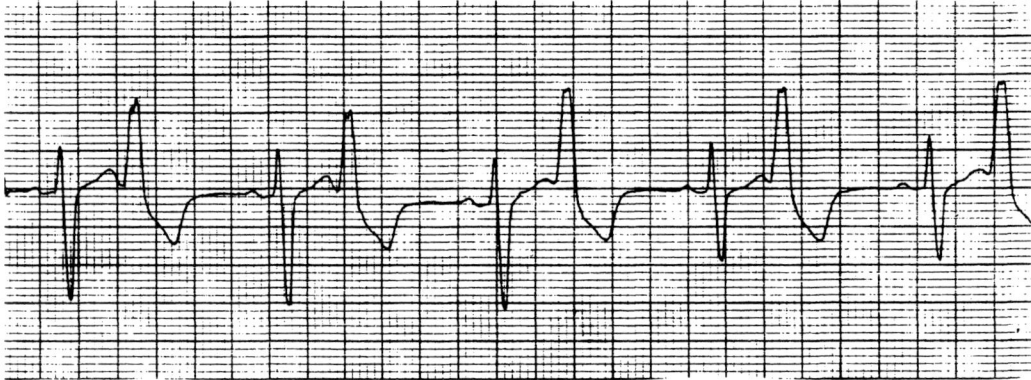

Fig. **39-2**   Premature ventricular contractions.

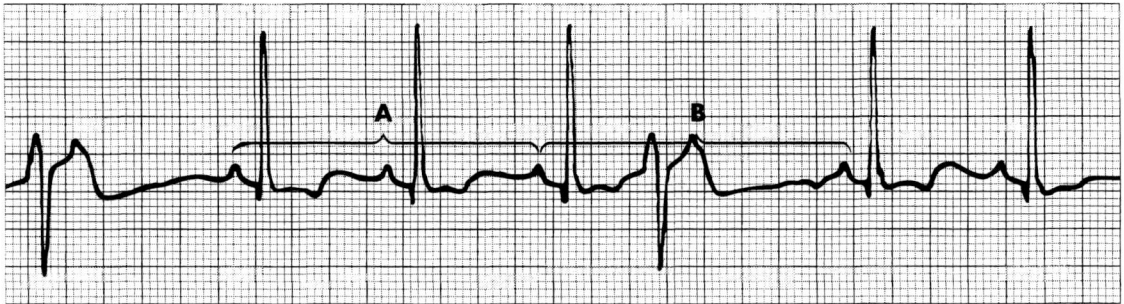

Fig. **39-3**   Premature ventricular contractions causing compensatory pause. Note that sinus P wave is seen in a T wave. Pause is equal to two sinus intervals. A equals B.

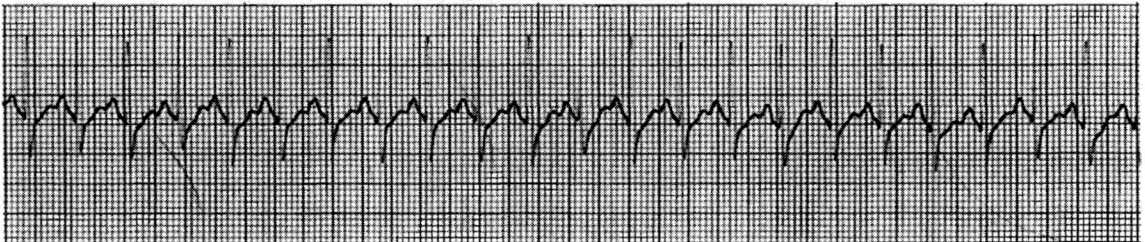

Fig. **39-4**   Sinus tachycardia, rate 176.

therapeutic dip in serum levels as a result of the early distribution phase.

Procainamide is a secondary agent. Administer procainamide IV at a rate less than 50 mg/minute until the PVCs are suppressed, the total dose reaches 15 to 17 mg/kg (12 mg/kg in patients with heart failure), or signs of toxicity develop with hypotension or QRS prolongation. The loading dose should be followed by a maintenance infusion of 2.8 mg/kg/hour (1.4 mg/kg/hour in patients with renal failure).

REGULAR NARROW-COMPLEX TACHYCARDIA

Regular narrow-complex tachycardia originates from above the AV node. The impulses are conducted normally (antegrade) down the conducting system, and the QRS complexes are usually normal (narrow).

Sinus Tachycardia

Sinus tachycardia results from an acceleration of the sinus node discharge to rates above 100 beats/minute but typically less than 160 beats/minute, with normal P-wave morphology, a normal PR interval, and a 1:1 AV conduction (Fig. 39-4). The rhythm may vary slightly rather than being precisely regular.

Sinus tachycardia represents a response to the following stimuli: (1) physiologic (infants and children, exertion, anxiety, fear), (2) pharmacologic (atropine, sympathomimetics, alcohol, caffeine), or (3) pathologic (fever, hypoxemia, anemia, hypovolemia, heart failure). A specific treatment is not usually indicated for sinus tachycardia, but the underlying disorder should be investigated and treated.

Paroxysmal Supraventricular Tachycardia

Paroxysmal supraventricular tachycardia (PSVT) results from sustained reentry over a circuit located above the bifurcation of the bundle of His.

The onset is typically sudden and is often initiated by a premature beat; hence the term *paroxysmal.* Approximately 60% of all patients with PSVT have the reentry circuit within the AV node, approximately 20% have a reentry circuit involving a bypass tract, and the remainder have reentry in other sites. Some cases of PSVT are associated with preexcitation syndromes, such as Wolff-Parkinson-White (WPW) syndrome. In a large number of cases, PSVT occurs without definable cardiac disease.

PSVT has several electrocardiographic characteristics: (1) a regular and rapid tachycardia with narrow QRS complexes, (2) a ventricular rate of typically 160 to 200 beats/minute, and (3) absent P waves, although they may be visible after or before the QRS complex (Fig. 39-5). Occasionally the QRS complex may be wide as a result of aberrancy or preexisting bundle branch disease. The onset and offset of PSVT is sudden (Fig. 39-6).

In a normal heart, PSVT at the typical rate of 160 to 200 beats/minute is often tolerated for hours to days. Nevertheless, cardiac output is always depressed regardless of blood pressure, and some patients become unstable, especially with preexisting cardiac disease. Synchronized cardioversion should be performed in the unstable patient. The initial setting should be 50 watt-sec, with succeeding shocks increased at increments of 25 watt-sec. Premedication with IV midazolam (1 to 2.5 mg) or diazepam (5 to 10 mg) is recommended before cardioversion.

Stable patients with PSVT can be treated with vagal maneuvers or IV antidysrhythmics. Performing the Valsalva maneuver in a supine position is reported to be the most effective vagal maneuver in treating PSVT. The strain phase must be adequate (at least 10 seconds), with slowing or conversion seen during the release phase.

Adenosine is an ultrashort-acting (20 seconds or less) agent that produces AV block and converts over 90% of all PSVT. The dose is 6 mg given as a rapid IV push. If no response is seen

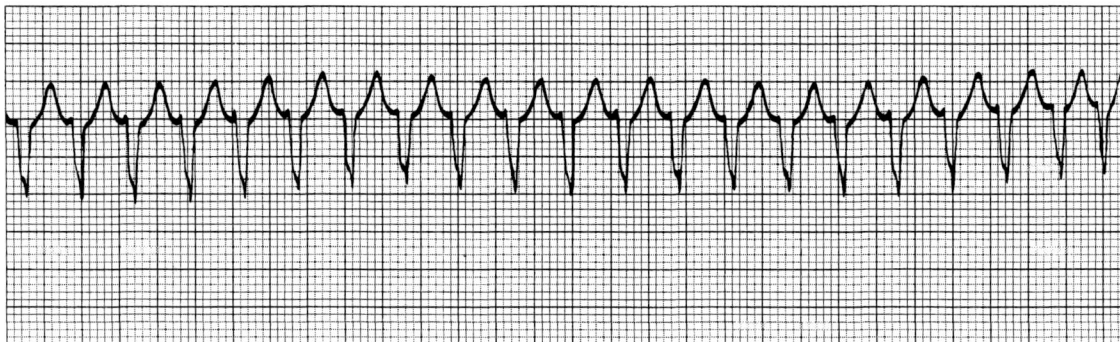

Fig.39-5   Supraventricular tachycardia. Exact origin of rhythm cannot be determined.

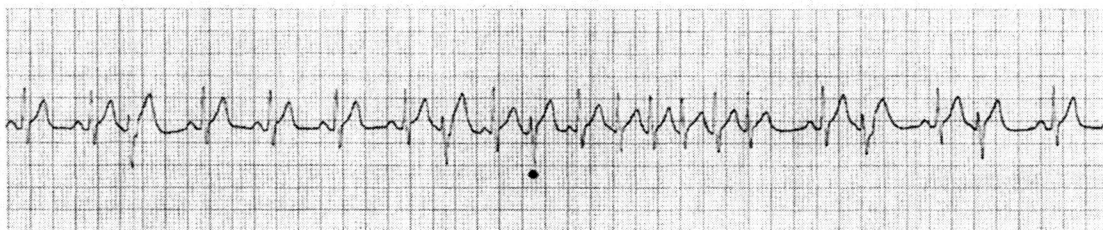

Fig.39-6   The sudden onset of paroxysmal supraventricular tachycardia after third premature atrial contraction *(dot)*.

within 2 minutes, a second dose of 12 mg can be given. There is no proven benefit to repeated doses or to doses above 20 mg. Many patients experience distressing but transient side effects, such as chest pain. Because adenosine has no sustained antidysrhythmic effect, recurrences of PSVT have been seen in as many as 25% of all cases. The major advantage of adenosine is its ultrashort effect, lack of hypotensive or myocardial depressive activity, and safety when given to patients with ventricular tachycardia.

Verapamil produces more sustained AV block and is effective in at least 90% of the cases of PSVT. The initial dose is 5 mg (0.075 mg/kg) IV over 1 to 2 minutes. The maximal therapeutic response is seen within 2 to 3 minutes. If necessary, a repeat dose can be given in 10 minutes. The total dose should not exceed 15 mg. In previously normotensive patients, IV verapamil almost always produces a drop in blood pressure. Excessive decreases in blood pressure can be treated with IV calcium chloride or calcium gluconate without reducing the antidysrhythmic effect of verapamil. The major disadvantages of verapamil are its sustained chronotropic effects, negative inotropic effects, and possible deleterious effects in ventricular tachycardia. IV verapamil should not be given concomitantly with IV ß-blockers and is relatively contraindicated in patients who are taking oral ß-blockers.

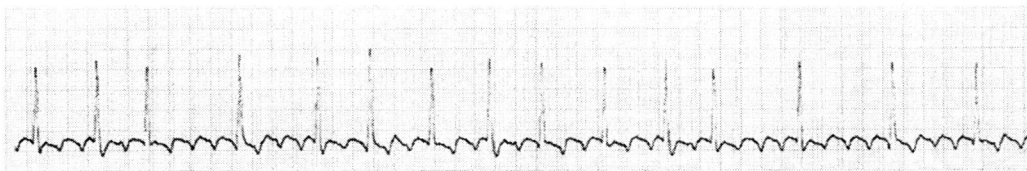

Fig.39-7   Atrial flutter.

Atrial Flutter

Atrial flutter originates from a small region of atrial myocardium, typically the inferior right atrium. Atrial flutter has several electrocardiographic characteristics: (1) a regular atrial rate between 250 and 350 beats/minute (most commonly 280 to 320 beats/minute); (2) sawtooth flutter waves directed superiorly and most visible in leads II, III, and aV_F; and (3) AV block, typically 2:1 but occasionally greater (Fig. 39-7). The ventricular rate is typically approximately 150 beats/minute, and because flutter waves may not be appreciated, the rhythm may be mistaken for sinus tachycardia. Vagal maneuvers such as carotid sinus massage or the Valsalva maneuver may temporarily increase AV block, slow the ventricular response, and make flutter waves more obvious. Rarely, atrial flutter may have 1:1 conduction with a ventricular rate of 300 beats/minute and wide QRS complexes resembling ventricular tachycardia.

Atrial flutter rarely occurs in the absence of heart disease; it is most commonly seen in patients with ischemic heart disease or acute myocardial infarction. Less common causes include congestive heart failure, pulmonary embolus, valvular heart disease, myocarditis, or myocardial contusion.

Unstable patients with atrial flutter should be treated with synchronized cardioversion starting at 25 to 50 watt-sec. More than 90% of all cases of atrial flutter can be converted to sinus rhythm with this dose.

Stable patients can be treated with digoxin, verapamil, diltiazem, esmolol, or propranolol to reduce AV conduction and slow the ventricular rate. After the ventricular rate has been controlled, procainamide or other antidysrhythmics can be used to convert atrial flutter. Verapamil occasionally converts atrial flutter to sinus rhythm (in approximately 30% of all cases) or to atrial fibrillation (approximately 20% of all cases).

Atrial Tachycardia With Block

Atrial tachycardia with block originates from a small portion of atrial tissue that acquires independent pacemaker activity and usurps control of the heart. This ectopic focus typically discharges at a rate of 150 to 250 beats/minute, is associated with AV block, and is sometimes variable (Fig. 39-8). The dysrhythmia is generally nonparoxysmal, with no sudden onset or offset. Atrial tachycardia with block is "classically" associated with digitalis toxicity, but there are other causes (e.g., acute myocardial infarction, chronic lung disease, pneumonia, alcohol intoxication), and other dysrhythmias are more common in the setting of digitalis toxicity.

Treatment of atrial tachycardia not associated with digitalis toxicity begins with agents for ventricular rate control: digoxin, verapamil, diltiazem, esmolol, or propranolol. Atrial tachycardia resulting from digitalis toxicity can be treated with the following: (1) correction of hypokalemia to reduce atrial ectopy, (2) IV phenytoin or magnesium to reduce atrial ectopy, and

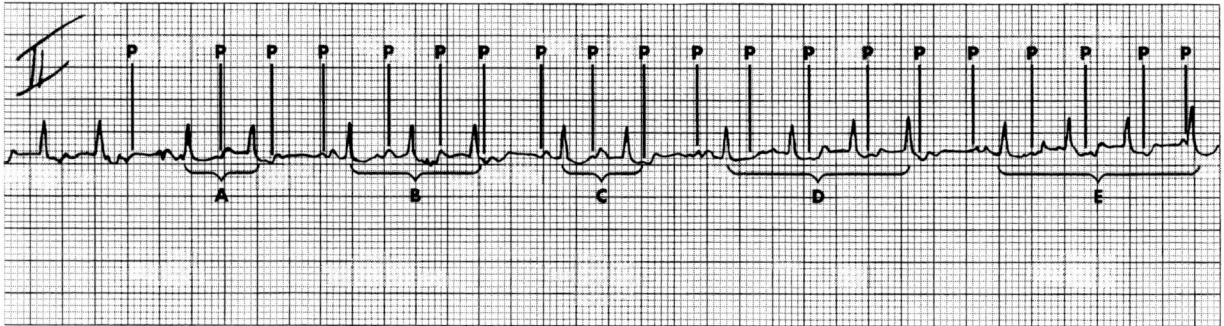

Fig. 39-8   Patient shows paroxysmal atrial tachycardia rate of 200 with Mobitz type I atrioventricular block. P wave is bifed (P mitrale). A to E group beating. This rhythm should not be confused with atrial fibrillation.

(3) digoxin-specific antibody fragments (Fabs). The latter should be reserved for patients with hemodynamic deterioration or serious ventricular dysrhythmias. Because atrial tachycardia with block originates from an ectopic focus, cardioversion is not effective.

IRREGULAR NARROW-COMPLEX TACHYCARDIA

Irregular narrow-complex tachycardia originates from above the AV node. Ventricular depolarization occurs via the normal conducting system, but the ventricular response is haphazard because of chaotic atrial activity.

Atrial Fibrillation

Atrial fibrillation occurs when multiple small areas of the atrial myocardium continuously depolarize and contract in a chaotic and disorganized manner. Atrial fibrillation has several electrocardiographic characteristics: (1) fibrillatory waves at a rate above 300 beats/minute, which are usually best seen in leads V_1 to V_3 or aV_F; or (2) an irregular ventricular response, typically around 160 to 180 beats/minute because of the refractory period of the AV node (Fig. 39-9).

Disease or drugs (e.g., digoxin) increases the AV nodal refractory period and markedly slows the ventricular response. More rapid ventricular rates are possible in patients with bypass tracks; rates above 200 beats/minute, often with wide QRS complexes, are possible. Occasionally irregularity may not be apparent; therefore careful measurement with calibers is necessary. The fibrillatory waves may not be easily seen; vagal maneuvers to slow the ventricular response are useful to enhance visibility.

Atrial fibrillation can be paroxsymal or sustained. The most common predisposing factor is increased atrial size and mass. Atrial fibrillation is usually found in association with rheumatic heart disease, hypertension, ischemic heart disease, or thyrotoxicosis. Less common causes are chronic lung disease, pericarditis, alcohol binging, or an atrial septal defect. In patients with heart failure, left atrial contraction provides an important contribution to cardiac output. The loss of atrial contraction seen with atrial fibrillation and rapid ventricular rates can cause sudden deterioration into pulmonary edema. Chronic atrial fibrillation predisposes an individual to peripheral venous and atrial thrombosis, with a risk of pulmonary or systemic arterial embolism.

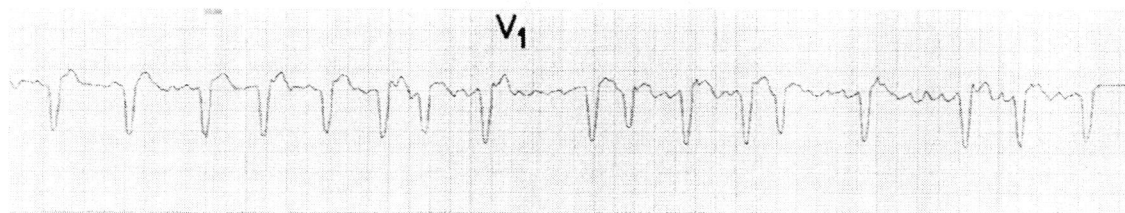

Fig.39-9   Atrial fibrillation.

In unstable patients, synchronized cardioversion is indicated. Over 60% of the cases of atrial fibrillation can be converted with 100 watt-sec, and over 80% can be converted with 200 watt-sec. Electrical conversion and maintenance in sinus rhythm is more likely when atrial fibrillation is of short duration and the atria are not greatly dilated.

In stable patients, ventricular rate control is the first therapeutic goal. This control can be achieved with IV digoxin, verapamil, diltiazem, esmolol, or propranolol. Digoxin is commonly used, with doses of 0.25 to 0.5 mg given intravenously and additional amounts given according to the response. The chief disadvantage with digoxin is the slow response; it typically takes 9 to 11 hours to achieve the desired ventricular rate. Verapamil in a dose of 5 to 10 mg IV effectively slows the ventricular response in 60% to 70% of all patients with atrial fibrillation and may convert 10% to 15% of them to sinus rhythm. Diltiazem 20 mg (0.25 mg/kg) IV over 2 minutes followed by an infusion of 10 mg/hour is also effective. A repeat dose of diltiazem 25 mg (0.35 mg/kg) may be given in 15 minutes. IV esmolol or propranolol is especially effective in atrial fibrillation resulting from thyrotoxicosis or rheumatic mitral stenosis. The major disadvantage of calcium or ß-adrenergic blockers is their negative inotropic effects, which makes them poor choices in patients with heart failure.

Once ventricular rate control has been obtained, chemical conversion can be considered. A wide variety of IV and oral antidysrhythmics have been used to chemically convert atrial fibrillation. Procainamide IV is often effective. Conversion of chronic atrial fibrillation carries as much as a 1% to 2% incidence of arterial embolism. Most physicians therefore anticoagulate 1 to 3 weeks before attempting electrical or chemical conversion in patients with atrial fibrillation that has lasted longer than 3 days.

Multifocal Atrial Tachycardia (MFAT)

Multifocal atrial tachycardia (MFAT) (also known as a "chaotic atrial rhythm" or "wandering atrial pacemaker") is caused by at least two different sites of atrial ectopy competing with the sinus node for ventricular pacing. MFAT has several electrocardiographic characteristics: (1) three or more differently shaped P waves; (2) varying PP, PR, and RR intervals; and (3) a ventricular rate between 100 and 180 beats/minute (Fig. 39-10). MFAT can be confused with atrial fibrillation or flutter.

MFAT is most commonly found in elderly patients with exacerbations of chronic lung disease, but it is also reported with heart failure, sepsis, and methylxanthine toxicity.

Specific antidysrhythmic treatment of MFAT is not sought; treatment of the underlying disorder usually resolves the dysrhythmia. Although IV magnesium, verapamil, esmolol, and metoprolol have been shown to reduce atrial ectopy and slow ventricular response in MFAT, the dysrhythmia is more dependent on the status of the underlying disease.

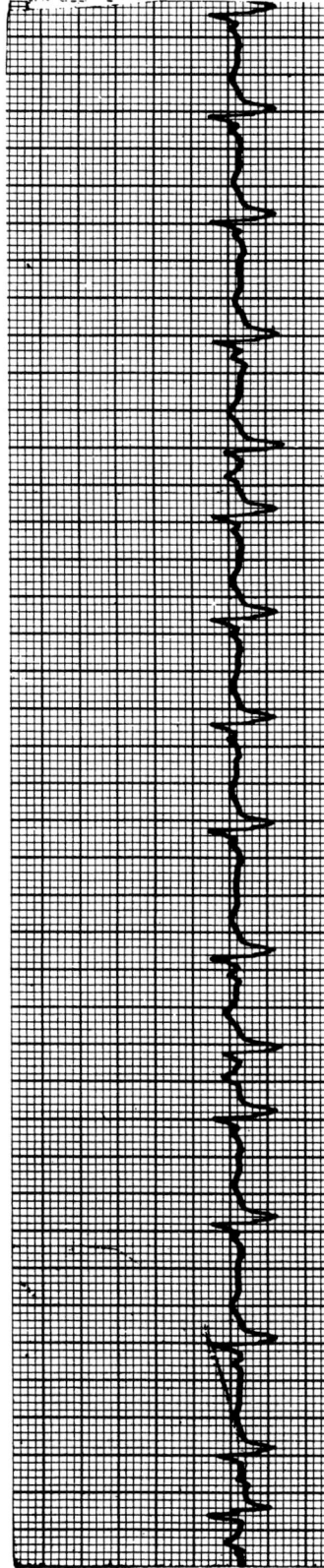

Fig. *39-10* Multifocal atrial tachycardia. Note that baseline shows no evidence of atrial fibrillation.

WIDE-COMPLEX TACHYCARDIA

Wide-complex tachycardia may be a result of ventricular tachycardia or supraventricular tachycardia (SVT) with aberrant conduction; the distinction can be difficult. Criteria that favor ventricular tachycardia are noted in the box below. In general, the majority of patients with wide-complex tachycardia have ventricular tachycardia and should be approached as such until proven otherwise. Unstable patients should be cardioverted regardless of the specific diagnosis. Stable patients can be safely treated with adenosine or procainamide intravenously.

Ventricular Tachycardia

Ventricular tachycardia results from an ectopic ventricular pacemaker that typically paces the ventricles at a rate faster than the sinus node rate. Ventricular tachycardia has several electrocardiographic characteristics: (1) wide, consistent QRS complexes; (2) at least three wide QRS complexes in succession without an intervening P wave; and (3) a regular ventricular rate greater than 100 beats/minute (typically 150 to 200 beats/minute) (Fig. 39-11). Variants of ventricular tachycardia may occur, usually with

---

FACTORS THAT FAVOR THE DIAGNOSIS OF VENTRICULAR TACHYCARDIA IN PATIENTS WITH WIDE-COMPLEX TACHYCARDIA

Clinical: age >35, history of myocardial infarction, congestive heart failure, or coronary artery bypass graft
QRS duration >140 msec
Consistently positive or negative QRS complex in all precordial leads
Extreme left axis deviation in the frontal plane
AV dissociation
Fusion beats

---

beat-to-beat variation in the QRS morphology.

Ventricular tachycardia is rare in patients who do not have underlying heart disease and is most commonly found with ischemic heart disease and acute myocardial infarction. Less common etiologies include hypertrophic cardiomyopathy, mitral valve prolapse, and drug toxicity. Hypoxemia, alkalosis, and other electrolyte abnormalities promote ventricular ectopy and may produce ventricular tachycardia.

Unstable patients should be treated with cardioversion. Awake patients can be converted with as little as 10 watt-sec; more than 100 watt-sec is rarely required. Pulseless ventricular tachycardia should be defibrillated (unsynchronized cardioversion) with 200 watt-sec.

Clinically stable patients with ventricular tachycardia can be treated with IV antidysrhythmics. Lidocaine or procainamide is usually effective in doses previously described. Bretylium 500 mg (5 to 10 mg/kg) IV over 10 minutes followed by an infusion of 1 to 2 mg/minute is also effective.

Supraventricular Tachycardia with Aberrancy

A SVT with aberrant conduction is suggested in cases of wide complex tachycardia when one of the following occurs: (1) a right bundle branch block pattern is present in lead V_1, (2) a varying bundle branch block pattern is present, (3) there is slowing or termination in response to vagal maneuvers, or (4) there is a history of pre-excitation or WPW syndrome.

BRADYCARDIAS

Bradycardias result from the depression of sinus node activity or conduction system blocks. Subsidiary pacemakers may take over and pace the heart with an escape rhythm, usually with a ventricular rate less than 60 beats/minute.

Sinus bradycardia occurs when the sinus rate falls below 60 beats/minute with a normal P-

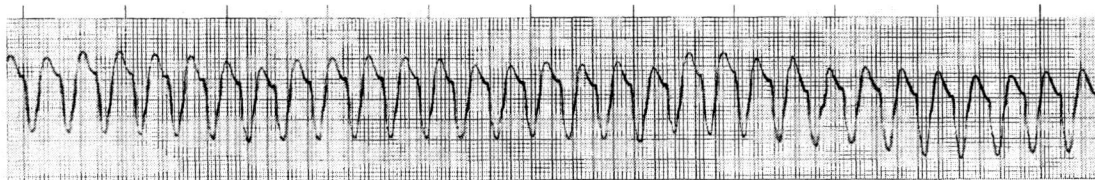

Fig.39-11   Ventricular tachycardia, rate 170.

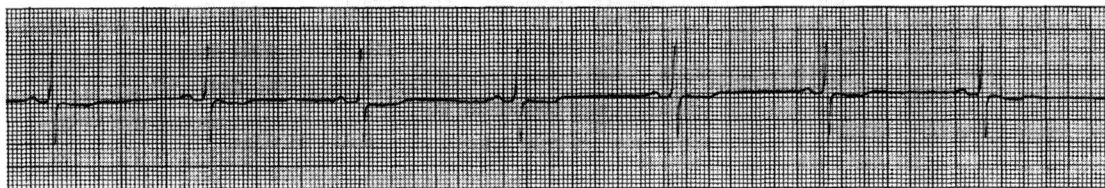

Fig.39-12   Sinus bradycardia, rate 45.

wave morphology, normal PR interval, and 1:1 AV conduction (Fig. 39-12).

Sinus bradycardia represents a response to the following stimuli: (1) physiologic (in well-conditioned athletes, during sleep, with vagal stimulation), (2) pharmacologic (digoxin, narcotics, ß-adrenergic blockers, calcium channel antagonists), or (3) pathologic (acute inferior myocardial infarction, increased intracranial pressure, hypothyroidism). A specific treatment is not usually indicated for sinus bradycardia unless the heart rate is below 50 beats/minute and there is evidence of hypoperfusion. Most patients readily respond to atropine.

PREEXCITATION SYNDROMES

Preexcitation occurs when some portion of the ventricle is activated by an impulse from the atria sooner than would be expected if the impulse were transmitted down the normal conducting system. The anatomic basis for preexcitation involves accessory conducting tracks that bypass the AV node. The most com-

mon form of preexcitation is the WPW syndrome, with a bypass path that directly links the atria and ventricles. WPW has several electrocardiographic characteristics during sinus rhythm: (1) a shortened PR interval; (2) initial distortion of the QRS complex (delta wave); and (3) because there is altered depolarization, altered repolarization with inverted T waves (Fig. 39-13). Patients with WPW have a high incidence of tachydysrhythmias: atrial flutter (approximately 5%), atrial fibrillation (approximately 10% to 20%), and PSVT (40% to 80%).

A PSVT occurs when an impulse is sustained around a loop composed of the bypass tract and the AV conducting system. Approximately 80% of the time, the impulse travels down the normal conducting system and up the bypass tract; the QRS complex is therefore narrow (orthodromic tachycardia). A minority of patients sustain PSVT with the impulse traveling down the bypass tract and up the AV conducting system; in these cases the QRS complex is wide (antidromic tachycardia).

When patients with WPW develop atrial flutter or fibrillation, the ventricles are activated by

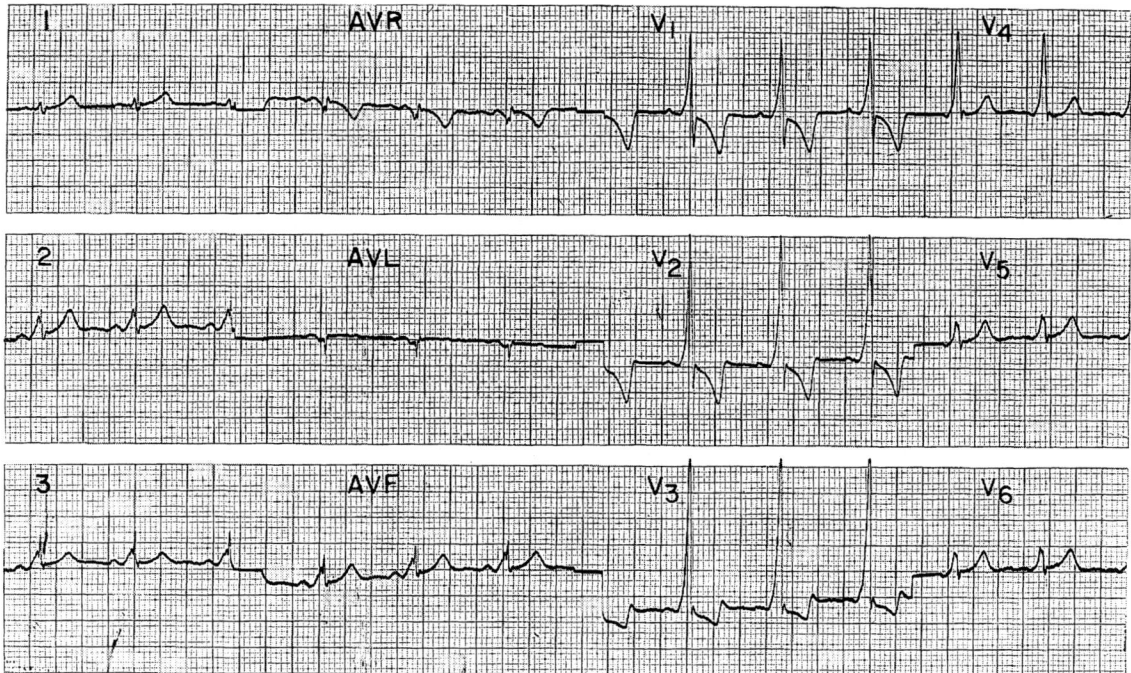

Fig.39-13 Wolff-Parkinson-White syndrome.

impulses that travel down the normal AV conducting system, the bypass tract, or both. In a minority of patients, more impulses are conducted through the bypass tracts; in such cases the QRS complexes are wide and the ventricular rate is often very rapid. These rhythms may resemble ventricular tachycardia, and excessive ventricular stimulation may degenerate into ventricular fibrillation.

A PSVT with narrow QRS complexes in patients with WPW (orthodromic tachycardia) can be treated with any maneuver or drug that slows conduction through the AV node; adenosine or verapamil are highly effective.

Stable patients with WPW and antidromic tachycardia (wide QRS complexes) should be treated with adenosine or procainamide IV; verapamil or ß-adrenergic blockers are to be avoided.

In patients with WPW, atrial fibrillation or flutter with a rapid ventricular response is best treated with cardioversion. Antidysrhythmics that prolong the refractory period of the bypass tract—such as procainamide—are preferred, whereas drugs that shorten the refractory period—such as digoxin, verapamil, phenytoin, esmolol, or propranolol—should be avoided.

ATRIOVENTRICULAR BLOCK

The nearly universally used classification for AV block is defined according to the relation between atrial and ventricular activity.

First-degree Atrioventricular Block

In first-degree AV block, each normal sinus beat is conducted into the ventricles but more slowly than normal. This condition is indicated by a PR

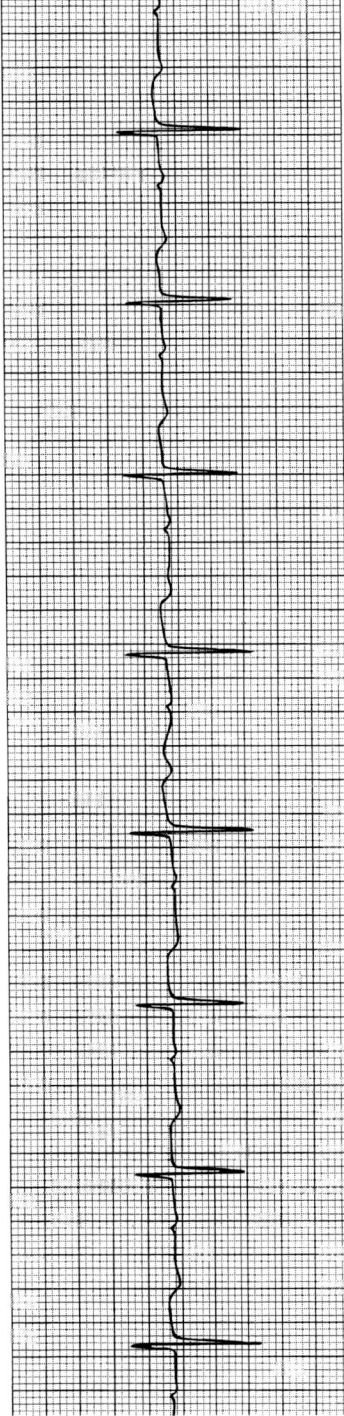

Fig. 39-14   First-degree atrioventricular block.

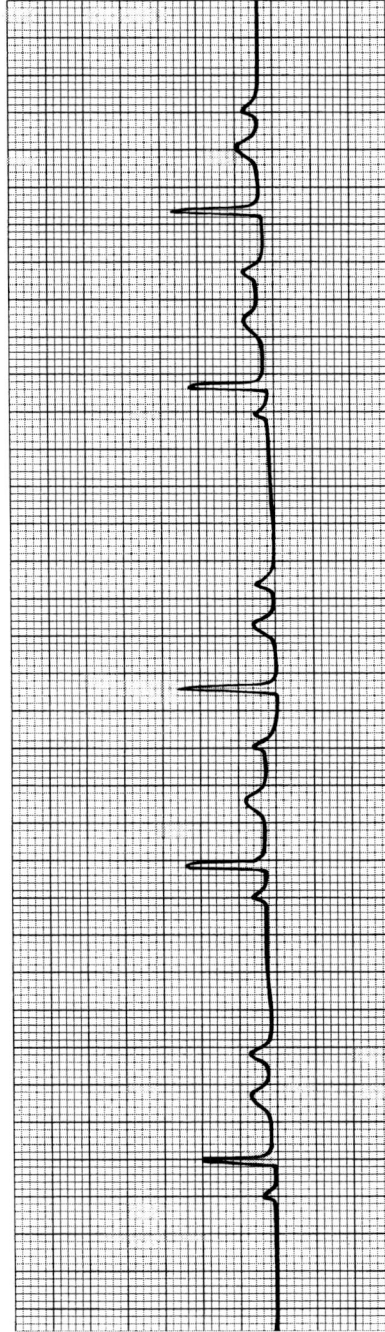

Fig. 39-15   Second-degree atrioventricular block. Mobitz type I (Wenckebach). PR interval of beat 1 is greater than PR interval of beat 2. PR interval of beat 3 is greater than PR interval of beat 4.

interval greater than 200 milliseconds on the surface ECG (Fig. 39-14). First-degree AV block is occasionally found in normal hearts, in situations of increased vagal tone, or with digitalis toxicity, myocarditis, or inferior myocardial infarctions. No treatment is indicated.

Second-degree Atrioventricular Block

Second-degree AV block is characterized by intermittent AV conduction; some P waves are not conducted. Second-degree AV block occurs in two varieties, Mobitz type I block and Mobitz type II block.

Mobitz type I block (Wenckebach block)

With a Mobitz type I block, there is progressive prolongation of AV conduction (and the PR interval) until an atrial impulse is not conducted (Fig. 39-15). Conduction ratios are used to describe the relation between atrial and ventricular beats. After the dropped beat, AV conduction returns to baseline, and the cycle usually repeats itself with the same conduction ratio (fixed ratio). The ventricular beats appear to be grouped with pauses on each side; "group beating" is characteristic of the Wenckebach phenomenon.

A Mobitz type I block is often transient and is usually associated with acute inferior myocardial infarction, digitalis toxicity, myocarditis, or post–cardiac surgery. Specific treatment is not necessary unless slow ventricular rates produce symptoms or signs of hypoperfusion. Atropine 0.5 mg IV, repeated every 5 minutes and titrated to the desired effect (or to a total dose of 2 mg), is usually effective.

Mobitz type II block

With a Mobitz type II block, the PR interval remains constant before and after the nonconducted atrial beat (Fig. 39-16). Mobitz type II blocks usually occur in the infranodal conducting system and often have associated bundle branch blocks with wide QRS complexes.

Mobitz type II blocks imply structural damage to the conducting system, are permanent, and may progress suddenly to complete heart block, especially with acute myocardial infarctions. In unstable patients, atropine may be temporarily effective until a pacemaker can be inserted. Stable patients should have a transcutaneous pacemaker applied on a stand-by mode until the need for an IV pacemaker can be assessed.

Third-degree Atrioventricular Block

There is no atrial-to-ventricular conduction with third-degree (complete) AV block. The ventricles are paced by a regular escape pacemaker that is located in the junction or ventricles (Fig. 39-17). Junctional escape rhythms are often stable with ventricular rates of 40 to 60 beats/minute. Ventricular escape rhythms are often unstable and slow, with rates below 40 beats/minute.

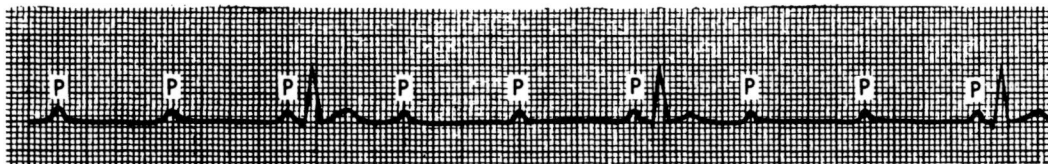

Fig.39-16 With Mobitz type II AV block, there is a series of nonconducted P waves followed by a P wave that is conducted. In this example, 3:1 AV block is present with three P waves for each QRS complex. (From Goldberger AL and Goldberger E: *Clinical electrocardiography*, ed 4, St Louis, 1990, Mosby.)

|← ———————————————————————— 6 SEC. ————————————————————————→|

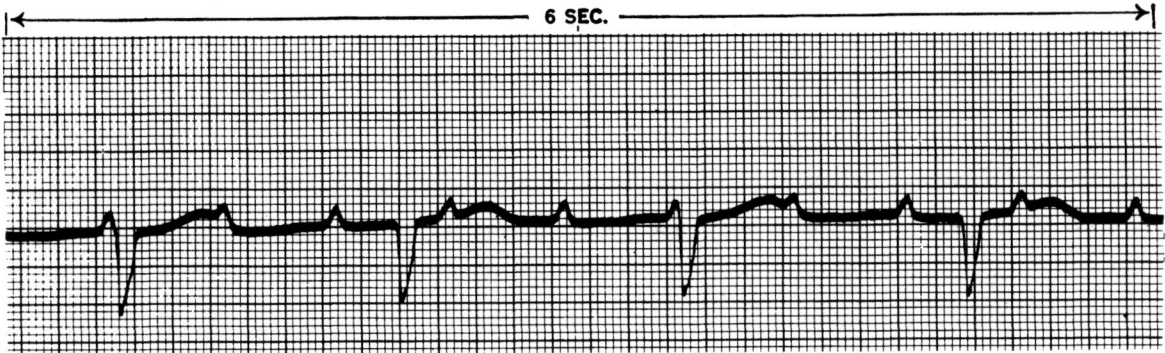

Fig.39-17 Complete third-degree atrioventricular block.

Third-degree AV block can be a result of acute infarction or degenerative disease of the conducting system. In symptomatic patients, atropine or a transcutaneous pacemaker should be used to temporarily maintain an adequate ventricular rate until a transvenous pacemaker can be placed.

SICK SINUS SYNDROME

Sick sinus syndrome (SSS) is a heterogenous disorder with abnormalities of supraventricular impulse generation and conduction that produce a variety of intermittent tachydysrhythmias and bradydysrhythmias. Typical tachydysrhythmias include atrial fibrillation, junctional tachycardia, PSVT, and atrial flutter. Common bradydysrhythmias are marked sinus bradycardia, prolonged sinus arrest, and sinoatrial block usually associ-

ated with AV nodal conduction abnormalities and inadequate AV nodal escape rhythms. Symptoms of SSS usually stem from cerebral or myocardial ischemia as a result of a heart rate that is either too fast or too slow: syncope, near-syncope, chest pain, dyspnea, or palpitations. Ambulatory ECG monitoring is usually necessary for diagnosis because a routine ECG cannot detect the intermittent dysrhythmias of this syndrome.

SUMMARY

The emergency physician must be able to manage life-threatening and symptomatic dysrhythmias with an analysis of hemodynamic stability, recognition of key electrocardiographic features, and the appropriate use of electrical cardioversion and IV antidysrhythmics.

||||||||||KEY CONSIDERATIONS

WHAT IS THE LIFE THREAT?

Life-threatening dysrhythmias that lead to cardiac arrest include ventricular fibrillation, pulseless idioventricular rhythm, asystole, and ventricular tachycardia without pulse. Serious dysrhythmias that could be life threatening include ventricular tachycardia, severe bradycardia, and complete heart block. Dysrhythmias causing increased atrial rate such as atrial fibrillation or atrial flutter become life threatening if the ventricular rate speeds up to approach the atrial rate.

Premature ventricular contractions following an acute myocardial infarction may herald more serious subsequent dysrhythmias. Sinus tachycardia may reflect a life-threatening, underlying condition such as acute blood loss, sepsis, pulmonary embolism, acute thyrotoxicosis, or poisoning.

DOES THE PATIENT NEED ADMISSION?

Many asymptomatic patients exhibit occasional PVCs (perhaps related to caffeine ingestion or fatigue). Such patients do not require admission. Athletes in great physical condition tend to have lower than normal heart rates that should not require treatment.

Patients with chronic atrial fibrillation or atrial flutter can be discharged if the ventricular rate is kept well controlled by a medication such as digoxin. Patients with supraventricular tachycardia who convert easily with adenosine or verapamil can usually be discharged if they are asymptomatic. Patients with other dysrhythmias and new dysrhythmias are typically admitted for evaluation and treatment as needed.

WHAT IS THE MOST SERIOUS DIAGNOSIS?

Ventricular tachycardia and severe bradycardia are the most serious diagnoses. Dysrhythmias tend to be more serious if they produce excessive oxygen demands.

HAVE I PERFORMED A THOROUGH WORK-UP?

Evaluate the patient for underlying causes of tachycardia, and explain any abnormal heart rate. Sometimes patients who are anxious or in pain exhibit tachycardia that returns to a normal range as the emergency stay progresses. Document such normal vital signs.

Recommended Reading

Ganz LI, Friedman PL: Supraventricular tachycardia, *N Engl J Med* 332:162, 1995.

Harken AH, Honigman B, VanWay CW: Cardiac dysrhythmias in the acute setting: pathophysiology or anyone can understand cardiac dysrhythmias, *J Emerg Med* 5:123, 1987.

Mehta D et al: Relative efficacy of various physical maneuvers in the termination of junctional tachycardia, *Lancet* 1:1181, 1988.

Yealy DM, Stapczynski JS: Dysrhythmias. In Rosen P et al, editors: *Emergency medicine, concepts and clinical practice,* ed 3, St Louis, 1992, Mosby.

Chapter Forty
UPPER GASTROINTESTINAL TRACT DISORDERS

MARCUS L. MARTIN AND LEONARD F. URBANSKI

GENERAL CONSIDERATIONS

Upper gastrointestinal (UGI) tract disorders are extremely common, and patients often come to the emergency department for evaluation. The difficulty with evaluating such complaints is not only that they may represent a life-threatening process but that many symptoms of UGI origin are vague, nonspecific and nonlocalizing. The evaluation of abdominal pain can be frustrating for the emergency physician; only 40% of all initial examinations make the correct diagnosis. This is due in part to atypical presentations in patients with abdominal pain. The clinician must be able to distinguish symptoms that are of UGI origin from those of cardiovascular (e.g., acute myocardial infarction, unstable angina, thoracic aortic dissection), musculoskeletal (e.g., costochondritis, arthritis, muscular), and pulmonary (e.g., pulmonary embolus, pneumothorax, pleuritis) origins. Many of the diagnostic studies performed in the emergency department involve these organ systems and need to be considered in every patient with UGI symptoms.

PHYSIOLOGY

The esophagus contains striated muscle in its upper third and smooth muscle distally. The cricopharyngeal muscle is striated and under some degree of voluntary control. No distinct lower esophageal sphincter exists, but manometry reveals evidence of a functional sphincter. Swallowing initiates primary peristalsis in the esophagus; a ringlike contraction carries food distally. Secondary peristalsis resists reflux of gastric material.

VOMITING

The neural stimulus for vomiting is located in the medulla, and many organ systems have receptors capable of stimulating this center (heart, peritoneum, stomach, small bowel, colon, biliary tract). *Nausea* generally precedes emesis and is associated with diminished gastric tone and peristalsis. *Retching* involves spasmodic contractions of the pyloric portion of the stomach while the fundus relaxes. During *emesis* there is a powerful sustained contraction of the abdominal muscles that elevates the intragastric pressure and opens the cardia, with evacuation of stomach contents.

Acute gastroenteritis is the most common cause of vomiting (diarrhea should be present to report this diagnosis in a patient with vomiting). Gastric outlet obstruction from peptic ulcer disease tends to cause emesis 30 to 60 minutes after a meal and tends to have a more insidious onset and slower progression. *Gastroparesis* is most commonly seen in diabetics and may cause vomiting more than 4 hours after food ingestion; it also tends to follow a more chronic presentation. *Pyloric stenosis* is a consideration in the infant who has progressive and eventually projectile emesis. This diagnosis is most common between the second and eighth weeks of life, and the risk in siblings of the patient with the disorder is 12 times greater than normal.

Metabolic abnormalities may either cause emesis (e.g., hyperglycemia, diabetic ketoacidosis, metabolic acidosis) or result from a patient's recurrent vomiting (e.g., metabolic alkalosis secondary to loss of hydrochloric acid, hypernatremia, hypokalemia). *Psychogenic emesis* deserves special mention. It is more common in women, is associated with a prolonged course, may be manifested by weight loss, and can be associated with metabolic abnormalities (typically metabolic alkalosis). Occasionally missed causes of vomiting that have potentially serious consequences include carbon monoxide poisoning and pregnancy. These causes need to be considered in every patient with unexplained vomiting.

Management of the patient with vomiting depends on the underlying cause. Those who are dehydrated from repeated emesis as reflected by examination, vital signs, or orthostatic findings benefit from intravenous (IV) hydration, usually beginning with 1L normal saline solution in adults or 20 ml/kg in children. If evidence of obstruction exists, nasogastric tube insertion and suction may help relieve symptoms.

Several agents may be used to prevent nausea and emesis. Prochlorperazine (Compazine) 5 to 10 mg may be administered in adults slow IV, IM, or PO; in children the single IM dose of prochloperazine is 0.13 mg/kg. Promethazine (Phenergan) 25 mg IM, IV, or rectal may be given to adults every 6 hours as needed; the pediatric dose is 0.25-0.50 mg/kg every 6 hrs IM, rectal, or PO. Trimethobenzamide (Tigan) 200 mg IM or rectal is recommended in adults every 6 to 8 hours or 250 mg PO every 6 to 8 hours. The pediatric dose for children weighing between 13 and 40 kg is 100 to 200 mg every 6 to 8 hours. Ondansetron (Zofran) is a 5-HT$_3$ receptor antagonist that has been approved for prevention of nausea and vomiting associated with chemotherapy; however, it is increasingly being used for emesis that is resistant to more conventional antiemetics. These antiemetics are contraindicated in cases of gastric outlet obstruction, and the parenteral route is faster and more effective than the oral or rectal route.

Infants with suspected pyloric stenosis need to have the diagnosis confirmed with a UGI contrast x-ray study or ultrasonography. Pyloromyotomy is the surgical treatment of choice once the diagnosis has been confirmed and the metabolic abnormalities have been corrected.

DYSPHAGIA

Dysphagia means "difficulty in swallowing" and can be classified on the basis of mechanism (motor disorder vs. a mechanical abnormality) and further subdivided by location (oropharyngeal and esophageal). Motor disturbances (neuromuscular) cause intermittent dysphagia, tend not to be progressive, and generally cause the patient as much difficulty swallowing liquid as solid foods (see the box on p. 474). Mechanical abnormalities such as obstruction are much more common than motor dysphagia and tend to be progressive (see the box on p. 474). Initially the patient may have difficulty swallowing

NEUROMUSCULAR CAUSES OF DYSPHAGIA

Vascular

Cerebrovascular accidents
  Basivertebral system
  Posterior inferior cerebellar artery

Immunologic (presumed)

Dermatomyositis
Polymyositis
Myasthenia gravis
Scleroderma
Multiple sclerosis

Infectious

Poliomyelitis
Diphtheria
Botulism
Rabies
Tetanus
Sydenham chorea

Metabolic

Lead poisoning
Magnesium deficiency

Other

Thyrotoxic myopathy
Parkinson disease
Amyotrophic lateral sclerosis
Myotonic dystrophy
Oculopharyngeal muscular dystrophy
Familial dysautonomia
Brain tumor

OBSTRUCTIVE CAUSES OF DYSPHAGIA

Carcinoma
Hypertrophic cervical spurs
Goiter
Vascular anomalies (dysphagia lusoria)
Foreign bodies
Esophageal webs
Esophageal ring (Schatzki ring)
Achalasia
Esophageal stricture
Zenker diverticulum
Aortic aneurysm
Left atrial enlargement
Benign tumors

only solid foods, but as the structural lesion evolves, liquids become difficult to swallow.

Oropharyngeal dysphagia occurs within 1 to 2 seconds of swallowing; patients have difficulty transferring a food bolus from the mouth to the upper esophagus (i.e., initiating swallowing). Clues to this problem may include complaints of aspiration or coughing with eating. Motor abnormalities are responsible for 80% of these types of dysphagia, with cerebrovascular accidents accounting for a large number of these cases.

Esophageal dysphagia is defined as a difficulty in transporting a food bolus through the body of the esophagus. Contrary to oropharyngeal dysphagia, it is associated with a structural abnormality in 80% of the cases. The patient is often able to precisely define the area of involvement. Depending on the degree of associated inflammation, pain may or may not be present with the dysphagia. Esophageal carcinoma, peptic stricture, and the Schatzki ring (a fibrous, diaphragm like stricture near the gastroesophageal junction that is present in 5% to 10% of the population but usually asymptomatic) are the more common causes of esophageal dysphagia. Achalasia, esophageal spasm, connective tissue diseases, amyloidosis, and extrinsic compression of the esophagus (mediastinal tumors, aortic arch aneurysm, and substernal thyroid) may also cause dysphagia, but these conditions are less common than carcinoma or peptic stricture. The dysphagia from a structural mass (intrinsic or extrinsic) is usually progressive, worse with solid food, and commonly associated with weight loss.

In children, acute infectious processes and the ingestion of a foreign body are the leading causes of dysphagia that appear in the emergency department and should be the focus of evaluation.

The evaluation of dysphagia usually requires endoscopy. In the emergency department, a chest x-ray study sometimes helps rule out compressive lesions, and a barium swallow may help rule out an obstruction. Evaluation for a foreign body obstruction is discussed later in this chapter.

ODYNOPHAGIA/ACHALASIA

Odynophagia refers to pain with swallowing and can result from any inflammation in the oropharyngeal area or esophagus (pharyngitis, aphthous ulcers, herpes, esophagitis, *Candida* organism). Odynophagia may or may not accompany dysphagi, worsens during food bolus transmission, and is relieved when the food leaves the esophagus. *Achalasia* is a special cause of dysphagia, with unknown pathogenesis; peak incidence is in the fourth to fifth decades of life. It is characterized by absent peristalsis in the esophagus and poor lower esophageal relaxation. Unlike other neuromuscular causes of dysphagia, achalasis tends to be more progressive, and structural abnormalities need to be ruled out. A chest x-ray study is sometimes suggestive with air fluid levels present in a dilated esophagus, but esophageal manometry is the definitive diagnostic test.

CHEST PAIN OF ESOPHAGEAL ORIGIN

Esophageal-induced chest pain is a common problem in the general population. It is difficult to determine if the pain is esophageal or cardiovascular origin. The nature of the pain may be identical in both esophageal spasm and coronary ischemia, and sublingual nitroglycerin is often effective in relieving the pain from either

of these sources. Fortunately, clues in the history are sometimes helpful in distinguishing which of the two organ systems are responsible for the pain (see Chapter 36).

An *esophageal reflux* typically causes a retrosternal burning sensation and is the most common cause of esophageal pain. A *hiatal hernia* is often present and contributes to the inability of the lower esophageal sphincter to prevent reflux. Pain from reflux is caused by mucosal irritation of the esophagus as a result of reflux of acidic gastric contents. It may be burning in nature or present as a dull, squeezing type of pain across the anterior side of the chest. Pain that is worsened or reproduced by lying flat suggests a diagnosis of esophageal reflux. Chest pain that is worsened after eating and relieved with antacids also suggest a diagnosis of esophageal reflux.

Esophageal spasm and *nutcracker esophagus* represent two motility disorders of the esophagus that appear as chest pain. In esophageal spasm, the patient's symptoms may be induced by reflux, stress, or drinking hot or cold liquids. Dysphagia is often present during the spasm. With nutcracker esophagus (hypertensive esophagus), the patient has normal peristaltic contractions in the distal esophagus, but the amplitude of the contractions is extremely elevated (which produces a pressure greater than 180 mm Hg) and sometimes prolonged in duration. Manometric studies are needed to confirm the diagnosis.

Treatment of esophageal reflux primarily involves lifestyle modifications, such as placing 6-inch blocks under the head of the bed, avoiding esophageal irritants, not eating for 3 hours before bed, and avoiding drugs that decrease the lower esophageal sphincter pressure. If such changes are unsuccessful, beginning pharmacologic therapy to decrease acid production with H_2 antagonists, augmenting lower esophageal pressure with metoclopromide, or improving gastric mucosal protection with sucralfate (Carafate) may be done. Patients with severe esophageal spasm or nutcracker esophagus respond to nitrates or calcium channel blockers. Some physicians have had success using various anticholinergics or tranquilizers in more difficult patients.

Esophagitis is inflammation of the esophagus and is usually caused by chronic reflux of acidic gastric contents. Patients with this condition usually have a history of frequent or severe heartburn. Esophagitis has some unique complications, including distal esophageal strictures and esophageal bleeding. Treatment of esophagitis is identical to the treatment previously discussed for esophageal reflux. Esophagitis caused by fungus (*Candida* organisms) is being seen often in HIV-positive patients and needs to be considered in any such patient with dysphagia or suspected esophageal pain.

An *esophageal perforation* may be spontaneous or iatrogenic. Patients who vomit blood, have a history of esophageal foreign bodies, or complain of severe chest pain after vomiting should be suspected of having an esophageal perforation. Boerhaave syndrome involves spontaneous esophageal rupture after forceful vomiting, followed by severe epigastric and retrosternal chest pain. An esophageal rupture may also be seen after severe coughing, weight lifting, auto accidents, or straining. The patient usually appears critically ill and may be in shock from the complicating mediastinitis. A diagnosis may be suggested by mediastinal or cervical emphysema. A left pleural effusion or pneumothorax is present in 80% to 90% of these patients on the chest x-ray study. A Gastrografin study or endoscopy may be done to confirm the diagnosis, and the chance of survival is proportional to the time between the perforation and operative repair.

ABDOMINAL PAIN OF GASTRIC/DUODENAL ORIGIN

Pain of gastric or duodenal origin accounts for approximately 10% of the cases of abdominal pain, with peptic ulcer disease (PUD) account-

able for the majority of these cases. Approximately 10% of all Americans will have peptic ulcer disease sometime in their life. Nonsteroidal antiinflammatory agents are well known for causing gastric inflammation and are the single most common types of drugs responsible for PUD. When found in the mucous gel layer *Helicobacter pylori* (previously called *Campylobacter pylori*) may also potentiate gastric ulcer formation. Smoking has been shown to increase the risk of ulcer formation and slows the rate of healing.

The pain in PUD is typically described as an "ache" or "burning"; rarely is it colicky in nature. Of most importance is the time of onset and the relieving factors. Gastritis pain is more often worsened shortly after eating, whereas patients with duodenal ulcer pain tend to have pain relieved by eating. Most patients with gastric or duodenal ulcers experience some pain relief with antacids.

Treatment of PUD begins by removing any of the previously mentioned offending agents. Agents that protect the mucosa include antacids, sucralfate, and bismuth-containing compounds (e.g., Pepto-Bismol). When used with antibiotics they are the only agents proven to decrease recurrence rates when no maintenance therapy is used. The H_2-receptor antagonists are another line of therapy often used and include cimetidine (Tagamet), ranitidine (Zantac), famotidine (Pepcid), and nizatidine (Axid). Omeprazole (Prilosec) is a H^+/K^+ adenosinetriphosphatase (ATPase) inhibitor and has been found to quickly relieve symptoms and speed healing of peptic ulcers when compared to H_2 antagonists; however, it is only approved for short-term use.

Ulcer perforation is a life-threatening complication of PUD and typically is manifested as a sudden, severe abdominal pain. The pain tends to be severe and boring and is often accompanied by abdominal rigidity. Fifty percent of the patients have associated vomiting. Any type of movement typically causes the patient severe pain, and rebound tenderness is present. A chest x-ray study and abdominal supine and upright x-ray studies may reveal free air under the hemidiaphragm in 50% to 80% of these patients. The definitive management of an acute perforation involves surgical repair, but a nasogastric tube should be placed immediately to evacuate the stomach, and antibiotics should be started immediately.

GASTROINTESTINAL BLEEDING

UGI bleeding has some unique features in terms of diagnosis and management (see also Chapter 13). Lesions proximal to the ligament of Treitz usually result in hematemesis and nasogastric aspirates that are positive for blood. Bright red hematemesis indicates little or no contact with gastric juices as a result of an active bleeding site at or above the cardia. Coffee-ground aspirate indicates gastric juice contact with the blood. Melena indicates a blood loss in excess of 50 ml/day. Common causes of UGI bleeding include duodenal or gastric ulcers, gastritis, esophageal varices, a Mallory-Weiss tears, esophagitis, and duodenitis.

In children, the cause of UGI bleeding is age specific. In premature infants, necrotizing enterocolitis (NEC) and swallowed maternal blood are causative. In the older child, PUD, gastritis, and esophagitis are common causes of UGI bleeding.

The rate of duration of UGI bleeding determines how the patient will come to the emergency department. If the patient is hypotensive, at least a 30% blood volume loss (approximately 2000 ml in an adult) has occurred and necessitates immediate blood product replacement in addition to IV crystalloid. Two large-bore peripheral IVs should be placed, and a nasograstic aspirate should be examined to determine if ongoing active UGI bleeding is present. There is no evidence that an iced saline lavage is of any benefit in stopping UGI bleeding.

An endoscopy needs to be performed to definitively identify the source of bleeding and, in the case of variceal bleeding, may be used to administer sclerotherapy. On admission the hematocrit and hemoglobin are often normal in face of acute GI blood loss and cannot be used early in the course of bleeding to determine the degree of blood loss. Hematochezia present from a UGI source reflects a massive GI bleed.

When transfusions are deemed necessary, packed red blood cells (RBCs) are the blood products of choice. Fresh frozen plasma and platelets should be given if the patient requires more than one circulatory volume of transfusions (ten or more units) or if there is a known clotting deficiency or thrombocytopenia.

Variceal bleeding as a result of portal hypertension has a notoriously high associated mortality rate (15% to 40%). As many as 60% of these patients will be dead within 1 to 5 years. IV vasopressin (.25 to .50 units/minute) has been the standard medical therapy in the United States. If the blood pressure is stable, nitroglycerin is sometimes used in conjunction with vasopressin to decrease the cardiovascular side effects.

FOREIGN BODIES

The ingestion of foreign bodies occurs in all age groups. Because of their inquisitiveness, children, usually between the age of 8 months and 3 years, commonly swallow foreign bodies. In adults it is more common for a large bolus of food (usually inadequately chewed meat) to become lodged in the esophagus. The five areas of physiologic narrowing are found at the cricopharyngeal muscle, the carina, the aortic arch, the Schatzki ring, and the cardioesophageal junction. Most episodes of obstruction occur proximally at the cricopharyngeal muscle, which may compress the trachea and cause respiratory distress. In "cafe coronary" a bolus of meat impacts at the cricopharyngeus, causing respiratory distress that may be misinterpreted as an acute myocardial infarction. Once any foreign body passes into the stomach, it usually passes through the remainder of the GI tract without difficulty.

Symptoms of foreign body ingestion range from experiencing severe dysphagia/odynophagia and respiratory distress to being totally asymptomatic. Perforation of the esophagus is uncommon but must be considered when a sharp pointed object is swallowed or even when blunt foreign bodies are present for an extended period. Button batteries deserve special mention because they may cause local tissue damage and lead to perforation as a result of corrosiveness. They also contain a heavy metal, often mercury with an alkaline electrolyte, that may be released and cause an esophageal perforation. Diagnosis is primarily by history. In young children, poor feeding may be the only symptoms. The posteroarterior (PA) and lateral neck and chest x-ray studies are occasionally helpful. Coins positioned in a sagittal plane are lodged in the trachea, and those in a frontal plane are more commonly in the esophagus. A barium swallow is seldom necessary and usually considered undesirable by the endoscopist because the barium may obscure visualization of the foreign body when removal is attempted. The use of gastrografin is not advocated because it is hypertonic, and aspiration can cause serious pulmonary complications. A CT scan of the cervical esophagus (C_3 to T_1) has been shown to be helpful in identifying foreign bodies when conventional x-ray studies are negative (particularly when minimally calcified chicken or fish bones are present). Treatment for esophageal foreign bodies is often not required because most foreign bodies pass spontaneously into the stomach (70% of all rounded objects initially in the lower esophagus pass spontaneously, and some advocate a 8- to 12-hour observation period).

Early removal of the foreign body is recommended if the obstruction is in the upper esophagus or if a button battery or sharp, pointed object is involved. A meat bolus obstruction also is usually removed early because it may become soft and difficult to remove in one piece if left impacted for a prolonged period of time.

Endoscopy is the most commonly used method to remove foreign bodies, but nonendoscopic techniques have been used by many centers in removing round, radiopaque foreign bodies that are not lodged in the proximal esophagus. IV glucagon has been used with a success rate of 50% or less in food bolus impaction. Meat tenderizer should never be used as a treatment modality. Foley-catheter extraction has been advocated by some and has been found to be safe and effective if the obstruction is less than 24 hours old, is associated with no respiratory distress and has occurred in patients with no history of esophageal disease or surgery. Because with Foley-catheter extraction the operator does not grasp the foreign body, there is a chance that the object could be dropped into the hypopharynx and aspirated. With the availability of flexible endoscopy and the ability to perform the procedure with IV sedation, many experts feel it is the treatment of choice.

The indication for removal of foreign bodies in the stomach or proximal duodenum is a failure of the object to progress down the GI tract in 5 to 7 days, a risk of perforation, or a risk of absorbing a dangerously toxic substance. Certain sharp objects in asymptomatic patients can be managed conservatively with daily observation. Button batteries that pass the pylorus virtually always pass through the GI tract without complications. Daily x-ray studies are recommended to document progression if managed conservatively. Body packers who transport condoms or balloons filled with drugs such as cocaine present a special problem. Observation for spontaneous passage, endoscopy, and laparotomy have all been described in treating these patients. Care must be taken not to rupture the cocaine packets during removal, because GI absorption of significant amounts of cocaine can lead to dysrhythmias, seizures, or even death. Diets, stool softeners, and laxatives play no role in the management of foreign body passage in the GI tract.

▌▌▌▌▌▌▌KEY CONSIDERATIONS

WHAT IS THE LIFE THREAT?

The underlying causes of epigastric pain or vomiting may be life threatening (e.g., acute myocardial infarction or carbon monoxide poisoning). Protracted vomiting can lead to electrolyte imbalance, hypovolemia, or bleeding.

Upper gastrointestinal bleeding can be life threatening, especially when there is bleeding from esophageal varices.

DOES THE PATIENT NEED ADMISSION?

Patients with vomiting as a result of a severe life-threatening underlying condition should be admitted. Patients with ongoing gastrointestinal bleeding and vomiting that is uncontrollable with antiemetics also require admission. Patients whose vomiting interferes with their ability to take medications (e.g., antibiotics prescribed for pyelonephritis) also need admission.

WHAT IS THE MOST SERIOUS DIAGNOSIS?

Vomiting resulting from a cardiovascular or pulmonary cause and/or a severe intraabdominal emergency (e.g., a perforated ulcer or acute appendicitis) or severe gastrointestinal bleeding are the most serious diagnoses.

HAVE I PERFORMED A THOROUGH WORK-UP?

Distinguish symptoms of upper gastrointestinal origin from those of life-threatening cardiovascular and pulmonary origins (acute myocardial infarction, unstable angina, thoracic aortic dissection, and pulmonary embolism).

Recommended Reading

Barsan WG, Wolf LR: Upper gastrointestinal tract disorders. In Rosen P et al, editors: *Emergency medicine: concepts and clinical practice,* ed. 3, St Louis, 1992, Mosby.

Berggreen PJ et al: Techniques and complications of esophageal foreign body extraction in children and adults, *Gastrointest Endasc* 39:626-630, 1993.

Blair SR et al: Current management of esophageal impactions, *Chest* 104(4)1205-1209, 1992.

Brady PG: Esophageal foreign bodies, *Gastroenterol Clin North Am* 20(4):691-700, 1991.

Linnik W: Gastrointestinal emergencies. In Kravis T-C et al, editors: *Emergency medicine: a comprehensive review,* ed 3, New York, 1993, Raven Press.

Peterson WL, Laine L: Gastrointestinal bleeding. In Sleisenger M et al, editors: *Gastrointestinal disease,* ed 5, Philadelphia, 1993, WB Saunders.

Sung JYJ: Octreotide infusion or emergency sclerotherapy for variceal haemorrhagia, *Lancet* 342:637, 1993.

Ziller SA, Netchvolodoff CV: Uncomplicated peptic ulcer disease. *Postgrad Med* 93(4):126-138, 1993.

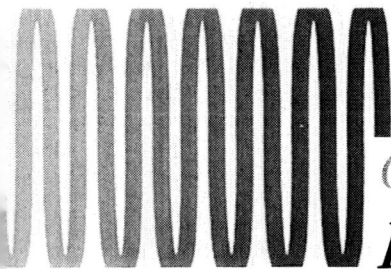

Chapter Forty-one

LOWER GASTROINTESTINAL TRACT DISORDERS

ROBERT A. BITTERMAN

Disorders of the lower gastrointestinal (GI) tract may manifest in the emergency department patient as signs and symptoms of primary GI disease, as well as systemic findings. These conditions are best approached from a symptomatic and anatomic perspective. Abdominal pain is covered in Chapter 12, acute gastroenteritis and diarrhea are discussed in Chapter 15, vomiting is discussed in Chapter 14, and GI bleeding is covered in Chapters 13 and 40.

INTESTINAL OBSTRUCTION

Mechanical small bowel obstruction may arise outside of the bowel, within its walls, or within its lumen. Obstruction distends the abdomen and retards absorption of intraluminal fluid. Lesions extrinsic to the bowel (most commonly postoperative adhesions and hernias) account for most pathologic findings (Table 41-1).

Lesions Responsible for Small and Large Bowel Obstruction

Intussusception and congenital lesions of the bowel wall are common causes of small bowel obstruction in children. Stenosis and atresia are present in 1 out of every 2700 live births and may occur throughout the GI tract. Meconium ileus occurs in 10% of all children born with cystic fibrosis. Postoperative adhesions, hernias, and neoplasms are the most common causes of small bowel obstruction in adults.

A common cause of colonic obstruction is carcinoma of the colon or rectum (usually initially in the left colon). Diverticulitis, either acute or chronic, may also produce obstruction, volvulus, and fecal impaction (Table 41-2).

Patients typically develop a gradual pattern of pain with accompanying vomiting and abdominal distension. Vital signs reflect volume status and bowel function. Many patients delay treatment for several days because of the insidious onset of symptoms. The hallmark of small bowel obstruction is intermittent, severe, colicky pain that occurs at regular intervals. With high obstruction, pain is perceived primarily in the upper abdomen, and cramps occur every 3 to 5 minutes. Pain from low ileal obstructions commonly is referred to the umbilical region; cramps occur less often. Vomiting is more common with high obstruction; a low obstruction may involve a 24- to 48-hour delay in vomiting. Abdominal bowel sounds are initially exaggerated, with a crescendo-decrescendo high-pitched sound dur-

Table **41-1**

LESIONS RESPONSIBLE FOR SMALL BOWEL OBSTRUCTION

Origin Within Bowel Lumen	Origin Within Bowel Wall	Origin Extrinsic to Bowel Wall
Congenital diaphragms	Stenosis	Adhesions
Tumor	Atresia	Surgical
Polyps	Strictures	Inflammatory
Meckel diverticulum	Crohn disease	Congenital
Carcinoma	Radiation	Crohn disease
Intussusception	Chemical	Diverticulitis
Gallstones	Anastomotic	Hernias
Bezoars	Traumatic	Inguinal
Feces	Endometriosis	Femoral
Meconium	Carcinoma	Umbilical
Intestinal parasites		Incisional
Foreign body		Internal
Enteroliths		Masses
		Tumor
		Abscess
		Hematoma
		Anomalous vessel
		Volvulus

ing peristalsis, but progressive distension may inhibit intestinal mobility. With total obstruction, obstipation may develop. Strangulation may occur. An incarcerated inguinal hernia is usually associated with a groin lump that becomes painful and tender.

Colonic obstruction is usually less severe than small bowel obstruction. Distension and vomiting are similarly less common. Feculent vomiting may occur.

Consider intestinal obstruction in any patient with abdominal pain, vomiting, and prior abdominal surgery. Laboratory evaluations will note hypokalemia and hypochloremia that reflect fluid shifts and extraintestinal loss. Alkalemia from ongoing vomiting, elevated anion-gap acidemia, and evidence of dehydration may be present. Abdominal radiographic findings that establish the diagnosis of small bowel obstruction include the following:

- Dilated loops of small bowel
- Air-fluid levels on upright or decubitus x-ray films
- Linear streaks of gas (stacked coins)
- String of beads

Moderate-to-severe gaseous distension of the transverse loops of the small bowel with little or no colon air and air-fluid levels on upright and decubitus views is typical of colonic obstruction. Colon gas is distinguished from gas in the small bowel by its peripheral location and the presence of haustrations, which are spaced further apart than the valvulae and do not involve the entire transverse diameter of the bowel.

Strangulation is a difficult radiographic diagnosis, but several plain x-ray film findings may suggest vascular compromise:

- Coffee bean sign, representing a single gas-distended loop whose lumen is separated by a broad dense band of edematous bowel

Table 41-2

CAUSES OF MECHANICAL COLONIC OBSTRUCTION

Disease	Features	Age (yrs)	Approximate Frequency
Major Causes			
Carcinoma of the colon	Change in bowel habits, rectal bleeding	>40	60%-65%
Volvulus	Institutionalized patient, psychoneurologic disorders	Any, but usually >75	10%-15%
Sigmoid diverticulitis	Repeated attacks of left lower quadrant pain	50	10%-15%
Less Common Causes			
Intussusception	Acute paroxysmal abdominal pain with rectal bleeding	2	Common in infants, rare in adults
Ischemic colitis	Stenosis from previous ischemic episode	50	Rare
Radiation colitis	Irradiation years ago	Any	Rare
Inflammatory bowel disease	Repeated attacks, toxic megacolon	20-40	Rare
Fecal impaction	History of severe, chronic constipation	Any	Occasional

- Pseudotumor, representing a closed loop whose lumen is filled with fluid
- Fixation of the loop in three views

Small bowel contrast studies may be of considerable diagnostic value. In general, perform the sigmoidoscopic examination, which may delineate mass lesions and mucosal abnormalities, before the barium enema. The latter contrast study may define further pathologic conditions.

Differential considerations must include other causes of adynamic ileus from extraperitoneal and intraperitoneal lesions, including appendicitis, pancreatitis, perforated ulcer, mesenteric ischemia, metabolic abnormalities (hypokalemia, diabetic ketoacidosis, uremia), systemic infections such as pneumonia, or acute myocardial infarction.

Fluid resuscitation should reflect deficits and electrolyte abnormalities. A nasogastric tube should be inserted. A surgical consultation is required, often on an emergent basis. Preoperatively, the administration of antibiotics is usually indicated.

APPENDICITIS

The appendix is a hollow muscular tube that arises from the apex of the cecum and is closed distally. Its cecal base is richly endowed with lymphoid tissue. Inflammation of the appendix commonly results from lumen obstruction with secondary bacterial invasion. The resultant distension causes edema and pain and, if undiagnosed, eventually leads to gangrenous appendicitis and perforation.

Appendicitis affects all age groups, with the highest incidence in the second and third decades of life. Although often difficult, diagnosis in the young and elderly presents a particular challenge. In children under 4 and in the elderly, rates of perforation exceed 50%; 94% of children under 2 years old are not diagnosed until perforation has occurred.

Classically, patients with appendicitis have a low-grade fever and loss of appetite. Symptoms quickly progress to include pain, vomiting, and changes in bowel habits. The cramping abdominal pain is initially in the area of the umbilicus, but over the ensuing 4 to 12 hours, the pain shifts to the right lower quadrant. Intensity peaks over the McBurney point, which is located 1½ to 2 inches from the iliac crest and along a line drawn between the iliac crest and the umbilicus. Children and the elderly are more apt to have only diffuse pain. With a retrocecal appendix or a gravid uterus, pain may be felt solely in the flank. A retroileal appendix may irritate the ureter and cause testicular pain, whereas suprapubic pain may occur when a pelvic appendix irritates the bladder. An inflamed appendiceal tip that reaches the right or left lower quadrant may cause pain in these areas initially or after localization. Most often the pain starts in one location and moves elsewhere.

Clinical signs and symptoms depend on the degree of inflammation and whether perforation has occurred. Localized deep tenderness to gentle abdominal palpation is common. The abdomen has diminished bowel sounds and associated tenderness, rebound, and guarding in the right lower quadrant. With perforation, more generalized peritoneal signs are present. A rectal examination may demonstrate tenderness (greatest on the right). The psoas sign, in which extending the right thigh while lying on the left side produces pain, indicates peritoneal irritation or pelvic inflammation. Pain with the obturator sign, which involves flexing the right thigh and internally rotating it while in a supine position, is consistent with pelvic inflammation. Cervical tenderness with motion may be present.

Complications of appendicitis include peritonitis and its incumbent problems: intraabdominal or pelvic abscess, ileus, or obstruction; pyelophlebitis; sepsis; and shock.

Diagnostic tests may suggest appendicitis. White blood cell counts over 15,000/mm³ occur in 40% of all patients, with 93% having a shift to the left. The percentage of neutrophils is >50% in children 1 to 5 years of age, >65% in those 5 to 10 years, and >75% in 10- to 15-year-olds. A urinalysis may differentiate appendicitis from a urinary tract infection. A serum pregnancy test is appropriate in women of childbearing age. Other laboratory tests may be useful as indicated.

A barium enema that fills an appendix is good evidence against appendicitis. A barium enema that does not fill the appendix or extravasation of barium from the appendix is suggestive of appendicitis.

Differential considerations may include a host of infectious, traumatic, and other conditions (Table 41-3).

Management should include initial hydration followed by early surgery. Antibiotic treatment is indicated before surgery and following exploration.

MESENTERIC VASCULAR OCCLUSION

The superior mesenteric artery and its extensive collaterals provide vascular supply from the ligament of Treitz to the midtransverse colon. Intestinal ischemia may be caused by a reduction in splanchnic blood flow as a result of local or systemic factors and mesenteric vasoconstriction. Interstitial fluid accumulates within 30 minutes of sudden vascular occlusion, followed by infarction and sloughing of the mucosal villi

Table 41-3

RIGHT LOWER QUADRANT PAIN: DIFFERENTIAL CONSIDERATIONS

	Infectious	Trauma	Congenital	Other
Systemic	Influenza	Black widow spider		Functional Diabetic ketoacidosis Porphyria, acute
Skin	Herpes zoster Cellulitis			
Abdominal wall		Contusion Muscle strain	Inguinal hernia	
Pulmonary	Pneumonia			
Gastrointestinal	Mesenteric adenitis Gastroenteritis Appendicitis Peritonitis	Impacted feces	Intussusception Obstruction Meckel diverticulum	Mesenteric infarct/ischemia Regional enteritis Ulcerative colitis
Gynecologic	Salpingitis		Ruptured ovarian cyst	
	Pelvic abscess			
Spine	Osteomyelitis			

over the next 30 minutes. Subsequent third-space accumulation leads to substantial fluid shifts; ischemia allows bacterial invasion and toxin production. Death from hypovolemia and sepsis may ensue.

Major arterial or venous occlusion can compromise the intestinal vasculature. A multifactorial syndrome of ischemia accounts for 30% to 50% of all cases of compromise.

Clinically, abdominal pain occurs in 75% to 90% of patients, the rapidity of which reflects the underlying pathophysiology of the ischemia. An incomplete occlusion may have preceding intermittent pain, vomiting, and diarrhea. Occult blood in diarrheal stool is common; gross rectal bleeding is occasionally the primary manifestation in patients without pain. Patients may exhibit mild diffuse or right lower quadrant tenderness that progresses to peritoneal findings. Cyanosis and mottling of the flanks may occur

with advanced disease, similar to hemorrhagic pancreatitis or a ruptured abdominal aneurysm. Circulatory instability may develop.

Laboratory findings are consistent with ischemia, fluid shifts, and blood loss. A significant base deficit without significant hypotension or peripheral hypoperfusion may be a helpful finding early in the disease. A radiologic evaluation may be useful for excluding other processes. Findings consistent with intestinal infarction include mucosal changes, bowel wall thickening, and gas in the bowel wall or portal venous system. Angiography establishes the diagnosis.

REGIONAL ENTERITIS

Regional enteritis, or Crohn disease, produces an inflammation of all layers of the intestine, which leads to a thickened, stenotic bowel.

Mononuclear infiltration produces granulomas, which leads to a matting of bowel loops with fibrotic bands that predispose the bowels to obstruction.

Variable clinical manifestations reflect the site of bowel involvement and disease progression. Differentiating initial right lower pain and tenderness from acute appendicitis may be difficult. Patients develop vomiting and a protracted course of diarrhea, crampy abdominal pain, fever, weakness, and weight loss with intermittent exacerbations. Obstruction, perirectal and enterovesical fistulas, and fistulas that end blindly in intraperitoneal or retroperitoneal abscess cavities are common complications. Occult and visible lower GI bleeding is common.

Extraintestinal manifestations are common. Those directly attributable to small bowel involvement include carbohydrate, fat, and vitamin B_{12} malabsorption; gallstones; and kidney stones. Arthritis occurs in as many as 23% of all patients; large joints are primarily affected. Cutaneous involvement (erythema nodosum and pyoderma gangrenosum are most common), recurrent uveitis, aphthous stomatitis, iritis, episcleritis, and conjunctivitis may be present. Perianal fissures and fistulae are common.

The diagnosis of regional enteritis is based on the presence of occult blood, fecal leukocytes, bacterial or parasitic infection, and an elevated white blood cell count (WBC) and sedimentation rate. Radiologic contrast studies, endoscopy, and a histologic examination are diagnostic.

Focus therapy on support, analgesia, and antidiarrheal agents. Antiinflammatory agents may be useful in ongoing management.

ULCERATIVE COLITIS

Primarily involving the mucosa and submucosa, ulcerative colitis is a chronic inflammatory and ulcerative disease of the colon and rectum. Disease severity increases as it progresses distally, with ultimate rectosigmoid colon involvement in most cases.

Presentation covers a spectrum of severity. Most patients have mild disease associated with less than four bowel movements per day and no systemic findings. More frequent stooling with significant anemia, fever, weight loss, and extraintestinal findings occurs with severe illness. Patients have exacerbations with complete remission between attacks.

Toxic megacolon may result from involvement of all colonic layers, with distension leading to perforation, peritonitis, and septicemia. Patients have toxic conditions and hypovolemia. Extraintestinal problems include arthritis, ankylosing spondylitis, episcleritis, posterior uveitis, and erythema nodosum. Liver disease may occur, including pericholangitis, chronic active hepatitis, fatty liver, or cirrhosis. Carcinoma of the colon may develop.

Examine the stool for ova and parasites, and culture blood and mucus. An endoscopy with rectal biopsy differentiates the entity from infectious colitis. Supplement supportive treatment by administering antidiarrheal agents, steroids, antiinflammatory agents, and antibiotics and by correcting fluid and electrolyte abnormalities. Surgical intervention may be indicated if acute attacks do not respond to medical intervention in 24 to 48 hours.

HERNIA

In a hernia, the intestines protrude into an abnormal location. Normally hernias are asymptomatic, but they may incarcerate or become irreducible. The incarcerated hernia cannot be returned to its normal position by manipulation and ultimately requires surgical intervention. Incarceration is most likely to occur in association with a small defect. Vascular compromise may strangulate the hernia.

A direct inguinal hernia occurs with protrusion through the Hesselbach triangle, which is bounded by the inguinal ligament, inferior epigastric vessels, and rectus abdominis muscle. Indirect inguinal hernias go through the inguinal canal and occur lateral to the inferior epigastric vessels. Femoral, umbilical, and other sites of hernias are common.

Treatment must reflect the presence of incarceration, strangulation, or other signs of decompensation.

STRUCTURAL COLON DISORDERS

Intussusception

The proximal bowel may invaginate into the distal bowel, which results in intussusception with infarction and gangrene of the inner bowel. Intussusception commonly occurs in children under 1 year of age but may occur in older patients if associated with a definable pathologic lead point. Lead points in older children include Meckel diverticulum, polyps, duplication, lymphoma, Henoch-Schönlein purpura, and those resulting from surgery. In 90% of adults a local lesion is responsible, with an overall malignancy rate of 42%.

Classically, patients have acute, intermittent episodes of sudden intense pain, with screaming and flexion of the legs. Episodes occur every 5 to 20 minutes. Vomiting, often bilious, is common and accompanied by the passage of blood and mucus ("currant jelly stool") via the rectum. This classic triad is actually present in less than half of patients, and the currant jelly stool is usually a late finding.

The abdomen is often distended and swollen, with a palpable mass in the right iliac fossa. Peristaltic waves may be present. Mental status may be altered and marked by lethargy, behavioral changes, irritability, somnolence, and listlessness that may precede abdominal findings. Occasionally, perforation of bowel with peritonitis, sepsis, and shock may develop.

Abdominal x-ray films are positive in 35% to 40% of patients and demonstrate the following:
- Decreased bowel gas and fecal material in the right colon
- An abdominal mass

- The apex of the intussusception outlined by gas
- Small bowel distension and air-fluid levels caused by mechanical obstruction

A barium enema may be both diagnostic and therapeutic, with a 75% success rate, particularly in younger children when seen in the first 14 to 24 hours. A barium enema is contraindicated in the hemodynamically unstable patient and in those in whom perforation is suspected. Involve a surgeon early in the decision-making process. If the barium enema is unsuccessful, surgery is indicated. Adults and children over 4 years of age commonly need surgery because of the high incidence of pathologic lead points.

Volvulus

Volvulus is a closed-loop obstruction with massive distension that results from the twisting of a section of the intestine on its own axis. Rotation occurs at the movable segment of the bowel, which in the colon is at the sigmoid and cecum.

Sigmoid volvulus occurs in patients who have severe psychologic or neurologic disease and, as well as in the elderly. Patients have a history of severe, chronic constipation, intermittent cramping, lower abdominal pain, and progressive abdominal distension with tympany. Fluid and electrolyte abnormalities may develop.

Plain radiologic films of the abdomen normally demonstrate a dilated single loop of colon in the lower half of the abdomen. Although generally not necessary, a barium enema shows a pathogenic twisted "bird's beak" or "ace of spades" deformity.

Treat nonstrangulated sigmoid volvulus with decompression and detorsion, using a rectal tube via the sigmoidoscope. Otherwise, surgery is necessary.

Cecal volvulus is common in 25- to 35-year-olds; chronic constipation is not an underlying factor. Cecal volvulus occurs with hypofixation of the cecum, a proximal ascending colon, and terminal ileum to the posterior abdominal wall. The incidence of previous surgery is relatively high. It is possible that the surgery disturbs normal fixation.

Patients have evidence of small bowel obstruction and severe, colicky abdominal pain associated with nausea, vomiting, and distension. An abdominal radiograph usually demonstrates an ovoid dilated segment of colon in the midabdomen, with distended small bowel loops and a relatively empty distal large bowel.

Immediate surgical consultation is indicated.

DISORDERS OF COLONIC MOTILITY

Hirschsprung Disease

Congenital megacolon, or Hirschsprung disease, results from congenital aganglionosis of the distal colon and rectum, which prevents effective peristalsis through the aganglionic segment.

Symptoms may begin at birth, with neonates failing to pass meconium in the first 24 hours of life. Constipation usually does not occur until 2 to 3 weeks of age. Bowel obstruction is usually present, with a distended, tympanitic abdomen; hyperactive or high-pitched bowel sounds; and a history of vomiting. A rectal examination reveals an absence of stool in the ampulla, often followed by evacuation of gas and liquid stool after the examiner withdraws his or her finger. Patients may develop acute necrotizing enterocolitis, malnutrition and failure to thrive, and septicemia.

Abdominal x-ray films may show distended and gas-filled proximal segments. A barium enema demonstrates a normal diameter in the aganglionic segment and a dilated proximal segment that tapers at the rectosigmoid. After defining the dilated segment, completing the study is not necessary and may in fact may be dangerous. A postevacuation film 12 to 48 hours later shows residual barium. Ideally, perform a rectal biopsy in the stable patient with an uncertain diagnosis, often following an equivocal barium enema.

Sample the tissue proximal to the anorectal junction, 2 to 3 cm above the rectal columns. Examine both the mucosal and muscular layers, and determine the acetylcholinesterase (AChE) level. Manometry may be helpful.

Stabilization and decompression are essential. Surgery remains the definitive therapy if the biopsy shows no ganglion cells and if AChE activity is high. Acute decompression with a loop colostomy may be required.

Diverticular Disease

Diverticulosis results from an increase in tone of the muscle layers of the bowel wall that causes these areas (particularly the taeniae coli) to shorten. Diverticula, which are saclike protrusions of the colonic mucosa through the muscularis, are most common in the sigmoid colon, and their incidence increases with age.

Although often asymptomatic, diverticulosis may become symptomatic, with a heightened response to stimuli. Patients may develop recurrent and colicky left lower quadrant pain (often after a meal), which is relieved by defecation or the passage of flatus. The tender, freely mobile, ropelike sigmoid is often palpable; signs of peritoneal inflammation are absent. A barium enema makes the diagnosis. Local application of heat or anticholinergics may relieve the pain and accompanying muscle spasm. Sedatives and a high-fiber diet may be useful.

Diverticulitis results from inflammation of the diverticula and is usually caused by mechanical obstruction with sequestered fecal matter in the diverticular sac. The inflammation may vary from a small intramural or periocolic abscess to generalized peritonitis. Pain is the predominant finding, with a varying severity that worsens during defecation. Anorexia, nausea, altered bowel habits, tenderness, and peritoneal irritation are common. A tender mass may be palpable. Complications include perforation, obstruction, and fistula formation.

With both diverticulosis and diverticulitis, radiologic studies may be diagnostic but sometimes raise the suspicion of carcinoma. Colonoscopy or a CT scan may be useful. Treatment includes bowel rest, fluids, antibiotics, and treatment of any complications. Because bleeding may complicate diverticulosis and develop into massive and life-threatening blood loss with rectal bleeding, vascular stabilization is essential.

ANORECTAL DISEASE

The rectum serves as the terminal portion of the colon. It is separated from the anus by the dentate line, which is the point of transition from the squamous epithelium of the anus to the columnar epithelium of the rectum. Vascular supply is via the superior, middle, and inferior hemorrhoidal arteries. The pupendal nerve cutaneously innervates the anus, which is sensitive to pain. The rectum receives sensation from parasympathetic fibers and is relatively insensitive to pain.

Three primary muscles control defecation. The external sphincter is striated muscle and is under voluntary control. This muscle prevents defecation when the urge is present. The internal sphincter consists of circular smooth muscle and involuntarily prevents stool from entering the anus and emptying the rectal ampulla. The puborectalis muscle reflexively initiates defecation after rectal dilatation and the expulsive process.

In addition to a physical examination, evaluation of the anorectum may include anoscopy and sigmoidoscopy.

Hemorrhoids

Hemorrhoids represent dilated venules and varicosities of the hemorrhoidal venous plexus. External hemorrhoids originate below the pectinate line and are covered by skin, whereas internal hemorrhoids are above the pectinate line and are covered by mucosa.

External hemorrhoids are painless unless associated with thrombosis, infection, or severe inflammation. Bleeding is typically not prominent. On physical examination, one or more dark blue nodules are covered with skin at the external anal orifice. Treatment is symptomatic with topical and later systemic analgesia/antiinflammatory agents. With severe pain that is secondary to thrombosis, the thrombosis may be excised.

Internal hemorrhoids may lead to acute thrombosis, prolapse, ulceration, and bleeding. Rectal examination reveals a tender mass with prolapse on straining. Permanent prolapse makes it difficult to differentiate internal hemorrhoids from acute external thrombosed hemorrhoids. Painless, bright red rectal bleeding is common and is often associated with defecation. Treatment of nonthrombosed internal hemorrhoids is symptomatic with gentle manual reduction.

Anal Fissure

A tear in the squamous epithelium–lined anal canal may cause severe pain that lasts for hours. Sphincter spasm and pain may lead to constipation. Symptomatic relief consists of sitz baths, the addition of bran to the diet, and hydrocortisone ointments.

Anorectal Infections

A perianal abscess produces erythema, tenderness, and fluctuation. Patients with a perianal abscess should be treated with early incision and drainage. An ischiorectal abscess produces greater toxicity, with fever and throbbing deep pain of the buttocks. The buttocks may be asymmetric. Submucosal, supralevator, and pilonidal abscesses may be present. Incision and drainage followed by sitz baths are appropriate.

Infections may relate to sexual activity. The gay bowel syndrome includes anorectal gonorrhea, herpes, chlamydia, syphilis, and amebiasis. Gonococcal disease may be asymptomatic in homosexual patients. The primary chancre of syphilis may be seen early in the course of the disease. *Chlamydia trachomatis* causes lymphogranuloma venereum (LGV), which manifests as a papule or rectal discharge, usually with massive inguinal adenopathy. Condyloma acuminatum may cause bleeding, itching, and irritation.

Rectal Prolapse

This problem may involve prolapse of the rectal mucosa alone or of all layers of the mucosa, or it may involve intussusception of the upper rectum into the lower rectum. The most common type of prolapse in younger patients is believed to be caused by a congenital absence of the mesentery and may not appear until the third decade of life.

Most episodes may be reduced manually, although sometimes analgesia and sedation are required. Surgical intervention may be needed, particularly if vascular compromise is present.

Fecal Impaction

Feces in the rectum and colon may become hard, dry, and immovable. Such patients may develop diarrhea, obstipation, or persistent rectal urgency. Diarrhea is a common symptom because only liquid stool can pass around the relative obstruction. In children this condition may cause encopresis. Management may include a number of modalities, including disimpaction, enemas, and oral laxatives.

Foreign Body

A wide range of objects may be present in the rectum. Diagnosis is primarily historical. Causes of rectal foreign bodies include autoeroticism, diagnostic or therapeutic instrumentation, criminal assault, or self-administered treatment. The location and type of foreign body determines treatment. Manual removal may be attempted transanally and is sometimes assisted by sedation and local anesthesia. Sharp objects present unique dangers. Glass may be removed by bimanual rectal and abdominal manipulation, obstetric forceps, tonsil snares, "super glue," and other methods. After extraction of the object, close observation, often supplemented by sigmoidoscopy to assess mucosal integrity, is required.

Neoplasm

Common neoplasms of the anorectum include adenocarcinoma, basal cell carcinoma, epidermal carcinoma, and malignant melanoma. Evaluate the patient's history of bleeding, change in stool character, weight loss, abdominal pain, or suspicious lesions.

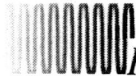

KEY CONSIDERATIONS

WHAT IS THE LIFE THREAT?

Small bowel obstruction, bowel ischemia, acute appendicitis, a strangulated hernia, and acute volvulus can be life threatening.

DOES THE PATIENT NEED ADMISSION?

Abdominal pain caused by a potentially life-threatening process in the lower gastrointestinal tract requires surgical consultation and admission.

WHAT IS THE MOST SERIOUS DIAGNOSIS?

Mesenteric infarction, volvulus, appendicitis, and a perforated viscus are the most serious diagnoses.

HAVE I PERFORMED A THOROUGH WORK-UP?

Perform a history and physical examination. Search for the most serious causes of lower gastrointestinal dysfunction and abdominal pain, especially in cases in which immediate surgery will be required.

Recommended Reading

Bitterman RA: Colon disorders. In Rosen P et al, editors: *Emergency medicine: concepts and clinical practice,* ed 3, St Louis, 1992, Mosby.

Kiernan CJ, Cales RH: Acute abdominal disorders, *Emerg Med Clin North Am* 7 (3), 1989.

Sawyers JL, Williams LF: The acute abdomen, *Surg Clin North Am* 68 (2), 1988.

Taylor MB: *Gastrointestinal emergencies,* 1992, Baltimore, Williams & Wilkins.

Wong RD: Gastrointestinal emergencies, *Med Clin North Am* 77 (5), 1993.

Chapter Forty-two

DISORDERS OF THE LIVER, BILIARY TRACT, AND PANCREAS

DAVID A. GUSS

HEPATIC DISORDERS

The liver weighs an average of 1500 gm in the adult and is one of the largest organs in the body. It receives approximately 30% of the resting cardiac output via the hepatic artery and portal vein. Disorders of the liver are common and can be quite varied. Because of the wide array of essential metabolic functions, the clinical manifestations of liver dysfunction can be highly variable.

Hepatitis

Hepatitis is a generic term referring to inflammation of the liver. It can be a consequence of infection with a number of different viruses, bacteria, fungi, or parasites; a result of toxin exposure; or secondary to immune-related diseases.

Many viruses have been associated with liver injury, but the most often incriminated include the hepatitis A virus, hepatitis B virus, hepatitis C virus, hepatitis D virus (also called delta hepatitis), non-A and non-B hepatitis virus, or hepatitis E virus. Other important causes in the United States include herpes simplex 1 and 2, cytomegalovirus, and the Epstein-Barr virus.

The hepatitis A virus (HAV) is an RNA virus and is most commonly spread by the fecal-oral route, either directly or secondary to ingestion of contaminated foodstuffs. It is the most common of the viral causes of hepatitis and has a typical incubation period of 15 to 45 days. The severity of clinical expression increases with age but is rarely associated with death and is never associated with chronic infectivity. Clinically occult or anicteric disease is common in children. A diagnosis is made by measuring the amount of IgM antibody to HAV, whereas a prior infection is identified by the IgG antibody. In the United States, approximately 50% of all adults are seropositive for the antibody for HAV; in other regions, the number of seropositive adults approaches 100%. Infection is associated with a very brief viremic phase and a more prolonged period of fecal shedding that begins as many as 2 weeks before symptom onset and wanes shortly after jaundice appears.

Hepatitis B (HBV) virus is a DNA virus that is spread via parenteral means or as a result of intimate personal contact. Blood transfusion is a historically important means of transmission that has been largely eliminated as a result of routine donors screening. The incubation period for hepatitis B is 60 to 90 days, but serologic evidence of infection can emerge within 1 to 3 weeks of infection. The clinical illness is variable but generally more severe than with HAV and is associated with a chronic carrier state in 10% of all adults. Diagnosis of acute infection is made by measurement of the IgM antibody to the hepatitis B core antigen. A variety of markers of HBV infection are available that relate to prior infection, ongoing infection, and relative infectivity (Table 42-1). Chronic infection with HBV is associated with a variety of illnesses, including hepatocellular cancer and periarteritis nodosa. Chronic carriers pose a potential risk to health care workers, but this risk

can be largely obviated by preexposure immunization. The risk of sexual transmission has resulted in the recommendation by the American College of Pediatrics for general HBV immunization during childhood.

The hepatitis C virus (HCV) is an RNA virus that spreads principally via parenteral means. It is the primary cause of transfusion-associated hepatitis, but only approximately 10% of all patients infected with HCV report a history of prior blood transfusion or parenteral exposure. There is a relatively new serologic test for HCV, but there may be a 6- to 12-month delay in developing the antibodies after infection. As a result, screening donated blood does not completely

Table 42-1

SEROLOGIC MARKERS IN HEPATITIS

Serologic Marker	Abbreviation	Interpretation
Antibody to HAV	Anti-HAV	A combination of IgG/IgM antibody that defines infection with HAV, acute or past
IgM antibody to HAV	Anti-HAV IgM	Antibody to HAV, indicating acute infection
Hepatitis B surface antigen	HBsAg	Surface antigen associated with acute or chronic HBV infection
Hepatitis B e antigen	HBeAg	Antigen associated with active infection, acute or chronic; indicative of high infectivity
Antibody to hepatitis B surface antigen	HBsAb	Antibody indicative of acute or past infection or immunization
Antibody to hepatitis B core antigen	HBcAb	A combination of IgG/IgM antibody that defines infection with HBV, acute or past
IgM antibody to hepatitis B core antigen	HBcAb-IgM	Antibody to B core antigen, indicating acute infection with HBV
Antibody to hepatitis B e antigen	HBeAb	Antibody to e antigen; may represent resolving HBV infection and decreased infectivity
Antibody to HCV	Anti-HCV	A new antibody that defines infection with HCV, acute or past
Antibody to HDV	Anti-HDV	Antibody that defines infection with HDV; HBsAg should be present

eliminate the transfusion risk associated with this virus. The incubation period for HCV infection is between 20 and 90 days. Fulminant disease is uncommon, whereas chronic hepatitis occurs in approximately 50% of the patients. Approximately 20% of the patients in this group develop cirrhosis within 10 years. Health care workers are at risk of parenteral exposure to chronically infected patients, but the magnitude of risk compared to HBV is unknown. Presently there is no immunization for HCV and no documented evidence to support postexposure treatment with γ-globulin.

The hepatitis D virus (HDV), or delta hepatitis, is a defective RNA virus that was discovered in 1977 by investigators working on liver specimens from patients with chronic HBV infection. Because this virus cannot produce its own envelope, it can only infect patients, with the HBV virus, which simultaneously produces hepatitis B surface antigen (HBsAg). The incidence of HDV in the United States is between 4% and 30% of all patients with chronic HBV infection. It is likely that many cases of HDV infection are misdiagnosed as acute or reactivated HBV infection. HDV is spread in a manner similar to HBV; HDV infection can occur concurrent with or subsequent to an HBV infection. In cases of coinfection there is evidence to suggest that HDV carries an increased risk of a more aggressive disease course. HDV infection can be prevented through immunization with an HBV vaccine.

The hepatitis E virus (HEV) is an RNA virus responsible for the hepatitis that is commonly encountered in parts of the former Soviet Union and Asia. It is not an important pathogen in the United States. It is spread through the fecal-oral route and has an incubation period and clinical course similar to HAV infection.

The pathogenesis of viral hepatitis is not completely understood. With a possible exception of HDV infection, it appears that the clinical illness is more likely a manifestation of an immune response to infection rather than a di-

rect cytopathic effect of the virus itself (Figure 42-1).

The clinical presentation of viral hepatitis is highly variable and generally not related to the inciting agent. The protean nature of the symptoms and the common occurrence of anicteric disease can result in misdiagnosis. The most common symptoms are fever, malaise, anorexia, nausea, vomiting, diarrhea, and abdominal discomfort. Often the first symptom that leads to physician consultation is scleral icterus or jaundice. HBV infection may be associated with a prodrome characterized by a rash that may be urticarial or macular, as well as by arthralgia or arthritis. Fulminant hepatitis, which is characterized by a progression over a period of days to hepatic failure and is associated with coagulopathy and encephalopathy, can develop in association with any of the hepatitis viruses. However it appears more commonly with HBV or HDV infection.

Physical manifestations of hepatitis include fever, scleral icterus, jaundice, and an enlarged and tender liver; gray or acholic stools are rarely identified. Diagnosis is supported by elevated liver transaminases, aspartate transaminase (AST or SGOT) and alanine transaminase (ALT or SGPT). Transaminases are typically 10 times normal, with ALT > AST. Hyperbilirubinemia is common but variable, is generally 5 to 10 mg/dl, and does not emerge until several days after the onset of symptoms. Alkaline phosphatase and lactic dehydrogenase are also elevated but rarely more than two to three times normal. Prothrombin time (PT) or the International Normalized Ratio (INR) are good measures of hepatic synthetic function. A prolonged PT may be an early sign of a complicated course or emerging hepatic failure. A definitive and viral-specific diagnosis is made by serologic means (see Table 42-1).

The protean nature of symptoms raises a broad differential diagnosis, but the presence of elevated liver transaminases tends to focus the considerations. Beyond the viruses mentioned,

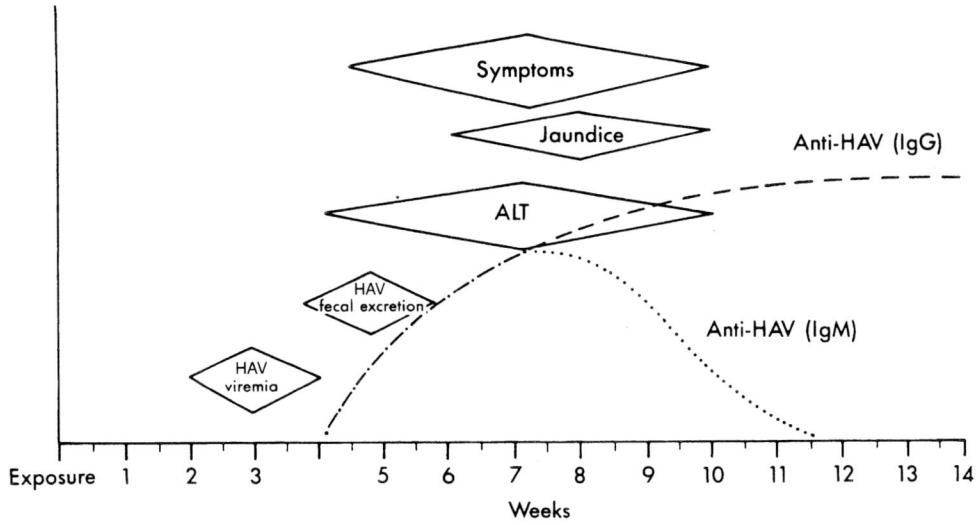

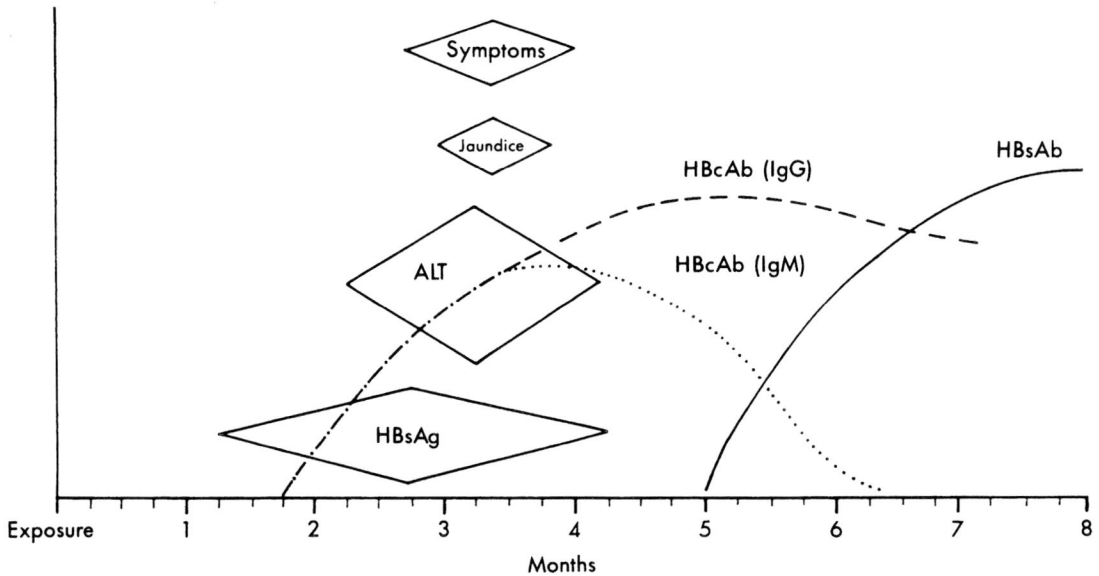

Fig. 42-1 Acute HBV infection. (From Guss DA: Disorders of the liver, biliary tract, and pancreas. In Rosen P, et al, editors: *Emergency medicine: Concepts and Clinical practice,* ed 3, St Louis, 1992, Mosby.)

other infectious causes of hepatic injury need to be considered. In most bacterial, fungal, or even mycobacterial infections, transaminase elevation is generally less dramatic. Toxin- or drug-induced hepatitis can be more difficult to eliminate on the basis of a laboratory profile, which necessitates greater reliance on exposure history, toxicology screening, and serologic testing. Obstructive etiologies are often suspected by the marked elevation of bilirubin relative to transaminase, the lack of hepatic enlargement, and the common lack of constitutional symptoms. Imaging with ultrasonography or CT scans is useful.

The management of patients with hepatitis is supportive. In most cases no specific therapy is required, whereas in other cases fluid and electrolyte replacement may be required. Antiemetics may allow restoration of oral intake and obviate the need for admission. Hospitalization is reserved for patients who have evidence of impending hepatic failure, a PT >5 seconds prolonged, encephalopathy, marked fluid and electrolyte imbalances, or unsuitable living arrangements. The emergency physician generally assumes responsibility for reporting cases of viral hepatitis to local health authorities and for making arrangements for immunoprophylaxis for family members or close personal contacts (Table 42-2).

Drug-Induced Liver Disease

Injury to the liver can occur as a result of a variety of commonly used medications or uncommonly encountered toxins. Hepatic injury may be secondary to direct cellular toxicity from the principal agent or its metabolite or as a consequence of a hypersensitivity or allergic reaction. For reasons that are not entirely understood, the incidence of drug-related liver injury appears to increase with age. This phenomenon is best exemplified by agents such as acetaminophen and isoniazid.

Many drugs cause injury only when taken in excess (acetaminophen), whereas others can induce damage with relatively small or therapeutic doses (isoniazid, halothane). A list of drugs commonly associated with hepatic injury, as well as the presumed mechanism, is found in Table 42-3.

The clinical presentation of drug-induced liver disease is highly variable and often offers little to distinguish it from other causes of hepatic injury. Patients may be entirely asymptomatic or display varying degrees of nausea, vomiting, abdominal pain, weakness, fatigue, and even fever. Transaminase levels are usually moderately elevated, but in cases of cholestatic presentation, the predominant abnormality may be hyperbilirubinemia. The presence of a rash or eosinophilia might provide clues for a chlorpromazine- or halothane-induced injury. Most often, the key to timely diagnosis lies in identifying a suspect drug in the medical history and in eliminating other concerns, either through serologic testing or hepatic imaging.

The emphasis in the management of the patient with drug-induced liver disease lies with eliminating the inciting agent and providing general supportive measures as outlined under viral hepatitis. A specific intervention is available in the case of acetaminophen overdose but is only effective if administered soon after ingestion and generally before the onset of detectable liver damage.

Alcoholic Liver Disease

Although ethanol and its metabolites are toxic to most organ systems, the liver is the organ most sensitive to these toxins and is thereby most often damaged. It is estimated that there are 10 million alcoholics in the United States; alcoholic liver disease ranks as the fourth leading cause of death in men between the ages of 25 and 64. Cirrhosis, most often a consequence of chronic alcohol ingestion, ranks as the ninth most common cause of death overall.

The pathogenesis of alcoholic liver disease is probably multifactorial and related to the accumulation of toxic metabolites (e.g., acetalde-

Table 42-2

POSTEXPOSURE HEPATITIS PROPHYLAXIS

Hepatitis A

Nature of Exposure	Recommended Treatment
Close personal contact	Immune serum globulin (ISG)—0.02 ml/kg IM
Day care center	
Employee	ISG—0.02 ml/kg IM
Attendee	ISG—0.02 ml/kg IM
School contacts	None
Hospital contacts	None
Workplace contacts	None
Foodborne source	
Within 2 weeks of exposure	ISG—0.02 ml/kg IM
After 2 weeks from exposure	None
After common source outbreaks have begun to occur	None

Hepatitis B

Nature of Exposure	Source	Recommended Treatment	
		Unvaccinated individual	**Vaccinated individual**
Percutaneous/mucosal	HBsAG positive	1. HBIG[*] 2. HB vaccine[†]	1. Test HBsAb; if negative, then HBIG and HB vaccine
	Known Source High risk for HBsAg positive	1. HB vaccine 2. Test source; if positive then HBIG	1. Test HBsAb; if negative and source is HBsAg positive, then HBIG and HB vaccine
	Low risk for HBsAg positive	1. HB vaccine	1. None
	Unknown Source	1. HB vaccine	1. None
Intimate sexual	HBsAg positive	1. HBIG 2. HB vaccine[‡]	1. None
Household/workplace	HBsAg positive	1. None	1. None
Perinatal	HBsAg positive	1. HBIG[§] 2. HB vaccine	NA

Modified from MMWR 39(RR-2), Feb 1990.

[*]HBIG—Hepatitis B immunoglobulin, dose 0.06 ml/kg IM.

[†]HB vaccine—Hepatitis B vaccine. Adequate vaccination requires three injections; therefore all patients should be referred for follow-up.

[‡]Vaccine required only if repeated sexual contacts are likely to occur over an extended period of time and the source becomes a chronic carrier.

[§]Dose of HBIG 0.5 ml/kg

Table 42-3

COMMON AGENTS INVOLVED IN HEPATIC INJURY

Agent	Injury Pattern
Acetaminophen	Cytotoxic
Amiodarone	Cytotoxic
Amphotericin	Cytotoxic
Anabolic steroids	Cholestatic/venoocclusive
Azathioprine	Cytotoxic/cholestatic/venoocclusive
Carbamazepine	Cytotoxic/cholestatic
Chlorpromazine	Cholestatic
Cisplatin	Cytotoxic
Contraceptive steroids	Cholestatic/hepatic vein thrombosis
Cyclophosphamide	Cytotoxic
Erythromycin estolate	Cholestatic
Gold salts	Cytotoxic/cholestatic
Haloperidol	Cholestatic
Isoniazid	Cytotoxic
Ketoconazole	Cytotoxic
Lovastatin	Cytotoxic
Methotrexate	Cytotoxic
Methoxyflurane	Cytotoxic
Methyldopa	Cytotoxic
Phenobarbital	Cholestatic
Phenytoin	Cytotoxic
Quinidine	Cytotoxic
Tetracycline	Cytotoxic/fatty infiltration
Salicylate	Cytotoxic
Valproic acid	Cytotoxic
Verapamil	Cholestatic

hyde), excessive production of nicotinamide adenine dinucleotide (NADH) leading to steatosis, induction of hepatic microsomal enzymes, alteration of immune function, and malnutrition. Although the risk of alcohol induced liver damage correlates to the quantity of alcohol ingested, susceptibility is genetically related.

Hepatic enlargement secondary to chronic alcohol ingestion is generally secondary to fatty infiltration. Hepatitic enlargement is often a benign disorder and can be reversible with the cessation of ethanol consumption. Alcoholic hepatitis is a potentially more severe disorder and a common cause of visits to the emergency department. It can occur after a single bout of heavy ingestion, or it may fail to appear despite excessive chronic consumption.

Clinical manifestations of alcoholic liver disease range from mild anorexia to severe abdominal pain, nausea, vomiting, diarrhea, and fever. The liver may be enlarged from coexistent steatosis, or it may be small secondary to underlying cirrhosis. Variable degrees of jaundice may be noted and may be either secondary to acute injury or a consequence of underlying cirrhotic changes. Differentiation from viral hepatitis may be difficult on the basis of clinical features alone. The presence of only a mild elevation of liver transaminases and the predominance of AST relative to ALT support a diagnosis of an alcohol-related process.

Management is supportive, with attention given to coexistent alcohol-related problems such as vitamin deficiencies, withdrawal syndrome, and gastric or pancreatic disorders. The severity of disease is highly variable; acute or first episodes can be fatal, but this consequence is rare. Guidelines for patient admission and the assessment of severity are similar to those for viral hepatitis.

Cirrhosis

Cirrhosis describes the end stage of chronic liver disease of any cause. It is characterized by the destruction of hepatocytes and the deposition of fibrous tissue with an attendant loss of normal hepatic architecture. The clinical manifestations are related to a loss of normal hepatic metabolic and synthetic function and to impaired portal blood flow. Symptoms include fatigue, anorexia, weight loss, gastrointestinal (GI) bleeding, and an altered mental status. Physical examination may reveal muscular atrophy, thinning of the skin, spider angiomata, palmar erythema, Dupuytren contracture and, in men, gynecomastia or testicular atrophy. Ascites and peripheral edema are commonly present. Ascites may be severe enough to limit ambulation or impair ventilation. Caput medusae, a prominent venous pattern over the anterior abdominal wall, may be apparent, particularly in cases with portal hypertension. Laboratory tests are not specific. Liver transaminase and bilirubin may be mildly elevated; albumin is usually diminished, and coagulation tests are prolonged.

Management is usually directed toward the common complications of cirrhosis, including GI bleeding from gastric or esophageal varices, marked ascites, hepatic encephalopathy, spontaneous bacterial peritonitis, and hepatorenal syndrome. Any GI bleeding should be treated aggressively with fluid resuscitation, blood transfusion, and fresh frozen plasma as indicated. Early consultation with a gastroenterologist for diagnostic endoscopy and consideration of laser or sclerotherapy is recommended. Mild degrees of hepatic encephalopathy can be treated on an outpatient basis with a low-protein diet and lactulose. This disposition assumes that a stable home environment can be ensured and that underlying precipitants, such as infection and electrolyte disorder, can be eliminated.

Spontaneous bacterial peritonitis (SBP) should be considered in any patient with ascites and either fever, abdominal pain, or hepatic encephalopathy. Diagnosis requires paracentesis with a cell count, Gram stain, and culture of peritoneal fluid. An emergency department diagnosis is generally made on the basis of an ascitic fluid granulocyte count of more than 500 cells/mm^3.

Treatment of SBP requires intravenous antibiotics with agents that cover the most common organisms involved: *Escherichia coli, streptococcus* organisms, and *Klebsiella* organisms. Hepatorenal syndrome is generally a fatal complication despite aggressive inpatient management of fluid and electrolyte disorders.

Hepatic Abscess

The most common causes of a hepatic abscess are *E. coli; Klebsiella, Pseudomonas,* and *Enterococcus* organisms; various *Bacteroides* organisms; and *Entamoeba histolytica.* A pyogenic abscess is generally a consequence of an underlying biliary obstruction but may also be seen in association with diverticulitis, omphalitis, pancreatic abscess, appendicitis, inflammatory bowel disease, or bacteremia of any cause. An amebic liver abscess is most commonly a complication of an antecedent intestinal infection.

The clinical presentation of hepatic abscesses is usually acute, but chronic courses are occasionally encountered with amebic infections. Typical symptoms include a high fever, right upper quadrant abdominal pain, nausea, and vomiting. An amebic abscess may appear at the same time as symptomatic intestinal disease, particularly in children. Laboratory tests include leukocytosis, elevated alkaline phosphatase and bilirubin, and mild elevation of ALT and AST. Significant elevation of bilirubin supports a pyogenic etiology and should suggest a biliary tract obstuction. A chest x-ray study may reveal a right-sided pleural effusion, elevated hemidiaphragm, or atelectasis.

A diagnosis is made with the assistance of either abdominal ultrasonography or a CT scan. A blood culture may identify the organism in pyogenic disease, and occasionally in the case of amebic abscess, ameba can be identified in the stool. Serologic tests such as agar gel diffusion and counterimmune electrophoresis are positive in the majority of cases of amebic infection.

The treatment for a pyogenic abscess includes fluid resuscitation and initially a triple-antibiotic regimen with (1) an aminoglycoside or third-generation cephalosporin, (2) metronidazole or clindamycin, and (3) ampicillin. Metronidazole alone, 750 mg orally or intravenously three times daily for 7 days, is generally sufficient for amebic abscesses.

Liver Diseases Associated With Pregnancy

Three types of liver disease are associated with pregnancy: cholestatic disease, an acute fatty liver, and spontaneous rupture. Cholestatic disease is not rare and seems to have a familial association. Onset is in the third trimester and is heralded by the onset of pruritus. Alkaline phosphatase, 5'-nucleotidase, and bilirubin are elevated but generally not dramatically. For the mother, the disorder is principally a physical nuisance, but for the fetus the consequences may be more grave. Malabsorption of vitamin K may lead to coagulopathy in the fetus, which predisposes it to spontaneous intracranial hemorrhage. Treatment is supportive with subcutaneous vitamin K. The illness resolves spontaneously in the postpartum period.

Acute fatty liver of pregnancy is a more aggressive process that can rapidly progress to maternal and fetal demise. This disorder emerges in the later portion of the third trimester with symptoms of anorexia, nausea, vomiting, and abdominal pain. Jaundice and hepatic tenderness are usually present. Liver transaminases are elevated 5 to 10 times above normal, bilirubin is abnormal, and blood glucose is depressed. Laboratory or clinical evidence of disseminated intravascular coagulation may be present. Treatment includes aggressive fluid and electrolyte resuscitation, glucose administration, and early delivery. The disease generally remits without sequelae after delivery.

Fortunately, spontaneous rupture of the liver is a rare disorder, but it can be potentially devastating if unrecognized. The vast majority of cases occur with preeclampsia. Patients experience acute abdominal pain, hypotension, and shock. A CT scan is useful in diagnosis. A peritoneal tap with the identification of gross blood narrows the diagnosis to a spontaneous rupture of either the liver, spleen, or uterus. Management is fluid resuscitation and acute surgical intervention.

Hepatic Cancer

Hepatocellular carcinoma is the most common variety of primary hepatic malignancy. In some regions the incidence approaches 100 out of every malignancy. In some regions the incidence approaches 100 out of every 100,000 people, whereas in the United States it is approximately 5 out of every 100,000 people. Worldwide, approximately 75% to 90% of those cases are associated with chronic HBV infection. Other important risk factors appear to be chronic alcoholic liver disease, hemochromatosis, primary biliary cirrhosis, infection with *Schistosoma* or *Clonorchis* organisms, and exposure to estrogens, androgens, thoratrast, and vinyl chloride. In the United States, metastasis to the liver from distant sources is encountered more often than primary hepatic carcinoma.

The clinical presentation of hepatocellular carcinoma is highly variable and nonspecific. Common symptoms include anorexia, weight loss, nausea, vomiting, jaundice, and abdominal pain. A variety of laboratory abnormalities may be encountered, none of which are specific. Although α-fetoprotein is often elevated with hepatocellular carcinoma, it is neither specific nor of utility in the emergency setting. Imaging with ultrasonography, a CT scan, or magnetic resonance imaging can identify a tumor mass, but a biopsy is required for a definitive diagnosis.

Management is supportive with provision of adequate analgesia. If not previously accomplished, screening for HBV infection is recommended in cases of suspected hepatoma.

GALLBLADDER AND BILIARY TRACT DISORDERS

Cholelithiasis

Approximately 20% of all women and 8% of all men have gallstones at some point in their lives, which leads to approximately 500,000 operations annually in the United States. There are two principal varieties of gallstones: cholesterol and pigmented. Cholesterol stones are the most common and occur when bile is supersaturated with cholesterol or contains insufficient quantities of solubilizing lecithin and bile salts. Risk factors for stone formation include female gender, increasing age, obesity, rapid weight loss, parity, cystic fibrosis, the use of drugs such as clofibrate, oral contraceptive agents, and a genetic predisposition. Pigmented stones segregate into two varieties: (1) black stones seen in conjunction with diseases that cause intravascular hemolysis, and (2) brown stones seen in patients with a biliary tract infection.

Passing a stone into the cystic duct or common bile duct may result in biliary colic. The term *colic* can be misleading, because many patients report a steady rather than an intermittent or cramping pain. Although the discomfort is most commonly perceived in the right upper quadrant, it may be noted in a wide region of the abdomen. Radiation of pain, when present, most commonly travels to the base of the scapula or shoulder. Associated symptoms include nausea and vomiting, which may be severe enough to result in fluid or electrolyte abnormalities. Many patients with biliary colic provide a history of similar symptoms that are usually precipitated by eating. Examination may reveal an ill-appearing individual, particularly if there is significant vomiting. Tenderness without guarding or rebound in the right upper quadrant or epigastrium is common. Laboratory tests are generally normal, but measuring ALT, AST, bilirubin, and lipase is important to rule out associated pancreatitis or common duct obstruction. The diagnosis is confirmed by imaging the gallbladder using ultrasonography.

Treatment involves fluid and electrolyte replacement in addition to symptom relief. Nausea and vomiting are managed with antiemetics and, if necessary, nasogastric suctioning. Pain can be treated with anticholinergics such as glycopyrrolate or parenteral analgesics. Ketorolac, an injectable nonsteroidal antiinflammatory agent, appears to be a very effective alternative to opiate analgesics. Most patients resolve their symptoms after several hours. Patients with symptomatic gallstones should be referred for definitive therapy. Treatment alternatives presently include extracorporeal shock wave lithotripsy, chemical dissolution, or cholecystectomy.

Cholecystitis

Cholecystitis is an acute inflammation of the gallbladder and occurs most often in patients with underlying cholelithiasis. Approximately 5% of all cases occur in patients without evidence of gallstones. Obstruction of the cystic duct appears to be the primary factor in cholecystitis. This obstruction is usually a result of an impacted gallstone but may be secondary to tumors, lymphadenopathy, fibrosis, or parasites. Symptoms are similar to patients with biliary colic, but fever may also be noted; fever is not, however a requirement for the diagnosis. Examination reveals right upper quadrant tenderness, often with some guarding or rebound. Tenderness in the right upper quadrant that is elicited with palpation during deep inspiration is referred to as the *Murphy sign* and is characteristic of cholecystitis. Abnormal laboratory tests include leucocytosis and a mildly elevated AST, ALT, bilirubin, and alkaline phosphatase. All of these tests may be normal in acute cases.

Ultrasonography is the most useful test in the emergency setting. The absence of gallstones has a very high negative predictive value, whereas the identification of gallstones, a thickened gallbladder wall, and pericholecystic fluid has a positive predictive value of more than 90%. Nuclear scanning with technetium 99 m–labeled iminodiacetic acid (IDA) or diisopropyl IDA is the most sensitive test for the diagnosis of cholecystitis. Failure to outline the gallbladder with common and hepatic duct visualization confirms cystic duct obstruction and, in the appropriate clinic setting, establishes the diagnosis of cholecystitis. Conversely, visualization of the gallbladder has a negative predictive value of 98%.

Important diagnostic considerations in patients with cholecystitis include cholangitis, pancreatitis, and hepatic abscess. Hepatic imaging, as well as the elevation of bilirubin, amylase, or lipase, helps bring clarity to the differential.

Treatment is initially identical to cases of biliary colic with the addition of parenteral antibiotics and admission to the hospital. A second- or third-generation cephalosporin is usually sufficient. Patients with cholecystitis should eventually undergo a cholecystectomy, which can generally be accomplished several days after admission, when the acute inflammation has subsided.

Acute Cholangitis

Central to all cases of cholangitis is biliary tract obstruction. The most common cause of acute cholangitis is choledocholithiasis; other causes include pancreatic or cholangiocellular carcinoma, cancer of the ampulla of Vater, metastasis to the porta hepatis, pancreatitis, and stricture of the common bile duct. Cholangitis was first described in 1877 by Charcot, who described the classic triad of clinical findings: right upper quadrant pain, fever, and jaundice. Although these signs and symptoms are commonly encountered, they are not specific to this disorder and may be encountered in cases of cholecystitis and hepatitis. Patients with cholangitis typically appear toxic. Hypotension (secondary to septic shock) and mental obtundation may be present. These findings in conjunction with the Charcot triad form the Reynolds pentad.

Laboratory findings for acute cholangitis include elevated bilirubin, alkaline phosphates, AST, and ALT. Leucocytosis is typical, but leukopenia may also be encountered, particularly in patients with septic shock. Ultrasonography is the imaging technique of choice because it offers rapid availability, a relatively low cost, and high sensitivity and specificity for biliary tract obstruction. Although transhepatic cholangiography (THC) and endoscopic retrograde cholangiopancreatography (ERCP) are somewhat more difficult imaging techniques, they are very sensitive and can have therapeutic value by decompressing the biliary tree.

Treatment involves restoring perfusion with fluids and vasopressors. Antibiotics should be started immediately after blood cultures have been obtained. Antibiotic choices should cover the most commonly encountered pathogens; *E. coli* and *Klebsiella, Enterococcus,* and *Bacteroides* organisms. Patients failing to respond to medical therapy require decompression of the biliary tree, which can be accomplished with THC, ERCP, or surgery.

PANCREATIC DISEASE

Pancreatitis

The pancreas is a retroperitoneal organ that serves a variety of digestive and endocrine functions. Except for diabetes mellitus, pancreatitis is the most common malady associated with the pancreas. The incidence of pancreatitis is estimated as 1.5 cases for every 100,000 people, but the incidence can vary considerably depending on the population being studied.

The pathophysiology of pancreatitis is incompletely understood. It may be a result of one or more of the following: bile or duodenal reflux, bacterial infection, pancreatic enzyme activation before acinar secretion, and pancreatic ductal hypertension. The most common associations are gallstones and alcohol ingestion; other causes are listed in the box at right. A variety of drugs have been implicated in acute pancreatitis (see the box on p. 503). A recent and important addition to this list is the antiretroviral drug dideoxyinosine (ddI).

With pancreatitis, abdominal pain is usually located in the midepigastric region and is the most common clinical manifestation. The pain often radiates to the back and is accompanied by nausea and vomiting. The severity of the symptoms is variable but is most often characterized as severe. Patients may display a low-grade fever and generally have tachycardia and tachypnea secondary to pain and fluid depletion. A physical examination reveals tenderness and voluntary guarding in the midabdomen. Peritoneal signs are uncommon because of the retroperitoneal location of the pancreas. The presence of ecchymosis in the flanks (Grey Turner sign) or a bluish discoloration around the umbilicus (Cullen sign) is associated with hemorrhagic pancreatitis.

Serum amylase and lipase are the most useful

CAUSES OF ACUTE PANCREATITIS

Alcohol (ethanol, methanol)
Biliary tract disease
Drugs (see the box on p. 503)
Hypercalcemia
Hyperlipidemia
Idiopathic
Infectious Agents
   Mumps
   Coxsackie virus
   Hepatitis B
   Mycoplasma
   Legionella organisms
   Ascariasis
Pancreas divisum
Penetrating peptic ulcer
Postoperative
Postpancreatography
Pregnancy
Scorpion bites
Trauma
Tumor

diagnostic tests. The ready availability of lipase measurements coupled with the high degree of sensitivity and specificity of this test has largely supplanted the need for the determination of amylase clearance. Despite their utility in establishing a diagnosis, enzyme measurements are of limited utility in assessing the severity of pancreatic inflammation or attendant prognosis. There are a number of scoring systems for pancreatitis; Ransom's system is most often cited (see the box on p. 503). These parameters were originally developed as a prognostic guide for patients with alcoholic pancreatitis but have been modified for nonalcoholic etiologies as well. The presence of fewer than three signs is associated with a mortality of 1%; three or four signs, 15%; five or six signs, 40%; and seven or more signs, 100%.

DRUG-INDUCED PANCREATITIS

Definite	Probable	Possible
Azathioprine	Acetaminophen	Bumetanide
Cisplatin	Cimetidine	Carbamazepine
L-asparaginase	Estrogens	Chlorthalidone
Furosemide	Indomethacin	Clonidine
Tetracycline	Mefenamic acid	Colchicine
Thiazides	Opiates	Corticosteroids
Sulfonamides	Phenformin	Co-trimoxazole
ddI	Valproic acid	Cyclosporine
		Cytarabine
		Diaxozide
		Enalapril
		Ergotamine
		Ethacrynic acid
		Isoniazid
		Isotretinoin
		Methyldopa
		Metronidazole
		Nitrofurantoin
		Pentamidine
		Piroxicam
		Procainamide
		Rifampicin
		Salicylates
		Sulindac

PROGNOSTIC SIGNS IN ACUTE PANCREATITIS

At admission	Within 48 hours
Age >55	Hematocrit fall >10%
WBC >16,000/mm^3	BUN rise more than 5 mg/dL
Blood glucose >200 mg%	Serum calcium <8 mg%
Serum LDH >350 IU/L	Arterial PO_2 <60 mm Hg
Serum AST >250 U/L	Base deficit >4 meq/L
	Fluid sequestration >6 L

Modified from Ransom JHC: Etiological and prognostic factors in human acute pancreatitis: a review, *Am J Gastroenterol* 77:663, 1982.

A variety of imaging techniques have been used with patients with presumed pancreatitis but gain their utility principally in the search for an alternative diagnosis or complication. Plain abdominal x-ray films may reveal a localized ileus in acute disease or pancreatic calcification in chronic pancreatitis. Ultrasonography is most useful in searching for gallstones as a potential cause of inflammation or for identifying a pseudocyst. A CT scan can visualize the pancreas directly and detect a peripancreatic spread of inflammation, hemorrhage, phlegmon, pseudocyst, or abscess formation.

Management is directed toward correcting fluid and electrolyte disorders and putting the pancreas at rest; the latter requires a cessation of oral intake. All patients with pancreatitis should be admitted to the hospital until there is clinical and laboratory evidence of resolving inflammation. A common fallacy is to attempt outpatient management of those patients who have a perceived mild disease and can tolerate oral intake; this approach invites the risk of precipitating more severe illness. Nasogastric suction helps control vomiting and can decompress an ileus but has not been demonstrated to otherwise affect the course of pancreatitis. Parenteral analgesics are often required for pain management. Meperidine may offer some advantage over morphine because with meperidine, there is reportedly less associated spasm of the sphincter of Oddi.

Chronic pancreatitis results from repeated episodes of acute disease and is most often a complication of alcoholic pancreatitis. The clinical presentation can be similar to acute pancreatitis, but the patient rarely appears as ill as in acute pancreatitis. Isolated abdominal pain is the principal symptom. If there are no complicating features, patients with chronic pancreatitis can be treated as outpatients with a clear liquid diet, antiemetics, and analgesics. Administration of a pancreatic enzyme not only treats any exocrine deficiency, but may help lessen the pain.

Pseudocysts and Abscesses

Pseudocysts, as the name suggests, are not true cysts but are collections of pancreatic debris and secretion within a fibrous lining. Pseudocysts occur in approximately 10% of all patients with chronic pancreatitis and may also appear in acute disease. Many pseudocysts resorb spontaneously, whereas others can persist or grow and cause symptoms related to their size or to compression of surrounding structures. Complications include bowel obstruction, intracystic hemorrhage, infection, or erosion into vascular structures. Examination may reveal a palpable abdominal mass and tenderness. Amylase and lipase levels are normal or abnormal with approximately equal frequency. Diagnosis is confirmed by ultrasonography or a CT scan. An uncomplicated pseudocyst can be managed with observation, whereas symptomatic cases can be referred for percutaneous drainage. Infections or hemorrhages require admission for antibiotics and fluid resuscitation, respectively.

Abscesses can occur as result of a bacterial infection of necrotic tissue during an episode of acute pancreatitis or as a result of seeding of a pseudocyst. The presentation of an abscess is that of acute pancreatitis, with the addition of

Table 42-4

PANCREATIC ENDOCRINE TUMORS

Tumor	Clinical Manifestation
Insulinoma	Hypoglycemia
Glucagonoma	Rash, hyperglycemia, venous thrombosis
Gastrinoma	Peptic ulceration, diarrhea
VIPoma	Diarrhea, hypokalemia, acidosis, hypovolemia, flushing
Somatostatinoma	Hyperglycemia
Carcinoid	Flushing, diarrhea

persistent fever and abdominal pain or evidence of clinical deterioration several days or a week after the onset of the initial illness. Diagnosis is aided with ultrasonography or a CT scan. Treatment includes parenteral antibiotics and a percutaneous or open surgical drainage.

Pancreatic Cancer

Cancer of the pancreas is the fourth most common cause of cancer deaths in the United States. The incidence has increased steadily and has more than doubled in the last half century. Malignancies can be of an endocrine or nonendocrine variety. Ductal adenocarcinoma is the most common type of pancreatic cancer, with a 3-year survival rate of 2%. Risk factors for this type of cancer include tobacco smoking, diabetes mellitus, and high-fat and high-protein diets. The most common manifestation is weight loss and pain. Examination may reveal inanition, abdominal tenderness, hepatic enlargement, an abdominal mass, or jaundice. Diagnostic aids include imaging with a CT scan or ERCP. Emergency department management is usually limited to correcting fluid and electrolyte management and providing analgesics.

Although uncommon, the endocrine tumors are an interesting group of disorders by virtue of the clinical syndromes they can produce. The most common endocrine tumors and their associated symptom complexes are presented in Table 42-4.

KEY CONSIDERATIONS

WHAT IS THE LIFE THREAT?

Because adequate liver functioning is necessary to sustain life, any severe liver disorder, including hepatitis and cirrhosis, can be a threat to life. Bleeding from esophageal varices as a result of cirrhosis can be fatal. Spontaneous rupture of the liver associated with preeclampsia can be fatal. Acute cholecystitis and cholangitis can be life threatening, especially in patients with diabetes.

Pancreatitis has a high mortality, especially when associated with the signs identified in the text, including hyperglycemia, hypocalcemia, a falling hematocrit, and hypoxemia.

DOES THE PATIENT NEED ADMISSION?

The patient with hepatitis requires admission if there is evidence of impending hepatic failure, a prolonged protime or elevated INR, encephalopathy, marked fluid and electrolyte imbalances, or unsuitable living arrangements. Patients with cirrhosis require admission for bleeding from gastric or esophageal varices, severe hepatic encephalopathy, spontaneous bacterial peritonitis, hepatorenal syndrome, and clinical deterioration. The patient with severe pancreatitis requires admission, especially if three or more signs listed in the box on p. 503 are present.

WHAT IS THE MOST SERIOUS DIAGNOSIS?

Fulminant hepatitis, end stage liver disease with gastrointestinal bleeding, severe cholecystitis, or pancreatitis with the presence of three or more adverse prognostic signs are the most serious diagnoses.

HAVE I PERFORMED A THOROUGH WORK-UP?

Measure transaminase and coagulation parameters in patients with liver disease. Consider cholangitis in patients with fever, jaundice, and right upper quadrant pain. In cases of pancreatitis, measure amylase, lipase, white blood cell count, glucose, and liver enzymes.

Recommended Reading

Diehl AM: Alcoholic liver disease., *Med Clin North Am* 73(4):815, 1989.

Kadakia SC: Biliary tract emergencies: acute cholecystitis, acute cholangitis, and acute pancreatitis, *Med Clin North Am* 77(5):1015, 1993.

Rosen P et al: *Emergency medicine: concepts and clinical practice,* ed 3, St Louis, 1992, Mosby.

Rustgi AK, Richter JM: Pyogenic and amebic liver abscess, *Med Clin North Am* 73(4):847, 1989.

Wilcox CM, Dismukes WE: Spontaneous bacterial peritonitis: a review of pathogenesis, diagnosis and treatment, *Medicine* 66(6):447, 1987.

Chapter Forty-three

ACUTE GENITOURINARY DISORDERS

ANN L. HARWOOD-NUSS

GENERAL PRINCIPLES OF URINARY TRACT INFECTIONS

Urinary tract infections (UTIs) are a common problem and affect all age groups (Table 43-1). The term *UTI* encompasses a variety of clinical entities in which microorganisms invade a portion of the urinary tract. It is estimated that between 10% and 20% of all women will experience a UTI. After men reach the age of 50, the incidence increases with the onset of prostatic hypertrophy. A nosocomial UTI is the most common type of hospital-acquired infection and accounts for significant morbidity and mortality. To better understand UTIs, several terms have been defined in the box at right.

Predisposing Factors

Abnormalities of the urinary tract that interfere with its natural resistance to infection include obstructions, stasis of urine, foreign bodies (stone, catheter), reflux in children, and incomplete bladder emptying secondary to mechanical or neurogenic malfunction. Conditions known to be associated with an increased frequency of UTI include diabetes, sickle cell traits, and immuno-

compromise. Catheterization carries a small risk of infection to a patient; in pregnant or debilitated patients, the risk increases to between 10% and 15%.

Bacteriology

The vast majority of UTIs are caused by gram-negative aerobic bacilli. *Escherichia coli* is the dominant pathogen in more than 80% of the

---

TERMINOLOGY

Bacteriuria: the presence of bacteria in the urine
Low count infection: $<10^{2-4}$ bacteria/ml
Urinary tract infection: an infection caused by microorganisms in the urinary tract; the infection may be in the upper tract (kidney) or the lower tract (urethra or bladder)
Cystitis: UTI of the bladder
Pyelonephritis: UTI of the kidney
Complicated UTI: UTI associated with underlying neurologic, structural, or medical problems

---

Table **43-1**

PREVALENCE OF URINARY TRACT INFECTION ACCORDING TO AGE AND SEX

Age Group	Prevalence (%)	Approximate Sex Ratio (Male:Female)
Neonatal	1	1.5:1
Preschool age	1.5-3	1:10
School age	1.2	1:30
Reproductive age	2.5	1:50
Geriatric	10-30	1:1

From Fang L: Pharmacotherapy 2(2):91-99, 1982. Modified from Rubin RH: Infections of the urinary tract. In Rubinstein E, editor: *The Scientific American textbook of medicine,* New York, 1981, The Scientific American Illustrated Library.

UTIs in men and women, and *Staphylococcus saprophyticus* is a common cause of UTIs in young women. Other causes include *Streptococcus faecalis,* as well as *Proteus, Klebsiella,* and *Enterobacter* organisms.

Screening Tests and Urinalysis

The leukocyte esterase test correlates well with chamber counts and is specific for pyuria. The nitrite test detects bacteria in the urine, but is unreliable in UTIs caused by *Staphylococcus, Enterococcus,* and *Pseudomonas* organisms. These tests are limited in low-count UTIs. A urinalysis should be performed if the patient is symptomatic. In unstained, uncentrifuged urine specimens, one organism/oil immersion field indicates more than 10^6 organisms/ml. If the urine has been Gram stained and centrifuged, it is possible to detect 10^4 bacteria/ml. The identification of more than 10 bacteria/high-power field (HPF) correlates closely with a UTI. A Gram stain may be negative in a UTI caused by a low-count bacterial infection and, in many cases, *S. saprophyticus* and *Chlamydia* organisms. The presence of more than 10^2 bacteria/ml in a patient with dysuria is the best indicator of UTI.

Urine collection

If a UTI is suspected in neonates and young children, either a suprapubic aspirate or a urethral catheterization is the preferred method for collecting urine. In women, either a clean catch urine or a sterile catheterization should be used. In men, a voided urine is appropriate; it is *not* appropriate to catheterize a male patient simply to obtain a urine specimen.

Urine culture

Most patients do not need a urine culture (see the box on p. 509).

Urinary Tract Infections in High-Risk Patients

The majority of UTIs are simple, uncomplicated lower tract infections in otherwise healthy women. Treatment and disposition are altered in pregnancy, diabetes, and sickle cell anemia, as well as with indwelling catheters and immunocompromised hosts. Patients with diabetes are at risk for papillary necrosis, perinephric abscesses, and pyelonephritis (see the box on p. 509).

INDICATIONS FOR URINE CULTURE

Children
Adult males
Immunosuppressed patients
"Treatment failures" (recently completed
course of antibiotics with persistent urinary
symptoms)
Patients with symptoms in excess of 4 to 6
days
Elderly patients at risk for developing
bacteremia
Toxic-appearing patients with signs and
symptoms suggestive of pyelonephritis or
bacteremia
Pregnant women
Patients with known chronic or recurrent
renal infection
Patients with known anatomic urologic
abnormalities
Patients in whom urinary tract obstruction is
suspected (e.g., stones, BPH)
Patients with serious medical diseases,
including diabetes mellitus, sickle cell
anemia, cancer, or other debilitating
diseases
Patients with alcoholism, drug dependence
Recently hospitalized patients
Patients recently on antibiotics
Patients recently instrumented (e.g.,
cystoscopy, catheterization)

From Harwood-Nuss AL, Holland RW III: Genitourinary disease. In Rosen P et al, editors: *Emergency medicine: concepts and clinical practice,* ed 3, St Louis, 1992, Mosby.

RISK FACTORS FOR PATIENTS WITH UTI

The existence of any of the following factors
places the patient at risk for a possible
complicated UTI:
Urban emergency department
Lower socioeconomic status
Hospital-acquired infection
Indwelling catheter
Recent urinary tract instrumentation
Known urinary tract abnormality or stone
disease
Relapse after treatment for UTI
UTI before age 12
Pyelonephritis or more than three UTIs in past
year
Symptoms occurred more than 7 days before
treatment
Recent antibiotic use
Diabetes
Immunosuppression (renal failure, chronic
illness, drug or alcohol abuse, cancer,
elderly)
Pregnancy
Sickle cell anemia and trait

Modified from Johnson J, Stamm W: Urinary tract infections in women: diagnosis and treatment, *Ann Int Med* 111:906-917, 1989. From Harwood-Nuss AL, Holland RW III: Genitourinary disease. In Rosen P et al, editors: *Emergency medicine: concepts and clinical practice,* ed 3, St Louis, 1992, Mosby.

Indications for Emergency Imaging

Most patients with cystitis or pyelonephritis do not need emergency imaging (usually either an intravenous pyelogram (IVP) or ultrasonography). However, the patient with an unusually severe presentation, symptoms that suggest an obstruction, or a fever that persists more than 72 hours after treatment should probably undergo urgent imaging. A CT scan is the best single test for assessing the kidney, but it is usually reserved for difficult diagnostic cases.

SPECIFIC PATIENT GROUPS

Urinary Tract Infections in Women

In women, dysuria is a common complaint and most often a result of a bacterial UTI. The differ-

Table 43-2

TREATMENT REGIMENS FOR BACTERIAL URINARY TRACT INFECTION

Condition	Characteristic Pathogens	Mitigating Circumstances	Recommended Empirical Treatment*
Acute uncomplicated cystitis in women	E. coli, S. saprophyticus, Proteus mirabilis, Klebsiella pneumoniae	None	3-day regimens: oral trimethoprim-sulfamethoxazole, trimethoprim, norfloxacin, ciprofloxacin, ofloxacin, lomefloxacin, or enoxacin[†]
		Diabetes, symptoms for >7 days, recent urinary tract infection, use of diaphragm, age >65 yr	Consider 7-day regimen: oral trimethoprim-sulfamethoxazole, trimethoprim, norfloxacin, ciprofloxacin, ofloxacin, lomefloxacin or enoxacin[†]
		Pregnancy	Consider 7-day regimen: oral amoxicillin, macrocrystalline nitrofurantoin, cefpodoxime proxetil, or trimethoprim-sulfamethoxazole[†]
Acute uncomplicated pyelonephritis in women	E. coli, Proteus mirabilis, K. pneumoniae, S. saprophyticus	Mild-to-moderate illness, no nausea or vomiting—outpatient therapy	Oral[‡] trimethoprim-sulfamethoxazole, norfloxacin, ciprofloxacin, ofloxacin, lomefloxacin, or enoxacin for 10-14 days
		Severe illness or possible urosepsis—hospitalization required	Parenteral[§] trimethoprim-sulfamethoxazole, ceftriaxone, ciprofloxacin, ofloxacin, or gentamicin (with or without ampicillin) until fever gone; then oral[‡] trimethoprim-sulfamethoxazole, norfloxacin, ciprofloxacin, ofloxacin, lomefloxacin, or enoxacin for 14 days

Complicated urinary tract infection	*E. coli, Proteus* species, *Klebsiella* species, *Pseudomonas* species, *Serratia* species, enterococci, staphylococci	Pregnancy—hospitalization recommended	Parenteral§ ceftriaxone, gentamicin (with or without ampicillin), aztreonam or trimethoprim-sulfamethoxazole until fever gone; then oral‡ amoxicillin, a cephalosporin, or trimethoprim-sulfamethoxazole for 14 days
		Mild-to-moderate illness, no nausea or vomiting—outpatient therapy	Oral‡ norfloxacin, ciprofloxacin, ofloxacin, lomefloxacin, or enoxacin for 10-14 days
		Severe illness or possible urosepsis—hospitalization required	Parenteral§ ampicillin and gentamicin, ciprofloxacin, ofloxacin, ceftriaxone, aztreonam, ticarcillin-clavulanate, or imipenem-cilastatin until fever gone; then oral‡ trimethoprim-sulfamethoxazole, norfloxacin, ciprofloxacin, ofloxacin, lomefloxacin, or enoxacin for 14-21 days

From Stamm W, Hooton TM: Management of urinary tract infections in adults, *N Engl J Med* 329(18):1328-1334, 1993.

*Treatments listed are those to be prescribed before the etiologic agent is known (Gram's staining can be helpful); they can be modified once the agent has been identified. The recommendations are the authors' and are limited to drugs currently approved by the Food and Drug Administration, although not all the regimens listed are approved for these indications. Fluoroquinolones should not be used in pregnancy. Trimethoprim-sulfamethoxazole, although not approved for use in pregnancy, has been widely used. Gentamicin should be used with caution in pregnancy because of its possible toxicity to eighth-nerve development in the fetus.

†Multiday oral regimens for cystitis are as follows: trimethoprim-sulfamethoxazole, 160-800 mg every 12 hours; trimethoprim, 100 mg every 12 hours; norfloxacin, 400 mg every 12 hours; ciprofloxacin, 250 mg every 12 hours; ofloxacin, 200 mg every 12 hours; lomefloxacin, 400 mg every day; enoxacin, 400 mg every 12 hours; macrocrystalline nitrofurantoin, 100 mg four times a day; amoxicillin, 250 mg every 8 hours; and cefpodoxime proxetil, 100 mg every 12 hours.

‡Oral regimens for pyelonephritis and complicated urinary tract infection are as follows: trimethoprim-sulfamethoxazole, 160-800 mg every 12 hours; norfloxacin, 400 mg every 12 hours; ciprofloxacin, 500 mg every 12 hours; ofloxacin, 200-300 mg every 12 hours; lomefloxacin, 400 mg every day; enoxacin, 400 mg every 12 hours; amoxicillin, 500 mg every 8 hours; and cefpodoxime proxetil, 200 mg every 12 hours.

§Parenteral regimens are as follows: trimethoprim-sulfamethoxazole, 160-800 mg every 12 hours; ciprofloxacin, 200-400 mg every 12 hours; ofloxacin, 200-400 mg every 12 hours; gentamicin, 1 mg per kilogram of body weight every 8 hours; ceftriaxone, 1 to 2 g every day; ampicillin, 1 g every 6 hours; ticarcillin-clavulanate, 3.2 g every 8 hours; and aztreonam, 1 g every 8 to 12 hours; imipenem-cilastatin, 250-500 mg every 6 to 8 hours.

ential diagnosis includes urethritis, vaginitis, and noninflammatory dysuria (trauma, irritants).

Bacteriology

E. coli is the dominant pathogen, followed by *S. saprophyticus.*

Classification

UTIs may be categorized into 4 groups: acute uncomplicated cystitis, acute uncomplicated pyelonephritis, complicated UTI, and asymptomatic bacteriuria. Upper tract infections include pyelonephritis, and lower tract infections include urethritis and cystitis. Both upper and lower UTIs may have elevated ($>10^5$ bacteria/ml) or low ($<10^{2-4}$ bacteria/ml) bacterial counts on a urine culture.

Urethritis. Coliforms cause the majority of infections, but *Chlamydia* organisms may cause as many as 20% of the cases. Urethritis should be suspected in the patient who has multiple sexual partners or a recent change in sexual partners. A pelvic examination with appropriate cultures is indicated. Other causes of urethritis include herpes simplex virus, *Trichomonas* organisms, and gonorrhea. Treatment options for urethritis from *Chlamydia* organisms include doxycycline 100 mg bid × 7 days, azithromycin 1 gm po once, erythromycin 500 mg qid × 7 days (in pregnancy), or ofloxacin 300 mg bid × 7 days.

Acute bacterial cystitis. Dysuria, frequency, urgency, and suprapubic discomfort are associated with significant bacteriuria in most women. A short-course therapy (3 to 5 days) is appropriate. Treatment options are outlined in Table 43-2.

Acute pyelonephritis. Acute pyelonephritis may range from occult pyelonephritis to uncomplicated and complicated pyelonephritis. If the factors listed in the box on p. 509 are present, be cautious about both treatment and disposition. The nontoxic patient with uncomplicated pyelonephritis can either be discharged or undergo a period of observation and treatment in the emergency department. The patient should be instructed to return if fever or chills persist or if nausea or vomiting preclude taking antibiotics. Outpatient antibiotic therapy is listed in Table 43-2. Hospitalization is indicated in the presence of toxicity, a complicated UTI, an inability to take oral medications, an immunocompromised host, pregnancy, and urologic abnormalities. See Table 43-2 for therapeutic options.

UTI in pregnancy

During pregnancy, untreated bacteriuria is associated with increased prematurity and fetal wastage. Maternal complications include a 20% to 40% incidence of pyelonephritis. It is recommended that *asymptomatic bacteriuria* be treated with either ampicillin 500 mg qid × 7 to 10 days, nitrofurantoin 100 mg qid (avoid use in the third trimester), or cephalexin 500 mg qid. Short-course therapy is not appropriate. The antibiotics appropriate for cystitis are the same as those for asymptomatic bacteriuria. If pyelonephritis is present, the patient should be admitted for parenteral antibiotics; cefazolin 1 gm IV qid is the drug of choice; ciprofloxacin is not recommended for use in pregnancy. Avoid aminoglycosides unless sepsis is present. Catheterization should be avoided.

Catheter-associated urinary tract infection

A level of $>10^2$ organisms/ml is evidence of infection. Symptomatic episodes of infection should be treated with those antibiotics recommended for complicated UTI (see Table 43-2). Treating asymptomatic bacteriuria has little benefit.

Caveats

The box on p. 509 identifies a special group of patients for whom caution is urged regarding all facets of care, including disposition and treatment choices. Do not use short-course therapy on such groups.

Urinary Tract Infections in Children

A UTI in a child is a major cause of bacterial disease but is often overlooked because of nonspecific findings. Most UTIs are uncomplicated and responsive to therapy, but be aware of certain features that suggest an underlying disease of the urinary tract: palpable bladder, hypertension, abnormalities of electrolytes, acidosis, elevated blood urea nitrogen/creatinine, dribbling, poor urinary stream, and straining to void.

Clinical presentation

The clinical presentation of a UTI is age dependent. Neonates can have nonspecific signs and symptoms that predominate with fever, feeding difficulties, jaundice, hypothermia, vomiting, diarrhea, seizures, irritability, dribbling of urine, and failure to thrive. Infants (1 to 24 months) tend to have many of the same signs and symptoms previously listed in addition to offensive or cloudy urine, hematuria, frequent urination, and dysuria. Preschoolers (ages 2 to 6) have abdominal, flank, and suprapubic pain; frequency or urgency of urination; dysuria; fever; or enuresis.

Pathogenesis and bacteriology

Most UTIs are thought to be hematogenous in origin during the first 3 months of life. In older children a UTI develops via the ascending route, with *E. coli* and *Proteus* and *Staphylococcus* organisms being the most common pathogens. Underlying abnormalities are found in as many as 50% of those children with first infections (vesicoureteral reflux, reflux nephropathy, or obstructive lesions).

Urine collection and urinalysis

Obtain a urine collection and urinalysis through suprapubic aspiration (if <age 2 or there is a palpable bladder), catheterization, or midstream voiding. A urine culture should be performed on all children with a suspected UTI. The same criteria for the urinalysis in adults apply to children.

Disposition

Disposition depends on the age and condition of the child. Infants between ages 3 and 6

ANTIBIOTIC REGIMEN: UTIS IN CHILDREN

Oral antibiotics

Amoxicillin 50 mg/kg/day × 5-7 days
Augmentin 20 to 40 mg/kg/day × 5-7 days
Trimethoprim 6 to 12 mg/kg/day × 5-7 days
Sulfamethoxazole 30 to 60 mg/kg/day × 5 to 7 days (do not use in infants <2 months of age)

Intravenous antibiotics

Ampicillin 200 mg/kg/day
and
Gentamicin 2.5 mg/kg/day
or
Cefotaxime alone 100 mg/kg/day

---

months with any symptoms, as well as older children with a high fever, toxicity, or signs or symptoms of an upper UTI, are generally admitted for parenteral antibiotics (see the box above). Imaging to assess for underlying urologic abnormalities can be done on an inpatient basis. Children over 6 months of age who have a lower UTI can be treated as outpatients, with oral therapy for 5 to 7 days and follow-up 2 to 3 days after the initiation of therapy.

Caveats

The child with symptoms of a UTI but no bacteriuria may be a victim of sexual abuse. All children should be evaluated for an anatomic abnormality after the first UTI.

Urinary Tract Infections in Men

Cystitis or pyelonephritis

It is unusual for either cystitis or pyelonephritis to occur in a man with normal host defenses and anatomy. If a UTI is suspected, the physician should actively seek predisposing factors. Any UTIs in men should always be considered serious and complicated. The route of infection is ascending, the pathogens are identical to those seen in women, and the clinical presentation is similar. Gram-negative sepsis should be considered because few UTIs occur in men in the absence of underlying abnormalities. A urinary obstruction at the level of the prostate is common in older men and must be identified and treated if present. An IVP or ultrasonography is indicated if an obstruction (from calculi, stricture, or prostatic hypertrophy) is suspected. Catheterization for residual urine or bladder drainage is indicated if urinary retention is suspected. Catheterization for specimen collection is not indicated unless the patient is experiencing urinary retention. Urine cultures should be obtained on all men who have symptoms of UTI. Antibiotic therapy should be started (see Table 43-2), and a urologic consultation is warranted.

Urethritis

Urethritis may be classified as either gonococcal or nongonococcal urethritis. Gonococcal urethritis is caused by *Neisseria gonorrhoeae*. *Chlamydia trachomatis* is the major etiologic agent for nongonococcal urethritis in heterosexual men. The two pathogens coexist in as many as 30% to 50% of all cases, and both can produce symptomatic urethritis. Gonococcal urethritis is associated with urethral discharge and dysuria. Chlamydial urethritis may produce minimal symptoms and discharge. Urethral secretions should be examined after a Gram stain for gram-negative intracellular diplococci. New diagnostic tests for Chlamydial urethritis are available. The decision to treat urethritis is made on the basis of dysuria and urethral discharge. Urethritis can be treated with doxycycline 100 mg bid × 7 days or azithromycin 1 gm po once *and* ceftriaxone 125 mg IM once. Sexual partners must be treated or referred for treatment.

Acute bacterial prostatitis

Acute bacterial prostatitis is a bacterial infection caused most commonly by *E. coli;* other less

common pathogens include *Klebsiella, Enterobacter, Proteus,* and *Pseudomonas* organisms. Prostatitis is a febrile illness with chills, lower back and perineal pain, and malaise. Frequency and urgency of urination, dysuria, and varying degrees of difficulty in voiding are present. The prostate examination reveals a tender, swollen gland that is firm and warm to the touch. Avoid vigorous massage in the acutely infected prostate. A urine culture will reveal the responsible organism. Treatment includes trimethoprim-sulfamethoxazole (TMP-SMX DS) bid × 14 days, ampicillin 500 mg qid × 14 days, or ciprofloxacin 500 mg bid × 14 days. If the patient is toxic and has fever, chills, or urinary retention, hospitalization is warranted for parenteral therapy with gentamicin 3 to 5 gm/kg/day and ampicillin 2 gm IV qid. Urology should be consulted.

Epididymitis

Epididymitis is the most common type of intrascrotal inflammation and is a disease of young adults. In men over the age of 35, *E. coli* is the dominant pathogen, and underlying urologic abnormalities are often seen. In men under the age of 35, epididymitis is most often a result of the sexually transmitted organisms *Chlamydia* and *N. gonorrhea*. The onset of pain is usually gradual, and pain and swelling in the scrotum progress over the course of hours to days. Fever and toxicity may occur; urethral discharge and voiding symptoms may also be present. The white blood cell count (WBC) is often elevated in the range of 10,000-30,000/mm^3. The urinalysis may or may not demonstrate bacteria and leukocytes. Treatment is based on identifiable pathogens (gonococcus, coliforms) and age. In general, men over the age of 35 with a probable *E. coli* or *Pseudomonas* infection should be treated with TMP-SMX or ciprofloxacin. Sexually transmitted epididymitis is the most common cause of epididymitis in men under the age of 35 and should be treated with ceftriaxone 250 mg IM once or ciprofloxacin 500 mg once *and* doxycycline 100 mg bid × 10 days. Sexual partners should also be treated. Scrotal ultrasonography is indicated if the patient is not responsive to medical therapy or if an epididymal abscess is suspected. Supportive measures include bed rest, scrotal support, analgesics, and sitz baths. A urologic referral is indicated for all cases of epididymitis. Resolution of the process occurs within 2 weeks, but it may be at least a month before the epididymis returns to its normal size.

Orchitis

Orchitis is an acute infection of the testicle and most often is the result of direct extension from an infected epididymis (epididymoorchitis). The patient is acutely ill with fever, pain, and swelling of the scrotum. Viral orchitis is most often caused by mumps and is rarely seen before puberty. In viral orchitis, testicular pain and swelling begin 4 to 6 days after the onset of parotitis but may occur without parotid involvement. The clinical course varies, but resolution usually occurs in 4 to 5 days. Testicular atrophy occurs in 50% of the patients. Less often, orchitis may be a result of granulomatous disease or syphilis.

THE ACUTE SCROTAL MASS

Testicular Torsion

The onset of acute unilateral scrotal pain and swelling can present a significant diagnostic challenge. The most important process to consider is testicular torsion. Torsion can occur at any age but is most common between ages 12 and 18 years. Epididymitis and testicular torsion account for 60% to 75% of all causes of acute scrotal mass.

Pathophysiology

The essential process of torsion is that of testicular ischemia. The testis and cord twist within the tunica vaginalis testis and cause occlusion of the venous system; arterial flow is de-

creased. The degree of damage relates to the duration and extent of the vascular obstruction. The time limit for viability is not firmly established, but the standard gauge is that a testicular salvage rate of 100% is possible if surgical detorsion occurs within 6 hours.

Clinical presentation

Acute onset of testicular pain and swelling is typical. More than 50% of all patients with testicular torsion report previous episodes. Nausea and vomiting are common, but voiding symptoms are rare. The examination reveals a painful, shortened testicle with a horizontal line within the scrotum; enlargement and swelling are variable. Unfortunately, these classic findings are not always present. Nearly half of all cases of testicular torsion have significant pain and swelling that make an adequate examination difficult to perform (amorphous mass or "missed torsion"). A useful finding is the ipsilateral loss of the cremasteric reflex.

Differential diagnosis

In diagnosing testicular torsion, the following diagnoses should also be considered: epididymitis, orchitis, torsion of the appendices of the testis and epididymis, tumor, hernia, hydrocele, or hematocele. Epididymitis is the most common misdiagnosis but is rare before puberty, generally has a more gradual onset, and is usually associated with voiding symptoms or urethral discharge. Fever may be seen in both testicular torsion and epididymitis but is higher in epididymitis.

Evaluation

A rapid consideration for the diagnosis of torsion is possible on the basis of history and physical examination. Color Doppler ultrasonography and nuclear testicular scintigraphy are excellent diagnostic tools but are not required to make the diagnosis nor to initiate a request for emergency urologic consultation. Color-coded Doppler ultrasonography is the test of choice with an acute scrotal mass because it provides information about both anatomic detail and arterial perfusion. Testicular scintigraphy is equally effective but is often unavailable during the night hours. A urologist should be consulted if testicular torsion is considered. Manual detorsion should be attempted; the success rate is 30% to 70%. Detorsion should be followed by surgical exploration.

Testicular Carcinoma

Testicular carcinoma is the most common type of cancer in boys and men between the ages of 15 and 35 years. Pain is usually not a prominent feature unless an intratesticular tumor hemorrhage has occurred. Examination typically reveals a painless testis that may or may not be enlarged; more often, a distinct, firm intratesticular mass is palpated. If a tumor is sus-

pected, an immediate urologic referral is indicated.

Torsion of Testicular Appendages

Vestigial appendages may undergo torsion and cause an acute, painful scrotal mass. The edema may mask the small, tender mass of a twisted appendage. The symptoms are usually less severe than those seen in testicular torsion. Transillumination may reveal a "blue-black dot." Excision remains the preferred treatment, but observation has also been successful.

ACUTE URINARY RETENTION

Most causes of urinary retention are obstructive (see the box below). The most common cause in men over the age of 50 is benign prostatic hy-

---

CAUSES OF ACUTE URINARY RETENTION IN ADULTS

Penis
  Phimosis
  Paraphimosis
  Meatal stenosis
  Foreign body
  External constriction (e.g., hair, rubber band)
Urethra
  Tumor
  Foreign body
  Calculus
  Urethritis (severe)
  Stricture
  Meatal stenosis (female)
  Hematoma
Prostate
  Benign prostatic hypertrophy
  Carcinoma
  Prostatitis (severe)
  Prostatic infarction

Neurologic causes
  Spinal shock
  Spinal cord syndromes
  Tabes dorsalis
  Diabetes
  Multiple sclerosis
  Syringomyelia
  Herpes zoster
Miscellaneous
  Drugs
    Antihistamines
    Anticholinergics
    Antispasmodics
    Tricyclic antidepressants
    Alpha-adrenergic stimulators
      "Cold" tablets
      Ephedrine derivatives
      Amphetamines
  Psychogenic problems

Modified from Sacknoff EJ, Dretler SP: Urologic emergencies. In Wilkins E, editor: *MGH textbook of emergency medicine,* Baltimore, 1978, Williams & Wilkins. From Harwood-Nuss A, Holland RW III: Genitourinary disease. In Rosen P et al, editors: *Emergency medicine: concepts and clinical practice,* ed 3, St Louis, 1992, Mosby.

perplasia (BPH). Other causes include prostate carcinoma, urethral stricture, and an atonic or neurogenic bladder. In women, a chronic decompensated bladder may result in urinary retention. Urinary retention may be an early manifestation of multiple sclerosis. Individuals with diabetes often develop a neurogenic bladder with retention. Drugs may induce urinary retention, particularly in susceptible patients (e.g., the elderly man who takes antihistamines, anticholinergics, or antispasmodics).

Clinical Presentation

Not all patients with urinary retention are acutely symptomatic, particularly if the process is long-standing and compensated. In this case, a midline mass or renal failure may be an incidental finding. If symptomatic, the patient may complain of progressive urinary hesitancy, decreased force and volume of the urinary stream, and nocturia. If infection has developed, irritative symptoms (dysuria, urgency, frequency) may be seen. The examination may reveal an enlarged prostate gland or a hard nodule that suggests prostatic carcinoma. Urinary obstruction is possible without a clinically enlarged prostate. There may be a midline abdominal mass.

Laboratory Evaluation

Obtain a urinalysis to assess for infection and hematuria; also obtain blood urea nitrogen (BUN), creatinine, and electrolytes. Postobstructive uropathy is seen occasionally with elevated BUN and creatinine; decompression of the bladder may be complicated by the development of a postobstructive diuresis.

Treatment

Treatment is best approached initially with a Foley catheter. Slow decompression (300 ml/hour) is probably prudent because some patients develop a bladder hemorrhage after long-

standing retention. A coudé catheter is useful if the Foley catheter does not pass. Further efforts at instrumentation should probably be performed under the direction of a urologist. If none is available, a percutaneous bladder stick may be used to decompress the bladder.

Disposition

If the patient is in good health and reliable with no UTI and an uncomplicated decompression, outpatient management is possible with a urologic follow-up. According to local practice, men with a mechanical obstruction may or may not be admitted. Patients with a UTI and retention, renal insufficiency, a neurogenic bladder, a serious medical illness, or those requiring extensive instrumentation to relieve the obstruction may need to be hospitalized.

Caveat

The act of decompressing the bladder does not address the underlying cause. A urologic consultation is recommended.

URINARY STONE DISEASE

Urinary stone disease is one of the most common diseases of the urinary tract. Most calculi originate in the kidney and pass into the ureter and bladder. Most ureteral calculi occur in men between the ages of 20 and 50 years. The majority of stones are composed of calcium oxalate or a mixture of calcium oxalate and calcium phosphate. The recurrence of calculi is the rule. Approximately 90% of all ureteral calculi smaller than 4 mm pass spontaneously; 75% of the stones first appear in the distal ureter (the narrowest portion of the ureter).

Clinical Presentation

Colicky pain classically occurs at night or in the early morning. The onset is abrupt, with a crescendo of pain that begins in the flank and radiates into the abdomen and groin. Nausea and vomiting are seen. A stone near the bladder may cause urgency to void, but voiding symptoms should otherwise not be prominent. As many as one third of all patients have gross hematuria. The patient is often in agony and is unable to find a comfortable position. There should be no fever and only a moderate elevation of pulse and blood pressure commensurate with the pain. Examination of the abdomen and flank are usually unremarkable. If the patient is elderly, consider a ruptured abdominal aortic aneurysm and search for masses and bruits.

Differential Diagnosis

The following entities should be considered: narcotic seeker (often claim IVP contrast allergy and drug allergies, factitious hematuria), rupture of abdominal aortic aneurysm, acute pyelonephritis, renal tumor, renal vascular compromise (renal vein thrombosis or renal artery embolism), and renal abscess.

Laboratory Studies

A urinalysis should be done. Most calculi cause microscopic hematuria, but this may be absent in cases of complete obstruction. Pyuria and bacteriuria are worrisome indicators of a possible coexisting infection. A urine culture should be done if an infection is suspected. Few other laboratory studies are indicated in the initial evaluation.

Radiographic Studies

The IVP remains the gold standard and is necessary regardless of whether a calcification is evident on a plain kidney, ureter, and bladder x-ray film. Ultrasonography is a good alternative if there are contraindications to the IVP (renal insufficiency with a creatinine >2.0 or a prior serious contrast reaction). Although ultrasonography

---

> **INDICATIONS FOR ADMISSION: URINARY STONE DISEASE**
>
> **Absolute**
>
> Obstruction with infection (urologic emergency)
> Pain not controlled by oral analgesics
> Persistent nausea and vomiting
> Urinary extravasation
> Hypercalcemic crisis
>
> **Relative**
>
> High-grade obstruction
> Solitary kidney
> Intrinsic renal disease
> Size of obstructing stone (5 to 8 mm)
> Social situation

---

effectively identifies an obstruction, it is less reliable than the IVP in detecting small ureteral stones. A CT scan provides an excellent demonstration of renal and ureteral calculi, the degree of hydronephrosis, and potentially important information about other retroperitoneal structures and conditions.

Management

Initial care includes appropriate analgesia, hydration, and diagnostic testing. Morphine and meperidine (Demerol) are the usual parenteral narcotics. Ketorolac (Toradol) is an excellent alternative and provides comparable pain relief with fewer side effects. Nausea and vomiting should be treated with an antiemetic agent and vigorous fluid replacement.

Disposition

Most patients can be discharged home after an appropriate consultation with a urologist. The patient should be instructed to strain their

THE MOST COMMON CAUSES OF HEMATURIA BY AGE AND SEX

Age 0-20 years
Acute glomerulonephritis
Acute urinary tract infection
Congenital urinary tract anomalies with obstruction

Age 20-40 years
Acute urinary tract infection
Bladder cancer
Urolithiasis

Age 40-60 years (women)
Acute urinary tract infection
Bladder cancer
Urolithiasis

Age 40-60 years (men)
Acute urinary tract infection
Bladder cancer
Urolithiasis

Age 60 years and older (women)
Acute urinary tract infection
Bladder cancer

Age 60 years and older (men)
Acute urinary tract infection
Benign prostatic hyperplasia
Bladder cancer

From Restrepo N, Carey P: Evaluating hematuria in adults. *Am Fam Phys* 40(2):149, 1989. Modified from Gillenwater J, editor: *Adult and pediatric urology,* St Louis, 1996, Mosby.

urine, follow-up with urology, and return if there is pain, fever, chills, or intractable nausea or vomiting (see the box on p. 518).

HEMATURIA

Gross or microscopic hematuria should be considered to be a harbinger of serious urologic disease. The box at left lists the most common causes of hematuria by age and gender. Approximately 60% of all cases of hematuria are caused by bleeding from the lower and middle urinary tracts. Hemorrhage from the prostate is most often a result of benign lesions; in fact, BPH is the most common cause of gross hematuria in men over the age of 60. Red or brown urine in the absence of red blood cells on the urinalysis may be caused by free hemoglobin or myoglobin. Myoglobinuria should be suspected when the urinalysis dipstick is positive but no red blood cells are seen on the microscopic examination. The patient with hematuria should generally be referred to a urologist for further evaluation, particularly if the patient is over 50 years of age.

Recommended Reading

Fihn SD: Lower urinary tract infection in women, *Curr Opin Obstet Gynecol* 4:571-578, 1992.

Harwood-Nuss A: Genitourinary Disorders, In Rosen P et al, editors: *Emergency medicine: concepts and clinical practice,* ed 3, St Louis, 1992, Mosby.

Lingemann J: Calculous disease of the kidney and bladder. In Harwood-Nuss A, editor: *The clinical practice of emergency medicine,* ed 2, Philadelphia, 1996, JB Lippincott.

Stamm WE, Hooton TM: Management of urinary tract infections in adults, *N Engl J Med* 329(18):1328-1334, 1993.

Chapter Forty-four
RENAL FAILURE AND DIALYSIS

ALLAN B. WOLFSON AND RICHARD L. MAENZA

Severe renal dysfunction ultimately results in disturbances in volume regulation, acid-base balance, and electrolyte metabolism, but patients with earlier stages of the disease often have the cardinal manifestations of hematuria, proteinuria, or azotemia. Azotemia is reflected clinically by elevated blood urea nitrogen (BUN) and serum creatinine levels. Urinalysis, serum and urine chemical determinations, and renal imaging studies are used in the emergency department to assess the degree of renal dysfunction and to take the first steps in determining its cause.

EMERGENCY DEPARTMENT DIAGNOSTICS

Urine Volume

Because urine flow does not diminish until the glomerular filtration rate (GFR) is quite markedly decreased, urine volume is a poor indicator of renal dysfunction. In fact, urine volume often *increases* as concentrating ability is lost with advancing renal dysfunction. Oliguria, which is defined as a urine volume of 100 to 400 ml/24 hours, may be seen with prerenal (blood-flow dependent), intrarenal (intrinsic), or postrenal (obstructive) causes of acute renal failure (ARF). Complete or near-complete anuria, and especially intermittent episodes of oliguria, should prompt a consideration of urinary tract obstruction.

Urinalysis

The standard urinalysis consists of a dipstick screening for heme pigment, protein, glucose, ketones, pH, leukocyte esterase, and nitrite reduction; there is also a microscopic examination of a spun specimen of urine. Of these tests, only heme and protein tests and microscopic examination are likely to be of direct utility in evaluating the patient with acute renal dysfunction.

Heme

The dipstick detects both free hemoglobin (or myoglobin) and hemoglobin that is contained in red blood cells. A positive dipstick result should prompt a microscopic examination of the urine. If red cells are seen, the diagnosis of hematuria is confirmed; if no red cells are seen, pigmenturia (myoglobinuria or hemoglobinuria) should be suspected.

Protein

The dipstick can detect protein at concentrations of 10 to 15 mg/dl but does not yield reliable positive results until the concentration is greater than 30 mg/dl.

The dipstick is three to five times more sensitive to albumin than to globulins and immunoglobulin light chains (e.g., Bence Jones protein); this limitation is significant. The addition of 20% sulfosalicylic acid (SSA) to the specimen (8 drops in 2 ml of urine) creates a more sensitive test for detecting proteinuria—turbidity is produced in the presence of as little as 5 mg/dl of nonalbumin or albumin protein. Urine specimens that produce a positive dipstick result should be retested using SSA; if the SSA result is significantly more positive than that of the dipstick, a urine electrophoresis should be performed to detect nonalbumin proteins such as the light chains associated with multiple myeloma.

Microscopic examination

After the urine has been spun, a slide of the resuspended sediment is scanned under high power for red blood cells, white blood cells, renal tubular epithelial cells, oval fat bodies, bacteria, and crystals (see the box below). The composition of a cast reflects the contents of the tubule. Hyaline casts, those that are devoid of formed elements, are seen with dehydration, after exercise, or in association with glomerular proteinuria. A sediment without formed elements or with only hyaline casts is characteristic of prerenal azotemia or obstruction. Red blood cell casts suggest glomerulonephritis or vasculitis. In acute tubular necrosis, the urinary sediment commonly shows granular casts and renal tubular epithelial cells.

Serum and Urine Chemical Analysis

Creatinine and blood urea nitrogen

The serum creatinine concentration is a function of the amount of creatinine entering the blood from muscle and its rate of excretion by the kidneys. Because the amount of creatinine entering the blood is usually constant, changes in the serum creatinine concentration generally reflect changes in the GFR. If the GFR is halved under steady-state conditions, the serum creatinine doubles. Abrupt cessation of glomerular filtration causes the serum creatinine to rise by 1 to 3 mg/dl/day. Rhabdomyolysis releases creatinine into the plasma and may cause the serum creatinine to increase by more than 3 mg/dl/day.

BUN also rises with renal dysfunction but is also influenced by many extrarenal factors. Increased protein intake, gastrointestinal bleeding, and the catabolic effects of fever, trauma, infection, or drugs such as tetracycline and corticosteroids all increase protein turnover and result in increased hepatic urea production and an elevated BUN. Conversely, the BUN tends to decrease in patients with liver failure or protein malnutrition.

Despite preservation of tubular function, urea clearance is decreased in patients with prerenal azotemia or acute obstruction. In such individuals the ratio of BUN to serum creatinine, which is normally approximately 10:1, is usually greater than 10:1; this ratio is usually not markedly increased in uncomplicated intrinsic ARF.

URINALYSIS—MICROSCOPIC EXAMINATION: ABNORMAL FINDINGS

Red blood cells: 5 or more/hpf (hematuria)
Hyaline casts: after exercise, with dehydration, glomerular proteinuria, (prerenal azotemia, obstruction)
Red cell casts: glomerular hematuria (glomerulonephritis, vasculitis)
White cell casts: glomerular inflammation (interstitial nephritis, pyelonephritis, papillary necrosis)
Granular casts: cellular debris
Fatty casts: with heavy proteinuria, glomerular renal disease (nephrotic syndrome)
Eosinophils: appreciable only after staining (acute interstitial nephritis)
Oxalic or hippuric acid crystals: ethylene glycol ingestion
Uric acid crystals: nonspecific (may suggest uric acid nephropathy)

Table 44-1

TYPICAL URINARY FINDINGS IN PRERENAL AZOTEMIA AND ACUTE TUBULAR NECROSIS (ATN)

Laboratory Test	Prerenal Azotemia	ATN
Urinalysis	Normal, or hyaline casts	Brown, granular casts, cellular debris
Urine Na (mEq/L)	<20	>40
U_{Cr}/P_{Cr} ratio	>40	<20
FE_{Na} (%)	<1	>1

Urine sodium and fractional excretion of sodium

The urine sodium (Na) concentration and the fractional excretion of sodium (FE_{Na}),* an additional measure of tubular sodium handling, provide information about the integrity of tubular resorptive function and help distinguish between the two most common causes of ARF: prerenal azotemia and acute tubular necrosis (ATN) (Table 44-1).

In general, patients with oliguria, a urine sodium concentration less than 20 mEq/L, and a FE_{Na} less than 1% should be considered to have prerenal azotemia. A U_{Na} greater than 40 mEq/L and a FE_{Na} greater than 1% suggest ATN (see the box on p. 523). The use of diuretics increases the urinary excretion of sodium, which makes these tests unreliable.

Imaging Studies

Intravenous pyelography (IVP) provides an anatomic image of the urinary tract but does not evaluate renal function. The classic findings of obstruction of the upper urinary tract are kidneys that are normal-to-large in size, nephrograms that become increasingly dense (for as long as 24 hours after contrast injection), de-

*FE_{Na} is a percentage defined as $[(U_{Na}/P_{Na})/(U_{Cr}/P_{Cr})] \times 100$.

layed excretion of contrast, and opacification of dilated collecting systems.

IVP carries the risk of causing contrast-induced ARF. Patients who already have azotemia and those who have diabetes or are dehydrated tend to tolerate this additional insult to the kidneys less readily than those with a normal baseline creatinine level, who have only approximately a 2% chance of experiencing a significant decrease in renal function after a contrast study. The newer nonionic contrast agents appear to have the same potential for nephrotoxicity as the ionic agents.

Ultrasonography has been reported to be 98% sensitive and 74% specific in demonstrating an obstruction (using IVP as the gold standard) but may also detect intrarenal and ureteral calculi.

A CT scan may be useful in the evaluation of some patients with azotemia. Hydronephrosis and often ureteral dilatation can be recognized without the use of contrast material and the level of obstruction determined. Moreover, the cause of obstruction (e.g., lymphoma, retroperitoneal hemorrhage, metastatic cancer, or retroperitoneal fibrosis) can often be delineated. The CT scan is the technique of choice for visualizing a ureteral obstruction at the level of the bony pelvis.

Occasionally an obstruction severe enough to result in renal failure may cause no detectable dilatation of the proximal urinary tract. A bilateral ureteral obstruction resulting from a malig-

CAUSES OF HIGH OR LOW FE$_{Na}$ AND U$_{Na}$ IN PATIENTS WITH ACUTE RENAL FAILURE

U$_{Na}$ <20 mEq/L, FE$_{Na}$ <1%
    Prerenal azotemia
    Acute glomerulonephritis
    Acute obstruction
    Contrast-induced ATN (some cases)
    Rhabdomyolysis-associated ATN (some cases)
    Early sepsis
    Nonoliguric ATN (10% of all cases)
U$_{Na}$ >40 mEq/L, FE$_{Na}$ >1%
    ATN (90% of all cases)
    Chronic obstruction
    Diuretic drugs
    Osmotic diuresis
    Underlying chronic renal failure

From Spiegel DM, Molitoris BA: *Textbook of internal medicine,* Philadelphia, 1989, JB Lippincott.

nancy or retroperitoneal fibrosis is the most important cause. When noninvasive studies produce negative results, the diagnosis must be made by retrograde pyelography or by antegrade pyelography via a percutaneous nephrostomy.

APPROACH TO HEMATURIA

As little as 1 ml of blood in 1 L of urine can produce grossly appreciable hematuria, an occurrence that usually causes the patient to seek medical attention (see the box at right). The emergency department evaluation of the patient who has gross or microscopic hematuria should begin with a complete history to define the pattern and character of the hematuria. Blood that is noted only during the initiation of voiding suggests a urethral source, whereas blood that is present only in the last few drops of urine suggests a prostatic or bladder neck source. Total hematuria (i.e., hematuria present throughout urination) suggests a source in the bladder,

CAUSES OF HEMATURIA*

Hematologic
Coagulopathy
Sickle hemoglobinopathies

Renal (glomerular)
Primary glomerular disease
Multisystem disease (e.g., systemic lupus erythematosus, Henoch-Schönlein purpura, hemolytic uremic syndrome, polyarteritis nodosa, Wegener granulomatosis, Goodpasture syndrome)

Renal (nonglomerular)
Renal infarction
Tuberculosis
Pyelonephritis
Polycystic kidney disease
Medullary sponge kidney
Acute interstitial nephritis
Tumor
Vascular malformation
Trauma
Papillary necrosis

Postrenal
Stones
Tumor of ureter, bladder, urethra
Cystitis
Tuberculosis
Prostatitis
Urethritis
Foley catheter placement
Exercise
Benign prostatic hypertrophy

*The most common causes of hematuria are stones, tumors, urethritis, cystitis.

ureter, or kidney. Brown or smoky-colored urine usually originates in the kidney. Blood clots indicate a nonglomerular renal or lower urinary tract source of bleeding. Flank pain suggests a calculus, neoplasm, renal infarction, obstruction, or infection as the cause. Symptoms of frequency, dysuria, or suprapubic pain suggest cystitis or urethritis; in adult men, perineal pain, dysuria, and terminal hematuria suggest prostatitis.

Other clues to the cause of renal failure should be sought through careful questioning. A history of familial disease, a recent infection (especially a sore throat), foreign travel, multisystem disease, or medication use may provide useful clues. Hematuria appears in 15% to 20% of otherwise healthy individuals after strenuous exercise; the mechanism is unclear, but the condition resolves spontaneously within a few days.

The evaluation of hematuria should include assessing the blood pressure and measuring the BUN and serum creatinine levels to gauge the patient's underlying renal function; a urinalysis can be expected to provide more specific information. A finding of red cell casts or other casts or of significant proteinuria in combination with hematuria suggests intrinsic renal disease and mandates appropriate referral. Hematuria in combination with pyuria or bacteriuria suggests a urinary tract infection; the infection should be treated and the hematuria reassessed after therapy has been completed. Even if the urinalysis does not show white blood cells or organisms, the urine should be cultured to rule out hemorrhagic cystitis, particularly when lower tract symptoms are present.

Blood studies should be ordered only as necessary to gauge renal function and to confirm causes suggested by the clinical presentation. Routinely ordering the full gamut of chemical and serologic studies to rule out all possible causes of hematuria is rarely appropriate. In particular, a platelet count and coagulation study are extremely unlikely to be helpful in the absence of a suggestive history or other specific clinical clues.

Patients with hematuria who have no other abnormality revealed by urinalysis, who are otherwise asymptomatic, who are not azotemic or hypertensive, and who have no evidence of intrinsic renal disease may be followed up as outpatients; a possible exception is the patient with a known bleeding disorder. Other patients should generally be admitted to the hospital for prompt evaluation. Extensive outpatient evaluation of an episode of hematuria is usually not undertaken in patients who are less than 40 years of age unless hematuria is persistent; most patients over the age of 40 should undergo a thorough evaluation after even a single episode of hematuria.

APPROACH TO PROTEINURIA

Abnormal proteinuria is defined as the excretion of more than 150 mg/24 hours in adults or more than 140 mg/m^2/24 hours in children. Proteinuria may be classified broadly as glomerular or tubular. *Glomerular proteinuria* is more common and results from increased permeability of the glomerular capillaries to plasma proteins. *Tubular proteinuria* occurs in patients with normal glomeruli when the smaller proteins that are normally filtered at the glomerulus and reabsorbed in the tubule appear in the urine because of tubular or interstitial abnormalities. The term *overflow proteinuria* refers to the urinary loss of small proteins that are present in the blood in excessive concentrations and appear in the glomerular filtrate in amounts exceeding the normal tubular resorptive capacity (e.g., the light chains produced in multiple myeloma). Miscellaneous causes of transient proteinuria include exertion, stress, or fever. The excretion of as much as 300 mg of protein/24 hours can occur during an otherwise normal pregnancy.

The excretion of more than 2 g of protein/24 hours is likely to be caused by a glomerular process, whereas less than 2 g is typical of tubular or overflow proteinuria. In the nephrotic syndrome, protein losses exceed the liver's capacity to synthesize albumin, resulting in hypoalbuminemia (see the box on p. 525). Edema is the clinical hallmark of the nephrotic syndrome and is often the presenting complaint of patients who have significant proteinuria. Nephrotic-range proteinuria is defined arbitrarily as exceeding 3.5 g/

CAUSES OF THE NEPHROTIC SYNDROME

Primary renal disease
Multisystem disease
  Diabetes mellitus
  Collagen vascular disease
    Systemic lupus erythematosus
    Rheumatoid arthritis
    Henoch-Schönlein purpura
    Polyarteritis nodosa
    Wegener granulomatosis
  Amyloidosis
  Cryoglobulinemia
Drugs and toxins
  Heroin
  Captopril
  Heavy metals
  Nonsteroidal antiinflammatory drugs
  Penicillamine
  Others
Malignancy
  Solid tumors
  Multiple myeloma

Lymphoma
Leukemia
Infection
  Bacterial
    Infective endocarditis
    Poststreptococcal
    Syphilis
  Viral
    Hepatitis B
    Human immunodeficiency virus
    Cytomegalovirus
  Protozoal
    Malaria
    Toxoplasmosis
Allergens
Miscellaneous
  Hereditary nephritis
  Preeclampsia
  Malignant hypertension
  Reflux nephropathy
  Transplant rejection

24 hours. Patients with the nephrotic syndrome are at an increased risk for thromboembolic events, including deep venous thrombosis of the lower extremity, renal vein thrombosis, and pulmonary embolism. This propensity may be related in part to urinary loss and decreased plasma levels of antithrombin III and other circulating normal anticoagulant or fibrinolytic factors. Hyperlipidemia is another feature typical of the nephrotic syndrome.

Evaluation of the patient with proteinuria involves not only gauging the severity of the proteinuria and the likelihood of complications but also identifying any associated signs of underlying renal disease or systemic illness. In young female patients, the possibility of pregnancy should be kept in mind because pregnancy can exacerbate a previously subclinical renal disease; in late pregnancy, proteinuria may be the first sign of preeclampsia.

Although the finding of isolated proteinuria may or may not be clinically important, it is always significant when it occurs in combination with hematuria. In the absence of edema, azotemia, hypertension, an abnormal urine sediment, or known systemic illness affecting the kidney, patients with proteinuria may be referred to their primary care provider for follow-up observation.

ACUTE RENAL FAILURE

Acute renal failure is a generic term used to describe a precipitous decline in kidney function (see the box on p. 526). The causes of ARF may

CLINICAL FEATURES OF ACUTE RENAL FAILURE

Cardiovascular
  Pulmonary edema
  Dysrhythmia
  Hypertension
  Pericardial effusion
  Myocardial infarction
  Pulmonary embolism
Metabolic
  Hyponatremia
  Hyperkalemia
  Acidosis
  Hypocalcemia
  Hyperphosphatemia
  Hypermagnesemia
  Hyperuricemia
Neurologic
  Asterixis
  Neuromuscular irritability
  Mental status changes

  Somnolence
  Coma
  Seizures
Gastrointestinal
  Nausea
  Vomiting
  Gastritis
  Gastroduodenal ulcer
  Gastrointestinal bleeding
  Malnutrition
Hematologic
  Anemia
  Hemorrhagic diathesis
Infectious
  Pneumonia
  Septiciemia
  Urinary tract infection
  Wound infection

From Brezis M, Rosen S, Epstein FH: *The kidney,* ed 3, Philadelphia, 1986, WB Saunders.

be divided into those that decrease renal blood flow (prerenal), produce a renal parenchymal insult (intrarenal), or obstruct urine flow (obstructive or postrenal ARF). The term *acute tubular necrosis* denotes a broad category of intrinsic renal failure that cannot be attributed to specific glomerular, vascular, or interstitial causes.

Prerenal Azotemia

Decreased renal perfusion that is sufficient to cause a decrease in the GFR results in azotemia. The possible causes can be grouped into entities causing intravascular volume depletion, volume redistribution, or decreased cardiac output (see the box on p. 527). Individuals who have a preexisting renal disease are particularly sensitive to the effects of diminished renal perfusion. Prerenal azotemia is characterized by increased urine specific gravity, a BUN/Cr ratio greater than 10:1, a urine sodium concentration less than 20 mEq/dl, and a FE_{Na} less than 1%. In all cases, the goal of treatment involves addressing the underlying problem that is leading to decreased renal blood flow.

Postrenal (Obstructive) Acute Renal Failure

Obstruction is an eminently reversible cause of ARF and should be considered in every patient with newly discovered azotemia or worsening renal function. As noted previously, oliguria should prompt a strong consideration of an obstruction. Obstruction may occur at any level of the urinary tract but is most commonly produced by prostatic hypertrophy or by functional bladder neck obstruction (e.g., secondary to medication side effects or a neurogenic bladder (see the box on p. 527). Treatment of postrenal

CAUSES OF PRERENAL AZOTEMIA
Volume loss
Gastrointestinal: vomiting, diarrhea,
nasogastric drainage
Renal: diuresis
Blood loss
Insensible losses
Third-space sequestration
Pancreatitis
Peritonitis
Trauma
Burn
Cardiac
Myocardial infarction
Valvular disease
Cardiomyopathy
Decreased effective arterial volume
Antihypertensive medication
Nitrates
Neurogenic
Sepsis
Anaphylaxis
Hypoalbuminemia
Nephrotic syndrome
Liver disease

CAUSES OF POSTRENAL ACUTE RENAL FAILURE
Intrarenal and ureteral
Kidney stone
Sloughed papilla
Malignancy
Retroperitoneal fibrosis
Uric acid, oxalic acid, or sulfonamide
crystal precipitation
Methotrexate or acyclovir precipitation
Bladder
Kidney stone
Blood clot
Prostatic hypertrophy
Bladder carcinoma
Neurogenic bladder
Urethra
Phimosis
Stricture

ARF consists of relieving the obstruction. In the absence of infection, full renal recovery is said to be possible even after 1 to 2 weeks of total obstruction; however, the serum creatinine level may not return to baseline for several weeks.

Intrinsic Acute Renal Failure

Of all of the specific intrarenal disorders that cause ARF, glomerulonephritis, interstitial nephritis, and abnormalities of the intrarenal vasculature are amenable to specific therapy and thus should be carefully considered as possible causes (see the box on p. 528). However, these entities are responsible for only 5% to 10% of all cases of

ARF in adult inpatients; the vast majority are a result of ATN. In adults who develop ARF outside the hospital, there is a much greater incidence of glomerular, interstitial, and small-vessel disease, and in children these entities account for approximately one half of all cases of ARF.

Glomerular disease

Acute glomerulonephritis (GN) may represent a primary renal process or may be the manifestation of any of a wide range of other disease entities. Patients may have dark urine, hypertension, edema, or congestive heart failure (secondary to volume overload); patients may also be completely asymptomatic, in which case the diagnosis results from an incidental finding on urinalysis. The hematuria associated with glomerular disease may be microscopic or gross and may be persistent or intermittent. Proteinuria, although often in the range of 500 mg to 3 g/day, is often in the nephrotic range (greater than 3.5 g/24 hours). Hematuria, proteinuria, or red cell casts are very

INTRINSIC RENAL DISEASES CAUSING ACUTE RENAL FAILURE

Vascular

Large vessel
  Renal artery thrombosis or stenosis
  Renal vein thrombosis
  Atheroembolic disease
Small and medium vessel
  Scleroderma
  Malignant hypertension
  Hemolytic uremic syndrome
  Thrombotic thrombocytopenic purpura

Glomerular

Systemic diseases
  Systemic lupus erythematosus
  Infective endocarditis
  Systemic vasculitis (e.g., periarteritis
    nodosa [PAN], Wegener granulomatosis)
  Henoch-Schönlein purpura
  Essential mixed cryoglobulinemia
  Goodpasture syndrome
Primary renal disease
  Poststreptococcal glomerulonephritis
  Other postinfectious glomerulonephritis
  Rapidly progressive glomerulonephritis

Tubulointerstitial

Drugs (many)
Toxins: heavy metals, ethylene glycol
Infections
Multiple myeloma

Acute tubular necrosis

Ischemia
  Shock
  Sepsis
  All causes of severe prerenal azotemia
Nephrotoxins
  Nonsteroidal antiinflammatory agents
    (reversible)
  Radiographic contrast agents
  Pigment (myoglobin, hemoglobin)

suggestive of GN; in fact, red cell casts are essentially diagnostic of active glomerular disease and are rarely seen with other types of renal disease. Conversely, the absence of red cell casts, proteinuria, and hematuria argues strongly against GN as the cause of ARF.

Interstitial disease

Acute interstitial nephritis (AIN) is most commonly precipitated by drug exposure or by infection. The most commonly incriminated drugs are the penicillins, diuretics, anticoagulants, and nonsteroidal antiinflammatory drugs (NSAIDs). It has been reported in association with bacterial, fungal, protozoal, and rickettsial infections.

AIN classically presents with a rash, fever, eosinophilia, and eosinophiluria, but it is common for one or more of these cardinal signs to be absent. Pyuria, gross or microscopic hematuria, and mild proteinuria are observed in some cases. A definite diagnosis can sometimes be made only by renal biopsy. Treatment is directed at removing the presumed cause; infections should be treated, and the offending drugs should be discontinued. Renal function generally returns to baseline over several weeks, but the development of chronic renal failure has been reported.

Intrarenal vascular disease

Vascular disease of the kidney can be classified according to the size of the vessel that is affected. Disorders such as renal arterial thrombosis or embolism, which affect large blood vessels, must be bilateral (or must affect a single functioning kidney) to produce ARF. Renal arterial embolism can cause acute renal infarction, which is generally manifested by sudden flank, back, chest, or upper abdominal pain. Urinary findings, including hematuria, are variable; fever, nausea, and vomiting are common. In some cases, evidence of embolization to other vessels provides a useful clue. The diagnosis is usually made by renal flow scanning or arteriography.

Several diseases affecting the smaller intrarenal vessels can cause ARF. Patients whose disease is severe enough to cause ARF generally also have hypertension, microangiopathic hemolytic anemia, and other systemic and organ-specific manifestations. Malignant hypertension, though much less common since the advent of more effective antihypertensive therapy, has by no means disappeared. Patients with scleroderma (systemic sclerosis) may have a "scleroderma renal crisis," which is characterized by malignant hypertension and rapidly progressive renal failure. Whereas vasculitis associated with glomerular capillary inflammation typically causes gross or microscopic hematuria and the formation of red cell casts, involvement of the medium-sized vessels, such as that produced by scleroderma, often spares the preglomerular vessels and tends not to produce an active urine sediment. However, extrarenal manifestations (rash, fever, arthritis, pulmonary symptoms) are usually evident.

Patients with malignant hypertension have been reported to recover renal function after aggressive antihypertensive therapy, with temporary maintenance on dialysis if necessary. For individuals who have a scleroderma renal crisis, specific therapy with angiotensin-converting-enzyme inhibitors has been shown to lead to an improvement in renal function.

Acute tubular necrosis

As previously stated, the term *acute tubular necrosis* refers to a deterioration of kidney func-

tion associated with any of a variety of renal insults. Oliguria may or may not be a feature of ATN. A diagnosis of ATN is made after prerenal and postrenal causes of ARF and disorders of the glomeruli, interstitium, and intrarenal vasculature have been excluded.

The most common precipitant of ATN is renal ischemia during surgery or after trauma. The remainder of the cases occur in the setting of medical illness, most commonly as a result of the administration of nephrotoxic aminoglycoside antibiotics or radiocontrast agents or in association with rhabdomyolysis. Hemolysis, which results in hemoglobinuria and the release of hemoglobin into the circulation, can cause ATN but usually only in the presence of coexisting dehydration, acidosis, or other causes of decreased renal perfusion. An ATN may be associated with the hemolysis of as little as 100 ml of blood (see the box below).

CAUSES OF PIGMENT-INDUCED ACUTE RENAL FAILURE

Rhabdomyolysis and myoglobinuria
    Vigorous exercise
    Arterial embolization
    Status epilepticus
    Status asthmaticus
    Coma- and pressure-induced myonecrosis
    Heat stress
    Diabetic ketoacidosis
    Myopathy
    Alcoholism
    Hypokalemia
    Hypophosphatemia
Hemoglobinuria
    Transfusion reactions
    Snake envenomation
    Malaria
    Mechanical destruction of RBCs by
        prosthetic valves
    G6PD deficiency

SYSTEMIC DISORDERS

ATN associated with rhabdomyolysis is often oliguric. It is characterized by rapid increases in the serum creatinine, potassium, phosphorus, and uric acid levels. The urine dipstick yields a positive result for heme in only 50% of those patients with rhabdomyolysis because myoglobin is rapidly cleared from the serum and may therefore be undetectable in the urine at the time of presentation. Therefore a negative urine dipstick result does not rule out the diagnosis. Serum creatine phosphokinase (CPK) is cleared much more slowly and is therefore a much more sensitive indicator.

Antibiotics and radiographic contrast agents are commonly implicated in the development of ATN. Clinically significant renal dysfunction usually occurs only after several days of aminoglycoside therapy and often after more than 1 week of therapy. However, renal failure can develop as long as 10 days after the drug has been discontinued.

ATN can occur after any procedure involving contrast, but the highest incidence occurs after arteriography. Contrast-induced ATN encompasses a spectrum that ranges from asymptomatic nonoliguric renal insufficiency to severe renal failure requiring dialysis; most cases are mild. The most important risk factors for contrast-induced ATN are preexisting renal insufficiency, diabetes mellitus, multiple myeloma, an age greater than 60 years, volume depletion, and higher doses of contrast material. Of these factors, preexisting renal insufficiency is the most important.

APPROACH TO THE PATIENT WITH AZOTEMIA OR ACUTE RENAL FAILURE

In attempting to identify the cause of azotemia, the general strategy is to rule out both prerenal and postrenal causes before considering the many intrinsic renal causes.

General Management

Management of ARF in the emergency department is directed at reversing decreases in GFR and urine output (if possible) while minimizing further hemodynamic and toxic insults, maintaining normal fluid and electrolyte balance, and managing other complications of ARF as required. After ensuring that the vital signs are adequate and that the patient is in no immediate danger from volume or metabolic derangements, the next step is identifying and correcting prerenal and postrenal factors, if any. Intravascular volume should be repleted in hypovolemic patients and maintained in euvolemic patients by matching input to measured and insensible output. Inadequate cardiac output should be augmented whenever possible. Postrenal or obstructive ARF is treated by restoring normal urine outflow. Bladder outlet obstruction may be relieved with a Foley catheter, whereas upper tract obstruction may require percutaneous nephrostomy. When prerenal and postrenal factors have been ruled out, the challenge to the clinician is in identifying the cause of intrinsic renal ARF and keeping in mind the multitude of known possible causes.

It has repeatedly been noted that patients who have oliguric ARF have a significantly higher mortality and a much greater risk of complications than those who are not oliguric. The difference in prognosis may simply reflect a more severe renal insult in patients who are oliguric. However, no controlled prospective human studies have been performed to determine whether interventions to convert oliguric ARF to nonoliguric ARF affect renal function or mortality. Nevertheless, an attempt to increase urine flow is warranted because nonoliguric patients are easier to manage. Mannitol, furosemide, and low-dose dopamine have all been used for this purpose.

Mannitol has been shown to prevent ARF in experimental models of myoglobinuria, presumably by inducing osmotic diuresis and decreasing intratubular deposition of pigment. On the other hand, furosemide has not consistently demonstrated a beneficial effect in pigmenturia. Other studies suggest that myoglobin precipitates in an acidic urine but not in an alkaline urine. Therefore aggressive volume repletion, alkalinization, and mannitol infusion are indicated after crush injuries to reduce the likelihood of ARF; this regimen also helps control hyperkalemia. Once ARF has occurred, management is similar to that of other forms of ARF, but early dialysis may be required to control rapidly developing hyperkalemia, hyperphosphatemia, and hyperuricemia.

Volume and Metabolic Complications

Hyperkalemia, the most common metabolic cause of death in patients with ARF, results from an inability to excrete endogenous and exogenous potassium loads. In oliguric patients, the serum potassium level typically increases by 0.3 to 0.5 mEq/L/day but may increase more rapidly in catabolic, septic, or traumatized patients and in the face of exogenous loads from diet or medications. Although some hyperkalemic patients note muscular weakness, the vast majority are generally asymptomatic until major manifestations of cardiotoxicity supervene. Mild hyperkalemia (K^+ < 6.0 mEq/L) may be cautiously observed without specific treatment at the same time that all exogenous sources of potassium are eliminated. Urgent intervention is necessary if the serum potassium level is greater than 6.5 mEq/L, particularly if ECG changes are present. When cardiotoxicity must be reversed immediately (e.g., when there is hemodynamic compromise), IV calcium (10 ml of 10% calcium gluconate or calcium chloride given over several minutes) is the treatment of choice. IV insulin (given with glucose to prevent hypoglycemia) and IV bicarbonate temporarily shift potassium to the intracellular space. Bicarbonate should be used with particular caution in patients

with renal failure because of its potential to cause volume overload and to provoke hypocalcemic tetany or seizures. Recent reports have documented the safety and efficacy of inhaled albuterol in hyperkalemic patients with chronic renal failure; like insulin and bicarbonate, this agent causes potassium to move into cells. The use of albuterol in patients with ARF has not yet been formally investigated but appears to be effective and safe. The elimination of potassium from the body is promoted by using a potassium-binding ion exchange resin (sodium polystyrene sulfonate [Kayexalate]), by enhancing urinary potassium excretion, or through dialysis.

Asymptomatic *hypocalcemia* requires no immediate treatment, but incipient or frank tetany should be treated with IV calcium (the initial dose is the same as for hyperkalemia).

Hyperphosphatemia resulting from decreased renal elimination of phosphate is another common feature of ARF. The serum phosphorus level usually ranges from 6 to 8 mg/dl but may be much higher with rhabdomyolysis or in catabolic states. A calcium-phosphate product greater than 70 may result in metastatic soft-tissue calcification. Hyperphosphatemia is often treated with oral calcium-based antacids that bind ingested phosphate in the gut.

Acids produced in normal metabolic processes accumulate in ARF and are buffered in part by serum bicarbonate, which results in a decrease in the serum bicarbonate level and a high-anion-gap *metabolic acidosis.* Compensatory hyperventilation may be mistakenly attributed to primary cardiac failure or to volume overload. The metabolic acidosis associated with ARF is usually mild, and treatment is not generally necessary if the serum bicarbonate level is greater than 10 mEq/L. Overzealous correction may result in hypokalemia, hypocalcemia, or volume overload.

Hypermagnesemia complicates ARF when patients are given magnesium-containing antacids or laxatives. Therefore these products should be avoided in the therapy of ARF.

Disturbances of volume regulation can be expected to occur in most patients with ARF. Some nonoliguric patients excrete salt and water well enough that intravascular volume depletion occurs if adequate fluid replacement is not provided, which prolongs recovery from ARF. Much more commonly, ARF is complicated by volume overload because sodium and water excretion may be inadequate to match even modest intakes. Volume overload is largely responsible for the hypertension often seen in ARF and often leads to congestive heart failure and pulmonary edema. Iatrogenic volume overload is particularly common and can be prevented only by giving careful attention to fluid intake and output and by using prudent estimates of insensible loss. Volume overload can be treated with diuretics or IV nitroglycerin while preparations are being made to initiate dialysis.

Organ System Effects

Uremia impairs host defenses, particularly leukocyte function. Infection occurs in 30% to 70% of all patients with ARF and is a significant cause of morbidity and mortality.

Pericarditis, which has a prevalence of 12% to 20% in dialyzed patients with end-stage renal disease (ESRD), may also occur in patients with ARF. Chest pain that is worse in a recumbent position is the most common symptom, and most patients have a pericardial friction rub. Fever is common. The ECG may show ST-T wave elevation, low voltage, or atrial fibrillation. The presence of pericardial effusion is identified most accurately by echocardiography, but tamponade, with the typical clinical signs, occurs in some patients. In contrast to the situation of chronic renal failure, pericarditis or pericardial effusion in the setting of ARF is generally an indication for the urgent initiation of dialysis. Patients who have hemodynamically significant tamponade require surgical drainage of the effusion or, occasionally, emergency pericardiocentesis.

Neurologic abnormalities in ARF may be precipitated by electrolyte abnormalities, medications, or uremia. Common symptoms in uremic patients include lethargy, confusion, agitation, asterixis, myoclonus, and seizures.

Anorexia, nausea, vomiting, gastritis, and pancreatitis are also associated with ARF. Gastrointestinal hemorrhage is seen in 10% to 30% of these patients and results from a combination of stress and impaired hemostasis. Gastrointestinal hemorrhage is the second leading cause of death in ARF.

Impaired erythropoiesis, shortened red blood cell survival, hemolysis, hemodilution, and gastrointestinal blood loss together play a role in the normocytic normochromic anemia that usually accompanies ARF. Although mild thrombocytopenia may be present, the qualitative defect in platelet function associated with ARF is more significant and contributes to these patients' bleeding tendency. In patients with active bleeding or in whom an invasive procedure is contemplated, the prolonged bleeding time can be corrected by administering cryoprecipitate or desmopressin acetate (DDAVP).

Disposition

Patients who have new-onset ARF should be admitted to the hospital. Decisions regarding dialysis are generally made by the nephrology consultant and take into account many factors, including laboratory test results and the presence or absence of symptoms of uremia such as nausea, vomiting, and a change in mental status. Intractable volume overload and life-threatening hyperkalemia are the two most common indications for emergency dialysis.

CHRONIC RENAL FAILURE

Patients with chronic renal disease commonly have experienced a slowly progressive course of decreasing renal function over a period of months or years. They are likely to come to the emergency department with either slowly progressive symptoms or with acute problems brought on by superimposed illness, trauma, or other physiologic stress. The focus in the emergency department must be first identifying and correcting any immediate life-threatening conditions and then returning the patient to a stable, chronically compensated status.

Pathophysiology and Clinical Presentation

The term *chronic renal insufficiency* denotes a condition in which GFR has been moderately reduced but not to a degree sufficient to cause clinical symptoms—in general, by no more than 75%. The term *end-stage renal disease* describes a condition in which renal function has diminished to a very low level and in which serious, life-threatening manifestations can be expected

to occur without dialysis or transplantation. At this stage, the kidneys are often shrunken and diffusely scarred.

As with ARF, the causes of chronic renal failure can be conveniently classified as prerenal (vascular), intrinsic renal (glomerular and tubulointerstitial), and postrenal (obstructive) (see the box below). Glomerular disease accounts for approximately one third to one half of all cases of ESRD, of which diabetic nephropathy forms the largest group. Hypertensive nephrosclerosis is another important cause, particularly among blacks, in whom it may be the cause of at least 25% of all cases of ESRD. Among children and adolescents, reflux nephropathy is the most common cause of ESRD. Renal failure related to IV drug use or to human immunodeficiency virus (HIV) infection is a major consideration in some populations. Clues to other specific causes may be gained from elements of the history, physical examina-

MAJOR CAUSES OF CHRONIC RENAL FAILURE

Vascular

Renal arterial disease
Hypertensive nephrosclerosis

Glomerular

Primary glomerulopathies
  Focal sclerosing GN
  Membranoproliferative GN
  Membranous GN
  Crescentic GN
  IgA nephropathy
Secondary glomerulopathies
  Diabetic nephropathy
  Collagen vascular disease
  Amyloidosis
  Postinfectious
  Heroin nephropathy

Tubulointerstitial

Nephrotoxins
Analgesic nephropathy
Mypercalcemia/nephrocalcinosis
Multiple myeloma
Reflux nephropathy
Sickle nephropathy
Chronic pyelonephritis
Tuberculosis
Polycystic kidney disease
Alport syndrome
Medullary cystic disease

Obstructive

Nephrolithiasis
Ureteral tuberculosis
Retroperitoneal fibrosis
Retroperitoneal tumor
Prostatic obstruction
Congenital

tion, or laboratory and imaging studies.

Regardless of the underlying etiology, a progressive loss of renal function eventually results in a recognizable syndrome called *uremia.* Despite the presence of often impressive laboratory abnormalities, the clinical manifestations do not generally appear until GFR has been reduced to perhaps 15% to 20% of normal. The uremic state is characterized by derangements in homeostasis and metabolism and by specific effects on multiple organ systems.

Disturbances in homeostasis generally develop gradually. As the patient becomes unable to excrete promptly an ingested salt or water load, the external balance of sodium and water is affected; volume overload, hypernatremia, or hyponatremia may result. An inability to concentrate the urine is an early manifestation of renal insufficiency and may be manifested as nocturia. Potassium homeostasis is also disrupted, and a relatively small potassium load may lead to dangerous hyperkalemia. Because of a decreased ability to excrete ammonium and phosphate, the acid-base balance is disturbed as the kidney fails to clear the daily metabolic acid load; the result is a non–anion-gap acidosis in the earlier stages of chronic renal failure and a superimposed anion-gap acidosis as GFR decreases further. Calcium and phosphate metabolism is affected early; retention of phosphate and a progressive loss of the capacity of the kidney to synthesize 1,25-dihydroxycholecalciferol (1,25-DHCC), the active form of vitamin D, lead to hypocalcemia, secondary hyperparathyroidism, and eventually to the development of renal osteodystrophy.

Uremia causes less dramatic but similarly serious derangements in protein, carbohydrate, and lipid metabolism. Nitrogenous by-products of protein catabolism are retained in the blood and are the presumed cause of many of the diverse abnormalities of organ function in renal failure. The majority of patients with ESRD show decreased glucose tolerance, but it is rarely severe enough to require treatment unless there is a history of overt diabetes. Incompletely under-

stood alterations in lipid metabolism result in a type IV hyperlipoproteinemia in many ESRD patients. Uremia has specific effects on a variety of organ systems; these systems are discussed in the following sections.

Cardiovascular

The cardiovascular system is perhaps the most dramatically affected by uremia. Many of the manifestations can be attributed to the effects of chronic volume overload, anemia, hyperlipidemia, and volume- and hormonally-mediated hypertension. Pericarditis, with or without pericardial fluid accumulation, is also fairly common in ESRD, particularly among patients who have not been dialyzed.

Pulmonary

Similarly, some patients develop uremic pleuritis, with or without associated pleural fluid collections. Pulmonary edema often occurs and is a result of volume overload or myocardial dysfunction.

Neurologic

Neurologic dysfunction is also a feature of advanced uremia and is usually manifested by lethargy, somnolence, difficulty concentrating, or a frank alteration in mental status. Hiccups, asterixis, or myoclonic twitching are also seen. The latter should not be confused with tetany resulting from hypocalcemia, which is also common in untreated patients with ESRD. Seizures may also occur, but causes other than uremia per se must be ruled out. Some patients on chronic dialysis therapy have developed "dialysis dementia"—a syndrome characterized by dementia, altered mental status, and movement disorders that appears to be related at least in part to aluminum overload associated with aluminum-containing medications (e.g., oral phosphate binders) or dialysate. In the peripheral nervous system, uremia often causes cramps and a distal sensorimotor neuropathy. A troublesome and very characteristic complaint is the "restless legs syndrome," in which there is persistent neuropathic discomfort in the legs that patients find can be relieved only by movement.

Gastrointestinal

Anorexia, nausea, and vomiting are nearly constant features of uremia. These symptoms are thought to be caused by an accumulation of nitrogenous wastes because they seem to correlate roughly with the BUN level and are often relieved, even in the undialyzed patient, by the introduction of a low-protein diet.

Dermatologic

The skin of patients with chronic renal failure has a characteristic yellowish tinge. "Uremic frost" is the result of deposition of urea from evaporated sweat on the skin and is a classic finding that, like "uremic fetor," is seen only rarely now with the widespread use of dialysis. Diffuse pruritus is often a major source of discomfort for the ESRD patient; in some cases it may be a result of calcium deposition in the skin related to derangements in calcium metabolism.

Musculoskeletal

The complex disturbances of calcium and phosphate metabolism in ESRD result in renal osteodystrophy, a term encompassing several overlapping varieties of bone disease that can cause symptoms of bone pain or frank fracture. Patients with chronic renal disease are generally treated with long-term oral calcium, vitamin D, and dietary phosphate binders in an effort to prevent both secondary hyperparathyroidism and uremic osteodystrophy. Occasionally patients have a poor response to therapy and require parathyroidectomy. A particular type of arthritis caused by the deposition of calcium hydroxyapatite or calcium oxalate crystals in joints is seen in some patients.

Immunologic

Patients with uremia have long been noted to have an increased susceptibility to infection, and infection remains a leading cause of mortality associated with renal failure. Both humoral and cellular immunity are affected. Although patients with renal failure should be considered to be immunocompromised, most infections in patients with ESRD are a result of common pathogens rather than opportunistic organisms.

Hematologic

End-stage renal disease leads to a rather severe normochromic normocytic anemia, with a hematocrit commonly in the range of 18% to 25%. Primarily a result of decreased renal production of erythropoietin, it is nearly universal in untreated ESRD, except among patients with polycystic disease. Administration of this hormone has proven to effectively maintain the hematocrit at a near-normal level and prevent the need for repeated blood transfusions. Other factors that may contribute to anemia are increased red cell hemolysis, nutritional deficiencies, and increased bleeding secondary to platelet dysfunction. Although platelet number is generally normal in uremia, the bleeding time is prolonged because of defective platelet adhesiveness and activation.

Evaluation

Patients with chronic renal failure, particularly those who are not yet on dialysis, are likely to come to the emergency department with one of the manifestations previously noted. Those in whom the diagnosis of renal failure has not previously been made most commonly have nonspecific complaints that are often of insidious onset: generalized weakness, poor appetite, or a deterioration of mental functioning. The initial laboratory finding of a reasonably well-tolerated but rather severe anemia may be the first clue to the diagnosis, which is subsequently confirmed by the finding of elevated BUN and serum creatinine levels. A prudent next step is to check the ECG for evidence of an immediately life-threatening hyperkalemia before proceeding with further laboratory and radiographic investigations. Although chronic renal failure is as a rule irreversible and slowly progressive, it is

REVERSIBLE FACTORS AND TREATABLE CAUSES OF CHRONIC RENAL FAILURE

Reversible factors

Hypovolemia
Congestive heart failure
Pericardial tamponade
Severe hypertension
Catabolic state/protein loads
Nephrotoxic agents
Obstructive disease
Reflux disease

Treatable Causes

Renal artery stenosis
Malignant hypertension
Acute interstitial nephritis
Hypercalcemic nephropathy
Multiple myeloma
Vasculitis (e.g., systemic lupus erythematosus, Wegener granulomatosis, polyarteritis nodosa)
Obstructive nephropathy (possibly)
Reflux nephropathy (possibly)

critical to exclude the possibility of potentially reversible factors (in effect, to rule out "acute on chronic" renal failure) and to be sure that disorders which, if treated, might allow for some return of renal function have not been overlooked. It is important to consider these potentially reversible and treatable causes of chronic renal failure because they represent the only potential opportunity to reverse rather than simply manage the patient's disease (see the box above).

Management

Individuals with chronic renal failure are susceptible to infections, bleeding, and numerous other complications associated with renal failure per se, as well as those that may be associated with the underlying disorder that caused the renal failure. Moreover, these patients are more than normally vulnerable to the effects of any intercurrent illness or trauma. Those who are maintained on chronic hemodialysis or peritoneal dialysis are also subject to complications entailed by the dialytic therapy itself.

Patients with chronic renal failure are also uniquely susceptible to iatrogenic illness. They are less able than normal individuals to handle fluid and solute loads. The presence of renal failure significantly alters the metabolism and action of many drugs, often in ways that are not predictable a priori. Therefore it is imperative that the dose and schedule of every administered agent, even apparently innocuous ones such as antacids and multivitamin preparations, be carefully considered.

In general, the emergency physician should consult with the patient's nephrologist once the initial evaluation has been completed, because the details of management and follow-up after the patient leaves the emergency department are often complex.

Hyperkalemia

The most rapidly lethal potential complication of chronic renal failure is severe hyperkalemia. It is critical to remember that this condition is usually clinically silent until it presents with potentially life-threatening manifestations. An ECG should be obtained whenever hyperkalemia is a possibility; if signs of hyperkalemia are found, appropriate therapy should be started immediately pending laboratory confirmation of a high serum potassium level (Table 44-2). However, ECG changes may be completely absent even when hyperkalemia is se-

Table *44-2*

TREATMENT OF HYPERKALEMIA

Drug	Dose	Onset/Duration	Mechanism	Comments
Ca Gluconate or CaCl (10%)	10 ml IV, may repeat × 2 prn q 5-10 min	1-5 min/1 hr	Antagonizes membrane effects of K^+	ECG Monitor Do not mix with bicarb
Sodium bicarbonate	50 mg IV, may repeat × 1 prn	10-15 min/1-2 hr	Intracellular movement of K^+	Beware: volume overload, hypertonicity alkalosis (seizures)
Albuterol	10-20 mg aerosol	30 min/2+ hr	Intracellular movement of K^+	Few side effects
Insulin and glucose	10-20 units regular insulin IV per 100 g glucose	30 min/during infusion	Intracellular movement of K^+	Beware: hypoglycemia or hyperglycemia. Use D50 for minimum volume
Kayexalate	25g in 25 ml 70% sorbitol po q6h ± 50 g in 50 ml 70% sorbitol enema q6h	Hours/while continued	Exchange of K^+ for Na^+	Beware Na^+ overload Enema must be retained 30-45 min
Dialysis	Hemodialysis Peritoneal dialysis	Minutes/while continued	Removal of K^+ from blood	May remove 50 mEq/h (HD); 15 mEq/h (PD) Beware: K^+ rebound
IV diuretics (with volume if hypovolemic)	Varies greatly depending on renal function	Minutes/while diuresis continues	Urinary K^+ excretion	Only in patients with residual renal function

From Wolfson AB, Singer I: Hemodialysis-related emergencies, Part II, *J Emerg Med* 6:61, 1988.

vere. A potassium level of 6 mEq/L should be considered potentially dangerous despite the fact that many ESRD patients chronically tolerate levels somewhat above this without ECG changes. A patient with chronic renal failure who presents in cardiac arrest should be assumed to be hyperkalemic and treated accordingly while the usual resuscitative measures are undertaken.

Pulmonary edema

Perhaps the most common emergency in the patient with chronic renal failure is pulmonary edema secondary to volume overload. Surprisingly, this diagnosis is not always straightforward. The patient may present with a suggestive history of increasing dyspnea on exertion or paroxysmal nocturnal dyspnea, but physical examination may not reveal the expected signs of congestive heart failure, and even chest radiography may be deceptive. A history of recent weight gain or of being considerably over "dry weight" (typically more than 5 pounds) is the most reliable clue. In the absence of convincing evidence of another cause for dyspnea, it should be assumed that volume overload is the cause and treat accordingly.

Treatment of pulmonary edema in the patient with chronic renal failure needs to be somewhat different from that used with other patients. Arrangements for the initiation of dialysis should be made as soon as possible because dialysis is the most rapidly effective way to decrease intravascular volume in the absence of renal function. However other measures should be instituted in the meantime (see the box above). The patient should be placed in the sitting position, and high-flow oxygen should be administered by mask. Sublingual or topical nitroglycerin, or both, can be administered immediately to help rapidly reduce both preload and afterload; an IV infusion can be started promptly and titrated to effect. IV nitroprusside may have an advantage in producing more arteriolar dilatation. IV morphine increases venous capacitance, but as with non–renal-failure patients, its

TREATMENT OF PULMONARY EDEMA IN RENAL FAILURE
Dialysis
Hemodialysis
Hemofiltration
Peritoneal dialysis
Oxygen
Morphine
Diuretics
Furosemide
Bumetanide
Nitroglycerin (sublingual, IV, topical)
Nitroprusside

use in pulmonary edema has become less routine. IV furosemide, although ineffective as a diuretic in patients with advanced renal failure, is a rather potent pulmonary venodilator and may provide additional relief. Patients with residual renal function may produce diuresis in response to high IV doses of some diuretics but much more slowly than in patients without renal compromise. However, there are reports that the use of ethacrynic acid has been associated with permanent deafness in some patients with renal failure.

Infection

The possibility of serious infection should be entertained even when the expected classic findings are not all present. For example, bacteremia may be manifested by fever alone, just as it is in other patients with impaired immunity. Pneumonia may present with only vague dyspnea or malaise, which are symptoms that may be attributed to volume overload or uremia. Upper and lower urinary tract infections can occur even in patients with minimal urine output or in those with long-standing renal failure. Therefore all diagnostic possibilities should be pursued; empiric broad-spectrum antibiotic coverage is often advisable until infection has been ruled out in the hospital.

DIALYSIS

Dialysis can normalize fluid balance, correct electrolyte and other solute abnormalities, and remove uremic toxins or drugs from the circulation when the patient's kidneys are unable to do so. To a lesser degree dialysis can also reverse some uremic symptomatology and permit better long-term control of hypertension, anemia, and renal osteodystrophy.

There are two major dialysis modalities: hemodialysis and peritoneal dialysis. Each is based on technology wherein the patient's blood comes into contact with a semipermeable membrane; on the other side of this membrane is a specially constituted balanced physiologic solution. Water and solutes diffuse across the membrane by moving along concentration and osmotic gradients, which effectively normalizes the composition of the blood.

Indications for Dialysis

The decision to initiate chronic dialysis in the patient with ESRD is generally made by the patient's nephrologist in the setting of gradually decreasing GFR and slowly progressive manifestations of renal failure. The absolute value of the BUN or serum creatinine levels is usually only a rough guide as to when chronic dialysis should be instituted. Provision of vascular or peritoneal access generally has been arranged weeks to months before the anticipated initiation of dialysis to allow the access to mature and to minimize any avoidable mechanical complications. However, for the patient who comes to the emergency department with acute renal failure, as well as for the patient with chronic renal failure who develops acute problems, the emergency physician must be prepared to decide to arrange for dialysis to be provided emergently

---

INDICATIONS FOR EMERGENCY DIALYSIS

Pulmonary edema
Hyperkalemia
Other severe electrolyte or acid-base
  disturbances
Severe uncontrollable hypertension
Some overdoses
Pericarditis (possibly)

(see the box above). How urgently dialysis must be initiated depends not only on the severity and acuteness of the presenting problem but also on the availability of appropriate facilities, trained dialysis personnel, and effective temporizing measures for the immediate problem at hand.

As mentioned, the serum creatinine and BUN levels themselves should not be considered indications for dialysis. The occurrence of uremic symptoms such as nausea, vomiting, lethargy, or itching indicates a need for dialysis but does not require that dialysis be initiated immediately. The appearance of pericarditis, even in the absence of cardiac tamponade, has been thought by some to be an exception. However, pericarditis can occur in well-dialyzed ESRD patients as well; pericarditis is not dangerous in itself, nor does it invariably lead to tamponade. In a previously undialyzed patient who has progressive renal insufficiency, the appearance of pericarditis indicates that it is time to initiate dialysis, although not emergently.

Hemodialysis

In *hemodialysis,* the patient's heparinized blood is pumped through an extracorporeal circuit, where it comes into contact with an artificial membrane. The amount of fluid transferred across this membrane can be controlled by adjusting the pressure under which the blood is pumped through the dialyzer. Because high blood-flow rates (typically at least 200 ml/minute) are necessary to achieve reasonable clearances, hemodialysis requires special access to the patient's circulation, generally through a surgically created *arteriovenous fistula* or an implanted *artificial graft.* Some patients are dialyzed through a specially designed chronic subclavian catheter (Uldall catheter). This type of catheter is most commonly used when hemodialysis must be performed before a peripheral access has had a chance to mature or after all of a patient's peripheral sites for access have been exhausted. Chronic hemodialysis is typically performed three times a week for 3 to 5 hours/treatment, either at home or at a specially staffed dialysis unit. The vascular access must be treated with care because hemodialysis cannot be performed without it. Careless manipulation or puncture can result in bleeding, infection, or thrombosis that may result in loss of the access. The involved arm should never be used for blood pressure determinations, and a tourniquet should never be applied.

Complications

Vascular-access–related complications. The performance of hemodialysis depends on reliable vascular access; complications related to the vascular access device most commonly require evaluation in the emergency department.

Bleeding from the dialysis puncture site can occur hours after a hemodialysis treatment, either spontaneously or after inadvertent minor trauma to the site. Patients are usually able to control the bleeding by applying pressure to the area but need to be evaluated to exclude significant blood loss. Care must be taken not to occlude and possibly thrombose the vessel by compressing it too vigorously, and the presence of a thrill immediately after the procedure should be documented on the chart.

A vascular surgeon should be consulted immediately if the patient complains that the thrill in the access has been lost. Success in reopening a clotted access appears to depend on the amount of time since thrombosis has occurred. The access device should not be forcefully manipulated or irrigated because vessel rupture or venous embolization may result.

Infection of the vascular access has the potential to cause persistent or recurrent bacteremia, as well as loss of the access. Infection appears to result from contamination at the time of puncture; most infections result from the staphylococci typical of skin flora. Infections are more likely to occur in artificial grafts than in native fistulas. The signs and symptoms of access infection—redness, warmth, and tenderness over the site—are often rather obvious. However, in many cases patients manifest no localizing findings and have only fever or a history of recurring episodes of fever and bacteremia. For this reason, it is common practice to draw blood cultures on all hemodialysis patients who have fever without an obvious source of infection and to treat them presumptively for access infection. Before concluding that inapparent access infection is the cause, a careful search for other sources of infection should be made.

IV vancomycin is generally the drug of choice for presumed access infections because the great majority of infections are staphylococcal and because this drug is not hemodialyzable and can therefore be given to the dialysis patient only every 5 to 7 days. Its major toxicity is also renal. If a gram-negative infection is also thought to be reasonably likely, as for example in a patient who has had recent episodes of gram-negative bacteremia, a third-generation cephalosporin or a loading dose of an aminoglycoside (e.g., tobramycin) can also be administered. Aminoglycosides are hemodialyzable and have a half-life of approximately 2 days in ESRD; therefore patients can be reloaded at the end of the next hemodialysis if cultures prove to be positive.

Non–vascular-access-related complications. Hypotension that occurs after dialysis is most commonly the result of an acute reduction in circulating intravascular volume. Most episodes of hypotension that occur during hemodialysis either resolve spontaneously or are readily managed by a decrease in blood-flow rate or the infusion of small volumes of saline (to effect transient volume expansion) or hypertonic solutions (to transiently reverse acute hypoosmolality). Patients with significant hypotension who do not respond to these maneuvers are often brought to the emergency department for further evaluation (see the box below).

Dialysis patients should be considered to be at high risk for acute myocardial infarction, acute dysrhythmia, and sepsis. These causes of hypotension are common among all emergency patients, and consideration should first be given to these entities. Acute hemorrhage is also common in dialysis patients, particularly in view of the anticoagulation required for dialysis and the platelet dysfunction characteristic of renal failure. Gastrointestinal bleeding, often a result of angiodysplasia or peptic disease, can be quite

DIFFERENTIAL DIAGNOSIS OF HYPOTENSION IN HEMODIALYSIS PATIENTS

Hypovolemia
  Excessive fluid removal
  Hemorrhage
Septicemia
Cardiogenic shock
  Dysrhythmia
  Pericardial tamponade
  Myocardial infarction
  Myocardial or valvular dysfunction
  Anaphylactoid reaction
Electrolyte disorders
  Hyperkalemia or hypokalemia
  Hypercalcemia or hypocalcemia
  Hypermagnesemia
Vascular instability
  Drug-related
  Dialysate-related
  Autonomic neuropathy
  Excessive access arteriovenous flow
Air embolism

dramatic. Occult hemorrhage (e.g., spontaneous retroperitoneal or pleural bleeding) may create a confusing picture because symptoms and signs of volume loss may be overshadowed by the local manifestations of bleeding.

Occasionally, acute hypotension may be caused by anaphylaxis or an anaphylactoid reaction to some component of the dialyzer or dialysate. Acute pulmonary embolism and acute air embolism are two other less likely possibilities. The latter was reported occasionally in the past but has been almost eliminated by improved dialysis monitoring equipment and safety mechanisms.

Two additional entities should always be considered in the differential diagnosis of hypotension in the dialysis patient. The first is acute pericardial tamponade, which may result from either a sudden pericardial hemorrhage or from a compensated pericardial effusion that suddenly becomes symptomatic in the face of rapid correction of volume overload. Emergency pericardiocentesis must occasionally be performed in the emergency department to relieve acute tamponade, but there is often enough time for the patient to be transported to the catheterization suite or operating room for safer and more definitive therapy in a controlled setting.

The second major concern in the differential diagnosis of hypotension is severe life-threatening hyperkalemia, which is unusual in a dialyzed patient but can occur in the presence of underlying catabolic illness or with a prolonged period of hypotension and low flow.

Shortness of breath in dialysis patients is often a result of volume overload. If the patient becomes short of breath while being dialyzed other causes must be sought, particularly sudden cardiac failure, pericardial tamponade, or pleural effusion or hemorrhage. Often, pneumonia or underlying airway disease is responsible. Air embolism and anaphylactoid reactions are unusual causes.

Chest pain during dialysis must be taken quite seriously because more than half of all

ESRD patients die of cardiovascular causes, and it is likely that the majority of episodes of chest pain that occur during dialysis are ischemic in origin. The presence of renal failure does not obscure the usual electrocardiographic changes of acute myocardial infarction. The pattern of the change of serum cardiac enzymes with acute infarction is also not altered by ESRD. The treatment of ischemic chest pain and myocardial infarction is the same as for other populations. The possibility of pericarditis should always be considered, even in the well-dialyzed patient and especially if heparinization or thrombolytic therapy is contemplated.

Neurologic dysfunction during or immediately following hemodialysis is most often a result of disequilibrium syndrome, which is a constellation of symptoms and signs that is thought to be produced when serum osmolality is lowered rapidly during dialysis, leaving the brain relatively hyperosmolar relative to the extracellular fluid. Patients typically have headache, malaise, nausea, vomiting, and muscle cramps; in more severe cases there may be an altered mental status, seizures, or coma. These symptoms resolve over a period of several hours as fluid and solutes are redistributed across cell membranes.

It is dangerous to attribute an altered mental status to disequilibrium syndrome unless other potential causes have been satisfactorily ruled out, particularly when symptoms persist, fluctuate, or become worse during a reasonable period of observation (see the box above). Likewise, when seizures occur during dialysis it is tempting but unwise to attribute them to disequilibrium syndrome without considering other potentially serious causes, even in patients who have had seizures in the past. In particular, the finding of any new focal neurologic abnormality mandates at a minimum an immediate head CT scan to rule out an intracranial hemorrhage. Meningitis must be a serious consideration if there is fever or other evidence of infection. One should also consider hyperglycemia, hypoglycemia (especially in the patient with diabetes), electrolyte abnormalities, hypoxemic

DIFFERENTIAL DIAGNOSIS OF ALTERED MENTAL STATUS IN DIALYSIS PATIENTS
Structural
Cerebrovascular accident (particularly hemorrhage)
Subdural hematoma
Intracerebral abscess
Brain tumor
Metabolic
Disequilibrium syndrome
Uremia
Drug effects
Meningitis
Hypertensive encephalopathy
Hypotension
Postictal state
Hypernatremia or hyponatremia
Hypercalcemia
Hypermagnesemia
Hypoglycemia
Severe hyperglycemia
Hypoxemia
Dialysis dementia

states, hypotension of any cause, and other toxic or metabolic causes. The treatment of seizures in patients with ESRD is essentially the same as in other populations.

Peritoneal Dialysis

In *peritoneal dialysis* the patient's peritoneum functions as the dialysis membrane. Water and solutes diffuse from the peritoneal capillaries across this membrane to equilibrate with sterile dialysate, which has been infused into the peritoneal cavity. In chronic ambulatory peritoneal dialysis (CAPD), a technique in which patients with ESRD perform dialysis themselves at home, dialysate is infused through a surgically implanted Silastic catheter (Tenckhoff catheter) that penetrates the peritoneum and abdominal musculature, passes through a subcutaneous tunnel, and exits through the skin of the lower abdominal wall. The catheter is attached externally to sterile plastic tubing, which is connected to a sterile bag of dialysate. Dialysate is allowed to dwell in the peritoneal cavity for 4 to 8 hours; during this time the dialysate bag is still attached to the sterile tubing and is kept rolled under the patient's clothing or belt. The patient typically exchanges the fluid four times a day, 7 days a week and discards the bag of drained fluid and attaches (using sterile technique) a bag of fresh fluid, which is then infused. This form of dialysis is truly continuous and, although it is substantially less efficient on an hourly basis than hemodialysis, achieves a total weekly clearance comparable to that obtained with thrice-weekly hemodialysis.

In contrast to hemodialysis, in which a relatively isosmolar dialysate is used and excess intravascular fluid is removed by adjusting the pressure under which the blood is pumped, CAPD uses a hyperosmolar dialysate to remove intravascular fluid by osmotic forces. The typical 1.5% glucose solution continues to remove fluid for at least 4 hours before it has substantially equilibrated with the blood. Patients generally use a more concentrated solution (e.g., 4.25% glucose) for fluid removal during the long overnight exchange.

CAPD offers patients with ESRD greater independence than hemodialysis, avoids the dangers of anticoagulation, and achieves smoother control of volume and hypertension without the intermittent rapid shifts of solute that are typical of hemodialysis. In addition, medications such as insulin and antibiotics can be administered intraperitoneally, which allows for smoother absorption and more stable blood levels. The main disadvantage of CAPD is a significant incidence of bacterial peritonitis, but this condition is usually readily treated.

Complications

Peritonitis. As with hemodialysis, most of the complications of peritoneal dialysis are related to the dialysis access device, in this case

the Tenckhoff catheter. Peritonitis is the most common complication of CAPD. Fortunately, it is generally much less severe than other types of peritonitis and usually can be treated quite readily on an outpatient basis despite the continued presence of a foreign body (the Tenckhoff catheter) in the peritoneal cavity. Occasionally, an episode of peritonitis will respond poorly to antimicrobial therapy or a patient will suffer repeated episodes of peritonitis caused by the same organism; in such cases the catheter must be removed and the patient sustained on hemodialysis until the infection is completely cleared and a new catheter can be placed. Repeated infections carry the risk of permanently altering peritoneal permeability or effective surface area, which would necessitate a permanent switch to hemodialysis.

Peritonitis in patients using CAPD is presumably a result of inadvertent bacterial contamination of the dialysate or tubing during an exchange or to the extension of an infection of the exit site or subcutaneous tunnel into the peritoneal cavity. Approximately 70% of these cases are caused by *Staphylococcus aureus* or *Staphylococcus epidermidis;* most of the other cases (approximately 20%) are caused by gram-negative enteric organisms. Fungal infections are rare but are generally refractory to medical therapy and are often considered an indication for catheter removal. Polymicrobial infection suggests direct contamination from the gastrointestinal (GI) or genitourinary (GU) tract and mandates a search for a site of perforation or fistula.

The diagnosis of peritonitis is usually made when the patient notices a cloudy dialysis effluent, which corresponds to the appearance of white blood cells (WBCs) in the dialysate. Peritonitis is often accompanied by nonspecific abdominal pain, malaise, or fever.

In the emergency department the diagnosis of peritonitis is confirmed by the finding of more than 100 WBC/mm^3 in the peritoneal fluid with a predominance of neutrophils or by a positive Gram stain. A CAPD-associated peritonitis can usually be treated with an initial intraperi-

Table *44-3*

ANTIBIOTIC DOSAGES FOR TREATMENT OF CAPD-ASSOCIATED PERITONITIS

Drug	Loading Dose	Maintenance Dose
Vancomycin	30 mg/kg IP	30 mg/kg IP q5-7d
Ceftazidine	1 g IP or IV	1 g IP in one exchange daily
Gentamicin*	2 mg/kg IP or IV	20 mg/L IP in one exchange daily

*Caution: ototoxicity

toneal loading dose of an antibiotic, followed by a course of intraperitoneal antibiotics that the patient self-administers at home (Table 44-3). All patients using CAPD are taught during training how to inject antibiotics into the dialysis bags. After making the diagnosis, it is advisable to contact the patient's nephrologist or dialysis nurse specialist.

Individuals who have severe abdominal pain, vomiting, ileus, chills, high fever, or hypotension should be admitted to the hospital. Patients with severe underlying illness and those who cannot reliably perform exchanges or administer antibiotics at home also require inpatient management. Perhaps the most serious potential pitfall in caring for the patient who is using CAPD and who has abdominal pain or other signs of peritonitis is to overlook other serious intraabdominal conditions that may mimic peritonitis (e.g., appendicitis, diverticulitis, pancreatitis).

Infection. Infections of the catheter exit site are another relatively common problem. These infections tend to be caused by typical skin flora and are manifested by the usual local signs of infection. Although not serious in themselves, they should be taken seriously because they may lead to infection of the subcutaneous tunnel, in which a persistent infection can cause repeated episodes of peritonitis and ultimately necessitate removal of the catheter. Any visible exudate should be cultured and gram

stained, and an oral antibiotic such as cephalexin should be started pending the availability of culture and sensitivity results. The patient should be instructed to cleanse the site meticulously several times a day with a povidone-iodine or peroxide solution.

Tunnel infections can be difficult to detect on physical examination and may be suspected only after the patient suffers several bouts of peritonitis caused by the same organism. As with other closed-space infections, tunnel infections tend to be difficult to eradicate unless the tunnel is partially unroofed and drained.

Other complications. The patient using CAPD may also come to the emergency department with any of several basically mechanical problems; the most common problem is an inability to drain the dialysate completely at the time of an exchange. Occasionally this is simply because of kinking or inadvertent clamping of the external catheter or tubing; more often it is the result of catheter obstruction by fibrinous debris or kinking or migration of the catheter within the peritoneal cavity. Radiologic evaluation and surgical consultation are necessary.

Although patients using CAPD are instructed to weigh themselves daily and to measure their pulse and blood pressure often, some become progressively volume overloaded. The result may be only minor worsening of blood pressure control, but occasionally a patient develops acute pulmonary edema and requires immediate attention in the emergency department.

A patient using CAPD can also become volume depleted, particularly when volume continues to be removed by dialysis despite poor oral intake or significant GI fluid loss. Oral or IV rehydration and further instruction on maintaining normal volume status are generally all that is necessary.

Severe metabolic disturbances are much less common among patients using CAPD than patients using hemodialysis because with CAPD, dialysis is being performed essentially continuously and the blood remains in near-equilibrium with the dialysate. However, significant disturbances do occasionally occur, usually in association with hypercatabolic states, major dietary indiscretions, or significant gastrointestinal fluid loss.

MISCELLANEOUS PROBLEMS AMONG PATIENTS WITH END-STAGE RENAL DISEASE

Nausea and vomiting unattributable to medications, underdialysis, or the dialytic procedure itself occasionally occurs without apparent cause in many patients with ESRD. Once anatomic disease of the GI tract has been ruled out, symptomatic relief can often be obtained with standard antiemetics such as prochlorperazine or trimethobenzamide. Diabetic gastroparesis often responds to metoclopramide, but dystonic reactions may occur unless the dose has been adjusted for renal failure.

Constipation is common among patients who take aluminum- or calcium-containing antacids to bind dietary phosphate. Oral sorbitol or lactulose is generally effective in relieving constipation and does not have the potential danger of magnesium-containing cathartics.

Muscle cramps, particularly those occurring at night, are thought to be a manifestation of uremic myopathy or neuropathy that is not improved by dialysis. Cramps are usually effectively treated with oral quinine at bedtime or with a benzodiazepine.

KEY CONSIDERATIONS

WHAT IS THE LIFE THREAT?

The most lethal acute complication of renal failure is hyperkalemia. Volume overload can result in life-threatening pulmonary edema. Acute pericardial tamponade can also be life threatening.

DOES THE PATIENT NEED ADMISSION?

Patients who have acute renal failure should be admitted to the hospital. Intractable volume overload and life-threatening hyperkalemia are the most common considerations for emergency dialysis. Patients with acute or chronic renal failure who have pulmonary edema, pericardial tamponade, severe infection, severe anemia (especially with superimposed acute blood loss), or an acute mental status change are also admitted.

Acute loss of the vascular access site requires surgical consultation.

WHAT IS THE MOST SERIOUS DIAGNOSIS?

Volume overload, hyperkalemia, and hypervolemia associated with renal failure are the most serious diagnoses.

HAVE I PERFORMED A THOROUGH WORK-UP?

In cases of acute renal failure, consider prerenal, postrenal and intrarenal causes. Examine the urine sediment. Obtain BUN, creatinine, and electrolytes. Evaluate cardiac status and lungs with an ECG and a chest x-ray study.

When hyperkalemia is suspected in renal failure, obtain an ECG and measure serum potassium.

Do not assume that acute changes in mental status following dialysis are a result of disequilibrium syndrome. Be alert for infection, electrolyte abnormalities, hypoxemic states, hypotension of any cause, intracranial hemorrhage, or other toxic or metabolic causes.

Recommended Reading

Bennett WM et al: *Drug prescribing in renal failure: dosing guidelines for adults,* ed 3, Philadelphia, 1994, American College of Physicians.

Israel RS, Wolfson AB: Acute renal failure. In Rosen et al, editors: *Emergency medicine: concepts and clinical practice,* ed 3, St Louis, 1992, Mosby.

Wolfson AB: Chronic renal failure and dialysis. In Rosen et al, editors: *Emergency medicine: concepts and clinical practice,* ed 3, St Louis, 1992, Mosby.

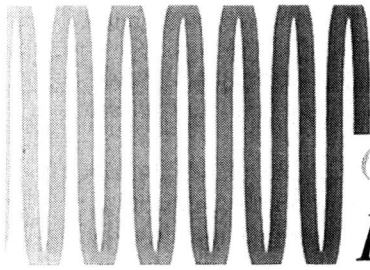

Chapter Forty-five

PREGNANCY

JEAN ABBOTT

The pregnant patient may come to the emergency department for problems specific to either early or late pregnancy. In early pregnancy, the major emergency department issues usually concern the diagnosis, location, and viability of the pregnancy. The most common complications of early pregnancy include bleeding, pain, and vomiting. After 20 weeks, bleeding and seizures are the most common urgent complications and may be life threatening to both the mother and the fetus. After 24 weeks, two patients—both mother and baby—must be considered in assessment and management.

COMPLICATIONS OF THE FIRST HALF OF PREGNANCY

General Patient Assessment

Pregnancy should be considered in all women ages 14 to 50 years who come to the emergency department with abdominal or vaginal complaints. Clinical clues include amenorrhea, breast tenderness, nausea, and increasing abdominal girth. After 12 weeks the uterus is usually palpable in the lower abdomen, and fetal heart tones may be heard with an obstetric Doppler. After 15 to 18 weeks gestation, the fetal heartbeat is usually audible by fetoscope.

Pregnancy testing is mandatory in the absence of fetal heart tones if a pregnancy-related diagnosis is being considered or if radiography

or drug administration is part of the patient's care in the emergency department. Current qualitative urine and blood tests are very accurate if they detect the beta-subunit of human chorionic gonadotropin (hCG) at levels less than 50 mIu/ml. (International Reference Preparation, or IRP). Because less accurate tests are also available to the public and to health clinics, a pregnancy should always be confirmed in the emergency department with a sensitive test that has known reliability.

The most serious complication of early pregnancy is an ectopic pregnancy. From the patient's perspective, the threat of miscarriage often is also an important concern. Because of these possibilities, the patient who experiences pain or bleeding in early pregnancy requires an assessment of the location and viability of the pregnancy (see the box on p. 548). Whether this assessment is completed at the time of the emergency department visit or is scheduled for follow-up depends on the clinical urgency of the patient's symptoms and signs.

Ultrasonography is the standard method of locating a pregnancy, particularly in a stable patient. With transabdominal ultrasonography, normal intrauterine pregnancies (IUPs) can be detected by 5 to 6 weeks gestation (time measured from the last menstrual period) or at an hCG level of 6000 to 10,000 mIu/ml (IRP). An ectopic gestation is rarely seen by transabdominal imaging. Better resolution is achieved with newer trans-

CAUSES OF BLEEDING IN PREGNANCY

Early pregnancy

Ectopic pregnancy
Miscarriage
  Threatened
  Inevitable
  Incomplete
  Complete
Gestational trophoblast (hydatidiform mole)

Late pregnancy

Placenta previa
Abruptio placentae
Vaginal/cervical infections and lesions
Bloody show (release of cervical plug)

vaginal technology; IUPs can be detected approximately 1 week sooner at an hCG level of approximately 1000 to 2000 mIu/ml IRP. Viability is diagnosed by seeing a beating fetal heart in the uterus with ultrasonography; a miscarriage is much less common with a viable fetus than with a gestation in which growth never progresses to fetal heart activity.

The other method of assessing the health of a pregnancy is to follow the stable patient with serial *quantitative hCG levels* before 6 weeks gestation and until the time in which the pregnancy is visible by ultrasonography. HCG is secreted from the time of implantation (20 to 22 days after the last menstrual period). Levels double every 2 to 3 days until approximately 6 to 7 weeks of gestation. From this time, the quantitative hCG level plateaus at approximately 100,000 mIU/ml or even drifts downward for the duration of the pregnancy.

Ectopic Pregnancy

An ectopic pregnancy (EP) accounts for approximately 10% of all maternal deaths. Hemor-

rhagic shock from EP is sometimes preventable, but delays in recognition and intervention are common.

The incidence of EP is approximately 2 cases for every 100 reported pregnancies, and this incidence has been increasing in the past several decades. Risk factors that predispose the patient to the development of EP include increased age, prior salpingitis, a previous EP, the presence of an intrauterine device (IUD), prior tubal ligation, infertility and, more recently, in vitro fertilization procedures.

The natural history of EP is quite variable. As the abnormally implanted pregnancy grows, the most dreaded complication is rupture into the peritoneal cavity with diffuse peritonitis and maternal hemorrhagic shock. However, in most cases frank rupture is preceded by irregular growth of the ectopic gestation accompanied by several days of intermittent contained hemorrhage into the surrounding tissues. Less commonly, the EP may end in abortion via the endometrial cavity or even through resorption into the fallopian tube itself.

Clinical characteristics

A wide spectrum of presentations occurs with EP, from hemorrhagic shock with diffuse peritonitis as a result of frank rupture to painless vaginal bleeding or intermittent lower abdominal cramping. The patient usually complains of lower abdominal pain, but the characteristics are quite variable: the pain may be crampy, intermittent, midline, or unilateral; peritoneal irritation may be absent, transient, or severe. Light or moderate vaginal bleeding is common and is thought to be caused by fluctuations and declines in hormone levels associated with the erratic growth of a pregnancy not supported on endometrial tissue. Eighty-five percent of those women with an EP have a history of missed menses, and more than half have at least one risk factor for EP (see the box on p. 549).

The physical findings of an EP are also nonspecific. Tenderness, either midline or unilat-

Amenorrhea
Breast tenderness
Nausea
Vaginal spotting, bleeding
Lower abdominal pain or cramping
Risk factors
   Prior ectopic pregnancy
   Prior pelvic inflammatory disease
   Tubal ligation
   Intrauterine device
   Infertility
   Fertility procedures
   Increased age

eral, is commonly noted. A mass is felt in only approximately half of all patients. Cervical motion tenderness can be a sign of peritoneal irritation, and significant hemoperitoneum may be accompanied by alterations in vital signs, which suggests blood loss. Anemia is rare. Sensitive qualitative pregnancy tests are positive in more than 98% of women with an EP.

Diagnostic strategy

Intravenous (IV) fluid resuscitation, transfusions if needed, and rapid surgical intervention are indicated in the rare patient with hypovolemic shock, diffuse peritonitis, and a suspected ruptured EP. A qualitative pregnancy test should be performed promptly, but treatment and diagnosis must sometimes be accomplished simultaneously.

A culdocentesis is the most rapid technique for confirming the diagnosis of free blood within the peritoneum. Aspiration of fluid from the posterior cul-de-sac, the most dependent portion of the peritoneal cavity, is an invasive procedure that has been superceded in stable patients by ultrasonography. However, in the unstable patient the finding of unclotted intraperitoneal blood, as

contrasted to the normal small amount of serous fluid, rapidly confirms hemoperitoneum and implies a need for surgery. Approximately 20% of all culdocenteses are nondiagnostic, with an aspiration of either no fluid or of clotted blood, which is believed to originate from pelvic veins in the noncritical patient. Further diagnostic tests are required in patients with a nondiagnostic culdocentesis.

In the stable patient, the urgency of diagnosis of an EP depends on the degree of symptomatology. Transabdominal ultrasonography is most useful in diagnosing an IUP and thus excluding an ectopic location. A positive pregnancy test and empty uterus as detected with ultrasonography raises the suspicion of an ectopic pregnancy. With transvaginal ultrasonography, a definitive diagnosis of intrauterine or ectopic gestation is more common. Serial ultrasonography or quantitative hCG levels may be required to clarify the diagnosis. Patients with an ectopic pregnancy should be discussed with a gynecologic consultant to form a treatment plan. Patients who are discharged when the diagnosis of EP is still possible should always be given careful instructions to return if pain increases or if dizziness or other signs of progressive intraabdominal bleeding develop.

Spontaneous Miscarriage

A spontaneous miscarriage or abortion is the loss of a pregnancy before the twentieth week of gestation. Approximately 15% to 25% of all pregnancies that are detectable by newer sensitive pregnancy tests end in miscarriage, and 80% to 90% of these miscarriages occur in the first trimester. Risk factors for miscarriage include multiple prior miscarriages, increased age, and increased parity. The pathologic examination of the products of miscarriage reveals a number of possible causes: fetal genetic defects, failure of the embryo to develop (anembryonic gestation), or abnormal host factors such as an inadequate endometrium.

Classification

A *threatened* miscarriage is defined as uterine bleeding associated with an IUP of less than 20 weeks gestation. The internal cervical os is closed, and the risk of miscarriage in such women is 50% to 80%. An *inevitable* miscarriage occurs when the internal os opens; the expulsion of the conceptus can be expected. An *incomplete* miscarriage occurs when there has been a partial expulsion of the products of conception and may be associated with a severe vaginal hemorrhage through the open cervical os. The hemorrhage may often be slowed by removing the tissue in the os with a ring forceps at the time of the pelvic examination, which allows the cervix and uterus to contract and control bleeding.

A *completed* miscarriage occurs when the entire fetus, placenta, and decidual lining are completely evacuated from the uterus. A spontaneous complete miscarriage occurs most often in the second trimester. To ensure prompt completion of the miscarriage, a dilatation and curettage (D and C) is usually performed if the cervical os is open. When no D and C is performed, a completed miscarriage is confirmed by the relief of cramping and bleeding and the fall of quantitative hCG measurements to zero within 2 to 4 weeks. A history of tissue passage is difficult to interpret, because clots and slough of the endometrial lining can appear similar to pregnancy tissue and because the cervical os can close intermittently during expulsion of the pregnancy. In the emergency department the diagnosis of a completed miscarriage should be made only if the intact fetus can be identified either visually or by pathologic analysis. In unclear cases, completion is diagnosed at follow-up with a gynecologist if the bleeding and cramping resolve and the pregnancy test converts to "negative."

A *missed abortion* is a relatively obsolete term for the diagnosis of fetal death or a failure of uterine growth before clinical miscarriage symptoms occur. With the extensive use of ultrasonography in modern first-trimester diagno-sis, it is now known that fetal death often occurs at least 1 or 2 weeks before bleeding and cramping start. A more appropriate diagnosis for women who have fetal death detected by ultrasonography but have no or few symptoms would be "first- (or second-) trimester fetal demise." Management consists of a gynecologic referral for confirmation of the fetal demise and timely evacuation of the pregnancy.

Hydatidiform Mole

A hydatidiform mole (gestational trophoblastic disease) occurs when abnormal villi develop (usually without fetal development), which creates a cystic cluster of placental tissue that fills the uterus. Malignant degeneration of the trophoblast can occur. Symptoms of this disease usually occur early in the second trimester and include abdominal cramping and bleeding. The uterus may be larger than would be expected, and hCG levels are usually extremely high. Early pregnancy-induced hypertension can be seen, and the passage of the grapelike abnormal placental tissue may occur. Ultrasonography shows the absence of a fetus and a snowstorm appearance resulting from the proliferation of abnormal villi in the uterus. Treatment consists of obstetric consultation for evacuation of the pregnancy tissue and close monitoring by a gyncologic specialist for signs of malignant change.

Hyperemesis Gravidarum

Nausea and vomiting occur in more than 70% of all pregnant women. The incidence peaks at the end of the first trimester (between 8 and 14 weeks of gestation). Hyperemesis gravidarum is the term given to a condition in a small subset of women who develop severe dehydration, prolonged ketosis, and weight loss. Incidence is increased in younger, nulliparous females and in those who have an increased body weight. Circulating hormone levels appear to be increased in this group of patients. The fetal outcome of women with this condition is probably at least as good as that in women who do not have significant nausea as long as their ketosis and starvation physiology can be controlled.

Treatment in the emergency department consists of IV fluid repletion by the administration of dextrose-containing crystalloid (D5NS or D5LR) and the use of parenteral antiemetics (almost all are considered safer than prolonged ketosis in pregnancy). Fluid repletion usually continues until IV volume is restored and the patient can take adequate fluids by mouth. Consideration should be given to alternative diagnoses, such as pyelonephritis or hepatitis, particularly in women with a sudden onset of vomiting or symptoms that begin in the second or third trimester. Women should be taught to develop strategies for retaining fluids and calories, including eating small meals, ingesting simple carbohydrates, and consuming protein-containing snacks before bed.

EMERGENCIES IN THE SECOND HALF OF PREGNANCY

Physiologic Changes

Physiologic changes in pregnancy particularly affect the assessment and patient management in the second half of pregnancy. Normal maternal vital signs reflect the hypermetabolism and vasodilatation characteristic of pregnancy. The baseline pulse is usually in the 80 to 90 beats/minute range. Blood pressure during pregnancy is never normally higher than the patient's prepregnancy normal; elevations suggest chronic hypertension or preeclampsia. Respirations are usually slightly increased, at 18 to 20 per minute, with an increased tidal ventilation. There is a mild respiratory alkalosis, and PCO_2 measurements of 32 to 36 mm Hg are common. The alveolar-arterial oxygen gradient is increased, but measurements greater than 20 are considered abnormal. With high diaphragms, residual volume is reduced. Pregnant women are less able to compensate for respiratory or cardiovascular in-

sults related to trauma or medical illnesses.

Blood analysis shows an anemia, with hematocrits running approximately 32% to 34%, even with iron supplementation. The white blood cell count gradually increases through pregnancy to a normal of 15,000/mm^3 in the third trimester and 25,000/mm^3 during delivery. Pregnancy is a hypercoagulable state, and plasma proteins and fibrinogen levels (pregnancy normals are approximately 450 mg/dl) are increased.

Smooth muscle relaxation as a result of increased progesterone levels causes ureteral dilatation, an increased risk of both gastric and ureteral reflux, and slower bowel motility.

In response to hypovolemia and other physiologic stresses, the pregnant woman has a compromised ability to compensate, and much of the physiologic compensation is at the expense of the fetus. Hypovolemia causes early constriction of uterine vascular beds to maintain the maternal circulation. Hypoxemia and hypercarbia also cause uterine vasoconstriction and early impairment of fetal well-being.

Supine hypotension is another physiologic consideration during the second half of pregnancy. Supine positioning results in the compression of the inferior vena cava by the mass of the uterus. In some women, abdominal collaterals allow adequate venous return to the heart. However, in other women, a 20% to 30% decrease in cardiac output can result from supine positioning. To prevent this problem, women of more than 20 weeks gestation should always be kept on their side or be tilted at least 15 degrees toward their left side during treatment in the emergency department.

Bleeding in the Second Half of Pregnancy

Major causes of bleeding during the second half of pregnancy include placenta previa (20%) and abruptio placentae (30%) (see the box on p. 548). Other causes include cervical or vaginal inflammation or infection, bloody show (a mucous plug released by the cervix usually just before the onset of labor) or early labor, and polyps or other local lesions. In many cases, the cause is not determined, but small marginal separations of the placenta (marginal abruptio placentae) are believed to be a major cause.

Abruptio placentae

Abruptio placentae refers to the separation of the placenta from its normal implantation site on the uterine wall before delivery. Separation may occur at the margins or centrally, and it may involve only a small portion of the placental surface area or the entire placenta. Because the placenta functions to allow the transfer of maternal red blood cells and oxygen to the fetus, fetal distress or death can occur if a sufficient amount of placenta is separated from the uterine wall. Factors that predispose a woman to abruptio placentae include maternal hypertension, increased maternal age and parity, and a history of smoking. Abruptio placentae is also more common in women who use cocaine and other vasospastic drugs. Traumatic placental separation is associated with blunt forces to the abdomen that shear all or part of the nonelastic placenta from the elastic uterine wall.

Symptoms of abruptio placentae include variable uterine bleeding that is often dark and not usually severe. Uterine pain is also common. Signs include bleeding on examination and firmness and tenderness of the contracting uterine muscle. Because blood loss can be hidden, maternal signs of shock may exceed the degree of visible vaginal bleeding. Fetal heart rate may be decreased or absent if the fetus is distressed or dead.

Emergency management includes establishing IV access, continually monitoring the fetal heart rate to determine fetal health, and assessing and restoring the maternal blood volume. In addition to being occult, blood loss may be aggravated by coagulopathy, which can develop from the consumption of coagulation factors at the uterine wall–placental interface. Ultrasonography can be used to monitor visible subplacental hemorrhages but only detects approximately half of all significant placental abruptions.

Placenta previa

Placenta previa refers to the implantation of the placenta over the cervical os. Placenta previa is common in the midtrimester but is seen in less than 1% of pregnancies at term. Risk factors include a prior cesarean section and multiparity.

The characteristic symptom of placenta previa is bright red, painless vaginal bleeding. Bleeding tends to be minor and intermittent and persists throughout the third trimester. The bleeding usually becomes severe only during labor or when the placenta has been dislodged by a vaginal examination.

The identification of placenta previa by ultrasonography is highly accurate. When the diagnosis is suspected and bleeding is present, the patient should be transported to an operating room for vaginal evaluation, where it is possible to proceed to emergent cesarean section if necessary. The possibility of placenta previa is the reason that *no* cervical probing is indicated after 20 weeks of gestation. A perineal examination and cautious examination of the vagina is indicated in the stable woman with scant bleeding to identify other sources of bleeding, such as hemorrhoids or local lesions, and to identify the cervical os as the source of bleeding.

Management of bleeding in the second half of pregnancy

The management of the patient who is of more than 20 weeks gestation involves consideration of both the mother and a potentially viable fetus. The patient should be resuscitated if necessary and transported to the Labor Deck immediately. The box on p. 552 outlines the steps in management when an immediate obstetric examination is not possible or the patient requires transfer.

Eclampsia or Pregnancy-Induced Hypertension

Eclampsia is a vasospastic disease of unknown cause and is unique to pregnant women. Uncontrolled vasospasm can lead to ischemia and thrombosis in the small vessels of a wide variety of organs, which causes renal failure, liver dam-

<table>
<tr><td>

EMERGENCY MANAGEMENT OF VAGINAL BLEEDING IN THE SECOND HALF OF PREGNANCY

Intravenous access and maternal fluid resuscitation

Fetal heart rate monitoring

Baseline hematocrit, coagulation studies, Rh

Ultrasonography in the stable patient to diagnose placenta previa

Immediate obstetric consultation for significant bleeding

Careful external perineal examination in stable patient to exclude local lesions

Fresh whole blood or fresh frozen plasma for patients with signs of disseminated intravascular coagulation

Rh immunoglobulin for Rh-negative mother and Rh-positive (or unknown) father

Transfer to obstetrics care or high-risk referral

</td><td>

SIGNS AND SYMPTOMS OF PREECLAMPSIA IN PREGNANCY

Hypertension

Exaggerated peripheral edema

Proteinuria

Visual disturbances

Headache, apprehension

Epigastric or right upper quadrant pain

Hyperreflexia

</td></tr>
</table>

age, hemolysis, thrombocytopenia, and central nervous system injury (see the box above, right).

Hypertension is defined as an absolute blood pressure of 140/90 mm Hg or higher. This includes readings that are well within the "normal" range of the general nonpregnant population, yet a rising blood pressure must not be taken lightly. The risk of preeclampsia and eclampsia is increased in young women (<20 years of age), primagravid women, those with a family history of eclampsia, those with a history of hypertension (either associated with prior pregnancies or when not pregnant), and those with twin or molar pregnancies.

Diagnosis

Hypertension, exaggerated edema, and proteinuria that develop during pregnancy or the puerperium are the most well-recognized signs of preeclampsia. Headache, apprehension, liver tenderness, hyperreflexia, or visual disturbances are especially significant warning signs that

preeclampsia is severe and that eclampsia may be imminent.

Eclampsia is defined as the development of seizures or coma in the woman with preeclampsia. Seizures can occur in the third trimester, peripartum, or in the first postpartum week. Both preeclampsia and eclampsia are associated with significant maternal and fetal mortality.

Management

The patient with mild preeclampsia should be referred promptly to an obstetrician for ongoing care. Emergency treatment is the same for both severe preeclampsia and eclampsia. Initial laboratory studies should be drawn to assess end-organ injury: liver and renal function studies, a complete blood count, and coagulation studies. IV access should be established. The preferred drug to treat eclamptic seizures or severe preeclampsia is magnesium sulfate, a peripheral vasodilator and membrane stabilizer, 6 grams IV over 15 minutes, with a 2 gm/hour maintenance drip. Although not a specific antihypertensive, magnesium sulfate treatment is often associated with a decrease in blood pressure to a safe range (<160/110). Benzodiazepines such as diazepam (Valium) have also been used to control eclamptic seizures.

If hypertension does not readily decrease, hydralazine 5 mg IV repeated every 20 minutes is recommended to keep the diastolic blood pressure below 110 mm Hg. Nifedipine and labetalol can also be used. Because a fall in blood pressure may result in decreased fetal perfusion, these medications should be used only to titrate the diastolic pressure reading to between 100 and 110 mm Hg. The blood pressure should be monitored continuously, and a CT scan of the head may be indicated if the patient does not respond promptly to the above management.

Women with severe preeclampsia or eclampsia should be hospitalized. The definitive treatment of eclampsia involves delivery of the baby once the mother has been stabilized; a vaginal delivery is usually recommended. The management of the woman with a very premature fetus is still debated because both delivery and observation can be associated with significant morbidity to mother and baby.

Premature Rupture of Membranes

Premature rupture of membranes is associated with increased rates of premature labor, peripartum infection (with associated increases in fetal morbidity and mortality), and postpartum hemorrhage.

Amniotic fluid leakage can be tested and confirmed by the presence of vaginal fluid with a pH of 7.0 to 7.5. Because of the sodium chloride content of the amniotic fluid and the paucity of protein, drying amniotic fluid on a laboratory slide gives a typical ferning crystal pattern. Visualizing the cervix during a cough or Valsalva maneuver is also useful and may direct fluid sampling to test for amniotic fluid. Women with a premature rupture of membranes should have an obstetric consultation and be monitored for fetal heart rate and uterine contractions.

⫸KEY CONSIDERATIONS

WHAT IS THE LIFE THREAT?

During the first half of pregnancy the major life threat is a ruptured ectopic pregnancy. During the second half of pregnancy, threats involve both the mother and the unborn child and include placenta previa, abruptio placentae, preeclampsia, and eclampsia.

DOES THE PATIENT NEED ADMISSION?

Admit patients with a known or ruptured ectopic pregnancy. Asymptomatic patients in whom the diagnosis has not been established can be discharged with the assurance of close gynecologic follow-up. Patients with a threatened miscarriage can usually be discharged unless bleeding is excessive, hemoglobin is low, or vital signs suggest significant hemorrhage. Those with incomplete miscarriages can be admitted for dilatation and curettage.

Patients with hyperemesis are usually managed as outpatients, but those with intractable vomiting that is unresponsive to antiemetics may require admission. During the second half of pregnancy, admit patients with vaginal bleeding, preeclampsia, or eclampsia.

WHAT IS THE MOST SERIOUS DIAGNOSIS?

In the first 20 weeks, ectopic pregnancy is the most serious diagnosis. In the second 20 weeks, placenta previa and abruptio placentae are the most serious diagnoses.

HAVE I PERFORMED A THOROUGH WORK-UP?

Consider an ectopic pregnancy in women with abdominal pain. In women of childbearing age, order a pregnancy test if low abdominal pain is present. Evaluate the severity of bleeding in the early pregnancy with a good history and assessment of vital signs.

Evaluate fetal heart tones.

Recommended Reading

Abbott JT: Complications related to pregnancy. In Rosen P et al, editors: *Emergency medicine: concepts and clinical practice*, ed 3, St Louis, 1992, Mosby.

Abbott JT et al: Ectopic pregnancy: ten common pitfalls in diagnosis, *AM J Emerg Med* 8:515, 1990.

Barnhart K et al: Prompt diagnosis of ectopic pregnancy in an emergency department setting, *Obstet Gynecol* 84:1010, 1994.

Cunningham FG et al: Hypertension in pregnancy, *N Engl J Med* 326:927, 1992.

Hod M et al: Hyperemesis gravidarum: a review, *J Reprod Med* 39:605, 1994.

Chapter *Forty-six*
HEMATOLOGIC DISORDERS

GLENN C. HAMILTON

To facilitate the approach to hematologic disorders, the hemogram is divided into its components: red blood cells, the hemostatic elements—vascular integrity, platelets, and coagulation factors—and white blood cells. Approaching any hematologic problem by categorizing it into one of these three components generally allows a focused diagnostic pursuit early in the course of care.

RED BLOOD CELL DISORDERS

Red blood cell (RBC) disorders are manifest as an alteration in the absolute numbers of red cells or as changes in RBC morphology, which results in complications. Normal values of red blood cell number measurements and red blood cell morphologic indices must be understood (Tables 46-1 and 46-2).

Anemia

Anemia is defined as an absolute decrease in circulating red blood cells. It is usually diagnosed when hemoglobin concentrations fall below the normal range for a patient's age group (see Table 46-2). Anemia is caused by several mechanisms (Table 46-3).

Clinically, anemia may result in impaired oxygen transport. Oxygen transport is influenced by the amount of hemoglobin, its oxygen affinity, and blood flow. Anemia may produce compensatory changes in cardiac function and stimulate erythropoiesis. The patient's presentation reflects the rapidity of the evolution of the anemia. A rapid onset of anemia (blood loss or sudden hemolysis) is accompanied by headache, dizziness, postural hypotension, tachycardia, hypovolemia, and high-output failure. The attenuated history of and physical examination for rapid onset or severe anemia is listed in the box on p. 558.

The insidious onset of anemia from a nutritional deficiency, underlying disease, leukemia, or a gastrointestinal or menstrual blood loss may cause pallor, fatigue, and decreased exercise tolerance. Vital signs may be normal, but orthostatic changes may also be noted. Ultimately,

Table **46-1**

CONCENTRATIONS OF HEMOGLOBIN BY AGE

Age	Hemoglobin	Hematocrit
3 months	10.4-12.2	30-36
3-7 years	11.7-13.5	34-40
Adult men	14.0-18.0	40-52
Adult women	12.0-16.0	35-47

Table 46-2

CALCULATION OF RED BLOOD CELL INDICES AND NORMAL VALUES

Index	Formula for Calculation	Normal Range
Mean corpuscular volume	Hematocrit (%) divided by red blood cell count ($10^6/\mu L$)	81-100 μm^3
Mean corpuscular hemoglobin	Hemoglobin (g/dl) divided by red blood cell count ($10^6/\mu L$)	26-34 pg
Mean corpuscular hemoglobin concentration	Hemoglobin (g/dl) divided by hematocrit (%)	31%-36%

Modified from Maslow WC et al: *Practical diagnosis: hematologic disease*, Boston, 1980, Houghton-Mifflin.

Table 46-3

CAUSES OF ANEMIA

Disease	Mechanism
Impaired Red Blood Cell Production, Maturation, or Release from the Bone Marrow	
Malignancy, storage disease	Infiltration
Fanconi anemia drugs, Diamond-Blackfan anemia, transient erythroblastopenia of childhood (TEC), aplastic anemia	Aplasia, hypoplasia
Folate, B_{12}, B_6, copper deficiency	Impaired maturation of red cell precursors in bone marrow
Thalassemia syndromes, lead poisoning, sideroblastic anemia, pyridoxine deficiency	Impaired hemoglobin production, intramedullary hemolysis (thalassemias)
Chronic disease, inflammation, renal disease, hypothyroidism	Impaired erythropoiesis
Destruction, Sequestration, or Acute Loss of Circulating Red Blood Cells	
Sickle cell disease, vitamin E deficiency, autoimmune hemolytic anemia, RBC enzyme deficiency, RBC membrane defect, hemolytic-uremic syndrome (HUS), disseminated intravascular coagulation (DIC), hemangioma, cardiac defect, prosthetic heart valve	Hemolysis
Portal hypertension, sickle cell disease	Splenic sequestration
Trauma, surgery, bleeding disorder, peptic ulcer disease	Hemorrhage

---

HISTORY AND PHYSICAL EXAMINATION FOR EMERGENT ANEMIA

History

General
  Prehospital status, therapy, and response to
    therapy
  Bleeding diathesis
  Previous blood transfusion
  Underlying diseases, including allergies
  Current medications, especially those causing
    platelet inhibition
Trauma
  Nature and time of injury
  Blood loss at scene
  Tetanus immunization
  Time of last meal
Nontrauma
  Skin: petechiae, ecchymoses
  Gastrointestinal: hematemesis, hematochezia,
    peptic ulcer
  Genitourinary: menorrhagia, metorrhagia, last
    menstruation, hematuria

Physical examination

Vital signs measured serially
  Blood pressure, pulse, respiratory rate
  Orthostatic blood pressure and pulse
    (contraindicated with severe hypotension)
Level and content of consciousness
Skin
  Pallor
  Diaphoresis
  Jaundice
  Cyanosis
  Purpura, ecchymoses, petechiae
  Examine completely for penetrating wounds
Cardiovascular
  Murmurs, S_3, S_4
  Quality of femoral and carotid pulse
Abdomen
  Hepatosplenomegaly
  Pain, guarding, rebound on palpation
Rectal and pelvic examination
  Masses
  Pain, guarding, rebound on palpation
  Stool hemoglobin testing

---

high-output failure and other evidence of volume deficit may be evident.

Differential considerations require an initial laboratory investigation, including a complete blood count (CBC) with a hemoglobin (Hb), hematocrits (Hct), and RBC indices; a peripheral smear, and a reticulocyte count. Microcytic anemia manifests as a reduced mean corpuscular volume (MCV) (see Table 46-2). It suggests an iron deficiency because this is the most common cause of this type of anemia. Microcytic anemia is often associated with a decreased mean corpuscular hemoglobin (MCH). The evaluation of a suspected iron deficiency anemia includes measuring serum iron, total iron binding capacity (TIBC), free-erythrocyte protoporphyrin (FEP), or serum ferritin. An iron satura-

tion (serum iron/TIBC $\times$ 100) of less than 20% is indicative of an iron deficiency but is subject to greater error because of diurnal and acute diet-related fluctuations in serum iron. An FEP greater than 35 µg/dL of whole blood is typical of an iron deficiency. An FEP greater than 100 µg/dL of whole blood strongly suggests lead poisoning. Serum ferritin levels are the best means of assessing iron stores. The normal range in adult men is 20 to 500 µg/L, with a mean of 90 µg/L. In women, the range is 10 to 200 µg/L, with a mean of 35 µg/L. Mean serum ferritin levels in patients with an iron deficiency are 3 to 6 µg/L. The emergency physician should evaluate the patient's urine and stool for blood, examine the patient for other sources of blood loss, and assess underlying chronic physical conditions.

Sickle Cell and Hemolytic Anemia

Sickle cell anemia is an important hemolytic anemia for emergency physicians. Hemolytic anemias are defined by the shortened life span of the RBC. Other hemolytic anemias are listed in the box below).

CLASSIFICATION OF HEMOLYTIC ANEMIAS

Intrinsic

Enzyme defects
  Glucose-6-phosphate dehydrogenase
    deficiency
  Pyruvate kinase
Membrane abnormality
  Spherocytosis
  Elliptostomatocytosis
  Paroxysmal nocturnal hemoglobinuria
  Spur-cell anemia
Hemoglobin abnormality
  Hemoglobinopathies
  Thalassemias (discussed with microcytic
    anemias)
  Unstable hemoglobin
  Hemoglobin M

Extrinsic

Immunologic
  Alloantibodies
  Autoantibodies
Mechanical
  Microangiopathic hemolytic anemia
  Cardiovascular, such as prosthetic heart
    valve disease
Environmental
  Drugs
  Toxins
  Infections
  Thermal
Abnormal sequestrations as in hypersplenism

From Hamilton GC, Braen GR: Anemia and white blood cell disorders. In Rosen P et al, editors: *Emergency medicine: concepts and clinical practice*, St Louis, 1992, Mosby.

Sickle cell disease is an inherited disorder of hemoglobin synthesis and results from a single amino acid substitution in the beta subunit of the hemoglobin molecule. Homozygotes for the sickle gene produce a predominance of sickle hemoglobin and develop symptomatic sickle cell anemia. Sickle cell–(SC) hemoglobin C disease and ß-thalassemia are less common variants with similar but less significant clinical manifestations. Heterozygotes for the sickle gene produce both sickle (S) and normal adult (A) hemoglobin and remain symptomatic carriers of the sickle trait, except with severe hypoxemia.

The clinical presentation of sickle cell and hemolytic anemia is one of a chronic progressive illness punctuated by acute episodes. Anemic crises result from a sickling of erythrocytes with acute hemolytic anemia. A splenic sequestration crisis occurs in young children between the ages of 6 months and 6 years who suddenly pool peripheral blood volume in the spleen. This pooling results in massive splenomegaly, severe anemia, and hypovolemic shock that evolves over a period of hours to days. An aplastic crisis may result from the impairment of red blood cell production in the bone marrow after an infection and can lead to profound anemia and congestive heart failure.

Vasoocclusive crises occur because of the less deformable nature of the erythrocytes, which leads to recurrent thromboses of the microvasculature. Local ischemia and tissue infarction result. Sickling is enhanced by dehydration, hypoxemia, acidosis, and hypertonicity. The potential for organ damage in patients with recurrent vasoocclusive injury is unlimited.

With sickle cell and hemolytic anemia, infection is common because of altered immune competence and functional asplenia. The likelihood of bacterial infection is increased when there are more than 1000/mm^3 nonsegmented neutrophils in the CBC. Causative organisms include the following:

- **Sepsis (nonfocal):** *Streptococcus pneumoniae, Haemophilus influenzae*

Table 46-4

HEMATOLOGIC VALUES IN SICKLE CELL ANEMIA

	Normal Values	Sickle Cell (SS) Disease	
		Average	Range
Hemoglobin (g/dl)	12	7.5	5.5-9.5
Hematocrit (%)	36	22	17-29
Reticulocytes (%)	1.5	12	5-30
WBC count (per mm^3)	7500	20,000	12,000-35,000

From Pearson HA, Diamond LK: In Smith CA, editor: *The critically ill child*, Philadelphia, 1985, WB Saunders.

- Meningitis: *S. pneumoniae, H. influenzae*
- Pneumonia: *S. pneumoniae, H. influenzae, Mycoplasma pneumoniae*
- Osteomyelitis: *Salmonella organisms, Staphylococcus aureus, S. pneumoniae*

Laboratory evaluation should include a CBC, reticulocyte count (Table 46-4), hemoglobin electrophoresis, and specific studies for clinical presentation. Basic treatment measures for vasoocclusive crises that appear in the emergency department include oxygenation, hydration, adequate analgesia, and a search for precipitating factors and evolving organ damage. A small population of patients with sickle cell disease are frequent visitors to the emergency department. This group must be managed with constant vigilance for serious complications and with a mutually acceptable approach to pain therapy.

Polycythemia

Increased red blood cell content causes excessive blood viscosity. As the hematocrit rises to above 60%, the viscosity increases in an exponential fashion, which leads to reduced tissue flow, thrombosis, and hemorrhage. Polycythemia may be relative and caused by dehydration or by stress associated with hypertension or obesity.

Primary polycythemia vera is a myeloproliferative disorder that occurs predominantly in middle-aged or older patients. Secondary polycythemia may be caused by increased erythropoietin in response to relative hypoxemia (right-to-left shunt, pulmonary disease, high altitude) or on an autonomous basis (renal carcinoma or hydronephrosis, uterine fibroids, hepatoma, cerebellar hemangioma).

Clinically, patients may develop hypervolemia (vertigo, dizziness, blurred vision, headache), hyperviscosity (venous thrombosis), and platelet dysfunction (epistaxis, spontaneous bruising, and gastrointestinal bleeding). Plethora, engorged conjunctiva, and venous congestion (splenomegaly, congestive heart failure) may be noted. Treatment of symptomatic patients requires a phlebotomy, usually to lower the hematocrit below 60%. Polycythemia vera may require alkylating agents or radioactive phosphorus.

HEMOSTATIC DISORDERS

Abnormal bleeding may appear as prolonged bleeding associated with minor injuries, diffuse petechiae or ecchymoses, or spontaneous bleeding from mucous membranes. Many of the he-

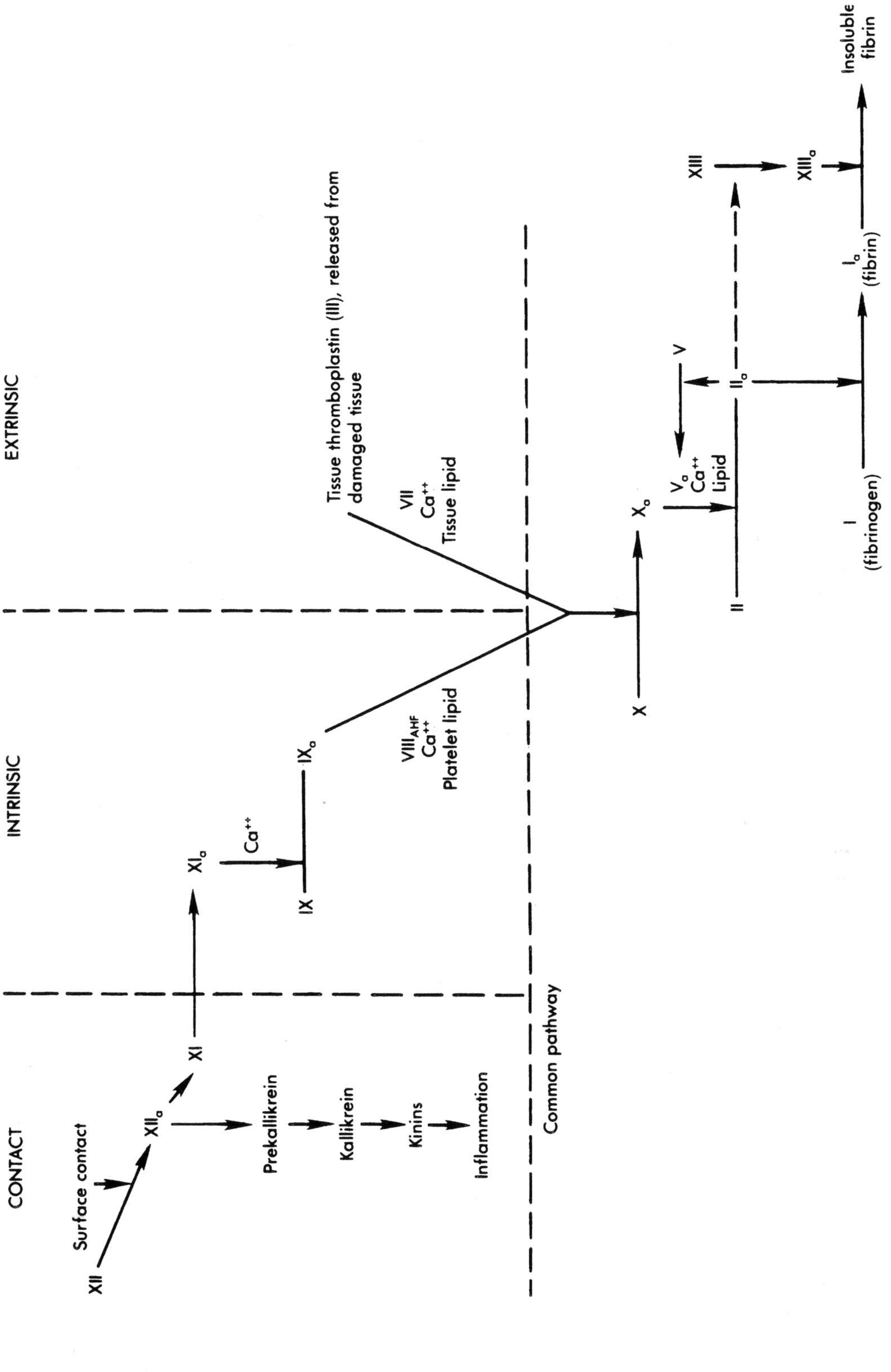

Fig. 46-1 Coagulation pathway.

Table 46-5

PATTERNS OF BLEEDING

Diagnostic Findings	Small-vessel Hemostasis Defect (Platelet or Capillary)	Intravascular Defect (Coagulation)
Bleeding Pattern		
Spontaneous	Small, superficial, diffuse bleeding involving mucous membranes (epistaxis, GI, menorrhagia)	Major bleeding (musculoskeletal, CNS)
Superficial cut or abrasion	Profuse, prolonged	Minimal
Deep cut or tooth extraction	Immediate; good response to pressure	Delayed; poor response to pressure
Hemarthrosis	Rare	Common
Petechiae	Common	Rare
Ancillary Data	Prolonged bleeding time Abnormal platelets	Prolonged PTT, PT

From Barkin R, Rosen P: *Emergency pediatrics: a guide to ambulatory care,* ed 4, St Louis, 1994, Mosby.

mostatic disorders seen in the emergency department are medication related (e.g., aspirin or Coumadin).

Hemostasis requires the integration of vasculature, platelets, and coagulation factors. Vascular integrity is maintained by a lining of nonreactive, overlapping endothelial cells. Platelets participate in primary hemostasis and serve to stop blood loss when reinforced by a fibrin clot. The coagulation pathway controls the formation of fibrin clots on the basis of a complex system of enzymatic stimuli and inhibitions (Fig. 46-1).

As noted in Table 46-5, the history of bleeding is useful in differentiating the two major categories of hemostatic disorders. The pattern of bleeding, its location, and whether it is spontaneous or a response to minor or major trauma are central factors. A family history of similar problems may indicate a hereditary basis for the bleeding disorder. A focused history and physical examination are essential for a clear understanding of the problem and its potential origin (see the box on p. 563).

A laboratory evaluation is the best method for determining the nature and origin of any bleeding diathesis. Laboratory tests to evaluate disordered hemostasis must include the following:
- CBC, blood smear, and platelet count
- Partial thromboplastin time (PTT)
- Prothrombin time (PT)
- Bleeding time
- Adjunctive tests (such as fibrinogen level and factor assay)

A diagnostic application of these tests for screening the bleeding patient is outlined in Table 46-6.

Vascular Disorders

Vascular disorders may be inherited abnormalities of connective tissue, such as Ehlers-Danlos syndrome or osteogenesis imperfecta, or of blood vessels such as hemorrhagic telangiectasia. Acquired conditions may include scurvy, steroid use, or vascular damage such as that found in meningococcemia, azotemia, hypox-

---

EVALUATION OF THE BLEEDING PATIENT

History

Nature of bleeding
   Petechiae
   Purpura
   Ecchymosis
   Significant bleeding episodes
Sites of bleeding
   Skin
   Mucosa: oral or nasal
   Muscle
   Gastrointestinal
   Genitourinary
   Joints
Pattern of bleeding
   Recent onset or lifelong
   Frequency and severity
   Spontaneous or postinjury
   Challenges to hemostasis: tooth extraction,
     operative procedures
   Association with medication, particularly
     aspirin
Medications
Associated diseases
   Uremia
   Liver disease
   Infection
Malignancy
Previous transfusion
Family history

Physical examination

Vital signs
Skin: nature of bleeding, signs of liver disease
Mucosa: oral or nasal
Lymphadenopathy
Abdomen: liver size and shape, splenomegaly
Joints: signs of previous bleeding
Other sites of blood loss: pelvic, rectal, urinary
   tract

Laboratory tests (see text)

Complete blood count and smear (EDTA—
   purple top)
Platelet count (EDTA—purple top)
Bleeding time
PT (citrate—blue top)
PTT (citrate—blue top)
Other coagulation studies: fibrinogen level,
   thrombin time, clot solubility, factor levels,
   inhibitor screens
As necessary: electrolytes, glucose, blood urea
   nitrogen, creatinine, type and crossmatch

---

emia, snakebites, and thrombotic thrombocytopenia purpura. Vascular disorders are manifest with signs and symptoms similar to thrombocytopenic conditions.

Platelet Disorders

Thrombocytopenia is caused by a decreased production, a pooling, or an increased destruction of platelets (see the box on p. 565). Immune thrombocytopenia is associated with increased peripheral destruction of platelets and a shortened survival time. It is caused by an antibody associated with collagen-vascular diseases (sys-temic lupus erythematosus), drugs (quinine, quinidine, digitoxin, sulfonamides, phenytoin, heparin), infections (postrubella, rubeola, varicella). It can also follow transfusions and can have an idiopathic autoimmune basis.

Idiopathic thrombocytopenic purpura (ITP) in its acute form occurs most commonly in children following a viral prodrome. Bleeding complications may include intracranial hemorrhage, gastrointestinal (GI) bleeding, and hematuria. The course is self-limited, with a 90% rate of spontaneous remission. Chronic ITP is primarily found in adults, more commonly in women, and it is often associated with autoimmune, collagen-

Table 46-6

SCREENING OF THE BLEEDING PATIENT

Condition	Platelet Count 150-400,000/ml	BT 4-9 min	PTT 25-35 sec	PT 12-13 sec	TT 8-10 sec	Comments Fibrinogen 190-400 mg/dl
Normal (WNL) (varies with laboratory)						
Hereditary Disorders						
Hemophilia						
Factor VIII (classic: A)	WNL	WNL	↑	WNL	WNL	Factor assay
Factor IX (Christmas: B)	WNL	WNL	↑	WNL	WNL	Factor assay
Factor XI	WNL	WNL	↑	WNL	WNL	Factor assay
Factor XII	WNL	WNL	↑	WNL	WNL	Factor assay
Factor II, V, X	WNL	WNL	↑	↑	WNL	Factor assay
Factor VII	WNL	WNL	WNL	↑	WNL	Factor assay
von Willebrand (many variants)	WNL	↑	↑	WNL	WNL	VIII antigen, VIII cofactor, ristocetin cofactor
Platelet dysfunction	WNL/↓	↑	WNL	WNL	WNL	Platelet aggregation studies
Acquired Disorders						
Disseminated intravascular coagulation	↓	↑	↑	↑	↑	↓Fibrinogen, ↑fibrin split products
Idiopathic thrombocytopenic purpura	↓	↑	WNL	WNL	WNL	
Henoch-Schönlein purpura	WNL	WNL	WNL	WNL	WNL	
Liver failure (severe)	WNL/↓	WNL/↑	↑	↑	WNL/↑	↓Fibrinogen, ↑fibrin split products
Uremia	WNL/↓	↑	WNL	WNL	WNL/↑	Caused by hepatic dysfunction or protein loss
Anticoagulants						
Heparin	WNL	WNL	↑	WNL/↑	↑↑	Also lupus-like and inactivating anticoagulant
Coumadin	WNL	WNL	WNL/↑	↑	WNL	
Aspirin	WNL	↑	WNL	WNL	WNL	

From Barkin RM, Rosen P: *Emergency pediatrics: a guide to ambulatory care,* ed 4, St Louis, 1994, Mosby.

DIFFERENTIAL DIAGNOSIS OF PLATELET DISORDERS

Thrombocytopenia

Decreased production
   Decreased megakaryocytes caused by drugs,
      toxins, or infection
   Normal megakaryocytes with megaloblastic
      hemopoiesis or hereditary origin
Platelet pooling and splenic sequestration
Increased destruction
   Immunologic
      Related to collagen-vascular disease,
         lymphoma, leukemia
      Drug related
      Posttransfusion
      Infection
      Idiopathic (autoimmune)
         thrombocytopenic purpura
   Mechanical or toxic
      Disseminated intravascular coagulation
      Thrombotic thrombocytopenic purpura
      Hemolytic uremic syndrome
      Vasculitis
Dilutional resulting from massive blood
   transfusion

Abnormal platelet function

Adhesion defects such as von Willebrand disease
Acquired and drug-related release defects
Aggregation defects such as in thrombasthenia

Thrombocytosis

Autonomous (primary thrombocythemia)
Reactive (secondary thrombocythemia)
   Iron deficiency
   Infection/inflammatory
   Trauma
   Nonhematologic malignancy
   Postsplenectomy
   Rebound from alcohol, cytotoxic drug
      therapy, folate/vitamin B_{12} deficiency

vascular, or malignant diseases. Its onset is insidious and usually is manifest with easy bruising, prolonged menses, and mucosal bleeding. Platelet counts usually range from 30,000 to 100,000/ mm^3. Treatment of the chronic presentation may require platelet transfusion, steroids, splenectomy and, in refractory cases, immunosuppressive therapy.

Nonimmune thrombocytopenia is caused by excessive destruction from consumption or mechanical problems. Thrombotic thrombocytopenic purpura is associated with extensive subendothelial and intraluminal deposits of fibrin and platelet aggregates in capillaries and arterioles. Classically patients have purpura, microangiopathic hemolytic anemia, fluctuating neurologic symptoms, renal disease, and fever. Anemia is common, and the platelet count ranges from 10,000 to 50,000/mm^3. The triad of anemia, purpura, and neurologic abnormalities is seen in 75% of all cases. A combination of steroid infusion and plasma exchange is currently the recommended treatment.

Abnormal platelet function may result from impaired adhesion, release, and aggregation. Von Willebrand disease is the classic inherited adhesion problem and partially reflects a factor VIII deficiency. Aspirin blocks the aggregation of platelets. It is the most commonly acquired platelet function disorder. Thrombocytosis represents a platelet count more than 1×10^6/mm^3. It is usually secondary to iron deficiency, infection,

Table 46-7

RECOMMENDED FACTOR VIII THERAPY FOR SPECIFIC PROBLEMS IN HEMOPHILIA

Type of Bleeding	Initial Dosage	Duration	Comment*
Skin			
Abrasion	None	None	Treat with local pressure and topical thrombin
Laceration Superficial	Usually none; if necessary treat as minor	None	Local pressure and anesthetic with epinephrine may benefit; watch 4 hours after suturing, reexamine in 24 hours
Deep	Mild bleed (12.5 units/kg)	Single-dose coverage	May need hospitalization for observation; repeat may be necessary for suture removal
Nasal Epistaxis			
Spontaneous	Usually none; may need to be treated as mild bleed	None	Uncommon; consider platelet inhibition; treat in usual manner
Traumatic	Moderate bleed (25 units/kg)	Up to 5-7 days	Trauma-related bleed can be significant
Oral			
Mucosa or tongue bites	Usually none; treat as minor if persists	Single dose	Commonly seen
Traumatic (laceration) or dental extraction	Moderate (25 units/kg) to severe (50 unit/kg)	Single dose; may need more	Saliva rich in fibrin lytic activity; oral ε-aminocaproic acid (Amicar) may be given 100 mg every 6 hours for 7 days to block fibrinolysis; check contraindications; hospitalize patients with severe bleeds
Hematomas			
Soft tissue/muscle hematomas	Moderate (25 units/kg) to severe (50 units/kg)	2-5 days	May be complicated by local pressure on nerves or vessels, such as iliopsoas, forearm, calf

*Desmopressin increases factor VIII levels three to five times baseline in patients with a mild-to-moderate deficiency; may be considered in mild dose situations.

Table **46-7**

RECOMMENDED FACTOR VIII THERAPY FOR SPECIFIC PROBLEMS IN HEMOPHILIA—cont'd

Type of Bleeding	Initial Dosage	Duration	Comment
Hemarthrosis			
Early	Mild (12.5 units/kg)	Single dose	Treat at earliest symptom (pain); knee, elbow, ankle more common
Late or unresponsive cases of early	Mild-to-moderate (25 units/kg)	3-4 days	Arthrocentesis rarely necessary, and only with 50% level coverage; immobilization is a critical point of therapy
Urine			
Hematuria	Mild (12.5 units/kg)	2-3 days	Urokinase, the fibrinolytic enzyme, if in urine; with persistent hematuria an organic cause should be ruled out
Major Bleeding			
Gastrointestinal severe bleeding Neck/sublingual Retroperitoneal Intraabdominal Major trauma Head injury Central nervous system bleed Surgical procedure	Major bleed (50 units/kg)	7-10 days or 3-5 days after bleeding ceases	In head trauma, therapy should be given prophylactically; in severe head trauma or with associated neurologic signs, early CT scanning recommended

postsplenectomy, or trauma. Primary forms may be seen in polycythemia rubra vera and chronic myelogenous leukemia.

Coagulation Disorders

Abnormalities in the complex coagulation enzymatic cascade produce the pattern of bleeding noted in Table 46-5. These deficits in absolute factor level or activity prolong either the PT (extrinsic pathway), PTT (intrinsic pathway), or both (common pathway) (see Fig. 46-1). The most common disorder is hemophilia, which is primarily an X-linked recessive condition that results from deficits in factor VIII (classic) or factor IX (Christmas). Patients are classified by their factor activity level: mild (5% to 25%), moderate (1% to 5%), or severe (0% to 1%). Bleeding commonly occurs in deep muscles or joints, either spontaneously or as a result of minimal trauma. Sites typically involved include the following:

- Musculoskeletal, producing joint injury (elbow, knee, or ankle) or muscle bleeding
- Subcutaneous with hematoma or ecchymoses
- Intracranial—a major cause of death in these patients
- Spinal cord hematoma
- Upper or lower GI bleeding—rare unless patient has peptic ulcer disease or platelet inhibition
- Retropharyngeal hematoma
- Mild hematuria

Complications of hemophilia include hepatitis caused by factor replacement, the presence of factor VIII or IX inhibitor, acquired immunodeficiency syndrome (AIDS), or death from CNS injury.

Blood coagulation studies should include the PTT, PT, thrombin time (TT), and bleeding time (BT). Assays of factors VIII and IX define the deficiency (see Table 46-6). Other studies are indicated to define specific causes.

Stabilization may require IV fluids or blood. Factor replacement may be graded, as outlined in Table 46-7. Immediate administration of fluids is essential once the decision has been made. For a mild bleeding risk, the desired factor VIII level should be at least 5% to 10%; for a moderate risk the level should be raised to at least 20% to 30%; and with a severe bleeding risk, a 50% level or higher is protective. One unit of factor VIII or IX equals the activity of the factor contained in 1 milliliter of plasma. This factor is currently available as a plasma-derived or recombinant factor. Calculations follow for replacement in specific conditions and ages. In emergency therapy, the initial factor level is assumed to be zero:

1. Number of units of factor VIII required = 0.5 × weight (kg) × desired increment (%) of factor VIII level. The half-life is 12 hours.
2. Number of units of factor IX required = 1.0 × weight (kg) × desired increment (%) of factor IX level. The half-life is 24 hours.

Use factor VIII to treat mild hemophilia A, as well as children with hemophilia A who are less than 5 years of age to decrease secondary complications. The use of vasopressin or desmopressin (DDAVP) increases factor VIII levels three to five times the baseline levels in patients with a mild-to-moderate deficiency. Aminocaproic acid (Amicar) is considered in conjunction with factor replacement for oral (mouth, lip, and tongue) bleeding. Prednisone may be useful in the management of hematuria. Patients with inhibitors require hematologic consultation for optimal care.

TRIGGERS OF DISSEMINATED INTRAVASCULAR COAGULATION

Infection
  Bacterial: gram-negative sepsis, meningococcemia, gram-positive sepsis (*S. pneumoniae* and *S. aureus*)
  Viral: herpes simplex, measles, chickenpox, cytomegalovirus, influenza
  Rocky Mountain spotted fever
Shock
Respiratory distress and asphyxia
Trauma: burns, multiple trauma, snake bites, heat stroke, head injury
Neoplasm
Obstetrics: amniotic fluid embolism, abruptio placentae, eclampsia of pregnancy, hydatidiform mole
Necrotizing enterocolitis (NEC)
Hemangioma
Intravascular hemolysis: incompatible blood transfusion, autoimmune hemolytic anemia

Disseminated Intravascular Coagulation

Disseminated intravascular coagulation is an acquired coagulopathy that may occur in multiple clinical settings in which the clotting cascade is triggered. The abnormal coagulation sequence involves the following:

- Platelet and coagulation factors are consumed, particularly fibrinogen and factors V, VIII, and XIII.
- Thrombin is formed.
- Fibrin is deposited in small vessels.
- Fibrinolytic system may lyse fibrin and impair thrombin formation.
- Fibrin degradation products are released and affect platelet function and inhibit fibrin polymerization.

A number of conditions may trigger DIC; infection is the most common condition (see the box on p. 568).

The clinical presentation of DIC reflects causative factors as well as specific findings related to DIC (Table 46-8). Simultaneous diffuse bleeding and thrombosis, including petechiae, purpura, peripheral cyanosis, ischemic necrosis of the skin and subcutaneous tissues, hematuria, and melena are often seen. Prolonged bleeding from venipunctures and organ damage may be noted. A GI hemorrhage, hematuria, and CNS bleeding may complicate the clinical condition. Purpura fulminans appears as a patchy hemorrhagic infarction of the skin and subcutaneous tissue.

Treatment of DIC primarily focuses on treat-

Table 46-8

LABORATORY DIAGNOSIS OF DISSEMINATED INTRAVASCULAR COAGULATION

Test	Finding	Pathophysiology
Peripheral smear	Low platelets, schistocytes, red blood cell fragments	Red blood cell fragmentation on fibrin strands; schistocytes not always seen
Platelet count	Low (usually <100,000/mm^3)	Consumed in clotting; lower numbers are reflected in bleeding time
Prothrombin time	Prolonged	Factors II and IV consumed
Partial thromboplastin time	Prolonged	Factors II, V, and VIII consumed
Thrombin time	Prolonged	Decrease in factor II and fibrin degradation products
Fibrinogen level	Low	Factor II consumed; may be difficult to interpret because this is an acute-phase reactant
Fibrin degradation products	Zero to large	Dependent on amount of secondary fibrinolysis
Serum creatinine or urinalysis	May be abnormal	Functional assessment of organ most commonly injured by fibrin deposition

From Hamilton GC: Disorders of hemostasis and polycythemia. In Rosen P et al, editors: *Emergency medicine: concepts and clinical practice,* ed 3, St Louis, 1992, Mosby.

Table **46-9**

CAUSES OF LEUKOCYTOSIS

	Neutrophilia	Lymphocytosis
Infection	Bacteria	Viral, tuberculosis
Inflammation	Rheumatoid arthritis	
Metabolic	Diabetic ketoacidosis, thyrotoxicosis	Hyperthyroidism
Stress	Exercise, pain	
Neoplasm	Chronic myelogenous leukemia, polycythemia vera	Chronic lymphocytic leukemia, acute lymphoblastic leukemia

ing the underlying condition. Replacement of depleted coagulation factors with fresh frozen plasma (fibrinogen; factors II, V, and VIII), cryoprecipitate (factors I and VIII), and platelet concentrates may be useful. Heparin is rarely indicated but may be beneficial in the presence of widespread thrombosis or active bleeding that cannot be controlled by the replacement of clotting factors and platelets coupled with aggressive treatment of the triggering condition.

WHITE BLOOD CELL DISORDERS

Leukocytosis and Leukopenia

Because of the wide range of normal values, the emergency physician must interpret abnormal white blood cell (WBC) values within the context of the patient. Neutrophil leukocytosis with blood neutrophil counts of more than $7500/mm^3$ is com-

monly associated with infection or inflammation. Lymphocytosis is age specific ($>9000/mm^3$ for children 1 to 6 years, $>7000/mm^3$ for those 7 to 16 years, and $>4000/mm^3$ for adults) and similarly reflects infection or lymphoproliferative disease (Table 46-9).

Leukopenia is defined as an absolute WBC count of less than 4000 cells/mm^3. It may be caused by infiltrative proliferation in the bone marrow as a result of leukemia, aplastic anemia, or other bone marrow suppression. Bone marrow maturation of WBCs may be impaired because of a folic acid or B_{12} deficiency. Splenomegaly may cause sequestration. Increased destruction is seen with autoimmune disease or severe infection and is often viral in origin. Neutropenia of less than 500 cells/mm^3 is a potentially life-threatening condition because the patient is markedly susceptible to overwhelming infection.

||||||||||KEY CONSIDERATIONS

WHAT IS THE LIFE THREAT?

Severe anemia can cause high output cardiac failure and even myocardial infarction. Patients with a headache and coagulation disorder such as hemophilia may have a life-threatening intracranial hemorrhage.

Neutropenia with an absolute neutrophil count (ANC) less than 500 cells/mm^3 predisposes the patient to the risk of life-threatening infections.

DOES THE PATIENT NEED ADMISSION?

Admit patients with severe anemia or ANC of less than 500 cells/mm^3.

Admit patients with sickle cell disease who have an anemic crisis, splenic sequestration crisis, and aplastic crisis or severe infection. Patients with a vasoocclusive crisis may require admission if pain cannot be controlled with hydration and oral analgesics at home.

Patients with intracranial, spinal cord, or gastrointestinal hemorrhage associated with the exacerbation of a bleeding disorder require admission.

WHAT IS THE MOST SERIOUS DIAGNOSIS?

Severe life-threatening anemia, bleeding in a vital organ associated with a coagulation disorder, or a neutrophil count less than 500 cells/mm^3 are the most serious diagnoses.

HAVE I PERFORMED A THOROUGH WORK-UP?

With a bleeding disorder, determine the nature, site, and pattern of bleeding. Obtain a history of medication, associated disease, and family history. Examine the patient for the site of bleeding. Obtain CBC, platelet count, and coagulation studies.

In evaluating severe anemia, consider current medications and underlying disease.

Following trauma, evaluate the patient for external or internal blood loss. Examine skin, heart, abdomen, rectum, and pelvis.

Recommended Reading

Bell WR: *Hematologic and oncologic Emergencies,* New York, 1993, Churchill Livingstone.

Chen H: *Advisory council on newborn screening for hemoglobinopathies: the resource manual for hemoglobinopathies,* Columbus, 1992, Ohio Department of Health.

College of American Pathologists: Practice parameter for the use of fresh-frozen plasma, cryoprecipitate, and platelets, *JAMA* 271(10):777-781, 1994.

Harmening DM: *Clinical hematology and fundamentals of hemostasis,* ed 2, Philadelphia, 1992, FA Davis.

Hoyer LW: Hemophilia A, *N Engl J Med* 330(1):38-47, 1994.

Lee GR et al: *Wintrobe's clinical hematology,* ed 9, Philadelphia, 1993, Lea & Febiger.

Moore GP, Jorden RC: Hematologic/oncologic emergencies, *Emerg Med Clin North Am* 11(2):273-555, 1993.

Ruggenenti P, Remuzzi G: Thrombotic thrombocytopenic purpura and related disorders, *Hematol Oncol Clin North Am* 4:219-241, 1990.

Tardio DJ, McFarland JA, Gonzalez MF: Immune thrombocytopenic purpura: current concepts, *J Gen Intern Med* 8:160-163, 1993.

Chapter Forty-seven
ONCOLOGIC EMERGENCIES

MARC BORENSTEIN

Cancer is the second leading cause of death in this country; however, contemporary effective treatments have led to increased survival rates and cures for many patients. Larger numbers of patients and older patients are receiving more aggressive therapy. Emergency department visits often stem from complications that produce serious morbidity and mortality if left unrecognized or inadequately treated. Fears and denial surrounding cancer may cause patients, family members, or health professionals to minimize symptoms. Many patients have multiple concurrent clinical findings; complications may arise from the cancer, its treatment, or both. Evaluation requires careful history collection, thorough diagnostic testing, and rapid institution of therapeutic measures.

FEVER AND NEUTROPENIA

Fever can be caused by infection, inflammation, transfusion, medications, and tumor necrosis. Cancer patients with a temperature above 38° C and diminished polymorphonuclear leukocytes ($<500/mm^3$) must be presumed to have an underlying infection that requires rapid evaluation and antibiotic treatment. Infection remains the number-one cause of cancer-related deaths; untreated infections have a mortality of 20% to 50% in the first 48 hours. Influencing the evaluation may be the prior use of antimicrobials, the degree of immunocompromise, and recent chemotherapeutic maneuvers. Although fever may be caused by the underlying disease, in the emergency department it is usually not possible to differentiate patients with bacteremia-induced fever from those with fever of tumor or chemotherapeutic origins.

Granulocytopenia that accompanies chemotherapy impairs the response to infection, whether bacterial, fungal, viral, or parasitic. Gram-negative bacteria, especially *Klebsiella* organisms and *Escherichia coli,* are common. The incidence of *Pseudomonas aeruginosa* is decreasing. The increased use of indwelling catheters has led to a rising incidence of Gram-positive pathogens, including *Staphylococcus aureus, Staphylococcus epidermidis, Corynebacterium* organisms, and JK-diptheroids. Frequently noted fungal organisms are *Candida albicans, Histoplasma capsulatum, Cryptococcus, Aspergillus,* and *Phycomycetes. Pneumocystis carinii* is a major parasite, and herpes simplex, varicella zoster, and cytomegalovirus are commonly encountered viral agents.

Empiric treatment must be initiated immediately after an initial evaluation with a complete blood count (CBC), chest radiograph, blood cultures, and other appropriate cultures. Approximately 85% of all initial pathogens are bacterial and require treatment with broad-spectrum antibiotics, including a semisynthetic penicillin with antipseudomonas activity (ticarcillin, carbenicillin, or piperacillin) and an aminoglycoside (gentamicin, tobramycin). Some centers add specific antistaphylococcal activity (nafcillin or oxacillin) to this regimen. The use of vancomycin is reserved for settings in which the incidence of methicillin-resistant *S. aureus* is prevalent. A third-generation cephalosporin (e.g., ceftazidime), alone or in combination with an antipseudomonal penicillin, is being increasingly recommended.

SUPERIOR VENA CAVA SYNDROME

Superior vena cava syndrome (SVCS) results from compression, infiltration, or thrombosis of the superior vena cava. The superior vena cava rises from the innominate vein; an obstruction may be bypassed through chest wall collaterals that rejoin the superior vena cava via the azygos. If the obstruction falls below the entrance to the azygos, blood may traverse down the azygos in a retrograde fashion. Of the patients with cancer of the lung or lymphoma, 3% to 8% may develop SVCS; benign causes underlie 10% to 25% of all cases. Of the malignant causes, 75% are a result of cancer of the lung and 15% are a result of lymphoma; 10% are metastatic (primarily breast and testicular carcinoma).

Clinical findings reflect venous hypertension within the area drained by the superior vena cava; many of the findings are more evident in the recumbent position. Signs may include periorbital edema, conjunctival suffusion, and facial swelling. Shortness of breath, coughing, dysphagia, and chest pain may also be noted. Progression leads to thoracic and neck vein distension, facial edema, tachypnea, tightness of the shirt collar, plethora of the face, edema of the upper extremities, and cyanosis.

The severity of the findings is related to the rapidity of the developing obstruction and the development of collaterals. In general, this process is not immediately life-threatening, and time is available to obtain a tissue biopsy and a specific *histologic* diagnosis. If left untreated, SVCS can ultimately lead to headache, blurred vision, and altered mental status. Increased intracranial pressure and airway obstruction do not occur in the absence of intracranial metastases or tracheal compression.

Differential considerations must initially exclude nephrotic syndrome, pericardial tamponade, and congestive heart failure. In a large majority of patients, chest radiographs reveal a mass, which is associated with pleural effusion. Venous contrast studies have an inherent risk because of the elevated intraluminal pressures. All venous access should be limited to the lower extremities and used only when absolutely necessary. Invasive diagnostic procedures, including bronchoscopy, mediastinoscopy, scalene node biopsy, and limited thoracotomy are often necessary to establish the diagnosis and extent of disease.

Radiation therapy has previously been the primary therapeutic modality, with high-dose radiation (300 to 400 rad for 3 days) followed by fractionated radiotherapy at lower doses (180 to 200 rad/day) in symptomatic patients. However, chemotherapy has supplanted radiation therapy as the primary treatment of SVCS because of its efficacy in small-cell lung cancer, lymphoma, and breast and testicular carcinoma.

ACUTE TUMOR LYSIS SYNDROME

Acute tumor lysis syndrome may occur 1 to 5 days after instituting chemotherapy or radiotherapy for rapidly growing tumors that are sensitive to antineoplastic drugs. The most common types of these tumors are hematologic malignancies (acute leukemia and lymphoma); solid tumors are rarely causative. Acute renal failure, cardiac dysrhythmias, neuromuscular symptoms, and sudden death may develop. Initial biochemical findings include hyperuricemia, hyperkalemia, and hyperphosphatemia with secondary hypocalcemia.

Treat patients at risk for this syndrome prophylactically; chemotherapy may be delayed until metabolic complications can be treated. Allopurinol, diuretics, and alkalinization of urine may all be helpful; hemodialysis may be lifesaving.

HYPERVISCOSITY SYNDROME

Excessive viscosity can result from marked leukocytosis or elevated paraproteins; the latter are associated with dysproteinemias. Sludging, decreased perfusion of the microcirculation, and vascular stasis may develop. The underlying pathologic condition is commonly multiple myeloma, Waldenström macroglobulinemia, or chronic myelocytic leukemia.

Clinically, patients have visual disturbances that are associated with retinopathy and characterized by venous engorgement. Neurologic findings may include headache, dizziness, jacksonian and generalized seizures, somnolence, lethargy, coma, auditory disturbances, and hypotension. Fatigue, anorexia, and weight loss are noted. Complications may include respiratory, cardiac, and renal failure.

Initial therapy for hyperviscosity syndrome should include hydration, pending leukapheresis or plasmapheresis. Partial volume exchanges may be used as immediate temporizing measures in patients who are comatose and have an established dysproteinemia.

HYPERURICEMIA

Hyperuricemia results from either increased production or decreased excretion of uric acid. The necrosis of neoplastic tissues results in production of uric acid following chemotherapy or radiation therapy. Decreased excretion may follow from renal insufficiency or precipitation of urates in the renal tubules, parenchyma, or ureters. Specific problems associated with hyperuricemia may include acute hyperuricemia nephropathy, uric acid nephrolithiasis, and gouty nephropathy that progresses to renal failure.

Institute treatment with allopurinol, fluids, and alkalinization of urine if the uric acid is at least 9 mg/dl in association with chemotherapy or radiotherapy. Prevention is key. Impaired renal output may be improved with diuretics or mannitol. Peritoneal dialysis or hemodialysis are useful at times.

HYPERCALCEMIA

Metastatic bone disease or tumor-produced parathyroid hormone–like polypeptides may produce elevated calcium levels. Hypercalcemia is particularly associated with malignancies of the breast, ovary, or lung (squamous cell only); multiple myeloma; lymphoma; and epidermoid tumors of the head and neck.

The clinical presentations of hypercalcemia often reflect the rapid rate of rise and high levels of ionized blood calcium typically associated with the hypercalcemia of malignancy. The rapid onset of hypercalcemia is commonly associated with CNS effects that range from personality changes (depression, paranoia, lethargy, somnolence) to coma. With a slower onset, anorexia, nausea, vomiting, constipation, polyuria, polydipsia, loss of memory, and shortened QT intervals on the ECG may be evident.

Treatment reflects the clinical status of hypercalcemia but generally includes encouraging ambulation, increasing calcium excretion, decreasing calcium bone mobilization, and reducing calcium intake. Manage levels below 14 mg/dl with hydration and ambulation. High levels of calcium require aggressive fluid and furosemide therapy.

CARDIAC TAMPONADE

Cardiac decompensation may result from cardiac tamponade caused by an accumulation of malignant fluid within the pericardial sac. The clinical findings in this situation are identical to those of cardiac tamponade resulting from non-neoplastic causes (see Chapter 22). The most common causes of neoplastic cardiac tamponade with malignant pericardial effusion are malignant melanoma, Hodgkin lymphoma, acute leukemia, and carcinoma of the lung, breast, and ovary. Involvement may be primary or secondary. Cardiac tamponade may also be caused by postradiation pericarditis with effusion. Emergency intervention may include pericardiocenteses. Additional therapy may include pericardial window, radiotherapy, intrapericardial chemotherapy, and pericardiectomy.

NEUROLOGIC FINDINGS

Of the patients with cancer, 15% to 20% have neurologic findings during their illness that reflect the nature of the lesion.

Cerebral herniation primarily occurs in patients with primary or metastatic brain tumors and intracerebral hemorrhage. Brain abscesses, subdural hematomas, acute hydrocephalus, and radiation-induced brain necrosis may be causative, but only rarely. Uncal, central, and tonsillar herniation may occur. Emergency management includes hyperventilation, diuresis, and surgical intervention. A CT scan may be obtained in the stable patient.

Seizures commonly are caused by brain metastases, toxic or metabolic disturbances (usually hyponatremia or uremia), coagulation or vascular problems (intracerebral hemorrhage or subdural hematoma), and infections. Obtain a CBC, electrolytes, glucose, blood urea nitrogen (BUN), calcium, and magnesium, as well as a CT scan as indicated. Focus on airway, ventilation, and management of seizures (see Chapter 18).

Epidural spinal compression from metastatic involvement of lymphoma and lung, breast, and prostate carcinoma requires urgent recognition. Back pain typically precedes clinically apparent neurologic findings by weeks to months. Plain radiographs of the vertebral spine are mandatory in oncologic patients with cancer who come to the emergency department with back pain. Neurologic findings, including weakness and autonomic or sensory dysfunction, that eventually progress to symmetric flaccidity and hyperreflexia are late manifestations of spinal cord compression. Plain radiographs that demonstrate vertebral metastases require an emergency myelography or magnetic resonance imaging (MRI) to rule out spinal cord compression. If a malignant etiology is in doubt, surgery is indicated to establish a histologic diagnosis. Radiation therapy should be planned as soon as possible in conjunction with surgery.

Encephalopathy on a toxic or metabolic basis may be associated with electrolyte and nutritional abnormalities or paraneoplastic syndromes. An appropriate diagnostic work-up is indicated, with therapy reflecting the findings.

SYNDROME OF INAPPROPRIATE ANTIDIURETIC HORMONE

Syndrome of inappropriate antidiuretic hormone (SIADH) most often associated with small-cell lung cancer and, less commonly, the brain, pancreas, and prostate is a result of the elaboration of ectopic ADH. The clinical presentations, diagnostic approach, and emergency management of hyponatremia in the patient with cancer parallels that in the nonmalignant setting (see Chapter 57). With mild hyponatremia, water restriction and demeclocycline are useful. Severe hyponatremia is a true medical emergency that requires monitoring (cardiac, hemodynamic, input, output), frequent electrolyte determinations, and the induction of a saline/furosemide free water clearance. In general the rate of rise in serum sodium concentration should not exceed 1 mEq/hour to prevent the complication of central pontine myelinolysis. Seizures are best managed with diphenylhydantoin.

KEY CONSIDERATIONS

WHAT IS THE LIFE THREAT?

Cardiac tamponade can cause acute cardiac decompensation, which leads to hypotension and irreversible shock. Cerebral metastases can cause sufficient cerebral edema to create uncal herniation and death. Fever and neutropenia create a risk for a life-threatening infection.

Depending on the level of the lesion, cord compression from a tumor creates an acute threat to bowel and bladder function and to motor function of lower and upper extremities.

Acute tumor lysis can create marked disturbances of electrolytes that place the patient at risk for lethal cardiac dysrhythmia.

DOES THE PATIENT NEED ADMISSION?

Patients requiring admission include those with fever and an absolute neutrophil count below $500/mm^3$, superior vena cava syndrome, acute tumor lysis syndrome, hyperviscosity syndrome, acute hyperuricemia, severe hypercalcemia, cardiac tamponade, cord compression, and cerebral edema.

WHAT IS THE MOST SERIOUS DIAGNOSIS?

Cardiac tamponade, severe cerebral edema, acute electrolyte derangement, and cord compression are the most serious diagnoses.

HAVE I PERFORMED A THOROUGH WORK-UP?

Consider life-threatening complications that can arise from cancer and its treatment. Look for a source of fever in the patient with neutropenia. If the patient has an altered level of consciousness, consider electrolyte disturbances, brain metastases, cerebral edema, hyperviscosity syndrome, and hypercalcemia. Consider tumor lysis syndrome in patients with dysrhythmia. Cardiomegaly on a chest x-ray study may reflect pericardial effusion. Consider the risk of tamponade.

Recommended Reading

Berger NA: Oncologic emergencies, *Sem Oncol* 16:6, 1989.

Hamilton GC, Braen GR: Anemia and white blood cell disorders. In Rosen P et al, editors: *Emergency medicine: concepts and clinical practice,* ed 3, St Louis, 1992, Mosby.

Hamilton GC: Disorders of hemostasis and polycythemia. In Rosen P et al, editors: *Emergency medi-* cine: concepts and clinical practice, ed 3, St Louis, 1992, Mosby.

Moore GP, Jordan RC: Hemalologic/Oncologic emergencies, *Emerg Med Clin North Am* 11:2, 1993.

Silverman S, Borenstein MA: Oncologic emergencies. In Rosen P et al, editors: *Emergency medicine: concepts and clinical practice,* ed 3, St Louis, 1992, Mosby.

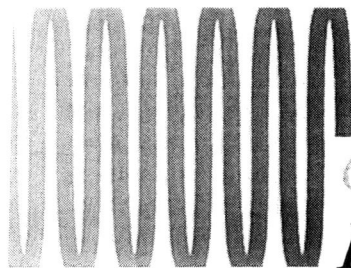

Chapter Forty-eight

RHEUMATOLOGY AND CONNECTIVE TISSUE DISEASES

BRUCE K. NEELY AND DOUGLAS A. RUND

Musculoskeletal problems may be manifestations of rheumatologic or connective tissue diseases that have not been identified. The emergency physician should consider such conditions in the differential diagnosis of musculoskeletal pain.

RHEUMATOID ARTHRITIS

Rheumatoid arthritis (RA) is one cause of polyarticular arthritis. The polyarthritis is caused by the formation of immune complexes within the synovium and joint cartilage, which ultimately results in the release of enzymes from leukocytes; these enzymes injure and eventually destroy the joints. Women develop RA more commonly than men, with a peak age of incidence between 40 and 60 years of age.

At the onset of disease, the patient may experience a prodrome of fatigue, weakness, and myalgia. Eventually the patient experiences painful swelling of the smaller joints of the hands and feet in a symmetrical pattern. The proximal interphalangeal (PIP) and metacarpophalangeal (MCP) joints of the finger, wrist, elbows, and feet are the joints most commonly involved. The distal interphalangeal (DIP) joints of the hands are typically not involved in cases

of rheumatoid arthritis and therefore help differentiate rheumatoid arthritis from psoriatic arthritis.

As rheumatoid arthritis progresses, the joint cartilages are eventually destroyed, and the patient develops the deformities characteristic of the disease, including ulnar deviation of the fingers, limited dorsiflexion of the wrist, and enlargement of the MCP and PIP joints. Morning joint stiffness is a common clinical feature.

Serious complications that are of particular importance to the emergency physician include the possibility of involvement of the transverse ligament of the first cervical vertebra, C1. Degeneration of the ligament can lead to subluxation of the atlantoaxial joint, which can in turn lead to compression of the cervical cord by the odontoid. Other possible complications include arthritis of the cricoarytenoid joints, which causes hoarseness and even airway obstruction. Stiffness of the temporomandibular joints can interfere with mastication, and popliteal cysts associated with the disease may mimic thrombophlebitis. Serious pulmonary complications can include interstitial fibrosis. Pericarditis with tamponade can also occur.

The evaluation of the patient with new-onset joint inflammation involves a consideration of the many causes of arthritis, including gout, septic joint, Lyme disease, viral illnesses, and other connective tissue diseases such as systemic lupus erythematosus.

Rheumatoid arthritis treatment includes salicylates or other nonsteroidal antiinflammatory drugs (NSAIDS), corticosteroids, gold salts, penicillamine, azathioprine, and methotrexate. Patients with new-onset disease should be referred for treatment; a short course of NSAIDS relieves many of the symptoms.

ANKYLOSING SPONDYLITIS

Ankylosing spondylitis is a seronegative spondylopathy characterized by arthritis of the sacroiliac joints and lumbosacral spine. Patients with ankylosing spondylitis are typically men under the age of 40 who experience a gradual onset of back discomfort and morning back stiffness that improves with exercise. Lumbosacral spine films eventually show a symmetric squaring of the margins of the vertebral bodies that resembles a "bamboo spine." Peripheral joints and tendons may be involved.

Of special concern is the involvement of the cervical and lumbar spine. This condition causes back and neck stiffness and may predispose such patients to spinal cord injury following trauma. Any trauma, even minor, to the ankylosed spine should be considered an unstable spinal fracture until proven otherwise. Ankylosis of the cervical spine is also of concern in airway management for these patients. The stiffened neck does not move properly, which hinders intubation. Applying excessive force to the head in an attempt to position the airway can fracture the ankylosed segments and lead to spinal cord damage. Therefore extreme care must be taken when intubating such patients.

POLYMYALGIA RHEUMATICA

Polymyalgia rheumatica is a syndrome of pain and stiffness in the neck, shoulder, and hip girdle and is generally accompanied by a systemic reaction such as a low-grade fever, fatigue, and weight loss. This syndrome occurs primarily in the elderly; in the 70- to 79-year-old group it is as common as rheumatoid arthritis. Polymyalgia rheumatica is twice as common in women as in men and is uncommon in blacks.

Clinical Features

Polymyalgia rheumatica is characterized by polymyalgia, and the symptoms may be gradual or abrupt in onset. Patients may become quite disabled. Simple acts of dressing, grooming, and other activities of daily living become an ordeal; many patients require help in performing such activities. When questioned, patients localize pain to the muscles, and the pain is generally described as aching in character and often worse at night. Movement makes the pain worse, and most patients state that nothing they have been able to do makes the pain any better. Constitutional symptoms include anorexia, weight loss, fever, and malaise. Symptoms of synovitis are often present (Table 48-1).

Physical examination reveals a normal or near-normal range of motion in the affected areas. Despite pain with muscular effort, muscle strength is normal.

Laboratory Studies

The erythrocyte sedimentation rate (ESR) is typically elevated above 50 mm/hour and may be greater than 100 mm/hour in some cases. As many as half of the patients with polymyalgia rheumatica have evidence of anemia of chronic disease. The rheumatoid factor is generally negative, and antinuclear antibodies (ANAs) are positive in approximately 19% of all cases. Radiographs of the affected areas are normal.

Differential Diagnosis

The differential diagnosis of diffuse muscular pain includes malignancy, (lung, breast, genital,

Table *48-1*

CLINICAL FEATURES OF POLYMYALGIA RHEUMATICA

Features	Frequency
Musculoskeletal	
Proximal myalgias	
Shoulders	96%
Neck	66%
Arms	63%
Thighs	54%
Distal arthralgias	83%
Knee down	73%
Elbow down	56%
Tenderness	39%
Systemic Symptoms	
Malaise	30%
Depression	15%
Anorexia	14%
Weight loss	15%
Low-grade fever	13%

colon, or renal cancer; multiple myeloma; and leukemia) infection, rheumatic diseases, endocrine disorders, and neurologic disorders. Infectious causes of myalgias include subacute bacterial endocarditis, chronic viral infection, and trichinosis. Rheumatic diseases that can appear similar to polymyalgia rheumatica include rheumatoid arthritis, polymyositis, polyarteritis nodosa, systemic lupus erythematosus, Wegener granulomatosis, and fibromyalgia. Endocrine disorders that result in a similar presentation include thyrotoxic myopathy, hypothyroidism, and hyperparathyroidism. Parkinsonism is a neurologic cause of myalgias and should also be considered.

Management

Treatment includes low-dose corticosteroids. NSAIDs are occasionally effective, but a rapid symptomatic response to steroids strongly supports the diagnosis. Generally the dose is started at 10 to 20 mg/day in either a divided or single daily dose. After 3 to 4 weeks the dosage is slowly tapered to 5 to 7.5 mg/day. The dose should be slowly tapered further as symptoms allow. The goal of therapy should be adequate control of symptoms with the lowest possible dose of corticosteroids.

GIANT CELL ARTERITIS

Giant cell arteritis is a disseminated vasculitis of large- or medium-sized elastic arteries. The disease may involve the temporal arteries, which produces tender induration and a distinctive headache. Giant cell arteritis has a peak incidence among patients in their 80s. Women are affected more often than men, and the disease is uncommon in blacks.

Giant cell arteritis classically affects the branches of the internal and external carotid arteries. Because the disease has a tendency to affect the elastic arteries of the head and neck region, it is also called temporal arteritis. However, autopsy studies have shown that any large- to medium-sized artery can be involved.

Clinical Features

A classic symptom of giant cell arteritis is a continuous, sharp, boring headache that radiates to the neck, face, and jaw. Scalp tenderness is often associated. Other symptoms include jaw claudication and visual disturbances. Sudden blindness in association with a bitemporal headache suggests the possibility of giant cell arteritis. Sudden blindness often occurs after a period of certain transient visual disturbances, including diplopia, ptosis, and amaurosis fugax. Other symptom complexes include limb claudication; ear, nose, or throat pain; visual hallucinations; confusion; and systemic complaints of fever, weight loss, and malaise. Physical findings can include visual field cuts, ophthalmoplegia, and funduscopic changes of ischemia. Paralysis that affects any of the cranial nerves, seizures, and hemiparesis can also be seen. The inflammation of elastic arteries can cause aortic valve insufficiency from aortic dissection or thoracic aortic aneurysm.

Laboratory Studies

An elevated ESR is present in nearly 100% of all cases of giant cell arteritis. Other findings include anemia of chronic disease, as well as abnormal liver function studies from granulomatous hepatitis. The rheumatoid factor and ANA are positive in only 10% of these patients.

A diagnosis of giant cell arteritis is made by visualizing granulomatous arteries (particularly in the media of the artery) on microscopic sections of a temporal artery biopsy. Often there is also smooth muscle necrosis and occasional destruction of the internal elastic lamina. Other findings on microscopic inspection of the biopsy specimen can include a panarteritis of the vessel wall and intimal fibrosis with occlusion of the vessel by fibrous tissue.

Treatment

In contrast to the low doses of corticosteroids used to treat polymyalgia rheumatica, high doses of corticosteroids are used to treat giant cell arteritis. Dosages between 60 and 80 mg/day are given for 4 to 6 weeks and then decreased to between 25 and 40 mg/day. Further reductions in the steroid dose (of approximately 10% of the total dose each week) can be attempted; the slow taper can be stopped if symptoms recur. The duration of treatment is usually 1 year.

Treatment with corticosteroids normalizes the ESR and may help restore some vision if the loss was not total before the onset of treatment. In many cases vision does not increase, but there is usually no further reduction in vision after treatment. Nonsteroidal medications do not have any role in the treatment of giant cell arteritis.

SYSTEMIC LUPUS ERYTHEMATOSUS

Systemic lupus erythematosus (SLE) is manifested as damage to tissues and cells as a result of the deposition of autoantibodies and immune complexes. The exact etiology of the disease is unknown. The deposition of autoantibodies and immune complexes can affect any organ system, which makes diagnosis and recognition difficult.

The prevalence of this disease is 15 to 50 cases for every 100,000 people. SLE is more common in women than men. Approximately 90% of all cases occur in women; usually these women are of child-bearing age, but any age group can be affected. The disease is more common in blacks than whites.

Clinical Features

The clinical features of SLE depend on which organ system is affected. Many, if not all, patients with SLE develop myalgias and arthralgias. Often the pain that patients report is out of proportion to their physical findings. Fusiform swelling of the fingers, especially around the PIP and MCP joints, is common.

One of the common physical findings in SLE is a malar rash. The rash is often raised and typically occurs in a "butterfly" pattern across the cheeks, bridge of the nose, and often the ears. Exposure to ultraviolet light worsens the rash.

Renal involvement, characterized by a nephritis that is caused by deposition of immune complexes in the glomeruli, is common in SLE. Urinalysis shows proteinuria and blood in the urine. The renal failure is often not responsive to treatment, and the complications of chronic renal failure in conjunction with the chronic illness from the SLE itself can be devastating.

SLE can affect areas of the brain, and the presentation can range from mild mental status changes to seizures. Cerebritis, aseptic meningitis, organic brain syndromes, and migraine-type headaches are also common.

Chest pain is a common complaint in patients with an acute exacerbation of SLE. The chest pain may be a result of pericarditis, myocarditis, or ischemia; pericardial pain is one of the most common symptoms of SLE. Chest pain can also be caused by pulmonary disease. Lupus pneumonitis and pleural effusions are often seen. Lupus pneumonitis can cause recurrent episodes of fever, coughing, and shortness of breath. Chest x-ray studies may show single or multiple infiltrates, which may be a result of lupus pneumonitis; however, the most common cause of infiltrates is infection.

Laboratory Studies

ANA is the best screening test in patients without a known diagnosis of SLE but in whom the disease is suspected, because 95% of all patients with SLE have a positive ANA. Hematologic abnormalities are often seen. Anemia, leukopenia, and thrombocytopenia are the most common types of such abnormalities. An elevated ESR signifies an acute flare-up of the disease.

Management

High-dose corticosteroids remain the mainstay of treatment for an acute exacerbation of SLE. Dosages between 1 and 2 mg/kg/day are given initially. After the disease has been under control for several days, the steroids should be tapered as rapidly as allowed. Cytotoxic agents, especially cyclophosphamide, are also used to treat SLE and seem to be especially effective in cases of renal involvement.

Hospital admission is indicated for acute relapses of SLE. Cerebritis, worsening nephritis, and pericarditis all need close monitoring to follow the response to treatment. Minor relapses may be managed on an outpatient basis if the patient receives close follow-up.

EMERGENCY CONDITIONS ASSOCIATED WITH VARIOUS OTHER CONNECTIVE TISSUE DISEASES

Hypertension is a well-known complication of scleroderma. The hypertension in scleroderma is thought to result from changes in blood vessel walls, especially in the kidney. Such changes result in sclerosis of the vessels and impaired glomerular perfusion. An acute hypertensive crisis was the leading cause of death from scleroderma before the development of angiotensin-converting-enzyme (ACE) inhibitors. Any patient with scleroderma who is diagnosed with a hypertensive crisis should be treated promptly with ACE inhibitors and hospitalized for close control of blood pressure.

Marfan syndrome is characterized by unusually tall height and unusually long limbs. Many of these patients have chest wall deformities resulting from scoliosis and rib overgrowth. The combination of a chest wall deformity and scoliosis can result in respiratory impairment. Patients with Marfan syndrome are also prone to having hypermobile joints and tend to suffer from recurrent joint dislocations.

Marfan syndrome often affects the cardiovascular system. Mitral valve prolapse and aortic dilatation are common complications. Patients with this syndrome are particularly prone to aortic dissection as a result of the progressive dilatation of the aortic root. It is important to remember the very real possibility of dissection in any patient with chest pain and a typical Marfanoid body habitus. Echocardiography, especially transesophageal echocardiography, is valuable in rapidly diagnosing aortic dissection in such patients.

Ehlers-Danlos syndrome is a connective tissue disease characterized by abnormal collagen fibers, hypermobile joints, and frequent joint dislocation. The disease may also affect the cardiovascular system. Such patients are prone to valvular heart disease, particularly mitral valve prolapse. Patients with type IV Ehlers-Danlos syndrome are also prone to rupturing the large arteries of the bowel, which leads to massive gastrointestinal bleeding. There is no specific treatment for the underlying condition, and complications need to be treated as they would be for any other patient, with attention given to the ABCs and resuscitation as needed.

Relapsing polychondritis is an inflammatory disease that affects cartilage, and it affects the airway in approximately 50% of all cases. Patients often complain of throat soreness, hoarseness, and tenderness over the cartilagenous structures of the throat. Such patients may also have shortness of breath, coughing, and stridor. Particular attention should be paid to maintaining an adequate airway, and an emergency cricothyrotomy may be needed if the airway becomes completely compromised. Relapsing polychondritis that affects the airway requires hospital admission for high-dose steroids and careful observation.

Impaired ventilation is most commonly caused by weakness of the respiratory muscles. Dermatomyositis and polymyositis are particularly prone to causing respiratory difficulty in chronic and poorly controlled cases. Emergent intubation is indicated for overt or impending respiratory failure. Admission for disease control and careful monitoring of respiratory status is indicated for any patient with inflammatory muscle disease and respiratory involvement.

An acute pulmonary hemorrhage can complicate many rheumatic diseases, including Goodpasture syndrome, hypersensitivity vasculitis, Wegener granulomatosis, and SLE. A pulmonary hemorrhage should be managed by controlling the airway, positioning the patient with the affected side down (if the affected side can be identified), and aggressively resuscitating any previous and ongoing blood loss. Emergent bronchoscopy may also be a consideration to help control the hemorrhage.

Osteogenesis imperfecta is a disorder of bone structure that makes the bones uncommonly brittle. This diagnosis is often first considered in the emergency department when children sustain multiple fractures from a seemingly minor trauma. Treatment for these patients includes stabilization of the fractures, adequate pain control, and a referral to an appropriate specialist for further evaluation and long-term care.

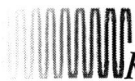

KEY CONSIDERATIONS

WHAT IS THE LIFE THREAT?

Patients with rheumatoid arthritis can develop subluxation of the atlantoaxial joint, arthritis of the cricoarytenoid joints, or pericarditis with pericardial effusion and tamponade, all of which are potentially life threatening. Systemic lupus erythematous (SLE) can cause cerebritis, pericarditis, and pneumonitis. Patients with scleroderma can develop a hypertensive crisis; and patients with Marfan syndrome can develop aortic root dissection. An acute pulmonary hemorrhage can complicate Goodpasture syndrome, hypersensitivity vasculitis, Wegener granulomatous, and SLE.

DOES THE PATIENT NEED ADMISSION?

Some acute complications of rheumatoid diseases require inpatient treatment. Severe exacerbations of SLE, including cerebritis, pneumonitis, and pericarditis typically require admission. A hypertensive crisis associated with scleroderma, gastrointestinal bleeding associated with Ehlers-Danlos syndrome, and aortic dissection associated with Marfan syndrome are all emergencies that require admission.

WHAT IS THE MOST SERIOUS DIAGNOSIS?

Complications of rheumatic diseases that threaten airway, ventilation, and cardiac, cerebral, or spinal cord function are the most serious diagnoses.

HAVE I PERFORMED A THOROUGH WORK-UP?

Consider rheumatologic and corrective tissue diseases in patients who have pain and inflammation in muscles, joints, and tendons. Consider giant cell arteritis in elderly patients who have headaches or visual disturbances. Consider SLE in patients with an unexplained facial rash, joint pain, anemia leukopenia, or thrombocytopenia.

Recommended Reading

Allen NB, Studenski SA: Polymyalgia rheumatica and temporal arteritis, *Med Clin North Am* 70(2):369-384, 1986.

Kyle V, Hazelman BL: Treatment of polymyalgia rheumatica and giant cell arteritis, I. Steroid regimens for the first two months, *Ann Rheumat Dis* 48(8):658-661, 1989.

Morgan MC, Ragsdale CG: Musculoskeletal disorders in adults and children. In Tintinalli JE, editor: *Emergency medicine: a comprehensive study guide,* New York 1992, McGraw-Hill.

Olhagen B: Polymyalgia rheumatica, *Clin Rheumat Dis* 12(1):33-47, 1984.

Chapter Forty-nine
DERMATOLOGIC PROBLEMS

GEORGE L. STERNBACH

Skin lesions traditionally are categorized by their morphology. *Macules* are flat, nonpalpable areas of color change. *Papules* are small palpable masses elevated above the skin surface. Elevated patches of papules are known as *plaques*. *Wheals* are edematous papules, and *vesicles* are fluid-filled, translucent papules. Large vesicles, or blisters, are called *bullae*. When leukocytes accumulate within vesicles, the translucent appearance is lost, and *pustules* are produced. Because morphologic appearance is key to identifying various dermatologic entities, this chapter presents dermatologic problems according to this characterization.

MACULAR LESIONS

Brown Macules

Fungal infection

Scaling and pruritus characterize superficial fungal skin infections (ringworm).

Appearance. Scalp involvement (*tinea capitis*) occurs primarily in children and may produce circular patches of partial baldness. Infected hairs fluoresce greenish-yellow under the Wood lamp. *Tinea corporis* affects the trunk and extremities and is classically a sharply marginated annular lesion with raised or vesicular margins and central clearing (Fig. 49-1). *Tinea pedis,* or athlete's foot, displays scaling, maceration, vesiculation, and fissuring between the toes and on the plantar surface of the foot.

Assessment. With any eruption that appears to be a fungal infection, first sponge the lesion with alcohol and allow it to dry. With a scalpel, gently scrape a specimen from the border of the lesion onto a microscope slide. Apply a drop of 10% potassium hydroxide solution to this specimen and place a cover slip over it. Heat the slide and examine the specimen for the long, thin, branching hyphae that are characteristic of a fungal infection.

Management. Infections of the body and extremities usually respond to topical measures alone. A number of effective topical antifungal agents are available, including clotrimazole (Lotrimin, Mycelex), miconazole (MicaTin), and tolnaftate (Tinactin). Applying such agents two to three times daily results in healing of most superficial lesions in 1 to 3 weeks.

Infections of the scalp require additional treatment with oral micronized griseofulvin (5 to 10 mg/kg/day for patients with tinea capitis) until complete clearing of lesions occurs (usually 3 to 6 weeks). Applying only a topical therapy to the nails in tinea unguium rarely produces a cure; this infection usually requires the administration of griseofulvin (0.5 to 1.0 g/day) for 6 to 12 months.

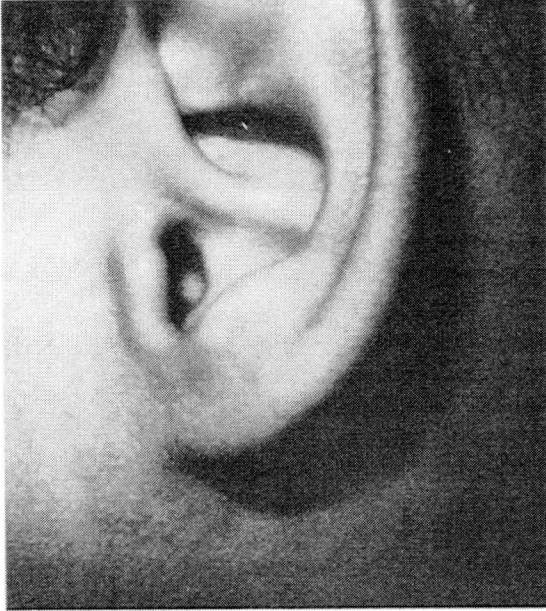

*Fig.*49-1   Tinea corporis.

Red Macules (Table 49-1)

Candidiasis

A number of conditions predispose the patient to infection of the skin or mucous membranes with *Candida albicans.* These conditions include infancy, old age, pregnancy, obesity, malnutrition, diabetes and other endocrine imbalances, malignancy and other debilitating diseases, and treatment with corticosteroids, antibiotics, and immunosuppressive agents.

Appearance.   Cutaneous lesions tend to occur in the interdigital web spaces, groin, axilla, and intergluteal and inframammary folds. Lesions appear as moist, red plaques with scalloped borders. Small vesicles or pustules just peripheral to the main body of the rash ("satellite lesions") are characteristic.

Management.   The treatment of intertriginous lesions requires the removal of excessive moisture and maceration. Expose lesions to circulating air several times a day. Soak inflamma-tory lesions or cover them with compresses of cool water or Burow solution. Apply nystatin dusting powder, lotion, or cream; clotrimazole and miconazole also are effective as topical agents.

Cellulitis

Cellulitis is a bacterial infection of subcutaneous tissue. The causative organism may be *Streptococcus* or *Staphylococcus.* Erysipelas is a streptococcal infection of the skin and subcutaneous tissue.

Appearance.   Cellulitis is denoted by erythema, swelling, and local tenderness. In erysipelas, the involved area is red, indurated, and edematous. The borders of the lesion are elevated and sharply demarcated. The face is the most commonly involved area. The patient may experience fever, chills, and systemic toxicity.

The appearance of facial cellulitis in children 6 months to 2 years of age suggests an infection with *Haemophilus influenzae.* A bluish or purplish-red discoloration is accompanied by marked temperature elevation and irritability.

Management.   Treatment of cellulitis includes antibiotics. Severe or extensive cases may require hospitalization for parenteral administration of penicillin or nafcillin. Treat erysipelas with oral administration of 250 to 500 mg of phenoxymethyl penicillin four times a day. Severe cases may require hospitalization and parenteral antibiotics. Manage *H. influenzae* infection with parenteral antibiotics; a third-generation cephalosporin may be required.

Atopic dermatitis

Although not itself an allergic disorder, atopic dermatitis is associated with allergic diseases such as asthma and allergic rhinitis.

Appearance.   In atopic dermatitis, skin lesions appear as inflammatory macules or papules with indefinite borders. The skin is typically dry and scaly, but lesions may be vesicular, weeping, or oozing in the acute phase. Distribution of lesions varies with the patient's age. In

Table 49-1

COMMON MACULOPAPULAR EXANTHEMS

	Measles (Rubeola)	Rubella (German, 3-day Measles)	Roseola (Exanthem Subitum)
Incubation	10-14 days	14-21 days	10-14 days
Prodrome	3 days high fever, cough, conjunctivitis, and coryza; child appears toxic, lethargic	May be none; lymphadenopathy (especially post-auricular, suboccipital), malaise, variable low-grade fever	3-4 days high fever in otherwise well child, preceding rash
Exanthem	Reddish-brown; begins on face and progresses downward; generalized by third day; confluent on face, neck, upper trunk; lasts 7-10 days; desquamates; atypical measles: maculopapular, purpuric, petechial, or vesicular rash	Pink; begins on face and progresses rapidly downward; generalized by second day; discrete; lasts 2-3 days, fades in order of appearance	Appears after defervescence; rose, discrete; initially on chest, spreads to involve face and extremities; fades quickly
Enanthem	Koplik spots (2 days before rash, on buccal mucosa opposite molars)	None	None
Complications	Pneumonia Encephalitis Otitis media Thrombocytopenia Hemorrhagic measles Pneumothorax Hepatitis Exacerbation of tuberculosis	Arthritis (common in women) beginning after 2-3 days of illness; knee, wrist, finger Congenital rubella syndrome Encephalitis Thrombocytopenia	Febrile seizure
Management	Supportive; may require hospitalization; active immunization of contacts; immune serum globulin (0.05 ml/kg) for children <1 yr; reportable	Supportive; isolate from pregnant women; active immunization of contacts; reportable	Supportive; good fever control
Comments	Rare with immunization	Rare with immunization; serologic diagnosis	Usually 1- to 4-yr-olds Probably caused by human herpesvirus-6 (HHV-6)

From Barkin RM, Rosen P: *Emergency pediatrics: a guide to ambulatory care,* ed 4, St Louis, 1994, Mosby.

Fifth Disease (Erythem Infectiosum)	Enterovirus	Scarlet Fever
7-14 days None	Variable (short) Variable; fever, malaise, vomiting, sore throat, rhinorrhea	2-4 days 1-2 days fever, vomiting, sore throat; often toxic
Erupts in 3 stages: (1) red-flushed cheeks with circum-oral pallor (slapped cheek), (2) maculopapular eruption on extremities (lacelike), (3) may recur secondary to heat, sunlight, trauma	Maculopapular, discrete, non-pruritic, generalized; rubella-like; hand, foot, and mouth distribution	Erythematous, punctate, sandpa-per texture; appears first in flexion areas, then general-ized; most intense on neck, axilla, inguinal, and popliteal skin fold; circumoral pallor; lasts 7 days, then desquamates
Variable	Variable	Red pharynx, tonsils; palatal petechiae; strawberry tongue
Transient arthritis	Aseptic meningitis Myocarditis Hepatitis	Rheumatic fever Acute glomerulonephritis
Rarely needs care	Supportive	Penicillin
Caused by human parvovirus B19	Concurrent family illness, gastro-enteritis, herpangina	Group A streptococci

infants, inflammatory exudative plaques appear on the cheeks and in the diaper area. Older children have lesions in the antecubital and popliteal flexion areas. In adults the disorder involves the hands, feet, forearms, groin, and scalp. Intense pruritus is a hallmark of atopic dermatitis. Repeated scratching and rubbing produces lichenification, which consists of hyperpigmentation, thickening of the skin, and accentuation of skin furrows.

Management. To treat exudative areas, apply two to three layers of gauze soaked in Burow solution for 15 to 20 minutes four times daily. Also consider using antihistamines for their antipruritic, sedative, and soporific effects. Topical corticosteroids are the cornerstone of therapy. An effective medication is 0.025% or 0.1% triamcinolone ointment. Apply small amounts to involved areas 3 to 6 times daily.

Drug eruption

Drugs may cause skin lesions of virtually any morphology.

Appearance. Urticarial, exanthematous, and eczematous lesions are common drug reactions. Drug eruptions, however, may take many other appearances.

Management. Discontinue the inciting agent. Control itching as needed by applying a drying antipruritic lotion such as calamine. Cool compresses or tepid water baths with colloidal oatmeal (Aveeno), emollients, or cornstarch may be useful. Also consider diphenhydramine (Benadryl) in a dosage of 50 mg every 6 hours.

If the condition is severe, institute systemic corticosteroid therapy (such as 25 mg of prednisone every 6 hours) until the patient improves. This treatment is most likely to be necessary for severe erythema multiforme, drug-induced toxic epidermal necrolysis, or vasculitis.

Toxic epidermal necrolysis

Two forms of toxic epidermal necrolysis (TEN) exist, both of which are characterized by an acute loosening of large areas of epidermis from underlying layers of tissue. One form is associated with *Staphylococcus aureus* infections, has an excellent prognosis when managed appropriately, and is often referred to as staphylococcal scalded skin syndrome. The other form is related to medication, infection, or medical illness, or it is idiopathic. The non-staphylococcal form is associated with a substantial mortality. Drugs are an important cause of nonstaphylococcal TEN. Drugs implicated as inciting agents include the long-acting sulfonamides, penicillin, aspirin, barbiturates, phenytoin, and allopurinol. The mechanism of production of nonstaphylococcal TEN is not known.

Appearance. Staphylococcal scalded skin syndrome generally occurs in children 6 years of age or younger. Exotoxin-producing staphylococci cause the illness, which begins with erythema and crusting around the mouth. The erythema spreads down the body, and bullae formation and desquamation follow. Mucous membranes are not usually involved. After desquamation, clinical resolution occurs in 3 to 7 days.

Non–staphylococci-induced TEN has as its main feature the full-thickness separation of large sheets of epidermis from the underlying dermis. The onset is usually on the face, and mucous membrane involvement is the rule.

Assessment. When the two forms of TEN cannot be distinguished on clinical grounds, recall that the two conditions are histologically distinguishable at skin biopsy.

Management. For intravenous therapy of staphylococcal scalded skin syndrome, administer 50 to 100 mg/kg of nafcillin daily. If the patient is able to take an oral medication and is nontoxic, administer 50 mg/kg/day of dicloxacillin instead. For nonstaphylococcal TEN, administer fluids and systemic corticosteroids. The benefit of corticosteroids is controversial; physicians have used prednisone, up to 300 mg daily or its equivalent, but deaths occur even with patients receiving corticosteroids in high doses.

Toxic shock syndrome

Toxic shock syndrome is an acute febrile illness characterized in part by the appearance of a diffuse desquamating erythroderma. The syndrome classically is composed of high fever, hypotension, constitutional symptoms, and rash.

Appearance. The rash is typically a diffuse, blanching, macular erythroderma. An accompanying nonexudative mucous membrane inflammation is common. The patient may have pharyngitis, conjunctivitis, or vaginitis. As a rule, the rash fades within 3 days of its appearance, and desquamation follows.

Meningococcemia

The severity of meningococcemia runs the gamut from a transient mild febrile illness to an acute, fulminant infection that may be fatal within hours.

Appearance. The rash initially consists of macular, nonpruritic, erythematous lesions that appear on the trunk or extremities. They may be 2 to 15 mm in diameter and blanch on pressure. Petechiae may appear and occasionally coalesce to form large intracutaneous hemorrhages.

Urticaria

Substances that can cause urticaria through contact with the skin include foods, textiles, animal dander and saliva, plants, topical medications, chemicals, and cosmetics. The role of drugs in the production of urticaria is well known. Almost any drug may produce urticaria, with penicillin and aspirin being the most commonly implicated.

A variety of food allergies may result in urticaria. Hereditary forms include familial cold urticaria and hereditary angioneurotic edema. Infections are an uncommon cause, but occult infections with fungi, bacteria, viruses, and parasites may trigger hives. Urticaria is occasionally associated with internal disease and malignancies.

Appearance. Urticaria is among the most commonly seen skin lesion in emergency practice. It appears as circumscribed raised wheels,

or hives, which may be erythematous and display central clearing.

Management. Remove the inciting factor (when applicable), and administer antihistamines or other antipruritic agents. We recommend hydroxyzine (Atarax, Vistaril). When anaphylaxis accompanies urticaria, give precedence to treating this life-threatening condition.

Exanthems

The exanthems of various infectious illnesses are erythematous macular or maculopapular eruptions. The following discussion details some of the more commonly encountered exanthems (see Table 49-1).

Measles. Measles is a viral illness; the onset usually involves fever and malaise. The fever usually increases daily in a stepwise fashion until it reaches 40.5° C on the fifth or sixth day of the illness. Coughing, coryza, and conjunctivitis begin within 24 hours of the onset of symptoms.

Appearance. On approximately the second day, Koplik spots appear on the buccal mucosa. These small, irregular, bright red spots with bluish-white centers are pathognomonic of the disease. Beginning opposite the molars, Koplik spots spread to involve a variable extent of the oropharynx.

The cutaneous eruption begins on the third to fifth day of the illness. Maculopapular erythematous lesions involve the forehead and upper neck and spread to involve the face, trunk, and extremities.

Management. Treatment for measles is symptomatic only.

Rocky Mountain spotted fever. Rocky Mountain spotted fever is an acute infectious disease caused by *Rickettsia rickettsii,* an organism harbored by a variety of ticks. The onset of the illness is usually abrupt, with headache, nausea, myalgias, chills, and a fever spiking to 40° C. Occasionally the onset is more gradual, with progressive anorexia, malaise, and fever.

Appearance. The rash develops on the second

to sixth day of the illness. It begins with erythematous macules that appear first on the wrists and ankles and blanch on pressure. They spread rapidly and may become petechial or hemorrhagic. The presence of lesions on the palms and soles is particularly characteristic (Fig. 49-2).

Assessment. Although the latex agglutination test is more readily available, the best serologic test is the indirect immunofluorescent antibody assay. Begin treatment as soon as the diagnosis is suspected on clinical grounds.

Management. Tetracycline is the preferred antibiotic in patients over 8 years of age; administer the drug orally, 25 to 30 mg/kg daily, in divided doses. If the patient is unable to take oral medications, administer tetracycline intravenously. Use chloramphenicol for patients who are allergic to tetracycline.

Roseola infantum. Roseola infantum is a self-limited illness characterized by fever, a skin eruption, and a paucity of other physical findings. Nearly all cases occur in children 6 months to 3 years old, and most often in infants younger than 2 years. The fever typically has an abrupt onset, is as high as 41° C, and is present for 3 to 4 days.

Appearance. The appearance of the rash typically coincides with the subsidence of the fever. The lesions are discrete pink or rose-colored macules or maculopapules 2 to 3 mm in diameter that blanch on pressure and rarely coalesce. The trunk is involved initially, with subsequent spread to the extremities.

Assessment. Despite the presence of a high fever, the child may not appear particularly ill. The physical findings are nonspecific, the cause is unknown, and no diagnostic tests exist for the illness.

Management. The prognosis for roseola infantum is excellent, with the most common com-

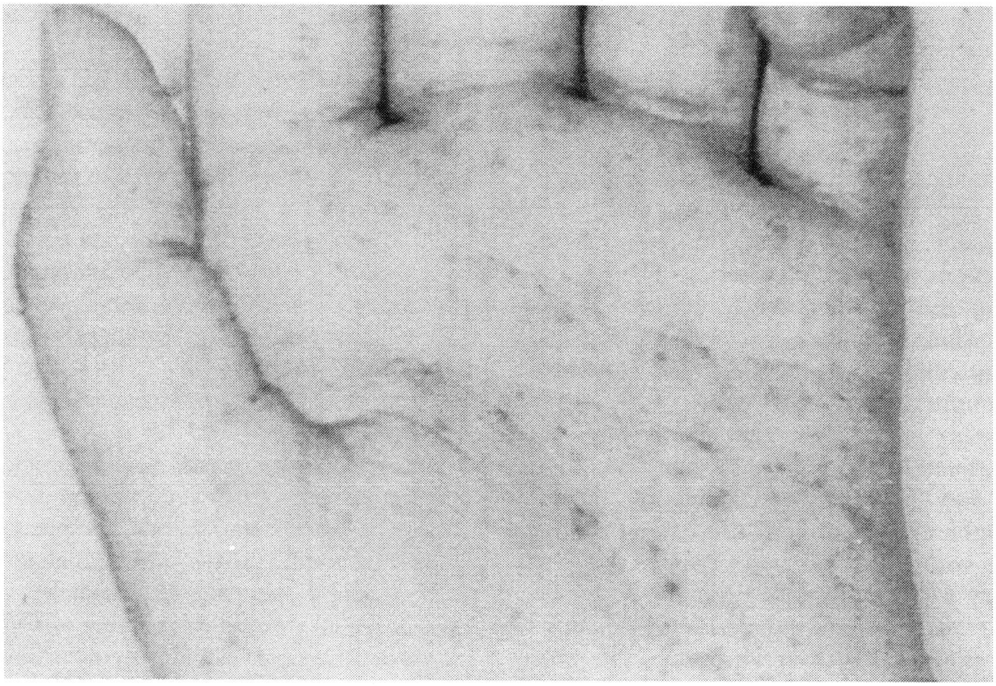

Fig. **49-2** Rocky Mountain spotted fever.

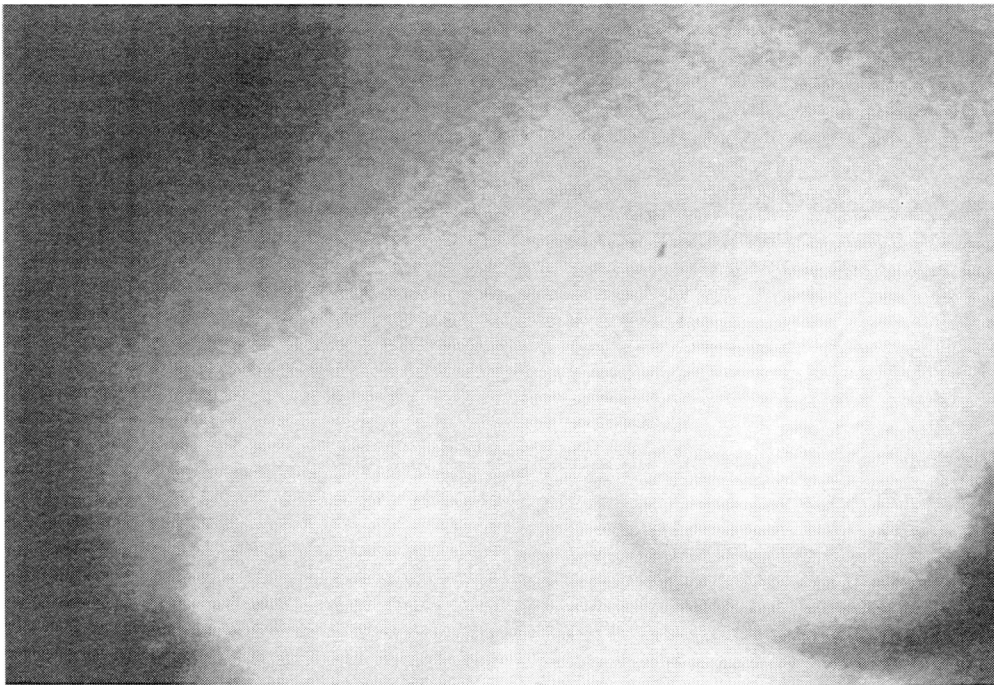

Fig.49-3 Rubella.

plication being the occurrence of febrile convulsions.

Rubella. Rubella (German measles) is a viral illness characterized by fever, skin eruption, and lymphadenopathy.

Appearance. The rash appears first on the face and spreads rapidly to the neck, trunk, and extremities. The pink or red maculopapules (Fig. 49-3) remain for 1 to 5 days and disappear at the end of 3 days.

Although the lymphadenopathy is generalized, the nodes most apparent are the suboccipital, postauricular, and posterior cervical.

Management. The most severe complication of rubella is fetal damage in pregnant women. No treatment is necessary in most cases of rubella.

Scarlet fever. Scarlet fever is caused by a group A beta-hemolytic streptococcal infection. The illness has an abrupt onset, with fever, chills, malaise, and sore throat followed by a distinctive rash.

Appearance. Scarlet fever includes a generalized papular eruption that overlays a hyperemic base that may spare the perioral areas. The skin has a rough "sandpaper" texture, which is produced by the many pinhead-sized lesions. The pharynx is infected, and erythematous lesions or petechiae may occur on the palate. Following the resolution of symptoms, desquamation of the involved areas occurs and is characteristic of the disease.

Management. Late complications include the development of rheumatic fever and acute glomerulonephritis. Penicillin is the preferred drug. Aim treatment at providing adequate antistreptococcal antibiotic levels for at least 10 days. For children less than 60 pounds, administer 600,000 units of penicillin G benzathine and 200,000 units of aqueous penicillin G procaine intramuscularly. For older children, the dose of benzathine penicillin is 900,000 units, with 300,000 units of aqueous penicillin G procaine intramuscularly (available as Bicillin C-R 900/300). Adults receive 1.2 million units of penicillin G benzathine intramuscularly. For patients who are allergic to penicillin, give 250 mg of erythromycin four times a day (or 40 mg/kg/day) orally for 10 days.

PAPULAR LESIONS

Red Papules

Drug eruptions (see the previous discussion) are commonly papular.

Contact dermatitis

Contact dermatitis is an inflammatory reaction of the skin to chemical, physical, or biologic agents. Caustics, industrial solvents, and detergents are common causes of irritant contact dermatitis. A skin eruption may result from a brief contact with a potent caustic agent or from repeated or prolonged contact with milder irritants.

Clothing, jewelry, plants, cosmetics, and medications contain allergens that commonly cause allergic contact dermatitis. The most common allergens include rubber compounds, nickel, and plants of the *Rhus* genus (poison ivy, oak, and sumac).

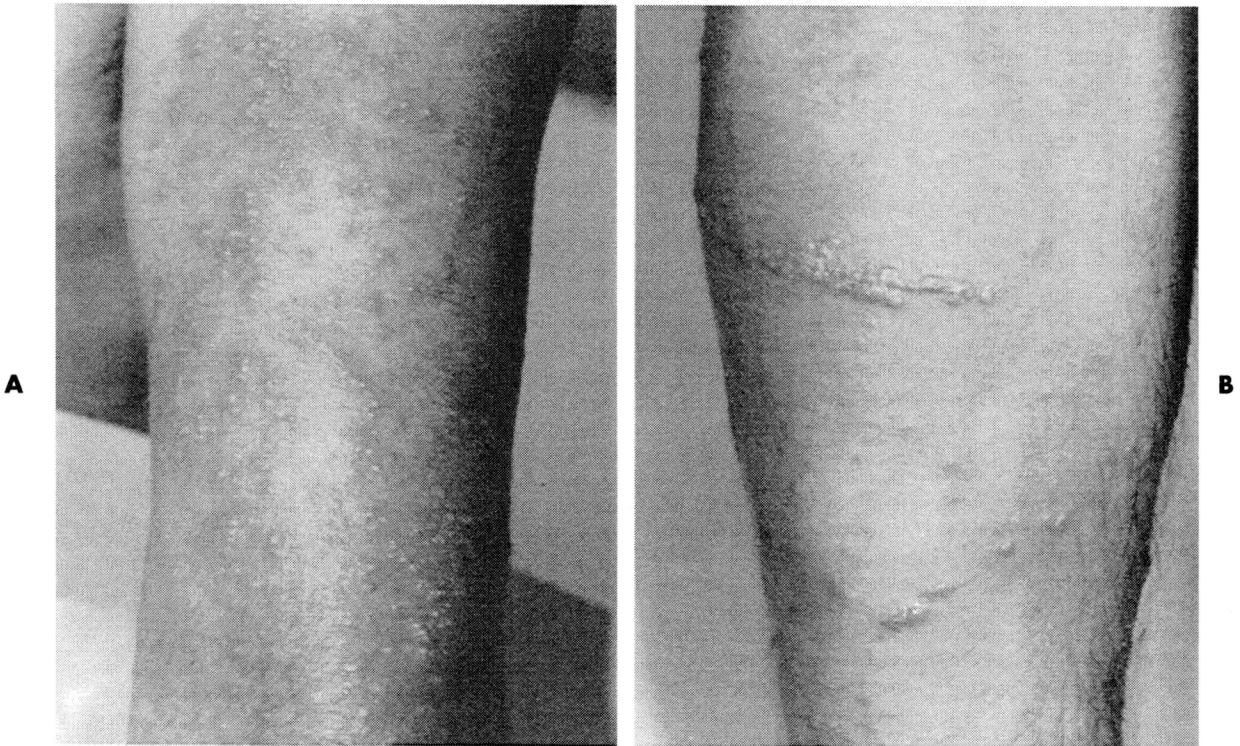

Fig. 49-4 **A,** Contact dermatitis secondary to nickel. **B,** Typical linear lesions of contact dermatitis secondary to poison ivy. (From Cydulka RK: Dermatologic disorders. In Rosen P et al, editors: *Emergency medicine: concepts and clinical practice*, ed 3, St Louis, 1992, Mosby. Photographs by David Effron, MD.)

Appearance. The primary lesions of contact dermatitis are papules, vesicles, or bullae on an erythematous bed (Fig. 49-4).

Management. Treat oozing or vesiculated lesions with cool wet compresses of Burow solution applied three to four times daily. Topical corticosteroid creams or ointments help reduce inflammation and pruritus. In some instances, such as severe cases of *Rhus* contact dermatitis, a 10- to 14-day tapering dose of systemic corticosteroids (beginning with a dose of prednisone of 30 to 80 mg daily) is necessary.

Erythema multiforme

Erythema multiforme is an acute, usually self-limiting disease precipitated by a variety of factors, the most common of which are drug exposure and herpes simplex infection. Other causes include other viral infections (especially hepatitis and influenza A), group A streptococcus, and a variety of illnesses. In approximately half of the cases, no provacative factor is apparent.

Appearance. Skin lesions are erythematous or violaceous macules, papules, vesicles, or bullae (Fig. 49-5). Their distribution is often symmetric and most commonly involve the palms and soles, backs of the hands and feet, and the extensor surfaces of the extremities.

The target lesion is the hallmark of erythema multiforme. Commonly occurring on the hand or wrist, this papule or vesicle is surrounded by a zone of normal skin and a halo of erythema.

The Stevens-Johnson syndrome is a severe form of erythema multiforme that is occasionally fatal. It is characterized by bullae, mucous membrane lesions, and multisystem involvement. The patient may be in a toxic condition; complaining of chills, headache, and malaise; and displaying fever, tachycardia, and tachypnea. Systemic involvement may occur, including renal, gastrointestinal, or respiratory tract lesions. Death results from infection and dehydration.

Management. Begin treatment of erythema multiforme with a search for the underlying cause. Severe cases (including Stevens-Johnson syndrome) require hospital admission for intravenous hydration and systemic corticosteroid therapy.

Pediculosis

Pediculosis consists of lice infestation and usually affects the hair-bearing areas of the body.

Appearance. Except with excoriations, no rash occurs. Louse eggs (nits) in the pubic hair and occasionally in the hair of other parts of the body are the identifying sign. *Pediculosis capitis* appears more commonly in small children

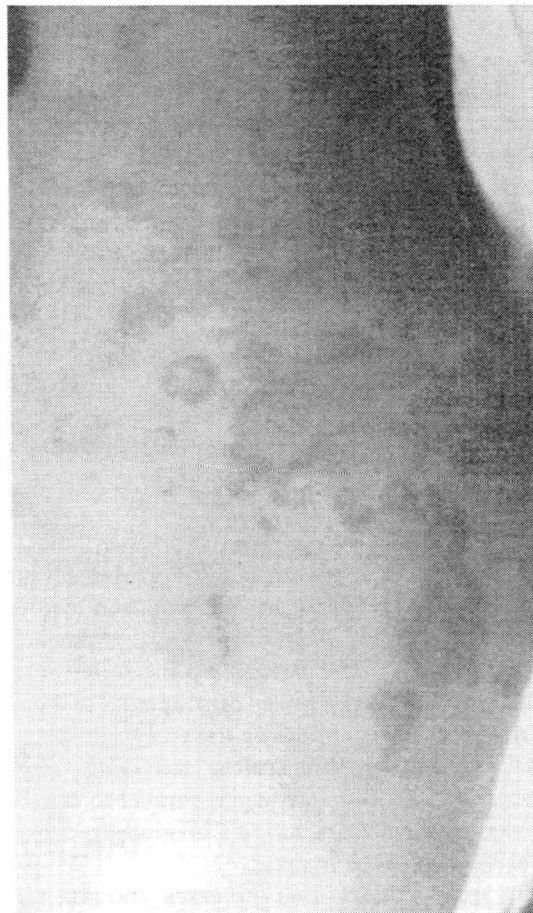

*Fig.*49-5 Erythema multiforme.

than in adults. Nits attach to the bases of hair shafts and appear as white dots. Adult forms look like blue or black grains. The patient complains of intense itching and scratching.

Management. Apply lindane (Kwell) lotion or cream to the infested and adjacent hairy areas. Also treat sexual partners.

Scabies

Scabies is a mite infestation characterized by severe itching that is usually worse at night.

Appearance. The areas of the body most commonly involved are the interdigital web spaces, the flexion areas of the wrists, the axillae, buttocks, lower back, scrotum, and breasts. Lesions may be papular, but the characteristic lesion is an elongated burrow.

Management. The transmission of scabies involves close personal contact. Treatment forms include lindane and crotamiton (Eurax) lotion and cream and permethrin (Elimite) cream. Apply the scabicide to the entire body (except the face and scalp), even though the lesions may be localized. Treat all family members and sexual contacts.

Scaly Papules

Fungal lesions (see the previous discussion) are typically scaly.

Pityriasis rosea

Pityriasis rosea is a benign skin eruption that occurs predominantly in children and young adults.

Appearance. The lesions are multiple, oval, pink or pigmented papules or plaques 1 to 2 cm in diameter. They appear on the trunk and proximal extremities. Mild scaling may occur (Fig. 49-6). The lesions are arranged parallel to the direction of the ribs, forming a Christmas tree–like distribution on the trunk.

In approximately half the cases, the generalized eruption is preceded by the appearance of a "herald patch," a larger (2 to 6 cm diameter) le-

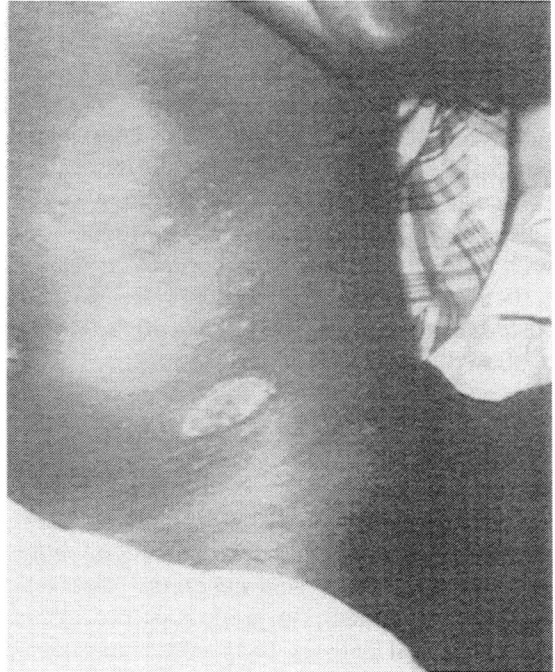

Fig. 49-6 Pityriasis rosea.

sion that resembles the smaller lesions in other respects.

Management. Pityriasis rosea is a self-limited condition of unknown cause that usually resolves in 8 to 12 weeks.

VESICULAR LESIONS (TABLE 49-2)

Pemphigus Vulgaris

Pemphigus vulgaris is an uncommon disorder and has a mortality rate of 10% to 15%. It is a bullous disease that affects men more commonly than women and is most common in patients 40 to 60 years of age.

Appearance

The typical skin lesions are small flaccid bullae that break easily and form superficial erosions and crusted ulcerations. The disorder may

Table 49-2

VESICULAR EXANTHEMS

Varicella (Chickenpox)	Herpes Zoster (Shingles)	Herpes Simplex
Diagnostic findings		
Rapid progression of erythematous macules, developing into papules and vesicles; vesicles are thin-walled and superficial, surrounded by an erythematous area; pruritic; distribution is central with relative sparing distally; marked variability in severity of exanthem—may only have a few lesions; usually febrile; enanthem—shallow mucosal ulcers; different ages of lesions; may initially resemble insect bites	Erythema followed by red papules that become vesicular in 12-24 hr, become pustular in 72 hr, and crust in 10-12 days; distribution is unilateral after peripheral dermatome or cranial nerve; preeruptive pain with hyperesthesia over involved skin	Multiple presentations **Gingivostomatitis:** fever; irritability; pain in mouth, throat, and with swallowing; shallow ulcers on mucosa (buccal, tonsillar, and pharyngeal); crusts on lips; cervical lymphadenopathy; lasts 1-14 days **Vulvovaginitis:** similar shallow ulcers on vagina and vulva; pain on urination **Keratoconjunctivitis:** corneal ulceration
Complications		
Pneumonia Secondary bacterial infections: cellulitis, bacterial pneumonia Encephalitis, myelitis Hepatitis Reye syndrome	Ophthalmic: neuralgia, corneal dendrites, iritis Postherpetic neuralgia	Ophthalmic: corneal ulceration Encephalitis Neonatal viremia with encephalitis
Management		

Antipruritic agents
  Topical: calamine lotion; cold baths with small amount baking soda (⅓ tsp) in water
  Systemic: diphenhydramine
Antipyretics—Do *not* use aspirin
Treatment of complications
Acyclovir 80 mg/kg/24 hr (max: 3200 mg/24 hr) po qid for 5 days; begin within 24 hr onset of rash in high-risk patients*
Varicella-zoster immune globulin (VZIG) for exposure in high-risk patient; 125 units/10 kg (max: 625 units)
	Support, analgesia
	Eye involvement needs ophthalmology consultation
	Acyclovir may have a role in specific circumstances
	Steroids or amitriptyline may reduce postherpetic neuralgia
		General support
		Gingival: topical analgesia—antacid or mixture of viscous lidocaine (Xylocaine), diphenhydramine, Kaopectate; acyclovir (Zovirax): topical, IV, po for initial and recurrent lesions

Comment		
Incubation: 14-21 days Vaccine Particularly dangerous in newborns, pregnant females, immunosuppressed or immunodeficient individuals	Common history of chickenpox	Sexual spread of vulvovaginitis Potentially life threatening to newborn, immunodeficient, or immunosuppressed; consider systemic acyclovir

From Barkin RM, Rosen P: *Emergency pediatrics: a guide to ambulatory care,* ed 4, St Louis, 1994, Mosby.
*Nonpregnant patients ≥13 yr, children >12 mo with chronic cutaneous or pulmonary disorders, as well as children receiving short, intermittent, or aerosolized courses of corticosteroids. The use in children of household contacts is controversial.

involve any area of the body. Applying firm tangential pressure to the intact epithelium may extend blisters or form new bullae; this sign is characteristic of the condition. Approximately half of the patients with pemphigus vulgaris have oral lesions, which are bullous but commonly break, leaving painful, denuded areas of superficial ulceration.

Management

The cause of pemphigus vulgaris is unknown. Treat this condition with oral glucocorticoids (in the initial dose of 100 to 300 mg of prednisone or an equivalent). Most deaths are related to uncontrolled spread of the disease. Secondary infection, dehydration, thromboembolism, and other illness also contribute to the mortality.

Herpes Simplex Infection

Appearance

The hallmark of skin infection with herpes simplex virus (HSV) is the presence of grouped vesicles on an erythematous base. The lesions are usually localized in a nondermatomal distribution, but the distribution may be more gener-

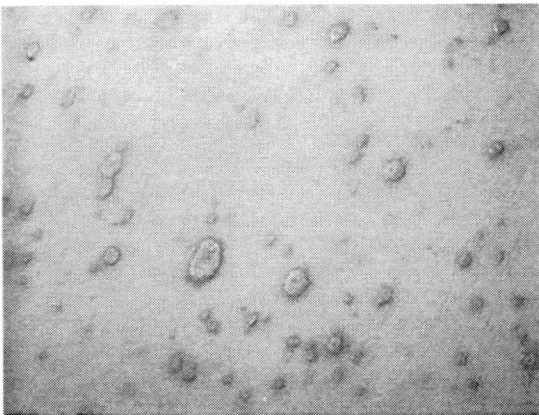

Fig. 49-7 Varicella. (From Stratte EG: Common exanthems. In Noble J et al, editors: *Textbook of primary care medicine*, St Louis, 1996, Mosby.)

alized in patients with atopic dermatitis or other dermatoses.

Genital infections in men appear with either single or multiple vesicles on the shaft or glans penis. The patient may experience fever, malaise, and regional lymphadenopathy. The vesicles erode after several days, become crusted, and heal in 10 to 14 days. Infections in women may involve the introitus vaginae, cervix, or vagina. Herpetic cervicitis or vaginitis may cause severe pelvic pain, dysuria, or vaginal discharge. Recurrence of HSV infection is common, but recurrent episodes tend to be less severe. In immunocompromised patients, the HSV infection may become disseminated to diffuse areas of the skin or viscera.

Management

For either primary or recurrent genital herpes, administer acyclovir 200 mg five times per day. This treatment is not curative nor has it been shown to prevent recurrences. However, it does produce a significant reduction of symptoms, viral shedding, and time for lesions to heal.

Varicella

Varicella (chickenpox) is an infection caused by the varicella-zoster virus.

Appearance

The vesicle of varicella is 2 to 3 mm in diameter and is surrounded by an erythematous border. Drying of the vesicle begins centrally, producing umbilication. Skin lesions rapidly (sometimes within hours) progress from macules to papules to vesicles to crusting (Fig. 49-7). The hallmark of varicella is the appearance of lesions in all stages of development in one region of the body.

Management

The illness is usually self-limited, and treatment is symptomatic only. Pneumonia, encephalitis, and bacterial secondary infections must be considered. Because varicella infection is more serious in adolescents and adults, treatment with acyclovir (800 mg qid for 5 days) may be considered. Treatment is only effective if initiated within 24 hours of disease onset.

Herpes Zoster

Herpes zoster (shingles) is also an infection caused by the varicella-zoster virus. The majority of cases occur in healthy individuals, but the association of the eruption with various malignancies is well known.

Appearance

The rash consists of grouped vesicles on an erythematous base and involves one or several contiguous dermatomes. The thorax, abdomen, or face is the usual site of involvement (Fig. 49-8). Before the appearance of the rash, the patient typically develops pain in the dermatomal distribution.

Herpes zoster has a low mortality, even when dissemination occurs. Ocular involvement occurs in half of the cases and involves the ophthalmic division of the trigeminal nerve. Postherpetic neuralgia (pain that persists after the lesions have healed) occurs more commonly in elderly and immunocompromised patients. It may last a number of months and is often resistant to treatment with standard analgesic medications.

Management

Treatment of herpes zoster is rarely necessary. Prescribe analgesics as needed. Early corticosteroid therapy may shorten the duration of postherpetic neuralgia but does not affect the rate of the healing of skin lesions. Acyclovir 600 to 800 mg five times daily may be useful in patients with immune system compromise. The use of acyclovir in uncomplicated cases is controversial. Acyclovir appears to shorten the duration of skin lesions, but there appears to be little effect on postherpetic neuralgia.

PUSTULAR LESIONS

Impetigo

Impetigo is a slowly evolving pustular eruption that is most common in preschool children. In this group, group A *Streptococcus* has long been

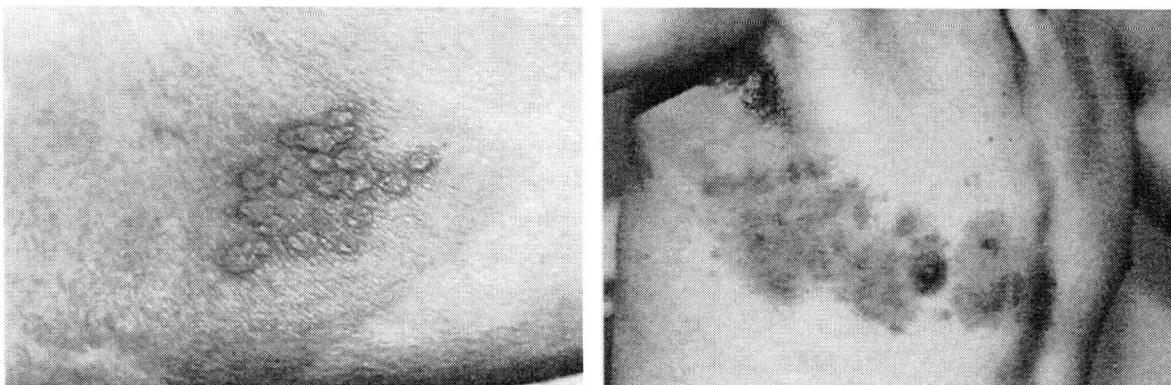

Fig. 49-8   **A,** Herpes zoster. **B,** Herpes zoster infection. (From Cydulka RK: Dermatologic disorders. In Rosen P et al, editors: *Emergency medicine: concepts and clinical practice,* ed 3, St Louis, 1992, Mosby. Photographs by David Effron, MD.)

Fig. 49-9   Impetigo.

considered to be the primary pathogen. However, there is increasing evidence that *S. aureus* is a major pathogen in impetigo, either alone or in conjunction with streptococcus. Bullous impetigo is caused by staphylococcal infection and is a less common form than streptococcal impetigo.

Appearance

Impetigo occurs most often on the face and other exposed areas. It begins as vesicles 1 to 2 mm across with erythematous margins. When these vesicles break, they leave a red erosion covered with a golden, yellow crust (Fig. 49-9). Regional lymphadenopathy is common. Postinfection glomerulonephritis is a recognized complication.

Bullous impetigo appears primarily in infants and young children. The initial skin lesions are thin-walled bullae 1 to 2 cm across. When these bullae rupture, they leave a thin serous crust.

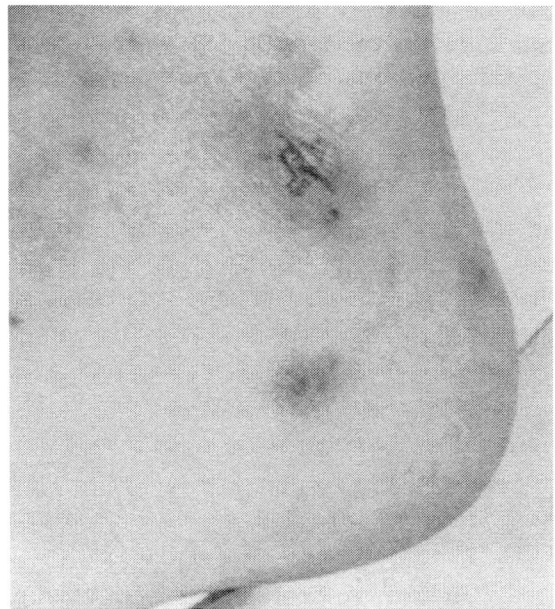

Fig. 49-10   Disseminated gonococcemia.

Management

Treat localized impetigo with a topical application of mupirocin, three times/day. Do not use if there is significant local lyphadenopathy. Treat widespread lesions with erythromycin 30 to 50 mg/kg/day, cephalexin 25 to 50 mg/kg/day, or dicloxacillin 25 to 50 mg/kg/day.

Gonococcal Dermatitis

The arthritis-dermatitis syndrome is the most common presentation of disseminated gonococcal disease and primarily affects young women. Fever and migratory polyarthralgias commonly accompany the rash.

Appearance

Skin lesions are often multiple and have a predilection for periarticular regions of the distal extremities. The lesions begin as erythematous or hemorrhagic papules that evolve into pustules and vesicles with an erythematous halo (Fig. 49-10). These lesions are tender and may have a gray necrotic or hemorrhagic center.

Management

The patient should be hospitalized for initial treatment of disseminated gonococcal infection (a 7-day course of treatment). Initial treatment should be parenteral, with one of the following agents: ceftriaxone (1 g IV or IM every 24 hours) or ceftizoxime or cefotaxime (dosage for either is 1 g IV every 8 hours). Patients with beta-lactam allergies should be given spectinomycin 2 g IM every 12 hours.

Recommended Reading

Levine N: Management of life-threatening dermatoses, *Emerg Med Clin North Am* 4:747, 1985.

Parker CW: Drug allergy, *N Engl J Med* 292:511, 957, 1975.

Sternbach GL: Dermatologic problems. In Rosen P et al, editors: *Emergency medicine: concepts and clinical practice,* ed 3, St Louis, 1992, Mosby.

Sternbach GL, Callen JP: Dermatitis, *Emerg Med Clin North Am* 4:677, 1985.

Weston WL, Morelli JG, Lane AT: *Color textbook of pediatric dermatology,* ed 2, St Louis, 1996, Mosby.

Chapter Fifty
STROKE

RASHMI U. KOTHARI AND WILLIAM G. BARSAN

Strokes are the third leading cause of death and the leading cause of brain damage in the United States. The hallmark of a stroke is the abrupt onset of focal neurologic deficits as a result of a disruption of regional cerebral blood flow. Strokes are classified as either ischemic or hemorrhagic. Ischemic strokes are caused by the occlusion of arteries by a thrombus or embolus, whereas a hemorrhagic stroke results from the rupture of a cerebral vessel.

More than 80% of all strokes are ischemic in nature. The majority are caused by vessel thrombosis, which occurs when clot formation is superimposed on gradual vessel narrowing or alterations in the luminal lining of the vessel. Atherosclerotic disease is the most common cause of thrombotic strokes in the United States. In an embolic stroke, intravascular material that is released from a proximal source occludes a distal vessel. The most common sources of emboli are the heart or neck vessels (common vascular sites include the carotid bifurcation and the junction of the vertebral and basilar arteries). The heart becomes a major source of emboli when intracardiac flow is impaired or valves are damaged. Conditions involving impaired flow include atrial fibrillation and recent myocardial infarction (MI) with a dyskinetic left ventricle. Among other lesions, valve emboli may result from rheumatic heart disease, prosthetic valves, bacterial endocarditis, or mitral valve prolapse.

A hemorrhagic stroke is categorized according to the location of the bleeding. An intracerebral hemorrhage (ICH) occurs when there is bleeding into the brain parenchyma; a subarachnoid hemorrhage (SAH) is a result of bleeding on the brain surface within the subarachnoid space. An ICH is twice as common as an SAH and is commonly caused by the rupture of weakened arterioles resulting from chronic systemic hypertension. Bleeding is usually localized to the putamen, thalamus, pons, or cerebellum. Amyloid angiopathy may be an important cause of ICH in the elderly who have recurrent or lobar hemorrhages. An SAH is primarily caused by an aneurysmal rupture, which most commonly arises at an arterial bifurcation and occurs in a somewhat younger population than does an ICH. A substantial proportion of SAHs occur in patients younger than 55 years of age.

CLINICAL PRESENTATION

Ischemic Stroke

A cerebral artery occlusion results in the sudden appearance of focal neurologic deficits. With an embolism, these deficits can occur within seconds or minutes; with a thrombus, such deficits develop over minutes to hours. Although the patient may be confused or drowsy after stroke onset, significant obtundation is unusual unless the patient has had a massive stroke, a stroke that involves both cerebral hemispheres, or a brainstem stroke.

Ischemic strokes can usually be clinically described as involving either the anterior (carotid) circulation or the posterior (vertebrobasilar) circulation. Anterior circulation strokes produce contralateral motor and sensory deficits; aphasia may occur if the dominant hemisphere is involved. Pathologic neglect and an inability to identify right from left are often seen with nondominant hemispheric lesions. The posterior circulation supplies blood to the brainstem, cerebellum, and visual cortex. The hallmarks of a posterior circulation stroke are crossed neurologic deficits (e.g., ipsilateral cranial nerve deficits with contralateral motor weakness). Other signs and symptoms attributable to vertebrobasilar stroke include dizziness, vertigo, diplopia, dysphagia, ataxia, and cranial nerve palsies.

Transient ischemic attacks (TIAs) manifest as temporary focal neurologic deficits as a result of an occlusion in either the anterior or posterior circulation and are most commonly associated with thrombotic lesions. They are different from strokes because the deficits completely resolve within 24 hours. Most TIAs occur rapidly over minutes and usually resolve within an hour. There is a 5% to 6% increased risk for a stroke each year after a TIA.

Strokes and TIAs that involve specific cerebral arteries often appear in classical patterns (Table 50-1). Occlusions of the middle cerebral artery are often associated with contralateral sensory and motor deficits, in which the arm and face are more affected than the leg. In addition, such patients are often aphasic or exhibit neglect, depending on the hemisphere involved. In contrast, lesions of the anterior cerebral artery produce leg weakness that is more prominent than arm weakness, mild contralateral cortical sensory deficits, and dyspraxia. Lacunar strokes represent a special subset of thrombotic stroke that is seen almost exclu-

Table *50-1*

PHYSICAL FINDINGS SUGGESTING SPECIFIC STROKE SYNDROMES

Stroke Syndrome	Findings
Embolus	Sudden onset of deficits, atrial fibrillation or recent MI, history of multiple TIAs or strokes in multiple vascular distributions
Thrombus	Deficits developing over minutes to hours, carotid bruit, history of TIAs in the same vascular distribution
MCA* occlusion	Motor deficits of arm and face greater than leg, aphasia with dominant hemispheric involvement, neglect with nondominant hemisphere involvement
ACA* occlusion	Motor deficits of leg greater than arm, cortical sensory deficit, dyspraxia
Vertebrobasilar syndrome	Ipsilateral cranial nerve deficits with contralateral motor weakness, dysphagia, ataxia, diplopia
ICH	Sudden onset of neurologic deficit, headache, vomiting, markedly elevated blood pressure, and rapid clinical deterioration
SAH	Sudden onset of severe headache, nuchal pain or rigidity, mental confusion, relatively nonfocal examination, preretinal hemorrhage
Cerebellar hemorrhage	Sudden onset of severe vertigo, truncal ataxia, and vomiting

*MCA, Middle cerebral. ACA, anterior cerebral.

sively in hypertensive patients. These strokes are small, well-localized infarcts that primarily involve the basal ganglia and pons. They are abrupt in onset, stabilize over days, and do not affect higher language function or consciousness. Unilateral pure motor or pure sensory deficits are the most common presentations in patients with lacunar strokes.

Hemorrhagic Stroke

An ICH may be clinically indistinguishable from a cerebral infarction; patients with ICH may experience contralateral hemiplegia, hemianesthesia, hemianopsia, and aphasia. The presentation may differ from an infarction in that patients are more commonly lethargic, have marked hypertension, can quickly deteriorate, and often require emergency intubation. Headache, nausea, and vomiting often precede or occur concomitantly with the neurologic deficit. Such symptoms are less common in patients with ischemic stroke. Large hemorrhage volume, intraventricular hemorrhage, and deep (versus lobar) hemorrhage are associated with a lower 30-day survival rate.

A lack of focal findings, as well as the patient's age, help distinguish SAH from ICH. Lateralizing findings are notably absent with SAH except for the occasional visual field cut, oculomotor palsy (caused by aneurysmal compression), or focal seizure. The cardinal SAH symptom is an excruciating headache that is maximal at onset and often accompanied by vomiting and nuchal rigidity. Premonitory headaches caused by leakage of blood (sentinel headache) occur in 15% to 31% of all patients with SAH and may precede a significant hemorrhage by hours or days.

ASSESSMENT

The initial evaluation for a stroke should follow the same sequence used in any critically ill pa-

tient and should start with the ABCs of resuscitation. After the initial stabilization, a more focused examination should be performed. The neurologic examination is obviously the most important part of the assessment but can be done quickly in a focused manner. Examination of the cranial nerves is important, particularly with reference to cranial nerves II through VII. The pupils and extraocular movements often reveal important information regarding cerebral herniation. Third- or sixth–cranial nerve palsy may be the first sign of impending herniation. Central facial weakness can be distinguished from peripheral causes of weakness by observing the patient's ability to wrinkle the forehead; patients with upper motor neuron involvement (i.e., stroke) retain the ability to wrinkle the forehead.

After assessing the cranial nerves, a motor and sensory examination is appropriate. Muscle tone can be assessed by moving a relaxed limb. Proximal and distal strength in the extremity should be measured against resistance and gravity. Arm drift is a particularly sensitive sign of motor weakness and is performed by having the patient close his or her eyes and stretch out both hands with the palms up. Observe the distance the arms drift from the original position and any difference between the two extremities. Leg strength is best assessed by walking if the patient is able to do so. Even subtle motor weaknesses are evident on attempted gait. If the patient cannot walk, leg strength can be assessed by having the patient hold the leg above the bed at 45 degrees for 5 seconds and by observing for any weakness. The neurologic examination should always test cerebellar function, reflexes, and gait. Finger-to-nose testing, heel-to-shin testing, and the observation of rapid alternating movements can be used to assess cerebellar function in the nonambulatory patient. If the patient is able to stand and walk, it is important to observe ambulation and heel-and-toe walking. Deep tendon reflexes and the Babinski sign should also be tested.

Speech assessment is a particularly important part of the neurologic examination. The distinction should be made between aphasia (dysphasia) and dysarthria. Dysarthria is a disturbance in articulation resulting from paralysis or incoordination of the muscles used for speech; the content of speech is appropriate and normal. In contrast, aphasia is a result of a disturbance in language processing and appears as an inability to understand speech or communicate effectively using speech.

Although a complete physical examination should be performed in all patients with stroke, there are some particular areas that should be thoroughly assessed. An examination for signs of trauma is important for detecting the patient who may have a subdural or epidural hematoma. A funduscopic examination may reveal papilledema, a preretinal hemorrhage of SAH, hypertensive changes, or diabetic retinopathy. The cardiac examination should specifically assess heart rate and rhythm, cardiac murmurs, and large vessel bruits, particularly in the carotid area. Clinical evidence of cardiac failure should also be sought because poor cardiac output may contribute to brain hypoperfusion.

DIFFERENTIAL DIAGNOSIS

Although a stroke is the most common cause of unilateral weakness, other causes must be considered (see the box above). All patients with neurologic deficits should have a blood sugar determination to rule out hypoglycemia. Bell palsy (peripheral seventh–cranial nerve palsy) usually occurs in younger patients, is associated with upper and lower facial paralysis, and does not involve the extremities. Evidence of trauma should be sought because an epidural or subdural hematoma can mimic an acute stroke. Although a stroke can appear with marked hypertension, a stroke can usually be differentiated from hypertensive encephalopathy by the history and physical examination. Unlike a stroke, the onset of

DIFFERENTIAL DIAGNOSIS OF ACUTE STROKE
Hypoglycemia Postictal (Todd) paralysis Bell palsy Hypertensive encephalopathy Epidural/subdural hematoma Brain tumor/abscess Complicated migraine

hypertensive encephalopathy is more gradual, and focal neurologic deficits, if present, are superimposed on a more global cerebral dysfunction (e.g., decreased level of consciousness) rather than isolated to one brain region. Papilledema, flame-shaped retinal hemorrhages, and acute renal failure are all indicative of hypertensive encephalopathy. A hemiplegic or ophthalmoplegic migraine can also be mistaken for stroke, and either of these migraines can cause focal neurologic deficits that last for hours. Postictal (Todd) paralysis, demyelinating processes, vasculitis, and brain tumors are other diseases that can mimic a stroke.

GENERAL APPROACH TO MANAGEMENT

When managing patients who have had a stroke, priority should be given to airway, oxygenation, stabilization, and comfort. Patients should be placed on oxygen, a monitor and intravenous line established, and the head of the bed should be slightly elevated. A determination of blood glucose and a noncontrast CT scan should be ordered early in the patient's evaluation. Fluids should usually be run at a minimum rate to prevent cerebral edema. Hypotension, if present, should be treated immediately to prevent brain hypoperfusion. Dextrose-containing solutions should be avoided in patients who are suspected of having a stroke, except in those with documented hypoglycemia. In patients with ischemic strokes, hyperglycemia has been associated with an increase in infarct volume and poor long-term outcome. Blood samples for a complete blood count, platelet count, blood chemistry, and coagulation studies should also be obtained.

A noncontrast CT scan of the head is essential because it can quickly differentiate an ischemic from a hemorrhagic infarction. Most ischemic strokes are undetectable by a CT scan until 24 to 48 hours following the event. A CT scan can identify almost all ICHs greater than 1 cm in diameter and as much as 95% of all SAHs. A lumbar puncture (LP) is required in all patients who are suspected of having an SAH when the CT scan is normal. In fact, if the patient is young and complains of "the worst headache of my life," it is acceptable to start with the LP and skip the CT scan, because the LP can detect smaller bleeds.

Ischemic Stroke

Emergency physicians should take a cautious approach to the management of elevated blood pressure in patients with an acute ischemic stroke. Only sustained severe hypertension (≥220 mm Hg systolic or ≥120 mm Hg diastolic) should be treated; pharmacologic lowering of systemic blood pressure may reduce perfusion to areas of the brain that are already marginally perfused. A sudden reduction in systemic pressure can convert an area with reversible injury to an area of infarction.

Transient ischemic attacks

Although the effectiveness of heparin is unproven in the management of acute stroke, its use should be considered for patients with recent TIAs who are at high risk for recurrence. Such patients include those with: (1) a known high-grade stenosis in the appropriate vascular distribution for the symptoms, (2) a cardioembolic source, (3) TIAs of increasing frequency

(crescendo TIAs), and (4) TIAs that occur despite antiplatelet therapy.

An urgent carotid endarterectomy should be considered for anterior circulation TIAs that resolve within the first 6 hours and are associated with 70% to 99% stenosis of the appropriate carotid artery. An endarterectomy has been shown to significantly reduce the risk for a future stroke in these patients.

Embolic stroke

Patients who have had an embolic stroke and are experiencing minor deficits should be anticoagulated. Approximately 10% to 15% of all recurrent emboli occur within 2 weeks of the initial event, and some within 24 hours. Because of the increased risk of spontaneous hemorrhagic changes associated with heparin, anticoagulation with heparin should be withheld for 3 to 4 days following a large cardioembolic stroke.

Thrombotic stroke

Treatment for a stable, completed thrombotic stroke is largely supportive. Anticoagulation has not proven to be beneficial and should not be used in patients with completed strokes. Large randomized stroke trials are currently underway to study the efficacy of thrombolytic therapy within 3 to 6 hours of symptom onset, and the results appear promising. Immediate heparinization should be considered in patients with stuttering or progressively worsening symptoms.

Emergency thrombectomies or endarterectomies for patients with persistent neurologic deficits resulting from cerebral ischemia are controversial and unproven. Some authors suggest that emergency surgery be considered for a progressive anterior circulation stroke with extracranial arterial disease when there are favorable angiographic findings such as stenosis greater than 90%, carotid dissection, aortic dissection, or an intraluminal clot attached to a plaque.

The use of agents that prevent platelet aggregation, such as aspirin and ticlopidine, has been suggested for acute treatment of a recent stroke. It is unlikely that these agents would be effective if given in the first few hours after a stroke, but when given chronically are useful in preventing recurring strokes in patients who have had TIAs and small strokes.

Vertebrobasilar infarction

Unfortunately, no study definitively establishes the advantages or disadvantages of a specific therapy for patients with an acute, well-defined, occlusive vascular disease within the posterior circulation. Most authors suggest the use of heparin in patients with posterior circulation TIAs or progressive vertebrobasilar strokes.

Cerebellar infarction

Symptoms and signs of a cerebellar infarction include the sudden onset of severe vertigo, truncal ataxia, and vomiting. An early neurosurgical consultation is needed for all patients with a cerebellar infarction. Cerebellar swelling can lead to rapid deterioration with herniation, and a neurosurgical consultation is required to determine the need for an emergency posterior fossa decompression.

Management of Hemorrhagic Strokes

After appropriate attention has been given to the ABCs, early management of hemorrhagic stroke should focus on the regulation of blood pressure, the control of brain edema, and prompt neurosurgical evaluation.

Intracerebral hemorrhage

To date, there are no randomized studies to evaluate the appropriate management of blood pressure after an intracerebral hemorrhage. Current published guidelines recommend treatment only for severe hypertension (i.e., ≥200 mm Hg systolic or >120 mm Hg diastolic). When treated,

blood pressure should be gradually lowered to prehemorrhage levels with either labetalol or nitroprusside. Exceptions to this rule are cases of intracerebral hemorrhage associated with cardiac failure or aortic dissection, in which more rapid reduction is required. Treatment with hyperventilation, mannitol, and furosemide is recommended for patients with evidence of increased intracranial pressure when mass effect, midline shift, or herniation are present.

The role of acute surgical intervention remains controversial except in patients with cerebellar hemorrhage (in which surgical decompression is strongly recommended). Surgical intervention for noncerebellar hemorrhages depends on the neurologic status of the patient, as well as the size and location of the hemorrhage.

Subarachnoid hemorrhage

Rebleeding and vasospasm are the major morbid complications in SAH; the risk of re-

Table *50-2*

HUNT AND HESS CLASSIFICATION OF SUBARACHNOID HEMORRHAGE

Classification	Symptoms
Grade I	Asymptomatic or minimal headache and mild nuchal rigidity
Grade II	Moderate-to-severe headache, nuchal rigidity, no neurologic deficit other than cranial nerve palsy
Grade III	Drowsiness, confusion, or mild focal deficit
Grade IV	Stupor, moderate-to-severe hemiparesis, possible early decerebrate rigidity and vegetative disturbance
Grade V	Deep coma, decerebrate rigidity, moribund appearance

bleeding is greatest in the first 24 hours. Lowering systolic blood pressure to 160 mm Hg or maintaining a mean arterial pressure of 110 mm Hg has been associated with a lower risk of rebleeding and a decreased mortality. Current guidelines recommend that blood pressure be maintained at prehemorrhage levels.

Cerebral ischemia resulting from vasospasm occurs 2 days to 3 weeks after an aneurysm rupture. Nimodipine 60 mg PO every 6 hours has been found to reduce the incidence and severity of vasospasm and should be given to all patients with SAH who are in good neurologic condition (Hunt and Hess Grades I to III) (Table 50-2). Seizures and persistent vomiting can cause elevations in systemic and intracranial pressure

(ICP). Phenytoin loading is recommended as a prophylaxis against seizures. Nausea and vomiting should be promptly treated with an antiemetic.

Management of increased ICP is an important aspect of therapy in SAH. Increased ICP may be caused by mass effect, infarction with edema, or blockage of cerebrospinal fluid (CSF) absorption that results in hydrocephalus. Hyperventilation and osmotic agents are useful temporizing measures. Ventricular drainage is effective in treating hydrocephalus. Candidates for early angiography and surgical intervention usually are stable patients in good neurologic condition (Hunt and Hess Grades I to III). However, there is little published evidence that this regimen reduces long-term morbidity or mortality.

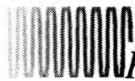

KEY CONSIDERATIONS

WHAT IS THE LIFE THREAT?

Hemorrhagic stroke, subarachnoid hemorrhage, or massive ischemic strokes can be lethal.

DOES THE PATIENT NEED ADMISSION?

Patients with stroke and TIA generally require hospital admission for continuing evaluation and treatment, including life support following a massive stroke.

WHAT IS THE MOST SERIOUS DIAGNOSIS?

Severe intracranial or subarachnoid hemorrhage and a massive ischemic stroke that involves either anterior or posterior cerebral circulation are the most serious diagnoses.

HAVE I PERFORMED A THOROUGH WORK-UP?

Perform a CT scan.

Carefully evaluate and control blood pressure after an ischemic and hypertensive stroke. To maintain cerebral perfusion, blood pressure must not be lowered too aggressively.

Recommended Reading

Adams HP et al: Guidelines for management of patients with acute ischemic stroke: a statement for health professionals from a special writing group of the stroke council, American Heart Association, *Stroke* 25(9):1901-1913, 1994.

Barnett HJM: *Stroke: Pathophysiology, diagnosis, and management,* ed 2, New York, 1992, Churchill Livingstone.

Brott T, Broderick JP: Intracerebral hemorrhage, *Heart Dis Stroke* 2:59, 1993.

Caplan LR: *Stroke: a clinical approach,* ed 2, Stoneham, Mass, 1993, Butterworth-Heinemann.

Emergency Brain Resuscitation: A working group on emergency brain resuscitation, *Ann Intern Med* 122:622-627, 1995.

Kase CS: Diagnosis and management of intracerebral hemorrhage in elderly patients, *Clin Geriatr Med* 7:549, 1991.

Kassell NJ et al: The international cooperative study on the timing of aneurysm surgery, Part I: Overall management results, *J Neurosurg* 73:18, 1990.

National Stroke Association Consensus Statement: Stroke: the first six hours, *Stroke Clin Update* 4:1, 1993.

Powers WJ: Acute hypertension after stroke: the scientific basis for treatment decisions, *Neurology* 43:461, 1993.

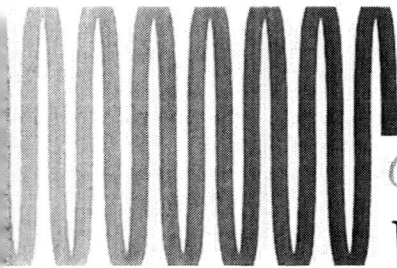

Chapter *Fifty-one*

VERTIGO

JONATHAN S. OLSHAKER

Most patients who experience "dizziness" have an organic basis for their symptoms. The diagnostic process is consistently based on two basic concepts: deciding whether the patient has true vertigo and, if vertigo exists, whether the cause is central or peripheral.

Patients use the term *dizzy* to describe a variety of experiences. Ask the patient to describe the sensation without using the word *dizzy*. True vertigo is defined as a sensation of disorientation in space combined with a sensation of motion. There is a hallucination of movement of either the self (subjective vertigo) or the external environment (objective vertigo). Descriptions of lightheadedness or feeling faint should lead the physician to consider a differential diagnosis for presyncope that includes dysrhythmias, hypovolemia, and vasovagal episodes. For some patients, dizziness is simply a metaphor for malaise and represents a variety of other causes such as anemia, viral illness, and depression.

If the patient has true vertigo, determine whether the cause is a peripheral lesion (e.g., of the inner ear) or a central process such as cerebrovascular disease or a neoplasm. In most cases peripheral disorders are benign, whereas central processes have more serious consequences that warrant an aggressive, urgent work-up and, in most cases, admission to the hospital. Occasionally, as in the case of a cerebellar bleed, immediate therapeutic intervention is indicated.

Cases of centrally caused vertigo share several typical characteristics: gradual onset, continuous symptoms, all varieties of nystagmus, the absence of hearing loss and positional symptoms, and the presence of associated neurologic abnormalities. Peripherally caused vertigo is typified by a sudden onset, intermittent episodes, horizontorotary positional nystagmus, and a normal neurologic examination. An associated hearing loss is sometimes present. Table 51-1 summarizes the characteristics of peripheral and central vertigo.

PATHOPHYSIOLOGY

The maintenance of equilibrium and an awareness of the body in relationship to its surroundings depends on the interaction of three systems: visual, proprioceptive, and vestibular. The sense organs of these systems are connected with the cerebellum by way of the vestibular nuclei in the brainstem (Fig. 51-1). Any disease that interrupts the integration of these three systems, such as lesions or ischemia in the brainstem or cerebellum, may give rise to symptoms of vertigo and disequilibrium.

Visual impulses are mediated through the higher brain centers and provide information about body position in space. Impulses from proprioceptors of the joints and muscles supply data about the relative positions of the parts of the body.

Table 51-1

CHARACTERISTICS OF PERIPHERAL AND CENTRAL VERTIGO

	Peripheral	*Central*
Onset	Sudden	Gradual
Intensity	Severe	Mild
Duration	Usually seconds or minutes; occasionally hours, days (intermittent)	Usually weeks, months (continuous)
Direction of nystagmus	One direction (usually horizonto-rotary), never vertical	Horizontal, rotary, or vertical (different directions in different positions)
Effect of head position	Worsened by position, often a single critical position	Little change, associated with more than one position
Associated neurologic findings	None	Usually present
Associated auditory findings	May be present, including tinnitus	None

The vestibular apparatus consists of three semicircular canals with their cristae and two otolithic structures, the utricle and saccule. The semicircular canals provide information about body orientation with respect to gravity. The semicircular canals are paired structures on each side of the head and normally respond to motion symmetrically. With inner ear disease, the resting discharge or the discharge stimulated by motion can be altered in one ear, which produces asymmetric responses and results in the perception of vertigo.

Impulses leave the vestibular apparatus by the vestibular part of the acoustic (VIII) nerve, enter the brainstem just below the pons and anterior to the cerebellum, and proceed to the four vestibular nuclei of the brainstem and to the cerebellum. From there impulses travel along two pathways that contribute to the clinical manifestations of vertigo: the medial longitudinal fasciculus and the vestibulospinal tract.

The medial longitudinal fasciculus coordinates the contraction of the ipsilateral medial rectus muscle (cranial nerve III) and the contralateral lateral rectus muscle (cranial nerve VI).

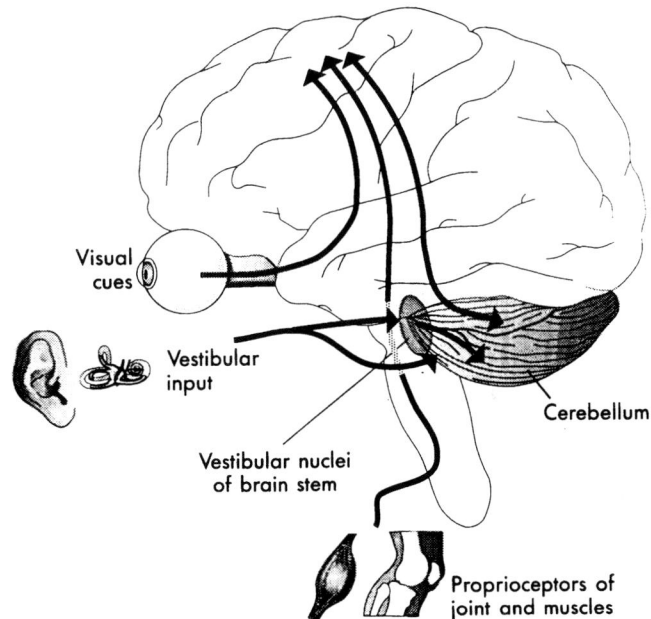

Fig. 51-1. Interaction of input from eyes, muscles and joints, and otic labyrinths. From Olshaker JS: Vertigo. In Rosen P et al, editors: *Emergency medicine: concepts and clinical practice,* ed 3, St Louis, 1992, Mosby.

In individuals with healthy vestibular systems, these connections allow the eyes to compensate for body movement in different directions and to maintain a visual axis that is stable with respect to the environment. Nystagmus occurs when the synchronized vestibular information becomes unbalanced. Nystagmus typically results from unilateral vestibular disease, which in turn causes asymmetric stimulation of the medial and lateral rectus muscles.

By convention, the direction of nystagmus is denoted by the direction of the fast "cortical" component. Nystagmus caused by vestibular disease tends to be unidirectional and horizontal. If the nystagmus is vertical, a central lesion, either brainstem or cerebral, is usually the cause.

The vestibular nuclei send information to the lateral vestibulospinal tract, where they connect with motor neurons that supply the muscles of the extremities. This phenomenon explains the false steps or other body movements made by people who have a defective vestibular apparatus and attempt to correct for an imagined change in position. Connections between the vestibular nuclei and the autonomic system account for the perspiration, nausea, and vomiting that commonly accompany an attack of vertigo. Connections between the vestibular nuclei and the cerebellum bring the modulating influence of this organ on motor activity into play.

DIAGNOSTIC CONSIDERATIONS

History

The patient history reveals (1) whether true vertigo is present, (2) the pattern of onset and duration of the vertigo, (3) if auditory disturbances are present, and (4) whether other associated neurologic symptoms are present that would suggest a central process as the cause of the vertigo.

Almost all but the mildest forms of vertigo are accompanied by some nausea, vomiting, pallor, and perspiration. The presence of such symptoms without symptoms of vertigo should lead the physician to consider such entities as myocardial ischemia. Conversely, just after an attack of severe vertigo the patient can be nauseated, pale, and diaphoretic and take on the look of a patient who is experiencing an acute myocardial infarction. Syncope suggests a nonvestibular disease process.

The time of onset and the duration of vertigo are important clues to the cause. Episodic vertigo that is severe, lasts several hours, and has symptom-free intervals between episodes suggests a peripheral labyrinth disorder. Vertigo produced primarily by a change in position also suggests a peripheral disorder. A medical history may uncover the use of drugs that have direct vestibulotoxicity (see the box below).

Vertiginous symptoms are common after whiplash injuries, and any history of head or neck trauma, whether recent or remote, should be explored. Most patients with posttraumatic vertigo have a specific organic cause for their symptoms. In addition, traumatic perilymphatic fistulas can cause vertigo months to years after the initial injury.

DRUGS CAUSING VERTIGO AND NYSTAGMUS

Alcohol
Antibiotics
    Aminoglycosides
    Chloramphenicol
    Vancomycin
    Minocycline
    Erythromycin
Barbiturates
Phenytoin (Dilantin)
Diuretics
    Ethacrynic acid
    Furosemide
Phencyclidine
Quinine
Quinidine
Salicylates

The presence of auditory symptoms suggests a peripheral cause of vertigo, such as in middle and inner ear problems, or a peripheral cause that progresses centrally, such as an acoustic neuroma. Hearing loss, vertigo, and tinnitus form the characteristic triad of Ménière disease.

Vertigo is a prominent symptom of vertebrobasilar artery insufficiency (VBI) and can therefore be an indicator of serious cerebrovascular disease. The majority of such patients experience other signs and symptoms within 1 to 2 weeks: visual disturbances, weakness, clumsiness in the arms and legs, dysphagia, dysarthria, facial palsy, or disturbances of consciousness. A few patients with VBI have vertigo as the sole manifestation. The older the patient, the greater the likelihood that the patient's vertigo is caused by VBI.

Question the patient or family members about the coexistence and time of onset of ataxia or gait disturbances. Ataxia of recent and relatively sudden onset suggests a cerebellar hemorrhage or a cerebellar infarction in the distribution of the posteroinferior cerebellar artery. The salient feature of chronic cerebellar disorders is a slowly progressive ataxia that usually begins in the legs.

Physical Examination

The physical examination should include auscultation of the carotid and vertebral arteries for bruits, which suggest atherosclerosis. The neck is auscultated along the course of the carotid artery from the supraclavicular area to the base of the skull. The pulse and blood pressure should be checked and measured in both arms. The majority of patients with subclavian steal syndrome, which can cause VBI, have pulse or systolic blood pressure differences between the two arms.

The ears should be carefully inspected. Vertigo can be caused by impacted earwax or a foreign object in the ear canal. Mild vertigo may be caused by an accumulation of fluid behind the eardrum secondary to a middle ear infection or by occlusion of the eustachian tubes associated with an upper respiratory tract infection. A perforated or scarred eardrum may indicate a perilymphatic fistula, especially if the history includes past trauma.

Examination of the ears should include an evaluation of hearing. Two simple and rapid tests, the Weber and Rinne tests, can be performed with a tuning fork and indicate whether any gross deafness is present and suggest whether the failure is in air or bone conduction.

Examination of the eyes is key in examining the patient with vertigo or disequilibrium. First note any pupillary abnormalities that may include involvement of the third cranial nerve or descending sympathetic tract, and look for any signs in the optic disc of early increased intracranial pressure, such as decreased or absent venous pulsations. The integrity of the extraocular movements should be carefully assessed; relatively subtle ocular movement abnormalities may be the only clue to a cerebellar hemorrhage. A sixth–cranial nerve palsy ipsilateral to the hemorrhage may result from early brainstem compression by the expanding hematoma. Bilateral internuclear ophthalmoplegia indicates brainstem disease and is virtually pathognomonic of multiple sclerosis.

The presence and quality of spontaneous and induced nystagmus provides key information to help distinguish central from peripheral causes of vertigo. Abnormal nystagmus is the cardinal sign of inner ear disease and the principal objective evidence of abnormal vestibular function. Nystagmus associated with peripheral vertigo is typically horizontorotary, is affected by position and head motion, fatigues over time, and is suppressed by visual fixation. Nystagmus of central vertigo can be in any direction, is not affected by position, does not fatigue, and is either unchanged or enhanced by visual fixation (Table 51-2).

If nystagmus is not present at rest, positional testing can help determine its existence and characteristics. The patient is moved quickly from an upright seated position to a supine posi-

Table *51-2*

___

DISTINGUISHING NYSTAGMUS CHARACTERISTICS OF CENTRAL AND PERIPHERAL VERTIGO

Characteristic	Central	Peripheral
Direction	Any direction	Horizontal or horizontorotary
Laterality	Unilateral or bilateral	Bilateral
Position testing effects		
Latency	Short	Long
Duration	Sustained	Transient
Intensity	Mild	Mild to severe
Fatigability	Nonfatigable	Fatigable
Effect of visual fixation	Not suppressed; may be enhanced	Suppressed

___

tion, and the head is turned to one side and extended approximately 30 degrees from the horizontal plane off the end of the stretcher. The eyes should be observed for nystagmus, and the patient should be queried for the occurrence of symptoms. This test should be repeated with the head turned to the left. Care should be taken not to perform this test if VBI is suspected, because sudden twisting movements can dislodge atheromatous plaques.

The physical examination should include observation for other cranial nerve abnormalities that provide strong evidence of a central cause of vertigo. The corneal reflex is a sensory fifth–cranial nerve circuit, and its diminution or absence can be one of the early signs of an acoustic neuroma. Vertigo caused by involvement of the eighth cranial nerve is likely to be accompanied by a unilateral perceptual hearing loss; patients cannot hear a tuning fork when it is held against the mastoid process. Involvement of the eighth cranial nerve should also raise suspicion of an acoustic tumor. Seventh–cranial nerve involvement causes facial palsy that affects the entire side of the face. In supranuclear facial paralysis, the forehead is spared because these muscles receive bilateral cortical innervation.

The patient should be specifically evaluated for evidence of cerebellar dysfunction. The essence of dysmetria should be assessed using finger-to-nose pointing movements. The gait must be evaluated when the patient gives a history that suggests ataxia, but such an examination may be impossible during an attack of vertigo. Any marked abnormality, such as consistent falling or a grossly abnormal gait, should arouse suspicion of a central lesion, especially in a patient whose vertiginous symptoms have subsided.

Ancillary Data

If a cerebellar hemorrhage, cerebellar infarction, or other central lesions are suspected, emergency CT scan of the brain is indicated. Glucose testing and ECG monitoring can also be useful emergency department studies in evaluating a patient who is experiencing dizziness, but such tests usually just confirm the clues provided by the patient's history.

Angiography may be necessary in cases of suspected VBI. Audiology and electronystagmography (ENG) are rarely available to the emergency physician but are extremely helpful in the follow-up and work-up of the patient with vertigo.

DIFFERENTIAL DIAGNOSIS

Labyrinth Disorders

Disorders of the labyrinth are the most common causes of true vertigo and consist of four diagnostic entities: (1) benign paroxysmal positional vertigo and nystagmus, (2) acute labyrinthitis, (3) Ménière disease, and (4) vestibular neuronitis.

Benign paroxysmal positional vertigo

Benign paroxysmal positional vertigo is an extremely common form of dizziness that often has no specific cause. It consists of short-lived episodes of true vertigo that are brought on by rapid changes in head position. After the head movement, a latency period of several seconds is followed by symptoms of vertigo, which are accompanied by a crescendo-decrescendo pattern of horizontorotary nystagmus. The nystagmus and vertigo usually subside in less than several minutes and are less pronounced with repeated stimuli, which demonstrates the fatigability characteristic of this disorder. The nystagmus is often rotatory and can typically be induced at the bedside by positional maneuvers.

Labyrinthitis

Labyrinthitis is a disorder of the inner ear and is associated with hearing loss. True labyrinthitis involves both the cochlear and vestibular systems. The onset is usually sudden, with patients experiencing vertigo and nystagmus and often some degree of hearing loss and tinnitus. The symptoms are usually continuous. Four classes of labyrinthitis have been described: serous labyrinthitis, acute suppurative labyrinthitis, toxic labyrinthitis, and chronic labyrinthitis.

Serous labyrinthitis is an inflammatory response to an adjacent or nearby infection of the ear, nose, throat, or meninges. Symptoms include mild-to-severe vertigo, nausea, and vomiting. A mild-to-severe hearing loss can occur.

Acute suppurative labyrinthitis is an acute bacterial exudative infection of the inner ear and is usually secondary to chronic otitis media or meningitis. The presentation is usually a dramatic combination of severe hearing loss, fever, and vertigo. An antecedent infectious cause and any coexistent CNS involvement are important markers of this condition.

Toxic labyrinthitis results from the toxic effects of medications on the cochlear and vestibular systems. The most commonly implicated drugs are the aminoglycosides. Clinically, the toxicity signs—mild tinnitus and high-frequency hearing loss—usually begin gradually. However, rapid and severe hearing loss may soon ensue unless the offending medications are stopped.

Chronic labyrinthitis is characterized by a local inflammatory process of the inner ear secondary to a fistula from the middle to the inner ear. Fistula formation usually occurs in the horizontal semicircular canal and is most often the result of destruction by a cholesteatoma.

Ménière disease

The classic triad of Ménière disease was first described in 1861 and consists of episodes of severe rotational vertigo, tinnitus, and sensorineural hearing loss in the involved ear. Patients with this disease have recurrent episodes of severe rotational vertigo that usually last for hours. The attacks may occur in clusters and have long, symptom-free remissions. During an attack, horizontorotary nystagmus is usually present, but nystagmus rarely occurs between attacks. Neither positional nystagmus nor signs of CNS dysfunction are present.

Vestibular neuronitis

Vestibular neuronitis is characterized by the sudden onset of severe vertigo that increases in intensity for several hours and gradually subsides over several days. A mild persistent positional vertigo often lasts for several weeks to several months. Patients sometimes have a history of infection or toxic exposure that precedes the initial attack. Unlike Ménière disease, associated auditory symptoms do not occur, but spontaneous nystagmus toward the inner ear may be present.

Other Differential Diagnoses

Acoustic neuroma is a cause of peripheral vertigo that ultimately has central manifestations. An acoustic neuroma is a tumor of the Schwann cells that envelop the eighth cranial nerve, and it produces vertiginous symptoms that are accompanied by unilateral sensorineural hearing loss and unilateral tinnitus. In the early stages, when the tumor is small, the only clinical symptoms may be those related to auditory or vestibular functions. However, as the tumor enlarges and enters the cerebellopontine angle, additional neurologic signs follow, the earliest usually being a depressed corneal reflex secondary to pressure on the brainstem.

Vascular disorders are extremely important central causes of vertiginous symptoms. Vertigo occurs when there is a decrease in blood flow to the vestibular nuclei in the lower pons and to the rest of the brainstem. Vertigo can be a prominent symptom of ischemia or infarction occurring in the territory of the basilar arteries, but it is unusual for vertigo to be the only manifestation of ischemia to these areas.

The signs and symptoms of brainstem ischemia that most commonly accompany vertigo are dysarthria, ataxia, facial numbness, hemiparesis, headache, and diplopia. Tinnitus and deafness are unusual manifestations of VBI. Vertical nystagmus is characteristic of a central (superior colliculus) brainstem lesion.

The subclavian steal syndrome is a rare central cause of vertigo. Exercising the arm on the side of the stenotic subclavian artery usually produces fatigue and crampy pain in the arm. Blood is shunted away from the brainstem and into the arms by retrograde flow through the ispsilateral vertebral artery. This "stealing" of blood from the vertebral and basilar arteries into the subclavian artery causes VBI and syncope. The classic picture of this disease is the occurrence of syncopal attacks during arm exercise, but such a phenomenon occurs in only a small percentage of patients. In the vast majority of patients, diminished or absent radial pulses or systolic blood pressure differentials between the two arms occur.

A cerebellar hemorrhage is a treatable neurosurgical emergency. This diagnosis should be sought in any patient with a sudden onset of headache, vertigo, vomiting, and ataxia. Early vi-

---

CAUSES OF VERTIGO

Peripheral causes

Foreign body in ear canal
Cerumen or hair against tympanic membrane
Acute otitis media
Labyrinthitis (serous, acute suppurative, toxic, chronic)
Benign positional vertigo
Ménière disease
Vestibular neuronitis
Perilymphatic fistula
Trauma (labyrinth concussion)
Motion sickness
Acoustic neuroma*

Central causes

Infection (encephalitis, meningitis, brain abscess)
Vertebral basilar artery insufficiency or occlusion
Subclavian steal syndrome
Cerebellar hemorrhage or infarction
Vertebral basilar migraine
Posttraumatic injury (temporal bone fracture)
Postconcussive syndrome
Temporal lobe epilepsy
Tumor
Multiple sclerosis
Cervical spine muscle and ligamentous injury

Systemic causes

Diabetes mellitus
Hypothyroidism

*Cause of peripheral vertigo that proceeds centrally.

sual findings, which have previously been discussed, may be present. Gaze preferences may be apparent, and the patient may have difficulty looking to the side of the lesion.

Head trauma may result in injury to the inner ear, the central vestibular nuclei, or both. Vertigo may also occur as the result of a neck injury. Because the vestibular nuclei are closely linked to muscle and joint sensors throughout the body, a musculoskeletal neck injury can account for nystagmus and vertigo without labyrinth end-organ involvement.

Metabolic abnormalities may cause vertigo. Hypoglycemia should be suspected in any patient with vertigo and diabetes or in a patient whose vertigo is accompanied by tachycardia, anxiety, or headache. Hypothyroidism can also cause vertigo. The clinical picture is one of unsteadiness, with falling, truncal ataxia, or generalized clumsiness.

The disease entities just mentioned, as well as other peripheral and central causes of vertigo, are mentioned in the box on p. 614.

MANAGEMENT

Management of vertigo is made on the basis of an accurate diagnosis. In combination with other neurologic symptoms, vertigo suggests a CNS process that requires an aggressive workup. Occasionally, immediate surgical intervention is necessary, such as with cerebellar hemorrhage.

Any patient of advanced age with isolated, new-onset vertigo without an obvious cause should be suspected of having VBI. Because of the possibility of progression of new-onset VBI in the first 24 to 72 hours, hospital admission for observation is probably warranted, even for stable patients.

Other specific causes of vertigo require surgical intervention, and the early identification of such causes is essential in reducing patient morbidity. The treatment for acoustic neuroma is surgical removal. The smaller the tumor, the

better the chance of preserving hearing and neurologic functioning. Early treatment of a posttraumatic perilymphatic fistula is important both for ameliorating patient symptoms and for closing a route for the direct spread of infection to the central nervous system.

Several conditions producing vertigo require specific interventions. Acute bacterial labyrinthitis requires admission, intravenous antibiotics, and occasionally surgical drainage and debridement. In cases of toxic labyrinthitis, the offending medication should be immediately discontinued.

The treatment for acute attacks of vertigo caused by peripheral disorders is mainly symptomatic. Several medications are useful in controlling symptoms through sedation, anticholinergic effects, or nausea control.

Intravenous diazepam in 2- to 10-mg doses is extremely effective in stopping vertigo quickly. It has a sedative effect and acts on the limbic system, the thalamus, and the hypothalamus. It can be used in similar doses orally every 8 hours. There is considerable evidence that the neurons involved in vestibular reactions are mediated by acetylcholine; anticholinergic drugs or antihistamines with anticholinergic activity have been extremely useful in the treatment of vertigo. Meclizine (Antivert), 25 mg every 8 to 12 hours, or diphenhydramine (Benadryl), 25 to 50 mg every 6 to 8 hours, are effective oral medications. If the patient is unable to take oral medications, transdermal scopolamine is often useful. Promethazine (Phenergan) 25 mg orally or rectally every 6 to 8 hours is effective because of its strong antiemetic and mild anticholinergic properties. It can also be used intravenously in doses of 12.5 to 25 mg.

Most patients with peripheral causes of vertigo can be discharged home from the emergency department. However, some patients may have such severe symptoms (vomiting, inability to walk) despite a trial of medication that they require hospital admission, intravenous fluid hydration, and observation. Sometimes the exact diagnosis is unclear, especially in older patients.

When VBI remains a likely diagnosis, the patient should usually be hospitalized.

One of the most useful tools the physician has is patient reassurance. The majority of patients with vertigo are not hysterical, anxious, or depressed. Most have self-limited disease processes that have a specific organic cause. By combining patient education and reassurance with the judicious use of medications, treating the patient with dizziness can be rewarding for both the patient and the physician.

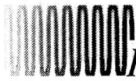

KEY CONSIDERATIONS

WHAT IS THE LIFE THREAT?

In the patient with vertigo, cerebellar hemorrhage and acute vertebrobasilar occlusion are life threats.

With presyncope, pulmonary embolism, cardiac dysrhythmia, and myocardial infarction are potentially life threatening.

DOES THE PATIENT NEED ADMISSION?

An acutely life-threatening medical illness that appears with presyncope requires inpatient treatment. Patients who are unresponsive to medical therapy and those who have severe vertigo, nausea and vomiting, or an inability to walk may require hospitalization.

Acoustic neuroma and acute bacterial labyrinthitis typically require hospitalization.

WHAT IS THE MOST SERIOUS DIAGNOSIS?

With vertigo, the most serious diagnoses are cerebellar hemorrhage, cerebellar infarction, cerebellar tumor, and acute vertebrobasilar occlusion.

With presyncope, the most serious diagnoses are pulmonary embolism, cardiac dysrhythmia, myocardial infarction, acute blood loss, hypoglycemia, and subclavian steal syndrome.

HAVE I PERFORMED A THOROUGH WORK-UP?

Differentiate vertigo from presyncope.

Perform a neurologic evaluation, including cranial nerves and tests for positional nystagmus, mental status, and gait.

Evaluate pulses, carotid artery, and vital signs.

Recommended Reading

Busis, SN: Diagnostic evaluation of the patients presenting with vertigo. *Otolaryngol Clin North Am* 6:3, 1973.

Eviatar, L: Dizziness in children, *Otolaryngol Clin North Am* 27(3):557-571, 1994.

Froehling DA et al: Does this dizzy patient have a serious form of vertigo? *JAMA* 271(5):385-388, 1994.

Herr RD, Zun L, Matthews JJ: A directed approach to the dizzy patient, *Ann Emerg Med* 18:664, 1989.

Linstrom, CJ: Office management of the dizzy patient, *Otolaryngol Clin North Am* 25(4):745-780, 1992.

Olsky M, Murray J: Dizziness and fainting in the elderly, *Emerg Med Clin North Am* 8(2):295-307, 1990.

Skiendzielewski JJ, Martyak G: The weak and dizzy patient, *Ann Emerg Med* 9:353, 1980.

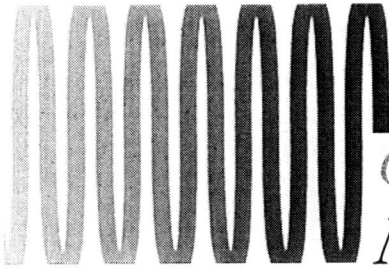

Chapter Fifty-two

MENINGITIS AND ENCEPHALITIS

DAVID W. OLSON AND JAY LANCE KOVAR

PATHOPHYSIOLOGY

Meningitis and encephalitis refer to an inflammatory process that involves the brain, spinal cord, and their membranes. Such a response is most commonly caused by a bacterial or viral infection but may also occur as a result of a fungal or parasitic infection. Vasculitic or immunologic processes may also cause such inflammation. Bacterial infection usually results from a hematogenous spread but may arise from a traumatic or surgical dural defect. A parameningeal spread from sinusitis or otitis has not been shown to occur without antecedent bacteremia.

Host-organism reactions play a major role in the development of CNS infection and place certain population groups at increased risk (see the box at right). The CNS is an area with relative immunodeficiency because of low concentrations of complement and immunoglobulin. The choroid plexus is a common portal for hematogenous entry into the cerebrospinal fluid (CSF). Depending on the number and virulence of the organisms, either clearance by the arachnoid or infection occurs. Bacterial inflammation reduces glucose transport into the CSF and increases the glucose requirement for the brain. Vascular and cell membrane permeability are altered with an influx of protein, and cerebral edema can result. Unless immunocompromise is present, cerebrospinal infection produces chemotaxis of polymorphonuclear (PMN) leukocytes early in the process. The spread of infection throughout the

---

HOST FACTORS ASSOCIATED WITH MENINGITIS

Demographic factors

Under 5 years or over 60 years of age
Male
Black
Low socioeconomic status
Crowding (e.g., military recruits)

Underlying medical conditions

Immunocompromised, malignancy
Sickle cell disease or thalassemia major
Splenectomy
Alcoholism and cirrhosis
Diabetes mellitus
Bacterial endocarditis
Ventriculoperitoneal shunt
Dural defect (trauma, surgery, congenital)

Exposure

Recent colonization
Household contact with case

subarachnoid space may lead to obstruction of CSF flow, edema, vasculitis, focal deficits, severe morbidity, and death. Even with rapid detection and treatment, the mortality rates associated with bacterial or fungal meningitis range from 10% to 50%. The use of antibiotics is effective against infecting organisms but may not prevent permanent brain damage. The severity and mortality of meningitis and encephalitis may represent the consequences of the host's response to the invasion and of the release of endotoxins associated with bacterial degradation.

ETIOLOGIC AGENTS IN MENINGITIS

Bacteria

Streptococcus pneumoniae
Neisseria meningitidis
Haemophilus influenzae
Gram-negative bacilli
Mycobacterium tuberculosis
Staphylococcus organisms
Group B streptococcus
Group C streptococcus
Bacillus organisms
Listeria monocytogenes
Treponema pallidum
Mycoplasma organisms
Others

Viruses

Mumps virus
Enteroviruses
Arboviruses
Herpes simplex types I and II
Hepatitis viruses
Others

Fungi

Cryptococcus species
Coccidioides species
Candida species
Blastomyces species
Histoplasma species
Cladosporium species
Paracoccidioides species
Others

Parasites

Ameba
Others

ETIOLOGY

Bacterial and viral pathogens are the most common causes of meningitis and encephalitis. Fungal and parasitic pathogens are less common (see the box at left). An acute and rapidly progressing presentation is often bacterial in origin and carries an associated mortality rate as high as 50%. Subacute meningitis that develops over 1 to 7 days is generally viral but may be bacterial or fungal. The death rate from a subacute bacterial infection is much lower than that from the acute presentation. Chronic meningitis is

Table **52-1**

BACTERIAL ETIOLOGIES OF MENINGITIS BY AGE

Age	Bacteria
Child less than 2 months	*Escherichia coli*
	Group B streptococcus
	L. monocytogenes
	H. influenzae
	N. meningitidis
	S. pneumoniae
Child 2 months to 9 years	*H. influenzae*
	N. meningitidis
	S. pneumoniae
Adult	*N. meningitidis*
	S. pneumoniae
	Group A streptococcus
Adults over 60 years	*N. meningitidis*
	H. influenzae
	Enterobacter organisms

caused by viral, tuberculous, fungal, or syphilitic disease. Noninfectious origins include neoplasm, sarcoid, systemic lupus erythematosus, rheumatoid arthritis, encephalitis, toxic encephalopathies, multiple sclerosis, and granulomatous angiitis.

Bacterial causes of meningitis and encephalitis in individuals without specific underlying conditions vary by age (Table 52-1); other specific host factors that may increase the range of causative organisms are listed in Table 52-2. Bacterial meningitis may be acquired from a contagious source or from colonization of existing body flora. The occurrence is more common in men, and the incidence peaks in late winter and early spring. *Streptococcus pneumoniae*, followed by *Neisseria meningitidis,* is the most common bacterial cause of meningitis. In the preantibiotic era, the mortality rate was almost 100%. Treatment with antibiotics has reduced

the mortality rate to between 10% and 70%. This wide variability reflects the importance of age and underlying conditions in determining mortality. Pneumococcal meningitis associated with endocarditis or pneumonia has a relatively poor prognosis. Residual neurologic defects are seen in 20% to 30% of the survivors of this condition. Meningococcal meningitis may occur at any age but is most common in children and young adults. The mortality rate of meningococcal meningitis is still approximately 20%. Complications are less common than with pneumococcal meningitis, but fulminant meningococcemia (Waterhouse-Friderichsen syndrome) is universally fatal.

Hemophilus influenzae is a casual bacteria that is less common in adults than in children, but it may predominate in the elderly. Bacteremia may be present in 90% of all *H. influenzae* disease and may lead to meningeal involvement. Children under 1 year of age with facial cellulitis are at high risk of developing *H. influenzae* meningitis. The current mortality rate is 10%, and adult sequelae are rare.

Other bacteria may also produce meningitis. *Listeria monocytogenes* may be seen in immunocompromised individuals, including neonates. *Staphylococcus epidermidis* is a common entity in patients with a CSF shunt.

Viral meningitis is largely season dependent. Enteroviruses are the most common cause of meningitis during the summer and fall, whereas the mumps virus is more common during the winter and spring. Most cases of viral meningitis are self-limited and do not require therapy beyond symptom relief. In contrast, viral meningoencephalitis can be a devastating disease process. Children and the elderly are the most vulnerable. Certain infections are treatable; therefore clinical distinction is important.

Arboviruses and herpes simplex viruses (HSVs) are the most common cause of endemic and sporadic cases of viral encephalitis. Arbovirus encephalitis requires an insect vector for transmission; the virus is neuropathic and

Table **52-2**

HOST FACTORS ASSOCIATED WITH BACTERIAL MENINGITIS

Host Factor	Bacteria
Alcoholism	*S. pneumoniae*
	L. monocytogenes
	H. influenzae
	Gram-negative rods
CNS shunt,	*S. aureus*
dural tear,	*S. epidermidis*
neurosurgery	*Enterobacter* organisms
Splenic dysfunction	*S. pneumoniae*
	H. influenzae
Immunosuppressed	*L. monocytogenes*
	S. aureus
	S. epidermidis
	Enterobacter organisms
Sickle cell disease	*S. pneumoniae*
	Enterobacter organisms

may not produce a precedent viremia. Because of the vector requirement, arbovirus encephalitis is commonly seen in the spring and summer months. The clinical disease develops in only a small percentage of those bitten by infected mosquitoes. Fungal infections are often associated with an immunocompromised state, trauma, surgery, or a foreign body. Parasite infection can follow exposure, especially in malnourished or immunocompromised patients.

Brain abscesses tend to occur regardless of season or age, but they do have a higher incidence in men than in women. The development of a brain abscess is associated with chronic sinusitis, otitis, a dental abscess, neurosurgical procedures, a penetrating head injury, or seeding from remote sources.

Postinfectious encephalitis is a syndrome of allergen-mediated perivenous neural tissue demyelination that follows a seemingly benign viral illness. The measles virus is the most common pathogen; postinfectious encephalitis syndrome develops in 1 out of every 1000 infections. The onset occurs 5 or more days after the onset of the rash. The mortality rate is 40%, and neurologic sequelae are high.

The differential diagnosis of meningitis is broad, and a definitive diagnosis is rarely made in the emergency department. However, a differentiation between bacterial meningitis, viral meningoencephalitis, HSV encephalitis, and a brain abscess must be presumptively made, because the treatments for each are distinctly different. A diagnosis of bacterial meningitis requires rapid assessment and treatment.

CLINICAL PRESENTATION

History and Symptoms

The chief complaint and symptoms of meningitis may appear similar to other bacterial and viral illnesses. The presentation of a patient who appears toxic and who is experiencing a headache, photophobia, nuchal rigidity, altered mental status, or a seizure strongly suggests bacterial meningitis, but the presentation may be more subtle. Viral meningitis may have a less dramatic or slower onset than a bacterial infection, but the rapidity of onset is unreliable as a differentiating characteristic (Table 52-3). The headache associated with meningitis is described classically as continuous and throbbing, located most prominently over the occiput, and increased by shaking the head, compressing the jugular vein, coughing, or straining.

Elderly patients and infants often have nonspecific findings such as fever, poor feeding, irri-

Table 52-3

COMPARISON OF BACTERIAL VERSUS VIRAL MENINGITIS

Clinical Findings	Percentage of Patients With Clinical Findings	
	Bacterial	Viral
Acute presentation (symptoms <24 hr)	25	5
Headache	Common	Common
Meningeal signs (stiff neck, Kernig sign, Brudzinski sign)	80	60-70
Fever (>38.9° C)	80	30-40
Focal neurologic findings	50	10
Impaired mental status	80-90	25-50
Seizures	30	5

tability, or lethargy. Often the only finding is an altered mental status, which may be difficult to differentiate from the progression of underlying CNS degeneration or from concurrent pneumonia, urinary tract infection, dehydration, or psychosis.

The presentation of meningitis in children less than 1 year old is commonly nonspecific and includes fever, hypothermia, dehydration, a bulging fontanelle, lethargy, irritability, anorexia, vomiting, seizures, respiratory distress, or cyanosis. Fever may be present in only one half of all infants with meningitis. A failure of the febrile infant to improve clinically following appropriate doses of acetaminophen and defervescence suggests a serious illness. Less than 50% of all infants with meningitis have a bulging fontanelle, irritability, or seizures; a bulging fontanelle is a late and ominous sign. The distinction between a simple febrile seizure and a seizure-complicating meningitis is difficult to make in younger children and often requires a diagnostic lumbar puncture. A child seen by another physician within 48 hours has been identified as a major risk factor.

Immunosuppressed patients also present a diagnostic challenge because the only findings may be a fever with a nonspecific headache and stiff neck. An infection with the human immunodeficiency virus (HIV) may mute the febrile response to infection. Fungal and tuberculous meningitis have a subacute course. Headache, low-grade fever, lassitude, and weight loss may be the presenting complaints. Meningoencephalitis may appear with similar findings but may also be manifest as hallucinations or personality changes.

Patients with ventriculoperitoneal (VP) or other shunts may have symptoms associated with low-grade ventriculitis, including headache, nausea, minimal fever, and malaise. The shunting device commonly consists of three components: the ventricular catheter, which is located in the anterior horn of the lateral ventricle; a reservoir, which may be tapped percutaneously; and a distal catheter, which contains a pump and one-way value to regulate pressure and flow. To assess shunt function, pump the reservoir; if it cannot be depressed, there is a distal block. If it pumps but does not refill, it is blocked proximally at the ventricular end. If it pumps poorly, there may be a relative dysfunction. Withdrawing fluid from the shunt for analysis or as a result of abnormal pumping requires consultation.

Physical Examination

Assess mental status, which may be greatly diminished and reflect inflammation and cerebral edema. Nuchal rigidity that occurs with attempted flexion of the neck is a classic sign of meningitis. The Kernig sign is present if the patient is unable to allow passive straightening of the leg to full-knee extension while lying on the back with the hip flexed at a right angle. The Brudzinski sign is present if passive flexion of the neck is accompanied by flexion of the hips.

Petechiae and cutaneous hemorrhages suggest meningococcemia and disseminated intravascular coagulation (DIC), but these symptoms have also been seen in infections caused by *H. influenzae,* pneumococcus, *L. monocytogenes,* and echovirus infections. Meningococcemia may be fatal within hours, even without concomitant meningitis.

Deep tendon reflexes may be normal or increased. Focal neurologic findings and ophthalmoplegia (particularly involving cranial nerve VI) are variably present; papilledema is unusual. Cryptococcal meningitis may trigger cerebellar signs such as ataxia or involuntary movements. Evidence of sepsis may accompany meningitis and if untreated can lead to endotoxic shock, DIC, and vascular collapse.

ASSESSMENT

Because the consequences of a missed CNS infection are severe, the patient with suspected meningitis must be approached from a standpoint of probability for disease. A CNS infection exists until it has been excluded from the differential. The detection of an alternative source for fever and symptoms does not exclude the diagnosis of meningitis. The presence of a non-CNS infective focus in an immunocompromised patient who has symptoms of meningitis constitutes an indication for a lumbar puncture.

Lumbar Puncture

Obtaining CSF is essential for evaluating the patient who has clinical signs of meningitis. A lumbar puncture (LP) was described by Quincke in 1878. In adults, the puncture is performed between L3 and L4. In infants and children, the puncture is performed between L4 and L5. Asphyxiation in infants resulting from excessive constraint or tracheal obstruction from cervical hyperflexion must be avoided. Absolute contraindications to the procedure include infection over the site of needle introduction, uncorrected clotting disorders, and acute spinal trauma. Painful sequelae can include backache, pain, nausea and vomiting, headache, or a stiff neck. Infrequent complications are temporary paralysis, bleeding into the subarachnoid space, epidural hematoma, and epidermoid tumors. No evidence exists to suggest that an LP in a bacteremic patient causes meningitis.

Serious complications as a result of an LP are uncommon. Disabling or permanent neurologic sequelae occur in 0.2% to 0.4% of all LP procedures. The risk of cerebral herniation from an LP performed in the setting of increased intracranial pressure (ICP) is very low. Only one third of all patients with an elevated ICP may have papilledema. Most case reports have occurred in the moribund or in patients with signs of preexisting herniation. If an intracranial mass is suggested by focal neurologic findings or history, the LP should be delayed until after a CT scan of the head has been performed. If a diagnosis of bacterial meningitis is suspected, a delay in performing an LP to obtain a CT scan should not delay antibiotic administration.

Following entry into the subarachnoid space, the opening pressure should be measured. The opening pressure of normal CSF varies from 5 to 19 cm of water when obtained in a lateral recumbent position. The following factors affect CSF pressure:

- **Decreased pressure:** circulatory collapse, dehydration, hyperosmolality, obstruction above the puncture site, hypocapnia, or hyperventilation.
- **Increased pressure:** sitting position, excessive flexion, cerebral edema, CNS mass lesion, subarachnoid hemorrhage, meningitis, congestive heart failure, obstruction of venous outflow from the CNS, hyperosmolality, and the Valsalva response.

The CSF is normally clear and colorless. Cloudiness is usually associated with leukocytosis and less commonly with the presence of red blood cells. Xanthochromia, or a yellowish discoloration, results from the lysis of red blood cells. Xanthochromia is evidence of pathologic bleeding but may appear as a false-positive result in delayed CSF analysis or in premature infants as a result of bilirubin crossing the blood-brain barrier. Crenation of red blood cells occurs in vitro and is of no diagnostic value.

Three to four separate sterile tubes are collected and sent for specific studies. Tube one is sent for a culture and Gram stain. The Gram stain generally reveals the offending organism in at least 80% of all cases of bacterial meningitis. In children this number may be as high as 95%. Prior antibiotic treatment may reduce the probability of detecting an organism by a Gram stain by 20% and reduce the culture probability by 30%. If the Gram stain is negative, a methylene blue stain may distinguish intracellular bacteria from nuclear material.

The second tube is sent for protein and glucose measurement. Elevated CSF protein is associated with meningitis, subarachnoid hemorrhage, CNS vasculitis, neoplasm, and demyelinating processes. CSF glucose and serum glucose are normally in a ratio of 0.6:1 unless there is marked hyperglycemia. Infants normally have a ratio between 0.74:1 and 0.96:1. Impaired glucose transport, and therefore decreased CSF glucose, is noted with infection or other inflammatory processes. A CSF glucose below 20 mg/dl is highly correlated with bacterial meningitis. Prior treatment with antibiotics (within 48 to 72 hours of the LP) has little effect on glucose or protein concentrations.

A white blood cell (WBC) count and differential are obtained from the third tube. Normal adult CSF contains less than 5 leukocytes/mm^3, whereas children have a more variable pattern. Cell counts in bacterial meningitis are markedly elevated, whereas abnormal cell counts are also seen with inflammatory processes in the CSF. The leukocyte differential cell count is important for differentiating between bacterial and nonbacterial meningitis. A differential cell count with more than 50% PMNs indicates a bacterial cause, whereas the presence of more than 50% mononuclear cells indicates a viral or other nonbacterial source. CSF with less than 1000 cells/mm^3 is not reliable because PMN pleocytosis may be delayed or failed. Other studies may also be indicated in specific conditions (Table 52-4).

Table 52-4

ANALYSIS OF CSF

Test	Normal Value	Significance of Abnormality
Cell count	<5 WBC/mm^3 <1 PMN/mm^3 <1 eosinophil/mm^3	Increased WBC counts are seen in all types of meningitis; increased PMN count suggests bacterial pathogen
Gram stain	No organisms	Offending organism identified 80% of the time in bacterial meningitis, 60% if patient has been pretreated
Turbidity	Clear	Increased turbidity with leukocytosis, blood, or high concentrations of microorganisms
Xanthochromia	None	Presence of RBCs in spinal fluid for 4 hours before LP; occasionally results from a traumatic tap (if protein >150 mg/dl) or hypercarotenemia
CSF/serum glucose	0.6:1 (adults) 0.74-0.96:1 (children)	Depressed in pyogenic meningitis or hyperglycemia; lag time if glucose is given IV
Protein	15-45 mg/dl	Elevated with acute bacterial or fungal meningitis; also elevated with vasculitis, syphilis, encephalitis, neoplasms, and demyelination syndromes
India ink stain	Negative	Positive in one third of all cases of cryptococcal meningitis
Cryptococcal antigen	Negative	90% accuracy for cryptococcal disease
Lactic acid	<35 mg/dl	Elevated in bacterial and tuberculous meningitis
CIE	Negative	Greater than 95% specific for organism tested; 30% false-negative rate
Limulus lysate	No clot	Clot indicates the presence of a gram-negative endotoxin
Acid-fast stain	Negative	Positive in 80% of all cases of tuberculous meningitis if >10 ml of fluid

Traumatic LPs make the cell count and protein level difficult to interpret. Although the interpretation may be inexact, the WBC count can still be estimated with the following calculations:

1. 100 RBC/mm^3 contributes 1 to 2 WBC/mm^3
2. Number of WBC introduced/mm^3 =
$$\frac{(Peripheral\ WBC) \times (RBC\ in\ CSF)}{Peripheral\ RBC\ count}$$
3. 1000 RBC/mm^3 in the CSF raises the protein level approximately 1.5 mg/dl

Blood Cultures

Even if there has been preceding antibiotic therapy, two or three blood cultures should be obtained before antibiotic administration. Causative organisms may be identified in 50% to 80% of all bacterial infections. A culture of the margins of purpuric lesions may yield meningococcus.

Countercurrent Immunoelectrophoresis

Perform countercurrent immunoelectrophoresis (CIE) on urine, blood, and CSF, particularly in treated patients with negative cultures and a negative Gram stain. Easily available tests for pathogens include those for *S. pneumoniae,* *H. influenzae,* and Group B streptococcus.

Additional Studies

Additional studies (electrolytes, glucose, creatinine, chest x-ray film) should be done as indicated by the patient's condition or by potential underlying conditions or complications. The complete blood cell count and differential is a nonspecific adjunct and may be normal in the face of significant disease, particularly in the elderly. Therefore a normal leukocyte count does not rule out meningitis. A platelet count, prothrombin time, and partial thromboplastin time are necessary in the presence of hypotension or hemorrhagic lesions.

MANAGEMENT

Initial stabilization must focus on the airway, ventilation, and circulation, all of which may be significantly altered by systemic infection. Seizures or an altered mental status should always be initially treated with naloxone (Narcan) and dextrose (if the fingerstick test reveals hypoglycemia). Alcoholics or nutritionally deficient patients should also receive thiamine 50 to 100 mg IV. Specific underlying conditions that may have been predisposing must be concurrently treated.

A definitive diagnosis of the responsible bacterial agent requires culture results that may take several days. However, antibiotic therapy must not be delayed for these results. The emergency department evaluation of a patient with a potential CNS infection should be expedient, and an antibiotic selection based on the most probable pathogen should begin within 30 to 60 minutes of the diagnosis of meningitis. The chosen antibiotics must cross the blood-brain barrier and be effective against the suspected organisms.

Penicillin G is the treatment of choice for meningitis caused by *N. meningitidis, S. pneumoniae,* and *Streptococcus pyogenes.* Ampicillin-resistant strains of *H. influenzae* are encountered more often. Chloramphenicol or third-generation cephalosporins such as ceftriaxone are recommended, but chloramphenicol should be avoided during pregnancy. Ampicillin should be added to cephalosporin during the neonatal period to provide coverage for Enterococcus organisms or *L. monocytogenes* (Tables 52-5 and 52-6).

Viral meningitis is generally treated only with supportive measures unless HSV is suspected; in such a case, acyclovir should be given. Fungal meningitis is treated with amphotericin B, 5-fluorocytosine, miconazole, or ketoconazole. Multiple drug therapy is indicated for tuberculous meningitis.

Cerebral edema is an uncommon complication of meningitis but may develop with evi-

Table *52-5*

ANTIBIOTIC THERAPY FOR BACTERIAL MENINGITIS

Organism	Therapy
N. meningitidis	Penicillin G 5 million IU IV stat then 2 million IU IV q2h; child: penicillin G 250,000 IU/kg/24 hr IV q1h
S. pneumoniae	Penicillin G 5 million IU IV stat then 2 million IU IV q2h; child: penicillin G 250,000 IU/kg/24 hr IV q4h
H. influenzae	Cefotaxime 2 g IV stat then q4h; *or* cefuroxime 3 g IV stat then q4h; *or* ampicillin 50 mg/kg/dose IV stat then q4h *and* chloramphenicol 25 mg/kg/dose IV stat then q6h; child: cefotaxime 200 mg/kg/24 hr IV q6h *or* ceftriaxone 100 mg/kg/24 hr IV q12h
S. aureus	Nafcillin 50 mg/kg/dose IV stat then q6h *or* vancomycin 20 mg/kg/dose IV stat (<1 g) then 10 mg/kg/dose IV q6h
L. monocytogenes	Ampicillin 2 g IV stat then q4h; child: 200 mg/kg/24 hr IV q4h
Gram-negative bacteria	Ampicillin 50 mg/kg IV stat then q4h *and* gentamicin 1.7 mg/kg IV stat then 1.5 mg/kg/dose IV q8h

Table *52-6*

INITIAL ANTIBIOTIC THERAPY WHEN CAUSATIVE ORGANISM IS UNKNOWN

Patient Characteristic	Therapy
Child <2 months	Ampicillin and cefotaxime, *or* ampicillin and gentamicin
Child 2 months-9 years	Cefotaxime (or another third-generation cephalosporin, such as ceftriaxone), *or* ampicillin *and* chloramphenicol
Young adults and adolescents	Penicillin *or* chloramphenicol
Recent surgery, VP shunt	Nafcillin, gentamicin, and cefoperazone (or another third-generation cephalosporin, such as ceftriaxone); *or* vancomycin and amikacin (7.5 mg/kg/dose) IV stat then q12h
Immunocompromised	Ampicillin, gentamicin, and nafcillin

dence of focal neurologic signs or evidence of herniation. If the patient is intubated, hyperventilate the lungs to maintain the $PaCO_2$ at approximately 25 mm Hg. Diuretics, including mannitol (20% solution) or furosemide (Lasix), may be useful.

Seizures should be treated with diazepam or lorazepam, followed generally with mainte-nance therapy of phenytoin or phenobarbital. *Fluid therapy* should reflect the hydration status and should ensure that there is no evidence of hyponatremia caused by inappropriate antidiuretic hormone (ADH) secretion. Avoid overhydration because it may worsen CNS edema.

Steroid administration is a useful therapy in the treatment of meningitis; the effect of steroids is to lessen the inflammatory response to the release of endotoxin from bacterial degradation. Clinical trials with dexamethasone 0.6 mg/kg/day divided into 4 doses given for 4 days have demonstrated earlier defervescence and a reduction in the incidence of neurologic deafness in children. The use of dexamethasone in adults, as well as the effects of preantibiotic and postantibiotic dosing, are under investigation.

Chemoprophylaxis is indicated for those individuals who have come in contact with patients with meningococcal meningitis. Individuals who have had intimate contact with a patient with meningitis caused by *N. meningitidis* should receive rifampin (adults: 600 mg; children older than 1 month: 10 mg/kg/dose; children less than 1 month: 5 mg/kg/dose) every 12 hours PO for a total of four doses.

Prophylaxis for *H. influenzae* exposures is recommended for all members of a household if children older than 2 years are in contact for at least 25 hours a week with the index case. Prophylaxis is also used if two or more cases of invasive disease occurred in contacts within 60 days. Prophylaxis is not indicated if the exposure is over 7 days. The dosage of rifampin for adults is 600 mg/dose (children: 20 mg/kg/dose; neonates: 10 mg/kg/dose) every 24 hours PO for four total doses. In addition, contacts should be advised of the warning signs of an impending infection and should be hospitalized if such signs develop. Vaccines are now available for the prevention of *H. influenzae, S. pneumoniae,* and *N. meningitidis.*

Admission is obviously indicated for patients with suspected or proven meningitis. Viral meningitis may be treated at home with appropriate follow-up care and well-informed, capable caretakers.

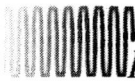

KEY CONSIDERATIONS

WHAT IS THE LIFE THREAT?

Bacterial meningitis is associated with considerable morbidity and potential disability. If untreated, the mortality rate approaches 100% for meningitis caused by *S. pneumoniae* and *N. meningitidis.* Antibiotic treatment should begin as soon as possible in such cases.

Meningitis caused by other organisms (including viruses and fungi), as well as brain abscesses and encephalitis, are also serious diagnoses.

DOES THE PATIENT NEED ADMISSION?

In general, most patients with an acute CNS infection require admission. Patients with bacterial meningitis require the administration of appropriate antibiotics within 30 to 60 minutes of diagnosis.

WHAT IS THE MOST SERIOUS DIAGNOSIS?

All CNS infections are considered serious. Rapidly progressing bacterial meningitis is the most serious in terms of an immediate threat to life.

HAVE I PERFORMED A THOROUGH WORK-UP?

Perform a lumbar puncture and obtain the following: opening pressure, culture, Gram stain, protein, glucose, cell count, differential, and closing pressure. Obtain a blood culture and urine cultures.

Do not delay antibiotic treatment to perform a lumbar puncture if a diagnosis of meningitis can be made on clinical grounds. Such a case might include a stiff neck, headache, fever, and rapidly spreading petechiae or purpura. Treat household contacts with rifampin and warn close contacts about the signs and symptoms of meningitis.

Recommended Reading

Barkin RM: Neurologic disorders. In Barkin RM, Rosen P, editors: *Emergency pediatrics*, ed 3, St Louis, 1992, Mosby.

Rennie C: Meningitis, encephalitis, and brain abscess. In Tintinalli J et al, editors: *Emergency medicine: a comprehensive study guide*, ed 3, St Louis, 1992, McGraw-Hill.

Simon HB: Infectious disease in the emergency department. In Wilkins E et al, editors: *Emergency medicine: scientific foundations and current practice*, ed 3, Baltimore, 1989, Williams & Wilkins.

Walls RM, Harrison DW: Adult meningitis, encephalitis, and intracranial abscess. In Rosen P et al, editors: *Emergency medicine: concepts and clinical practice*, ed 3, St Louis, 1992, Mosby.

Zeccardi JA: Bacteremia, sepsis, and meningitis. In Tintinalli J et al, editors: *Emergency medicine: a comprehensive study guide*, ed 3, St Louis, 1992, McGraw-Hill.

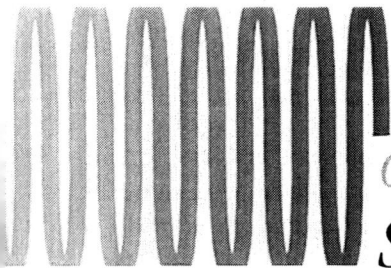

Chapter Fifty-three

SPECIAL NEUROLOGIC PROBLEMS

NEAL LITTLE AND MICHAEL G. MIKHAIL

PERIPHERAL NEUROPATHY

With the exception of the optic and olfactory nerves, the peripheral nervous system consists of all the neuroanatomic structures that lie outside the pial membrane of the spinal cord and brainstem. Those structures include the spinal nerve roots, the cranial nerves, and the peripheral nerves themselves. The vast extent of the peripheral nervous system and the multiple ways in which it can be affected make the subject of peripheral neuropathy one of the most extensive and difficult in neurology. A multitude of medical conditions can affect the peripheral nervous system in one or many places, which leads to tremendous variability in etiology, pathogenesis, clinical manifestations, treatment, and prognosis. Peripheral neuropathies can affect any or all of the functions of the peripheral nervous system and can result in motor, sensory, sympathetic, parasympathetic, and trophic changes.

The peripheral neuropathies can be categorized according to whether they involve predominantly motor, sensory, or autonomic systems. The most common categorization scheme involves the evolution time and the pattern of the neurologic symptoms. The term *polyneuropathy* refers to the involvement of multiple areas of the peripheral nervous system, *mononeuropathy* refers to involvement of a single defined peripheral nerve, *mononeuropathy multiplex* refers to involvement of multiple individual peripheral nerves, and *plexopathy* refers to involvement of multiple nerves in a plexus.

Many disease entities cause peripheral neuropathy, and these entities can be differentiated with a variety of classification systems. These classification systems overlap significantly (see the boxes on p. 629).

Pathophysiology and Etiology

The pathophysiology of most disorders of the peripheral nervous system is at best incompletely understood. Pathologic processes may involve Schwann cells, which produce the myelin sheath; the fibrous astrocytes that surround axons as they penetrate the central nervous system; the cerebrospinal fluid (CSF), which bathes the spinal roots; or the axons themselves. Circulatory disorders, such as polyarteritis nodosa (with widespread occlusion of the vasa nervorum, which causes direct ischemic neuropathy); bacterial or viral toxins; noxious agents such as heavy metals, industrial solvents, and other chemicals; and immunologic disorders may all affect the peripheral nervous system.

PERIPHERAL NEUROPATHIES	SUBACUTE SENSORY MOTOR NEUROPATHIES
Acute ascending motor paralysis with variable sensory disturbance Acute idiopathic polyneuritis (Landry syndrome, Guillain-Barré syndrome) Collagen vascular polyneuropathy Diphtheritic polyneuropathy Hepatic polyneuritis Infectious mononucleosis polyneuritis Porphyric polyneuropathy Toxic polyneuropathies Vaccinogenic polyneuropathy	Symmetrical Poisoning with industrial solvents and heavy metals Deficiency states: alcoholism: B_{12} deficiency Drug intoxication Uremia asymmetric neuropathies (mononeuropathy multiplex) Diabetes Polyarteritis nodosa Inflammatory angiopathies Ischemic neuropathy

Clinical Presentation

Patients with disorders of the peripheral nervous system have a combination of historical and physical findings of motor, sensory, autonomic, and trophic changes. The distribution of the weakness typically occurs in the legs and feet first and most severely, with later and lesser involvement of the hands and forearms. There are exceptions to this typical presentation, because some acute neuropathies tend to affect the upper extremities first, such as lead neuropathy, which involves muscles innervated by the radial nerve.

The spectrum of potential causes for peripheral neuropathy is so vast that a definitive evaluation in the emergency department is usually neither possible nor appropriate, even in acute presentations. The most important historical features of the patient's condition are the time course and pattern of involvement. A history of exposure to chemicals, solvents, toxins, infections, and immunizations may be relevant to the cause. Underlying metabolic disorders such as diabetes and alcoholism should be noted. A family history may be helpful.

The physical examination should focus on documenting the distribution and extent of motor, sensory, reflex, and autonomic loss. Atro-

phy of the affected muscles is a variable finding. Patients with acute neuropathies have no atrophy, whereas chronic neuropathy tends to produce a parallel degree of weakness and atrophy. Loss or diminution of tendon reflexes is a classic sign of peripheral nerve disease. The tendon reflex loss may be out of proportion to the weakness involved. Fasciculations and cramps are unusual findings. Sensation tends to be lost first and most profoundly in the distal segments of the limbs, and more in the legs than in the arms. All sensory modalities may be impaired or lost, but one modality may predominate over another. Sense of vibration tends to be affected more than sense of position.

As the condition progresses, the sensory loss tends to spread from a distal location to a proximal location. Paresthesias and dysesthesias may occur and are typically worse in the hands and feet. Some sensory neuropathies produce only paresthesias or dysesthesias, and others may produce varying degrees of pain. With diabetic and alcoholic neuropathy, a burning pain in the feet typically occurs. Loss of proprioceptive sensation may result from ataxia of gait and limb movement.

The most common autonomic disorders are orthostatic hypotension and anhidrosis. Other autonomic manifestations, such as unreactive pupils, lack of tears and saliva, sexual impotence, and sphincter disturbance, may occur.

SELECTED ACUTE PERIPHERAL NEUROPATHIES

Guillain-Barré Syndrome

Pathophysiology and etiology

The manifestations of Guillain-Barré syndrome (GBS) appear to be related to an immunologic reaction against peripheral nerves.

Clinical presentation

GBS is the most common syndrome of acute idiopathic polyneuritis. Patients typically experience a motor weakness that develops symmetrically over a period of several days or a week. The weakness typically occurs in the legs initially and involves the distal and then the proximal muscles. With time, the paralysis ascends to involve the muscles of the trunk, intercostals, upper extremities, and neck, as well as the muscles innervated by the cranial nerve. Respiratory paralysis can lead to death within hours to days. Pain, which is sometimes severe, and muscle aches commonly occur. Sensory symptoms occur, but the objective sensory loss is variable. Reduced and then absent tendon reflexes are considered classic findings; muscle tenderness may be present. Autonomic disturbances such as tachycardia, facial flushing, fluctuating blood pressure, and disturbances of sweating are common early in the course of the disease. Urinary retention is rare.

There are common variants to the typical picture of GBS. The paralysis may begin or develop quickly in the arms and cranial muscles. There may also be a development of complete ophthalmoplegia.

GBS occurs during all seasons of the year, does not occur in an epidemic fashion, affects men and women equally, and affects individuals of all ages. Most patients with GBS recover spontaneously and completely. The disease tends to occur suddenly and rapidly, and 6 to 18 months may be required for recovery.

Differential diagnosis

Few acute peripheral neuropathies have such an acute course as GBS. Poliomyelitis may appear with prominent, rapidly developing motor paralysis, but the fever, meningeal signs, and purely motor phenomena usually distinguish it from GBS. Severe hypokalemia may cause motor weakness similar to GBS. Acute transverse myelitis is characterized by an unchanging level and sphincter paralysis, which tends to distinguish it from GBS. A polyneuropathy (critical illness polyneuropathy [CIP]) similar to GBS may accompany a variety of critical illnesses. Tick paralysis mimics GBS but responds readily to removal of the tick.

Management

The primary concern in the emergency department is determining whether a rapidly ascending polyneuropathy has in fact occurred. Early symptoms, such as vague heaviness, weakness, or numbness in the legs, may not be sufficiently diagnostic of GBS. It is only after rapid progression of weakness and paralysis develop that the diagnosis becomes possible. Early loss or diminution of tendon reflexes is a typical early finding, but the presence of brisk tendon reflexes associated with severe weakness excludes GBS. Once the diagnosis has been considered, repeated examination and frequent measurement of respiratory effort are indicated. If the diagnosis is seriously considered, admission and evaluation for eventual respiratory support are necessary. The CSF shows a characteristic albuminocytologic dissocation (few or no cells with elevated protein), but this characteristic may take days or weeks to develop fully. Supportive respiratory and nursing care constitutes the most important component of treatment for this self-limited condition. Plasmapheresis, if initiated within 2 weeks of onset, may help shorten the course of mechanical ventilation and hospitalization. Steroids have not been found useful.

Bell Palsy

Pathophysiology and etiology

Bell palsy is a seventh nerve paralysis of unknown cause and by definition is idiopathic. Many authors believe this condition results from swelling of the nerve within the stylomastoid foramen. Bell palsy affects men and women equally and occurs at all ages, but it is more common in the third to fifth decade of life. Bell palsy involves the structures innervated by the seventh cranial nerve: motor fibers to facial muscles and the stapedius muscle, secretory fibers to the lacrimal gland, and taste fibers to the anterior two thirds of the tongue. Some authors believe that Bell palsy is a polycranial neuropathy that predominantly affects the seventh nerve, but in a subclinical fashion it may also affect the fifth and ninth cranial nerves in as many as two thirds of all cases. The detailed manifestations of a seventh nerve palsy are defined by its anatomy. Cortical motor fibers to the forehead muscles progress from both motor cortices to each seventh nerve nucleus; therefore a cortical lesion does not produce paralysis of forehead muscles. However, a lesion of the seventh nerve at the level of its nucleus in the brainstem, or peripheral to that, causes paralysis of forehead muscles on the ipsilateral side. If the lesion occurs at the level of the seventh nerve nucleus in the brainstem, the long motor tracts and the sixth nerve are usually involved as well (the sixth nerve fibers loop around its nucleus before exiting the pons).

The seventh nerve has two main divisions, the motor root and the nervus intermedius. The nervus intermedius conducts taste sensation from the anterior two thirds of the tongue and supplies autonomic fibers to the submaxillary and sphenopalatine ganglia, which innervate the salivary and lacrimal glands. A little known motor function of the seventh nerve is innerva-

tion of the stapedius muscle, which dampens the transmission of loud, low tones through the ear; paralysis of this muscle results in hyperacusis. Therefore in general, cortical lesions involving the face typically spare the forehead; nuclear lesions involving the seventh nerve typically involve gaze paralysis and other brainstem findings; and pure peripheral seventh nerve weakness may involve some combination of gustatory, auditory, and lacrimal findings along with unilateral upper and lower facial weakness.

Clinical presentation

The onset of Bell palsy is typically acute; half of all cases develop maximum deficit within 48 hours; in almost all cases, the deficit reaches the maximum within 5 days. The symptoms are almost always unilateral. Facial weakness may be mild and is best demonstrated by less frequent blinking on the affected side, possible sagging of the lower lid, and a possible asymmetry of smile. Bell phenomenon, an upward rolling of the eyeball that occurs during attempted lid closure, may be seen. More complete lesions involve great weakness of the facial muscles, which leads to incomplete eyelid closure with possible corneal exposure, drooling from the affected side of the mouth, weakness of the platysma muscle, and diminished lacrimation on the affected side. Although the seventh nerve is not definitively known to convey sensory information, patients with Bell palsy may complain of a "vague numbness" on the affected side of the face just before or as the weakness is developing; objective sensory loss rarely occurs. A fullness or pain behind the mastoid is felt in 61% of all cases. The patient may experience hyperacusis (29%), welling up of tears in the eye if the lacrimal gland has not been affected by the less frequent blinking (68%), or dryness of the eye (16%) if there is involvement of the lacrimal gland. Taste may seem unusual to the patient (57%) and is usually the first symptom to recover. Incomplete eyelid closure may cause corneal drying. A seeming deviation of the tongue is an illusion that results from the asymmetry of the face.

The principal focus of the initial examination is to certify the facial palsy as peripheral in nature; to document the extent of weakness, particularly eyelid closure; and to exclude any other neurologic deficit that would imply a diagnosis other than Bell palsy. Specifically, the corneal reflex should be intact; corneal sensation should be present on the involved side and produce contralateral eyelid closure. Cranial nerves V, VI, and VIII should the tested. Inspection of the eardrum and palpation of the parotid gland are necessary to exclude obvious causes of peripheral facial weakness.

There are many potential causes of acute facial nerve weakness, including basilar artery aneurysms, GBS, meningeal infection, trauma (skull fracture, penetrating facial injury), middle ear surgery, and infection. Many tumors can produce progressive facial weakness (acoustic neuromas; parotid, bone, and metastatic tumors). It is uncommon for the seventh nerve to be involved in the peripheral neuropathy of either diabetes or alcoholism. An increased incidence of Bell palsy occurs in pregnancy. Ramsey Hunt syndrome consists of a peripheral seventh nerve palsy in the presence of herpetic vesicles on the ear canal and tympanic membrane and may or may not involve tinnitus and vertigo.

When the typical history, physical examination, and neurologic findings of Bell palsy occur in a patient who enters the emergency department, little else is necessary to establish the diagnosis. Other testing is not indicated at that time unless special features of the history or examination suggest the possibility of a defined cause. A meticulous and well-documented neurologic examination that demonstrates only a peripheral seventh nerve lesion is all that is necessary to render the diagnosis. Follow-up testing may include electromyography.

The prognosis for Bell palsy is excellent, and recovery is usually complete or near-complete in 50% to 86% of all cases within 2 weeks to 2 months.

Management

Some authors believe that corticosteroids hasten the speed or completeness of recovery of Bell palsy, especially if prescribed early in the course of treatment. Prednisone 60 mg/day orally for 5 days, with a taper to 5 mg/day over the next 5 days, is commonly used. Considerable controversy exists concerning surgical therapy for Bell palsy to decompress the bony canal where the seventh nerve exits the skull. An important component of therapy is eye protection. Paralysis of eyelid closure may result in corneal drying and injury. Lubricating ointments and eye patches should be used for protection. There appears to be no benefit, and some theoretical risk, from electrically stimulating the facial muscles to promote recovery.

The critical issues in the diagnosis and management of a patient with suspected Bell palsy are the identification of a truly peripheral cause and the exclusion of any obvious treatable cause. Follow-up observation is important in patient management. The key diagnostic imperative involves ascertaining that no other cranial nerve deficits develop and that the signs or symptoms appear to suggest a specific cause.

Herpetic Neuralgia and Herpes Zoster

The varicella-zoster virus (VZV, or herpes zoster) may acutely inflame a peripheral nerve. Typical symptoms include itching or burning followed by pain in the distribution of peripheral nerve. A rash characterized by vesicles on an erythematous base develops along the course of the peripheral nerve within several days to 2 weeks and the pain typically intensifies. Before the rash develops, the condition cannot be definitively diagnosed but may be suspected. Patients with immunocompromise may develop disseminated herpes zoster, which involves more than one dermatome or peripheral nerve. If the ophthalmic branch of the fifth cranial nerve is affected, the cornea can become involved and cause vision loss. Involvement of the tip of the nose, which is innervated by the nasociliary branch of the ophthalmic division of the fifth nerve, not the maxillary division, may be a marker for potential corneal involvement.

Pathophysiology and etiology

VZV is thought to be present in latent form in the dorsal nerve root ganglia. Reactivation of the virus occurs for unknown reasons, affects the nerve, and causes the early "neuritic" symptoms. Migration of the virus along the course of the peripheral nerve and through the skin causes the skin eruption.

Management

Patients typically seek care because of the severe pain involved with this condition. Narcotic analgesics may be required. Acyclovir may shorten the course of the illness and improve healing in immunocompetent patients. It can be given intravenously 5 mg/kg three times per day for 5 days or orally at 800 mg five times per day. Administration of acyclovir within 48 to 72 hours of pain onset is more effective than later administration. Disseminated herpes zoster can be a life-threatening condition, and patients with involvement of more than one dermatome require admission to the hospital and treatment with intravenous (IV) acyclovir. In immunocompromised patients with herpes zoster, such as those who have human immunodeficiency virus (HIV) infection or those on chemotherapy or immunosuppressive therapy, IV acyclovir used within 72 hours of onset is recommended. Close household contacts who have not had chickenpox may develop the acute form of that infection through contact. Patients with herpes zoster should avoid close contact with anyone who is immunocompromised.

Postherpetic Neuralgia

Postherpetic neuralgia (PHN) is a syndrome that follows herpes zoster, is characterized by pain along the course of a nerve, and lasts longer than 1 month. It develops in 9.7% to 14.3% of patients, but after 1 year affects 3%. The incidence of pain increases with age, and for patients 70 years and older it is persistent in 75% of patients at 1 month. It is most common in thoracic dermatomes. The pain may be steady and described as "burning" or "nagging," or it may be paroxysmal and described as "sharp" or "shooting." Contact with clothing may aggravate it. Touch and pin sensation may be reduced, and hyperesthesia may be present in affected and nearby dermatomes. Prednisone, 60 mg/day with tapering over 2 weeks and given at the onset of herpes zoster in immunocompetent patients, may decrease the incidence of PHN. Acyclovir has been reported to be effective in preventing PHN in some studies but not in others. The combination of prednisone and acyclovir has not been proven effective.

Treatment of established PHN is difficult. Antidepressants, such as amitriptyline, or phenothiazines (perphenazine, fluphenazine decanoate, or thioridazine) may be effective. Anticonvulsants, such as phenytoin and carbamazepine, are probably ineffective. A variety of other therapies such as repeated nerve blocks, ethyl chloride spray, use of a hand vibrator, and transcutaneous electrical nerve stimulation (TENS) units are variably effective. A variety of neurosurgical pain procedures have been used for this disabling condition.

PSYCHOGENIC NEUROLOGIC SYNDROMES

Individuals may enter the emergency department with what appears to be an organically caused neurologic disorder but is subsequently determined to be a psychogenic illness. The following sections attempt to provide a frame of references for distinguishing these disorders.

Hysteria and Malingering

Hysteria has been identified as a clinical entity since ancient times, and the disease process as it is known today was first described by Briquet in 1859. A number of explanations have been proposed for the symptoms produced in hysteria, and most authors believe that unconscious psychic conflicts are converted into physical symptoms. This concept of conversion has been widely used, and such terms as *conversion reaction, conversion hysteria,* and *conversion disorder* (hysterical neurosis, conversion type) have been used to describe the condition. Used in this technical sense, the term *hysteria* refers to a condition in which the patient is not aware of the unreality of symptoms.

Conversion reaction

Conversion reactions must be distinguished from malingering, which describes a willful, deliberate imitation or exaggeration of illness that is intended to deceive others for a consciously desired end. Munchausen syndrome is an extreme form of malingering in which individuals present a variety of physical symptoms and sometimes self-inflict various injuries to gain hospitalization.

A conversion disorder, or hysterical neurosis of the conversion type, typically has symptoms that suggest a neurologic disease. These symptoms usually occur suddenly, and although they may usually occur during adolescence and early adulthood, they may also be manifested in middle age or even in the later decades of life.

General approach to the patient

Be extremely wary in assigning a diagnosis of hysteria or malingering on the basis of vague or inexplicable symptoms. Many symptoms that initially are labeled hysteria or malingering are later attributable to an underlying organic dis-

ease of the nervous system. An organic illness is subsequently diagnosed in 13% to 30% of patients with conversion disorder. Approach all patients with intellectual humility and be aware that some seemingly inexplicable sign or symptom may later be explained organically. However, be able to recognize hysteria and malingering so that inappropriate diagnostic testing and treatments are not provided.

In general, to establish a diagnosis of psychogenic neurologic syndromes, positive signs that are inconsistent with the known functioning of the nervous system must be demonstrated; do not simply document the lack of defined deficits. An example of a neurologic sign that is not organically possible is a midline split in vibratory sense, in which a patient feels a vibrating turning fork on one side of the skull but not on the other; this is a physically impossible situation because vibrations are transmitted through bone across the midline.

Weakness or Paralysis

A psychogenic weakness or paralysis typically affects a particular function that the patient may need to carry out in the absence of paralysis. For example, a patient may complain of inability to pick up or care for a sick child although the actual muscle groups involved in such an action are functioning normally. Such patients may complain of an inability to walk or move yet have driven themselves to the emergency department. They may exhibit an indifferent attitude toward an obvious deficit (la belle indifference). During the examination they may not be able to perform fine-motor–coordinated acts, but previously they were observed dressing and undressing in a normal fashion.

The key to examining the patient with a presumed psychogenic weakness or paralysis is skilled observation of stereotypical acts. Complex functions such as dressing and signing one's name provide key information. Supporting one's self with a supposedly paralyzed arm for balance may be noted during casual observation. When formal strength testing is done, the weakness may in fact be of a giveaway type and produce a ratchety feeling as the patient tries to simulate less than complete motor function. However, this ratchety type of weakness may also occur in conditions in which the patient is unable to give full cooperation for motor testing because of genuine pain. It is often found when palpating the limb that an antagonistic muscle is being contracted at the time an agonist is being tested. If a supposedly weak limb is dropped, it may fall at less than the speed dictated by gravity, may fall with greater force than expected, or may briefly hover in the air before the patient realizes that the limb should be set down.

There are several classic tests for psychogenic weakness, all of which are really tests of cooperation and not of true weakness. In the abduction test, the patient lies supine and is asked to abduct a supposedly weak leg. If the patient is indeed trying, the examiner will feel resistance from the "normal leg" as the patient uses that to counterbalance the action in the weak "abducting" leg, because abduction is usually a bilaterally innervated function. If no resistance is felt, it may be concluded that the patient is not trying. However, this lack of resistance does not exclude true weakness. Lack of effort is likewise the basis of the Hoover sign, in which the patient lies supine and the examiner places his or her hands under the patient's heels. As the patient attempts to raise a truly weak right leg, the examiner will feel increased pressure under the patient's left heel in an attempt to counterbalance the effort expended in raising the right leg. If that pressure is not felt, then the patient is not trying to lift the supposedly weak leg. It must be emphasized again that these are tests of cooperation and not of true weakness.

Hysterical paralysis or malingering commonly spares the face and tongue. Muscular wasting is uncommon except in longstanding processes. Patients with hysterical or malingered weakness in one leg typically have an ostentatious gait wherein the weak limb is dragged along the ground and not circumducted as in typical upper motor neuron disease. There may be a very bizarre character to the gait. Falling is a common problem and often occurs only in the direction of the examiner or the examination stretcher, where assistants can prevent a fall to the ground. However, truncal ataxia caused by true midline cerebellar disease may sometimes be difficult to distinguish from falling caused by hysterical paralysis.

Psychogenic Numbness

Impairment of sensation on a conversion basis is common and may be on the same side as a limb affected by hysterical weakness or paralysis. Occasionally this impairment is part of a pansensory loss involving all sensory modalities, including vision, hearing, taste, smell, and touch, which is obviously impossible on the basis of organic neurologic disease. The sensory loss associated with hysteria or malingering typically occurs as a numbness in a glove-and-stocking distribution, in which there is a very sharp line of transition from normal to anesthetic. This distribution is in contrast to the glove-and-stocking distribution of peripheral neuropathy, in which there is a gradual diminution of sensibility that typically does not stop at joint lines. Split vibratory sense, wherein a vibrating tuning fork is not felt over half of the skull or sternum, is a classically described sign of psychogenic sensory loss. Other such signs are islands of preserved sensation within large areas of sensory loss and sensory loss that begins and ends at the exact midline of the body, which is not common in organic disease. Classic psychogenic locations of sensory deficit that involve exactly half of the genitalia or rectum do not occur in organic disease because of crossover at the midline.

The patient's sensory loss must be defined as a complete lack of sensation, anesthesia, a lack

of painful sensation, analgesia, or some other alteration of sensory modality. Withdrawal from a
pin prick is probably one of the least useful
modalities to try to elicit because some patients
may withstand great pain without withdrawal.
Sensation can be tested with crossed and inter-
locked fingers.

Deafness

Psychogenic hearing loss is not common in the
emergency department. It may be part of a
pansensory or hemisensory loss, as previously
described. It is commonly a malingered problem. Extensive and sophisticated tests can distinguish true unilateral deafness from psychogenic
deafness.

Psychogenic Vision Loss

Vision loss on the basis of malingering is often
unilateral, whereas hysterical blindness is typically bilateral. Patients may also embellish a vision loss. During the clinical examination, a
patient with a true organic bilateral vision loss
attempts protection from the environment as
one would do if awakened in the middle of the
night in the dark. The truly blind patient assumes a wide-based gait with the hands for protection and does not purposely run into doors,
examiners, or other people. Because of auditory
tracking, a blind person typically can look at the
face of someone who is talking. Truly blind patients can look at parts of their own body, such
as a hand. Response to threat whereby the hand
of the examiner is quickly thrust toward the eye
may induce a blink response. Care must be
taken not to elicit a corneal reflex by a gust of
air. Optokinetic nystagmus is a useful and sophisticated test in which a series of stripes on a
cloth or drum are rapidly passed in front of the
patient's eyes to produce a rapid beating nystagmus opposite the direction of the stripes. This
response is normal in sighted individuals and in
feigned or hysterically blind individuals. Sophisticated testing, such as placing different colored

lenses over either eye, can be done. Tests with
prisms to isolate the images of the two eyes can
also be administered. Visual evoked responses
on EEG can be made to aid in diagnosis.

In nonorganic blindness, clinical examination
of the eye usually reveals a normal direct and
consensual light response. However, patients
with true cortical blindness may have intact
pupillary responses; therefore the presence of
pupillary light reflexes does not rule out an organic basis of blindness. Patients who are malingering may instill mydriatic drops in their eyes,
and these pupils will then not respond to pilocarpine. Patients with psychogenic vision loss
may only be able to read the top line on the
Snellen chart, regardless of its distance. Monocular diplopia may be psychogenic because it is
rare in organic lesions, with the exception of
lens dislocation (either natural or artificial),
corneal involvement, or a condition secondary
to buckling of the retina. Be aware of Anton syndrome, an organic visual loss syndrome that results from an infarction in the parietal and
occipital lobe and in which the patient is not
aware of, or denies, vision loss and therefore
may bump into objects.

Pseudoseizures

The diagnosis of pseudoseizures can present
great difficulty. Patients may have an established
organic diagnosis of seizures but may be embell-
ishing the true organic problem. Patients may
be medically sophisticated to the point of passing urine or biting the tongue during a pseudoseizure, but such behaviors are unusual. Many
pseudoseizures are very unsophisticated; during
observation of the spell, it is usually clear that
the event is very theatrical and bizarre. Purpose-
ful movements may occur, and the patient may
retain the ability to speak or act voluntarily.
Many times the shaking results in movement
away from the midline, which is unusual in true
seizures. There may be repetitive behavior,
which sometimes must be distinguished from
the repetitive behavior of temporal lobe

seizures. The shaking movements may simulate the tremulousness of delirium tremens (DTs) or high fever.

During pseudoseizures, it may be productive to observe the eyes because the usual pupillary dilation that accompanies seizures may not occur. Patients may communicate voluntarily during the pseudoseizure. Although it is true that focal motor seizures may result in no impairment of consciousness, generalized tonic-clonic seizures typically should cause a loss of voluntary abilities. Although patients may bite the tongue or become incontinent of urine during a pseudoseizure, the loss of bowel control is extremely unusual. Cyanosis is likewise unusual; but patients may hold their breath. Pseudoseizures may represent an embellishment on a true seizure disorder and should be interpreted as a cry for help.

Psychogenic Coma and Disorders of Consciousness

Psychogenic disorders of consciousness may be more common in the emergency department than is appreciated in the neurologic literature. There may be an embellishment on mild alcohol or other drug intoxication. Questioning first-hand witnesses and directly observing the patient are the best methods by which to establish the diagnosis. Obviously, true organic and rapidly treatable disorders that result in an alteration of consciousness, particularly hypoglycemia, must be quickly excluded. In a psychogenic coma, the patient may assume a trancelike state and may have normal posture and tone. Voluntary eyelid closure and Bell phenomenon typically occur. Increased eyelid resistance may be felt when attempting to open the eyes of a patient in psychogenic coma, which indicates an alert state. The Bell phenomenon consists of upward deviation of the eyes in response to forced voluntary contraction of the eyelids. If the examiner is able to open the eyes and the patient has voluntary resistance, the eyes exhibit the Bell phenomenon and are up-

wardly deviated. The eyes may show downward deviation regardless of the position of the patient, which indicates hysterical unconsciousness. Opening the patient's eyes may in fact establish visual contact and an opportunity to "reverse the problem."

A nasal tickle may cause the patient to raise the hand to the nose voluntarily, open the eyes, and thereby interact with the physician. If it is clear that there is no potential for cervical spine injury, patients with a psychogenic coma may be raised to a sitting position. This position makes it difficult to preserve the pseudounconscious state. Dropping the patient's hand toward the face may or may not be helpful; some patients allow it to fall in the face, which limits the diagnostic usefulness of this test. If the eyelids of a patient with psychogenic unconsciousness are opened by the examiner, they do not close in the very slow fashion of patients who are truly unconscious but blink shut abruptly. Patients with psychogenic unconsciousness may have voluntary limb resistance.

Management of the patient with psychogenic coma

Minimally provocative tests, such as nasal tickle or testing for voluntary eyelid resistance, may be all that is necessary to establish the diagnosis. Once the diagnosis is certain, the patient should be allowed time to reverse the "psychogenic coma." A trusting, reassuring, and comforting discussion by the physician that indicates a willingness to help the patient may go much further toward establishing a therapeutic alliance than painful and provocative procedures. If there is doubt, laboratory glucose testing may be necessary.

Disorders of Speech

Psychogenic disorders of speech may be such that the patient is not able to speak in a full voice but may be able to whisper. There is no known organic neurologic disease that results in a whisper. Hysterical patients may move the mouth without producing sound. There may be an abrupt onset and cessation of the ability to speak. The patient may speak in a slow, garbled, or "baby-talk" fashion. Stuttering may occur. Patients with true aphasia often make an attempt to speak, even if they are unable to do so.

Disposition of Patients With Psychogenic Neurologic Syndromes

The more difficult part of the patient encounter begins once a diagnosis of a psychogenic syndrome has been rendered. A thorough general physical and neurologic examination and any indicated laboratory testing must have already been conducted. The interaction with the patient must in no way compromise a therapeutic, trusting, and caring relationship.

The patient who is obviously malingering may be confronted with the conflicting facts found on examination, or the conflicting facts may be obvious to the patient without specific mention by the physician. Adequate documentation in the medical record and communication of findings to the patient are important. To obtain a satisfactory disposition, another opinion may need to be sought from another physician.

In less than obvious cases, a frank discussion of what can be explained on the basis of the examination and the physician's knowledge may be necessary. The fact that there may be unexplained components to the patient's illness, especially in the case of exaggeration, may provide the necessary avenue to seek consultation.

The emergency department should not be the last contact with the medical system for such patients, and it is often only through ongoing evaluation and treatment of both potentially organic and nonorganic symptoms that all of the applicable diagnoses can be reached. It is beyond the scope of this chapter to discuss specific psychiatric therapy for such patients.

DEMYELINATING DISEASE

Definitions

The term *demyelination* refers to a disease process in which the prominent feature is loss of the myelin sheath that surrounds axons in the central nervous system. Multiple sclerosis (MS) is the most common example of a demyelinating disease. It is characterized by CNS lesions that are "scattered in time and space." This description refers to clinical symptoms that wax and wane over a period of time and are referable to separate areas of the CNS. MS may be nearly impossible to diagnose definitively in its early stages because of the tremendous variation in the clinical presentation and course of this disease. The great variety of clinical manifestations of the disease mandates that strict definitions be used, particularly when assessing the results of studies on MS. "Clinically definite" MS is predominately a white-matter disease involving two or more areas of the CNS with two or more separate episodes, each lasting at least 24 hours, at least 1 month apart or in a progressive course over at least 6 months, and beginning between the ages of 10 and 50 years. This definition requires the passage of time, has a tendency to exclude mild cases, and does not rely on laboratory or radiographic data.

Pathophysiology, Etiology, and Epidemiology

Women develop MS 1.8 times as often as men, and whites twice as often as blacks. MS in a family member occurs in 10% to 15% of all cases. First-degree relatives of affected individuals have a fifteen to twenty fold increased risk of developing MS. MS rarely develops before age 20 or after age 50. Although immunologic changes have been found in the CSF and in the CNS plaques of patients with MS, the cause of MS is unknown. However, it is surmised that environmental and genetic factors may combine to increase vulnerability to the disease.

The CNS in patients with MS has scattered areas of demyelination, called *plaques*. Plaques occur in gray matter four times as often as in white matter but are more difficult to visualize on gross examination of gray matter. Plaques are common in the optic tracts, spinal cord, brainstem, and basal ganglia. Demyelinated axons conduct action potentials poorly or not at all. Edema and inflammation may result in reversible defects in action-potential propagation (conduction) and thus produce neurologic deficits or "negative" symptoms. Demyelinated axons may become hyperexcitable and generate action potentials with minimal stimuli to produce "positive" symptoms of MS such as the Lhermitte sign, an electric-shock–like feeling in the torso or extremities precipitated by neck flexion.

MS follows an exacerbating and remitting course in 80% to 90% of the patients. Of all patients with MS, 10% to 20% have a chronically progressive course from the start, and in an additional 10% the course becomes progressive after the first few attacks. After 10 years, 50% of all patients develop a chronic progressive course. In 80% of the cases, an exacerbation is characterized by the reappearance of previously present signs rather than the development of new signs. A relapse is defined as an episode that lasts more than 24 hours. Early in the disease process, remission may result in a complete resolution of symptoms. With time, irreversible deficits occur.

The extreme clinical variability of MS makes it difficult or impossible to predict the future course in individual cases; this disease is therefore an extremely difficult one for patients, clinicians, and researchers.

Clinical Presentation and Differential Diagnosis

Patients who have established MS may enter the emergency department because of an exacerbation of previous deficits, a development of new deficits, or an appearance of medical complications of the disease. Elevated body temperature may augment subclinical features of the disease or bring out new ones. Infectious complications that result from the neurologic lesion, such as urinary tract infection, infected decubitus ulcers, and pneumonia may transiently worsen a patient's neurologic status because of fever. Only anecdotal evidence supports the importance of other potentially exacerbating factors such as trauma, allergic responses, stress, and emotions.

The development of new focal deficits in a patient without known MS represents a diagnostic challenge to the clinician. The appearance of symptoms and signs typical of MS (see the box below) usually does not present a diagnostic difficulty. However, patients with established MS are not immune from other CNS insults, and before any new symptom or sign is attributed to MS, other common and treatable causes should be considered. Seizures and dementia are uncommon early neurologic manifestations of MS.

Medical problems that commonly complicate MS are those that accompany any chronic neurologic disease and produce bladder dysfunction, an impaired swallowing or cough reflex, prolonged immobilization, or poor nutrition.

COMMON NEUROLOGIC PRESENTATIONS IN MS

Internuclear ophthalmoplegia
Optic neuritis
Transverse myelitis
"Cerebellar signs," scanning speech, intention tremor
Diplopia (usually sixth nerve paresis)
Trigeminal neuralgia
Vertigo
Nystagmus
Lhermitte sign
Ill-defined sensory symptoms
Bladder dysfunction

MS should be the last consideration for the patient who has an undiagnosed acute focal neurologic deficit (see the box below). It is impossible to make such a diagnosis clinically at initial presentation. A few entities are "classic" for MS, such as optic neuritis, transverse myelitis, and internuclear ophthalmoplegia, but MS can at best be "suspected" in those circumstances. Even a patient with these entities should be evaluated for other, and potentially

more treatable, diseases; a patient should not be burdened with a diagnosis of a chronic, untreatable disease without solid evidence.

Of all patients who develop optic neuritis of unknown cause, only 15% to 40% later have other symptoms that suggest MS. Retrobulbar neuritis, in which inflammatory changes occur behind the optic nerve head within the eye, produces symptoms identical to those of optic neuritis, but the characteristic optic nerve head changes seen on ophthalmoscopy are absent. Unilateral internuclear ophthalmoplegia is produced by the interruption of fibers in the medial longitudinal fasciculus connecting the sixth nerve and third nerve nuclei and consists of weakness when adducting the ipsilateral eye, nystagmus on abduction of the contralateral eye, and preservation of convergence. Eye position at rest is normal, and diplopia is rare.

Acute transverse myelitis is an inflammation of a spinal cord segment resulting in loss of function (motor, sensory, autonomic, reflex, and sphincter) below the level of the lesion. The clinical symptoms of acute transverse myelitis have many potential causes, including potentially treatable compressing mass lesions, and should never be presumed to indicate MS until other causes have been appropriately excluded.

There are a large number of causes to consider in the differential diagnosis of an acute

CAUSES OF ACUTE FOCAL NEUROLOGIC DEFICIT

Traumatic: intracranial, intraspinal
Subdural hematoma
Intraparenchymal hemorrhage
Epidural hematoma
Traumatic hemorrhagic necrosis

Infectious
Brain abscess
Epidural and subdural abscesses
Meningitis

Neoplastic
Primary CNS tumors
Metastatic tumors
Syringomyelia

Vascular
Thrombosis
Embolism
Spontaneous hemorrhage from arteriovenous malformation, aneurysm, or hypertension

Metabolic
Hypoglycemia
B_{12} deficiency
Postseizure
Hyperosmolar hyperglycemic nonketotic coma

Other
Migraine
Bell palsy
Psychogenic

CAUSES OF MULTIFOCAL NEUROLOGIC DEFICIT

Acute disseminated encephalomyelitis
Postviral or postimmunization
Infectious encephalomyelitis
Poliovirus, enteroviruses, arbovirus, herpes zoster, Epstein-Barr virus
Granulomatous encephalomyelitis
Sarcoid
Autoimmune
Systemic lupus erythematosus
Familial spinocerebellar degenerations
Other

focal neurologic deficit (see the box on p. 640). This field of potential etiologies may be significantly narrowed by history and neurologic examination. The box on p. 640 lists a variety of disease entities that can cause multiple deficits. Patients who have symptoms that can be explained by MS require a consideration of other entities, including spinal cord compression by mass lesions or hematomas, expanding intracerebral lesions such as subdural hematomas, and metabolic abnormalities such as hypoglycemia and hyponatremia.

Management

When a patient with known MS enters the emergency department, measures such as airway management, urinary drainage, skin care, and treatment and prevention of hyperthermia constitute the initial priorities.

The issue of treatment for MS is extremely controversial. The scientific evaluation of treatment for MS also is extremely difficult because of the great clinical variability in the course; the lack of reliable markers for extent, progression, or regression of disease; and the possibility that complete deficits may mask the development of new lesions. For an acute exacerbation, corticosteroids in varying doses are commonly given despite the lack of definitive studies to support their efficacy. The issue of preventing progression of the disease is even more complex, and many treatment modalities such as immunosuppression, plasmapheresis, and the administration of hyperbaric oxygen are being evaluated. Patients and doctors who manage MS are confronted with many uncontrolled trials and a large number of charlatans who prey on desperate patients with chronic disease.

PSEUDOTUMOR CEREBRI

Pathophysiology and Etiology

The mechanism of intracranial pressure elevation in pseudotumor cerebri is unknown. Many factors have been implicated, most anecdotally, but a recent weight gain, menstrual irregularities, hypervitaminosis A, oral retinoids, and tetracycline administration have been found in many patients. Despite a preponderance of this condition in obese women, hormone levels are normal. The condition tends to be a self-limited process, with the only potential sequela being vision loss.

Clinical Presentation

Pseudotumor cerebri, or idiopathic intracranial hypertension, is a condition characterized by elevated intracranial pressure, headache, and papilledema. It typically occurs in obese women during late adolescence or early adulthood, but it may also occur in adult men (who are usually obese) and in children. The clinical syndrome can mimic that of the elevated intracranial pressure from a brain tumor. The headache typically develops over weeks to months, and the condition may last for many months. The headache typifies that of increased intracranial pressure in that it tends to be worse in the morning, better after rising, and worse with maneuvers that increase intracranial pressure, such as the Valsalva maneuver, coughing, and bending. There are usually no neurologic findings other than papilledema, but sixth nerve palsy may occur. Prolonged papilledema may lead to optic atrophy and vision loss. Patients appear to be surprisingly well.

Diagnosis

Pseudotumor cerebri is a diagnosis of exclusion. By definition, other causes of elevated intracranial pressure must be excluded, namely mass effect and chronic meningeal reactions (e.g., sarcoid, tuberculous, carcinomatous). Although intracranial venous thrombosis also can result in elevated intracranial pressure, this condition typically occurs in the setting of a hypercoagulable state, infection, and seizures. Hydrocephalus as a cause of elevated intracranial pressure should be easily distinguished on a CT scan. The spinal fluid is typically under a pressure of 250 to 400 mm of CSF but should otherwise be normal. A lumbar puncture is used to document the elevated pressure and to obtain spinal fluid for analysis to exclude meningeal infections. Removing CSF by lumbar puncture is therapeutic.

Management

Pseudotumor cerebri is a rare condition, and an initial presentation in the emergency department would be unusual. Patients who have headache, papilledema, and an absence of other neurologic findings (except, rarely, sixth nerve palsy) raises suspicions of a pseudotumor but should prompt an investigation to exclude an intracranial mass. A normal imaging study (CT scan or magnetic resonance imaging [MRI]) and a lumbar puncture confirming an elevated intracranial pressure and otherwise normal spinal fluid are all that are required to establish a diagnosis of pseudotumor cerebri.

The treatment of pseudotumor cerebri consists of eliminating potentially causative agents, such as medications, and repeating the lumbar puncture to decrease intracranial pressure and to prevent progressive papilledema and vision loss. Other medications to decrease intracranial pressure, including corticosteroids, glycerol, and acetazolamide, have been used with variable and debatable success. Weight reduction is commonly advocated. Shunting procedures from the lumbar subarachnoid space to the peritoneal cavity can be performed if repeated lumbar punctures fail and if visual changes become progressive. Optic nerve sheath decompression can also be done. None of these treatments are usually an issue for the emergency management of a patient with pseudotumor cerebri. However, close follow-up observation is essential, particularly with monitoring of visual fields and acuity.

NORMAL PRESSURE HYDROCEPHALUS

Pathophysiology and Etiology

Normal pressure hydrocephalus may follow subarachnoid hemorrhage, meningitis, or head trauma. Usually the cause is unknown. Although there may be an initial increase in intracranial pressure early in the course of ventricular dilatation, the pressure stabilizes in a normal range. However, the effect of this normal pressure over an enlarged ventricular surface area is sufficient to produce clinical effects.

Clinical Presentation

Normal pressure hydrocephalus is a condition characterized by dementia, ataxia, and incontinence of urine. The term refers to the characteristic dilatation of the ventricular system without any sustained increase in intracranial pressure. Drop attacks may occur. Headache and papilledema are absent. Neurologic findings include progressive intellectual loss simulating senile dementia, urinary urgency and frequency progressing to incontinence, and a gait disturbance that is maximally visible at curbs and on stairs. Grasp reflexes may occur. Dementia without ataxia or urinary incontinence may occur, but these patients tend to be least responsive to shunting procedures.

A variety of illnesses associated with dementia, primarily Alzheimer's disease, are the chief considerations in the differential diagnosis. The diagnosis is based on CT scan features that include dilatation of the ventricular system without significant evidence of cerebral-cortical atrophy, but it is sometimes difficult to establish the diagnosis with certainty on the basis of a CT scan alone.

Patients with normal pressure hydrocephalus may exhibit a combination of the typical symptoms of ataxia, dementia, and incontinence. They may have been presumed to have "senile dementia," but the course is usually more rapid with normal pressure hydrocephalus. The chief management issues concern establishment of the diagnosis and an appropriate referral. A lumbar puncture is performed to document the normal pressure and obtain spinal fluid for analysis. The issue of shunting procedures for normal pressure hydrocephalus is controversial, and the response to shunting procedures is variable.

AMYOTROPHIC LATERAL SCLEROSIS

The pathophysiology and etiology of amyotrophic lateral sclerosis (ALS) are unknown. ALS is a condition characterized pathologically by degeneration of the upper motor neuron tracts in the spinal cord and by deterioration of the lower motor neurons in the anterior horn cells. The symptoms and signs are therefore exclusively motor, and there is no sensory loss, except from compressive neuropathies secondary to immobility. There is no loss of sphincter control. A combination of both upper and lower motor neuron involvement causes atrophy and fasciculations, which is typical of anterior horn cell loss, and spasticity and long tract signs (e.g., the Babinski sign), which is typical of upper motor neuron damage.

ALS is one variant of a group of diseases categorized as motor neuron disease. When both lower motor neuron signs (atrophy, fasciculations, amyotrophia) and long tract (corticospinal) signs (hyperactive tendon reflexes and the Babinski signs) predominate in the extremities and trunk, the acronym *ALS* is used to describe the condition. When muscles of the tongue, jaw, face, and larynx are affected, the term *progressive bulbar palsy* is used. When only corticospinal processes are affected, the term *primary lateral sclerosis* is used. The term *progressive spinal muscular atrophy* applies when only lower motor neurons are affected. ALS is a slowly progressive condition that eventually becomes fatal because of involvement of respiratory muscles, aspiration pneumonia, general inanition, and medical problems associated with immobility.

It is distinctly uncommon for a new onset of ALS to be an emergency department diagnostic issue. The condition is not one that lends itself to definitive diagnosis in the emergency department, nor is that necessary. A recognition of the potential process and a referral to a neurologist should, however, be effected in a suspected case. More commonly, patients with ALS who have already been diagnosed enter the emergency department with complications of immobility, such as pneumonia, urosepsis, or respiratory failure. Management of the sequelae of immobility is the chief concern of the emergency department.

PARKINSON SYNDROME

Pathophysiology and Etiology

Parkinson syndrome, also called Parkinson disease or parkinsonism, is not one distinct disease but a collection of signs and symptoms resulting from diverse causes. The syndrome consists of tremors, rigidity, postural changes, and diminution of spontaneous motor activity. Parkinsonism occurs in 20 out of every 100,000 people, and men and women are affected equally. Of all Americans over age 50, 1% have parkinsonism, and 1 out of every 40 adults develops it. Symptoms of parkinsonism usually develop in the sixth decade of life, and the incidence increases with increasing age. Clinical variants of the syndrome may appear in younger patients, including those in their twenties.

Virtually all cases of parkinsonism that occur today are of the degenerative type (idiopathic: 49% to 86%) or are secondary to the use of prescription drugs (7% to 51%) or street drugs. The most common prescription drugs that cause parkinsonism are the phenothiazines and butyrophenones. Parkinsonism may rarely develop as a result of trauma. Parkinsonian features that occur in patients with brain tumors are usually unilateral and coexist with other features of the tumor—hemiparesis, visual field defects, seizures, and pyramidal signs—that are not typical of parkinsonism. With parkinsonism, pathologic changes occur in the extrapyramidal system and the cerebral cortex. Loss of pigment in the substantia nigra occurs macroscopically and corresponds to cell loss in that area. Diffuse cerebral cortical atrophy, more than expected for the patient's age, may occur. The cells of the basal ganglia (substantia nigra, caudate, and putamen) have a decreased amount of dopamine, a neurotransmitter; decreased amounts of the other neurotransmitters norepinephrine, serotonin, and γ-amino-butyric acid also occur. The way in which these changes result in parkinsonism is not completely understood. Typically the onset of parkinsonism is imperceptibly gradual, and the symptoms slowly worsen with time, with or without treatment; the course lasts many years.

Clinical Presentation

The clinical manifestations of parkinsonism vary widely (see the box above). The patient with parkinsonism typically walks with a stooped posture and with little or no automatic swinging of the arms. The patient may have postural instability, which causes falls or retropulsion. The slowness and loss of spontaneous movements lead to the masked facies with infrequent blinking. Drooling may result from the loss of automatic swallowing. Seborrhea is commonly present. Although a bilateral resting tremor is typically present, it is absent 20% of the time and may be unilateral at onset. The tremor typically becomes worse with excitement or agitation, lessens with active motion or sedation, and disappears with sleep. Rigidity and slowness of movement are the most functionally disabling components of the syndrome. Dementia is present in 30% to 40% of the patients but is usually not profound. Depression is reported in 37% to

---

CLINICAL FEATURES OF PARKINSONISM

Motor

Increased tone
Hypobradykinesia
"Masked facies"
Postural instability
Tremor: three to four seconds
Stooped posture
Drooling

Mental

Depression
Dementia

Other

Seborrhea
Constipation
L-dopa effects
"Freezing"
"On-off" phenomenon

90% of these patients. Patients with parkinsonism may also have a diminished upward gaze, limited convergence, the Myerson sign (a reflex consisting of persistent eye blinks with repeated tapping at the base of the nose), snout and sucking reflexes, and cogwheel rigidity. Tendon reflexes are usually normal but may be increased. Extensor toe signs (the Babinski sign) are usually absent. Sensory testing reveals normal findings. The spinal fluid is usually normal, and EEGs yield normal or nonspecific results. The CT scan may reveal generalized cortical atrophy and calcification of basal ganglia.

Some patients on levodopa (L-dopa) may exhibit marked fluctuations in motor ability over seconds to minutes, the so-called "on-off phenomenon," and a sudden brief inability to carry out certain movements, called *freezing*.

The diagnosis of parkinsonism is a clinical one, and no laboratory or other tests can confirm the diagnosis. When a patient has all the typical features of parkinsonism, the diagnosis presents little difficulty, and laboratory and other evaluations such as a CT scan are unnecessary. The chief feature that may cause difficulty in diagnosis is tremor. The tremor of parkinsonism typically is somewhat coarse and slow, lessens with active motion, and worsens with excitement. However, tremors may also be caused by other conditions: alcoholism, hyperthyroidism, senile tremors, and essential or familial tremors. The tremor of hyperthyroidism is usually of low amplitude and fast; that of alcoholism is also faster than that of parkinsonism and worse on movement. A senile tremor typically involves the head, and a familial tremor is usually an intention tremor. None of these conditions is associated with rigidity, and each is worse with movement. When a tremor is present in a young patient, hepatolenticular degeneration (Wilson disease) should be considered.

Once carbon monoxide exposure and manganese poisoning have been excluded by history, the chief differential diagnostic consideration for the patient with obvious features of parkinsonism is whether the parkinsonism is secondary to drugs or is idiopathic. Street drugs, especially the so-called designer drugs such as MPTP (a derivative of meperidine), produce a picture typical of parkinsonism. Psychotropic drugs, such as the phenothiazines and butyrophenones, may produce parkinsonism during or after treatment. Drug-induced parkinsonism may be dose-related and responds to antiparkinsonism drugs; a sudden worsening of parkinsonism may be caused by the cessation of those antiparkinsonism drugs.

Management

Drug therapy for parkinsonism is used to relieve symptoms; it does not arrest the course of the disease and is not required in mild cases. The decision to administer antiparkinsonism therapy to a patient with newly diagnosed parkinsonism is best made in conjunction with the physician who will be treating the patient. The medications used in parkinsonism include anticholinergics such as trihexyphenidyl, benztropine mesylate, L-dopa, L-dopa combined with a peripheral dopa-decarboxylase inhibitor (carbidopa), amantadine, and bromocriptine. Patients who have parkinsonism usually need hospitalization only for concomitant medical problems, such as dehydration or pneumonitis, and rarely for parkinsonism itself. Full-time nursing care may be required with severe manifestations or during the late stages of this disease.

KEY CONSIDERATIONS

WHAT IS THE LIFE THREAT?

In Guillain-Barré syndrome, an ascending polyneuropathy may progress rapidly to invade the thoracic musculature and impair respiration.

Airway and ventilation are major concerns in the assessment of patients with multiple sclerosis and amyotrophic lateral sclerosis.

DOES THE PATIENT NEED ADMISSION?

Admit patients with neuropathies who need airway and ventilatory support. Skin breakdown, urinary infections, or pulmonary infections may require inpatient treatment.

Admit patients with parkinsonism for concomitant medical problems such as dehydration or pneumonitis.

WHAT IS THE MOST SERIOUS DIAGNOSIS?

In patients with multiple sclerosis and other paralyzing illnesses, airway management, assurance of urinary drainage, and skin care are priorities.

HAVE I PERFORMED A THOROUGH WORK-UP?

Do not assume that sensory-motor symptoms have a psychogenic component until potentially life-threatening neurologic disorders such as cord compression have been considered.

Evaluate patients with a loss of sensation or motor function for skin breakdown, urinary infections, pulmonary infections, and sepsis.

Recommended Reading

Adour KK et al: The true nature of Bell's palsy: analysis of 1000 consecutive patients, *Laryngoscope* 88:787, 1978.

Colomba A et al: Pseudotumor cerebri: clinical features in evolution, *RIV Neurol* 59(4):164-166, 1989.

Gebarski S et al: The initial diagnosis of multiple sclerosis: clinical impact of magnetic resonance imaging, *Ann Neurol* 17:469, 1985.

Ireland B, Corbett JJ, Wallace RB: The search for causes of idiopathic intracranial hypertension: a preliminary case control study, *Arch Neurol* 47(3):315, 1990.

Kirshner H et al: Magnetic resonance imaging and other techniques in the diagnosis of multiple sclerosis, *Arch Neurol* 42:859, 1985.

Martin RA, Guthrie R: Office evaluation of dementia: how to arrive at a clear diagnosis and choose appropriate therapy, *Postgrad Med* 84(3):176, 1988.

May M, Klein SR, Taylor FH: Idiopathic (Bell's) palsy: natural history defies steroid or surgical therapy, *Laryngoscope* 95:406, 1988.

Miller J: Involuntary movements in the elderly, *Postgrad Med* 79(4):323, 1986.

Turner DA, McGeachie RE: Normal pressure hydrocephalus and dementia: evaluation and treatment, *Geriatr Med* 4(4):815, 1988.

Watson CPN: Post herpetic neuralgia, *Neurol Clin* 7(2):231, 1989.

Chapter Fifty-four
ACUTE PSYCHOSIS

EUGENE E. KERCHER

When confronted by a psychotic patient, the role of the emergency physician is to diffuse the immediate situation by facilitating the control of abnormal behavior, treat any life-threatening condition, determine whether the cause of the acute psychosis is functional or organic, and provide a proper medical and psychiatric disposition.

Psychosis is a dysfunction in the capacity for thought and information processing. There is an incapacity to be coherent in perceiving, retaining, processing, recalling, or acting on information in a consensually validated way. There is a decreased ability to mobilize, shift, sustain, and direct attention at will. A major feature of the psychotic state is a failure to rank the priority of stimuli. The ability to act on reality is unpredictable and diminished because the patient is unable to distinguish internal from external stimuli. The psychotic patient may act on any stimulus and become violent, combative, depressed, catatonic, or manic. For the emergency physician, the most easily recognized symptoms lie in observing that the patient is experiencing hallucinations and delusions.

Psychoses have traditionally been grouped as either organic or functional. Although the current diagnostic classification system for psychiatric disorders as published in the fourth edition of the *American Psychiatric Association Diagnostic and Statistical Manual of Mental Disorders* (DSM-IV) acknowledges the biologic and neurophysiologic basis of a mental disorder and eliminates specific reference to the terms *organic* and *functional,* such concepts are still clinically useful.

Examples of organic disorders include delirium, dementia, amnestic syndrome, and mental conditions caused by specific medical conditions. Characteristics of organic mental disorders typically include impaired consciousness, impaired thinking, disorientation, and memory deficits. Such elements can be contrasted against those of functional disorders as shown in Table 54-1 (the MADFOCS mnemonic). Most acute psychoses that have an organic basis result from intoxication, withdrawal states, and dementias. Functionally related psychoses usually result from one of the schizophrenic disorders or from an affective disorder.

APPROACH TO THE PATIENT WITH PSYCHOSIS

Assess the situation in terms of potential danger to self or staff. If the situation is potentially explosive, security forces should be on hand, and restraint may be required. Initial contact with the patient should be reassuring, firm, and in a quiet setting. A psychosis associated with an acute medical condition such as a drug overdose or hypoglycemia may also involve life-threatening symptoms or signs. In such settings the importance of attention to airway, breath-

Table 54-1

MADFOCS MNEMONIC (KEY POINTS TO BE CONSIDERED IN DIFFERENTIATING ORGANIC AND FUNCTIONAL PSYCHOSES)

	Organic	*Functional*
Memory deficits impaired	Recent memory impaired	Remote memory
Activity	Psychomotor retardation	Repetitive activity
	Tremor	Posturing
	Ataxia	Rocking
Distortions	Visual hallucinations	Auditory hallucinations
Feelings	Emotional lability	Flat affect
Orientation	Disoriented	Oriented
Cognition	Islands of lucidity	Continuous scattered thoughts
	Perceives occasionally	Unfiltered
	Attends occasionally	Unable to attend
Some other findings	Age >40	Age <40
	Sudden onset	Gradual onset
	Physical examination often abnormal	Physical examination normal
	Vital signs may be abnormal	Vital signs usually normal
	Social immodesty	Social modesty
	Aphasia	Intelligible speech
	Consciousness impaired	Alert, wake

WHHHIMP: (A MNEMONIC THAT PRESENTS VARIOUS LIFE-THREATENING CAUSES OF ACUTE PSYCHOSIS)

Wernicke encephalopathy
Hypoxemia or hypoperfusion of the central
    nervous system
Hypoglycemia
Hypertensive encephalopathy
Intracerebral hemorrhage
Meningitis/encephalitis
Poisoning

ing, and circulation cannot be overemphasized. Other potentially life-threatening causes of psychosis can be remembered with the use of the mnemonic "rule of the WHHHIMP" (see the box at left). Various rules of thumb in evaluating the psychotic patient with a given physical parameter are presented in the box on p. 649.

Various reversible medical causes of psychoses are listed in the box on p. 649. Specific clues that suggest an organic cause of illness include abnormal vital signs, disorientation, recent memory loss, incontinence, tremors and ataxia, a change in pupil size, onset of illness past age 50 or before age 12, visual or tactile hallucinations, sudden onset, and evidence of toxins that are either in the environment or have been previously ingested.

RULES OF THUMB IN THE CLINICAL EVALUATION OF THE PATIENT WITH PSYCHOSIS

Fever + psychosis = meningitis
Psychosis + alcoholism = Wernicke encephalopathy
Headache + psychosis = tumor; subdural or intracranial hemorrhage
Abdominal pain + psychosis = porphyria
Sweating + psychosis = hypoglycemia or delirium tremens
Autonomic signs + psychosis = toxic or metabolic encephalopathy

---

REVERSIBLE CAUSES OF PSYCHOSIS (DEMENTIA MNEMONIC)

Drug toxicity
Emotional disorders
Metabolic disorders
Endocrine disorders
Nutritional disorders
Tumors and trauma
Infection
Arteriosclerotic complications

MENTAL STATUS EXAMINATION

The Mini-Mental Status Examination is one of the easiest and most reliable bedside tests that can be administered in the emergency department. An assessment of orientation, memory, attention, concentration, constructional tasks, special discrimination, arithmetic ability, and writing must be included. These aspects of cognitive functioning can be assessed in less than 5 minutes.

Disorientation to the environment typically begins with an inability to recall the date; this inability is followed by disorientation to day, week, time, month, year, and eventually place. Memory assessment requires testing the patient's ability to repeat a short series of words or numbers, learn new information, and retrieve previously stored information. Constructional apraxia is the inability to perform constructional tasks, such as drawing geometric figures or clockfaces or connecting dots. Dysnomia (the inability to name objects correctly) and dysgraphia (impaired writing ability) are two of the most sensitive indicators of delirium. An example of a quantifiable mental status examination is shown in the box on p. 650.

PHYSICAL EXAMINATION

The physical examination focuses first on the patient's general appearance and vital signs. The general appearance can sometimes provide information about social supports, hygiene, and level of activity. For example, a neatly groomed psychotic individual is experiencing either an abrupt onset of psychosis or a functioning social support system. Vital sign abnormalities are an important clue and point to a diagnosis of psychosis resulting from a medical condition. In general, the further or more extreme the vital signs deviate from normal, the greater the likelihood that a medical illness is present.

An examination of the patient's head determines whether head trauma is present. The extraocular movements and pupillary responses provide information regarding nystagmus, intracranial pressure, and possible poisoning syndromes. Nystagmus suggests a medical disorder such as a cerebellar tumor, cerebellar bleed, or

MINI-MENTAL STATUS EXAMINATION

Maximum score	Orientation
5	What is the (year) (season) (date) (day) (month)?
5	Where are we (city) (state) (country) (hospital) (floor)?

Registration

3	Names three objects: one second to say each. Ask the patient for all three after you have said them. Give one point for each correct answer. Repeat them until all three are learned. Count trials and record number.

Attention and calculation

5	Serial sevens backward from 100 (stop after five answers). Alternatively, spell WORLD backward.

Recall

3	Ask for the three objects repeated above. Give one point for each correct answer.

Language and praxis

2	Show a pencil and watch, and ask subject to name them.
1	Ask the patient to repeat the following: "no ifs, ands, or buts."
3	Three-stage command: "Take this paper in your right hand, fold it in half, and put it on the floor."
1	Read and obey the following: "Close your eyes." (Written on a piece of paper)
1	Write a sentence. (Must contain a noun, a verb, and be sensible. Ignore grammar and punctuation.)
1	Copy this design (interlocking pentagons). Must contain all angles and must intersect.

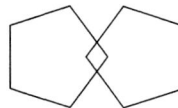

From Folstein et al: *J Psychiat Res* 12:189, 1975.

PCP intoxication. Paresis of gaze suggests a brainstem infarction, an intracranial mass effect, or Wernicke encephalopathy. The ears and surrounding mastoid area should be examined for evidence of trauma, such as hemotympanum or mastoid ecchymoses, either of which suggests basilar skull fracture.

Suppleness of the neck is important in helping to rule out a subarachnoid hemorrhage or meningitis. A complete examination also includes an evaluation of the chest, heart, abdomen, extremities, skin, and neurologic system. The neurologic examination should include an evaluation of cranial nerves, motor skills, reflexes (deep tendon and pathologic), coordination, sensation, and mental status.

TREATABLE CAUSES OF ORGANIC MENTAL DISEASE

Cardiac

Dysrhythmias
Congestive heart failure
Myocardial infarction

Pulmonary

Chronic obstructive pulmonary disease
Pulmonary emboli

Hepatic

Cirrhosis
Hepatitis
Wilson disease

Renal

Worsening of mild nephritis by urinary tract
    infection
Dehydration with elevation of BUN >50 mg/dl

Vascular

Subdural hematoma
Cerebrovascular accident

Infection

Endocrine disease

Thyroid disease
Cushing disease
Diabetes
Addison disease
Hypoglycemia

Electrolyte imbalance

Hyponatremia
Hypernatremia
Hypercalcemia

Vitamin deficiencies

Thiamine
Niacin
Riboflavin
Folate
Ascorbic acid
Vitamin A
Vitamin B_{12}

Drug-induced

Alcohol
Tranquilizers
Over-the-counter preparations
Any drug used to treat medical illness (e.g.,
    phenytoin [Dilantin], aminophylline, digitalis,
    steroids)

Exogenous toxins

Carbon monoxide
Bromide
Mercury
Lead

Tumors

Normal pressure hydrocephalus

Depression

LABORATORY AND RADIOGRAPHIC EXAMINATION

For most purposes the acute onset of psychosis or a sudden mental status change can be evaluated in the emergency department with the following studies: complete blood count and differential, electrolyte, glucose, blood urea nitrogen (BUN), creatinine, urinalysis, and some form of toxicology screen. An ECG is helpful, especially in elderly patients who may have sustained a myocardial infarction, heart block, or some other cardiac abnormality that has caused the abrupt onset of the mental status change. Pulse oximetry provides a rapid approximation of oxygen saturation, but arterial blood gases provide additional information about ventilation and acid-base status. The psychiatric inpatient faculty often requests a complete toxicology screen, with the results to be reported at a later date. A somewhat comprehensive list of medical conditions that cause abnormal thoughts or behaviors is presented in the box on p. 651.

TREATMENT

The treatment goal in the emergency department is to decrease the patient's discomfort, anxiety, and disruptive behavior. For an acute, reversible, organic psychosis, treat the underlying disequilibrium. For the safety of the patient and staff, functional psychoses and many of the organically caused psychoses often require immediate tranquilization in the emergency department.

The standard medical treatment for an acute psychosis is haloperidol. Haloperidol is a safe major tranquilizer to use in the emergency department and produces minimal hemodynamic or respiratory side effects. Rapid tranquilization with haloperidol has proven to be safe and effective when given intramuscularly (IM) or intravenously (IV). Haloperidol 5 to 10 mg IM/IV every 30 to 60 minutes is suggested when de-

creased agitation, clarity of thought, or a reduction of confusion is desired. Haloperidol 5 mg, with 2 mg of lorazepam given IV every 30 minutes until the appropriate sedation has been reached, has also been suggested for controlling acutely psychotic behavior. The administration of haloperidol (5 to 10 mg IM or IV) plus 25 to 50 mg of diphenhydramine (Benadryl) given IM or IV not only increases the sedative effect but also counteracts the extrapyramidal side effects of haloperidol.

DISPOSITION OF THE ACUTELY PSYCHOTIC PATIENT

Hospitalization of the acutely psychotic patient is recommended under the following circumstances: (1) this is the patient's first psychotic episode, (2) the patient is a danger to self or others (i.e., suicidal, homicidal, or influenced by command hallucinations), or (3) the patient is unable to appropriately care for himself or herself. Hospitalization is also recommended if the functionally psychotic patient does not sufficiently improve under initial emergency department tranquilization or if an acute organic psychosis is present and does not resolve in the emergency department.

THOUGHT DISORDERS (SCHIZOPHRENIC AND DELUSIONAL DISORDERS)

Schizophrenic and delusional disorders are marked by the presence of psychotic symptoms, primarily delusions and hallucinations. Delusions are defined as fixed false beliefs that are not amenable to arguments or facts and are not shared by others of a similar cultural background. The most prevalent functional psychosis is schizophrenia, which is one of the most serious public health problems in the world. It accounts for 25% of all admissions to psychiatric hospitals. A summary of DSM-IV cri-

SUMMARY OF DSM-IV CRITERIA FOR SCHIZOPHRENIC DISORDERS

A. *Characteristic symptoms*: Two (or more) of the following, each present for a significant portion of time during a 1-month period (or less if successfully treated):

(1) Delusions

(2) Hallucinations

(3) Disorganized speech (e.g., frequent derailment or incoherence)

(4) Grossly disorganized or catatonic behavior

(5) Negative symptoms (e.g., affective flattening, alogia, or avolition)

Note: Only one Criterion A symptom is required if delusions are bizarre or if hallucinations consist of a voice keeping a running commentary on the person's behavior or thoughts, or two or more voices conversing with each other.

B. *Social/occupational dysfunction*: For a significant portion of the time since the onset of the disturbance, one or more major areas of functioning such as work, interpersonal relations, or self-care are markedly below the level achieved before the onset (or, when the onset is in childhood or adolescence, failure to achieve an expected level of interpersonal, academic, or occupational achievement).

C. *Duration*: Continuous signs of the disturbance persist for at least 6 months. This 6-month period must include at least 1 month of symptoms (or less if successfully treated) that meet Criterion A (i.e., active-phase symptoms) and may include periods of prodromal or residual symptoms. During these prodromal or residual periods, the signs of the disturbance may be manifested by only negative symptoms or by two or more symptoms listed in Criterion A present in an attenuated form (e.g., odd beliefs, unusual perceptual experiences).

D. *Schizoaffective and Mood Disorder exclusion*: Schizoaffective Disorder and Mood Disorder With Psychotic Features have been ruled out because either (1) no Major Depressive, Manic, or Mixed Episodes have occurred concurrently with the active-phase symptoms; or (2) if mood episodes have occurred during active-phase symptoms, their total duration has been brief relative to the duration of the active and residual periods.

E. *Substance/general medical condition exclusion*: The disturbance is not due to the direct physiologic effects of a substance (e.g., a drug of abuse, a medication) or a general medical condition.

F. *Relationship to a Pervasive Developmental Disorder*: If there is a history of Autistic Disorder or another Pervasive Developmental Disorder, the additional diagnosis of Schizophrenia is made only if prominent delusions or hallucinations are also present for at least 1 month (or less if successfully treated).

From American Psychiatric Association: *Diagnostic and statistical manual of mental disorders,* ed 4(DSM-IV), Washington, DC, 1994, American Psychiatric Press.

teria for schizophrenic disorders is presented in the box on p. 653.

Hallucinations and delusions are typically the emergency physician's first indication that the patient is psychotic. Bizarre delusions, such as thought broadcasting or being controlled by a dead person (not explained by patient's culture), and prominent hallucinations of a voice with content (not related to mood) are most typical.

A marked deterioration from a higher level of functioning subsequent to the disturbance (e.g., work, self-care, social relations) often occurs. Schizoaffective disorders and mood disorders with psychotic features must be ruled out, and the symptoms must not be secondary to any organic mental disorder or mental retardation. A *schizophreniform disorder* is diagnosed when the patient meets the criteria for schizophrenia but the symptoms have been present continuously for less than 6 months. A rapid onset over a few days and good premorbid functioning are more common with a schizophreniform disorder than with schizophrenia. A *brief psychotic disorder* is the diagnosis for individuals who become acutely psychotic following an exposure to an extremely traumatic life experience; such an episode lasts for less than 2 weeks. Precipitants of the psychosis may include the death of a loved one or a life-threatening situation such as combat or a natural disaster. Emotional turmoil, confusion, and extremely bizarre behavior and speech are common symptoms.

A *delusional disorder* is a syndrome distinct from schizophrenia and is characterized by persistent, nonbizarre delusions. Unlike schizophrenia, delusional disorders rarely are characterized by an impairment in daily functioning, and aside from the strange ideas expressed, the patient may appear outwardly normal. The onset occurs during middle or late adulthood, and the delusions develop over months or years. Several subtypes of delusional disorders have been identified. The most common is the persecutory type, in which the delusions follow themes of being conspired against, cheated, followed, poisoned, or harassed. With delusional jealousy, the patient has an unsubstantiated conviction that his or her partner is being unfaithful. Somatic delusions cause patients to believe that they emit a foul odor or are infected with parasites.

•   •   •

An acute psychosis is a true emergency and is a manifestation of multiple organic and functional disorders. The emergency physician's role when dealing with the acutely psychotic patient is to control the patient's behavior, delineate the cause of the psychosis, and provide appropriate initial treatment and disposition.

████████KEY CONSIDERATIONS

WHAT IS THE LIFE THREAT?

Death can occur from an undetected medical illness that is causing the abnormal thoughts or behaviors.

DOES THE PATIENT NEED ADMISSION?

Patients with an acute onset of psychosis require admission for medical and psychiatric evaluation and treatment.

WHAT IS THE MOST SERIOUS DIAGNOSIS?

Poisoning, CNS infection, sepsis, intracranial hemorrhage, alcohol or drug withdrawal, hypoxemia, hypertensive encephalopathy, and hypoglycemia are the most serious diagnoses.

HAVE I PERFORMED A THOROUGH WORK-UP?

Obtain an adequate history. Perform a physical examination, including a mental status and neurologic examination. Obtain targeted laboratory tests depending on the patient's history and physical (e.g., complete blood count, electrolytes, BUN, creatinine, glucose, liver function tests, toxicology screen, arterial blood gases).

Perform an ECG and targeted imaging studies (as needed) such as a head CT scan and a chest x-ray examination.

Recommended Reading

American Psychiatric Association: *Diagnostic and statistical manual of mental disorders,* ed 4, revised, Washington, DC, 1994, The Association.

Anderson EH, Stern TA: Psychiatric emergencies. In Wilkens EW, editor: *Emergency medicine: scientific foundations and current practice,* Baltimore, 1989, Williams & Wilkins.

Frame DS, Kercher EE: Acute psychosis: functional vs organic, *Emerg Med Clin North Am* 9(1):123-136, 1991.

Jorden RD: Initial evaluation of the patient with altered mental status, *Topics Emerg Med* 13(2):1-9, 1991.

Lucke WC: Thought and affective disorders. In Rosen P et al, editors: *Emergency medicine: concepts and clinical practice,* ed 3, St Louis, 1992, Mosby.

Rund DA: Evaluating and managing the violent patient. In Rosen P et al, editors: *Emergency medicine: concepts and clinical practice,* ed 3, St Louis, 1992, Mosby.

Shy J, Rund DA: Psychotropic medications. In Tintinalli JE et al, editors: *Emergency medicine: a comprehensive study guide,* 1995, McGraw-Hill.

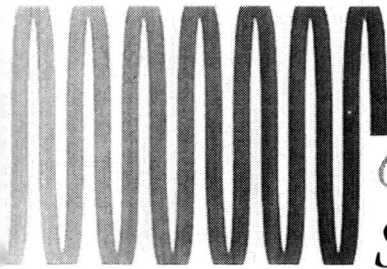

Chapter *Fifty-five*

SUICIDE

PHILLIP I. BIALECKI

Suicide is the tenth leading cause of death in the United States and results in 40,000 deaths each year. However, because many suicides are erroneously attributed to accidental deaths, the true number is probably higher. Suicide ranks as the second leading cause of death among those aged 15 to 24 years, and the incidence has increased more than 300% since 1960. For every one completed suicide, there are 50 to 150 suicide attempts, or approximately 3 to 6 million attempts each year.

Approximately 50% of those persons who commit suicide saw a physician within the preceding month. Of those who successfully overdose, 50% received a prescription for the lethal medication within 1 week of the final act. Important clinical findings that suggest the possibility of suicide are often subtle; for example, a patient can appear with vague physical complaints.

The suicidal state is an acute and treatable condition and represents a cry for help. Suicidal patients are looking for a way out of the emotional or physical pain they are experiencing. They may come to the emergency department because of a suicide attempt or because they have run out of available coping mechanisms and see suicide as the only answer to what is an acute crisis.

STABILIZATION AND EVALUATION

Suicidal patients should be searched and never left unattended. Suicidal precautions, including a treatment room that is free of potentially harmful medical equipment and allows for adequate patient observation, should be in place. A history of current medications, doses, and the amount of drug available to the patient is essential. Patients may require observation either in the emergency department or as an inpatient so that the effects of alcohol or drugs can diminish to enable a more accurate evaluation.

Patients who are depressed can have a variety of complaints such as being "sick all over," "weak and dizzy," or "tired all the time." Screening for depression includes asking about symptoms of depression, such as a loss of appetite and sleep disturbance. The mnemonic *IN SAD CAGES* shown in the box on p. 657 is useful for remembering the common features of depression.

A history of a recent loss, a current ambivalence about living, and a general sense of hopelessness about life should all be "red flags" and are often subtly offered by patients who are feeling depressed and suicidal. Although the degree of depression has not been shown to correlate directly with the seriousness of an attempt, the degree of "hopelessness" or "helplessness" does.

From Rund DA, Hutzler JC: *Emergency psychiatry,* St Louis, 1983, Mosby.

Concerns expressed by family and friends need to be given serious attention in evaluating the suicidal patient because such individuals often provide key information not offered by the patient. Recent changes in the patient's personality, as well as activities such as giving personal items away (often a last act) or purchasing a firearm, are all clues to suicide risk.

FEATURES OF SUICIDAL PATIENTS

A previous suicide attempt, however remote, should be taken very seriously because 50% of those who go on to complete a suicide had made at least one previous attempt. Of special concern are those individuals who used serious medical means in a previous attempt. However, do not trivialize even the most medically in-

significant attempt because such patients are still at risk, and the next attempt may be both medically and psychiatrically serious.

Alcoholic patients, those with a severe psychiatric illness, or those who have suffered severe physical or psychologic trauma must be considered as high risk. Statistically, women attempt suicide more often than men, but men complete suicide more often than women and use more lethal devices such as firearms.

The suicide rate for whites is two times that for any other group. The incidence of suicide increases with age and peaks for women between the ages of 40 and 60 years. Males have a bimodal distribution, with peaks during adolescence and a steady increase from age 45 into the geriatric age group. The "typical" suicidal patient is a divorced, unemployed, middle-aged white man who has suffered a recent loss. The highest suicide rate exists for those between the ages of 75 and 84 years (approximately 22 out of every 100,000). Suicide is uncommon in children and usually involves acting on a desire to hurt the parents for some perceived wrongdoing.

In evaluating a suicidal attempt, perform a quick and simple Mini-Mental State Examination to assess orientation, mood, affect, and thought. Evaluate the patient's orientation to place, time, and person; evaluate both long- and short-term memory. *Mood* is the patient's subjective experience of self; *affect* is the objective observation of how the patient appears. Both mood and affect are assessed for type (sad, angry, elated) and intensity (flat, blunted, constricted, exaggerated). Thought content and means of expression should be noted: Is the patient delusional, paranoid, scattered, or nonsensical? Is the story organized, and how fast or slow is the patient's speech? The presence of psychosis is an indication for psychiatric admission. Determining suicidal risk requires gathering adequate information about suicidal ideation; ask about the patient's thoughts, means, and actions preceding the attempt.

A common myth in both the lay and medical

communities is that asking a depressed person if he or she is suicidal may introduce the idea to him or her. In reality, most patients feel relieved when asked this question and see the question as a sign that someone appreciates the amount of pain that they are experiencing. Simply ask the patient, "Have you been thinking about killing yourself?" If the answer to this question is "yes" or is ambiguous, the patient should be questioned about the means by which he or she would carry out the thought. If a plan is present, it is necessary to assess the detail of the plan and what if any action has been taken to complete it. Finally, the patient must be asked directly if he or she has attempted to harm himself or herself at any time in the recent or distant past.

Given the information gathered, the patient can be placed into one of four categories on a risk/rescue rating scale. Risk is denoted as either high or low on the basis of the perceived lethality of the attempt. Rescue is the likelihood of rescue as perceived by the patient. A high-risk patient might have used (or have readily available) a loaded firearm, whereas a low-risk patient has not decided what type of pills he or she would use or where he or she might attain them. A low-rescue rating is assigned when the attempt has been planned in a setting in which there is little likelihood of rescue. Those judged to be in the high-risk/low-rescue category need admission, whereas those in the low-risk/high-rescue category may be appropriate for outpatient follow-up. The patient who has planned to hang himself or herself in a lonely motel room is at a much greater risk than the patient who takes a few cold tablets in front of witnesses.

Important criteria for admission include suicidal intent, symptoms and signs of severe major depression, an age over 45 years, and psychosis. The patient with psychosis cannot distinguish reality from internal thoughts, delusions, or hallucinations and may react to an otherwise unseen or unheard stimulus and terminate his or her own life.

Disposition of the possibly suicidal patient is often difficult in ambiguous cases; the use of a sensitive numeric scoring system may help. The modified SAD PERSONS scale is one such test; the mnemonic stands for ten high-risk factors (see the box below). The risks are weighed by assigning two points to each of four variables that correlate highly with the need for hospitalization and one point for each of the remaining lower risk variables. Those with a score of 0 to 2 can be sent home with outpatient follow-up. Those with a score of 7 or greater need hospitalization. A score between 3 and 6 must be carefully evaluated, with consideration given to the patient's reliability and access to support and follow-up.

PREDICTING LIKELIHOOD OF SUICIDE

1. **S**ex: male (1 pt)
2. **A**ge: less than 19 or more than 45 years old (1 pt)
3. **D**epression or hopelessness: may use the IN SAD CAGES criteria (2 pts)
4. **P**revious attempts: no previous attempt is too trivial to be included; previous psychiatric care is also included here (1 pt)
5. **E**xcessive alcohol or drug use: in the present or past (1 pt)
6. **R**ational thinking loss: delusional or frankly psychotic (2 pts)
7. **S**eparated, divorced, or widowed (1 pt)
8. **O**rganized plan or serious attempt (2 pts)
9. **N**o social supports: the patient must not only have the support but must also be able to use the support (1 pt)
10. **S**tated future intent: includes those ambivalent or determined to *repeat the attempt* (2 pts)

Score two points if present for items 3, 6, 8, and 10
Score one point if present for items 1, 2, 4, 5, 7, 9

From Hockberger RS, Rothstein RJ: Assessment of suicide potential by nonpsychiatrists using the "sad persons" score, *J Emerg Med* 6:99, 1988.

INDICATIONS FOR HOSPITALIZATION

Patients who present a danger to themselves or others must be hospitalized—involuntarily if necessary. An estimated 15% of all suicides occur after a patient has been allowed to refuse hospitalization. All states have provisions for the involuntary admission of such patients.

Any patient who refuses to answer questions or to make a commitment to follow the treatment plan must be admitted. Adolescents who have been brought to the emergency department by concerned parents are notorious for refusing to answer questions; by age alone they fall into the high-risk category. Patients who have previously shown an inability to control impulses or those who are still in the midst or immediate aftermath of their crisis also warrant hospitalization.

The use of a written "No suicide" contract that includes alternatives for coping with hopeless feelings and also lists sources of support with phone numbers is very helpful. A patient who refuses to sign such a contract must be considered actively suicidal and cannot be discharged. A high level of concern by either family members, friends, or the physician should be taken very seriously. When in question, err on the side of caution.

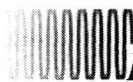

KEY CONSIDERATIONS

WHAT IS LIFE THREAT?

A possible completion of suicide constitutes the life threat.

DOES THE PATIENT NEED ADMISSION?

Important criteria for admission include an expression of suicidal intent, a high-risk suicide attempt, clinical signs of depression, being an adolescent, being over age 45, and being psychotic.

WHAT IS THE MOST SERIOUS DIAGNOSIS?

Physical risks from the suicide attempt, being actively suicidal, experiencing a major depression, or experiencing a psychosis are the most serious diagnoses.

HAVE I PERFORMED A THOROUGH WORK-UP?

Ask the following questions:

Have I treated the patient adequately from a medical standpoint (e.g., gastric decontamination in drug overdose)? Have I asked about future suicide plans? Have I screened for major depression? Have I instituted suicide precautions?

Recommended Reading

Hockberger RS, Rothstein RJ: Assessment of suicide potential by nonpsychiatrists using the "sad persons" score, *J Emerg Med* 6:99, 1988.

Hofmann DP, Dubovsky SL: Depression and suicide assessment. In Kercher EE, Moore GP, editors: *Emergency medicine clinics of North America: psychiatric aspects of emergency medicine*, vol 9, Philadelphia, 1991, WB Saunders.

Rund DA, Hutzler JC: *Emergency psychiatry*, St Louis, 1983, Mosby.

Schmidt T: Suicide. In Rosen P et al, editors: *Emergency medicine: concepts and clinical practice,* ed 3, St Louis, 1992, Mosby.

Tintinalli JE, Peacock FW, Wright MA: Emergency medical evaluation of psychiatric patients, *Ann Emerg Med* 23:4, 1994.

Weissberg MP, Suskauer SH: The suicidal crisis: preventing the final act, *Emerg Med Rep* 10:7, 1986.

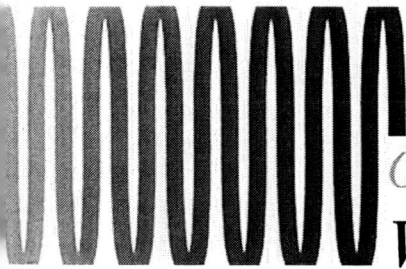

FRANK W. LAVOIE

The evaluation and management of all acute medical, surgical, and psychiatric conditions is the inherent task of emergency services. Therefore nonorganized acts of individual violence, which are sometimes associated with medical and psychiatric conditions, come to the attention of emergency clinicians, other health care specialists, and law enforcement personnel.

Studies performed in the emergency department and hospital demonstrate significant concerns with respect to assaultive and combative behaviors in the emergency department. As many as one third of all emergency departments may experience verbal threats on a daily basis, and many high-risk facilities often experience batteries of emergency department staff members, including physicians. This chapter addresses the causes and presentations of violent behavior, as well as the general management considerations in dealing with such behavior in emergency situations.

CAUSES OF VIOLENCE

Both organic and psychiatric conditions can be responsible for behavioral changes, including aggression, combativeness, and directed violence (see the box on p. 661). Combative and aggressive acts in the emergency department are most commonly related to acute psychotic conditions and to drug and alcohol intoxication

and withdrawal. However, general metabolic disorders that cause delirium and other CNS conditions are also common causes and should not be overlooked. It is important to consider and address serious and reversible conditions such as hypoxemia and hypoglycemia immediately on presentation.

PRESENTATION OF VIOLENCE

Although the victims of violence are seen in the emergency department more often than the perpetrators, three typical presentations of such patients are common.

The overtly violent patient is easy to spot and recognize. Physical restraint is immediately used to control the situation. Fortunately, most combative patients arrive with police or EMS personnel and have been restrained in the prehospital setting; in such a case, gathering prehospital data from the EMS or police can be invaluable. Details of violent acts, threats, the use of weapons, and the circumstances leading to patient transport and restraint should be sought. The presence of medication containers, drugs, or chemicals near the scene should also be noted. The use of tranquilizing medications may be indicated once the patient's condition has been assessed.

Agitated individuals who are not overtly violent present the greatest threat to the clinical

DIAGNOSES AND CONDITIONS ASSOCIATED WITH VIOLENCE

Intoxication

Alcohol
Barbiturates
Amphetamines
Cocaine
Phencyclidine
Hallucinogens

Withdrawal

Alcohol
Barbiturates
Other drugs

Organic mental disorder

Drug effects and side effects
  Metabolic: hypoglycemia,
  hyperthyroidism, electrolyte
  imbalance
Anoxia
Infection
  Sepsis
  Encephalitis
  Meningitis

Traumatic disorders

Head injuries
  Basilar skull fracture
  Subdural hemorrhage
  Subarachnoid hemorrhage
  Intracerebral hemorrhage

Functional disorders

Schizophrenia
Affective disorders
  Mania
  Depression
Personality disorders
  Antisocial
  Borderline
  Paranoid
Dementia
  Senile
Intermittent explosive disorder
Adjustment disorder

Seizure disorder

Postictal status
Complex postictal seizures
Temporal lobe epilepsy

From Rund DA: Evaluating and managing the violent patient. In Rosen P et al, editors: *Emergency medicine: concepts and clinical practice,* St Louis, 1992, Mosby.

staff and the physical environment. Recognizing the premonitory signs of impending violence is a critical skill. Behavioral intervention before a state of crisis develops is distinctly beneficial to the patient and the emergency department staff. Classical clues to impending violence include changes in posture, speech, and motor activity. Such changes traditionally involve sitting anxiously on the edge of the bed and gripping the armrails intensely; using an angry, loud voice or aggressive statements; changes in body position; and pacing. Depending on the degree of agitation, physical restraint may need to be used with such individuals. More often, however, psychologic and chemical management are used together with patient evaluation.

Additional patients may come to the emergency department for an evaluation after a violent outburst that occurred before arrival. Such patients may be calm and even remorseful. As with other presentations, this group of patients requires a mental status examination and an evaluation for organic causes. The emergency physician must also try to determine the potential for further violence if the patient is released; there may be a duty to warn any individuals whom the patient intends to harm.

STABILIZATION AND MANAGEMENT CONSIDERATIONS

Interviewing Patients

Assume that any patient has the potential for violent behavior, especially patients with neurologic and psychiatric complaints. When interviewing patients who are unrestrained, pay particular attention to the signs of impending violence described previously.

Several additional considerations are required when approaching potentially violent patients. Have physical assistance, such as security guards, nearby to provide a "show of force," which can help keep some patients under control. Sit in a manner that allows both the examiner and the patient to use the exit if tempers flare. Avoid eye contact because it may be perceived as threatening. Allow the patient to ventilate by providing nonjudgmental support.

Physical Restraint

Physical restraint is used to prevent imminent harm to the patient, to others, or to the physical environment. It is usually used involuntarily but occasionally is used at the request of a patient who fears loss of control. To prevent injuries to either the patient or staff members, restraints are applied using a coordinated team approach. The patient should be informed that the restraints are for protection and to control behavior.

Once restrained, the patient should be searched for weapons, drugs, and dangerous items. Restraints should not be removed if the patient pleas or barters. The restraints can be removed only after it is apparent that the behavior is well controlled. It may be necessary to medicate patients to achieve this behavior.

Seclusion

The use of a "quiet" room may benefit patients who are psychotic yet controlled. Seclusion de-creases patient stimulation and prevents the patient from wandering off without the use of physical restraint. Seclusion should never be used for patients with acute organic problems.

Chemical Restraint

Most patients who are physically restrained for violence require tranquilization to achieve long-term control. Major tranquilizers are the drugs used most often to control agitation and violent behavior. The butyrophenones, such as haloperidol or droperidol, are most commonly used and may be given intravenously, intramuscularly, or orally. Rapid-acting benzodiazepines, such as lorazapam, are also advocated but are stronger respiratory depressants than the butyrophenones. Because of cross-tolerance, the benzodiazepines are the preferred agents in alcohol withdrawal.

Droperidol (Inapsine) has a rapid onset of action, especially when administered intravenously. A dose of 2.5 to 5 mg produces rapid tranquilization and permits further evaluation. Mild hypotension is predictable when droperidol is used and can be treated effectively with volume infusion and head-down positioning. In most settings, lorazepam (Ativan), 2 mg intramuscularly, can be given along with 5 mg of intramuscular haloperidol (Haldol) to facilitate rapid tranquilization. Larger doses may occasionally be necessary.

Weapons

Patients with weapons present an increased threat to clinicians. Because most health care workers are unable to predict which patients carry weapons, routine searches may be advisable. The safest approach is to withdraw and allow the security personnel or police to intervene. The use of metal detectors in high-risk facilities may help control weapon-oriented violence in the emergency department.

KEY CONSIDERATIONS

WHAT IS THE LIFE THREAT?

Lethal injury to the staff or to other patients and suicide in the violent patient who directs anger toward self constitute life threats.

DOES THE PATIENT NEED ADMISSION?

Violent and agitated or near-violent patients require admission if an undetected and potentially life-threatening medical condition causes the symptoms. Continued violent ideations in the psychotic patient warrant admission.

WHAT IS THE MOST SERIOUS DIAGNOSIS?

Undetected and potentially life-threatening physical conditions that cause violence, agitation, or delirium are the most serious diagnoses.

HAVE I PERFORMED A THOROUGH WORK-UP?

Obtain a weapons search as needed.

Perform a medical assessment for hypoglycemia, alcohol or drug syndromes, anoxia, infection, head injury, and a postictal state.

Perform a mental status examination to test orientation, memory, and affect.

Recommended Reading

Clinton J et al: Haloperidol for sedation of disruptive emergency patients, *Ann Emerg Med* 16:319-322, 1987.

Lavoie FW et al: Emergency department violence in United States' teaching hospitals, *Ann Emerg Med* 17:1227-1233, 1988.

Rund DA: Evaluating and managing the violent patient. In Rosen P et al, editors: *Emergency medicine: concepts, and clinical practice,* ed 3, St Louis, 1992, Mosby.

Rund DA, Hutzer JC: *Emergency psychiatry,* St Louis, 1983, Mosby.

Schmidt T: An overview of psychiatric emergencies. In Rosen P et al, editors: *Emergency medicine: concepts and clinical practice,* ed 3, St Louis, 1992, Mosby.

Smith J: Organic brain syndrome. In Rosen P et al, editors: *Emergency medicine: concepts and clinical practice,* ed 3, St Louis, 1992, Mosby.

Chapter Fifty-seven

FLUIDS AND ELECTROLYTES

COREY M. SLOVIS

BODY FLUID DISTRIBUTION

Approximately 60% of the body weight consists of water, which is distributed into compartments that normally maintain their individual compositions within precise limits. Total body water (TBW) as a percentage of weight declines over time as a result of an increase in the percentage of body fat. As men age, their percentage of body weight due to TBW declines from approximately 60% to 50%. For adult women, their TBW declines only minimally and, in general, can be calculated at approximately 50% of their body weight.

There are two major fluid compartments in the body: (1) the intracellular fluid (ICF) compartment, and (2) the extracellular compartment (ECF), which can be subdivided into (a) plasma and (b) interstitial fluid. The ICF compartment accounts for 30% to 40% total body weight (or approximately two thirds of TBW). Potassium and magnesium are the two major intracellular cations; sulfates, phosphates, and proteins are the major intracellular anions (Table 57-1). The ECF compartment accounts for approximately 20% of total body weight (or approximately one third of TBW). Sodium is the predominant extracellular cation, and chloride and bicarbonate are the major extracellular anions. The major difference between plasma and the interstitial fluid is the significantly higher protein content of the plasma.

The distribution of the TBW is determined by osmotic forces. Although the cell membrane is freely permeable to water and various small uncharged molecules, it is relatively impermeable to many solutes, including sodium ions. Sodium ions do diffuse into the cell at a slow rate, but they are actively transported out of the cell.

Concentrating sodium ions outside the cell and other nondiffusible solutes (such as cellular proteins) inside the semipermeable cell membrane creates electrical and chemical gradients that determine the distribution of the freely permeable solutes and water between these compartments. Because of osmosis, the osmolarity within one compartment is equal to that in all others.

Osmotic forces may be counteracted by applying a pressure gradient across the membrane in a direction opposite that of the osmotic gradient. An illustration of the action of such opposing forces is the balance between the osmotic effect of plasma proteins and the hydrostatic pressure in the vascular system.

OSMOLARITY

Osmolarity refers to the concentration of a solution. As an expression of osmoles per liter of solution for relatively dilute solutions such as body fluids, osmolarity is roughly equivalent to osmolality, which is expressed in terms of osmoles

Table **57-1**

OSMOLAR SUBSTANCES IN EXTRACELLULAR AND INTRACELLULAR FLUIDS

	Plasma (mOsm/L of H₂O)	Interstitial (mOsm/L of H₂O)	Intracellular (mOsm/L of H₂O)
Na^+	146	142	14
K^+	4.2	4.0	140
Ca^{++}	2.5	2.4	0
Mg^{++}	1.5	1.4	31
Cl^-	105	108	4
HCO_3^-	27	28.3	10
HPO_4^-, $H_2PO_4^-$	2	2	11
SO_4^-	0.5	0.5	1
Phosphocreatine			45
Carnosine			14
Amino acids	2	2	8
Creatine	0.2	0.2	9
Lactate	1.2	1.2	1.5
Adenosine triphosphate			5
Hexose monophosphate			3.7
Glucose	5.6	5.6	
Protein	1.2	0.2	4
Urea	4	4	4
TOTAL (mOsm/L)	302.9	301.8	302.2
Correct osmolar activity (mOsm/L)	282.6	281.3	281.3
Total osmotic pressure at 37° C (mm Hg)	5453	5430	5430

From Guyton AC: *Textbook of medical physiology*, Philadelphia, 1976, WB Saunders.

per *kilogram* of solute. The osmolarity of the body fluids in a healthy person is maintained between 285 and 295 mOsm/L. The contributions of various substances to the osmolarity of the various fluid compartments are listed in Table 57-1. Plasma osmolarity can be calculated as follows:

Calculated serum osmolarity (cOsm/L) =

$$2\,[Na^+]^* + \frac{[glucose]^\dagger}{18} + \frac{[BUN]^\dagger}{2.8}$$

*mEq/L.
†mg/dl.

A change in the concentration of any solute that is preferentially contained in either the ICF or the ECF causes a change in that compartment's osmolarity and alters the compartmental distribution of the TBW. A change in the osmolarity of one compartment always results in a redistribution of water, and possibly solutes, between the various compartments until the osmolarity is again equivalent at a new level. However, when osmolarity rises because of an increase in the concentration of a substance that freely permeates cell membranes, such as urea, no significant intercompartmental fluid shift occurs.

BASAL FLUID REQUIREMENTS

Approximately 6% of the TBW is turned over daily for the average adult in a temperate climate. The percentage is higher in infants because of their relatively larger surface area. Losses to TBW are usually replenished by exogenous fluid intake. An additional 300 to 500 ml is produced daily as water of oxidation from the metabolism of nutrients.

Normally, water losses occur primarily in the urine and to a lesser degree in feces and sweat and as insensible losses from the skin and respiratory tract. Insensible loss, normally approximately 800 ml daily, is increased by low atmospheric humidity, fever, hyperventilation, and hypermetabolic states. Normal fecal water averages 100 ml every day. Sweat losses are highly variable.

Under normal circumstances, the kidneys in adults are able to produce hypertonic urine with a maximum osmolarity of approximately 1400 mOsm/kg. Urinary water losses are a function of water intake, antidiuretic hormone (ADH) secretion, effectiveness of renal function, and the solute load. In a maximum antidiuretic state, the average daily solute excretion necessitates a urine volume of at least 500 ml every day. Increases in the excreted solute load (such as occurs with osmotic diuresis caused by glycosuria) significantly increase obligatory renal water excretion. Renal concentrating ability is impaired in infants, in ADH deficiency, or with renal unresponsiveness to ADH.

REGULATORY MECHANISMS FOR WATER AND SODIUM

The major regulators of water homeostasis are thirst and ADH.

Thirst

The cells that regulate thirst reside in the hypothalamus. Their sensing mechanism involves cellular osmoreceptors. Normally, even small increases (as little as 1%) in the osmolarity of the fluid bathing these cells stimulates thirst. A deficit of total body fluid volume also stimulates thirst by a nonosmotic mechanism.

Antidiuretic Hormone

ADH is synthesized in the hypothalamus. Its major actions are on the renal medulla and collecting ducts, where it causes a more concentrated urine by increasing water reabsorption. ADH secretion is stimulated by increased plasma osmolarity, reduced blood volume, reduced arterial blood pressure, or an increased serum sodium. An increase in plasma osmolarity of as little as 1% to 2%, which is equivalent to a change as little as 1 to 2 mEq of sodium, is sufficient to stimulate maximum release of ADH. Normally, ADH secretion is inhibited by hypoosmolarity or an increase in left atrial pressure.

Disorders of ADH homeostasis include diseases in which there is oversecretion of the hormone (commonly referred to as the syndrome of inappropriate antidiuretic hormone [SIADH]), states in which ADH is deficient (diabetes insipidus), or states in which the kidneys do not respond to ADH (nephrogenic diabetes insipidus).

In SIADH, there is a failure of the normal negative feedback systems on ADH secretion. Characteristically, there is continued ADH secretion despite a continued decline in osmolarity. Decreased water excretion leads to ECF expansion, which in turn causes renal salt wasting. The ultimate result is hyponatremia combined with a relatively concentrated urine.

Because the urine of a hypoosmolar patient should be maximally dilute, the relatively concentrated urine of patients with SIADH is often referred to as "nonmaximally dilute." Unlike an otherwise normal individual with hyponatremia, the urinary sodium in SIADH is relatively high and is usually greater than 20 mEq/L.

The most common causes of SIADH are listed in the box on p. 667. The most common causes of ectopic ADH production are neoplasms, espe-

MOST COMMON CAUSES OF SIADH

CNS

Tumor (primary and metastatic)
Hemorrhage
Infection
Postneurosurgery

Pulmonary

Tumor (especially small cell carcinoma)
Pneumonia
Lung abscess
Mechanical ventilation (especially with
    positive end-expiratory pressure)

Medications

Antipsychotic agents
Antineoplastic agents
Antihyperglycemic oral agents
Miscellaneous
Bromocriptine, nicotine
Oxytocin, desmopressin, NSAIDs
Carbamazepine, opiates

Cancer

Gastrointestinal malignancy
Hodgkin disease
Nasopharyngeal carcinoma
Leukemia

Miscellaneous

General anesthesia
Alcohol withdrawal
Psychosis
AIDS

cially bronchogenic carcinoma. Endogenous (pituitary) SIADH is most often the consequence of CNS trauma or disease.

The most prominent clinical manifestations of SIADH are neurologic. Symptoms are usually mild and consist of dizziness or headache. Mental status changes are common and range from apathy and irritability to confusion and disorientation. Patients are especially prone to seizures when the serum sodium level rapidly falls below 120 mEq/L. Laboratory findings typically include some degree of hyponatremia accompanied by a urinary specific gravity above 1.002 (nonmaximally dilute). Treatment consists of fluid restriction and attention to the underlying pathologic process. Infusion of hypertonic saline is reserved for severe or symptomatic hyponatremia, for patients with profound alterations in mental status, and for patients with hyponatremia and seizures.

Diabetes insipidus (DI) refers to a lack of ADH and the resultant loss of the ability of the kidney to reabsorb free water. Most cases of DI are of idiopathic origin. Hypophysectomy, tumors, vascular abnormalities, infections, granulomatous diseases, histiocytosis, and head trauma may also produce DI. Breast cancer is the most common metastatic tumor to cause DI.

Clinically, DI is characterized by polyuria and polydipsia of between 3 and 15 L each day. If the thirst mechanism is intact and water is available, such patients are usually otherwise asymptomatic. However, if thirst or the ability to obtain adequate amounts of water is impaired, excessive hypotonic fluid losses may result in a rapid development of dehydration and hypernatremia. Definitive diagnosis calls for analysis of urine output and osmolarity during a period of fluid restriction and after the administration of exogenous ADH.

Dehydration

The term *dehydration* technically refers to a deficit in TBW, but almost all forms of dehydration also involve some losses of electrolytes. The ratio of water to electrolyte losses is highly variable, and the serum sodium value should not be relied on when assessing the state of hydration. The serum sodium may be elevated, low, or normal in any state of hydration.

However, the serum sodium value *does* reflect the ratio of TBW to sodium stores. With hypernatremia, there is an increase in the ratio of body sodium level to water content that signifies excessive body losses of both elements, with a relatively greater loss of water. Likewise, hyponatremia that occurs in the setting of dehydration indicates that salt losses have occurred in excess of water losses (or that some water losses have been replaced).

Dehydration may result from inadequate fluid intake or from excessive fluid losses from the skin, lungs, kidneys, or gastrointestinal tract. The composition and degree of fluid loss differs somewhat, depending on the source of the loss.

Clinical findings

Clinically, the earliest signs of dehydration consist of thirst, weakness, diminished sweating, and (if renal disease is not the cause of dehydration) decreased urine output. In infants and young children, a lack of tears is a helpful early sign. Dry mucous membranes and poor skin turgor signify more pronounced fluid losses. Irritability, lethargy, or other changes in mentation may occur. Orthostatic hypotension cannot be relied on to indicate dehydration but when present may indicate a TBW deficit of at least 10%. Supine hypotension is usually associated with a blood volume deficit of at least 15% to 25% and with an even larger fluid deficit.

Management

The mode of treatment for dehydration depends on the underlying cause and the duration, severity, and type of fluid loss. When hypotension is present, the rapid administration of a plasma volume expander such as saline or lactated Ringer's solution is appropriate.

Hypernatremia

Causes of hypernatremia are outlined in the box above. Hypernatremia almost invariably results from a deficit in TBW in excess of total body sodium losses, which may occur in a number of ways. Because a certain minimal obligatory amount of water is lost daily from the lungs, skin, and kidneys, a simple lack of water intake to replace these losses eventually results in hy-

---

CAUSES OF HYPERNATREMIA

Diminished water intake with normal fluid losses

Disorders of thirst perception
Inability to obtain water
   Lack of environmental water
   Ability to communicate needs
      Infants
      Patients with coma or cerebrovascular
         accident
      Intubated patients

Hypotonic fluid losses with water losses in excess of sodium losses

Sweat—hot climate, exertion
Insensible—hot climate, fever, tachypnea
Gastrointestinal—vomiting, diarrhea, fistulas
Renal—diabetes insipidus, osmotic diuresis as
   from glycosuria, mannitol infusion, high-
   protein diets, postobstructive diuresis,
   diuretics

Acute salt poisoning

Ingestion of hypertonic saline, seawater, or
   salt tablets
Iatrogenic—$NaHCO_3$ during cardiac
   resuscitation, hypertonic saline infusions
"Essential" hypernatremia
Adrenocortical overactivity

---

pernatremic dehydration. Hypernatremic dehydration is even more likely to occur when insensible losses are greater than normal as is seen with burns, fever, hyperventilation, or high ambient temperatures.

Although hypernatremia may be caused by disorders of thirst perception, it is more often the result of a failure to ingest water. Excessive sweating may also cause hypernatremia. Renal losses of water in excess of sodium eventually result in hypernatremia and may occur in several ways. There may be failure to produce a concentrated urine caused by lack of ADH effect, which occurs with DI or nephrogenic DI.

Renal water loss in excess of sodium excretion also occurs with osmotic diuresis.

Hypernatremia with elevated total body sodium stores is much less common. It may occur with Cushing disease and primary hyperaldosteronism, in which a mild hypernatremia (sodium values of 145 to 150 mEq/L) may be seen as a result of the sodium-retaining effects of aldosterone.

A more severe hypernatremia with total body sodium excess may follow salt poisoning such as occurs in infants fed formulas in which salt is accidentally substituted for sugar.

The signs and symptoms of hypernatremia are attributable to hyperosmolarity and intracellular dehydration. Symptoms correlate not only with the serum sodium concentration but also with the rapidity with which the elevation develops. A very gradual onset of hypernatremia usually produces much fewer symptoms than if a comparable serum sodium level is achieved abruptly. With the rare exception of infants who have salt poisoning, patients with hypernatremia are dehydrated, and the clinical manifestations of dehydration are also present.

Clinical findings

Symptoms of hypernatremia primarily involve the CNS. Mental status changes range from lethargy and confusion to delirium and coma. If the progression of hypernatremia is gradual, consciousness may be preserved even when the serum sodium concentration exceeds 170 mEq/L. Seizures are a common manifestation of moderate-to-severe hypernatremia (a serum sodium level that exceeds 160 mEq/L). Hyperactive deep tendon reflexes and muscular weakness are common findings. Muscular rigidity and tremors are also sometimes seen. Mortality is directly related to the magnitude of the increase in serum sodium.

Management

Treatment for hypernatremia varies to some extent with the underlying cause, but the water deficit needs to be corrected in all cases. In situations such as DI, in which water losses are accompanied by little or no sodium losses, oral replacement with hypotonic oral fluids or intravenous D_5W is appropriate.

Because most cases of hypernatremia represent a loss of salt and water, therapy can usually be achieved with normal saline. If cardiac disease is present, rehydration can be pursued more slowly with half-normal saline. Oral water replacement is preferable to the parenteral route whenever feasible. During the first 24 hours of treatment, it is reasonable to return the serum osmolarity halfway toward normal. If the water replacement is too rapid, cerebral edema follows and may result in seizures. This reaction is particularly likely to occur in children and may be seen even while the patient is still hypernatremic. An estimate of the total body water deficit may be derived from the following formula:

Total Body Water Deficit =

$$\frac{\text{Patient's serum sodium} - 140}{140} \times \text{TBW}$$

Hyponatremia

Most authorities divide hyponatremia into three types on the basis of the patient's overall state of hydration and TBW: (1) hyponatremic dehydration (i.e., a patient who has lost sodium in excess of the TBW deficit), (2) euvolemic hyponatremia (i.e., SIADH), and (3) hyponatremia in patients with excess TBW (i.e., edematous states resulting from congestive heart failure, chronic renal failure, or cirrhosis). The causes of hyponatremia are outlined in the box on p. 670. Hyponatremia almost always indicates a total body excess of water relative to solute, except in the cases of hyperglycemia and pseudohyponatremia (such as is found in hyperlipemia). In hyperglycemia, the accumulation of solute within the ECF that does not readily diffuse into cells causes a shift of cellular water into the ECF, which dilutes the serum

CAUSES OF HYPONATREMIA

Pseudohyponatremia
   Hyperlipemia
   Hyperproteinemia
   Laboratory error
   Blood drawn proximal to hypotonic IV
      infusion
Accumulation of solute within the ECF
   Hyperglycemia
   Mannitol infusion
SIADH (see the box on p. 667)
Drug-induced causes
   Chlorpropamide
   Tolbutamide
   Vincristine
   Cyclophosphamide
   Thioridazine (Mellaril)
   Carbamazepine
   Thiothixene (Navane)
   Fluphenazine (Prolixin)
   Amitriptyline
   Diuretics
Volume depletion: sodium deficit in excess of
      water deficit
   Gastrointestinal
   Renal
   Third space losses
   Sweat
   Addison disease
Edematous states
   Congestive heart failure
   Hepatic cirrhosis
   Nephrotic syndrome
Miscellaneous
   Oliguric phase of acute tubular necrosis
   Chronic renal failure
   Psychogenic polydipsia
   Myxedema
   Pain or emotional stress
   Acute intermittent porphyria
   Chronic administration of exogenous
      vasopressin
   Severe metastatic carcinoma or leukemia
   Angioimmunoblastic lymphadenopathy

sodium level by increasing the total plasma water volume. Each increment of 100 mg/dl above the normal blood sugar concentration reduces the measured serum sodium level by approximately 1.5 mEq/L.

The mechanisms by which volume depletion leads to hyponatremia are multifactorial and not completely understood. When volume depletion becomes significant, ADH secretion increases in response to hypovolemic stimuli, and the water retention that results may produce hyponatremia. In this setting, ADH secretion continues even in the face of hypoosmolality, a stimulus that otherwise suppresses ADH release.

Hyponatremia may occur when a dehydrated patient who is both sodium and free water deficient is "volume repleted" with D_5W or large amounts of half-normal saline. Hyponatremia may also occur in edematous conditions such as congestive heart failure, cirrhosis, and nephrotic syndrome. In these cases, renal hypoperfusion causes the secretion of ADH and results in increased free water reabsorption.

Measuring the urinary excretion of sodium is one of the best ways to classify patients with hyponatremia. A low urinary sodium value (<10 mEq/L) reflects renal hypoperfusion and is indicative of TBW depletion or a decrease in effective plasma volume (in cases of edematous patients). Patients with hyponatremia and high urinary sodium values (>20 mEq/L) are considered salt wasters. Elevated urinary sodium values are usually a result of either intrinsic renal disease, diuretic use, or adrenal insufficiency.

Clinical findings

The severity of the clinical manifestations of hyponatremia correlates with the degree and rapidity with which they develop. In chronic hyponatremia, serum sodium concentrations above 120 mEq/L are associated with minimal symptoms. The signs and symptoms of hyponatremia are nonspecific. Early symptoms may include headache, dizziness, anorexia, nausea, and vomiting. Some patients may complain of only abdominal cramping or muscular weakness. The signs of severe or chronic hyponatremia are primarily neurologic and result from water shifting into cells, producing cerebral edema. Early signs of an altered mental status may be subtle and consist only of concentration difficulties, inattentiveness, apathy, or agitation. As the serum sodium level falls below 120 mEq/L, irritability, disorientation, and confusion are common. Although seizures may occur whenever the sodium concentration falls below 120 mEq/L, serum sodium levels as low as 110 mEq/L may be associated with only mild neurologic symptoms when the hyponatremia has developed gradually. Tremors and hypoactive deep tendon reflexes may be found during the physical examination.

Management

The treatment of hyponatremia is based on cause, severity, and the presence or absence of associated symptoms. Hyponatremia induced by diuretic use usually corrects within 3 to 10 days simply by discontinuing the medication. Water intake should be restricted to a level below urinary and insensible losses when hyponatremia is asymptomatic and not severe (a serum sodium level above 120 mEq/L), when there is an excess of TBW alone, or when there is an excess of both water and sodium. When a patient has both hyponatremia and hypovolemia, normal saline should be used to correct both deficits.

Patients with severe hyponatremia (serum sodium values below 120 mEq/L) need to be treated carefully to avoid the complication of central pontine myelinolysis (CPM). This often irreversible syndrome, also called the *osmotic demyelinating syndrome,* may cause neurologic findings, including lethargy, cranial nerve palsies, the locked-in syndrome, coma, and death. It has been reported most commonly in premenopausal women and in chronic alcoholics with serum sodiums below 120 mEq/L. Almost all reported cases have occurred when the serum sodium has been passed at a rate faster than 0.5 mEq/L/hour (12 mEq/L/day). Patients who also have hypokalemia appear to be at the greatest risk for this syndrome.

To minimize complications, patients with severe hyponatremia should have their serum levels corrected over days, not hours. An extremely low sodium level should never be returned to normal during emergency care. In general, water restriction supplemented with the judicious use of furosemide helps safely correct patients with SIADH or water intoxication resulting from psychogenic polydipsia.

Hypertonic saline (3%) should be used only in cases of hyponatremia in which the serum sodium is below 120 mEq/L and the patient has severe neurologic deficits, is comatose, or has seizures. These patients usually have serum sodium levels in the range of 100 to 110 mEq/L and need to have their sodium acutely elevated by only 3 to 5 mEq/L. In these rare cases, 3% hypertonic saline should be infused at 100 ml/hr for 2 to 3 hours, and the patient's serum sodium should be rechecked. Concomitant dosing of furosemide (20 to 40 mg intravenously) results in increased free water excretion and blocks the sodium-induced stimulation of ADH. Appropriate quantities of potassium should be added to the hypertonic saline whenever a patient with hyponatremia has a low or borderline serum potassium. Although not usually that clinically useful, a patient's estimated total body sodium deficit may be calculated by the following formula:

Sodium deficit in mEq/L =

(normal sodium concentration −

measured sodium concentration) × TBW (L)

TBW can be measured by multiplying body weight in kilograms by 0.6 in men and by 0.5 in women.

POTASSIUM

Potassium is the major intracellular cation, with an ECF normally between 3.5 and 5.0 mEq/L (compared with 150 to 160 mEq/L in the ICF). Intracellular potassium is contained predominantly in muscle tissue. Less than 2% of the total body potassium content is extracellular, and the measurement of serum potassium may not be an accurate indication of total body stores. Nevertheless, a deviation in the serum level from normal profoundly affects physiologic function, even when the total body potassium content is normal.

Changes in pH may exert a significant effect on serum potassium concentration. When the concentration of extracellular hydrogen ion increases, potassium ions leave cells in exchange for hydrogen ions, which move intracellularly. The resultant intracellular buffering thus partially corrects extracellular acidosis at the expense of an increase in the ECF/ICF ratio of potassium ion concentration. Conversely, the decrease in extracellular hydrogen ion concentration that occurs in alkalotic states promotes the movement of potassium into cells from the ECF. A change in plasma pH of 0.1 results in an inverse change in serum potassium concentration by as much as 0.6 mEq/L. This result is much more likely to occur in inorganic acidosis and in the organic acidosis of diabetic ketoacidosis.

Hyperkalemia

Because of the effects on cardiac excitability and conduction, hyperkalemia (potassium concentration greater than 5.5 mEq/L) may cause a life-threatening medical emergency. The causes of hyperkalemia are outlined in the box at right.

Acidosis may cause hyperkalemia without a change in total body potassium by causing the ion to move out of cells in exchange for hydrogen ions. This phenomenon partly explains why patients with diabetic ketoacidosis often display an initial hyperkalemia, even though total body stores of potassium are almost always diminished. The hyperkalemia of diabetic ketoacidosis is also a result of a lack of insulin, which

MOST COMMON CAUSES OF HYPERKALEMIA
Spurious (as a result of hemolysis during or after phlebotomy)
Thrombocytosis
Leukocytosis
Abnormal erythrocytes
Acidosis
Renal Failure
Iatrogenic (usually associated with renal failure)
Intravenous potassium containing medications
Amino acid infusions
Cell death
Rhabdomyolysis
Crush injuries
Burns
Tumor lysis syndrome
Addison disease (or any low aldosterone state)
In vivo hemolysis
Hematologic
WBC >100,000
Hct >55-65
PLTs >1,000,000
Tumor lysis syndrome
Hyperkalemic periodic paralysis
Drugs
Spironolactone (Aldactone) and potassium-sparing diuretics
Captopril and other angiotensin converting enzyme inhibitors
NSAIDs
Heparin
Succinylcholine
Glucagon
Beta blockers
Calcium channel blockers
Digitalis (acute overdose)

moves both glucose and potassium into the cell. Most forms of acidosis also promote the renal excretion of large quantities of hydrogen ions. Acute increases in osmolarity may also cause hyperkalemia. The hypertonicity produced in the

ECF causes a shift of water and various solutes (including potassium) out of cells.

In acute anuric or oliguric renal failure, hyperkalemia is the result of impaired excretion and, to a lesser extent, acidosis. Although hyperkalemia is very common with chronic renal failure, serum potassium levels above 6 mEq/L are relatively uncommon until significant azotemia occurs.

Any process that leads to the disruption of a large number of cells and leakage of their contents into the extracellular space results in hyperkalemia. This is the mechanism for hyperkalemia seen with severe burns, crush injuries, and ischemic insults to limbs and digits. Intravascular hemolysis may cause hyperkalemia by a similar mechanism.

Several drugs may cause hyperkalemia if used improperly. Spironolactone (Aldactone) is a competitive inhibitor of aldosterone. Amiloride and triamterene, in addition to being aldosterone antagonists, also inhibit potassium excretion by a mechanism independent of aldosterone. These drugs may be hazardous if used in the presence of renal failure or the excessive intake of potassium. Angiotensin converting enzyme (ACE) inhibitors may cause hyperkalemia in patients with renal insufficiency.

Clinical findings

The effects of hyperkalemia are primarily neuromuscular and cardiac. Hyperkalemia also affects the kidney and acid-base balance.

Most patients with hyperkalemia have symptoms related only to their underlying disease and not just a result of an elevated potassium level. Hyperkalemia may however on occasion produce paresthesias, muscle cramps, lethargy, and hypoactive deep tendon reflexes. A sudden rise in serum potassium level results in tetany only rarely. Weakness that progresses to a flaccid quadriplegia may also occur. However, in most instances of hyperkalemia, the physical examination is normal.

The electrophysiologic effects of hyperkalemia are somewhat unpredictable and are based on the patient's absolute serum level and whether the hyperkalemia is acute or chronic. In general, acute hyperkalemia is much more likely than chronic hyperkalemia to result in more pronounced ECG changes for a given serum potassium value.

As potassium levels rise, a mild acceleration in conduction and an acceleration in repolarization occurs. However, a progressive depression in conduction occurs as levels rise further. The ECG changes associated with hyperkalemia are usually related to serum potassium values, but patients with chronic renal failure may have few changes until their levels approach life-threatening values.

As serum potassium levels begin to rise above 5 to 5.5 mEq/L, patients may develop the subtle changes of PR- and QT-interval shortening. The more classic findings of hyperkalemia are peaked T waves, loss of the P wave, and widening of the QRS complex, which may progress to a sine wave.

Tall, peaked T waves may be seen as potassium values rise above 5.5 to 6.0 mEq/L. Hyperkalemia should always be considered whenever the T wave appears more pronounced than the QRS complex, especially when the T-wave amplitude is greater than the positive deflection of the QRS complex in more than one chest lead. As potassium levels rise to above 6.5 to 7.0 mEq/L, the P wave may be lost. QRS widening is an ominous ECG finding in hyperkalemia and may be seen as potassium levels rise above 7.0 mEq/L. Patients with hyperkalemia may suffer a cardiac arrest with a pulseless sine-wave in pulseless electrical activity-electromechanical dissociation (PEA-EMD), may develop refractory ventricular fibrillation, or may become suddenly asystolic.

Management

The treatment of hyperkalemia is based on as many as five variables: (1) the patient's overall cardiovascular stability, including blood pressure and pulse rate; (2) the severity of the patient's potassium-induced ECG changes; (3) the patient's serum potassium level; (4) whether the hyperkalemia is acute or chronic; and (5) whether the patient is on hemodialysis or is capable of making urine.

Three types of therapies may be used to treat hyperkalemia: (1) counteracting the electrical effects of hyperkalemia; (2) driving potassium into the cell and; (3) removing potassium from the body.

Counteracting electrical effects.   Calcium may temporarily reverse the conduction abnormalities of hyperkalemia and cause a more normalized electrical gradient across cardiac cell membranes. The use of calcium as calcium chloride or calcium gluconate should be reserved for severe hyperkalemia associated with QRS widening. A dose of 5 to 10 ml of calcium chloride or 10 ml of calcium gluconate usually narrows the QRS complex temporarily and increases myocardial contractility. Doses in excess of 20 ml calcium chloride or 30 ml of calcium gluconate should almost never be used.

Moving potassium intracellulary.   Potassium may be moved intracellulary by a number of therapies. Bicarbonate and glucose administration in conjunction with insulin are the two best studied and most widely used methods of shifting potassium into the cell. Bicarbonate is effective only in patients with acidosis and should be reserved for hyperkalemia in association with a low serum pH. Bicarbonate is usually given in a dose of approximately 1 mEq/kg of body weight or one to two 50 mEq ampules over 5 to 10 minutes. It should, however, be given as a rapid bolus to patients who are agonal or in hyperkalemia-induced cardiac arrest.

Glucose and insulin are an excellent means of moving potassium intracellulary. Potassium is moved into the cell in exchange for sodium by stimulating the insulin-mediated glucose transport system. The usual dose of glucose is 50 grams (two 50 ml ampules of $D_{50}W$) in conjunction with 10 units of intravenous insulin.

Other less universally accepted means of moving potassium intracellularly include inhaled or intravenous beta agonists, intravenous magnesium, and intravenous saline. Albuterol has been used at doses up to twenty times normal by inhalation and appears to be relatively safe in selected patients; 0.5 mg in 100 ml of saline infused intravenously over 30 minutes also appears safe. Magnesium at a dose of 1 to 2 grams (8 to 16 mEq) over 1 to 5 minutes has also lowered serum potassium levels by 0.5 mEq/L. Its routine use in patients with potentially hypermagnesemic chronic renal failure cannot be recommended.

TREATING HYPERKALEMIA

Step 1: Reversing electrical effects
Calcium chloride
    5-10 ml of 10% CaCl
    may repeat up to 20 ml

*Step 2: Driving K into the cell
a. Glucose and insulin
    1-2 amps of $D_{50}W$
    10 units regular insulin
b. Bicarbonate
    1-2 amps of $NaHCO_3$

Step 3: Removing K from the body
a. Forced diuresis
    250-500 ml/hr NaCl
    Supplement with furosemide
b. Ion Exchange Resin
    30-60 g Kayexalate
c. Dialysis
    Hemodialysis and/or peritoneal dialysis
*Optional additional therapies to drive K
   into the cell
• Saline infusion
       Normal saline solution wide open if
           patient is not anuric
• Albuterol
       Inhaled or IV
       1-20 mg inhaled
       0.5 mg in 100 ml IV over 10-20 minutes
• Magnesium sulfate
       2 grams IV over 5-20 minutes

Saline at doses of 250 ml to 1000 ml may be useful in moving potassium intracellulary. It should be used routinely in dehydrated patients but very judiciously in patients with heart or renal failure.

Removing potassium from the body. Potassium may be removed from the body by three major means: diuretics, ion exchange resins, and hemodialysis. If a patient is capable of making significant urine, a saline diuresis in conjunction with furosemide is an excellent way to remove potassium. Unfortunately, this event is unlikely and is usually reserved for dehydrated patients who have mild hyperkalemia. Ion exchange resins, such as sodium polystyrene (Kayexalate), exchange their sodium for the body's potassium and generally remove 1 mEq of potassium for each gram of resin administered orally or for each retention enema. It should be given with sorbitol to prevent constipation. Hemodialysis is the most effective way to remove potassium from the body and should be used as early as possible in any patient with anuria and life-threatening hyperkalemia (see the box on p. 674).

Hypokalemia

Hypokalemia is a relatively common condition with many causes (see the box on p. 676). Diuretic therapy is the most common cause. The potassium-losing effects of the thiazides and the loop diuretics ethacrynic acid and furosemide depend on the increase in sodium load delivered to the distal sodium-potassium exchange site. Hypokalemia develops in as many as 40% of those patients treated with hydrochlorothiazide and in more than half of those given chlorthalidone. Because the potassium concentration of gastrointestinal fluid is 2 to 3 times that of plasma, any process that leads to excessive enteric fluid loss may produce hypokalemia.

Clinical findings

Hypokalemia leads to symptoms that primarily involve the gastrointestinal tract, nervous system, skeletal muscles, and heart. Hypokalemia causes an impaired response to parasympathetic stimulation and weakness of the gastrointestinal smooth muscle, resulting in decreased intestinal mobility with varying degrees of distension, abdominal cramps, and eventually a paralytic ileus. Anorexia, nausea, and vomiting may also result.

Neuromuscular symptoms of hypokalemia rarely occur in patients unless potassium concentrations fall below 2.5 mEq/L. Muscle cramps and paresthesias may develop even in the absence of muscular weakness. Such weakness is usually more prominent in the lower extremities and proximal motor groups. In severe potassium deficiency (usually in association with hypomagnesemia and hypophosphatemia), it may involve the muscles of respiration and lead to respiratory failure. Involvement of the muscles innervated by the cranial nerves is rare. Severe weakness or true muscular paralysis is unlikely to occur at potassium levels above 2 mEq/L. Although changes in cerebral function, including drowsiness, lethargy, and coma have been reported with severe hypokalemia, it is unclear whether low potassium values alone directly cause alterations in mental status.

Changes in the ECG usually are not seen until potassium concentrations fall below 3 mEq/L, and these changes consist of a flattening or inversion of T waves and the presence of U waves. An ST segment depression, PR interval prolongation, and slight widening of the QRS complex may also occur. It appears that the ECG changes of hypokalemia are unpredictable and are most likely to occur in patients with both hypomagnesemia and hypokalemia.

Hypokalemia may cause a number of dysrhythmias. Severe hypokalemia may produce sinus bradycardia and first- or second-degree heart block. Because these rhythms often respond well to atropine, the mechanism is thought to involve an increased sensitivity to vagal stimulation. Atrial flutter, paroxysmal atrial tachycardia with block, atrioventricular dissociation, and (more rarely) ventricular fibrillation

CAUSES OF HYPOKALEMIA

Decreased intake

Decreased dietary potassium
Clay ingestion

Increased gastrointestinal losses

Vomiting
Nasogastric suction
Diarrhea
Malabsorption
Fistulas
Chronic laxative abuse

Increased renal excretion

Tubular disease
   Renal tubular acidosis
   Salt-losing nephropathies
   Fanconi syndrome
   Cystinosis
Hyperaldosteronism
   Primary (Conn syndrome, hyperplasia,
     idiopathic)
   Secondary (congestive heart failure, cirrhosis,
     hypoproteinemia)
   Hyperreninemia
     Bartter syndrome
     Renal artery stenosis
     Hemangiopericytoma
     Juxtaglomerular tumors
   Elevations in adrenocorticotropic hormone
     (ACTH)
     ACTH-secreting tumors
Excessive adrenal corticosteroids
   Cushing syndrome
   Congenital adrenal hyperplasia
Drugs
   Diuretics

Tubular effects
   Furosemide
   Ethacrynic acid
   Thiazides
   Chlorthalidone
Other
   Acetazolamide
   Aminophylline
Mineralocorticoid effects
   Glycyrrhizic acid (licorice, snuff, chewing
     tobacco)
   Carbenoxolone
   Deoxycorticosterone
Amphotericin B
Increased sodium intake
High load of nonreabsorbable anions

Transcellular shifts

Acute alkalosis
Insulin
Hypokalemic periodic paralysis
Thyrotoxic periodic paralysis
Stimulation of β_2-adrenergic receptors
   (epinephrine, terbutaline, salbutamol)

Increased losses in sweat

Strenuous exertion in hot climates

Pseudohypokalemia

Laboratory error
Same causes as pseudohyponatremia

Miscellaneous

Mountain sickness
Hypomagnesemia
Hypernatremia
Barium poisoning

---

may result from hypokalemia. Chronic digitalis toxicity is more likely to occur in a patient with a potassium deficiency.

Management

The treatment of hypokalemia is usually determined by the patient's ability to tolerate oral fluids and the magnitude of the patient's deficit. Mild hypokalemia is best treated orally. Patients with potassium levels of 3.0 to 3.5 mEq/L have total body deficits of approximately 100 mEq. Because they usually excrete almost 50% of what they receive, as much as 200 mEq may be required for total body repletion. As a patient's potassium level drops to between 2.0 and 3.0 mEq/L, the deficit ranges from 200 to 400 mEq, and intravenous potassium administration is required. At least 10 mEq/hr and probably up to 20 mEq/hr is safe to administer to unmonitored patients. Administration rates above 20 mEq/hr require constant monitoring of the patient, the ECG monitor, and the serum potassium level. Patients with any conduction abnormality resulting from hypokalemia are at great risk and should be in an area that has access to transcutaneous and intravenous pacemakers. Severe, chronic, or refractory hypokalemia indicates hypomagnesemia until proven otherwise.

CALCIUM

The average adult body contains between 1000 and 1400 g of calcium; approximately 99% is contained within bone. Of the remainder, nearly half is bound to plasma proteins, primarily albumins, and the remaining calcium is diffusible between the intracellular and extracellular compartments. Approximately 90% of the diffusible calcium exists in the ionized form; the remaining 10% is complexed with phosphates, citrates, and bicarbonate. Only the ionized form of calcium (approximately 0.5% of total body calcium) is physiologically active.

Serum levels are usually determined by methods that measure the total serum calcium level. Normal total serum calcium levels range from 8.5 to 10.5 mg/dl. Because half of the serum calcium is protein bound, changes in serum albumin (and to a lesser extent, globulin content) also alter total serum calcium levels without affecting the concentration of the physiologically active ionized fraction. Therefore the significance of a serum calcium level cannot be assessed without knowledge of the albumin content.

Normal calcium balance reflects a dynamic interplay between intestinal absorption, renal excretion, and the uptake or release from a large exchangeable pool in the skeleton. All of these processes are in turn modulated by parathyroid hormone (PTH), calcitonin, and metabolites of vitamin D.

Hypercalcemia

The causes of hypercalcemia are summarized in the box on p. 678. Malignancy and hyperparathyroidism account for approximately 80% of all cases of persistent hypercalcemia.

Primary hyperparathyroidism is the major cause of hypercalcemia in the general population. In contrast, malignancy is the predominant cause of hypercalcemia in hospitalized patients and accounts for almost one half of all cases. Breast, lung, and renal carcinomas are the neoplasms most commonly associated with hypercalcemia.

In primary hyperparathyroidism, elevated levels of PTH result in hypercalcemia, hypophosphatemia, and hyperphosphaturia. Elevated levels of PTH also increase renal bicarbonate excretion, which usually results in a hyperchloremic acidosis. Hyperparathyroidism may also occur as a component of the syndrome of multiple endocrine neoplasias or as a familial disorder. Although secondary hyperparathyroidism develops as a compensatory response in any chronic condition that produces hypocalcemia, it is most commonly seen in renal failure.

Hypercalcemia occurs in as much as one third of patients with thyrotoxicosis and resolves with successful treatment of the thyroid disorder. Intestinal absorption of calcium is decreased, and urinary excretion is increased. Thyroid hormone increases calcium release from bone.

Hypercalcemia occurs in 20% of all patients with sarcoidosis. Patients with sarcoidosis are susceptible to vitamin D intoxication. Hypercalcemia is also seen in other granulomatous diseases, including tuberculosis.

In some patients, thiazide diuretics increase the renal tubular reabsorption of calcium and may cause as much as a 70% decline in urinary calcium excretion. Combined with a contrac-

MOST COMMON CAUSES OF HYPERCALCEMIA

Malignancy
  Direct bony destruction
  Ectopic PTH
  Ectopic PTH-like substances
  Osteoclast activating factor
  Prostaglandins
  Cytokines
Endocrine
  Hyperparathyroidism (primary and
    secondary)
  Multiple endocrine neoplasias
  Hyperthyroidism
  Pheochromocytoma
  Myxedema, acromegaly, adrenal
    insufficiency
Granulomatous Diseases
  Sarcoid
  Tuberculosis
  Histoplasmosis, coccidioidomycosis,
    berylliosis
Pharmacologic Agents
  Calcium supplements
  Vitamin D intoxication
  Vitamin A intoxication
  Thiazide diuretics
  Estrogens
  Milk-alkali syndrome
  Lithium
Renal Diseases
  Pseudohyperparathyroidism
  Postrenal transplant
Miscellaneous
  Dehydration
  Prolonged immobilization
  Iatrogenic
  Hyperproteinemia
  Rhabdomyolysis
  Idiopathic infantile hypercalcemia
  Familial
  Laboratory error

tion of plasma volume, this phenomenon accounts for the mild hypercalcemia often seen during thiazide therapy. Although the hypercalcemia resulting from thiazide use is usually mild and asymptomatic, severe hypercalcemia may occur in some patients when this drug is used concurrently with calcium-containing antacids or by those with preexisting hypercalcemia.

The signs and symptoms of hypercalcemia are summarized in the box on p. 679. The rate at which hypercalcemia develops is probably as important as calcium concentration in determining which signs and symptoms occur. Serum levels often do not correlate predictably with the clinical picture, but levels above 15 mg/dl almost always cause marked CNS depression.

Clinical findings

Findings of hypercalcemia are primarily neuromuscular. Depression, fatigue, weakness, lethargy, or confusion may occur with only mild elevation in serum calcium levels. At higher calcium concentrations, hallucinations, disorientation, hypotonicity, and coma may develop. Correction of the serum calcium level leads to complete recovery.

Elevated levels of calcium result in increased cardiac contractility until the serum calcium levels reach 15 to 20 mg/dl. Higher levels result in myocardial depression, and mechanical ventricular systole is shortened. Slowed conduction and shortening of the refractory period may predispose a patient to dysrhythmias. The most reliable ECG change of hypercalcemia is shortening of the QT interval, which is almost always seen when the calcium concentration exceeds 13 mg/dl. The PR interval and QRS complex may also be slightly prolonged.

Varying degrees of atrioventricular block often occur, but complete heart block caused by hypercalcemia is rare if the serum calcium is below 15 mg/dl. Cardiac arrest may occur at higher levels. Hypercalcemia increases the susceptibility to digitalis toxicity, even at low serum levels of the drug.

SIGNS AND SYMPTOMS OF HYPERCALCEMIA

Neurologic

Altered mental status (personality change,
   depression, lethargy, confusion, somnolence,
   hallucinations, psychosis, coma)
Weakness
Fatigue
Hypotonicity
Diminished deep tendon reflexes
Ataxia
EEG changes

Cardiac

Increased contractility
Shortening of ventricular systole
Decreased automaticity
Slowed conduction
   PR prolongation
   QRS prolongation
Shortening of refractory period
   ST segment shortens → short QT interval
Dysrhythmias
   Bradycardia
   Bundle branch block
   Second-degree heart block
   Complete heart block (levels usually above 15
      mg/dl)
Cardiac depression (levels above 15 mg/dl)
Predisposes and accentuates digoxin toxicity

Gastrointestinal

Anorexia, nausea, vomiting
Weight loss
Constipation
Abdominal pain
Peptic ulcer disease
Pancreatitis

Renal

Hyposthenuria
Increased excretion of sodium, bicarbonate,
   potassium, magnesium
   Polyuria, polydipsia
   Dehydration
   Hypokalemia
Nephrolithiasis
Nephrocalcinosis
Renal failure
Glycosuria, proteinuria, aminoaciduria
Renal tubular acidosis (variable)

Skeletal

Arthralgias, bone pain
Demineralization
Cystic bone lesions
Spontaneous fractures
Metastatic (soft tissue) calcifications

Ocular

Conjunctivitis
Band keratopathy

Vascular

Hypertension

Constipation is common in hypercalcemia, primarily because of the effects of calcium on intestinal smooth muscle tone. Nausea, vomiting, and anorexia are common even in mild cases.

Management

No emergency treatment is necessary in asymptomatic patients with serum levels below 12 mg/dl, and efforts should be directed toward diagnosis and treatment of the underlying cause. Hospitalization for diagnosis and treatment is warranted for all other patients. Treatment is outlined in the box on p. 680.

For patients with symptomatic hypercalcemia, forced saline diuretics is the mainstay of the emergency treatment because calcium excretion directly parallels sodium excretion. A urine output of 300 ml/hr should be maintained. Normal saline should be infused at a rate of 500 to 1000 ml/hr once the patient's volume status has been restored to normal with 1 to 2 L of saline.

STEPWISE THERAPY OF SYMPTOMS OF HYPERCALCEMIA

Step 1: Begin saline diuresis

(saline inhibits proximal reabsorption of Ca)
- Start normal saline (0.9% NSS) at 300 to 500 ml/hr
- Insert Foley catheter
- Follow intake/output

Follow cardiopulmonary status closely.

Step 2: Supplement urine flow with furosemide

(furosemide inhibits distal reabsorption of calcium)
- Use 40-200 mg q 30-90 min
- Keep urine flow above 200 ml/hr
- Follow intake/output carefully

Step 3: Follow calcium, potassium and magnesium values

- Begin 10 mEq/hr of potassium once urine flow is adequate
- Add 0.5 g of $MgSO_4$ (4 mEq) to each L of NSS
- Obtain calcium, potassium, and magnesium values every 1-2 hours

- Other therapies include the following:

Steroids: excellent in sarcoid, myeloma, lymphoma

Calcitonin: excellent in CRF, CHF; takes 8 hours; fails 25% of the time

Mithramycin: for myeloma-induced osteoclast activation; takes 1-2 days

Diphosphonates: new, promising for blocking bone reabsorption

NSAIDs: blocks prostaglandin-mediated hypercalcemia

Dialysis: lifesaving in patients with CRF, pulmonary edema

Furosemide at a dose of 40 to 100 mg IV every 30 to 90 minutes should be used to maintain the desired high-flow diuresis and caluresis. Because many patients with hypercalcemia have underlying cardiac disease, close attention must be paid to the patient's cardiopulmonary status. Respiratory rate, pulse changes, and pulse oximetry should be followed closely in addition to intake and output measures.

Because forced diuresis may result in dramatic losses of potassium, magnesium, and phosphorous. The levels of these elements should be followed closely along with the patient's serum sodium and calcium levels.

Additional therapies to lower serum calcium levels include steroids, phosphates, diphosphonates, mithramycin, and calcitonin. These agents should not be started unless specifically recommended by the patient's oncologist or internist. Hemodialysis should be considered early in the course of renally impaired patients. Symptomatic patients with hypercalcemia should either be admitted or have their emergency department treatment eventually guided by their internist or oncologist (see the box at left).

Hypocalcemia

Hypocalcemia is uncommon in the general population; the causes of this condition are summarized in the box on p. 681.

Thyroidectomy results in hypoparathyroidism in 1% to 4% of all cases. Idiopathic hypoparathyroidism occurs sporadically and is a familial disorder. An autoimmune mechanism is postulated. DiGeorge syndrome is a developmental disorder characterized by the congenital absence of the thymus and parathyroid glands. Hypocalcemia may be a result of an absolute decrease or decreased sensitivity to PTH, or it may be a result of decreased intake or bioavailability of Vitamin D_3. Pseudohypoparathyroidism is a syndrome that occurs because of an insensitivity to normal, or even elevated levels of, PTH.

CAUSES OF HYPOCALCEMIA

Hypoparathyroidism

Following thyroid, parathyroid, or other neck
    surgery
Following neck irradiation or ^{131}I treatment
Autoimmune
Familial
Developmental
    Isolated
    DiGeorge syndrome
Neonatal resulting from maternal
    hyperparathyroidism
Nonsurgical glandular destruction
    Infarction, metastases, hemosiderosis

Pseudohypoparathyroidism

Vitamin D deficiency

Anticonvulsant therapy

Renal failure

Acute
Chronic
Renal tubular acidosis

Hyperphosphatemic states

Phosphate ingestion
Intravenous phosphate
Tumor lysis (leukemia, lymphoma)
White phosphorus burns

Magnesium deficiency

Calcium complex formation

Ethylenediaminetetraacetic acid (EDTA)
Citrate (transfusion)
Fluoride poisoning

Neonatal

Prematurity
Low birth weight
Maternal diabetes
Complicated delivery
With hyperphosphatemia from excessive
    amounts of cow's milk
Maternal hyperparathyroidism
Maternal osteomalacia (congenital rickets)
Developmental
Hypernatremic dehydration
Lactic acidosis

Miscellaneous

Malabsorption syndromes
Pancreatitis
Respiratory alkalosis
Malignancies
Postoperative
Magnesium infusions
Cadmium poisoning
Hypoproteinemic states
Mithramycin or calcitonin therapy
Toxic shock syndrome
Colchincine overdose
Pernicious anemia

Hypocalcemia may occur in patients taking anticonvulsant medications, especially phenytoin and primidone. A mild degree of hypocalcemia is usual, with serum levels above 7 mg/dl. Either a magnesium deficiency or an excess can cause hypocalcemia. Magnesium can suppress PTH secretion and renal responsiveness to the hormone, causing hypocalcemia. The hypocalcemia that results from hypomagnesemia is relatively refractory to correction with calcium administration and will correct only after magnesium repletion.

Chronic alcohol abuse may cause hypocalcemia via a number of mechanisms, including the ability of ethanol to suppress PTH. Alcoholics are also usually hypomagnesemic, hypoalbuminemic, and combine a low calcium–vitamin D intake with a generalized protein-calorie malnutrition. Alcoholics may also become acutely hypocalcemic as a result of pancreatitis.

Clinical findings

The symptoms of hypocalcemia are predominantly neurologic and are most likely to occur when ionized calcium falls below 2.5 mg/dl. As serum calcium falls, spontaneous nerve discharges occur. The first sign of this phenomenon is often manifest as paresthesias of the distal extremities and perioral area. Progressive degrees of neural hyperexcitability lead to muscle cramping, hyperreflexia, carpopedal spasm, tetany, and seizures. Changes in mental status may also occur.

The calcium level at which symptoms develop varies widely. Latent hyperexcitability can be elicited by the Chvostek sign (facial contractions elicited by tapping over the cheek) or by the Trousseau sign (carpal or pedal spasm induced by application of a tourniquet).

Hypocalcemia also affects the heart. Contractility is diminished, and the QT interval is prolonged. The ECG manifestations of hypocalcemia are exacerbated by hypomagnesemia. The loss of contractility that occurs with hypocalcemia often causes frank heart failure, which may be improved with intravenous calcium infusion.

Management

In all patients with hypocalcemia, obtain serum electrolytes, BUN, creatinine, albumin, magnesium, arterial blood gas levels, and an ECG. Use oral calcium therapy (Table 57-2) when patients are asymptomatic, and titrate the dose to suit individual needs. Use more specific treatment, depending on the underlying disease process. Treat symptomatic hypocalcemia with parenteral calcium.

Give calcium preparations intravenously. Initially give 10 ml of 10% calcium gluconate or 5 ml of 10% calcium chloride for symptomatic hypocalcemia. Titrate further treatment to the patient's symptoms. Make an estimate of the degree of hypocalcemia during treatment by following the changes in the QT interval. Assess serum calcium levels at frequent intervals during treatment. If the patient fails to respond to treatment with calcium, consider the possibility

Table 57-2

CALCIUM PREPARATIONS

Drug Name	How Supplied	Route of Administration	Dose
Calcium gluconate injection	10% aqueous solution (1 g in 10 ml vial)	IV	5-10 ml (10 ml = 4.6 mEq of Ca)
Calcium chloride injection	10% aqueous solution (1 g in 10 ml vial)	IV	5-10 ml (10 ml = 13.6 mEq of Ca)
Calcium gluceptate injection	One 5 ml vial contains 1.1 g calcium glucep- tate (90 mg calcium)	IV or IM	5-10 ml
Calcium lactate	5 or 10 g tablets	Oral	Variable—usually 4 g with each meal
Calcium gluconate	500 or 1000 mg tablets	Oral	Variable—usually 15 g daily
Calcium ascorbate	500 mg	Oral	Variable
Whole milk	8 oz. serving	Oral	288 mg calcium
Skim milk	8 oz. serving	Oral	303 mg calcium

that the symptoms are caused primarily by hypomagnesemia, which is discussed in the following section.

Because calcium can exacerbate or initiate digitalis toxicity, administer it with great caution in patients who are receiving digitalis preparations. If calcium must be given to such patients, give the smallest effective dose at a very slow rate, and institute continuous cardiac monitoring.

Asymptomatic hypocalcemia is usually a result of malnutrition or chronic alcoholism and does not require immediate calcium therapy. Patients should be nutritionally repleted and receive multivitamins and minerals. Calcium supplementation, if provided, should be given orally (Table 49-3). Although calcium-containing tablets and liquids are available, skim milk is an excellent source of calcium and is usually well tolerated. Lactase-deficient individuals should be instructed to drink specially formulated low-fat milk that has been lactase supplemented.

Symptomatic patients with hypocalcemia should be treated with intravenous calcium chloride or calcium gluconate. Calcium gluconate is preferred because it is less concentrated and less sclerosing to the peripheral veins. Calcium gluconate has 0.46 mEq/ml of free calcium as compared with 1.36 mEq/ml in calcium chloride. In general, one or two 10 ml ampules of 10% calcium gluconate over 1 to 2 hours reverses the signs and symptoms of hypocalcemia. Refractory, severe, or chronic hypocalcemia is similar to hypokalemia in that hypomagnesemia is commonly either a coexisting variable or a causative factor.

KEY MAGNESIUM CONVERSIONS

1 g $MgSO_4$ = 8.12 mEq Mg
1 mEq Mg = 0.5 mmol Mg = 12.3 mg Mg
1 mEq/dl Mg = 1.2 mg/dl
1 g $MgSO_4$ = 98 mg of elemental Mg
1 10 ml ampule of 50% $MgSO_4$ = 5 g Mg or
   40.6 mEq Mg

MAGNESIUM

Magnesium may be reported in terms of milligrams, grams, and millimoles (see the box above). It functions as a cofactor in almost every aspect of cellular metabolism (see the box below). Disorders of magnesium homeostasis can, therefore, impair many vital functions and produce a variety of clinical disorders. One half of the body's magnesium is contained in bone, and much of the remainder is distributed among the soft tissues. Only 1% to 1.5% is present in the ECF, and one third of this is protein bound. Consequently, serum levels (normal being 1.5 to 2.5 mEq/L) are often inaccurate indicators of total-body magnesium stores. As with calcium, the plasma protein content and state of hydration must be known to correctly interpret the significance of any given magnesium level.

Hypokalemia and hypocalcemia often develop as a result of magnesium deficiency. Hypomagnesemic-induced hypokalemia may occur

---

MAGNESIUM'S MAJOR FUNCTIONS

Enzymatic	Electrical and mechanical	Metabolic
ATP-mediated energy transfer	Neurochemical transmission	Protein metabolism
Activation of cyclic AMP	Muscle contraction	Fat metabolism
Na-K ATPase pump	Cardiac conduction	Carbohydrate metabolism

despite a normal intake of potassium and cannot be corrected with potassium administration alone. It may, however, be corrected with replacement of magnesium alone, if the patient is consuming a normal diet. Potassium losses probably result from a shift of potassium into the ECF with subsequent increased urinary losses.

Magnesium exerts a similar though less marked effect as calcium on parathyroid function. Both inhibit the release of PTH. When hypocalcemia develops as a result of hypomagnesemia, calcium infusion alone is not effective until magnesium is replenished. The mechanism of secondary hypocalcemia is a result of the effects on PTH.

Hypermagnesemia

Hypermagnesemia is relatively rare and certainly much less common than magnesium deficiency. Most cases result from severe renal failure or are iatrogenically induced. Patients with chronic renal disease usually have normal or only slightly elevated serum concentrations unless they are taking medications that contain magnesium. Patients receiving intravenous magnesium at rates higher than 1 g/hour may double their serum levels, but symptoms are not usually seen until levels exceed 5 mEq/L.

Hypermagnesemia following oral ingestion in the absence of either renal or intestinal disease is extremely rare. Rare causes of hypermagnesemia include lithium use, hypothyroidism, milk-alkali syndrome, and neoplasms.

Clinical findings

Hypermagnesemia is usually asymptomatic. Rapid rises in serum magnesium levels, such as are seen when 2 to 4 g are given over less than 10 to 20 minutes, may result in warmth and flushing. Levels higher than 5 mEq/L are usually symptomatic. Decreased deep tendon reflexes, hypotonia, and hypotension are the most common symptoms seen in patients as they progress

from levels of 5 to 10 mEq/L. Levels higher than 10 mEq/L may cause shock, respiratory insufficiency, and eventually result in respiratory or cardiac arrest.

Newborns whose mothers were treated with magnesium sulfate for eclampsia may be born with hypotonia and respiratory depression. Serum levels generally range from 3 to 11 mEq/L. Supportive care is usually all that is required.

Management

Manifestations of magnesium intoxication usually respond to intravenous calcium administration. Calcium chloride, 5 ml of a 10% solution given intravenously over 30 seconds, directly antagonizes the effects of hypermagnesemia. Patients who have adequate urine output and renal function should be treated with intravenous normal saline infusion and furosemide administration to promote magnesium diuresis. Dialysis is the preferred treatment when magnesium levels exceed 8 mEq/L, when patients are severely symptomatic, or when renal elimination is greatly impaired.

Hypomagnesemia

Although the incidence of hypomagnesemia in the general population is low, certain patient groups are at a considerably greater risk to develop this disorder (see the box on p. 685). Hypomagnesemia from malnutrition alone is not generally seen in the United States. However, malnutrition in association with chronic alcohol abuse is the single most common cause of hypomagnesemia in patients seen by emergency physicians.

Alcoholism is the most common cause of magnesium deficiency in this country. Although this deficiency is caused partly by the alcoholic patient's poor nutritional habits, the major mechanism is via urinary losses of magnesium as a result of the diuretic effects of the alcohol. Alcohol may increase urinary magnesium losses

CAUSES OF HYPOMAGNESEMIA

Dietary

Alcoholism
Chronic diseases
Hyperalimentation
Long-term IV hydration

Gastrointestinal

Malabsorption
Nasogastric suction
Fistulas

Renal

Glomerulonephritis
Tubular dysfunction
Interstitial disease
Acute tubular necrosis–diuretic phase
   secondary to endocrine disease

Drug

Common
   Diuretics
   Digitalis
   Aminoglycosides
Less common
   Amphotericin B
   Cisplatin
   Carbenicillin
   Thyroxin

Acute change
   Insulin
   Catecholamines
   Citrate
   Glucose
   Amino acids

Endocrine-metabolic

Acute diseases
   Diabetic ketoacidosis
   Alcoholic ketoacidosis
   Burns
   Sepsis
   Bypass
   Hypothermia
Chronic
   Pregnancy
   Lactation
   Sweating
   Mg-free dialysis
   Refeeding status post starvation
Endocrine
   Hyperaldosteronism
   Hypercalcemia
   Hyperthyroidism
   SIADH
   Hypophosphatemia

twofold to threefold, even in the presence of a total body magnesium deficit. Serum magnesium levels usually fall even further during periods of alcohol withdrawal because of increased levels of circulating catecholamines.

A number of drugs may cause an increased urinary loss of magnesium, but such losses rarely result in symptomatic deficiency. A subclinical deficiency may be relatively common in patients who are taking furosemide or a thiazide diuretic. In patients taking digitalis preparations, even mild deficits should be avoided via dietary supplementation or by using potassium- and magnesium-sparing diuretics.

Hypomagnesemia may develop in many renal disorders because of defective tubular reabsorption. Its occurrence in these disorders is sporadic and unpredictable. More than one half of all patients with diabetic ketoacidosis have initially elevated serum magnesium concentrations, which is probably caused by dehydration and resolves with fluid therapy.

Clinical findings

Symptoms attributed to hypomagnesemia are summarized in the box on p. 686. Hypomagnesemia is associated with the development of supraventricular and ventricular tachydysrhyth-

---

REPORTED SIGNS AND SYMPTOMS ATTRIBUTED TO HYPOMAGNESEMIA

Neuromuscular

Tremor, spasm, tetany
Confusion, psychosis, coma
Ataxia, nystagmus, seizures
Paresthesias, weakness

Cardiovascular

ECG changes
Congestive heart failure
Dysrhythmias
Vasospasm
Hypertension
Digitalis and quinidine sensitivity

Gastrointestinal

Nausea
Anorexia
Abdominal pain
Electrolyte disturbance
Hypokalemia
Hypocalcemia
Hypophosphatemia
Hyponatremia

---

mias. Such dysrhythmias may prove refractory to conventional therapyp but usually respond rapidly to intravenous magnesium infusion.

A number of ECG changes have been reported with hypomagnesemia but probably represent a combination of hypomagnesemia, hypokalemia, and hypocalcemia. The most common ECG manifestation of hypomagnesemia is a prolonged QT interval.

Hypomagnesemia results in CNS and neuromuscular hyperexcitability. Mental status changes ranging from irritability to depression or disorientation, as well as combative or psychotic behavior, ataxia, nystagmus, athetoid movements, and grand mal seizures, have all been attributed to hypomagnesemia. However, it is unclear whether isolated hypomagnesemia is responsible for most of these signs and symptoms.

Painful muscle cramps may be a relatively early sign of magnesium deficiency, especially when they occur in association with hypokalemia. At extremely low levels, hypomagnesemia in conjunction with hypokalemia or hypocalcemia may result in tremors, hyperactive deep tendon reflexes, hyperreactivity to mechanical or auditory stimuli, muscular fibrillations, positive Chvostek and Trousseau signs, and carpopedal spasm. Respiratory muscle weakness may also be produced.

Hypomagnesemia may be one of the factors responsible for many of the symptoms of alcohol withdrawal. Correcting the magnesium deficiency in alcoholics is likely to reduce the tendency to develop symptoms of withdrawal and lessen their severity when they do occur.

Management

Oral therapy usually suffices if the hypomagnesemia is mild and the patient is asymptomatic and able to eat. A number of magnesium preparations are available in tablet form. Adjust the dosage to the patient's needs. Alcoholic hypomagnesemia usually corrects within 2 weeks if the patient abstains from alcohol and follows a normal diet.

Parenteral therapy is indicated whenever hypomagnesemia is severe or symptomatic or whenever the patient is already receiving intravenous therapy. The loading dose of magnesium is 1 to 2 g over 30 to 60 minutes followed by 1 g/hr. This dosage raises the levels to normal without inducing hypermagnesemia. Critically ill patients may be safely loaded with 2 g over 1 to 5 minutes and may receive 2 g/hr as long as they have normal renal function and are well hydrated. Patients with renal failure should receive magnesium only if their serum levels can be followed during repletion; they should not receive more than 2 g without having their levels rechecked.

Cardiac dysrhythmias resulting from hypomagnesemia should be treated aggressively with magnesium. Torsades de pointes variant ventricular tachycardia should be treated with 2 g (4 ml of 50% MgSO₄) IV push. Patients with ventricular ectopy resulting from hypomagnesemia may safely receive a loading dose of 2 g magnesium sulfate over 1 to 5 minutes and should initially be started on an intravenous infusion of 2 g/hr.

Patients in acute alcohol withdrawal do not need serum magnesium levels performed to have magnesium therapy initiated. Their total body deficit is usually 5 to 10 g. Because of renal losses during therapy, they require 10 to 20 g over a few days for total body repletion.

KEY CONSIDERATIONS

WHAT IS THE LIFE THREAT?

Severe derangements of sodium, potassium, calcium, and magnesium can produce cardiac dysrhythmias; potassium elevation is particularly worrisome. Use the ECG to assess the severity of hyperkalemia and to provide appropriate treatment.

DOES THE PATIENT NEED ADMISSION?

Admit patients for severe electrolyte disturbances, especially those associated with cardiac dysrhythmia. Treatment of electrolyte abnormalities may require gradual adjustment and monitoring.

Patients with chronic renal disease and hyperkalemia can be discharged if dialysis corrects the hyperkalemia.

WHAT IS THE MOST SERIOUS DIAGNOSIS?

Acute severe hyperkalemia is probably the most immediately life-threatening electrolyte disturbance.

HAVE I PERFORMED A THOROUGH WORK-UP?

Consider a wide range of potential causes for fluid and electrolyte abnormalities, including diminished water intake, gastrointestinal losses, renal disease, adrenal disease, medications, psychiatric illness, alcoholism, thyroid disease, parathyroid disease, and laboratory errors. Obtain an ECG to determine cardiac effects if any are produced by the electrolyte disturbance.

Recommended Reading

Feldman HI, Wolfson AB: Disorder of calcium and magnesium. In Wolfson AB, editor: *Endocrine and metabolic emergencies,* New York, 1990, Churchill Livingstone.

Kruse JA, Carlson RW: Rapid correction of hypokalemia using concentrated intravenous potassium chloride infusions, *Arch Int Med* 150:613-617, 1990.

McLean RM: Magnesium and its therapeutic uses: a review, *Am J Med* 96:63-76, 1994.

Oh MS, Carroll HJ: Disorders of sodium metabolism: hypernatremia and hyponatremia, *Crit Care Med* 20:94-103, 1992.

Salem MM, Rosa RM, Battle DC: Extrarenal potassium tolerance in chronic renal failure: implications for the treatment of acute hyperkalemia, *Am J Kidney Dis* 18:421-440, 1991.

Zaloga GP, Chernow B: Hypocalcemia in critical illness, *JAMA* 256:1924-1929, 1986.

Chapter *Fifty-eight*
ENDOCRINE DISORDERS

RITA K. CYDULKA

Disorders of the endocrine system often appear insidiously, but patients with endocrine disorders may come to the emergency department with acute decompensation caused by an intercurrent stress. Such disorders may be potentially lethal and in their extreme stages are medical emergencies. Because a laboratory confirmation of an endocrinologic diagnosis is often not available, the clinical diagnosis is essential in focusing on management.

DIABETES

Diabetes is a disorder of carbohydrate metabolism and reflects pancreatic beta cell dysfunction. Glucose homeostasis is a key function of insulin. Insulin augments the glucose uptake and storage needed for the process of energy generation and for glycogen and fat synthesis. Insulin inhibits gluconeogenesis and glycogenolysis.

The release of insulin is triggered by elevated blood glucose, which is sensed by the beta cells of the pancreas. Orally ingested glucose evokes more insulin release than glucose administered parenterally. Certain amino acids and certain medications induce the release of insulin. Sulfonylurea oral hypoglycemic agents are effective in part by stimulating the release of insulin from the pancreas.

When insulin secretion is lacking or inadequate, the peripheral uptake of glucose, amino acids, and fats does not keep pace with their absorption from the intestine. In the peripheral tissues, a lack of insulin receptors or a lack of sensitivity at receptor or postreceptor sites leads to the same effect. Hyperlipemia, hyperaminoacidemia, and hyperglycemia commonly occur. When the hyperglycemia becomes marked, the renal threshold is surpassed, glucose is excreted, and an osmotic diuresis occurs. The cells are unable to receive fuel from the circulation and begin to break down protein, which leads to aminoacidemia. Long-chain fatty acids are partially oxidized and converted to ketoacids, acetoacetic acid, and beta-hydroxybutyric acid in the liver, which leads to acidosis.

Glucagon is released by pancreatic alpha cells. It increases the activity of adenyl cyclase in the liver, with a resultant increase in the breakdown of glycogen to glucose and an increase in hepatic gluconeogenesis. Glucagon is a catabolic agent that increases blood glucose and may be released in response to hypoglycemia; it is also increased in stress, trauma, infection, exercise, and starvation.

Diabetes mellitus and glucose intolerance have been classified to facilitate an understanding of glucose control (see the box on p. 689). The features of a patient with diabetes partially reflect the class of diabetes and the relative de-

CLASSIFICATION OF DIABETES MELLITUS AND OTHER CATEGORIES OF GLUCOSE INTOLERANCE

Diabetes mellitus

Insulin-dependent type (IDDM)—type I
Non–insulin-dependent type (NIDDM)—type II
  Nonobese
  Obese
Other types include diabetes mellitus
  associated with certain other conditions
  and syndromes, such as the following:
  Pancreatic disease
  Disease of hormonal etiology
  Drug- or chemical-induced condition
  Insulin-receptor abnormalities
  Certain genetic syndromes
  Miscellaneous

Impaired glucose tolerance

Nonobese
Obese
Impaired glucose tolerance associated with
  certain conditions and syndromes, such as
  the following:
  Pancreatic disease
  Disease of hormonal etiology
  Drug- or chemical-induced condition
  Insulin-receptor abnormalities
  Certain genetic syndromes
  Miscellaneous

Gestational diabetes

Statistical risk classes (subjects with normal
  glucose tolerance but a statistically
  increased risk of developing diabetes)
Previous abnormality of glucose tolerance
Potential abnormality of glucose tolerance

From Bennett PH: The diagnosis of diabetes: new international classification and diagnostic criteria, *Ann Rev Med* 34:295, 1983.

gree of insulin deficiency. A patient with type I diabetes may have weight loss; polydipsia; polyuria; polyphagia; complications of the renal, neurologic, or vascular systems; or diabetic ketoacidosis. The patient with type II diabetes

usually is an older person who is either asymptomatic or is experiencing the long-term side effects of diabetes. The major metabolic emergencies of the patient with diabetes mellitus (DM) include diabetic ketoacidosis, hyperglycemic nonketotic coma (HNKC), and hypoglycemia.

There is a significant morbidity and mortality related to the complications of diabetes, including cardiovascular disease, cerebrovascular disease, diabetic coma, and renal failure. Other long-term manifestations of diabetes mellitus include ophthalmologic changes with retinopathy, skin ulcers, dermal hypersensitivity, insulin lipodystrophy, and an array of neurologic abnormalities. Autonomic and peripheral neuropathies develop in 15% to 60% of all patients, which leads to peripheral symmetric neuropathy, mononeuropathy, truncal mononeuropathy, and amyotrophy. Rheumatologic and genitourinary manifestations, as well as a host of gastrointestinal and infectious complications, are common.

Laboratory assessment is crucial in making the initial diagnosis and determining the severity of an acute episode. In general, more than one fasting venous glucose over 140 mg/dl or a random plasma glucose of more than 200 mg/dl is diagnostic of DM. Patients with suspected diabetes should be referred for an evaluation of their glucose tolerance. The most important test in the assessment of diabetic control is the measurement of glycosylated hemoglobin (Hb A_{1c}); its value is a reflection of the quality of control over time. The percentage of Hb A_{1c} is directly proportional to the blood glucose concentration and to the period that the hemoglobin has been exposed to that concentration.

Rapid glucose-measuring dipsticks generally use glucose oxidase; urine ketone dipsticks use the nitroprusside reaction. Urine ketone dipsticks are a good test for acetoacetate but do not measure ß-hydroxybutyrate. Therefore, they do not adequately reflect the extent of ketosis when ketones are in the form of ß-hydroxybutyrate.

DIABETIC KETOACIDOSIS

Diabetic ketoacidosis (DKA) is produced by an insulin deficiency and is characterized by hyperglycemia, acidosis, and ketonemia. It is caused by new-onset diabetes, infection, decreased insulin dosage (by physician or patient), trauma, myocardial ischemia or infarction, pregnancy, or a multitude of other stressors. DKA is most common in type I diabetes. Patients typically complain of polydipsia, polyuria, polyphagia, visual blurring, weakness, weight loss, nausea, vomiting, and abdominal pain. Typical clinical findings include tachypnea with Kussmaul respirations (deep and rapid), tachycardia, hypotension or orthostatic blood pressure changes, acetone on the breath, vomiting, dehydration, and mental status changes, which may lead to obtundation and coma. Abdominal pain is common and often mimics an acute surgical condition. DKA resolves with treatment of the acidosis.

Initial laboratory tests allow for preliminary confirmation of the diagnosis and immediate initiation of therapy. An arterial blood gas measures pH and bicarbonate. Other blood samples should be analyzed for a complete blood count (CBC), electrolytes, blood urea nitrogen (BUN), creatinine, phosphorus, serum ketones, and lactate levels.

The patient with DKA typically has an elevated anion gap (greater than 14). The anion gap is calculated as follows:

$$[Na^+] - [(Cl^-) + (HCO_3^-)]$$

An ECG should be obtained to rule out myocardial infarction, and it may show signs characteristic of electrolyte abnormality. In addition, a urinalysis should be evaluated for signs of infection. The need for other tests should be guided by the patient's history and physical examination. The underlying precipitant and complications should be sought. The box on p. 691 lists the differential considerations in the patient with an impaired mental status associated with diabetes.

With DKA, fluids and insulin are the basic elements for resuscitation. The severely affected patient may have a fluid deficit of 5 to 6 L. In a patient without cardiac or renal disease, initial therapy should begin with 1 L (10 to 20 ml/kg) of normal saline wide open. Subsequent fluid resuscitation should reflect the initial response and estimated dehydration. Initial serum potassium levels are generally high because potassium is shifted to the extracellular space during acidosis, but the total body supply of potassium is usually depleted. Therefore immediately after ensuring that the patient has adequate renal function, potassium replacement should begin with potassium chloride, 20 mEq/hour intravenously (IV).

In addition to fluids to correct acidosis, insulin is needed to correct hyperglycemia. Administer an initial bolus of insulin (5 to 10 units IV) followed by an infusion rate of 5 to 10 units/hour of regular insulin. Adjust the rate as indicated to optimally produce a fall in glucose of 50 to 100 mg/dl/hour. In children, insulin is started at a rate of 0.1 to 0.2 units/kg/hour. The insulin solution should be run through the IV tubing before initiating therapy. Insulin infusion should be lowered to 2 to 4 units/hour when the glucose is less than 250 mg/dl and concomitant with the addition of glucose to the infusing solution. One unit of insulin causes intracellular movement of approximately 2 to 4 g of glucose.

If the patient is significantly acidotic with a pH less than 7 or a pH of 7.1 with cardiovascular instability, or if bicarbonate is less than 7 to 10 mEq/L, sodium bicarbonate 50 to 100 mEq can be given to partially correct any deficit. However, restraint should be exercised when correcting acidosis, because the acidosis may actually have a beneficial effect in enhancing red cell oxygen release. Bicarbonate administration may create a paradoxical CNS acidosis and increase the systemic potassium requirement.

Careful monitoring with a flow sheet should be initiated at the start of therapy. Electrolytes and glucose should be measured every hour

DIFFERENTIAL CONSIDERATIONS IN PATIENT WITH AN IMPAIRED MENTAL STATUS ASSOCIATED WITH DIABETES		
Metabolic	**Intoxication**	**Other**
Diabetic ketoacidosis	Salicylates	Postictal
Hyperosmolar hyperglycemic nonketotic coma	Methanol	Cerebrovascular
Hypoglycemia	Isopropyl alcohol	Trauma
Hyponatremia	Ethanol	Abdominal lactic acidosis
Uremic acidosis	Ethylene glycol	Sepsis
	Paraldehyde	
	Cyanide	
	Chloral hydrate	

while the patient remains acidotic in the emergency department.

HYPERGLYCEMIC HYPEROSMOLAR NONKETOTIC COMA

The presentation of marked hyperglycemia without ketosis represents approximately 10% to 20% of all cases of severe hyperglycemia. The classic patient with hyperglycemic hyperosmolar nonketotic coma (HHNC) is a middle-aged or elderly individual who has type II diabetes or who has no previous diagnosis of diabetes mellitus but has an underlying infection. Other common precipitating illnesses include gastrointestinal hemorrhage, pneumonia, renal insufficiency, and gram-negative sepsis. The patient has a depressed mental status, fever, thirst, polyuria, or oliguria. A variety of neurologic findings may be noted, including seizures, segmental myoclonus, nystagmus, hallucinations, and quadriplegia.

The differential diagnosis of HHNC includes DKA, alcoholic ketoacidosis, lactic acidosis, sepsis, underlying hepatic disease, uremia, toxic ingestion, and hypoglycemia. The initial laboratory tests are the same as for a patient with DKA, in addition to serum osmolality.

With HHNC, the glucose is typically over 600 mg/dl, with a serum osmolality over 350 mOsm/L. Osmolality is calculated as follows:

Serum osmolality (mOsm/L) =
$2 [(Na^+) + (K^+) mEq/L] + (blood glucose (mg/dl)/18) + (BUN (mg/dl)/2.8)$

The approach to fluid and insulin management is similar to that of DKA, but many physicians prefer using half-normal saline initially. Because patients are older and may have underlying cardiac or renal disease, careful monitoring is required to avoid hypoglycemia and fluid and salt overload. The mortality rate for patients with HHNC approaches 50%.

HYPOGLYCEMIA

Hypoglycemia is defined as a level of glucose below which symptoms are produced—generally 45 mg/dl. Excessive administration of insulin or oral hypoglycemic agents may result in hypoglycemia. Patients with hypoglycemia develop tachycardia, clammy skin, anxiety, and restlessness. The symptomatic response to hypoglycemia reflects the release of counterregulatory hormones and the lack of glucose substrate for the CNS. If the counterregulatory response fails to adequately raise the serum glucose, CNS manifestations of lethargy, confusion, seizures, and coma may develop. The differential diagnosis includes toxic ingestion, sepsis, uremia, trauma, hepatic failure, seizures, meningitis, and cerebrovascular accident (CVA).

With hypoglycemia, a Dextrostix should be obtained immediately, and a blood sample should be sent to the laboratory to determine serum glucose. Patients who are alert may be given oral solutions containing sugar; all other patients should be given an IV bolus of 50 ml of 50% dextrose followed by an IV infusion of 500 ml D_5W over 1 hour. Rapid recovery generally follows. The patient should be observed for at least 1 hour and given a meal. If IV access is unobtainable, glucagon 1 mg may be given IM or SQ; a response will be seen within 20 minutes. If an adequate explanation for hypoglycemia is found and a second glucose test reveals that the condition has been corrected, the patient may be discharged and followed up with his or her primary physician within 1 to 2 days.

Patients with hypoglycemia secondary to sulfonylureas and other oral agents pose a problem because of the long half-life of some of these drugs. These patients require hospitalization and treatment with a continuous IV infusion of $D_{10}W$.

HYPERTHYROIDISM/THYROTOXICOSIS

Excessive function of the thyroid may produce a continuum of disease that ranges from mild hyperthyroidism associated with thyrotoxicosis to life-threatening manifestations that cause a thyroid storm, or a thyrotoxic crisis. Approximately 1% to 2% of all patients with hyperthyroidism progress to thyroid storm.

Graves disease is the most common underlying condition causing hyperthyroidism, and it typically occurs in women during the third and fourth decades of life. Toxic multinodular goiter may produce a storm in somewhat older

---

> ### CAUSES OF THYROTOXICOSIS
>
> Toxic diffuse goiter (Graves disease)
> Toxic multinodular or uninodular goiter
> Factitious thyrotoxicosis
> T_3 toxicosis
> Hashimoto thyroiditis
> Malignancy
> Hypothalamic hyperthyroidism
> Thyroid-stimulating hormone (TSH)-
>   producing pituitary tumor

---

women. Factitious hyperthyroidism may result from exogenous ingestion of thyroid hormone. The causes of thyrotoxicosis are listed in the box above.

The signs and symptoms of thyrotoxicosis reflect end-organ responsiveness to thyroid hormone. The most common symptoms are nervousness, tremor, weight loss, palpitations, heat intolerance, muscle weakness, excessive defecation, and emotional lability. Physical examination demonstrates thyroid enlargement, warm and smooth skin, tremors, proximal muscle weakness, a hyperdynamic precordium, and a widened pulse pressure.

Apathetic hyperthyroidism may be seen in the elderly, is associated with few and subtle findings, and often reflects single organ dysfunction such as heart failure. The cause is usually multinodular goiter; weight loss, depressed mentation, tremors, and hyperactivity may exist. The signs and symptoms of thyrotoxicosis are listed in the box on p. 693.

Patients with signs and symptoms of thyrotoxicosis should be evaluated by obtaining a free T_4, a high sensitivity TSH, and an ECG. If free T_4 is not available, a total T_4 and resin T_3 uptake should be obtained. Any elderly patient with new-onset congestive heart failure (CHF), especially if complicated by atrial fibrillation or supraventricular tachycardia, should have thy-

SIGNS AND SYMPTOMS OF THYROTOXICOSIS	
Signs	**Symptoms**
Fever	Weight loss
Congestive heart	Palpitations
failure	Tremor
Thyromegaly	Psychosis
Tremor	Disorientation
Jaundice	Myalgia
Hyperkinesis	Dyspnea
Psychosis	Chest pain
Tachycardia	Weakness
Wide pulse pressure	Diarrhea
Shock	Abdominal pain
Weakness	Hyperdefecation
Tender liver	
Coma	
Thyrotoxic stare	

STRESSES THAT PRECIPITATE THYROID STORM
Infection
Hypoglycemia
Diabetic ketoacidosis
Hyperglycemic hyperosmolar nonketotic coma
Trauma
Burn
Drug reaction
Surgery
Vascular accident
Pulmonary embolism
Visceral infarction
Thyroid ingestion
Withdrawal from antithyroid medication
Emotional stress
Pregnancy

roid function tests performed. Because the results of the thyroid function tests will not be available to the emergency physician, treatment must be based on clinical judgment and on (1) suppressing the rate of thyroid hormone synthesis with thioureas, (2) decreasing hormone release by iodide, and (3) reversing the effects of the sympathetic outflow with ß-blockers. Unless minimally symptomatic, such patients are often admitted to the hospital for treatment.

THYROID STORM

A thyroid storm is a life-threatening condition with exaggerated signs and symptoms of thyrotoxicosis. This diagnosis should be suspected in any patient with a goiter who has extreme tachycardia and hyperpyrexia; disorientation and mental status changes are also common. Stresses that precipitate a thyroid storm are listed in the box above, right.

The laboratory evaluation should include a T_4 level, TSH, CBC with differential, electrolytes, BUN, creatinine, glucose, calcium, liver function tests, arterial blood gases, and an ECG. A search for the underlying etiology must be pursued.

The diagnosis of a thyroid storm is based on thyroid function tests. Both T_4 and T_3 are elevated in thyrotoxicosis. Treatment must be based on clinical judgment, because confirmatory laboratory data probably will not be available in the emergency department. Treatment of thyroid storm should have six goals:

1. *Inhibit hormone synthesis* using thionamides, including propylthiouracil (PTU) 300 mg every 6 hours by mouth or nasogastric tube.
2. *Block hormone release* using iodine in one of several forms: oral saturated solution of potassium iodide (SSKI) 5 to 10 drops, oral Lugol solutions every 6 to 12 hours, or sodium iodide 1 to 2 g, continuous IV drip. Thionamides should be given at least 1 hour before iodine therapy to prevent organification of the iodine.
3. *Prevent peripheral conversion* of T_4 to T_3 with PTU or with dexamethasone 2 mg IV

every 6 hours. The initial dose of PTU is 900 to 1200 mg followed by 300 to 600 mg daily.

4. *Block the peripheral effects of thyroid hormone* using the beta blockade effect of propranolol (1 to 2 mg IV repeated every 10 to 15 minutes until effective). Propranolol is contraindicated in patients with congestive heart failure, diabetes mellitus, and reactive airway disease.

5. *Provide general support* to reduce hyperpyrexia with acetaminophen, to control congestive heart failure, and to manage dehydration. Admit the patient to the ICU.

6. *Identify and treat the precipitating event.*

CAUSES OF HYPOTHYROIDISM

Primary

Congenital
Autoimmune hypothyroidism/thyroiditis/
    Hashimoto's disease
Idiopathic
Iatrogenic
    Postsurgical
    External radiation
    Radioiodine therapy
    Antithyroid drugs (such as iodides, lithium)
Inherited defect
    Aplasia
    Hypoplasia
    Enzymatic defect
    Ingestion of drugs or goitrogens during
        pregnancy
Neoplasm
    Primary (carcinoma) or secondary
        infiltration
Infection
    Viral (rarely aerobic or anaerobic bacteria)
Trauma
    Neck injury

Secondary

Pituitary tumor
Infiltrative disease (sarcoid) or tumor
Trauma

HYPOTHYROIDISM/MYXEDEMA COMA

Hypothyroidism is a syndrome resulting from a deficiency of thyroid hormone. Thyroid failure is primarily attributable to thyroid disease caused by an autoimmune process. Pituitary disease or secondary failure accounts for less than 4% of the cases (see the box below, left). Hypothalamic failure is a rare cause.

Hypothyroidism usually follows an indolent course, with specific stress factors leading to decompensation. The clinical presentation of hypothyroidism may be varied; common signs and symptoms are listed in the box below. Patients who are noted to have hypothyroidism should have oral thyroid hormone replacement therapy.

Myxedema coma is a poorly defined condition that occurs most commonly in patients more than 50 years of age. It involves a rare

---

SIGNS AND SYMPTOMS OF HYPOTHYROIDISM

Signs	Symptoms
Hypothermia	Paresthesia
Puffy eyelids	Weakness
Sparse pubic axillary	Emotional lability
hair	Mental status changes
Hoarse voice	Cold intolerance
Lateral one third of	Weight gain
eyebrows absent	Fatigue
Prolonged relaxation	Drowsiness
phase deep tendon	Headaches
reflexes	Dysarthria
Yellow-tinged skin	Myalgias
Dry skin	Menorrhagia
Weight gain	
Pallor	
Goiter	
Myxedema	
Bradycardia	
Hypertension	
Galactorrhea	

but life-threatening deficit of thyroid hormone. Factors that contribute to the development of myxedema coma include serious medical illnesses such as myocardial infarction, sepsis, CVA, gastrointestinal hemorrhage, trauma, and drugs (sedatives, hypnotics, anesthetics, and tranquilizers). Behavioral disturbances, including confusion, psychosis, mental slowing, depression, and dementia, may precede coma.

The patient with myxedema coma experiences hypoventilation, hypothermia, hypotension, hyponatremia, hypoglycemia, obtundation, coma, bradycardia, ileus, and the other manifestations of hypothyroidism previously noted. Myxedema coma should be suspected in all comatose patients who are hypotensive and hypothermic. The initial laboratory examination should include serum-free T_4, TSH, CBC with differential, electrolytes, BUN, creatinine, creatine phosphokinase (CPK), serum cortisol level, and arterial blood gases. An ECG and chest radiograph should also be performed. A search for the underlying cause of myxedema coma should also be conducted. Treatment must be initiated immediately, because the results of thyroid function tests will not be available in the emergency department.

Therapy includes the following: (1) respiratory support—intubation and ventilation, (2) intensive monitoring and blood pressure support with fluids (pressors are to be avoided because they precipitate dysrhythmias), (3) correction of hypothermia with passive rewarming, and (4) thyroid hormone replacement (load with IV L-thyroxine 300 to 500 μg followed by 50 to 100 μg IV daily). Smaller doses of thyroid hormone replacement may be used in the elderly or in patients with cardiac disease. Other measures include hydrocortisone 100 mg IV bolus to prevent Addisonian crisis, a bolus of 50 ml $D_{50}W$ in the case of hypoglycemia and, finally, correction of the underlying precipitant. All patients with myxedema coma should be admitted to an intensive care unit.

ADRENAL INSUFFICIENCY

Adrenal insufficiency occurs when there is inadequate hydrocortisone secretion to meet the needs of the body during stress. The causes of adrenal insufficiency are listed in the box below. Symptoms of adrenal insufficiency include anorexia, nausea, vomiting, lethargy, abdominal pain, malaise, myalgias, and dehydration (in primary adrenal insufficiency). Signs include sodium depletion, orthostatic blood pressure changes, frank hypotension, hyperkalemia, mental status changes, tachycardia, hyperpigmentation (in primary adrenal insufficiency), vitiligo, muscle atrophy, and fever. Acute adrenal insufficiency, or Addisonian crisis, is a life-threatening emergency and may be pre-

---

CAUSES OF ADRENOCORTICAL INSUFFICIENCY

Primary adrenal failure

Idiopathic: autoimmune
Infectious
    Granulomatous: tuberculosis
    Protozoal and fungi: histoplasmosis,
        coccidioidomycosis, candidiasis
    Viral: cytomegalovirus, herpes simplex
Infiltration: sarcoid, neoplasm,
    hemochromatosis, amyloidosis, iron
    depletion
Postadrenalectomy
Hemorrhage: sepsis, birth trauma, pregnancy,
    seizures, anticoagulants
Congenital adrenal hyperplasia
Congenital unresponsiveness to
    adrenocorticotropic hormone (ACTH)

Secondary adrenal failure

Pituitary insufficiency: infarction (Sheehan
    syndrome), hemorrhage, pituitary tumor,
    ACTH deficiency, infiltration
Hypothalamic insufficiency
Head trauma
Glucocorticoid administration

cipitated by intensification of chronic adrenal insufficiency, acute adrenal hemorrhage, or rapid steroid withdrawal. Stress resulting from pregnancy, surgery, trauma, infection, or dehydration can precipitate a crisis in patients previously requiring corticosteroids or those with mild preexisting adrenal insufficiency.

The patient with Addisonian crisis experiences hypotension and shock, hyponatremia, hypokalemia, and hypoglycemia. On physical examination there is hypotension that is poorly responsive to fluids or vasopressor agents, tachycardia, orthostasis, and mental status changes. In patients with primary adrenal insufficiency there is also hyperpigmentation of the skin, particularly on friction areas, surgical scars, and skin creases. The differential diagnosis includes sepsis, shock of any cause, and an acute abdominal emergency.

Initial laboratory tests include plasma cortisol, cosyntropin (ACTH, Cortrosyn) stimulation tests, CBC with differential, serum glucose, electrolytes, BUN, creatinine, and an ECG. A search for an underlying infection should be pursued and includes obtaining blood cultures, a chest radiograph, and urinalysis. A plasma cortisol level of less than 20 µg/dl in the setting of shock suggests adrenal insufficiency.

Glucocorticoid replacement and volume expansion are the mainstays of therapy for Addisonian crisis. Because the results of the serum cortisol will not be available before initiating therapy, therapy should begin on the basis of the clinical diagnosis. Intravenous glucocorticoid therapy (hydrocortisone 100 mg IV every 6 hours or dexamethasone 4 mg every 12 hours) should be administered immediately after obtaining the laboratory studies. Dexamethasone will not interfere with the results of the Cortrosyn stimulation tests. Dextrose and saline (D_5NS) at a rate of 500 to 1000 ml/hour for the first 3 to 4 hours aids with volume expansion. Care should be taken to note the patient's age, volume status, cardiac function, and renal function. If the patient has hypoglycemia, 50 ml of $D_{50}W$ 50% dextrose IV should be given. Life-threatening dysrhythmias secondary to hyperkalemia should be addressed in the usual manner. The patient should be admitted to an intensive care setting with continuous cardiac and blood pressure monitoring, continuous evaluation of volume status, and frequent monitoring of serum glucose and electrolytes.

KEY CONSIDERATIONS

WHAT IS THE LIFE THREAT?

Hyperosmolar coma, ketoacidosis, and hypoglycemia can be life threatening.

A thyroid storm may precipitate life-threatening cardiac ischemia, congestive heart failure, and severe hyperpyrexia. Severe hypothyroidism can cause myxedema coma and hypothermia, hypotension, respiratory depression, and death.

A severe adrenal crisis appears with life-threatening hypothermia and electrolyte abnormalities.

DOES THE PATIENT NEED ADMISSION?

Hospitalize patients with life-threatening endocrine disorders. Predictors of serious endocrine disorders include mental status impairment, marked abnormality of vital signs, and severe electrolyte abnormalities.

WHAT IS THE MOST SERIOUS DIAGNOSIS?

Hyperglycemic hyperosmolar nonketotic coma, untreated hypoglycemia, diabetic ketoacidosis, thyroid storm, myxedema coma, and adrenal crisis are the most serious diagnoses.

HAVE I PERFORMED A THOROUGH WORK-UP?

Evaluate diabetic patients for end-organ damage, including a clinical assessment of vision, cardiovascular status, renal function, and neurologic status. Consider hypoglycemia (and hyperglycemia) in all patients with coma or seizure. Consider ketoacidosis in patients with type I diabetes and symptoms of gastroenteritis such as vomiting or abdominal pain. Consider thyrotoxicosis in new cases of atrial fibrillation. Consider adrenal crisis in patients who have hypotension and are ill, especially those who have been taking corticosteroids.

Recommended Reading

Graber TW: Diabetes mellitus and glucose disorders. In Rosen P et al, editors: *Emergency medicine: concepts and clinical practice,* ed 3, St Louis, 1992, Mosby.

Holmes L, Lakshmanan M: The patient with chronic endocrine disease. In Herr RD, Cydulka RK, editors: *Emergency care of the compromised patient,* Philadelphia, 1994, Lippincott.

Wogan JM: Endocrine disorders. In Rosen P et al, editors: *Emergency medicine: concepts and clinical practice,* ed 3, St Louis, 1992, Mosby.

Chapter Fifty-nine
BACTERIAL INFECTIONS

THOMAS W. TURBIAK AND JOEL J. REICH

DIPHTHERIA

Diphtheria is an acute bacterial infection caused by *Corynebacterium diphtheriae* and is characterized by a local inflammation of the respiratory tract or by skin and systemic effects involving the heart and central nervous system. Once a widely feared disease with a high morbidity and mortality, diphtheria has been almost completely eradicated in the United States by an active immunization program.

Epidemiology

C. diphtheriae is transmitted primarily through person-to-person contact via nasopharyngeal secretions or direct contact with skin lesion exudate. Humans are the only known reservoir for *C. diphtheriae* and may transmit the infection while actively ill, as asymptomatic carriers, or in the convalescent stage following an acute clinical infection. The risk of transmission from diphtheria patients is greater than that of transmission from asymptomatic carriers.

Immunization against diphtheria is highly effective if done properly and completely. Routine immunization of children in the United States has resulted in a decreased incidence of diphtheria and a shift of cases to older age groups. Most patients who contract diphtheria have not been adequately immunized. Those who have

received three or more doses of the diphtheria toxoid have a lower mortality than unimmunized patients. There have been several large outbreaks of diphtheria in the United States. Risk factors for such localized epidemics include poor hygiene, crowded living conditions, season, underlying skin disease, alcoholism, contaminated fomites, pyoderma, and the introduction of new *C. diphtheriae* strains.

The incubation period for respiratory diphtheria is usually 2 to 4 days but may range from 1 to 8 days. Cutaneous diphtheria usually develops as a secondary infection of a primary skin lesion or wound. Signs of this infection develop within an average of 7 days but may develop within 1 to more than 21 days.

Pathophysiology and Etiology

Diphtheria is caused by *C. diphtheriae,* a club-shaped, gram-positive bacillus. This organism is named for its shape ("coryne," or club) and for its characteristic clinical appearance on the skin or mucous membranes ("diphtheria," or hide).

The primary sites of infection are the respiratory tract (pharyngeal, nasal, and laryngeal types) and skin. Many strains of *C. diphtheriae* produce a locally acting exotoxin that contributes to the formation of the diphtheritic membrane. The toxin is transported via the circulation to other parts of the body, where its effects are manifested. The degree of toxicity depends on the location and extent of membrane formation. Pharyngeal diphtheria generally has the greatest toxicity, whereas cutaneous diphtheria has the least toxicity. The diphtheritic membrane is composed of leukocytes, erythrocytes, fibrin, epithelial cells, and bacteria. The *C. diphtheriae* exotoxin acts by inhibiting protein synthesis in the cell. This circulating exotoxin affects all body cells, but its most serious effects involve the nervous system and heart.

Clinical Findings

The signs and symptoms of respiratory diphtheria may be indistinguishable from other upper respiratory tract infections. Common symptoms include a sore throat, fever, and dysphagia; other symptoms include nausea, vomiting, headache, chills, neck edema and tenderness, and nasal discharge. Fever is usually low grade, cervical adenopathy is present in approximately one third of the patients, and a diphtheritic membrane is observed in more than one half of the patients.

In patients with faucial (pharyngeal or tonsillar) diphtheria, the extent of a diphtheritic membrane usually parallels the clinical severity of the disease. If the membrane is limited to the tonsils, the disease is likely to be mild. If the membrane covers the entire pharynx, the onset of the illness is abrupt and the severity is usually high. Cases of nasal diphtheria appear with unilateral or bilateral serous or serosanguinous discharge from the nares; the diphtheritic membrane may be visible in the nose. This group of patients does not usually appear to be toxic and does not develop constitutional symptoms. Laryngeal (tracheobronchial) diphtheria may begin in the larynx or spread downward from a more cephalad primary site. Patients may develop respiratory tract edema with subsequent upper airway obstruction.

The diphtheritic membrane first appears as a localized erythema that progresses to grayish-white patches, which coalesce to form the membrane. When fully developed, the membrane appears thick and grayish-black with sharply defined borders. The membrane is quite adherent to the underlying tissues; bleeding occurs if attempts are made to remove it.

Systemic effects in diphtheria are caused by the action of a circulating exotoxin on the cardiovascular and nervous systems. The extent of cardiac or neurologic problems correlates with the severity of the primary infection. Signs of cardiac dysfunction usually appear 1 to 2 weeks following the onset of illness. Diphtheria toxin injures the heart muscle directly, which produces myocarditis. Clinically, congestive heart failure and cardiac conduction abnormalities are seen. The electrocardiographic changes suggestive of myocarditis occur commonly, whereas the clinical signs of cardiac dysfunction are less common.

Neurologic toxicity is manifested by a peripheral neuropathy associated with muscle weakness. The muscles of the palate are usually the first to become paralyzed. In severe cases, paralysis may develop within the first few days of the illness. In milder cases, its onset may be delayed as long as several weeks. Generally the paralysis does not last more than 10 days, and complete function returns.

Cutaneous diphtheria has been reported to occur mostly in the tropics; however, cases have been reported in temperate climates in patients with significant risk factors for infection. Patients with cutaneous diphtheria generally do not become systematically ill.

The most serious complications of diphtheria are airway obstruction (secondary to membrane formation and edema), congestive heart failure, cardiac conduction abnormalities, and muscle paralysis.

The diagnosis of diphtheria is based on clinical findings, with laboratory tests providing confirmation. The laboratory must be notified when diphtheria is a suspected pathogen because routine culture techniques will not identify *C. diphtheriae*. Other laboratory tests may be helpful in identifying complications of the disease.

Differential Diagnosis

The differential diagnosis of respiratory diphtheria includes streptococcal or viral pharyngitis, tonsillitis, Vincent angina, acute epiglottitis, infectious mononucleosis, laryngitis, bronchitis, tracheitis, monilial infection, and various common conditions with associated rhinitis. In the absence of a diphtheritic membrane, it may be impossible to differentiate diphtheria from some of these conditions, especially in the early phase of infection.

Cutaneous diphtheria may have an appearance that is similar to other ulcerated acute and chronic skin conditions. Because cutaneous diphtheria often exists as a secondary infection, it may coexist with an initial primary skin lesion.

Treatment

With diphtheria, the goal of treatment is (1) to interfere with the action of the toxin that has already been produced, and (2) to kill the organism. Equine serum diphtheria antitoxin is a cornerstone of therapy for diphtheria. Because the antibodies neutralize only circulating toxin, the antitoxin should be administered promptly following the clinical diagnosis of respiratory diphtheria. Because as many as 10% of all individuals may exhibit hypersensitivity to horse serum, conjunctival or intradermal sensitivity skin testing should be performed before administering the antitoxin. The dose antitoxin is based on the probable quantity of the toxin.

In addition to antitoxin therapy, antibiotics should be administered for 14 days. Antibiotic treatment eradicates the local infection, eliminates further production of the toxin, and reduces the spread of the infection to other individuals. Erythromycin or penicillin are generally recommended antibiotics.

Local wound cleansing and a course of antibi-otics are recommended as treatments for cutaneous diphtheria. The value of administering an antitoxin for cutaneous diphtheria is questionable. However, some experts recommend administering an antitoxin to prevent the toxic sequalae that have been reported in some cases.

Carriers with *C. diphtheriae* should receive 7 days of oral penicillin or erythromycin or be given intramuscular penicillin G benzathine if compliance is in question. Active immunization should be provided for unimmunized and partially immunized carriers. Cultures should be obtained after antibiotic therapy.

Patients with respiratory or cutaneous diphtheria should be isolated, hospitalized, and provided with supportive care. Close contacts of patients should be cultured for diphtheria and kept under surveillance for 7 days. Antibiotic treatment should be initiated for those whose cultures are positive. Previously immunized close contacts should receive a booster of diphtheria toxoid if the last booster was given more than 5 years ago. Close contacts who are unimmunized or whose immunization status is unknown should be cultured before and after therapy, treated with the same antibiotic therapy as carriers, and have age-appropriate active immunization initiated.

A universal program of primary immunization along with regular diphtheria boosters every 10 years is the most effective way to control diphtheria. For wound management, emergency departments should administer diphtheria toxoid along with tetanus toxoid.

Disposition

Patients with clinically suspected or proven diphtheria should be hospitalized and placed in isolation. The emergency physician should initiate an effort to locate and treat close contacts and to report the infection to the appropriate local health agency. Health care providers should review their own immunizations status and the degree of patient contact to determine if any action is necessary.

PERTUSSIS

Pertussis means violent cough, and it is this symptom that is the hallmark of the disease. The disease is also called *whooping cough* because of the progressive, repetitive, and severe episodes of coughing, which are followed by a forceful inspiration that creates the characteristic "whooping" sound.

Until a vaccine was developed in the 1940s, pertussis was a major cause of morbidity and mortality in the United States. Its incidence has been steadily declining since the vaccine has been widely used. However, in the last few years, a world-wide reduction in the use of the vaccine has led to an increased incidence of pertussis in all age groups.

Patients with pertussis are often inaccurately diagnosed. To avoid misdiagnosis, the emergency physician must be knowledgeable about pertussis.

Epidemology

Although pertussis can occur in any age group, it is predominantly an illness of pediatric patients. The age-specific attack rates are highest in children under 1 year of age and decline with advancing age.

The incubation period of pertussis is approximately 7 to 10 days but may range from less than 1 week to greater than 3 weeks. Pertussis is very contagious; attack rates vary from 50% to 100%. Transmission occurs through exposure to airborne droplet particles from infected persons. Neither a vaccination against pertussis nor natural immunity from the disease produces lifelong protection.

Pathophysiology and Etiology

Pertussis is caused by organisms of the *Bordetella* genus. Although there are four species of this genus, only *B. pertussis* and *B. parapertussis* are responsible for this disease in humans. These organisms are nonmotile, small, gram-negative coccobacilli that appear singly or in pairs. Isolation of the organism requires a special culture medium to which antibiotics have been added (to reduce overgrowth of competing bacteria) for as long as 7 days.

B. pertussis adheres to ciliated respiratory epithelial cells, where it produces several toxins that cause local tissue reactions and systemic illness. *B. parapertussis* can also cause disease but is generally milder, probably because it does not produce toxins.

Clinical Findings

Pertussis exists in three distinct and sequential clinical phases or stages: the catarrhal phase, the paroxysmal phase, and the convalescent phase.

The catarrhal phase begins after an incubation period of approximately 7 to 10 days and lasts approximately 1 to 2 weeks. Symptoms are indistinguishable from a nonspecific upper respiratory tract infection with a cough, low-grade fever, rhinitis, and anorexia. During this stage of the illness, patients are usually not diagnosed as having pertussis. Infectivity is greatest during this phase.

The paroxysmal phase begins as the cough increases and the fever subsides. This phase is named for the frequent paroxysms of coughing that occur as often as 50 times each day. The patient coughs repeatedly in short exhalations; after 10 to 15 coughs, the patient inhales forcefully. The single, sudden, large, and forceful inhalation produces the whooping sound. Although the whoop is the hallmark of this disease, many patients never develop it.

The convalescent phase is characterized by a residual cough and a recovery period that lasts from several weeks to several months.

Atypical presentations of pertussis may occur in young infants, who may have a cough, nasal congestion, and episodes of apnea. Older children and adults who have partial protection as a result of a vaccination or previous illness may have symptoms that are indistinguishable from those of a nonspecific bronchitis.

The emergency physician should explore the details of the coughing episodes, ascertain whether there has been exposure to people with pertussis, obtain a history of previous pulmonary illnesses, and review the patient's vaccination history. The physician should ask questions to evaluate the severity of illness, the degree of dehydration, and the presence of any complications. The physical examination should assess for signs of hypoxemia, dehydration, and systemic toxicity.

The major complications of pertussis are pneumonia, CNS sequelae, otitis media, and a variety of complications related to the paroxysms of coughing. Pneumonia as a complication of pertussis is a leading cause of death, especially among young children and infants. Possible mechanisms for the development of pneumonia are aspiration and secondary infection. CNS complications occur in a small percentage of cases and may result in severe disability or death. The most frequent CNS complications are seizures, encephalopathy, and intracerebral hemorrhage. Sudden increases in intrathoracic and intraabdominal pressures during the paroxsyms of coughing and whooping cause a multiplicity of other physical conditions that further complicate the illness. These complications include periorbital edema, subconjunctival hemorrhage, petechiae, epistaxis, hemoptysis, subcutaneous emphysema, pneumothorax, pneumomediastinum, diaphragmatic rupture, umbilical and inguinal hernias, and rectal prolapse.

Ancillary studies are of limited value in the emergency department evaluation of the patient who is suspected of having pertussis. During the paroxsysmal phase a marked leukocytosis is often present, with a characteristic lymphocytosis and a white cell count of 25,000 to 50,000/mm^3. Laboratory confirmation of the diagnosis is made with a culture of a nasopharyngeal specimen on a special culture medium. However, even under ideal laboratory conditions, only 80% of all suspected cases produce a positive culture.

Differential Diagnosis

Pertussis should be suspected in a patient with an upper respiratory infection and one or more of the following features: (1) a history of exposure, (2) a severe persistant cough, (3) vomiting, and (4) leukolymphocytosis.

A variety of respiratory illnesses must be considered in the differential diagnosis, including acute viral upper respiratory tract infections, various pneumonias, bronchiolitis, cystic fibrosis, tuberculosis, exacerbation of chronic obstructive pulmonary disease, and foreign bodies of the respiratory tract.

Treatment

The most important aspect of treatment for acute pertussis is good supportive care, including oxygenation, suctioning (as required), maintenance of hydration and nutrition, and avoidance of respiratory irritants. All severely ill patients and any child under the age of 1 year should be hospitalized. Antibiotics are recommended, and erythromycin is the drug of choice. Corticosteroids may reduce the severity and duration of the illness.

The most important aspect of prevention is adequate vaccination. A pertussis vaccine is available in combination with diphtheria and tetanus toxoids (DTP). The vaccine is 80% to 90% effective, but immunity is not lifelong. Complications and adverse reactions occur more commonly from the pertussis component of the DTP vaccine than from any other vaccine commonly administered to children. These complications have led to a reduction in the use of this vaccine in some countries. However, as mentioned earlier, a reduction in the use of the vaccine has led to major epidemics of pertussis. The Advisory Committee for Immunization Practices (ACIP) of the Centers for Disease Control and Prevention (CDC) presently recommends that the benefit of this vaccine outweighs its adverse effects. Acellular pertussis vaccines formulated with diphtheria and tetanus toxoids (DTaP) have been developed and licensed for use in the United States. These vaccines are currently recommended for use as booster doses in children who have been immunized with three primary doses of DTP. Currently no pertussis vaccines are licensed for use in adults.

TETANUS

Tetanus is a severe but fortunately rare illness and is characterized by uncontrolled muscle spasms and autonomic nervous system hyperactivity. The emergency physician plays a major role in preventing this disease by initiating or updating immunizations against tetanus.

Epidemiology

Tetanus is found throughout the world. In the United States, the incidence is approximately 50 to 100 cases each year. The majority of these cases occur in older adults who have never been adequately immunized. This age specificity is in contrast to the majority of the cases in other parts of the world, which occur in neonates and children in underdeveloped nations.

Tetanus most commonly develops after trauma causes a break in the skin. Tetanus may develop following an acute wound or as a complication of a chronic skin wound or lesion. Postoperative tetanus has also developed in patients following intestinal surgery. However, in as many as 30% of all cases of tetanus, no break in the skin can be found.

Most cases of tetanus occur in individuals who have not been adequately immunized against *Clostridium tetani*, but rare cases have occurred in which patients have received a complete immunization series.

Pathophysiology and Etiology

C. tetani is a gram-positive, anaerobic, spore-forming, rod-shaped, noninvasive organism. The

bacillus forms a single, round, terminal endospore, which gives the organism a drumstick appearance. The bacteria is ubiquitous. It exists in its sporulative form in soil, dust, and human and animal excrement. The spores are resistant to heat and chemical disinfectants.

If clinical tetanus is to occur, there must first be a break in the skin to allow entry of the *C. tetani* spores. Favorable local tissue conditions must also exist to promote germination of the spores and subsequent toxin production. Inadequate immunization and a lack of antibody production allows the organism to grow.

Three toxins are produced by the *C. tetani* organisms: tetanospasmin, tetanolysin, and nonconvulsive neurotoxins. Tetanospasmin causes the cascade of events that lead to clinical tetanus. It causes disinhibition of motor groups, which leads to excessive and uncontrolled muscle activity. Tetanolysin and nonconvulsive neutotoxin are of no clinical significance.

Clinical Findings

After an incubation period of approximately 3 to 14 days (with a range of 1 day to several months), clinical tetanus can be seen. There are four types of clinical tetanus: (1) generalized tetanus, (2) cephalic tetanus, (3) localized tetanus, and (4) neonatal tetanus.

Generalized tetanus is the most severe form. Spasm of the masseter muscles leads to trismus, which is the most common finding. Other signs and symptoms include risus sardonicus (a characteristic sardonic smile), irritability, weakness, myalgias, dysphagia, hydrophobia, and increasing muscle spasms. Generalized muscular rigidity can lead to opisthotonos and spasm of the muscles of respiration. Autonomic nervous system instability produces tachycardia, hypertension, hyperthermia, and cardiac dysrhythmias. Amazingly, the patient remains lucid throughout the course of these events.

Cephalic tetanus is manifest as trismus associated with cranial nerve palsies. The most commonly involved cranial nerve is the facial nerve

(VII). Two thirds of all cases of cephalic tetanus progress to generalized tetanus; the remaining one third of the cases resolve spontaneously.

Localized tetanus is rare. With this condition, persistent localized muscle spasms occur in close proximity to the site of the inoculation of *C. tetani*. The severity of the symptoms and the course of the illness are variable. Most cases of localized tetanus do not progress to generalized tetanus.

Neonatal tetanus is a variant of generalized tetanus that occurs in neonates. Most cases occur in underdeveloped nations, where poor hygiene and lack of maternal immunization are prevalent. Early symptoms are nonspecific and include irritability, poor sucking, and a weak cry. Symptoms progress quickly; mortality is high.

Major complications of tetanus include respiratory failure, dysrhythmias, cardiac arrest, orthopedic injuries, rhabdomyolysis, renal failure, dehydration, infection, hypothermia, venous thrombosis, pulmonary embolism, gastrointestinal ulceration or perforation, and complications of intensive care.

Tetanus is diagnosed on clinical grounds. Ancillary tests may aid in considering other diseases in the differential diagnosis, in assessing for complications, or in providing supportive care.

Differential Diagnosis

The differential diagnosis of tetanus is outlined in the box above. Because many of these conditions are more prevalent than tetanus, the physician must be knowledgeable about the diagnostic criteria for each of them.

Treatment

The treatment of tetanus can be summarized by four basic principles: provide supportive care, inactivate the circulating toxin, eliminate toxin production, and initiate active immunization.

Supportive care begins with monitoring cardiac and respiratory status. Endotracheal intubation should be performed if the patient exhibits

> **DIFFERENTIAL DIAGNOSIS OF TETANUS**
>
> Acute abdomen
> Black widow spider bite
> Dental abscess
> Dislocated mandible
> Dystonic reaction
> Encephalitis
> Head trauma
> Hyperventilation syndrome
> Hypocalcemia
> Meningitis
> Peritonsillar abscess
> Progressive fluctuating muscular rigidity (stiff-man syndrome)
> Psychogenic
> Rabies
> Sepsis
> Subarachnoid hemorrhage
> Status epilepticus
> Strychnine poisoning
> Temperomadibular joint dysfunction (TMJ) syndrome

From Turbiak, Reich JJ: Bacterial infections. In Rosen P et al, editors: *Emergency medicine: concepts and clinical practice*, ed 3, St Louis, 1992, Mosby.

signs of airway compromise or respiratory insufficiency. Patients should be handled gently to minimize reflex muscle spasms; benzodiazepines or paralytic agents may be needed to reduce muscle spasms. Autonomic instability requires close monitoring and treatment. Fluid and electrolyte status must be carefully maintained. Alpha and beta adrenergic blockers may be useful in treating sympathetic overactivity. Bradydysrhythmias may necessitate the use of a temporary pacemaker. Acute hypertension can be treated with a titratable agent that has a short half-life, such as esmolol or sodium nitroprusside.

Human tetanus immune globulin (TIG) is an antitoxin that serves to neutralize any circulating toxin; it does not inactivate a toxin already present within the central nervous system. Although current dosage recommendations vary, most experts recommend administering 3,000 to 10,000 units of TIG intramuscularly. If tetanus toxoid is given at the same time, the toxoid and TIG should be administered at different sites.

Toxin production is eliminated by eradicating the *C. tetani* organism. Wounds must be cleaned and debrided, and antibiotics should be administered. Antibiotics that are effective against *C. tetani* include penicillin, tetracycline, erythromycin, and metronidazole.

Because infection with tetanus does not confer immunity, active immunization should be initiated (Table 59-1).

Patients with suspected or confirmed tetanus should be admitted to an intensive care unit. If

no such unit is available, the patient's condition should be stabilized before being transferred to an appropriate facility.

Although emergency physicians must be knowledgeable in the diagnosis and treatment of tetanus, their major contribution is in the area of prevention. All patients who come to the emergency department with wounds should be questioned about their tetanus immunization status, and vaccinations should be updated according to Table 59-1.

BOTULISM

Botulism is a rare, life-threatening, and toxin-mediated illness caused by *Clostridium botulinum*. There are four forms of botulism: (1) foodborne, (2) infant, (3) wound, and (4) unclassified. The role of the emergency physician is to recognize and promptly notify public health authorities to prevent disease outbreaks.

Epidemiology

Fewer than 100 cases of botulism are reported in the United States each year. Because *C. botulinum* spores are found in soil throughout the United States, the geographic distribution of the disease is widespread.

Foodborne botulism results from the ingestion of preformed toxin, not from the ingestion of spores. This form of botulism usually results from the ingestion of improperly prepared or stored home-canned foods. Most commonly, large outbreaks can result from commercial sources of contaminated foods.

Infant botulism, the most common form of botulism, occurs in children under age 1. In this form of the disease, spores are ingested, followed by in vivo production of toxin. Dust and soil are probably the major source of the ingested spores. Honey and corn syrup have also been described as sources of botulinum spores, and therefore it has been recommended that these foods not be given to children under 1 year of age.

*Table **59-1***

SUMMARY GUIDE TO TETANUS PROPHYLAXIS IN ROUTINE WOUND MANAGEMENT, **1991**

History of Adsorbed Tetanus Toxoid (Doses)	Clean, Minor Wounds		All Other Wounds*	
	Td[†]	TIG	Td[†]	TIG
Unknown or < 3	Yes	No	Yes	Yes
≥ 3[‡]	No[§]	No	No[‖]	No

From CDC: Diphtheria, tetanus, pertussis: recommendations for vaccine use and other prevention measures, *MMWR* 40:21, 1991.

*Such as, but not limited to, wounds contaminated with dirt, feces, soil, and saliva; puncture wounds; avulsions; and wounds resulting from missiles, crushing, burns and frostbite.

[†]For children <7 years old; DTP (DT, if pertussis vaccine is contraindicated) is preferred to tetanus toxoid alone. For persons ≥7 years of age, Td is preferred to tetanus toxoid alone.

[‡]If only three doses of *fluid* toxoid have been received, then a fourth dose of toxoid, preferably an adsorbed toxoid, should be given.

[§]Yes, if >10 years since last dose.

[‖]Yes, if >5 years since last dose. (More frequent boosters are not needed and can accentuate side effects.)

Wound botulism is a rare disease and results from *C. botulinum* contamination of wounds. This form of illness has been reported in patients with traumatic or surgical wounds and in intravenous and intranasal drug abusers.

Unclassified botulism is a rare form of botulism that occurs in patients with underlying disorders of the gastrointestinal tract. Unclassified botulism may be similar to infant botulism, in which ingested spores are not destroyed and in which the toxin is produced in vivo.

Pathophysiology and Etiology

C. botulinum is an anaerobic, gram-positive, spore-forming, rod-shaped bacteria. Under certain conditions, the spores germinate and the bacteria can produce a potent exotoxin that causes the clinical illness. A temperature of $100°$ C for 10 minutes will destroy any toxin present. Therefore heating toxin-contaminated food before ingestion prevents foodborne botulism.

Once the toxin has entered or is produced within the body, it must travel from the wound or gastrointestinal tract to the neurons. The toxin binds to the presynaptic nerve membrane and enters the neuron. The toxin then blocks the release of acetylcholine, which leads to neuromuscular blockade. This neurotoxin acts selectively and interferes with neurotransmission at the cholinergic synapses of the cranial nerves, automonic nervous system, and neuromuscular junction. Affected patients exhibit cranial nerve palsies, parasympathetic blockade, and a descending flaccid paralysis.

Clinical Findings

In cases of foodborne botulism, symptoms first appear 12 to 36 hours after the ingestion of toxin-containing food (with a range of 2 hours to 14 days). Initial symptoms of foodborne botulism are nonspecific weakness, malaise, lightheadedness, nausea, vomiting, and constipation.

Neurologic symptoms may occur at the same time or be delayed in onset for several days. The cranial nerves are affected first. Ocular symptoms include diplopia, blurred vision, and photophobia. Bulbar involvement leads to dysphonia, dysphagia, and dysarthria. A symmetrical descending muscular paralysis develops, which involves the upper and lower extremities and the muscles of respiration. The parasympathetic autonomic blockade results in decreased salivation, which results in severe mouth dryness. Ileus and urinary retention may also occur.

During the physical examination, the patient is alert and afebrile unless a secondary infection is present. Ocular abnormalities include ptosis; extraocular muscle palsies; and fixed, dilated pupils. The absence of ocular findings does not exclude the diagnosis. Decreased salivation results in a dry and reddish appearance of the mucosa of the mouth and tongue. Muscular weakness is variable in its severity; upper extremity muscles are weaker than lower extremity muscles, and proximal muscles are more affected than distal muscles.

Infant botulism is manifested differently from the adult forms. The differences in presentation are largely related to the development of the illness in an infant as opposed to in an adult. Classic symptoms of infant botulism include constipation followed by weakness as manifested by a weak cry, poor suck, and poor head control. Cranial nerve palsies, descending muscular paralysis, and automonic nervous system abnormalities may also develop.

The major life-threatening complication of botulism is respiratory failure resulting from weakness of the muscles of respiration. The loss of protective airway reflexes can lead to aspiration of gastric contents.

The diagnosis of botulism is clinical, but ancillary tests may be useful in excluding other illnesses and in providing supportive care. Electromyography can be used to differentiate botulism from other paralytic illnesses. The diagnosis of botulism can be confirmed by detecting the botulinus toxin in the patient's blood or by detecting botulinus toxin or *C. botulinum* in the suspected food source or in the patient's gastric contents, stool, or wound.

Differential Diagnosis

Botulism must be distinguished from other illnesses that cause paralysis, including Guillain-Barré syndrome, tick paralysis, myasthenia gravis, poliomyelitis, diphtheria, the Eaton-Lambert syndrome, and cerebrovascular accidents. Certain toxins may also produce a clinical picture that must be distinguished from botulism.

Infant botulism has a more extensive differential diagnosis than the adult form of botulism. Common pediatric illnesses in the differential diagnosis include sepsis, meningitis, dehydration, and failure to thrive. Other illnesses to consider include paralytic neurologic diseases, toxins, hypothyroidism, Reye syndrome, congenital errors of metabolism, congenital muscular dystrophy, and cerebral degenerative diseases.

Treatment

There are three basic principles of treatment for botulism: supportive care, administration of an antitoxin, and elimination of further toxin production.

Because paralysis of the muscles of respiration is the major cause of death, ventilatory status must be closely monitored. Endotracheal intubation should be performed as signs of ventilatory failure appear.

In cases of foodborne botulism, cleansing saline enemas and cathartics may be administered to remove residual toxins from the gastrointestinal tract. Cathartics should be avoided if an ileus is present. Magnesium-containing cathartics should be avoided because hypermagnesemia can exacerbate the muscle weakness.

Botulism antitoxin is recommended for use in adult patients. The CDC can help locate a supply of the antitoxin. Because this antitoxin is effective against only circulating toxin, it should be given early and after appropriate laboratory specimens have been obtained. Because botulinus antitoxin is derived from horse serum, a test for hypersensitivity to horse serum should precede the administration of this drug. Antitoxins have not been shown to be beneficial in infant botulism.

All patients suspected of having botulism should be hospitalized in a hospital that has age-appropriate intensive care capabilities. The CDC should be contacted immediately to assist with the diagnosis, treatment, and prevention of major epidemics. If patient transfer is necessary, endotracheal intubation should be performed before the transfer, or personnel skilled in advanced airway management should accompany the patient during the transfer.

PNEUMOCCEMIA

Illness related to infection with *Streptococcus pneumoniae* exists on a continuum from mild illness to overwhelming infection. For the purposes of this chapter, the following definitions are provided: *Pneumococcemia* is the invasion of the bloodstream by *S. pneumoniae*. Occult *bacteremia* occurs as a febrile illness without focal signs and is discovered through a positive blood culture report subsequent to the clinical evaluation of the patient. *Septicemia* is a clinical syndrome that includes systemic toxicity, tachypnea, tachycardia, altered mental status, and fever as a consequence of bacteremia. Localized infections, including otitis media, pneumonia, or meningitis, may accompany bacteremia or septicemia related to pneumococcal infection.

Epidemiology

Despite the availability of effective antibiotics and vaccines, *S. pneumoniae* is a significant cause of morbidity and mortality. A pneumococcal infection occurs episodically in normal individuals or in those with defects in host defense mechanisms. Individuals at increased risk for infection include those with chronic or respiratory illness, a history of alcohol abuse, diabetes mellitus, an absent or functionally impaired spleen, chronic renal disease, organ transplantation, lymphoma, multiple myeloma, and acquired immunodeficiency syndrome (AIDS).

Pathophysiology and Etiology

S. pneumoniae is a lancet-shaped, gram-positive coccobacillus. The frequent appearance of this organism in pairs led to its former name of *Diplococcus pneumoniae*. The organism enters the upper respiratory tract and travels to the lung, where it multiplies in the alveoli. It spreads from the lung to the mediastinal lymph nodes, into the thoracic duct, and into the circulation. Alternately, it may spread from the upper respiratory tract to the subarachnoid space, to the venous sinus, and into the bloodstream.

Pneumococcemia results in a clinical syndrome of variable severity ranging from a minor febrile illness to life-threatening septicemia. The mechanism for the development of the septicemia has not been absolutely determined, but the acuity and widespread effects of the illness are suggestive of a toxin-mediated illness. The variability in individual patient response to the illness is also not well understood. Patients surviving the pneumococcal infection develop an immunity that is specific to the capsule serotype of the organism.

Clinical Findings

The presentation of clinical signs and symptoms of pneumococcemia is quite variable. Adults commonly have fever and nonspecific constitutional symptoms. Approximately one third of these patients exhibit coughing, rigors, and pleuritic pain. Physical examination findings vary depending on the presence of the local infection. Elderly patients may not exhibit a fever or other signs and symptoms that are commonly seen with infection. Children with pneumococcemia may be indistinguishable from those with less serious common viral illnesses.

The most serious complication of pneumococcemia is cardiovascular collapse, which leads to shock and death if left untreated. Other sequelae include end-organ damage, disseminated intravascular coagulopathy (DIC), septic emboli, and complications related to intensive care treatment.

Ancillary studies may be beneficial in diagnosing pneumococcal infection and bacteremia. The selection of diagnostic tests is made on the basis of the history and physical examination findings. Blood cultures are generally positive. A chest radiograph may reveal an infiltrate or pleural effusion. If meningitis is suspected, a lumbar puncture should be performed. If sputum is available, it should be prepared with a Gram stain and cultured.

A complete blood count most often reveals leukocytosis, with an increased number of neutrophils and band forms. Some studies have shown an increased risk of bacteremia in young children who have elevated white blood cell counts, but testing for leukocytosis is an unreliable screening test for bacteremia in all age groups. Leukopenia may be present in the elderly and in those with overwhelming infection.

Differential Diagnosis

The differential diagnosis of pneumococcemia includes other bacterial and viral infections, including bacteremia. Unless a localized infection is present, it may be impossible to distinguish pneumococcemia from other infections.

Treatment

The goals of treatment are to stabilize the patient and to eradicate the organism. Hypoxemia secondary to pneumonia, shock, or respiratory failure is treated with supplemental oxygen and ventilatory assistance as required. Hemodynamics require careful monitoring and treatment with crystalloid infusion.

Antibiotic administration is necessary to kill the pneumococcal bacteria. Patients with pneumococcemia should be admitted to the hospital for intravenous (IV) antibiotics and supportive care. After the appropriate cultures have been obtained, treatment should be started as soon as possible. The first antibiotic dose should be given in the emergency department instead of waiting until the patient has been transferred to an inpatient unit.

In most instances, patients with laboratory-proven pneumococcal infection can be treated effectively with IV penicillin G. In situations in which the infecting organism has not been identified, the physician initially chooses a broad-spectrum antibiotic regimen that includes antibiotics effective against the pneumococcus. If meningitis is present, the antibiotic chosen must be able to penetrate the cerebrospinal fluid (CSF).

In some geographic areas, the pneumococcus has developed a relative resistance to penicillin. Therefore it is essential for the physician to be cognizant of local patterns of antibiotic resistance and to be aware that penicillin may not be the drug of choice.

The pneumococcal vaccine is safe and effective in preventing infection. Patients who are at increased risk for infection should be considered for immunization. The CDC has specific guidelines for vaccine use.

MENINGOCOCCEMIA

Infection with *Neisseria meningitidis* can cause a fulminant infection that leads to death within hours. Many veteran emergency physicians have seen such patients literally deteriorate before their eyes. The emergency physician can play an integral role in the early recognition and treatment of this disease.

Certain definitions will be helpful in understanding this infection. *Meningococcemia* is the invasion of the bloodstream by *N. meningitidis.* The clinical manifestation of this infection ranges from bacteremia to overwhelming sepsis. *Occult bacteremia* exists as a febrile illness and is associated with positive blood cultures in the absence of a recognizable site of local infection. *Septicemia* is a clinical syndrome of toxicity characterized by fever, chills, and signs of shock; it is often associated with a characteristic rash. *Fulminant meningococcemia,* the *Waterhouse-Friderichsen syndrome,* is a form of meningococcemia and is characterized by rapid clinical deterioration, which leads to cardiovascular collapse, shock, and (often) death. *Chronic meningococcemia* is a less virulent form of meningococcemia; is characterized by fever, rash, and joint pains; and is associated with positive blood cultures for *N. meningitidis.*

Epidemiology

Meningococcal infections are a serious cause of morbidity and mortality in the United States and throughout the world; they may occur as isolated cases or in epidemics. In nonepidemic cases, infection is most common in children under age 5. In epidemics, the incidence increases in the 5- to 19-year-old age group. Epidemics may be seen in crowded living conditions, such as those among college students or military recruits.

Pathophysiology and Etiology

N. meningitidis is an aerobic, gram-negative diplococcus. The organism is classified into at least 13 serogroups. This classification is important in the epidemiology of the disease but is less significant in the individual clinical cases.

N. meningitidis enters the nasopharynx, where it may remain and either produce an asymptomatic state or cause an upper respiratory tract infection. In certain circumstances, the bacteria enter the circulation, which leads to symptomatic bacteremia, septicemia, pulmonary infection, or meningitis. The organism and host characteristics that determine whether the infection progresses are not known.

Clinical Findings

The clinical presentation of patients with a meningococcal infection is varied. Several clinical syndromes have been described but are not distinct. Individual cases may share elements of the different forms of the illnesses described in the following paragraphs.

Patients may have bacteremia without evidence of sepsis. Such cases often exhibit a mild upper respiratory tract infection associated with a fever. Febrile children who do not appear toxic have subsequently been found to have blood cultures that are positive for *N. meningitidis.* Of particular concern are those few patients who appear clinically well on an initial examination and then rapidly deteriorate and die.

A second form of illness is meningococcemia without meningitis. These patients are acutely ill and exhibit fever, skin rashes, systemic toxicity, and shock.

Another group of patients have meningitis that may or may not be accompanied by meningococcemia. Symptoms include headache, fever, and a stiff neck. The patient may be totally alert or may exhibit a depressed mental status. Fulminant meningococcemia is a dramatic form of the illness and is characterized by sepsis, shock, disseminated intravascular coagulation (DIC), renal failure, coma, and bilateral adrenal hemorrhage. Chronic meningococcemia is a rare form of disease and is characterized by a persistent fever, rash, and arthritis associated with positive blood cultures for *N. meningitidis.*

Dermatologic findings may be the only indication of a meningococcal infection. Early in the course of the illness, a transient nonpruritic maculopapular eruption may be seen; within 24 hours, petechial lesions can be found. Because these lesions can be subtle, careful examination of the febrile patient is necessary. Discreet red or blue macules that are 1 to 2 mm in diameter can be seen. Petechiae may be present anywhere on the skin or mucous membranes but are most commonly found on the trunk, lower extremities, or on areas of the skin subject to pressure from clothing. These lesions may coalesce to form larger macules or areas of ecchymosis. Pupura fulminans is a situation characterized by sudden and rapidly spreading ecchymosis and gangrene of the extremities and is associated with meningococcal or streptococcal infection. Although fever associated with a petechial rash should suggest a meningococcal infection, a variety of viral and bacterial infections may produce a similar clinical picture.

Complications of infection with *N. meningitidis* have been reduced by early recognition and prompt treatment with antibiotics. However, the following complications may be detected: myocarditis, myopericarditis, congestive heart failure, cardiac conduction abnormalities, acute respiratory failure, disseminated intravascular coagulation, arthritis, cranial nerve dysfunction, skin necrosis, and adrenal insufficiency.

Ancillary studies aid in confirming a clinical suspicion of meningococcal infection. The diagnosis is confirmed with a positive culture of normally sterile body fluids such as cerebrospinal, blood, or synovial fluid. A positive Gram stain of CSF, petechial scrapings, or a smear of the buffy coat of the blood may identify infection before culture results are available.

If meningitis is suspected, a lumbar puncture should be performed. Abnormal CSF findings include elevated pressure, increased protein, decreased glucose, and a pleocytosis with a predominance of polymorphonuclear leukocytes. However, early in the disease there may be an absence of inflammatory cells associated with positive cultures for *N. meningitidis.*

Differential Diagnosis

The differential diagnosis of meningococcemia includes a variety of viral infections, Rocky Mountain spotted fever, typhus, typhoid fever, endocarditis, vasculitis, toxic shock syndrome, and acute rheumatic fever.

Treatment

The foundation of treatment for meningococcemia is prompt antibiotic therapy and supportive care. The antibiotic of choice is penicillin G 300,000 units/day IV up to a maximum dose of 24 million units/day in divided doses every 2 to 4 hours. Patients who are allergic to penicillin can be given chloramphenicol or third-generation cephalosporins.

To prevent epidemics, close contacts of the source of infection should undergo chemoprophylaxis. Current recommended therapy for meningococcal prophylaxis is rifampin 10 mg/kg (up to 600 mg) orally every 12 hours for 2 days. Patients should be warned that rifampin may discolor their urine and contact lenses. A meningococcal vaccine may be used to prevent epidemics in certain circumstances. Unfortunately no vaccine exists for the group B serotype, which is the most common source of meningococcal infection in the United States.

All patients suspected of having a meningococcal infection should be admitted to the hospital and kept under isolation. Universal precautions should be strictly enforced. Intensive care monitoring may be needed.

KAWASAKI SYNDROME

Kawasaki syndrome is a diffuse vasculitis of unknown cause that primarily affects young children. The clinical features are well described and an effective treatment program has been discovered, but the precise etiology is not known and no specific diagnostic test has been developed. The emergency physician has a key role in the diagnosis and institution of therapy for Kawasaki syndrome.

Epidemiology

The incidence of Kawasaki syndrome is highest in Asians but is found in virtually every race throughout the world. Most cases appear in children between 1 and 2 years of age, and more than 80% of all cases occur in children under the age of 5. The male to female ratio is 1:5. Most cases of this syndrome occur sporadically, but epidemics have been reported to occur.

Pathophysiology and Etiology

Over the years a number of etiologies have been considered, but Kawasaki syndrome presently is believed to be caused by an infectious agent. Despite extensive investigation, the exact cause has not been discerned. It is postulated that an infectious agent initiates an immunologic response that leads to a multisystem vasculitis and produces the classic clinical features of the illness. The major cause of morbidity and mortality is a result of vasculitis of the coronary arteries, which results in myocardial ischemia or infarction.

Clinical Findings

The diagnosis of Kawasaki syndrome is based on well-developed clinical criteria. The CDC (1985) has provided a case definition:

Fever lasting 5 days or more without other more reasonable explanations and at least four of the following criteria:
1. Bilateral conjunctival injection
2. At least one of the following mucous membrane changes: injected or fissured lips, injected pharynx, or strawberry tongue
3. At least one of the following extremity changes: erythema of palms or soles, edema of the hands or feet, or generalized or periungual desquamation
4. Rash
5. Cervical lymphadenopathy (at least one lymph node 1.5 cm or greater in diameter)

These clinical diagnostic criteria should serve as a guide to the physician. However, atypical cases may not exhibit all of the clinical features of the disease.

Each of the clinical criteria in the case definition is present in a majority of cases. The fever is high, spiking, and lasts 1 to 2 weeks. The conjunctival injection involves the bulbar conjunctiva more than the palpebral conjunctiva, and no exudate is seen. Mucous membrane changes occur, including an injected pharynx and injected, dry, and fissured lips. Prominent tongue papillae produce a "strawberry tongue" appearance similar to that of scarlet fever. The skin of the palms and soles are erythematous and painful. Desquamation of the skin of the fingers and toes occurs 10 to 20 days after the onset of illness. The rash appears within 5 days after the onset of fever and varies in appearance. Skin lesions may be scarlatiniform, urticarial, morbilliform, or maculopapular with or without target lesions. The trunk, perineum, and extremities are predominantly involved. Cervical adenopathy is usually unilateral and is the least common of the clinical findings. Less frequent findings include arthritis, arthralgias, irritability, aseptic meningitis, urethritis with sterile pyuria, myositis, myalgias, hepatitis, diarrhea, pneumonia, and hydrops of the gallbladder.

The most serious complications of Kawasaki syndrome affect the cardiovascular system. Early cardiac problems include myocarditis, congestive heart failure, pericarditis, pericardial effusions, mitral and aortic insufficiency, and cardiac dysrhythmias. Twenty percent of the patients develop coronary artery aneurysms and are at risk for myocardial infarction secondary to thrombosis or (less commonly) coronary artery aneurysm rupture. The mortality rate is less than 1%.

Kawasaki syndrome can be divided into three distinct clinical phases. The acute phase lasts for approximately 10 days and is characterized by fever and the acute findings described previously. During the subacute phase, the fever, rash, and adenopathy resolve. Desquamation, joint pains, and cardiac complications may be seen. The subacute phase lasts for approximately 10 to 25 days from the onset of the illness. The conva-

lescent phase begins when most of the clinical symptoms have subsided. Cardiac complications may appear or recur during this phase.

Although there is no diagnostic test for Kawasaki syndrome, ancillary studies are helpful in caring for the patient. Patients who are suspected of having this syndrome should undergo an ECG and an echocardiogram to establish a baseline or to search for cardiac complications. Typical laboratory abnormalities include leukocytosis with a shift to the left, a normochromic normocytic anemia, and thrombocytosis. The sedimentation rate becomes elevated early and is used to follow the course of the illness. Other tests may be needed to exclude other illnesses.

Differential Diagnosis

The differential diagnosis of Kawasaki syndrome includes scarlet fever, staphylococcal scalded skin syndrome, toxic shock syndrome, Rocky Mountain spotted fever, Stevens-Johnson syndrome, juvenile rheumatoid arthritis, drug eruptions, measles, various viral infections, and mercury toxicity.

Treatment

Oral aspirin and IV immune serum globulin compose the current treatment regimen for Kawasaki syndrome. Aspirin is given for its antithrombotic and antiinflammatory properties, and immune serum globulin is used for its antiinflammatory effect. The goal of therapy is to reduce the risk of developing coronary artery abnormalities. Other treatments may be needed to treat the cardiac complications of the disease.

During the acute phase of the syndrome, hospital admission may be necessary to confirm the diagnosis of Kawasaki syndrome, stabilize cardiac complications, or initiate treatment. In the subacute or convalescent phases, admission may be needed for the treatment of cardiac dysrhythmias, congestive heart failure, or myocardial ischemia.

TOXIC SHOCK SYNDROME

Toxic shock syndrome is a clinical syndrome that is characterized by fever, rash, hypotension, and multisystem involvement. This illness was first reported to occur in children by Todd and others in 1978. Widespread national attention was given to this disease after it was recognized that young women contracted a life-threatening illness that was associated with tampon use during menses. Over the last decade, the incidence of toxic shock syndrome has decreased, and general interest in this disease has declined. However, cases continue to occur; the emergency physician must be knowledgeable about this condition to correctly diagnose and treat it.

Epidemiology

Toxic shock syndrome occurs in two clinical settings. Menstrual toxic shock syndrome occurs in young, menstruating women who use high-absorbency tampons. Nonmenstrual toxic shock syndrome occurs in men, women, or children secondary to surgical wounds, infections, or a variety of other clinical situations. In the first few years after this disease was initially recognized, the menstrual form was more prevalent. In recent years, the incidence of both forms has become approximately equal. Most cases occur between the ages of 15 to 34 years, but any age can be affected.

Pathophysiology and Etiology

For toxic shock syndrome to develop, colonization or infection with *Staphylococcus aureus* must first occur; certain local conditions favor bacterial overgrowth. *S. aureus* has been detected in virtually all cases of both forms of the illness. *S. aureus* produces one or more toxins that enter the bloodstream. The organism is usually not invasive, because blood cultures are often negative. Toxic shock syndrome toxin (TSST) has been found in more than 90% of the menstrual cases and in 60% of the nonmenstrual cases; however, other exotoxins probably exist.

CASE DEFINITION OF TOXIC SHOCK SYNDROME

- Fever: temperature ≥38.9° C (102° F)
- Rash: diffuse macular erythroderma
- Desquamation: occurs 1 to 2 weeks after onset of illness, particularly on palms and soles of feet
- Hypotension: systolic blood pressure ≤ 90 mm Hg for adults or below fifth percentile by age for children under 16 years of age; orthostatic drop in diastolic blood pressure ≥ 15 mm Hg from lying to sitting; orthostatic syncope; or orthostatic dizziness
- Multisystem involvement—three or more of the following symptoms occur:
  Gastrointestinal: vomiting or diarrhea at onset of illness
  Muscular: severe myalgia or creatine phosphokinase level at least twice the upper limit of normal
  Mucous membrane: vaginal, oropharyngeal, or conjunctival hyperemia
  Renal: blood urea nitrogen or creatinine at least twice the upper limit of normal, or urinary sediment with pyuria (≥5 leukocytes per high-power field) in the absence of a urinary tract infection
  Hepatic: total bilirubin, AST*, ALT[†] at least twice the upper limit of normal
  Hematologic: platelets ≤100,000/mm³
  Central nervous system: disorientation or alterations in consciousness without focal neurologic signs with fever and hypotension are absent
- Negative results on the following tests, if obtained:
  Blood, throat, or cerebrospinal fluid cultures (blood culture may be positive for *S. aureus*)
  Rise in titer to Rocky Mountain spotted fever, leptospirosis, or rubeola

*AST denotes serum aspartate transaminase.
[†]ALT denotes serum alanine transaminase.

The toxins are transported to various body sites via the circulation, where they cause a systemic vasculitis that leads to the multisystem manifestations of the disease.

Clinical Findings

The CDC has published a clinical case definition of toxic shock syndrome (see the box on p. 713). Cases that do not meet the case definition are described as probable.

The major symptoms of toxic shock syndrome are fever, rash, and hypotension. The fever is high and abrupt in onset. The classical rash is a nonpruritic, diffuse, blanching, macular erythroderma. It may be subtle, and the patient must be carefully examined to detect the rash. The rash is seen best on the trunk, perineum, extremities, and mucous membranes. Desquamation occurs after 5 to 12 days. The hypotension is the result of an absolute or relative hypovolemia. The magnitude of the hypotension varies from postural hypotension to profound shock.

Because toxic shock syndrome involves virtually every organ system, a wide constellation of symptoms are seen. Gastrointestinal involvement leads to profuse diarrhea and vomiting. Muscular involvement causes severe myalgias. Mucous membranes of the oropharynx, vagina, and conjunctiva are hyperemic. Neurologic symptoms include headache and altered mental status. Acute renal failure may be seen.

In nonmenstrual cases, the surgical wound may not appear grossly infected, but if the wound is opened, some purulent drainage can usually be seen.

Complications of toxic shock syndrome include adult respiratory distress syndrome (ARDS), shock, gangrene, DIC, renal failure, and a constellation of neuropsychiatric symptoms. Recurrence of the menstrual form has been reported to occur.

Ancillary testing may be useful in distinguishing toxic shock syndrome from other illnesses and in providing supportive care for the patient.

Nonspecific laboratory findings are common. A complete blood count (CBC) may reveal leukocytosis with a shift to the left, normochromic normocytic anemia, and thrombocytopenia. Coagulation studies may show evidence of DIC. Liver enzymes and bilirubin are commonly elevated, and the MM band of creatine phosphokinase is elevated in most cases. Renal insufficiency results in elevation of the blood urea nitrogen (BUN) and creatinine. Cultures of the vagina, cervix, surgical wound, or site of focal infection are usually positive for *S. aureus*.

Differential Diagnosis

The diagnosis of toxic shock syndrome is made on a clinical basis after a consideration of the differential diagnosis. Other diseases to consider include Kawasaki syndrome, staphylococcal scalded skin syndrome, scarlet fever, Stevens-Johnson Syndrome, Rocky Mountain spotted fever, leptospirosis, meningococcemia, atypical measles, viral illnesses, and drug reactions.

Treatment

The foundation of treatment for toxic shock syndrome is supportive care. Hypotension is treated with large volumes of crystalloid intravenous fluids. Central venous pressure or Swan-Ganz monitoring may be needed. Vasopressors may also be needed to treat the hypotension. Tampons or other foreign bodies should be removed, the infections should be drained, and the surgical wounds should be opened. Administration of a penicillinase-resistant antibiotic does not affect the clinical course but may prevent recurrence of the syndrome. One retrospective study suggests that corticosteroids may be beneficial. Intubation and mechanical ventilation may be needed if ARDS develops, and dialysis is indicated if renal failure ensues.

All patients with suspected toxic shock syndrome should be admitted for monitoring and treatment. If shock or multisystem failure is present, intensive care admission is recommended.

KEY CONSIDERATIONS

WHAT IS THE LIFE THREAT?

Untreated diphtheria can cause respiratory distress from airway swelling and edema. Cardiac effects can include heart failure and conduction abnormalities. Pertussis and pneumococcus can cause a life-threatening infection of the airway and lung parenchyma. Infection with *N. meningitides* can cause fulminant infection, leading to death within hours. Toxic shock syndrome associated with *S. aureus* infection and the release of exotoxins can cause life-threatening hypotension and organ failure. Infection with *C. tetani* or *C. botulinum* results in a potentially fatal release of neurotoxins. Many acute bacterial infections necessitate hospital admission because of the potential for serious complications and death.

DOES THE PATIENT NEED ADMISSION?

Admit patients with bacterial sepsis or meningitis or immunocompromised patients with severe bacterial infections. Patients with bacterial infections that impair ventilation, cause hypotension, or are associated with the release of neurotoxins require hospital treatment. Kawasaki syndrome can lead to a variety of serious cardiovascular consequences, including myocardial infarction, coronary artery aneurysm rupture, and cardiac dysrhythmias.

WHAT IS THE MOST SERIOUS DIAGNOSIS?

Sepsis, meningitis, and infections that interfere with oxygenation or tissue perfusion are the most serious diagnoses. Less severe infections such as pneumococcal pneumonia tend to be considered more serious in elderly and immunocompromised patients.

HAVE I PERFORMED A THOROUGH WORK-UP?

Consider underlying illnesses such as diabetes and immunocompromise when evaluating patients with bacterial infections. A Gram stain and appropriate cultures are important aspects of patient evaluation.

Recommended Reading

Centers for Disease Control: Diphtheria, tetanus, and pertussis: recommendations for vaccine use and other preventive measures, *MMWR* 40:1, 1991.

Centers for Disease Control: Multiple outbreaks of Kawasaki's syndrome in the United States, *MMWR* 34:33, 1985.

Centers for Disease Control and Prevention: Resurgence of pertussis—United States, 1993, *MMWR* 42:952, 1993.

Chesney PJ: Clinical aspects and spectrum of illness or toxic shock syndrome, *Rev Infect Dis* 2:51, 1989.

Mandel GL, Bennett JE, Dolin R: *Mandel, Douglas and Bennett's principles and practice of infectious diseases,* ed 4, New York, 1995, Churchill Livingstone.

Ruthman JC, Hendricksen DK, Bonefeld R: Emergency department presentation of type A botulism, *Am J Emerg Med* 3:203, 1985.

Todd J et al: Toxic-shock syndrome associated with phage-group-I streptococci, *Lancet,* 2:116, 1978.

Turbiak TW, Reich JJ: Bacterial infections. In Rosen P et al, editors: *Emergency medicine: concepts and clinical practice,* St Louis, 1992, Mosby.

Wong VK, Hitchcock W, Mason WH: Meningococcal infection in children: a review of 100 cases, *Pediatr Infect Dis* 8:229, 1989.

Wright SW, Trott AT: Toxic shock syndrome: a review, *Ann Emerg Med* 17:268, 1988.

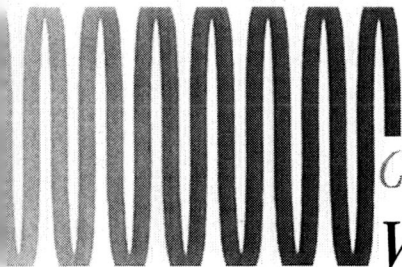

Chapter *Sixty*
VIRAL INFECTIONS

LINDA A. ROBINSON

Viruses are small particles of either DNA or RNA that are surrounded by a protein coat. Currently the classification of viruses is based on the type of nucleic acid present, the shape of the protein coat, and the presence of a lipid envelope.

Viruses are the cause of infections ranging from mild inconveniences to life-threatening illnesses. Therapy for such infections ranges from general supportive care to specific antiviral chemotherapy and active immunization (Tables 60-1 and 60-2).

A consideration of a range of viral infections according to disease type rather than viral classification should be helpful when evaluating and managing patients in the emergency department.

GASTROENTERITIS

In the United States, viral agents are an important cause of gastroenteritis. Rotaviruses are known for causing explosive diarrhea in infants, and adenoviruses are responsible for a milder illness in children and adults. The Norwalk virus has been responsible for localized epidemics of gastroenteritis. Vomiting and watery diarrhea are usually self-limited, but they can result in life-threatening dehydration in the pediatric patient. Spread of the infection occurs as a result of dissemination of infectious material via the fecal-oral route. Treatment involves providing supportive care through oral or parenteral hydration.

UPPER RESPIRATORY TRACT INFECTIONS

Colds

Adenoviruses, rhinoviruses, Coxsackie viruses A and B, and echoviruses are responsible for upper respiratory tract infections that are treated with supportive care. Patients with an underlying pulmonary disease, such as asthma, can have increased morbidity because of exacerbation of the underlying disease.

Croup

Croup is an infection of the upper airway in children less than 3 years of age; parainfluenza viruses are often the cause. Because of the variation in antigenic type, a past infection does not prevent recurrence of the disease. Typical upper respiratory tract symptoms are accompanied by a gradually worsening "croupy" cough. Symptoms last approximately 4 days, are worse at night, and can be treated with mist inhalation. Severe disease is marked by dyspnea and stridor. Some patients require hospitalization for treatment with supplemental oxygen and racemic epinephrine via aerosol. Intubation for

Table*60-1*

DRUGS FOR THE TREATMENT OF VIRAL ILLNESSES

Virus	Disease	Drug of Choice	Alternative Agents
Cytomegalovirus	Retinitis	Ganciclovir, 5 mg/kg IV bid for 14 to 21 days, then 5 mg/kg IV qd	Foscarnet,* 60 mg/kg IV tid for 14 to 21 days, then 90 to 120 mg/kg IV qd
	Colitis	Ganciclovir,* induction regimen as above, need for maintenance regimen not established	Foscarnet*
	Pneumonitis	Ganciclovir,* as above, with or without IV immune globulin, need for maintenance not established	Foscarnet*
Hepatitis B	Chronic hepatitis	Interferon alfa* dose to be determined	
Hepatitis C	Chronic hepatitis	Interferon alfa dose to be determined	
Herpes simplex virus	Genital herpes		
	Primary	Acyclovir, 200 mg PO 5 × d for 10 days	Acyclovir, 5 mg/kg q8h
	Recurrence	Acyclovir, 200 mg PO 5 × d for 5 days	
	Frequent recurrences	Acyclovir, 200 mg PO q8h to 5 × d for up to 1 year	
	Encephalitis	Acyclovir,* 10 mg/kg IV q8h	Vidarabine, 15 mg/kg IV qd for 10 days
	Mucocutaneous disease in immunocompromised patients	Acyclovir, 250 mg/m^2 IV q8h for 7 days, 400 mg PO 5 × d may be used,* oral regimens may provide effective prophylaxis	Foscarnet,* 40 to 60 mg/kg q8h
	Neonatal	Acyclovir,* 500 mg/m^2 IV q8h for 10 days	Vidarabine, 15 mg/kg IV qd for 10 days

Modified from Polis MA: Viral infections. In Rosen P et al, editors: *Emergency medicine: concepts and clinical practice*, ed 3, St Louis, 1992, Mosby.
*Not approved by the Food and Drug Administration for this indication.

Continued.

Table 60-1

DRUGS FOR THE TREATMENT OF VIRAL ILLNESSES—cont'd

Virus	Disease	Drug of Choice	Alternative Agents
Herpes simplex virus—cont'd	Keratoconjunctivitis	Trifluridine, 1% ophthalmic solution, 1 drop topically, q2h, up to 9 drops daily	Vidarabine, 3% ophthalmic ointment, 0.5 inch in lower conjuctival sac 5 × d for 7 to 21 days Idoxuridine, 0.1% ophthalmic solution, one drop q1h while awake, q2h at night; or 0.5% ophthalmic ointment, 5 × d
Influenza A virus	Influenza	Amantadine, 100 mg PO qd to bid for 5 to 7 days	Rimantadine,* 200 mg PO qd for 5 to 7 days
Respiratory syncytial virus	Severe bronchiolitis or pneumonia in infants and children	Ribavirin aerosol, 12 to 18 hours daily for 3 to 7 days with a 20 mg/ml concentration in reservoir	
Varicella-zoster virus	Varicella in immunocompromised patients	Acyclovir, 500 mg/m^2 IV q8h for 7 days	
	Herpes zoster in immunocompromised patients	Acyclovir, 10 mg/kg IV q8h for 7 days	Vidarabine, 10 mg/kg IV qd for 5 days
	Herpes zoster in normal hosts	Acyclovir, 800 mg PO 5 × d for 7 to 10 days	

airway maintenance is rarely necessary for croup but is indicated in the treatment of pediatric epiglottitis. Steroids have been found to be useful in the management of croup.

LOWER RESPIRATORY TRACT INFECTIONS

Bronchiolitis

Respiratory syncytial virus (RSV) is transmitted via infectious respiratory secretions and can cause bronchiolitis and pneumonia in infants.

Severe infection is more common in infants less than 6 months of age, and such patients often require hospitalization. Pneumonia can progress to respiratory failure. Treatment of severe disease involves supporting respiratory function. Ribaviran via aerosol has been used to treat hospitalized infants.

Flu

Influenza A and B can cause serious lower respiratory tract infections. Influenza A has been re-

Table 60-2

VIRAL VACCINES

Virus	Vaccine	Type	Indication	Recommended Schedule
Smallpox	Vaccinia	Live virus	None	None
Polio	Oral polio vaccine (Sabin) Salk vaccine	Live, attenuated virus	All normal infants and children	2, 4, 6, 15 months and at or before school entry
Measles	MMR*	Live, attenuated virus	All normal infants and children	15 months, repeat at preschool or at entrance to school after high school if no second dose had been given earlier
Mumps	MMR	Live, attenuated virus	All normal infants and children	15 months
Rubella	MMR	Live, attenuated virus	All normal infants and children	15 months
Hepatitis B	Inactivated Hepatitis B vaccine Recombinant Hepatitis B vaccine	Inactivated virus Recombinant viral component	Persons at risk for contracting hepatitis B sexually, occupationally, or perinatally	Three doses, given 1 month and 6 months after initial dose; hepatitis B immune globulin after perinatal, sexual, percutaneous exposure should also be given
Influenza A	Inactivated whole or split (disrupted) virus	Inactivated virus	Persons at high risk for complications Persons capable of transmitting influenza to high-risk persons Any person who wishes to reduce risk who has no contraindications to vaccination	1 dose yearly in adults of whole or split virus vaccine in adults in late fall or winter months 1 dose of split virus vaccine in children 2 doses in children who have not been previously vaccinated
Rabies	Human diploid cell vaccine Adsorbed rabies vaccine	Inactivated virus	Exposure to bite or scratch from infected or suspected animal	Five doses given on days 0, 3, 7, 14, and 28 after exposure Rabies immune globulin need also be given
Yellow fever	17D virus strain	Live, attenuated virus	Persons older than 6 months living in or traveling to endemic areas	Boosters every 10 years
Varicella-zoster	Varicella	Live, attenuated virus	Investigational	Investigational

From Polis MA: Viral infections. In Rosen P et al, editors: *Emergency medicine: concepts and clinical practice*, ed 3, St Louis, 1992, Mosby.
*Measles, mumps, rubella.

sponsible for epidemic and pandemic disease, whereas influenza B is responsible for more localized outbreaks. Mild episodes of either influenza A or B consist of fever, cough, sore throat, headache, and malaise. However, patients can also develop interstitial pneumonitis, which sometimes progresses to respiratory failure. Treatment of symptoms includes the use of antipyretics, decongestants, hydration, bronchodilators, supplemental oxygen, and ventilatory support as necessary. Mucosal and interstitial inflammation may lead to secondary bacterial pneumonia, which is often staphylococcal and requires specific antibiotic therapy.

Antiviral chemotherapy is available for influenza A infections. Amantadine must be started within the first 48 hours of infection to shorten the course of the illness. Treatment consists of 100 mg orally twice a day, but 100 mg orally only once per day should be considered for elderly patients and for patients with renal failure. Amantadine is not effective against influenza B infections.

Vaccinations against infections caused by influenza viruses are available and must be done on a yearly basis because of the antigenic variation of the responsible viruses from year to year. Such a vaccination is recommended for persons who are over the age of 65 years, those with cardiac or pulmonary disease, those who reside in institutions, and those who are immunosuppressed. Medical personnel who are in contact with those at risk for developing severe disease should also be vaccinated. The vaccine is derived from a whole attenuated or a split virus; the side effects of the vaccines currently in use are minimal.

VIRAL DISEASES OF CHILDHOOD

Measles

Rubeola is a highly contagious viral infection that is spread via respiratory secretions. The disease is characterized by a cough, conjunctivitis, a runny nose, fever, and finally a rash, which is erythematous, macular, and papular. The rash typically appears first on the head and face, spreads throughout the rest of the body, and finally becomes confluent. Koplik spots are pathognomonic of the disease; these spots are gray and are surrounded by erythema on the buccal mucosa. Acute complications of rubeola include pneumonitis, encephalomyelitis, and blindness. Death can occur in as many as 10% of the infants and malnourished children. A delayed complication of the infection is subacute sclerosing panencephalitis (SSPE). SSPE is a CNS disease of both white and gray matter, occurs in 1 out of every 100,000 cases, and is uniformly fatal. Infection during pregnancy may result in a stillbirth or in premature labor.

In general, treatment of rubeola is supportive. Passive immunization with immunoglobin for immunocompromised patients and infants less than 1 year of age is possible if given within 6 days of exposure.

Vaccination with a live attenuated virus is recommended at 15 months of age and is followed by a second dose before starting school. Between 2% and 5% of those vaccinated fail to seroconvert after a single dose. Persons engaged in patient care should be vaccinated if they are unable to document a past infection or two vaccinations.

German Measles

Rubella, also known as "three day measles," is a milder disease than rubeola and is characterized by fever, cephalgia, myalgia, rash, and adenopathy. Petechiae of the soft palate (Forchheimer's sign) may be seen. The most common complication of rubella is a temporary arthritis that involves the hands and knees.

Attempts are made to control this highly infectious but relatively benign disease because infection during pregnancy often results in birth defects or fetal death. If infection occurs during the first trimester, the probability that the fetus will be affected is 80% to 90%. Infection after the seventeenth week of pregnancy is unlikely to cause fetal problems. Associated birth defects include deafness, blindness, cardiac abnormalities, and mental retardation.

The rubella vaccine is made of live attenuated virus, and the seroconversion rate for a single dose is 95%. An initial vaccination is given at the age of 15 months and should be repeated when entering school. As in the case with rubeola, health care workers should be vaccinated if they are unable to document a previous infection or full immunization to rubella. Women should avoid pregnancy for 3 months if the vaccination is required.

Mumps

Mumps is typically characterized by fever and parotitis; other salivary glands may be involved to a lesser extent. As with rubella and rubeola, mumps is spread via respiratory secretions, and the patient is most infectious before the onset of symptoms. Mumps should be differentiated from bacterial parotitis because the treatment of mumps is purely supportive. Common complications of mumps include orchitis (10% to 15%), meningitis (10%), encephalitis (<0.15%), and fetal death in first-trimester infections. Myocarditis, deafness, transverse myelitis, pancreatitis, and arthritis can complicate mumps infections, but such an occurrence is rare.

Mumps is the third attenuated virus in the trivalent measles, mumps, rubella (MMR) vaccine. The vaccination is given at 15 months of age. Of those vaccinated, 95% will seroconvert. Testing for seroconversion is unnecessary if the immune status is in question, because there is no risk involved in vaccinating a person who is already immune.

Chickenpox

Varicella (chickenpox) is usually a childhood infection and is caused by the varicella-zoster

virus (VZV). VZV is a member of the herpes virus family. The infection is characterized by fever, malaise, and a pathognomonic rash that begins on the trunk and spreads peripherally. The lesions start as red papules, progress to vesicles on an erythematous base, and finally become crusted lesions. Typically, lesions of varying ages are present at the same time. Lesions of the mucosal membranes remain shallow ulcers.

Patients are infectious via their respiratory secretions for 5 days preceding the onset of the rash until 5 days after the onset of the rash, when all of the skin lesions have crusted over. A diagnosis of a varicella infection is usually made clinically, but a Tzanck preparation of the base of a vesicle should reveal multinucleate giant cells.

Although a varicella infection is a relatively mild illness, acute complications can include encephalitis, pneumonia, nephritis, and secondary bacterial infections of the skin lesions. Reye syndrome has been associated with varicella infections and the concomitant use of aspirin. Severe disseminated disease can occur in neonates and in the immunocompromised host. Persons considered to be at high risk for severe disseminated disease include those with AIDS, those with leukemia, or those who are undergoing chemotherapy. For the high-risk patient, the mortality rate is approximately 5%.

Shingles, or herpes zoster, is a late sequela of a varicella infection. Reactivation of the virus, which has been lying dormant in a dorsal root ganglion, results in painful vesicles along the dermatome of the dorsal root ganglion. Shingles usually appear in older individuals or in those with some degree of immunocompromise. Even after the lesions have healed, some patients experience severe pain that is difficult to treat. Of special concern is involvement of the dermatome surrounding the eye and tip of the nose, because the cornea can become involved, which can lead to blindness.

In the normal host, treatment for a varicella

infection is supportive. Aspirin should be avoided. Oral acyclovir has been investigated, but the cost outweighs the benefit. Hospital admission for administration of intravenous acyclovir is indicated for the patient who is immunocompromised or has complications such as varicella pneumonia. Persons at risk for developing severe disease who are not immune and have been exposed to a patient with chickenpox or shingles can be passively immunized with varicella zoster immune globin (VZIg) within 72 hours of exposure. A live attenuated viral vaccine has been developed but is not for routine use.

Treatment of shingles in the normal host includes oral acyclovir 800 mg five times daily for 7 days in addition to analgesia. Immunocompromised patients require intravenous therapy with either acyclovir or vidarabine.

SYSTEMIC VIRAL INFECTIONS

Infectious Mononucleosis

Epstein-Barr virus (EBV) is the causative agent of heterophile-positive mononucleosis, which is a syndrome characterized by fever, lymphadenopathy, fatigue, and exudative pharyngitis. In developed countries, this infection is usually seen in young adults and is spread via oral secretions. Symptoms last between 1 and 3 weeks. Hepatosplenamegaly is common, and the patient should be warned about the possibility of splenic rupture. Laboratory testing includes the monospot test for antibodies and the white blood cell differential smear, which should reveal atypical lymphocytes.

Treatment for mononucleosis consists of supportive care. Fewer than 1% of the patients develop a neurologic complication such as encephalitis, transverse myelitis, aseptic meningitis, and Guillain-Barré syndrome. The EBV has also been associated with lymphoma, carcinoma, and chronic fatigue syndrome.

Cytomegalovirus

Cytomegalovirus (CMV) is a herpes virus and in the normal host causes a mild viral syndrome or infectious mononucleosis. For children and adults, the infection is referred to as non-heterophile-positive mononucleosis. However, such an infection in the neonate and the immunocompromised patient is much more severe.

In the neonate, involvement of multiple organ systems is the rule; the central nervous system, liver, spleen, and lungs are involved. Neonates who survive are likely to have residual neurologic deficits. Immunocompromised patients start with a generalized infection, but most progress to a resistant single-organ involvement such as esophagitis, retinitis, or colitis.

Patients with a normal immune system do not require specific treatment or hospitalization, but neonates and patients who are immunocompromised do require hospitalization. Intravenous ganciclovir 5 mg/kg twice daily for 14 to 21 days followed by 5 mg/kg/day is the treatment of choice. Those with pneumonitis or multisystem involvement may benefit from the addition of immune globulin. Intravenous foscarnet is the alternate drug of choice.

Infectious Hepatitis

Hepatitis A virus (HAV) is the causative agent of infectious hepatitis, which is spread via the fecal-oral route and is common in children and adolescents. Most patients with infectious hepatitis have mild symptoms and never develop jaundice. As many as 50% of the adults in the United States test positive for past HAV infection. An HAV infection is not associated with a chronic carrier state, and infection results in lasting immunity. Passive immunization for HAV infection is also available. Susceptible individuals should receive a single intramuscular 0.02 ml/kg dose of immune globulin.

Serum Hepatitis

Hepatitis B virus (HBV) is the agent responsible for serum hepatitis, which is transmitted both percutaneously and via mucocutaneous contact with body fluids such as blood, saliva, and semen. The incubation period lasts 2 to 5 months. The infection may manifest as a mild viral syndrome, and the patient may not develop clinical jaundice. At the far end of the spectrum of disease is rapid onset of liver failure, encephalopathy, and coagulopathy with an 80% mortality rate. The overall mortality rate of serum hepatitis is 1%. A chronic carrier state exists for HBV infection.

Several tests are available to assess patient status and HBV infection. HBsAg is present during the initial infection with HBV and persists for several months after the jaundice has resolved. Anti-HB$_s$s appear in the serum several months after HBsAg has been cleared from the serum and indicates resolution of the infection and immunity to the disease. Chronic carriers have persistent HBsAg in the serum and do not develop anti-HB$_s$s. HBeAg is another marker of the chronic carrier state.

The outpatient treatment of serum hepatitis includes rest, adequate diet, avoidance of hepatotoxins (e.g., ethanol, acetaminophen), and follow-up care. Patients requiring admission include those with dehydration, hypoglycemia, coagulopathy, bilirubin >20 mg/dl, and an age over 45 years.

Both active and passive immunization are available for HBV infection. Active immunization consists of three intramuscular doses of a vaccine that is either derived from inactivated HBV or is produced via recombinant techniques. Adequate anti-HB$_s$ titers can be documented in more than 90% of those receiving the vaccine. Persons at high risk for contracting HBV through occupational or personal means should prophylactically receive the vaccine. Within 7 days of exposure to infectious material from an HBV-infected patient, hepatitis B immune globulin (HBIg) 0.06 ml/kg should be administered intramuscularly along with, but at a separate site from, the first dose of the HBV vaccine.

SEXUALLY TRANSMITTED VIRAL DISEASES

Herpes Simplex

Herpes simplex virus (HSV) type 1 is the causative agent of herpes labialis; HSV type 2 is the causative agent of herpes genitalis. However, depending on the mode of contact, either virus can be isolated from any mucous membrane lesion. HSV initially causes an infection in abraded skin or an intact mucous membrane. Lesions are vesicular on an erythematous base and appear in crops.

During the primary infection, the patient may experience fever, malaise, and lymphadenopathy. After the lesions heal, the virus lies dormant in the sensory nerve ganglia. Viral reactivation can occur by multiple triggers such as sunlight, stress, and fever. Infection resulting from reactivation usually results in a single lesion or very few lesions and no systemic symptoms.

Complications of HSV infection in the normal patient include keratitis, encephalitis, aseptic meningitis, and neonatal transmission. Neonatal herpes infection can result in a spectrum of illness that ranges from keratoconjunctivitis to systemic infection. Neurologic involvement is common in neonates and if untreated has a 70% mortality rate.

The treatment of choice for primary mucocutaneous herpes in the immunocompetent patient is oral acyclovir 200 mg five times daily for ten days. Mucocutaneous infection in an immunocompromised host, encephalitis, and neonatal herpes require intravenous acyclovir. Alternative agents include intravenous vidarabine and foscarnate. Herpes keratoconjunctivitis is treated with topical trifluridine or vidarabine. Acyclovir ointment is no longer used for mucocutaneous lesions.

Human Immunodeficiency Virus

Infection with the human immunodeficiency virus is discussed in Chapter 61.

VIRAL INFECTIONS OF THE NERVOUS SYSTEM

Polio

Poliovirus is the cause of paralytic poliomyelitis. Transmission occurs via the fecal-oral route and via respiratory secretions, and the infection is subclinical in as many as 95% of the patients. Paralytic disease is rare but the incidence increases with age. Type 1 and type 3 are more likely to cause paralytic disease. Paralytic polio occurs in four phases: viremic, recovery, meningitis, and paralysis. Paralysis should become apparent within 10 days of infection and lasts approximately 3 days. During that time, the patient is susceptible to aspiration pneumonia, pulmonary embolism, and respiratory failure. Myocarditis is a rare complication. Treatment consists of supportive care.

A vaccination for poliomyelitis is widely available in the United States and other developed countries. Inactivated poliovirus vaccine (IPV) prevents paralytic disease for the patient receiving it but does not contribute to herd immunity. Live attenuated oral poliovirus vaccine (OPV) confers immunity to the patient receiving it and contributes to herd immunity via secondary spread. Cases of paralytic polio have been associated with OPV.

Rabies

Rabies is a fatal infection of the central nervous system. Wild animals serve as a natural reservoir of this infection. Endemic areas in the United States include the middle and southern Atlantic, south central, and midwestern states. Animals implicated in rabies transmission include skunks, bats, raccoons, dogs, cats, foxes, and cows. Bites from rodents and rabbits do not carry a risk of rabies transmission. Contact with infectious secretions or tissue is sufficient for disease transmission.

Initial replication of the virus occurs in myocytes at the site of inoculation. Viral spread occurs via motor neurons to the dorsal root ganglia and finally to the central nervous system. After replicating in the brain, the virus spreads to the rest of the body via the peripheral nerves, and the patient's body fluids become infectious.

Incubation times average between 1 and 2 months. Initial symptoms are fever, malaise, cephalgia, anorexia, and painful paresthesia at the site of inoculation. After 4 days, symptoms relating to the central nervous system infection become apparent. Classically, patients are agitated and hypersensitive to sensory stimuli and have painful muscle spasms and hydrophobia. Coma and seizures precede death.

If left untreated rabies is uniformly fatal. No chemotherapy is presently available. Other than vigorous wound care, the only modes of therapy available are passive and active immunization. The decision to start the vaccination process is based upon the availability of the animal for observation, the history of animal vaccination, the likelihood of the presence of rabies in the area, the likelihood of rabies in the animal species involved, and the specific behavior of the animal. Because of the severity of the disease, the vaccination process should be initiated if there is a risk of transmission of rabies.

Passive immunization with rabies immune globulin (RIg) inactivates the virus and is used at the time of exposure. The patient receives 20 IU/kg of RIg; half of the dose is injected at the site of exposure and the rest is injected into the deltoid muscle. Active immunization with the human diploid cell rabies vaccine (HDCV) should be initiated in the opposite deltoid muscle at the time of exposure. The HDCV is given on days 0, 3, 7, 14, and 28. Postexposure vaccination is effective because of the long incubation time of the disease and the development of IgM antibodies by the third day and IgG antibodies by the seventh day. Preexposure prophylaxis consists of only three doses of HDCV and periodic boosters.

‖‖‖‖‖‖‖‖KEY CONSIDERATIONS

WHAT IS THE LIFE THREAT?

Certain viruses such as the Norwalk virus can cause gastroenteritis, vomiting, diarrhea, and life-threatening dehydration in children. Parainfluenza viruses that infect the airway can cause croup, which results in dyspnea and stridor. Viral infections of airways from the respiratory syncytial virus (RSV) can cause bronchiolitis in infants. Influenza viruses can result in pneumonitis, which can progress to respiratory failure.

Hepatitis B virus (HBV) can cause severe hepatitis and result in liver failure, encephalopathy, and co-agulopathy that can be fatal. Herpes simplex infection of the central nervous system can be fatal, especially in neonates. Rabies infection of the nervous system has a high mortality even if treated aggressively and is uniformly fatal if untreated.

DOES THE PATIENT NEED ADMISSION?

Hospitalize patients who have a respiratory impairment that is leading to hypoxemia and persists despite treatment. Infants with severe vomiting and diarrhea may require admission for symptomatic treatment and to correct fluid and electrolyte imbalances associated with dehydration. Admit patients with herpes simplex encephalitis or severe liver failure associated with hepatitis B infection. Admit patients with rabies.

WHAT IS THE MOST SERIOUS DIAGNOSIS?

Viral infections can be much more severe in immunocompromised patients and in neonates. Examples of such viral infections include cytomegalovirus (CMV), varicella virus, and herpes simplex virus infections. A rubella infection during the first trimester of pregnancy affects the fetus and results in associated birth defects; mumps infection in a pregnant patient during the first trimester has been associated with fetal death.

HAVE I PERFORMED A THOROUGH WORK-UP?

Evaluate oxygenation status in patients with respiratory distress caused by viral infection. Evaluate for dehydration in the neonate or infant who has viral gastroenteritis. Provide passive immunization within 6 days of exposure to infants and immunocompromised patients who have been exposed to rubeola (measles). If the patient develops mumps, evaluate for orchitis, meningitis, and encephalitis. With a varicella infection, consider such complications as encephalitis and pneumonia, especially in immunocompromised patients, neonates, and patients who are pregnant.

Recommended Reading

Barkin RM et al: *Pediatric emergency medicine: concepts and clinical practice*, St Louis, 1992, Mosby.

Polis MA: Viral infections. In Rosen P et al, editors: *Emergency medicine: concepts and clinical practice*, ed 3, St Louis, 1992, Mosby.

Sanford JP, Gilbert DN, Sande MA: *Guide to antimicrobial therapy 1995*, Dallas, 1995, Antimicrobial Therapy.

Tintinalli, Krome, Ruiz: *Emergency medicine: a comprehensive study guide*, New York, 1992, McGraw-Hill.

Chapter Sixty-one

HUMAN IMMUNODEFICIENCY VIRUS INFECTION AND AIDS

JOANNE WILLIAMS AND DOUGLAS A. RUND

Human immunodeficiency viruses type 1 (HIV-1) and type 2 (HIV-2) are RNA retroviruses that attach to CD4 T lymphocytes and to the cells of the central nervous system. In humans, infection with the HIV virus causes the acquired immunodeficiency syndrome (AIDS).

AIDS was first recognized in the United States in 1981 when the Centers for Disease Control (CDC) reported unusual occurrences of *Pneumocystis carinii* pneumonia (PCP) and Kaposi sarcoma in previously healthy homosexual men in California and New York. The recognition that AIDS could be transmitted through contaminated blood followed reports of the development of AIDS in intravenous (IV) drug users, recipients of blood transfusions, and patients with hemophilia who had received blood-derived coagulation factors. HIV has been isolated from blood, blood products, semen, vaginal secretions, saliva, tears, cerebrospinal fluid, synovial fluid, and amniotic fluid. It is transmitted through homosexual and heterosexual contact and via transplacental transmission in utero. The largest increase in AIDS infection is now occurring in teenagers and young adults, primarily from heterosexual contact. In the United States, AIDS is now the leading cause of death among those between the ages of 25 and 44 years.

The prevalence of HIV infection in the inner-city emergency department is estimated to be between 4% and 9%. Because the infection is unrecognized in many HIV-positive patients, universal precautions are necessary in the emergency department when dealing with procedures involving potential blood exposure.

An HIV infection ultimately causes the profound immunodeficiency that is the hallmark of AIDS. Continuing viral replication eventually results in functional impairment and eventual depletion of CD4 T lymphocytes. Counts for T lymphocytes that are lower than 200/mm^3 result in such impaired immunity that the host becomes susceptible to a variety of opportunistic infections, including mononucleosis, tuberculosis, tinea corporis, tinea pedis, *Candida albicans, Pneumocystis carinii, Mycobacterium avium-intracellulare* complex (MAI), and cytomegalovirus (CMV).

In association with known HIV infection, the presence of certain opportunistic infections and indicator conditions leads to a diagnosis of AIDS. Infection of CNS cells leads to cerebral atrophy and AIDS-dementia complex. The period from the initial infection with HIV to the development of AIDS is typically 7 to 9 years in adults and 2 years in children.

Initial infection with HIV results in a viremia

Table *61-1*

CDC CLASSIFICATION OF HIV INFECTION

Group	Description
I	Acute infection (either asymptomatic or resembling glandular fever) after which seroconversion occurs
II	Asymptomatic infection that leads either to an intermediate stage (Group III) or directly to AIDS (Group IV)
III	Characterized by palpable glands in two or more extrainguinal sites for >3 months
IV	AIDS

associated with a set of symptoms known as the "acute HIV syndrome." The syndrome resembles mononucleosis and includes symptoms such as fever, malaise, arthralgia, myalgia, and lymphadenopathy. This acute syndrome eventually subsides and is typically followed by a long asymptomatic period. As the infection continues, new stages develop (Table 61-1). Adenopathy in two or more extrainguinal sites for more than 3 months characterizes the stage of development preceding AIDS.

CD4 T-CELL COUNT AND STAGING OF HIV DISEASE

The CD4 T-cell count provides an important clue to the potential severity of HIV infection (Fig. 61-1). A CD4 count of 500 to 1000/mm^3 or greater is typically seen early in the infection. As the count drops close to 500/mm^3, certain opportunistic infections (e.g., tinea pedis, candidal vaginitis) and lymphadenopathy develop. Counts between 200 and 500/mm^3 are associated with thrush, oral hairy leukoplakia, and bacterial pneumonia. Counts of less than 200/mm^3 are associated with the advanced stages of the disease, including severe opportunistic infections (CMV, PCP, and MAC) and ultimate death.

The total lymphocyte count provides an esti-

mate of the CD4 count. A total lymphocyte count less than 2000/mm^3 may well be associated with a CD4 T-cell count of less than 200/mm^3. A total lymphocyte count of 1000/mm^3 or less indicates a strong likelihood that the CD4 T-cell count is less than 200/mm^3.

CLINICAL PRESENTATION AND TREATMENT

Pneumonia

The lung is the most common site of serious infection in patients who have AIDS, and *P. carinii* is the most common pathogen. With the advent of pneumocystis pneumonia prophylaxis (trimethoprim-sulfamethoxazole, or TMP-SMX), this pathogen appears to be occurring less commonly and at a more advanced stage of disease. Patients infected with HIV are also at an increased risk for acquiring pneumonia because of bacteria and mycobacteria.

Classically, pneumocystis pneumonia has a subacute presentation with symptoms such as fever, malaise, and fatigue. Shortness of breath and a dry cough may occur; the shortness of breath may only occur with exertion. The diagnosis of pneumocystis pneumonia depends on demonstrating the presence of *P. carinii* by staining induced sputum or performing a bronchoalveolar lavage.

"Typical" Course of HIV Infection

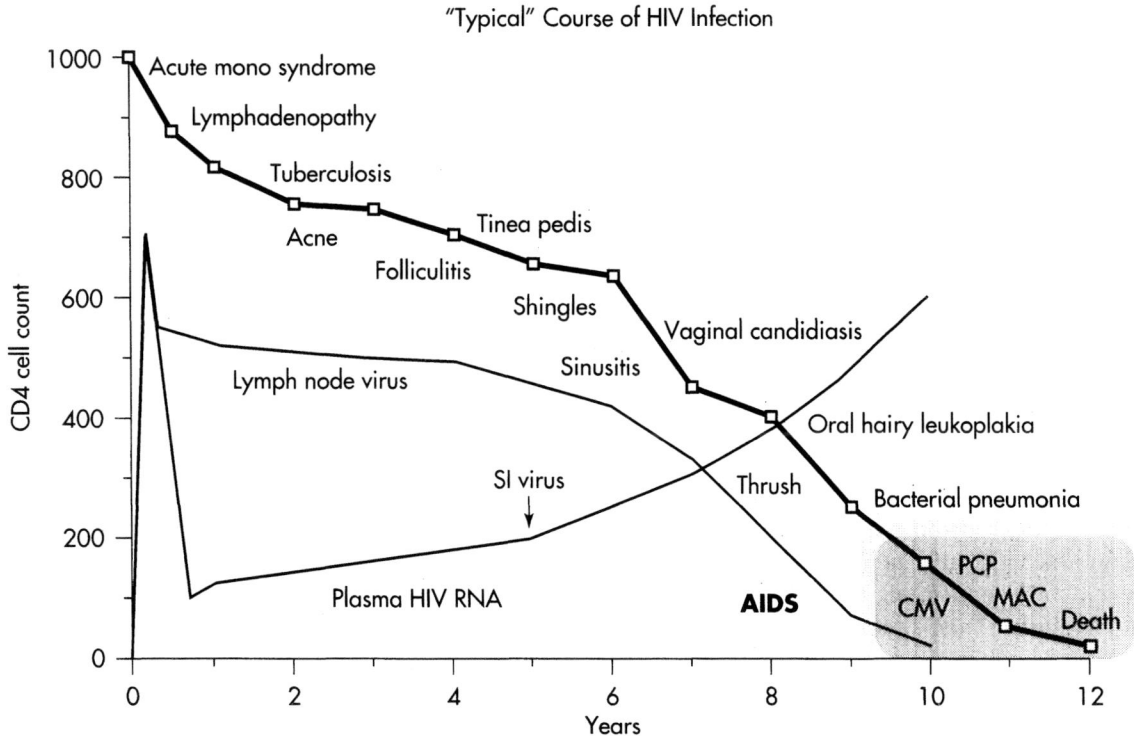

Fig. 61-1   Relationship of CD4 T-cell count to duration (in years) of HIV infection. Heavy line shows clinical features. Medium-heavy line shows plasma HIV RNA, and light line shows lymph node virus. (Courtesy of Michael Para, MD, Division of Infectious Diseases, The Ohio State University.)

Ordering a chest x-ray study is one of the first steps in diagnosing pneumocystis pneumonia. Unfortunately, the classic radiographic finding of a diffuse interstitial infiltrate may not be present. Findings can range from a normal chest x-ray film (early manifestation) to the appearance of nodular or lobar infiltrates, hilar lymphadenopathy, pleural effusion, apical infiltrates, spontaneous pneumothorax, and cavitation.

Patients with a PO_2 below 70 mm Hg, a low PCO_2, increased lactic dehydrogenase (LDH), an abnormal chest x-ray study, and rales on auscultation of the chest should be admitted to the hospital, because these findings are predictive of a poor outcome. Recurrent pneumocystis

pneumonia increases the risk of mortality; therefore such patients, as well as those deemed unreliable and at greater risk for lack of follow-up, should be admitted.

Treatment may begin in the emergency department, and oxygen supplementation should be provided. The drug of choice is IV trimethoprim-sulfamethoxazole. The usual therapy is 20 mg/kg of trimethoprim and 100 mg/kg of sulfamethoxazole in four divided doses; treatment is continued for 21 days. As many as 50% of the patients receiving this regimen develop side effects that may range from a mild skin rash to neutropenia and anemia. Treatment usually can be continued in the presence of mild adverse reactions.

An alternative drug for patients who are unable to tolerate trimethoprim-sulfamethoxazole is IV pentamidine 4 mg/kg/day. Because this drug may cause hypotension, it must be administered very slowly over the period of an hour. Pentamidine can also cause pancreatic islet-cell destruction that can result in irreversible diabetes mellitus; therefore blood glucose levels should be carefully monitored. A concomitant drug should be used with pentamidine because pentamidine does not provide bacterial coverage.

Patients who have a mild illness are managed on an outpatient basis with a 21-day course of trimethoprim-sulfamethoxazole (one double-strength tablet four times a day). Patients should be closely monitored because patients with AIDS are more prone to having adverse reactions to trimethoprim-sulfamethoxazole than patients who are not HIV-positive.

Bacterial pneumonia may not be distinguished from *P. carinii*, but trimethoprim-sulfamethoxazole is effective against the most common bacterial pathogens.

Tuberculosis (TB) is probably the most common secondary infection with HIV infection. It is more virulent than *P. carinii* and tends to occur at an earlier stage of AIDS. Many of the recent outbreaks of TB in the AIDS population have involved multidrug-resistant strains. To reduce the risk of transmission to health care workers, the patient should be given a mask and placed in isolation immediately. Ordinary surgical masks are not effective in blocking the transmission of TB. High-efficiency particulate respirator masks capable of filtering out the 1- to 5-micron tubercular organisms are the only masks currently recommended by the CDC.

If proper isolation facilities are not available, a room should be designated for the isolation of patients with suspected or confirmed TB. Circulating acid-fast bacilli may be reduced with air disinfection using portable high-efficiency particulate air filters or ultraviolet lamps. Patients should remain in isolation until TB has been ruled out. The current recommendation for

therapy is a four-drug regimen of isoniazid, rifampin, pyrazinamide, and either ethambutol or streptomycin.

Central Nervous System Disease

Central nervous system infections are the second most common infections in AIDS. Toxoplasmosis (by far the most common CNS infection) occurs in approximately 5% to 15% of all patients with AIDS. Cryptococcal meningitis is also commonly seen. Other opportunistic pathogens have been identified as causing CNS infections, including *Mycobacterium tuberculosis, Coccidioides immitis, Histoplasma capsulatum,* cytomegalovirus, and syphilis.

A CNS infection is typically evaluated with a CT scan and lumbar puncture. A CT scan with contrast should be considered for all AIDS patients with new CNS-related symptoms, such as headache, fever, or altered mental status. As with any patient, empirical antibiotic treatment should proceed immediately (before the CT scan and lumbar puncture) if the patient with AIDS has a fulminant, rapidly progressing illness indicative of an acute bacterial meningitis.

With toxoplasmosis, the CT scan typically shows multiple bilateral lesions in the cortical or subcortical regions of the brain. Administration of contrast typically demonstrates lesions with ring enhancement. If only a single lesion is visualized (as is seen in 20% of all toxoplasmosis cases), other diagnoses should be considered. Patients with toxoplasmosis should be admitted and treated empirically with pyrimethamine and sulfadiazine. It is not necessary to start therapy in the emergency department.

As with toxoplasmosis, cryptococcal meningitis may appear only as a fever or headache. Unlike bacterial meningitis, cryptococcal meningitis tends to develop slowly. The sensitivity of the cryptococcal antigen test is 91%. Because of the insidious nature of the illness, this antigen test may provide the only indication of cryptococcal meningitis. If the cryptococcal antigen is positive, the patient should be contacted for immediate follow-up. If symptoms are minimal, some specialists initiate outpatient therapy with oral fluconazole and close follow-up. Other specialists elect to admit such patients with IV therapy of amphotericin B.

When mass lesions have been ruled out by a CT scan, a lumbar puncture should be considered to evaluate new CNS symptoms. Spinal fluid cultures should be sent to rule out a bacterial infection, TB, meningitis, or other opportunistic pathogens. A Venereal Disease Research Laboratory (VDRL) test should be done on the cerebrospinal fluid because there is a high incidence of neurosyphilis among those who are HIV positive.

CMV retinitis must be considered when the patient with AIDS experiences a painless loss of vision. The lesions of CMV retinitis often cannot be identified through ophthalmoscopic examination in the emergency department. The HIV-positive patient who has suspected CMV retinitis should be evaluated by an ophthalmologist. A patient who has AIDS and confirmed CMV retinitis is admitted to the hospital for a 2- to 3-week course of induction therapy with ganciclovir or foscarnet. Unfortunately, lifelong IV therapy through an indwelling IV catheter is required to prevent relapses.

Gastrointestinal Disease

Diarrhea and dysphagia are the most common gastrointestinal complaints in the patient who is HIV positive. Diarrhea is often debilitating and is difficult to treat because the exact underlying cause is unknown or because the pathogens are resistant to therapy.

Antibiotic therapy in the HIV-positive patient with diarrhea is geared toward the causative pathogen. Stool samples should be cultured and examined for ova and parasites. Fluids and electrolytes should be closely monitored and corrected as needed.

Esophagitis in the patient with AIDS is often a result of *Candida albicans,* but it has also been caused by CMV and the herpes simplex virus. Patients with esophagitis who appear debilitated and are unable to tolerate oral intake should be admitted to the hospital for definitive treatment. For mild cases of esophagitis, patients can be treated with oral fluconazole 200 mg/day on an outpatient basis.

Table 61-2

ADVERSE EFFECTS OF MEDICATIONS USED IN HIV INFECTION

Drug	Effect
AZT	Granulocytopenia, anemia, nausea, fatigue, myositis
ddI	Pancreatitis, peripheral neuropathy, hypocalcemia, hypokalemia, diarrhea, dysrhythmias
ddC	Peripheral neuropathy, rash, fever, oral ulcers, neutropenia
Stavudine	Peripheral neuropathy, pancreatitis
TMP-SMX	Rash, neutropenia, anemia
Pentamidine	Hypotension, hypoglycemia, hyperglycemia, hyperkalemia, dysrhythmias
Dapsone	Anemia, hemolysis in patients deficient in glucose-6-phosphate dehydrogenase (G6PD)
Fluconazole	Drug interactions such as with warfarin, phenytoin, or antihistamines
Glanciclovir	Bone marrow suppression, increases in liver function test results

Patients may appear to have a suspected disease process associated with AIDS when in fact they may be suffering an adverse reaction to one of the drugs currently being taken. There-fore it is important to be aware of the potential toxicities associated with each drug being used in a patient's treatment (Table 61-2).

KEY CONSIDERATIONS

WHAT IS THE LIFE THREAT?

HIV infection progresses to AIDS, which is eventually fatal. A CD4 T-cell count of less than $200/mm^3$ predisposes the patient to severe opportunistic infections that are difficult to treat. Such infections include PCP, MAI, CMV, and drug-resistant tuberculosis. Certain neoplasms are associated with AIDS, including Hodgkin disease and non-Hodgkin lymphoma. Severe wasting, dementia, progressive weakness, anorexia, and serious infections often are terminal developments.

DOES THE PATIENT NEED ADMISSION?

It is recommended that patients with the initial onset of *Pneumocystis carinii* pneumonia (PCP) be admitted if they have a Po_2 less than 70 mm Hg, have an arterial-alveolar oxygen gradient greater than 35, an increased lactic dehydrogenase, and an abnormal chest x-ray study. Patients with recurrent PCP and those deemed unreliable in regard to obtaining follow-up are also admitted.

Isolate patients with drug-resistant tuberculosis who require admission. Admit patients with a CNS infection resulting from toxoplasmosis, tuberculosis, CMV, and cryptococcal meningitis.

Admit the patient who has esophagitis resulting from *Candida albicans* if he or she cannot tolerate oral intake. In general, patients who require admission include those who cannot sustain oral intake, those who cannot function as outpatients, and those with significant new alterations in vital signs or mental status. Patients with seizures, worsening hypoxemia, and severe volume depletion require admission.

WHAT IS THE MOST SERIOUS DIAGNOSIS?

The occurrence of opportunistic infections and neoplasms in the patient who has a CD4 count lower than $200/mm^3$ is a serious event in terms of life threat. Infections of the central nervous system, severe pulmonary infections, and advanced cachexia and dementia are serious conditions. Hodgkin disease and non-Hodgkin lymphoma are serious neoplasms associated with AIDS.

HAVE I PERFORMED A THOROUGH WORK-UP?

Suspect an undiscovered HIV infection in all emergency patients, and use universal precautions accordingly. An evaluation for opportunistic infections and neoplasms can include a complete blood count, electrolytes, a chest x-ray study, and an examination and culture of blood, urine, and CSF.

Liver function tests, a VDRL test, and serologic testing for *Toxoplasma, Coccidioides* and *Cryptococcus* antigens are appropriate. Consider a CT scan and lumbar puncture for those with a suspected CNS infection, including a brain abscess, encephalitis, and meningitis.

Recommended Reading

Bale AP, Gray JA: *Color guide to infectious diseases,* New York, 1993, Churchill Livingstone.

Centers for Disease Control and Prevention, AIDS Hotline.

Jewett JF, Hecht FM: Preventive health care for adults with HIV infection, *JAMA* 269:1144, 1993.

Kelen GD et al: Human immunodeficiency virus infection in emergency department patients: epidemiology, clinical presentations and risk to health care workers: the Johns Hopkins experience, *JAMA* 262:516, 1989.

Kelen GD, editor: HIV interface with emergency medicine, *Emerg Med Clin North Am*, 13(1):1-221, 1995.

Lane HC et al: Recent advances in the management of AIDS-related opportunistic infections, *Ann Intern Med* 120:945, 1994.

Talan DA, Kennedy CA: The management of HIV-related illness in the emergency department, *Ann Emerg Med* 20:1355, 1991.

Varghese GK, Crane LR: Evaluation and treatment of HIV-related illness in the emergency department, *Ann Emerg Med* 24(3): 503-511, 1994.

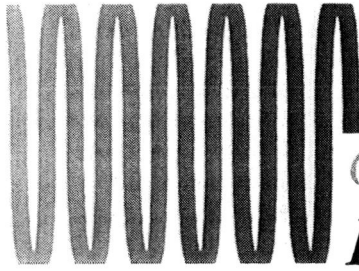

Chapter Sixty-two
PARASITIC DISEASE

RICHARD JOSEPH RYAN AND W. BRIAN GIBLER

Four groups of parasitic organisms cause disease in humans: protozoa, nematodes, cestodes, and trematodes. All diseases caused by these organisms can usually be diagnosed through methods available to most emergency physicians. Protozoan infestation may cause malaria, amebiasis, giardiasis, or a number of other maladies. Helminths, or worms, are responsible for a wide variety of human disease. These worms include the nematodes (roundworms), cestodes (tapeworms), and trematodes (flukes). Treatment for most parasitic diseases is usually effective and generally minimally toxic to the human host.

MALARIA

It has been estimated that 2 billion people live in areas of the world in which malaria is endemic. Each year 100 to 300 million new cases of malaria are reported, with 1 to 2 million deaths. Malaria has become resistant to various medical therapies; the *Anopheles* mosquito is resistant to certain insecticides; and international travel continues to expose a large number of nonimmune individuals to the malaria parasite. It is estimated that 30,000 American and European travelers contract malaria every year.

Four species of malaria are responsible for human disease: *Plasmodium falciparum, Plasmodium ovale, Plasmodium vivax,* and *Plasmodium malariae. P. falciparum* is respon-sible for approximately 50% of the cases of malaria and more than 95% of the fatalities.

The clinical signs and symptoms associated with malaria reflect the plasmodium life cycle. The female *Anopheles* mosquito ingests blood meals from dusk to dawn and is the vector responsible for malaria transmission. The mosquito ingests gametocytes from a malaria-infested human host. The gametocytes sexually reproduce within the gut of the mosquito and form *sporozoites*. Sporozoites are then released from the salivary glands of the mosquito and into a human host during a blood meal. Malaria may also bypass the mosquito vector and be acquired through needle sharing, congenital transmission, and blood transfusion.

Within minutes to hours, the sporozoites injected into the human bloodstream by the mosquito are sequestered in hepatocytes. During the asymptomatic exoerythrocytic phase, the uninucleate sporozoites mature and multiply asexually in the liver over a 1- to 2-week period. In the liver the sporozoites develop into *mature liver stage schizonts*. Each schizont develops into 10,000 to 40,000 uninucleate *merozoites*. With the eventual lysis of the hepatic cells, the merozoites enter the bloodstream and invade the erythrocytes. Once in the erythrocyte, each uninucleate merozoite develops into a trophozoite and finally to a mature *erythrocytic stage schizont* with 10 to 35 merozoites. The erythrocyte then lyses and releases merozoites into the bloodstream. Each merozoite can reinvade an erythrocyte, which initiates the cycle of amplification, rupture, and reinvasion. This cycle leads to increasing levels of parasitemia and the pathologic and clinical manifestations of malaria. After several erythrocytic cycles, the process may change, and male or female *gametocytes* may develop instead of merozoites. When a mosquito ingests blood that is infected with microgametocytes, the microgametocytes develop into sporozoites that can infect other humans.

The clinical manifestations of malaria occur after the rupture of infected erythrocytes and include shaking chills followed by fever. Such manifestations usually occur within 2 weeks after the mosquito bite. Few clinical manifestations are associated with the presence of sporozoites in the blood after inoculation by the mosquito or parasite development within the hepatocyte. The duration and cycling of clinical manifestations depends on the *Plasmodium* species involved. *P. vivax* and *P. ovale* are associated with rigors that occur at 48-hour intervals and last 1 to 8 hours, whereas the *P. malariae* manifestations occur at 72-hour intervals. The *P. falciparum* manifestations last 36 hours and occur every 36 to 48 hours. *P. vivax* and *P. ovale* sporozoites may take months or years to develop into merozoites, which explains the long relapses that are possible with infestation from these species.

Signs and symptoms of malaria develop within 2 weeks of exposure in the majority of patients and are related to the parasite-laden erythrocyte. Erythrocytes lose their membrane flexibility and may sludge, obstruct, and eventually infarct smaller blood vessels. Sludging in the cerebral vasculature can cause seizures, altered mental status, stupor, and coma. Occlusion of pulmonary vasculature can induce pulmonary edema and adult respiratory distress syndrome. Azotemia and acute renal failure may occur with sludging in the renal vessels. As a result of splenic sequestration of the abnormal erythrocytes, the spleen typically becomes engorged and may rupture. In addition, most patients develop anemia secondary to both acute and chronic hemolysis. Blackwater fever, which is hemoglobinuria that results from severe hemolysis, may be seen in patients with chronic falciparum malaria and may also present as a sudden, life-threatening event. Malaria should be sought in any patient with a febrile illness who has travelled to a malaria-infested area during the past 2 to 3 years or who has emigrated from such a locale. Malaria should be included in the differential diagnosis of any patient with a fever of unknown origin.

The diagnosis of malaria is made by the examination of thin and thick peripheral blood smears prepared with a Giemsa or Wright stain. The malaria parasite is usually visualized in the thick blood film within the erythrocyte; the thin smear is often used for species determination. Because parasitemia is usually greatest within 6 to 8 hours of a temperature spike, blood samples examined during this time may be more sensitive in identifying the parasite. To demonstrate the presence of the parasite, blood sample should be examined every 12 hours for several consecutive days.

The treatment of malaria is based on travel history and on the severity of the disease because different species are endemic to certain areas of the world. The treatment of straightforward attacks of malaria is often successful with chloroquine phosphate unless the parasite is resistant to chloroquine. A knowledge of the patient's travel history should allow the physician to determine whether chloroquine-resistant malaria may have been endemic at the locations visited during travel. Quinine sulfate plus pyrimethamine-sulfadoxine is recommended if chloroquine resistance is present. For severe cases that require parenteral therapy, quinidine gluconate is recommended for both chloroquine- and non–chloroquine-resistant malaria (Table 62-1).

Chloroquine is also used for the prevention

Table*62-1*

TREATMENT OF MALARIA

		Adult Dosage	Pediatric Dosage
Malaria			
Oral			
Drug of choice:	Chloroquine phosphate	600 mg base (1 gram), then 300 mg base (500 mg) 6 hr later, then 300 mg base (500 mg)/d × 2d	10 mg base/kg (max 600 mg base), then 5 mg base/kg 6 hrs later, then 5 mg base/kg/d × 2d
Parenteral			
Drug of choice:	Quinidine gluconate	10 mg/kg loading dose (max 600 mg) in normal saline slowly over 1 to 2 hrs, followed by continuous infusion of 0.02 mg/kg/min until oral therapy can be started	Same as adult dose
	or		
	Quinine dihydrochloride	20 mg salt/kg loading dose in 10 ml/kg 5% dextrose over 4 hrs, followed by 10 mg salt/kg over 2-4 hrs q8h (max 1800 mg/d) until oral therapy can be started	Same as adult dose
Chloroquine-resistant *P. falciparum*			
Oral			
Drugs of choice:	Quinine sulfate plus pyrimethamine-sulfadoxine	650 mg tid × 3d 3 tabs at once on last day of quinine	25 mg/kg/d in 3 doses × 3d <1 yr = ¼ tablet 1-3 yrs = ½ tablet 4-8 yrs = 1 tablet 9-14 yrs = 2 tablets
	or plus tetracycline	250 mg qid × 7d	20 mg/kg/d in 4 doses × 7d (>8 yrs)
	or plus clindamycin	900 mg tid × 3d	20-40 mg/kg/d in 3 doses × 3d
Alternatives:	Mefloquine	1250 mg × 1 dose	25 mg/kg × 1 dose (<45 kg)
	Halofantrine	500 mg q6h × 3 doses, repeat in 1 wk	8 mg/kg q6h × 3 doses (<40 kg); repeat in 1 wk
Parenteral Drug of choice:	Quinidine gluconate	Same as above	Same as above
	or		
	Quinine dihydrochloride	Same as above	Same as above
Prevention of relapses: *P. vivax* and *P. ovale* only			
Drug of choice	Primaquine phosphate	15 mg base (26.3 mg)/d × 14d or 45 mg base (79 mg)/wk × 8 wks	0.3 mg base/kg/d × 14d

Modified from *Med Lett Drugs Ther*, 35:111-122, 1993.

of malaria by those traveling to an area known to have endemic malaria. If chloroquine resistance has been reported in a particular area, mefloquine or doxycycline is instead recommended for prophylaxis.

Critically ill patients or those in which more than 3% of the erythrocytes contain parasites are best treated in the intensive care unit with intravenous (IV) medication. A transfusion may be necessary depending on the degree of anemia secondary to hemolysis. For severe parasitemia (more than 5% to 10% of the erythrocytes have parasites), exchange transfusion may be required. Serum glucose and acid-base status should be monitored carefully.

GASTROINTESTINAL INFESTATION

The gastrointestinal (GI) tract is often associated with parasitic disease. The diagnosis of many parasitic infestations relies on the identification of ova, cysts, ameba, larvae, or worms in the patient's stool. The stool is also used to monitor the effectiveness of therapy in the treatment of many parasitic diseases.

Gastrointestinal disease may be caused by many groups of parasites. Protozoans that infest the GI tract include *Giardia lamblia, Entamoeba histolytica,* and *Cryptosporidium* organism. The nematodes (roundworms) that cause GI disease include *Ascaris lumbricoides, Strongyloides stercoralis, Trichuris trichiura, Enterobius vermicularis,* and the hookworms *Necator americanus* and *Ancylostoma duodenale.*

Giardiasis

Giardiasis is a result of infestation with *G. lamblia* and currently infests more than 200 million people throughout the world. Transmission results from direct person-to-person contact or from fecal contamination of food or water. Several outbreaks of giardiasis in the United States have been traced to contaminated water supplies, and campers drinking untreated water in the Rocky Mountains have also become infested. Day-care facilities are also often responsible for large outbreaks.

Once the *Giardia* cysts are ingested they produce the active, motile-feeding trophozoite. These trophozoites reproduce by binary fission in the duodenum and adhere to the lumen of the small intestine by means of a concave sucking disk. Trophozoites that do not adhere to the small intestine are carried to the large intestine, where they form new cysts. Excretion of such cysts in the stool transmits the parasite to water supplies or to other individuals.

Although some patients with giardiasis may be asymptomatic, most experience an explosive, watery, nonbloody, and foul-smelling diarrhea associated with abdominal cramping. Malabsorption and steatorrhea result from the inability of the microvilli in the small intestine to properly absorb water and nutrients. Malaise, anorexia, nausea, flatulence, fever, and weight loss are also common clinical findings. The clinical course is usually self-limited, but some patients may develop a chronic, intermittent diarrhea.

Diagnosis of giardiasis is accomplished by identifying *Giardia* cysts in the stool. Because the stool samples often yield negative results, the diagnosis is often made by examining duodenal mucus or by performing a jejunal biopsy. To obtain duodenal mucus, the patient swallows a fuzzy string, which moves into the duodenum. The string is removed and the duodenal secretions are examined under the microscope for motile trophozoites. Treatment involves metronidazole, quinacrine, or various other medications (Table 62-2). Metronidazole is contraindicated in pregnancy because it is teratogenic.

Amebiasis

Approximately 10% of the world's population is infected with amebiasis, which causes almost

*Table*62-2

TREATMENT OF GASTROINTESTINAL PARASITIC INFECTIONS

Infection			Adult Dosage	Pediatric Dosage

Amebiasis (*Entamoeba histolytica*)

Asymptomatic

Drugs of choice:		Iodoquinol	650 mg tid × 20d	30-40 mg/kg/d in 3 doses × 20d
	or	Paromomycin	25-30 mg/kg/d in 3 doses × 7d	25-30 mg/kg/d in 3 doses × 7d
Alternative:		Diloxanide furoate	500 mg tid × 10d	20 mg/kg/d in 3 doses × 10d

Mild-to-moderate intestinal disease

Drugs of choice:		Metronida-zole	750 mg tid × 10d	35-50 mg/kg/d in 3 doses × 10d
	or	Tinidazole	2 g/d × 3d	50 mg/kg (max 2 g) qd × 3d

Severe intestinal disease

Drugs of choice:		Metronida-zole	750 mg tid × 10d	35-50 mg/kg/d in 3 doses × 10 d
	or	Tinidazole	600 mg bid × 5d	50 mg/kg (max 2 g) qd × 3d
Alternatives:		Dehydroeme-tine	1 to 1.5 mg/kg/d (max 90 mg/d) IM up to 5d	1 to 1.5 mg/kg/d (max 90 mg/d) IM in 2 doses up to 5d

Hepatic abscess

Drugs of choice:		Metronida-zole	750 mg tid × 10d	35-50 mg/kg/d in 3 doses × 10d
	or	Tinidazole	800 mg bid × 5d	60 mg/kg (max 2 g) qd × 3 d
Alternatives:		Dehydroeme-tine fol-lowed by	1 to 1.5 mg/kg/d (max 90 mg/d) IM for up to 5d	1 to 1.5 mg/kg/d (max 90 mg/d) IM in two doses for up to 5d
		Chloroquine phosphate	600 mg base (1g)/d × 2d, then 300 mg base (500 mg)/d × 2-3 wks	10 mg base/kg (max 300 mg base)/d × 2-3 wks

Ascariasis (*Ascaris lumbricoides*, roundworm)

Drugs of choice:		Mebendazole	100 mg bid × 3d	100 mg bid × 3d
	or	Pyrantel pamoate	11 mg/kg × 1 dose (max 1 g)	11 mg/kg × 1 dose (max 1 g)
	or	Albendazole	400 mg × 1 dose	400 mg × 1 dose

Modified from *Med Lett Drugs Ther*, 35:111-122, 1993.

Continued.

*Table*62-2

TREATMENT OF GASTROINTESTINAL PARASITIC INFECTIONS—cont'd

Infection			Adult Dosage	Pediatric Dosage
Enterobius vermicularis (pinworm) infection				
Drugs of choice:		Pyrantel pamoate	11 mg/kg × 1 dose (max 1 g); repeat in 2 weeks	11 mg/kg × 1 dose (max 1 g); repeat in 2 weeks
	or	Mebendazole	100 mg once; repeat in 2 weeks	100 mg once; repeat in 2 weeks
	or	Albendazole	400 mg once; repeat in 2 weeks	400 mg once; repeat in 2 weeks
Giardiasis (_Giardia lamblia_)				
Drug of choice:		Metronida-zole	250 mg tid × 5d	15 mg/kg/d in 3 doses × 5d
Alternatives:		Quinacrine	100 mg tid pc × 5d	6 mg/kg/d in 3 doses pc for 5d (max 300 mg/d)
		Tinidazole	2 g × 1 dose	50 mg/kg × 1 dose (max 2 g)
		Furazolidone	100 mg qid × 7-10d	6 mg/kg/d in 4 doses × 7-10d
		Paromomycin	25-30 mg/kg/d in 3 doses × 7d	
Hookworm infection (_Ancylostoma doudenale, Necator americanus_)				
Drugs of choice:		Mebendazole	100 mg bid × 3d	100 mg bid × 3d
	or	Pyrantel pamoate	11 mg/kg (max 1 g) × 3d	11 mg/kg (max 1 g) × 3d
	or	Albendazole	400 mg × 1 dose	400 mg × 1 dose
Schistosomiasis				
S. japonicum				
Drug of choice:		Praziquantel	60 mg/kg/d in 3 doses × 1 day	60 mg/kg/d in 3 doses × 1 day
S. mansoni				
Drug of choice:		Praziquantel	40 mg/kg/d in 2 doses × 1 day	40 mg/kg/d in 2 doses × 1 day
Alternative		Oxamniquine	15 mg/kg once	20 mg/kg/d in 2 doses × 1 day
Strongyloidiasis (_Strongyloides stercoralis_)				
Drugs of choice:		Thiabenda-zole	50 mg/kg/d in 2 doses (max 3 g/d) × 2d	50 mg/kg/d in 2 doses (max 3 g/d) × 2d
	or	Ivermectin	200 µg/kg/d × 1-2d	
Trichuriasis (_Trichuris trichiura_, whipworm)				
Drugs of choice:		Mebendazole	100 mg bid × 3d	100 mg bid × 3d
	or	Albendazole	400 mg × 1 dose	400 mg × 1 dose

110,000 deaths each year. It is estimated that 15% to 40% of all male homosexuals have asymptomatic *E. histolytica* infections. Transmission of amebiasis begins with the ingestion of cysts. Once ingested, the cyst exists in the distal ileum and undergoes binary fission to produce eight trophozoites, which enter the large intestine and either multiply and reencyst or invade the wall of the colon to produce intestinal and extraintestinal disease. Amebic cysts that do not invade the bowel are excreted in the stool. The most common sites of amebic infestation are the cecum, which is followed by the ascending colon, rectum, sigmoid colon, and appendix. Trophozoites may disseminate beyond the GI tract via the portal venous system. Extraintestinal infestation most commonly involves the liver, where amebic liver abscesses are formed.

The clinical presentation of intestinal infestation with *E. histolytica* may vary from being asymptomatic to having fulminant rectocolitis. Acute colonic invasion produces an explosive, bloody diarrhea that is associated with dehydration, fever, and occasionally a toxic megacolon with bowel perforation and peritonitis. Chronic liver abscesses that are usually located in the right lobe of the liver are formed. The rupture of these abscesses into the lung can cause a severe cough that is productive of trophozoites.

The diagnosis of intestinal amebiasis requires the identification of cysts or trophozoites in the stool. A variety of serologic tests, such as the amebic indirect agglutination test, are available to diagnose amebic infestation when stool samples are negative. Colonoscopy with biopsy may be useful in difficult cases. Radiologic examinations such as ultrasonography, computed tomography, and technetium liver scans are required to diagnose extraintestinal disease.

Cryptosporidiosis

Treatment of *E. histolytica* depends on the degree of infestation—whether the patient is asymptomatic or is experiencing mild-to-moder- ate intestinal disease, severe intestinal disease, or a hepatic abscess (see Table 62-2).

Cryptosporidium organisms were first identified in humans in 1976. In 1982, these organisms were found to produce a severe and sometimes fatal diarrhea in patients with AIDS. Human infestation begins with ingestion of an oocyst that liberates four motile sporozoites. The sporozoites undergo both asexual and sexual reproduction within the lumen of the gut. The life cycle is complete with the fecal excretion of infective oocysts.

The degree of severity of cryptosporidial infestation is determined by the immune competence of the patient. Immunodepressed patients may have a chronic, watery diarrhea with a 20 L/day output. In contrast, immunocompetent patients have a clinical syndrome similar to that of giardiasis: a nonbloody, self-limited diarrhea associated with abdominal cramps and fever.

The diagnosis of cryptosporidial infestation is made by an examination of the stool for fecal oocysts, which are plentiful in immunocompromised individuals. Stool-concentrating methods are used in immunocompetent patients because of the lower concentration of infecting oocysts in these individuals.

Because cryptosporidiosis is self-limited, treatment is unnecessary in immunocompetent patients. In immunocompromised patients with severe disease, octreotide 300 to 500 micrograms three times a day subcutaneously may control the diarrhea but not the infection. Paromomycin and azithromycin may sometimes be helpful.

Ascariasis

The nematode *Ascaris lumbricoides* infests approximately 1 billion people worldwide, with 1500 deaths every year a result of the intestinal obstruction. Infestation begins with the ingestion of eggs that hatch into larvae in the host's small intestine. The larvae penetrate the gut and migrate through the lungs, trachea, and pharynx, where they are swallowed. Maturation finally occurs in the proximal small intestine. Patients may vomit a large (as long as 35 cm) adult ascaris worm or pass one in the stool.

Although the majority of hosts infested with *A. lumbricoides* are asymptomatic, GI symptoms include nonspecific upper abdominal pain and diarrhea. Patients may develop pulmonary infiltration and peripheral eosinophilia (Löffler's syndrome) associated with the migratory course of the worm. Ascending cholangitis is a result of the death of migrating worms in the bile ducts. The decaying worms release their own bacterial gut flora into the sterile bile, which results in cholangitis. Occasionally liver abscesses are formed as a result of the migration of adult worms into the liver parenchyma.

Ascariasis is diagnosed by identifying the egg or worm in the stool of the patient. Mebendazole is effective in killing the worm, and the patient should be warned of the potential passage of large, dead worms with successful therapy.

Strongyloidiasis

Strongyloides stercoralis infests up to 35 million people worldwide. Although usually benign, *S. stercoralis* infestation (strongyloidiasis) may be fatal in the immunocompromised patient. Filariform larvae from contaminated soil penetrate the skin and gain entrance into the vascular system. The larvae migrate to the lung, mature, and crawl to the pharynx, where they are swallowed. Final maturation occurs in the duodenum. Adult females lay eggs in the duodenal crypts, where they become rhabditiform larvae that are passed in the stool. Such larvae develop into the infective filariform larvae that reside in the soil. In severe infestations, and in those of the immunosuppressed individual, the infective rhabditiform larvae may form within the gut itself and subsequently penetrate the gut mucosa. Infective larvae then disseminate to various organ systems. Patients with disseminated strongyloides, or hyperinfection syndrome, may experience ulcerations in their

small intestine, severe pneumonia, septicemia, disseminated intravascular coagulation, or overwhelming CNS infestation. This form of disseminated strongyloides has a 70% mortality rate. In immunocompetent patients, peripheral eosinophilia and malabsorption may be the only abnormality observed.

Diagnosis of strongyloidiasis in asymptomatic or mildly toxic patients requires the demonstration of rhabditiform larvae in the stool or duodenum. An enzyme-linked immunoabsorbent assay may also be used to diagnose strongyloidiasis. The treatment for this infestation is thiabendazole (see Table 62-2).

Trichuriasis

Trichuris trichiura (the whipworm) is the parasite commonly associated with rectal prolapse in overwhelming infestations. In young children, chronic dysentery, anemia, nausea and vomiting, and blood-streaked stools are signs of infestation. The life cycle involves the ingestion of eggs by the host and maturation of the eggs within the colon. Females lay distinctive, barrel-shaped eggs that are passed into the stool. Diagnosis is made by identifying these ova during the stool examination. Mebendazole is the treatment of choice for trichuriasis (see Table 62-2).

Enterobiasis

The pinworm, *Enterobius vermicularis,* is a common problem in the United States. As many as 80% of all U.S. children are infested with enterobiasis at some time during their school-age years. The patient usually complains of pruritus ani.

The infestation begins with the ingestion of *E. vermicularis* eggs that hatch in the duodenum and mature in the small intestine. The adults are usually located in the cecum. When the patient is asleep, female worms migrate to the anus and lay sticky-coated eggs on the perineum. It is this combination of female migration and sticky-egg coating that causes an intense anal pruritus. In addition to pruritus ani, *E. vermicularis* worms may be responsible for folliculitis and vulvovaginitis. Pinworms may also cause the clinical picture of appendicitis. The eggs may be spread via person-to-person contact, house dust, or family pets.

Diagnosis of enterobiasis is made by placing the adhesive side of clear cellophane tape against the anus and sticking the tape to a glass slide for microscopic examination. The ova will be readily identifiable. Mebendazole is the treatment of choice for children over 2 years of age (see Table 62-2).

Hookworm Infestation

The hookworms *Ancylostoma duodenale* and *Necator americanus* cause cramping epigastric pain in heavy infestations. Similar to strongyloidiasis, these hookworms penetrate the skin and migrate via the circulation through the lungs, trachea, and pharynx, where they are eventually swallowed by the host. The duodenum is the site of maturation. Eggs that are released in the host stool hatch into larvae in the soil and become potentially infective to humans. Clinical signs and symptoms include a pruritic dermatitis at the site of entrance and wheezing during worm migration. The major complaint of those infested with hookworms is severe, cramping, epigastric pain. Severe blood loss with resultant anemia may occur in the host as a result of the attachment of these worms to the gut mucosa via sharp cutting plates and the secretion of anticoagulants. The diagnosis of hookworm infestation is made through the identification of the eggs in a stool sample. Mebendazole, pyrantel pamoate, or albendazole may be used in treatment (see Table 62-2).

Schistosomiasis

Schistosomiasis afflicts more than 300 million people on three different continents. There are three species of schistosomes: *Schistosoma mansoni, Schistosoma japonicum,* and *Schistosoma haematobium. S. mansoni* and *S. japonicum* are responsible for intestinal schistosomiasis, whereas *S. haematobium* is responsible for urinary bladder schistosomiasis. The life-cycle begins when the infective larvae of the schistosomes, the cercariae, penetrate the human skin while the individual is swimming or bathing in parasite-infested freshwater. The cercariae enter the bloodstream and travel to the right side of the heart, to the lung, and finally to the liver, where they begin to grow. Adults migrate to the mesenteric venules, where the female lays her eggs. The eggs are extruded through the venule and gut wall and enter the gut lumen, where the eggs are excreted with the feces. The eggs hatch into miracidia in freshwater. These miracidia infect specific snail species that act as vectors for disease. Within the snail, miracidia evolve into cercariae that are released into the water to complete the life-cycle.

The symptoms associated with schistosomiasis may be numerous. Many patients who have been briefly exposed to schistosomiasis may be asymptomatic. Following penetration of the skin by cercariae, petechial hemorrhages occur. Localized edema and pruritus reach a maximum in 24 hours and disappear in approximately 4 days. Generalized malaise, fever, urticaria, and vague GI complaints follow. Coughing and hemoptysis occur during migration of the cercariae through the lungs. Acute hepatitis may develop when the cercariae reach the liver.

Acute infection causes high fever, weight loss, eosinophilia, arthralgia, myalgia, and abdominal pain. Copious blood and mucus may be present during severe dysentery. Once egg production begins, chronic schistosomiasis may develop. Many eggs remain in the bowel wall or are carried through the portal system and may lodge in the liver parenchyma, thus leading to granuloma formation. Eventual fibrosis of the liver leads to cirrhosis with its associated portal hypertension and splenomegaly. Fibrosis of the bowel wall is caused by eggs entrapped within the gut wall. In addition, eggs may enter the circulation and settle in other organ systems. Granulomas may be found in pulmonic tissue, the spinal cord, and the brain.

The diagnosis of schistosomiasis may be difficult. Diagnosis before egg formation occurs depends on an appropriate history of exposure, positive serodiagnostic tests, and peripheral eosinophilia. When eggs are actively being produced by the parasite, the eggs of the particular schistosome species may be identified. In the chronic stage of the disease, eggs may be trapped in the bowel wall, which makes rectal mucosal biopsy an important diagnostic tool. The current treatment for schistosomiasis is praziquantel (see Table 62-2).

• • •

It is evident that parasites may cause a variety of GI disturbances in the host. *G. lamblia, A. lumbricoides, S. stercoralis,* and the hookworms should be considered in patients who have upper abdominal pain. *S. stercoralis* should also be suspected in cases of malabsorption. *A. lumbricoides* may cause an obstruction of the biliary system. *E. histolytica* may cause a disabling diarrhea that contains blood and mucus. *G. lamblia* is strongly associated with a copious, steatorrheic, mucus-filled diarrhea and upper abdominal cramping. Rectal prolapse is caused by trichuriasis. Pruritus ani can be caused by infestation with *E. vermicularis.* Hepatomegaly may be associated with amebic and *A. lumbricoides* abscesses. Hepatosplenomegaly resulting from macrophage ingestion of erythrocyte pigment is a common finding in malaria-infested patients and may also be seen with infestation by schistosomes.

CENTRAL NERVOUS SYSTEM INFESTATION

Numerous parasites are able to infest the central nervous system. A potentially life-threatening complication of *P. falciparum* infestation is cerebral malaria. The sludging of parasitized red blood cells within cerebral capillaries may result in severe CNS dysfunction, such as a stroke or hemorrhage. Early diagnosis and therapy is very important in preventing such severe complications (see Table 62-1).

Infestation with *E. histolytica* may result in an amebic brain abscess. Once the parasite invades the bowel wall, it may be carried by the circulation to the CNS. Diagnosis is made by the identification of amebic trophozoites in the cerebrospinal fluid (CSF) or by biopsy of the affected brain tissue. Two other amebas, *Naegleria* and *Acanthamoeba,* are capable of causing CNS disease. These freshwater amebas invade the CNS via the cribriform plate and nasal mucosa and may cause meningoencephalitis. The antecedent events typically include a history of swimming and diving in freshwater lakes. Diagnosis of CNS infestation is made by identifying the mobile ameba in the CSF. Amphotericin B 1 mg/kg/day IV is the treatment of choice but both the duration of treatment and certainty of cure are as yet unknown.

Trypanosoma gambiense and *T. rhodesiense* are the parasites responsible for African sleeping sickness. These parasites are transmitted by the bite of the tsetse (*Glossina*) fly. Once the parasites have entered the host's bloodstream, they invade the lymph nodes and spleen and are then able to enter the intercellular spaces of the CNS. Severe headaches occur and are followed by sleepiness, lethargy, coma, and death. Diagnosis is made through the patient's clinical history and by the identification of the parasite in peripheral blood or biopsy tissue. Identification of trypanosomes in the CNS carries a very poor prognosis. Treatment is with suramin sodium, which is given as a 100 to 200 mg IV test dose and is followed by 1 g IV on days 1, 3, 7, 14, and 21. Suramin sodium is available by request from the Centers for Disease Control (CDC). Pentamidine isethionate is an alternative regimen.

The two main tapeworms capable of causing CNS dysfunction are *Taenia solium* (pork tapeworm) and *Echinococcus granulosus. T. solium* is acquired after eating pork products that contain the larval form of the parasite (*Cysticercus cellulosae*) or after ingesting eggs found in the food or water supply. The larval forms are capable of invading other tissues in the host, thus creating a condition termed *cysticercosis*. Cysts formed in the brain, termed *neurocysticercosis,* may result in seizures or produce symptoms by mass effect; new-onset seizures may be the first indication of neurocysticercosis. Both worldwide and in the United States, cysticercosis is the most common parasitic disease of the central nervous system.

The diagnosis of neurocysticercosis in the emergency department depends on an aggressive search. A laboratory examination is often not helpful, but peripheral leukocytosis and eosinophilia may be seen. Microscopic examination of the stool may be helpful in the diagnosis. A CT scan of the head may be helpful in identifying both calcified (nonactive) and uncalcified (active) cysts. The addition of IV contrast may identify ring-enhancing lesions. If the cysts are viable within the brain (uncalcified), albendazole or praziquantel is the treatment of choice. The dose of albendazole is 15 mg/kg/day in three divided doses for 28 days. Praziquantel is administered 50 mg/kg/day in three doses for 15 days. Pediatric doses are the same. Calcified and nonactive cysts may need to be surgically removed.

E. granulosus is transmitted through the ingestion of the ova that are found in the feces of sheep, cattle, and sheepdogs. *E. granulosa* forms loculated structures called *hydatid cysts,* which contain scolices (heads) and remains of germinal epithelium (hydatid sand). After penetration of the gut mucosa, the larval form of the parasite travels in the bloodstream and becomes encysted in multiple body locations. Although the liver is the primary site of encystment, the CNS may be involved in approximately 7% of the cases. Symptoms of *E. granulosa* CNS involvement are similar to that of neurocysticercosis. Serologic tests are used for making the

diagnosis. Albendazole 400 milligrams twice a day for 28 days is the treatment of choice for hydatid cysts. The pediatric dosage is the same as for neurocysticercosis.

PULMONARY INFESTATION

The life cycles of certain parasites involve passage through the pulmonary system. Pneumonitis is commonly seen with the passage of the roundworm *A. lumbricoides,* the hookworms *N. americanus* and *A. duodenale,* and the threadworm *S. stercoralis* through the pulmonary vasculature. Signs and symptoms of their passage through the lungs include coughing, dyspnea, and eosinophilia. *E. granulosus* may cause hydatid cyst disease of the lung, which appears as a unilocular lung cyst on the CT scan. The diagnosis and treatment of these infestations has been discussed previously.

CARDIOVASCULAR INFESTATION

The parasite most often responsible for cardiovascular disease in humans is *Trypanosoma cruzi,* which produces Chagas disease. Chagas disease is found in the southern United States, Mexico, Central America, and South America and is transmitted by the reduviid "kissing bugs" that usually bite at night. The patient scratches at the location of the bite, which introduces the feces of the bug into the bite. This excrement contains the trypanosome epimastigote. At the site of infestation the trypanosomes proliferate and produce an indurated, erythematous area known as a *chagoma.* The organisms spread rapidly to regional lymph nodes, which may become palpable in 3 days. Romaña sign, a unilateral swelling of the upper and lower eyelids associated with preauricular lymph node swelling and conjunctivitis, is sometimes seen with Chagas disease. Symptoms of generalized infestation occur 4 to 14 days after the bite. The acute phase is characterized by malaise, chills, fever, and muscle aches. Generalized lymphadenopathy and hepatosplenomegaly may be present. Infestation may spread to the central nervous system and cardiovascular system.

In acute Chagas disease, the invasion of the myocardium by trypanosomes leads to myocarditis. Electrocardiographic changes are seen in more than 40% of the acute cases. The conducting system of the heart is often involved, which leads to conduction defects such as right and left bundle branch blocks (right greater than left), and atrioventricular blocks of varying degrees. Death may be caused by cardiac dysrhythmias or cardiac insufficiency that results in pump failure. Chronic Chagas disease may result in cardiomegaly with resultant ventricular aneurysmal formation at the apex. Sudden death may occur with the rupture of this aneurysm.

Definitive diagnosis of *T. cruzi* infestation is made by identifying the parasite in the blood during the acute stage. In chronic illness, however, the trypanosome is very difficult to identify in a thick blood smear. The organism may be identified by special concentrating techniques, by culture, or by the method of xenodiagnosis (an uninfected reduviid bug takes a blood meal from a patient with probable Chagas disease). Complement fixation tests, indirect hemagglutination, and indirect immunofluorescence may also be used to diagnose *T. cruzi* infestation.

Treatment for cardiac infestation may require diuretics for acute pump failure and a pacemaker for conduction disturbances. Drugs that suppress the atrioventricular node should be avoided. The drug of choice for the treatment of *T. Cruzi* is nifurtimox given in a dose of 8 to 10 mg/kg/day and divided into four doses for 120 days. Children require slightly higher doses of nifurtimox (15 mg/kg/day) but are given the drug for only 90 days.

Infestation with *Trichinella spiralis* may also lead to cardiovascular disease. Larvae may penetrate duodenal and jejunal mucosa and invade both striated and cardiac muscle. Infestation within the myocardium leads to inflammation, necrosis, and fibrosis. The myocarditis is so severe that death may result within 2 weeks after infestation. The diagnosis of *T. spiralis* is made by identifying the larvae in a muscle biopsy sample; intradermal testing using trichinella antigens is also used to diagnose this infestation. The treatment of *T. spiralis* consists of steroids and mebendazole. Mebendazole is administered 200 to 400 milligrams three times a day for three days, followed by 400 to 500 milligrams three times a day for 10 days.

GENITOURINARY INFESTATION

The two parasites most responsible for genitourinary infestations are *Trichomonas vaginalis* and *Schistosoma haematobium*. *T. vaginalis* is a very common sexually transmitted protozoa acquired by sexual intercourse, and it inhabits the vaginal and urethral tissues. Vaginal discharge and pruritus are the most common complaints associated with this type of infestation. The discharge is often profuse and frothy greenish-yellow in appearance and may be associated with burning, itching, and chafing. The vaginal examination often reveals the classic "strawberry cervix." Dysuria and frequency are common associated symptoms, but cystitis is unusual. In men, infestation is often asymptomatic. In addition to dysuria, a thin discharge that often contains trichomonads may be visualized at the urethral meatus. In advanced cases the prostate may become tender and enlarged, and epididymitis may be present.

The diagnosis is made by viewing saline-prepared vaginal or urethral secretions under the light microscope. Motile protozoa are identified by the active movement of their flagella. Treatment with metronidazole may be given in one 2-gram dose, or as 250 mg three times a day for 7 days. The patient must be warned about a potential disulfiram-like reaction when taken with alcohol. Pregnant patients should not take metronidazole because it is teratogenic.

Unlike trichomoniasis, *S. haematobium* infestation (schistosomiasis) is not sexually transmitted. After invading the skin and circulation, *S. haematobium* migrates to the small venules in the bladder, where it matures into the adult. The eggs formed by the adults migrate through the wall of the urinary bladder into the bladder lumen, and the eggs are excreted in the urine. Dysuria, frequency, hematuria, and eosinophiluria are early signs and symptoms of infestation; terminal hematuria is usually the first sign. Obstructive uropathy may occur in those infested with large egg burdens. Squamous cell carcinoma of the bladder may occur in areas of the bladder where a large egg burden is located. The presence of schistosome eggs in the urine confirms the diagnosis. A one-day course of praziquantel, 40 mg/kg in two doses, is an effective therapy for urinary schistosomiasis.

DERMATOLOGIC INFESTATION

There are currently 1.2 million persons infested with cutaneous and mucocutaneous leishmaniasis. New world cutaneous leishmaniasis is caused by *Leishmania mexicana* and *Leishmania braziliensis.* Old world cutaneous leishmaniasis is caused by *Leishmania tropica.* The various species of *Leishmania* are transmitted by sandflies of the genus *Phlebotomus* during their blood meals. The parasite then resides in the macrophages of the host's skin and subcutaneous tissue. In Old world cutaneous leishmaniasis, *L. tropica* produces a chronic infestation characterized by dry lesions that may ulcerate. The lesions are usually single and are located primarily on the face. In New World cutaneous leishmaniasis, skin papules and nodules are identified soon after the bite of the sandfly. The papules may develop into a macule with a central ulceration and a raised border. A secondary bacterial infection may lead to increased scar-

ring. The subspecies of *L. braziliensis, L. braziliensis braziliensis,* is responsible for mucocutaneous lesions in the mouth, nose, larynx, and trachea. These lesions may lead to the destruction of cartilage and result in mutilation of the face and may also lead to airway compromise. Diffuse nodules and papules resembling leprosy may be found in disseminated cutaneous leishmaniasis. Individuals with such disseminated disease should be suspected of having a defect in their cell-mediated immune system.

Diagnosis of leishmaniasis may be accomplished in various ways. One method of diagnosis is by the Montenegro immunologic test, in which injection of dead leishmania produces a delayed hypersensitivity reaction within 72 hours if the patient is infested. Other methods of diagnosis include indirect fluorescent antibody tests and culturing the ulcer edge for the parasite. Stibogluconate sodium is the most effective compound presently available for the treatment of cutaneous leishmaniasis. The dose is 20 mg/kg IV or intramuscularly (IM) daily for 20 to 28 days. Coughing, headache, and vomiting are common side effects. Amphotericin B has been used in patients who are unresponsive to the other treatments.

The hookworm *Ancylostoma braziliense* is responsible for cutaneous larva migrans, or the "creeping eruption." The patient is infected through the skin while walking on warm soils or beaches. The diagnosis is made by visualizing the characteristic wandering skin rash that results from larval migration of the parasite. Treatment is with topical or oral thiabendazole together with oral antipruritics.

ECTOPARASITE INFESTATION

Ectoparasites, which are defined as living on the surface of the body, are a common problem. They may appear as a pruritic rash, localized pruritus, or simply as a visual nuisance. The lo-

*Table*62-3

TREATMENT OF ECTOPARASITE INFECTIONS

Infection		Adult Dosage	Pediatric Dosage
Lice (*Pediculus humanus, Phthirus pubis*)			
Drugs of choice:	1% Permethrin	Topically	Topically
	0.5% Malathion	Topically	Topically
Alternatives:	Pyrethrins with piperonyl butoxide	Topically	Topically
	Lindane	Topically	Topically
Mites (*Eutrombicula splendens*) **and scabies** (*Sarcoptes scabiei*)			
Drug of choice:	5% Permethrin	Topically	Topically
Alternatives:	Lindane	Topically	Topically
	10% Crotamiton	Topically	Topically

Modified from *Med Lett Drugs Ther*, 35:111-122, 1993.

cation of the patient's symptoms helps to identify the ectoparasite properly. *Sarcoptes scabiei* (scabies), *Eutrombicula alfreddugèsi* and *Eutrombicula splendens,* (chigger mites), *Pediculus humanus* (the human body or head louse), and *Phthirus pubis* (the pubic louse) are all commonly seen and may appear with any of these signs or symptoms.

S. scabiei burrows under the superficial epidermis to cause the formation of minute vesicle-like lesions. These lesions are most common between the digits and popliteal folds and are spread by scratching these vesicles. A secondary bacterial infection may occur as a result of this scratching. *E. splendens* (chigger mites), how-

ever, do not invade the epidermis. These mites attach to skin surfaces where clothing may be tight, such as the waistline and ankles, and feed on tissue fluid. This feeding causes a severe pruritus and dermatitis.

The diagnosis of scabies is made by examining skin scrapings of the vesicles immersed in potassium hydroxide (KOH) under low magnification. The Wood light examination is used to diagnose the body louse, because the eggs fluoresce under ultraviolet light. Ectoparasites are readily treated with topical lotions (Table 62-3). All clothing should be thoroughly cleaned, and contacts should be treated as needed.

KEY CONSIDERATIONS

WHAT IS THE LIFE THREAT?

Acute hemolysis associated with a malarial infection can be life threatening. Parasites that infect the brain, liver, or myocardium can cause life-threatening complications.

DOES THE PATIENT NEED ADMISSION?

Admit patients with life-threatening complications of parasitic disease.

WHAT IS THE MOST SERIOUS DIAGNOSIS?

Serious complications of malaria caused by sludging of erythrocytes in blood vessels of vital organs include seizures and coma, respiratory distress, renal failure, and splenic rupture. Acute hemolysis can be sudden and life threatening. Amebiasis can cause brain abscesses and liver abscesses. Ascending cholangiolitis and liver abscesses can be caused by ascariasis.

Hookworm infestation can cause severe epigastric cramping, pain, and significant blood loss.

Naegleria and *Acanthamoeba* organisms are capable of causing life-threatening meningoencephalitis. Chagas disease may result in cardiac dysrhythmia, pump failure, or death from the rupture of an aneurysm.

HAVE I PERFORMED A THOROUGH WORK-UP?

In patients with unexplained fever, examine thick smears of peripheral blood that have been prepared with the Giemsa or Wright stain, especially if the patients relate a history of travel to an area where malaria is endemic. Consider giardiasis and amebiasis in patients with abdominal cramping, intermittent diarrhea, and associated nonspecific symptoms such as flatulence, fever, weight loss, and malaise.

Obtain stool samples and examine them for ova and parasites in cases of unexplained diarrhea and abdominal cramping.

Recommended Reading

Drugs for parasitic infections, *Med Lett Drugs Ther* 35:111-122, 1993.

Gibler WB: Parasitology. In Rosen P et al, editors: *Emergency medicine: concepts and clinical practice*, ed 3, St Louis, 1992, Mosby.

Hoffman SL: Diagnosis, treatment, and prevention of malaria, *Med Clin North Am* 76:1327-1355, 1992.

Markell EK, Voge M, John DT: *Medical parasitology*, ed 7, Philadelphia, 1992, WB Saunders.

Panosian CB: Parasitic diarrhea, *Emerg Med Clin North Am* 9:337-354, 1991.

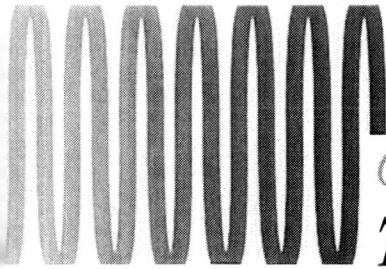

Chapter Sixty-three

TICKBORNE ILLNESSES

MICHAEL L. VORBROKER

Ticks are found almost worldwide. In the United States, they are the major arthropod vector of human disease. Ticks belong to the class Arachnida, which contains spiders and scorpions. There are three families of ticks: Ixodidae (hard ticks), Argasidae (soft ticks), and Nuttalliellidae. Tickborne illnesses are caused by both hard and soft ticks; the Nuttalliellidae family is of little medical importance. Ticks are the vectors of well-known diseases such as Lyme disease, tularemia, Rocky Mountain spotted fever, and tick paralysis. Other more obscure tickborne diseases include relapsing fever, Eastern spotted fever, Q fever, ehrlichiosis, babesiosis, and Colorado tick fever. Such illnesses are the result of bacterial, viral, parasitic, or toxin transmission from the tick to the human as the parasite feeds off human blood (Table 63-1).

Tickborne illnesses account for 95% of the vectorborne illnesses in the United States. The number of reported cases of Lyme disease doubled between 1987 and 1989 (from 2368 to 4572 cases). In 1992, there were nearly 10,000 reported cases in the United States.

TICK LIFE CYCLE

The life cycle of the ixodid tick involves four stages that complete a 2-year cycle: egg, larva, nymph, and adult. The eggs are deposited in the spring, and the larvae emerge in approximately 1 month. The larvae, nymphs, and adults are obligated blood feeders; they feed before molting. The larvae molt into nymphs the next spring and into adults later that summer. The larvae and nymphs prefer small mammals for their blood meal, such as the white-footed mouse. The adult prefers the white-tailed deer as its host, thus the origin of the popular name "deer tick." The white-footed mouse is the primary reservoir for the spirochete that causes Lyme disease. The nymph and adult can attach to a human who is walking through tall grass and brush, which establishes a route of transmission.

LYME DISEASE

Lyme disease is a relatively new illness that was first recognized in the mid 1970s in Old Lyme, Connecticut. Steere described this as Lyme arthritis, an oligoarticular arthritis that affects children and adults and is preceded by an unusual circular target rash. Some of these early patients remembered having a tick bite before the rash and actually saved the tick, which was identified as *Ixodes dammini*. Specimens of these ticks were found to harbor a spirochete that Burgdorfer later isolated from patient's sera; thus the spirochete was named *Borrelia burgdorferi*.

Epidemiology

Lyme disease is the most common tickborne illness in the United States. In 1992, it was reported in 49 states, with the highest rates in the northeastern states (Fig. 63-1). Men and women are equally affected, and the median age is 34 years.

Lyme disease is primarily a summertime illness that occurs with the emergence of the arthropod vector and outside activity. The peak incidence is in July; 80% of the cases occur between May and August. There are three areas where the majority of the cases arise: the coastal Northwest and Midwest, with *I. dammini* as the principal vector; and the West, with the *Ixodes pacificus* as the tick vector. Less than one third of the patients recall having had a tick bite because the nymph is responsible for the majority of disease transmission and is approximately the size of a pinhead.

Pathophysiology

Lyme disease is contracted when an individual is bitten by the feeding tick, which is usually a nymph. Spirochetes are inoculated beneath the skin, and after an incubation period of days to weeks, a three-stage multisystem illness develops.

Clinical Presentation

Stage I disease is heralded by the characteristic rash of Lyme disease, called erythema chronicum migrans (ECM). This rash appears at the site of the bite as a circular red lesion that mi-

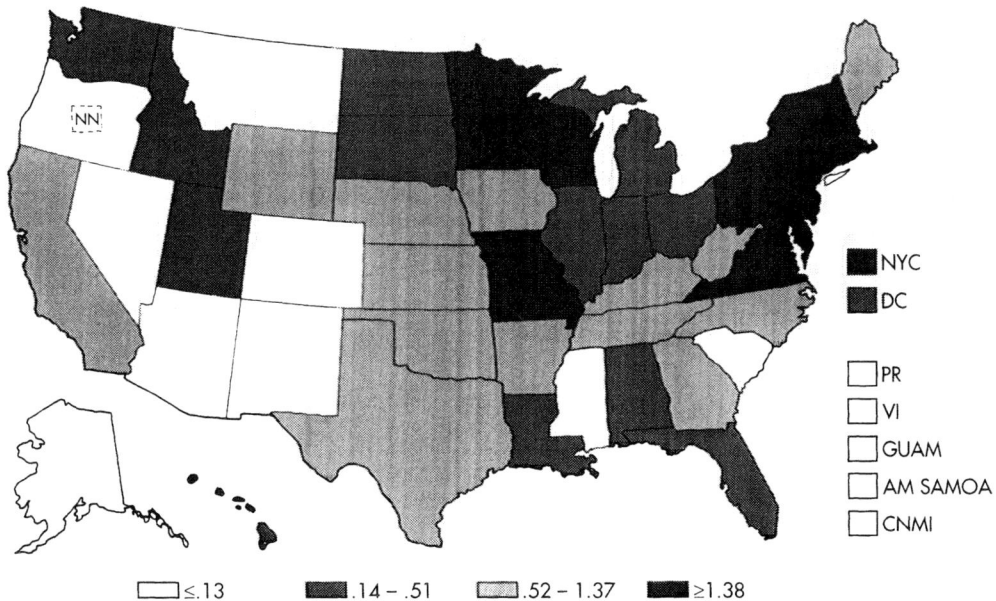

Fig.63-1 Lyme disease. Reported cases per 100,000 population, United States and territories—1992. (Courtesy Centers for Disease Control and Prevention: *MMWR,* September 24, 1993.)

Table 63-1

TICKBORNE ILLNESSES

Illness/ Pathogen	Tick Vector	Geography	Incubation Period	Clinical Presentation	Diagnosis	Treatment
Lyme disease/ *Borrelia burgdorferi* (spirochete)	*Ixodes dammini* *Ixodes pacificus*	Northwest coast and Midwest West	3-7 days	Stage I: Erythema chronicum migrans (ECM); flulike symptoms: fever, malaise, lethargy, myalgias, arthralgias	Early: clinical diagnosis	Stage I: doxycycline 100 mg bid for 10-21 days (if older than 8 years and nonpregnant)
			4 weeks after ECM	Stage II: Neurologic and cardiac; meningoencephalitis, cranial neuritis, AV block, myopericarditis	ELISA	Stage II: mild doxycline for 30 days Severe: ceftriaxone 2 mg IV for 30 days
			Weeks-months	Stage III: arthritis, oligoarthritis affecting large joints		Stage III: May use PO or IV as above
Relapsing fever/ *Borrelia* organisms (spirochete)	*Ornithodoros* organisms (soft tick) Lice (causes epidemic)	Western mountain states	4-18 days	Fever, chills, vomiting, arthralgias, myalgias, hepatosplenomegaly; resolves in 3 days to relapse in 1 week	Examine peripheral smear for spirochetes	Tetracycline 500 mg q6h for 5-10 days Erythromycin (alternative choice)
Tularemia/ *Francisella tularensis*	*Dermacentor variabilis*	Midwest South	2-5 days	Tender ulcer at bite, lymphadenopathy, cough, exudative conjunctivitis or pharyngitis, fever, headache, malaise, tender hepatosplenomegaly	Fourfold rise in antibody titers over 2-4 week period	Spectinomycin 15-20 mg/kg/d IM for 3 days, then 10-20 mg/kg/d IM for 10 days Tetracycline (alternative choice)

Disease	Vector/Organism	Distribution	Incubation	Clinical features	Diagnosis	Treatment
Rocky Mountain spotted fever (RMSF)/ *Rickettsia rickettsii*	*Dermacentor variabilis* *Dermacentor andersoni*	Southern and Eastern states	3-7 days	Abrupt onset of fever, severe headache, myalgias, vomiting, malaise; rash begins on wrist and forearms on fourth febrile day	Acutely: skin biopsy; Antibody titers	Tetracycline 25-50 mg/kg/d q6h; Chloramphenicol 50 mg/kg/d IV or PO q6h; Treat for 48 hours after fever resolves
Q fever/ *Coxiella burnetti* (rickettsia)	Unknown	Worldwide	2-14 days	Flulike illness with fever, headache, myalgias, cough	Fourfold rise in complement-fixing antibody titers	Supportive care; Tetracycline or chloramphenicol
Ehrlichiosis/ *Ehrlichia canis* (rickettsia)	*Ixodes dammini*	Southeast Midwest West	12 days (median)	Fever, chills, vomiting, headache, myalgias; 20% of those affected have nonspecific symptoms: fever, malaise, lethargy, myalgias, arthralgias	Fourfold rise in antibody titers	Tetracycline
Babesiosis/ *Babesia* organisms (intraerythrocyte protozoan)	*Ixodes dammini*	Same as Lyme disease	1-4 weeks	Gradual onset of malaise, fatigue, anorexia followed by more severe fever, sweats, myalgias; **no rash**	Blood smear; rise in antibody titers	Clindamycin 600 mg IV q6h and Quinine 650 mg PO q6h for 7-10 days
Colorado tick fever/ *Orbivirus* organisms	*Dermacentor andersoni*	West	3-5 days	Abrupt onset of fever, chills, anorexia, nausea, headache, myalgias; biphasic in half with fever and myalgias returning after a 2-3 day recovery period	Immunofluorescent staining of virus in the RBC; rise in titer	Self-limited; must rule out RMSF
Tick paralysis/ Toxin	*Dermacentor* organisms (females); causes epidemic	Southeast Northwest	4-7 days after attached	Restlessness, irritability, paresthesias progress to acute ataxia or ascending flaccid paralysis	Clinical presentation and finding the tick	Tick removal, supportive care, recovery in 48 hrs

grates outward to form a target, or bull's-eye, appearance. The ECM may be absent in one fourth of those infected, or it may be multiple with secondary lesions (Fig. 63-2). Stage I symptoms are difficult to distinguish from influenza because malaise, fatigue, and lethargy are the most common symptoms (80% of all patients). Headache, fever, chills, a stiff neck, myalgias, and arthralgias are common. Multiple annular lesions and lymphadenopathy occur in approximately 50%

of the patients, with pharyngitis and conjunctivitis occurring in approximately 10%. Stage I usually remits spontaneously, and the ECM fades in approximately 1 month.

Stage II begins an average of 4 weeks after onset of the ECM and is characterized by neurologic and cardiac manifestations. Neurologic manifestations include meningoencephalitis, cranial neuritis, and peripheral neuritis. Cranial neuritis most commonly involves the facial

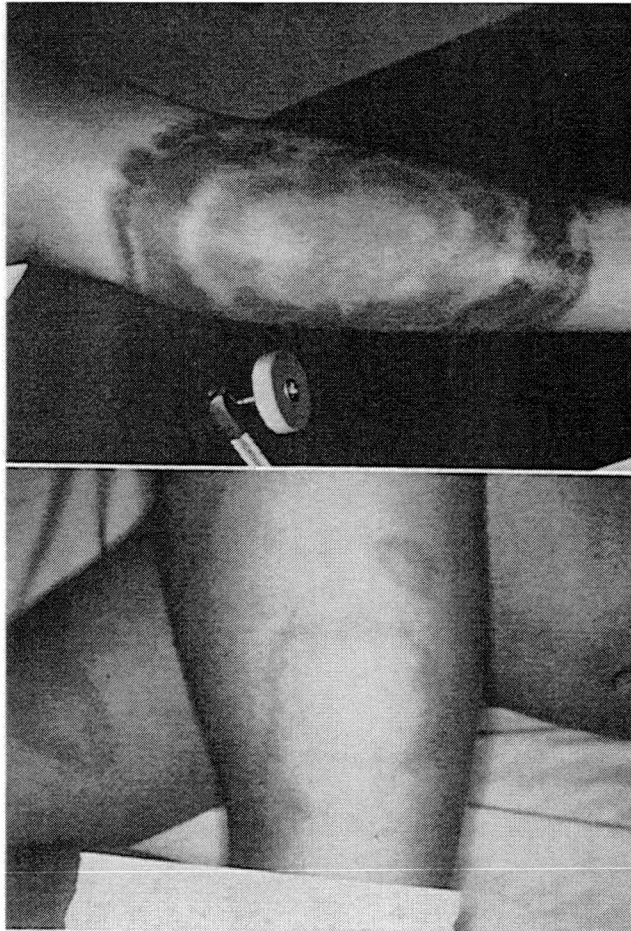

Fig. 63-2 Erythema chronicum migrans. (From Rosen P et al: *Emergency medicine: concepts and clinical practice,* ed 3, St Louis, 1992, Mosby.)

nerve, which leads to Bell palsy. Involvement of motor and sensory nerves causes weakness, pain, and dysesthesia in the affected distribution. There have been reports of cerebral vasculitis and subsequent infarcts secondary to Lyme disease; such neurologic manifestations may occur alone or in combination. With treatment, the neurologic manifestations completely resolve in 8 weeks; without treatment, they may persist for at least 30 weeks.

Cardiac abnormalities occur in approximately 8% of those with Lyme disease. The most common abnormality is a fluctuating degree of atrioventricular (AV) block. First degree, Wenckebach-type second degree, and complete heart block have been observed. The complete block would require a pacemaker. More diffuse cardiac involvement may produce myopericarditis, left ventricular dysfunction, or frank congestive heart failure. Cardiac involvement usually lasts only a few weeks, but a recurrence is possible.

Musculoskeletal pain is also common during Stage II. Ocular involvement, including conjunctivitis, keratitis, retinal detachment, and optic neuritis, have also been reported.

Stage III is the chronic phase and is characterized by arthritis. It is typically oligoarticular and affects large joints, especially the knee. It may last weeks or months, with intermittent recurrences in the same or other joints. Chronic arthritis with erosions of cartilage and bone occurs in 10% of all untreated patients. Interestingly, a peculiar skin rash can be the initial manifestation of Stage III disease: acrodermatitis chronica atrophicans, a chronic skin disorder that initially begins with reddish-violaceous lesions and becomes sclerotic and atrophic over a period of years. In untreated patients, the long-term remission rate is 10% to 20% each year.

Diagnosis

Lyme disease is best diagnosed through a careful history and physical examination. Early in the disease, the diagnosis is strictly based on historical and clinical findings and may be quite difficult without the characteristic ECM lesion. Enteroviral disease, erythema multiforme, erythema marginatum of acute rheumatic fever, encephalitis, Guillain-Barré syndrome, juvenile rheumatoid arthritis, Reiter syndrome, acute gouty arthritis, septic arthritis, and gonococcal arthritis all share symptoms similar to the various stages of Lyme disease and represent the differential diagnosis. Except for the serologic immunofluorescent antibody titers to *B. burgdorferi,* laboratory studies are not helpful. Immunoglobulin M (IgM) develops in 2 to 4 weeks, but immunogloblin G (IgG) may not develop for 2 months. The enzyme-linked immunosorbent assay (ELISA) for detecting IgM and IgG anti-*B. burgdorferi* antibodies (with a Western blot to confirm questionable ELISA results) offers the greatest sensitivity and specificity for the laboratory diagnosis of Lyme disease.

Treatment

The treatment of Lyme disease depends on the stage of the illness and on the severity of the symptoms. Doxycycline 100 mg PO twice daily for 10 to 21 days is the drug of choice in Stage I disease for nonpregnant women and for children older than 8 years of age. Amoxicillin, erythromycin, and cefuroxime may also be used.

A Stage II illness that displays mild neurologic or cardiac symptoms (Bell palsy or first-degree heart block that lasts less than 0.30 seconds) may be treated with the previously described oral regimen, with a duration of 1 month for neurologic and 3 weeks for cardiac symptoms. More severe neurologic and cardiac symptoms should be treated with intravenous (IV) ceftriaxone 2 g/day or penicillin G 20 to 24 million units/day. It should be noted that there is an increased risk of biliary disease and pseudolithiasis with prolonged ceftriaxone use.

In Stage III arthritic disease, oral or parenteral regimens may be equally effective in durations of 21 to 30 days. For Stage III neurologic disease, the IV regimen previously described should be used. It should be noted that a Jarisch-Herxheimer-type reaction may occur within the first day of treatment, with hyperpyrexia, tachycardia, and even hypotension. It is believed this reaction is caused by the killing of spirochetes and the release of pyrogens.

Lyme disease during pregnancy causes great concern because of the reports of fetal hydrocephalus, prematurity, heart disease, blindness, and even death. Because *B. burgdorferi* can be passed transplacentally, the pregnant woman with suspected Lyme disease must be treated aggressively with antibiotics to prevent harm to the fetus.

Prognosis

Antibiotic treatment shortens the duration of Lyme disease in all stages, but the best response occurs early in the illness. Approximately 50% of all patients have minor recurrences of headache, musculoskeletal pain, or fatigue irrespective of the antibiotic treatment. Morbidity or mortality results from cardiac, neurologic, ocular, and arthritic complications that develop in unrecognized cases. The majority of the patients treated with antibiotics eventually make a complete recovery.

RELAPSING FEVER

Epidemiology

Relapsing fever is an acute borrelial disease caused by various spirochetes. It is characterized by episodes of fever and spirochetemia with intervening asymptomatic periods. There are two forms of relapsing fever: the epidemic form (transmitted by lice), and the endemic form (transmitted by ticks). The tick vector is the argasid, or the soft tick that belongs to the genus *Ornithodoros*. The ticks become infected

by feeding on rodent reservoirs; adult ticks can also pass the infection to their offspring. The endemic area of the western mountain states is responsible for most of the cases.

Clinical Presentation

The incubation period of relapsing fever is 4 to 18 days, with the abrupt onset of fever, chills, nausea, vomiting, arthralgias, and myalgias. Hepatosplenomegaly and jaundice may be seen, but nuchal rigidity, peripheral neuropathy, and delirium are rare. Such nonspecific findings resolve in 3 days, which makes it nearly impossible to diagnose this condition on the initial visit. A relapse occurs in approximately 1 week but is usually less severe; this cycle repeats an average of three times. It is believed that the relapses occur as a result of an antigenic variation in the spirochetes. The variants are not cleared by the initial immune response, and clinical symptoms are produced when the spirochetes reach critical numbers—usually 1 week after the initial symptoms appear.

Diagnosis

Laboratory findings in relapsing fever are nonspecific. The definitive diagnosis is made by examining the peripheral smear for spirochetes. The history and knowledge of the epidemiologic factors may aid in the diagnosis.

Treatment

Treatment of relapsing fever involves tetracycline or erythromycin. A dose of 500 mg orally for 5 to 10 days is effective. However, a Jarisch-Herxheimer-type reaction may occur and be life threatening. This reaction usually occurs approximately 4 hours after antibiotic treatment and may be so severe that hypotension develops. Because of this reaction, it has been suggested that patients with relapsing fever be given the first dose of antibiotics in a monitored setting with good IV access in case hypotension does develop. Bad prognostic indicators include jaundice and hypotension, but 95% of the patients with relapsing fever recover completely with antibiotics.

TULAREMIA

Epidemiology

Tularemia, which is also known as rabbit fever, is an infectious disease caused by the pathogen *Francisella tularensis.* Many mammals have been found to harbor the infection, with the rabbit being the most notorious vector historically. However, it is now believed that the tick is the most common vector for transmission in the United States. The human becomes infected after being bitten by the tick *Dermacentor variabilis* at which time the infected feces of the tick enters the bite wound. (Interestingly, the saliva of the tick is not infectious.) The clinical symptoms develop after an incubation period of 2 to 5 days. Most cases of tularemia are reported from the midwestern, western, and southern states, with the peak incidence for tickborne tularemia occurring in the summer and rabbit fever occurring in the winter (Fig. 63-3).

Clinical Presentation

The clinical presentation of tularemia usually begins at the site of inoculation, which leads to the development of an erythematous papule that progresses to an ulcer. Fever, chills, headache, malaise, and tender hepatosplenomegaly are

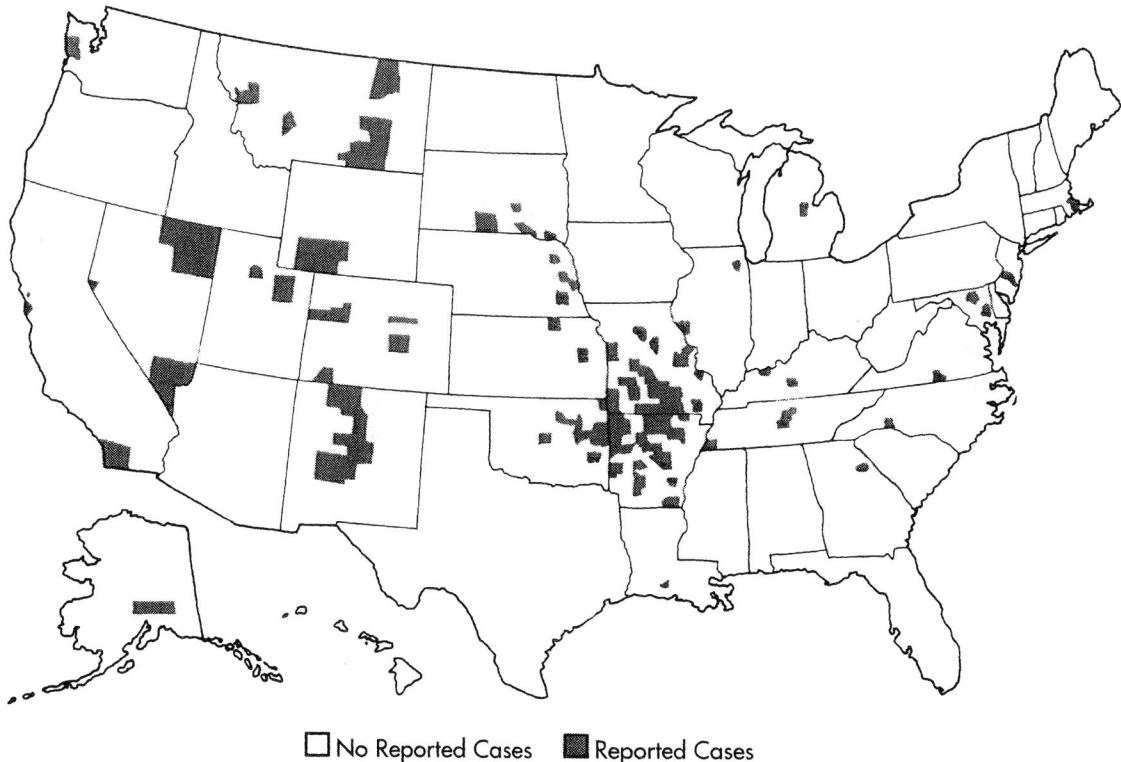

□ No Reported Cases ■ Reported Cases

Fig. 63-3   Tularemia. Counties reporting cases, United States—1992. (Courtesy Centers for Disease Control and Prevention: *MMWR,* September 24, 1993.)

common findings in all forms of tularemia. With the tickborne disease, there is pronounced tender lymphadenopathy, especially inguinal and femoral. This condition is known as *ulceroglandular tularemia* and is the first and most common of the six clinical presentations of tularemia. Glandular tularemia is the second most common form and lacks the characteristic ulcer formation. It occurs in approximately 20% of the cases. Pulmonary tularemia occurs in approximately 15% of the cases of tularemia and results from bacteremic spread or inhalation of the organisms. This condition usually occurs in laboratory workers and is characterized by a nonproductive cough, dyspnea, pleuritic chest pain, and bilateral patchy infiltrates. Typhoidal tularemia occurs in approximately 10% of the cases, and fever is the only manifestation. Skin lesions are absent, and therefore the diagnosis is difficult without any historical clues. The ocularglandular and oropharyngeal forms of tularemia occur rarely and are characterized by exudative conjunctivitis with regional lymphadenopathy and by exudative, membranous pharyngitis, respectively.

Diagnosis

A fourfold rise in paired specimens of agglutinating antibodies over a 2- to 3-week period is diagnostic of tularemia.

Treatment

Spectinomycin is the drug of choice for the treatment of tularemia. A dose of 15 to 20 mg/kg/day IM in two divided doses for three days followed by 10 to 20 mg/kg/day IM for a total of 7 to 10 days is sufficient. Tetracycline is the alternative choice, with a dosage of 50 to 60 mg/kg/day. Relapses may occur in as many as 20% of the patients treated with tetracycline. The overall mortality rate for tularemia is less than 8% but may be as high as 30% for those with the untreated pulmonary form.

ROCKY MOUNTAIN SPOTTED FEVER

Epidemiology

Rocky Mountain spotted fever (RMSF) is one of a group of illnesses caused by obligate intracellular parasites of the family Rickettsiaceae. There are several types of tickborne rickettsioses, with RMSF being the most prevalent. It is caused by *Rickettsia rickettsii* and is the second most common tickborne illness that afflicts humans. Female dog ticks (*D. variabilis*) and female wood ticks (*D. andersoni*) are the main vectors of disease transmission. The majority of the cases occur in the southern and eastern states, not in the Rocky Mountains, where it was prevalent in the early 1900s. Nearly all of the cases of RMSF occur between April and October (Fig. 63-4).

Clinical Presentation

Human infection occurs as the tick ingests a human blood meal. Clinical symptoms develop after a mean incubation period of 7 days. There is usually an abrupt onset of high fever, severe headache, myalgia, nausea, vomiting, and malaise. The parasites invade and multiply in the vascular endothelium and produce a vasculitis that becomes evident on approximately the fourth day of fever. As many as 15% of the cases may be spotless. The rash begins as pink macules on the forearms, palms, soles, and ankles. It spreads centripetally and becomes maculopapular and petechial by the fourth day of the rash. The vasculitis may lead to shock, adult respiratory distress syndrome (ARDS), disseminated intravascular coagulopathy (DIC) and, ultimately, even death.

Diagnosis

The diagnosis of RMSF can be quite easy if there is a history of a tick bite. It must be considered in anyone with an unexplained febrile illness and must be differentiated from other febrile

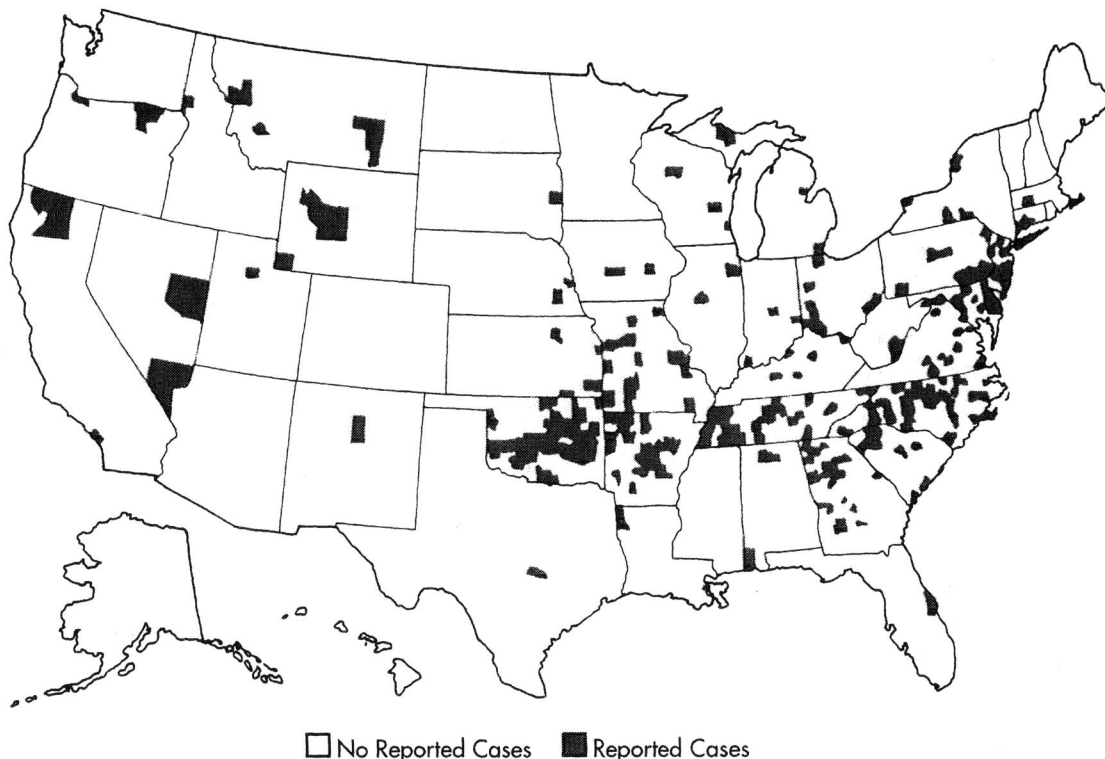

Fig. 63-4   Rocky Mountain spotted fever. Counties reporting cases, United States—1992. (Courtesy Centers for Disease Control and Prevention: *MMWR,* September 24, 1993.)

exathems such as rubeola, meningococcal infections, mononucleosis, enteroviral infections, and toxic shock syndrome. The presence of even a small petechial rash should prompt a consideration of RMSF.

The laboratory tests available in the emergency department are of little help in the acute setting. Abnormalities exist in any organ affected by the vasculitis but are nonspecific. The most specific serologic test available is the detection of the antigen by immunofluorescent antibodies. A titer of more than 1:64 or a fourfold rise in antibody titers of two samples obtained immediately and after 5 to 7 days is diagnostic of RMSF. In the acute setting, the diagnosis is expediently made by detecting the organism with an immunofluorescent study of a skin biopsy of the rash. Laboratory isolation of the rickettsias is considered too dangerous and is seldomly performed.

Treatment

The treatment of RMSF requires early institution of antibiotics and supportive care. Mortality increases as the delay in antibiotic therapy lengthens. Tetracycline or chloramphenicol are recommended therapies. Because they are rickettsiostatic, treatment must be continued for at least 2 days after the resolution of the fever to ensure that the immune system has cleared the infection. Tetracycline may be used in children older than 8 years of age and in nonpregnant women at a dose of 25 to 50 mg/kg/day up to 2 g/day in four divided doses for the adult. Chloramphenicol may be given at 50 mg/kg/day IV or PO in four divided doses up to 1 g/day.

Supportive care is directed at the complications of RMSF, such as shock, DIC, and ARDS. Steroids are controversial but may be used in those with complicating encephalitis or cerebral edema. Even with supportive care, the mortality rate remains at 5%.

EASTERN SPOTTED FEVER

Mediterranean spotted fever, North Asian tick typhus, and Queensland tick typhus are three tickborne rickettsial illnesses that resemble RMSF. The clinical presentation consists of the abrupt onset of fever, headache, malaise, and myalgias. There is a black eschar present at the site of the tick bite and, as with RMSF, tetracycline or chloramphenicol are used in treatment.

Q FEVER

Q fever is an infection caused by the rickettsia *Coxiella burnetti*. It has been transmitted by tick vectors, but the most common form of transmission is through aerosolized particles. Cattle, sheep, and goats are the primary reservoirs, and therefore farmers are most likely to be infected. Q fever appears as a flulike illness, with fever, headache, myalgias, and coughing. A diagnosis is made by detecting two specific complement-fixing antibodies during the first and second week of the illness. Treatment is with tetracycline or chloramphenicol. If untreated, most Q fever infections resolve, but a chronic infection may develop and require treatment for as long as 1 year. The mortality rate is less than 1%, even in those who remain untreated.

EHRLICHIOSIS

Epidemiology and Clinical Presentation

Ehrlichiosis is a tickborne illness caused by a rickettsial organism. The human infection was first described in 1986 and resembles RMSF, but there is no rash. It is unknown what tick species causes the human illness. Chronically infected dogs and rodents are possible reservoirs, but there has been no evidence of direct transmission to humans. The clinical illness occurs after an average incubation period of 12 days, with the onset of flulike symptoms. Fever, chills, nausea, vomiting, headache, and myalgias are common and nonspecific; approximately 20% of those affected may have a nonspecific rash. Splenomegaly, scrotal edema, and aseptic meningitis have been reported.

Diagnosis and Treatment

The diagnosis of ehrlichiosis is confirmed by demonstrating at least a fourfold increase in antibody titers against *Ehrlichia canis* in serum samples taken 2 to 4 weeks apart. This increase is detected with an indirect immunofluorescent antibody assay. Tetracycline is the drug of choice for the treatment of ehrlichiosis and produces defervescence in 24 to 48 hours.

BABESIOSIS

Epidemiology and Clinical Presentation

Babesiosis is caused by intraerythrocyte protozoan organisms from the genus Babesia, such as malarial organisms. The tick vector is *I. dammini*, which is also the vector for Lyme disease. The geographic distribution and seasonal prevalence of babesiosis is also similar to Lyme disease. Humans are infected when bitten by the tick. After an incubation period of 1 to 4 weeks, there is a gradual onset of malaise, fatigue, and anorexia followed by fever, sweats, and myalgias; a rash is not present. A history of tick bite is usually not obtained. Patients who have had a splenectomy may develop severe disease with hemolytic anemia, hemoglobinuria, and death.

Diagnosis and Treatment

The diagnosis of babesiosis may be made with the demonstration of intraerythrocyte parasites on the blood smear. Confirmation is made by a rise in immunofluorescent antibody titers to *Babesia microti.* Clindamycin 600 mg IV every 6 hours and quinine 650 mg PO every 6 hours is the regimen of choice for a severe infection. Treatment should be continued for 7 to 10 days.

COLORADO TICK FEVER

Epidemiology and Clinical Presentation

There are a myriad of viruses transmitted by the tick vector. In the United States, the *Orbivirus* organism is the only one of significance. It is the causative agent of Colorado tick fever and is transmitted through the bite of *D. andersoni,* the wood tick. The disease is found mainly in the western states, with a peak incidence from April to October.

After the human is bitten by the infected tick, a 3- to 5-day incubation period ends with the abrupt onset of a flulike illness. Fever, chills, anorexia, nausea, headache, myalgias, and lethargy are common, but a maculopapular rash may be present in only 5% to 12% of the patients. A biphasic illness occurs in half of the patients, with the initial symptoms resolving in 2 to 3 days. Fever and myalgias return after a 1- to 2-day asymptomatic period, and this phase is more severe. The illness usually resolves spontaneously within 2 weeks, but meningoencephalitis and coagulopathy have been reported to complicate the course in children.

Diagnosis and Treatment

Because a history of tick bite is not usually obtained and the clinical presentation is nonspecific, diagnosing Colorado tick fever may be difficult. Confirmation of the diagnosis may be made by acute and convalescent titers or by direct virus isolation through direct immunofluorescent staining of red blood cells.

Colorado tick fever is a self-limited illness; there is no specific therapy except supportive care. Antibiotics may be initiated until RMSF can be ruled out.

TICK PARALYSIS

Epidemiology

Tick paralysis has been recognized since the early 1800s. It is thought to be caused by a toxin that is secreted by the salivary glands of the tick. Most cases occur in the southeastern and northwestern areas. Many tick species have been implicated as causing tick paralysis, but *Dermacentor* organisms are the principal vectors in the United States. The peak incidence occurs during the spring and summer months.

Clinical Presentation

Symptoms of tick paralysis usually begin after the female tick has been attached for 4 to 7 days. Girls are more commonly affected than boys, which is probably because longer hair allows the tick to be concealed for an extended period of time and therefore to produce symptoms. Restlessness, irritability, and paresthesias are seen early and progress to ascending flaccid paralysis, acute ataxia, or both. Respiratory failure may lead to death if support is not given.

Diagnosis

The diagnosis of tick paralysis is made by clinical presentation and by finding the offending tick. This condition must be differentiated from Guillain-Barré syndrome, myasthenia gravis, poliomyelitis, botulism, and diphtheria.

Treatment

Treatment is accomplished by removing the tick. The action of the neurotoxin is not understood, but recovery occurs within 48 hours. Supportive care is the mainstay of therapy after tick removal, especially if respiratory paralysis is present. Mortality occurs in approximately 10% of those affected; deaths in adults are uncommon.

Prevention

It is nearly impossible to completely avoid ticks. Ticks may be found not only in the outdoor grassy environment, but pets and children may also unknowingly bring the pests home. Therefore everyone must know simple preventive measures to lessen the risk of tick exposure. Checking animals and children at least twice daily in tick-infested areas may reveal the parasite before it attaches. The insecticide permethrin and the insect repellent diethyltoluamide (deet) have been used successfully to repel ticks when applied *to clothing*. It should be noted that allergic and toxic side effects, including encephalitis, have been reported if deet is allowed to absorb into the skin. Permethrin is poorly absorbed and is quickly inactivated even if it enters the skin. It does, however, occasionally cause skin irritation as a side effect.

METHOD FOR REMOVING TICKS FROM THE SKIN

1. Grab at attachment point with blunt forceps, tweezers, or protected fingertips.
2. Provide gentle, steady, upward traction until the tick releases.
3. **Don't** twist, jerk, squeeze, or crush the tick.
4. Wear gloves to handle the tick, and dispose of it in the toilet or in alcohol.
5. Clean and disinfect the bite site with soap and water.

Modified from Needham GR: Evaluation of five popular methods for tick removal, *Pediatrics* 75(6):997-1002, 1985.

Once the tick has attached, it is important to properly remove it to avoid the needless spread of infectious material. Studies using petroleum jelly, isopropyl alcohol, fingernail polish, and hot matches have not proven to be effective in accomplishing tick release. It is recommended that an embedded tick be removed by steady upward traction as close as possible to the point of attachment with a blunt forceps, tweezers, or gloved fingertips (see the box above). Squeezing or crushing the tick may inject infectious material into the patient. The tick may be placed in alcohol for disposal or for preservation if identification or further study is warranted.

KEY CONSIDERATIONS

WHAT IS THE LIFE THREAT?

Untreated tularemia and Rocky Mountain spotted fever can result in serious illness and death. Untreated Lyme disease can result in serious cardiac complications. Tick paralysis can cause respiratory failure and death.

DOES THE PATIENT NEED ADMISSION?

Admit patients with serious complications of Lyme disease and advanced tularemia. Patients with untreated Rocky Mountain spotted fever can develop a vasculitis that leads to adult respiratory distress syndrome, disseminated intravascular coagulopathy, and shock. Such patients require admission.

WHAT IS THE MOST SERIOUS DIAGNOSIS?

Untreated Lyme disease can result in severe neurologic and cardiac manifestations, including meningoencephalitis, peripheral and cranial neuritis (such as Bell palsy), and stroke.

Cardiac abnormalities include heart block and myopericarditis. Left ventricular dysfunction can result and can cause congestive heart failure.

HAVE I PERFORMED A THOROUGH WORK-UP?

Consider Lyme disease in patients with an unexplained rash, arthralgia, or neuropathy. Consider Rocky Mountain spotted fever in patients with an unexplained petechial skin rash or an unexplained febrile illness.

In cases of unexplained paralysis, search the skin for ticks.

Recommended Reading

Bolgiano EB: Tick-borne illnesses. In Rosen P et al, editors: *Emergency medicine: concepts and clinical practice,* ed 3, St Louis, 1992, Mosby.

Gentile DA: Tick-borne diseases. In Auerbach PS, Geehr EC, editors: *Wilderness medicine: management of wilderness and environmental emergencies,* ed 3, St Louis, 1995, Mosby.

Rahn DW, Malawista SE: Lyme disease, recommendations for diagnosis and treatment, *Ann Intern Med* 114:472-481, 1991.

Schlesinger PA: Update on lyme disease, *Hosp Med* 29(8):53-64, 1993.

Steere AC: Lyme borreliosis. In Isselbacher KJ et al, editors: *Harrison's principles of internal medicine,* ed 13, New York, 1994, McGraw-Hill.

Woodward TE: Rickettsial diseases. In Isselbacher KJ et al, editors: *Harrison's principles of internal medicine,* ed 13, New York, 1994, McGraw-Hill.

Chapter *Sixty-four*

TOXICOLOGY: GENERAL MANAGEMENT PRINCIPLES

MICHAEL T. KELLEY

It is estimated that 7 million toxic exposures occur in the United States each year. Accidental exposures account for more than 5000 deaths annually, whereas intentional poisonings account for 7000 deaths. Patients with poisoning from a variety of sources are typically taken first to the emergency department when they require treatment. Management may require that the physician focus on early stabilization and support of vital signs before performing a detailed history and physical examination and before the results of laboratory tests (including the toxicologic screen) are available.

INITIAL STABILIZATION

One of the major causes of morbidity and mortality in a drug overdose is aspiration of stomach contents. Drugs and toxins that cause lethargy and coma when taken in excess can interfere with the reflexes that protect the airway. The overdose of many drugs causes nausea and vomiting and increases the risk of aspiration. Therefore the oral cavity should be cleared of vomitus and other debris. Intubation is indicated in any patient who lacks respiratory drive. It may be necessary to protect the airway in other situations, such as the performance of oral gastric decontamination in a lethargic or semicomatose patient.

Intoxication is often associated with instability and incoordination with subsequent trauma. Patients can lose consciousness, lose their balance, or crash their automobiles. In all suspected trauma cases, the cervical spine should be protected.

Ventilation and oxygenation must be assessed and supported as needed. The rate and depth of respirations can provide diagnostic clues about agents involved in the poisoning. All drugs in the sedative-hypnotic class (e.g., alcohol, narcotics, barbiturates, benzodiazepines) depress the respiratory centers and decrease sympathetic output from the brain; respiratory arrest is the usual cause of death. Sedative-hypnotic overdoses usually do not produce coma without signs of respiratory depression. In contrast, aspirin and dinitrophenol uncouple oxidative phosphorylation and directly stimulate the brainstem centers to increase respirations. Salicylates produce a metabolic acidosis that also increases respiratory rate.

Oxygen is the first therapeutic drug administered to any patient who has compromised ventilation. It should be given in as high a concentration as possible until a blood gas analysis is available. Oxygen is also the major antidote for carbon monoxide poisoning.

All serious intoxications require intravenous (IV) access to administer fluids, antidotes, and other medications. With many types of poisonings, a patient's condition can deteriorate rapidly after presentation. For example, patients who overdose on cyclic antidepressants can look well and have only a mild tachycardia when they enter the emergency department but develop cardiac arrest within a short period. It is much easier to establish an IV line in a patient with a normal blood pressure than in one with severe hypotension. Obtain a 12-lead ECG and provide continuous ECG monitoring.

Dextrose administration or the evaluation of blood glucose levels is indicated for any patient who has changes in mental status. Overdoses of various drugs can cause hypoglycemia; the most obvious drugs are the oral hypoglycemic agents and insulin. Other drugs and poisons can lower blood sugar to a dangerous level. Alcohol can cause a dangerously low blood glucose, especially in young children.

Narcotic drugs such as heroin, morphine, and meperidine cause death by depressing the respiratory center of the brain. Naloxone, a narcotic antagonist, is a specific antidote for opiate compounds because it competes with narcotics for the opiate receptors. Current recommendations are to administer 2 mg of naloxone IV to reverse respiratory depression. A full dose of naloxone need not always be given if the source of the overdose is known and intubation and respiratory control are successful. The use of less than a full dose should be considered in a situation in which the patient needs to be transported to another center or in which the patient is violent and some sedation is preferred.

HISTORY

Obtaining a good patient history is the next step after providing initial stabilization. Prehospital emergency care personnel are particularly important in this step because the patient may be awake at the scene but become unconscious on arrival to the emergency department. Such personnel should be questioned about the initial appearance of the patient at the scene, as well as about the scene itself. They should also be asked to retrieve all medications and any suspicious household chemicals from the scene if the source of the overdose is unknown.

Even if the patient is able to provide a history, it may not be accurate. The suicidal patient may deny ingesting anything. Alternatively, patients may exaggerate the amount taken or report taking one drug when in fact another was taken. With over-the-counter preparations, the patient may not even know the agent. The patient may think that he or she took an aspirin product when it actually was acetaminophen. When available, the history provided by a relative or friend supplements the history provided by the patient.

One of the most important pieces of information is the time that the poisoning or ingestion occurred. Treatments for acute aspirin and acetaminophen toxicity depend on a nomogram that determines toxicity on the basis of drug-blood concentrations at a given time. All drugs go through a period of distribution in the body. For example, a digoxin level of 20 ng/ml drawn shortly after overdose may not be as predictive of toxicity as a level of 5 ng/ml drawn 4 to 6 hours after ingestion. Count the number of tablets in each prescription container to determine the amount possibly taken.

Remember that alcohol is the most common secondary drug that is taken in the overdose setting. The addition of alcohol to the overdose may produce a confusing clinical picture.

PHYSICAL EXAMINATION

The physical examination in the toxicologic emergency concentrates in part on signs and symptoms that are pertinent to the autonomic nervous system. By noting changes in the autonomic nervous system, the toxicologist often can classify the patient into toxic syndromes, or "toxidromes." Changes in vital signs provide critical information. Skin and mucous membrane moisture is noted, and pupil size and reactivity and bowel activity are considered. The patient's level of consciousness should be examined at regular intervals. The remainder of the examination is similar to that for any emergency patient and includes a search for signs of trauma.

TOXIC SYNDROMES (TABLE 64-1)

Alpha-Adrenergic Syndrome

Drugs that stimulate the α-adrenergic receptors in the peripheral vasculature cause vasoconstriction and hypertension. If there is no direct stimulation of the heart, a compensatory reflex bradycardia occurs. The pupils dilate, and there is increased output from the sweat glands. Vasoconstriction of the blood vessels in the mucous membranes causes relatively dry oral and conjunctival tissues. Patients may be agitated as a result of stimulation of the dopamine system. Temperature, respiratory rate, and bowel sounds are not typically affected.

Beta-Adrenergic Syndrome

Stimulation of the β-adrenergic receptors in the peripheral vasculature causes vasodilatation. Hypotension is accompanied by a reflex tachycardia. Stimulation of the β-adrenergic receptors also increases heart rate and produces hyperglycemia and hypokalemia.

Mixed Alpha- and Beta-Adrenergic Syndrome

Cocaine, amphetamines, and over-the-counter decongestants and stimulants such as pseudoephedrine and ephedrine cause a mixed syndrome when taken in overdose. Blood pressure rises because of α-adrenergic stimulation to the peripheral vasculature. Instead of a reflex slowing of the heart rate as in the pure α-adrenergic syndrome, the β-adrenergic effects of the drug drive the heart rate and further increase the blood pressure. Hyperthermia is often present and can be life threatening. Alpha-adrenergic receptor stimulation causes dilated pupils, an increase in sweat production, and decreased mucous membrane secretions. An overdose causes agitation, and massive overdose may cause coma and respiratory arrest.

Table 64-1

TOXIC SYNDROMES

	Alpha	Beta	Mixed	Sympatholytic	Cholinergic	Anticholinergic
Blood pressure	Inc	Dec	Inc	Dec	Inc/dec	Inc
Heart rate	Dec	Inc	Inc	Dec	Inc/dec	Inc
Temperature	±	±	Inc	Dec	Ne	Inc
Respiratory rate	±	Ne	±	Dec	Dec	Ne
Level of consciousness	Ag	Ne	Ag	Dec	Ne	Dec/Ag
Pupils	Dil	Ne	Dil	Con	Con	Dil
Skin	Sweat	Ne	Sweat	Ne	Sweat	Dry
Mucous membranes	Dry	Ne	Dry	Ne	Wet	Dry
Bowel sounds	±	Ne	±	Ne	Inc	Dec

Inc, Increased; *Dec,* decreased; *Ne,* no effect; *Ag,* agitated; *Dil,* dilated; *Con,* constricted.

Sympatholytic Syndrome

The sympatholytic syndrome is produced by drugs that decrease sympathetic output from the brain. Included in this group are the alcohols, opiates, barbiturates, benzodiazepines, and other sedative-hypnotic drugs. These agents cause hypoventilation and respiratory arrest. Decreased sympathetic stimulation to the peripheral vasculature causes vasodilatation and hypotension. In the heart, unopposed vagal stimulation slows the heart rate. The level of consciousness is decreased. With only a few exceptions, the drugs that produce this syndrome cause small pupils.

Most patients with this syndrome are hypothermic. The sympatholytic drugs disrupt the ability of the body to regulate temperature. The patient becomes poikilothermic and assumes the temperature of the environment. Most of the time patients are in environments that are less than body temperature, but if the patient is in an area where the temperature is greater than body temperature, hyperthermia will occur.

Mixed Cholinergic Syndrome

Stimulation of nicotinic and muscarinic receptors produces the mixed cholinergic syndrome. The organophosphate insecticides inhibit the metabolism of acetylcholine and are the most common toxins that cause this syndrome. Because both the sympathetic and parasympathetic ganglia have nicotinic receptors, both bradycardia with hypotension and tachycardia with hypertension may be seen. Stimulation of the muscarinic receptors in the various glands causes increased glandular output. Salivation, lacrimation, spontaneous urination, and defecation (SLUD) are common in this syndrome. The pupils are small.

Anticholinergic Syndrome

Drugs such as atropine, scopolamine, and antihistamines, as well as plants such as jimsonweed and certain mushrooms, have anticholinergic effects. The blocking of vagal stimulation to the heart causes tachycardia and hypertension. The pupils are dilated, and the mucous membranes are dry. The skin is also dry and warm. The patient's temperature may be elevated and needs to be closely monitored. Bowel motility is slowed; therefore these substances delay their own absorption. Agitation is common.

Laboratory Tests

Certain laboratory tests are needed in the work-up of the poisoned patient to help identify the substance and treatment. The least important aspect of the initial patient management is the drug screen. Drug screens take time to complete, and the results are typically not immediately available. When ordering a drug screen, the physician should communicate to the laboratory the type of drug that is suspected.

The complete blood count (CBC) can provide clues to the diagnosis of unknown ingestions. Some drugs, such as iron and theophylline, cause the white blood count to increase when taken in overdose.

Electrolytes, glucose, blood urea nitrogen (BUN), creatinine, and osmolarity are obtained to rule out nontoxic disease, provide clues to the diagnosis of unknown ingestions, and calculate anion and osmolar gaps. Certain drugs affect laboratory values directly. Digoxin increases serum potassium levels, whereas acute theophylline ingestion decreases serum potassium levels. Acute theophylline ingestion causes hyperglycemia, whereas the sulfonoureas decrease blood glucose levels.

An anion gap is calculated by adding the serum cation concentrations (Na^+ and K^+) and then subtracting the serum anion concentrations (Cl^- and HCO_3^-). The normal anion gap is 8 to 12 mEq/L. Drugs or toxins produce an anion-gap metabolic acidosis by causing an increase in lactic acid, by being acids themselves, or by having acid metabolites. Almost every drug can cause lactic acidosis if the ingestion is large enough to disrupt respiration or cardiac function. The resultant hypoventilation and hypotension causes lactic acidosis.

Drugs and toxins can also produce lactic acidosis by disrupting or inhibiting cellular metabolism. Cyanide interferes with cytochrome oxidase activity, and the salicylates uncouple oxidative phosphorylation.

Certain drugs such as the salicylates and the barbiturates are weak acids. Other drugs have acid metabolites. Methanol (formic acid) and ethylene glycol (glycolic acid) are two alcohols that are metabolized to acids. In contrast, isopropyl alcohol is metabolized to acetone and does not produce an acidosis unless it is ingested in a quantity large enough to cause respiratory depression or hypotension and a subsequent lactic acidosis.

The osmolar gap is the difference between the *calculated* osmolarity and the *measured* osmolarity. The measured osmolarity must be determined by the freezing point of serum; the alternative method is to measure osmolarity by the vaporization point. In toxicology, the major use for the osmolar gap is in estimating the concentration of the alcohols. If the vaporization-point method is used, the alcohols boil off before the vaporization point is determined, which gives a falsely low osmolarity. The osmolarity is calculated by the following formula:

$$2Na^+ + \frac{BUN}{2.8} + \frac{Glucose}{18} = 290 \pm 10$$

Multiplying the osmolar gap by the molecular weight gives a close approximation of the concentration of the alcohol in mg/L. For example, if the measured osmolarity is 350 mOsm and the calculated osmolarity is 300 mOsm, the osmolar gap is 50 mOsm. If the suspected alcohol is methanol (molecular weight 32), the estimated concentration of methanol would be 1600 mg/L, or 160 mg/dl.

Although some disease states, such as sepsis, can cause both an osmolar gap and an anion gap, the only drugs that cause both are methanol and ethylene glycol. Because the treatment for methanol or ethylene glycol poisoning should begin as soon as possible and because determining the serum concentrations for these types of alcohols is difficult, calculating the osmolar gap and anion gap is useful if such poisoning is suspected.

The ECG is important in the initial evaluation of poisoning. Many drugs, especially cardiac medications, affect the rhythm and duration of the cardiac intervals (PR, QRS, QT). Sodium channel blockers such as the type Ia antidysrhythmics, the cyclic antidepressants, and cocaine prolong the QRS duration. Beta-adrenergic blockers prolong the PR interval, and the phenothiazines increase the QT duration.

Arterial blood gases are helpful in determining the degree of acidosis or alkalosis and the contribution of the respiratory and metabolic processes.

After initial stabilization and the collection of information through the history, physical, and laboratory tests, discuss the toxicology case with a regional poison control center. The trained poison information specialists can help with the identification of the drug or poison and can provide advice for patient management.

TREATMENT

General

The basic treatment for any drug or poison is to separate the patient from the substance. If there is exposure to a toxic gas, move the patient to fresh air and give oxygen to him or her. If the patient has a toxic substance in the eyes, rinse the eyes thoroughly. If the patient is covered with a toxic substance, brush or wash off the substance with copious amounts of water and remove all contaminated clothing.

In the case of an ingestion, separating the toxic substance from the patient can be accomplished in one of two ways. One way to remove the toxin from the stomach is with gastric lavage. When preparing for the gastric lavage, assess the patient's airway, level of consciousness, and gag reflex. Unconscious patients or patients with consciousness levels so impaired that they cannot protect their airway require endotracheal intubation before the lavage to protect the airway. Awake patients can be safely lavaged in a "head-down" position. To perform a gastric lavage, insert a large-bore lavage tube (36-40 Fr) into the stomach.

Even with a 40 Fr tube, many time-released medications and large capsules cannot fit through the end of the tube. For adults, water can be used, as the lavage fluid, but for children normal saline should be used because hyponatremia may be produced with the use of tap water. The lavage should be continued until the effluent is clear. Esophageal tears and aspiration of gastric contents are complications of this procedure.

A second way to separate a drug or toxic substance from the patient after an ingestion is to prevent absorption by keeping the substance inside the bowel and allowing or encouraging it to pass through the rectum. Activated charcoal adsorbs most drugs and toxins; smaller molecules such as alcohols and metals (e.g., lithium, iron) are poorly adsorbed. A cathartic such as sorbitol is often added to the activated charcoal. However, there is no evidence that cathartics reduce the toxic effects of any drug, and there have been cases of cathartic-induced hyponatremia. The major benefit of cathartics is to hasten transit of charcoal through the bowel. The presence of a charcoal stool can almost ensure the end of drug absorption. Use only one dose of cathartic in an ingestion. The dose of activated charcoal is based on the amount of drug ingested; at least 10 times the ingested amount should be administered. In most cases 70 to 100 grams in adults and 1 g/kg in children is sufficient. However, for large ingestions multiple doses of charcoal are necessary to completely prevent absorption of the drug. Multiple doses of charcoal have also

been used to hasten the elimination of certain drugs such as theophylline and phenobarbital. For such drugs the gut wall acts as a dialysis membrane, and the drugs in the system can diffuse into the bowel and be trapped there by the charcoal. Other drugs have extensive hepatoenteric recirculation. Multiple doses of charcoal are useful in preventing reabsorption and hastening elimination of the drug.

For drugs that are not adsorbed to charcoal (e.g., lithium, iron), whole-bowel irrigation with substances such as Golytely has successfully eliminated the drugs from the gastrointestinal tract. Hemodialysis and hemoperfusion are other ways to remove drugs from patients. The effectiveness of such procedures depends on the pharmacokinetic properties of the ingested toxin.

Seizures

For drug-induced seizures, the treatment of choice is a benzodiazepine, such as diazepam (Valium) or lorazepam (Activan). Many seizures stop spontaneously without therapy, and thus there should not necessarily be a rush to treat the first sign of seizure. Airway protection and protecting the patient from injury should be the first concern. Seizures caused by certain medication overdoses, such as theophylline, often require large doses of benzodiazepines. For example, it is not unusual to administer 50 mg or even 100 mg of diazepam in a severe theophylline overdose. It may also be necessary to add a barbiturate to the regimen. If a barbiturate is necessary, phenobarbital is a good agent for treating medication-induced seizures; however, it does not reach a sufficiently high concentration in the brain as rapidly as the benzodiazepines. If multiple doses of a benzodiazepine have been required to control the seizure, it is appropriate to begin a loading dose (15 mg/kg) of phenobarbital. The use of both benzodiazepines and phenobarbital in such high quantities has some intrinsic problems. Diazepam, like phenytoin, is mixed in propylene glycol, and there is a potential for cardiac dysrhythmias if diazepam is given too rapidly. Treatment with high doses of benzodiazepines and barbiturates also undoubtedly causes respiratory depression, and intubation is usually necessary.

Unresponsive seizures are very serious and often lead to death unless the causative drug can be eliminated by other measures, such as hemodialysis or hemoperfusion. Some drug-induced seizures are resistant to treatment with benzodiazepines. Isoniazid, for instance, produces seizures that are poorly responsive to benzodiazepines but are successfully treated with pyridoxine (vitamin B_6). Consultation with a medical toxicologist or poison control center can be helpful in these circumstances.

Hypotension

Drug- or toxin-induced hypotension is usually caused by a decrease in peripheral vascular resistance or by a decrease in myocardial contractility. Other drugs (e.g., iron) can cause gastrointestinal bleeding and fluid loss. If there are no signs of pulmonary edema or congestive heart failure, the initial therapy is to administer a bolus of normal saline or Ringer's lactate. The dose is 200 to 400 ml for adults and 20 ml/kg for children. Patients with drug overdoses that do not respond to bolus fluid therapy usually require pulmonary artery catheterization with cardiac monitoring. Overdoses of toxins that cause hypotension by decreasing cardiac output need specific therapy depending on the drug. The use of vasopressors also depends on the drug ingested.

Hypertension

Drugs such as amphetamines, cocaine, and over-the-counter decongestants can cause hypertension when taken in excess. The initial therapy for patients who have taken drugs that cause hypertension is to place the patient in an upright or sitting position. The gravitational re-distribution of blood often helps lower the blood pressure and reduces the cerebral pressure. Drug therapy can be either specific or general. A pure α-adrenergic agonist such as phenylpropanolamine (Entex LA, Dexatrim) can be treated with the alpha antagonist phentolamine. Labetalol has both alpha- and beta-agonist actions and is appropriate for mixed agonists such as amphetamine and cocaine. In general, the treatment of hypertension with nitroprusside is also appropriate.

Dysrhythmias

Ventricular fibrillation and cardiac arrest should be treated according to the usual advanced cardiac life support (ACLS) guidelines. Drug- or poison-induced cardiopulmonary arrests are very serious and usually fatal. Prolonged cardiopulmonary resuscitation (CPR) may be required until the drug can be removed or until the effects subside. Some patients have survived by being placed on cardiopulmonary bypass.

The treatment of ventricular tachycardia depends on the drug ingested. For example, chloral hydrate has a toxic metabolite that sensitizes the myocardium to circulating catecholamines. Ventricular dysrhythmias can develop, and treatment is with a β-adrenergic blockade. Cyclic antidepressants produce toxicity by blocking the sodium channels of the myocardium. This action is similar to that caused by class Ia antidysrhythmic drugs (e.g., quinidine, phenytoin). Therefore it would not be appropriate to use a class Ia antidysrhythmic to treat dysrhythmias caused by cyclic antidepressants. Instead the first-line therapy would involve administering sodium bicarbonate and then lidocaine if needed. Cardiac dysrhythmias caused by drugs that produce myocardial infarction can be treated with lidocaine.

Agitation

Hospital security personnel should be sought to deal with an agitated patient. For example, phencyclidine (PCP) can cause wild and bizarre behavior. Such patients are difficult to control because they do not experience any pain after an overdose of PCP. Be extremely cautious when approaching such individuals. Four or five persons often are necessary to apply four-point restraints. Agitation is often seen in patients who are hypoxemic; this fact is particularly true in children.

Body temperature rises rapidly in a patient who is agitated. Muscle damage can also occur, leading to rhabdomyolysis and kidney failure. A presumptive diagnosis of myoglobinuria can be made if the urine dipstick is positive for hemoglobin but no red blood cells are present. In most cases, agitation can be successfully treated with a benzodiazepine or an antipsychotic such as haloperidol.

Temperature

Overdoses with drugs such as those of the sedative-hypnotic class decrease the ability of the body to regulate temperature. The patient eventually assumes the temperature of the environment. Hypothermia is seen even in warm climates. In contrast, stimulants cause the body temperature to increase, and agitation or seizures can raise the body temperature to fatal levels. Emergent, rapid cooling is necessary to protect these patients against irreversible brain damage.

Child Abuse

Children who are intoxicated may actually represent child abuse. There are many unfortunate cases of adults who have given children drugs "just to see what would happen." Children are also given drugs to keep them quiet or to make them go to sleep. When a child accidentally ingests a parent's illicit drugs, child neglect may be present.

SUMMARY

Swift appropriate treatment of the intoxicated or poisoned patient by the emergency physician can greatly decrease morbidity and mortality. After the initial stabilization, determine what was ingested and what time the ingestion occurred. Note the vital signs, examine the pupils, look for mucous membrane moisture and sweat, and listen for bowel sounds. This evaluation can aid in determining what drug was ingested. Know the appropriate decontamination techniques, because these can prevent unnecessary complications. Understanding the specific therapies can be life saving.

KEY CONSIDERATIONS

WHAT IS THE LIFE THREAT?

Poisoning from sedatives, hypnotics, and narcotics cause death from respiratory depression and hypotension. In addition, the comatose patient who has an unprotected airway can vomit and aspirate gastric contents, which can result in respiratory distress and death.

DOES THE PATIENT NEED ADMISSION?

Patients requiring medical admission include those with lethal blood levels of overdosed drugs or poisons, those who remain comatose, and those who require ventilation and IV support.

Patients require psychiatric evaluation and admission if the poisoning was the result of a suicide attempt and the patient remains suicidal.

WHAT IS THE MOST SERIOUS DIAGNOSIS?

The most serious developments of overdoses and poisoning are acute loss of airway from aspiration and respiratory or circulatory failure.

HAVE I PERFORMED A THOROUGH WORK-UP?

Evaluate the patient's airway, and intubate the patient who remains comatose and cannot protect his or her own airway with the gag reflex. Protect the cervical spine during this procedure if there has been traumatic injury. Establish IV access and provide fluid to support blood pressure and tissue perfusion as needed. Give glucose and thiamine. Administer naloxone for clinical indications of a narcotic overdose. Consult with the regional poison center for all serious poisonings. Establish the airway and perform a gastric lavage. Administer activated charcoal and a cathartic.

Recommended Readings

Flomenbaum NE et al: General management of the poisoned or overdosed patient. In Goldfrank LR et al, editors: *Goldfrank's toxicologic emergencies,* ed 5, Norwalk, Conn, 1994, Appleton & Lange.

Olsen KR: Emergency evaluation and treatment. In Olsen KR, editor: *Poisoning & drug overdose,* ed 2, Norwalk, Conn, 1994, Appleton & Lange.

Olsen KR, Pentel PR, Kelley MT: Physical assessment and differential diagnosis of the poisoned patient, *Med Tox* 2:52-81, 1987.

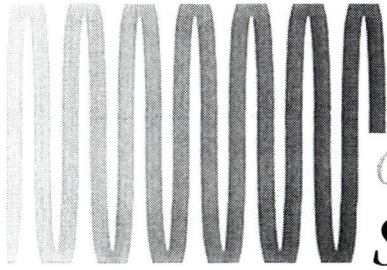

Chapter *Sixty-five*
SPECIFIC TOXINS

DONNA SEGER AND LINDSAY MURRAY

ACETAMINOPHEN

Acetaminophen, a widely used antipyretic and analgesic, is found in numerous over-the-counter preparations.

At therapeutic doses, acetaminophen is conjugated in the liver to form glucuronides and sulfates. Smaller amounts are excreted unchanged in the urine or metabolized via the P-450 mixed-function oxidase system to form a reactive intermediary, *N*-acetyl-*p*-benzoquinonimine (NAPQI). This substance is normally detoxified by glutathione, but with an overdose hepatic glutathione stores are overwhelmed, and this toxic metabolite binds covalently with hepatocytes, which results in centrizonal hepatic necrosis.

A single ingestion of 150 mg/kg of acetaminophen is potentially hepatotoxic in adults. The higher the dose, the greater the likelihood of hepatotoxicity, but there is great individual variation in susceptibility. Children are less susceptible and chronic alcoholics are more susceptible.

The clinical signs of acetaminophen toxicity are minimal during the first 24 hours following ingestion and consist mainly of mild gastrointestinal (GI) irritation. The signs may be completely absent or obscured by the presence of co-ingestants. The elevation of hepatic enzymes may occur 24 to 48 hours after ingestion. With severe intoxications, a coagulopathy and progressive hepatic encephalopathy may develop. If fulminant hepatic failure does not ensue, a gradual normalization of liver function occurs and is followed by complete recovery. Poor prognostic factors in the patient with hepatic coma include acidosis, a partial thromboplastin time (PTT) of longer than 100 seconds, and impaired renal function.

The diagnosis is made early if a serum acetaminophen level is obtained. A level obtained between 4 and 24 hours after ingestion predicts the risk of hepatotoxicity and can be interpreted using the Rumack-Matthew nomogram (Fig. 65-1). Activated charcoal should be administered to all patients who appear within 4 hours of a potentially toxic ingestion.

The outcome in the patient who is at risk for toxicity is greatly improved by the administration of the antidote *N*-acetyl-L-cysteine (NAC). The maximum benefit is obtained when NAC is administered within 8 hours of ingestion, but some benefit is obtained when it is administered within 24 hours. The initial oral dose is 140 mg/kg followed by further doses of 70 mg/kg every 4 hours for a total of 17 doses. If vomiting precludes NAC administration, ondansetron 0.15 mg/kg intravenously (IV) may be given and NAC repeated after 20 minutes. Liver function tests and a coagulation profile should be performed daily during the hospital admission until

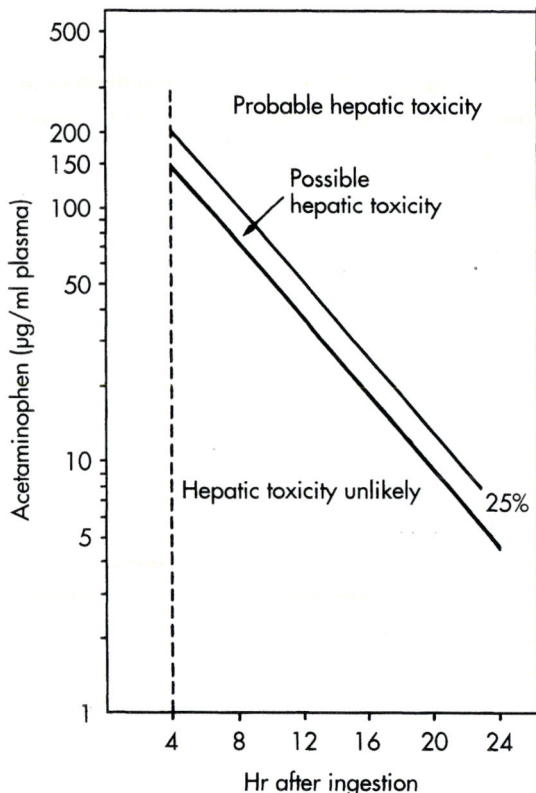

Fig 65-1 Rumack-Matthew nomogram for acetaminophen poisoning. (From Rumack BH, Matthew H: Acetaminophen poisoning and toxicity, *Pediatrics* 55:871, 1975.)

they show improvement. Patients developing a hepatic coma need appropriate intensive supportive care; if the poor prognostic signs are present, consideration should be given to liver transplantation.

ALCOHOLS

Ingestion of any of the alcohols (ethanol, isopropyl alcohol, methanol, ethylene glycol) by a nontolerant individual results in dose-dependent CNS depression, with respiratory failure

Table 65-1

ESTIMATION OF ALCOHOL LEVEL FROM CALCULATED OSMOLAL GAP*

Alcohol	Conversion Factor
Ethanol	4.3
Ethylene glycol	5.0
Isopropyl alcohol	5.9
Methanol	2.6

*To estimate the serum alcohol concentration (mg/dl), multiply the osmolal gap (mOsm/L) by the conversion factor.

and death as the ultimate potential complications. In addition, methanol and ethylene glycol form metabolites, which results in significant intrinsic toxicity. Ethanol abuse is well known as a widespread problem and is responsible for innumerable emergency department visits throughout the world.

Because the alcohols are rapidly and completely absorbed from the (GI) tract, gastric lavage is of little value when performed more than 30 minutes after ingestion. Activated charcoal does not significantly bind the alcohols and need not be administered unless there is suspicion of a co-ingestion. Specific alcohol levels are often useful in guiding therapy or excluding the ingestion of a toxic alcohol. If not readily obtainable, alcohol levels can be estimated from the osmolal gap (Table 65-1). Laboratory studies in seriously intoxicated patients should include arterial blood gases (ABGs), serum electrolytes, and glucose. Further evaluation may be required to exclude other causes of metabolic acidosis.

Isopropyl alcohol is widely used as a solvent and disinfectant and may be ingested as an ethanol substitute. As a CNS depressant, it is twice as potent as ethanol. It is metabolized by alcohol dehydrogenase to acetone, which contributes to and prolongs the CNS depression but does not share the metabolic, renal, cardiac, or retinal toxicity of ethylene glycol or methanol metabolites.

The clinical manifestations of isopropyl alcohol intoxication are similar to those of ethanol and include CNS depression and GI tract irritation. The characteristic odor of acetone may be a clue in distinguishing isopropyl alcohol from ethanol intoxication. Laboratory investigations reveal an elevated osmolal gap and acetonuria. Metabolic acidosis is not caused by isopropyl alcohol. Management is supportive, and all symptomatic patients should be admitted for observation. Watch for hypoglycemia. Hemodialysis effectively removes isopropyl alcohol and acetone and should be considered for severe intoxications (serum isopropyl alcohol >500 mg/dl or hypotension that is refractory to fluids and inotropes).

Methanol is widely used as a solvent and antifreeze. The ingestion of as little as 30 ml is potentially lethal. It is metabolized to formaldehyde and formic acid by alcohol dehydrogenase and aldehyde dehydrogenase, respectively. These two metabolites are highly toxic and accumulate to cause a progressive anion-gap metabolic acidosis, as well as ocular and CNS toxicity. Laboratory investigation reveals an osmolal gap and an anion-gap metabolic acidosis. Intravenous ethanol should be administered to competitively block the metabolism of methanol. A loading dose of 700 mg/kg (equal to 7 ml/kg of 10% ethanol in 5% dextrose solution) is followed by a maintenance infusion of 70 to 130 mg/kg/hr. The rate of infusion is titrated to maintain a serum ethanol level of greater than 100 mg/dl. Higher infusion rates are required in alcoholics and during hemodialysis. If an intravenous ethanol solution is unavailable, the same dose may be administered orally in the awake patient. Methanol and its metabolites are effectively removed by hemodialysis; this intervention is indicated if the methanol level is greater than 50 mg/dl or if there is severe or worsening metabolic acidosis, renal failure, or visual symptoms.

Ethylene glycol is a common ingredient of antifreeze. The minimal lethal dose in an adult is 100 ml. It is also metabolized by alcohol dehydrogenase and aldehyde dehydrogenase and forms glycolic, glyoxylic, and oxalic acids. The production of these metabolites together with lactate results in an anion-gap metabolic acidosis and CNS depression. If the condition is left untreated, acute tubular necrosis may follow but is usually reversible. Laboratory abnormalities include elevated osmotic and anion gaps, metabolic acidosis, calcium oxalate crystals in the urine and, rarely, hypocalcemia.

Management, which should be initiated as early as possible to ensure the best outcome, includes supportive care and the administration of IV ethanol to competitively inhibit ethylene glycol metabolism. The dosage regimen for IV ethanol is identical to that used in methanol poisoning. Hemodialysis is effective and indicated for ethylene glycol levels that are greater than 50 mg/dl, renal failure, significant or worsening metabolic acidosis, or any deterioration in clinical status.

ANTICHOLINERGICS

A wide variety of drugs and naturally occurring substances have anticholinergic properties (see the box on p. 774) and may cause the anticholinergic syndrome, which is characterized by tachycardia, hypertension, hyperthermia, mydriasis, ileus, urinary retention, dry flushed skin, dry mucous membranes, and delirium.

Care is supportive and may include intubation and ventilation for coma, sedation with a benzodiazepine for delirium, and cooling for hyperthermia. Physostigmine, a reversible acetylcholinesterase inhibitor, may be indicated to confirm the diagnosis and to treat severe intoxications that are unresponsive to supportive care. In particular, physostigmine administra-

AGENTS WITH ANTICHOLINERGIC PROPERTIES

Antihistamines
Belladonna alkaloids
  Atropine
  Homatropine
  Scopolamine
Benztropine
Butyrophenones
  Haloperidol
Cyclic antidepressants
Cyclobenzaprine
Phenothiazines
Plants
  Jimsonweed
  Mushrooms (certain species)

tion may be useful for severe delirium or hyperthermia. The potential side effects include seizures, bradydysrhythmias, and asystole, and for this reason physostigmine should always be administered in small dosage increments, in a monitored situation, and under direct physician supervision. The dose is 0.5 mg slow IV push, which may be repeated in 10 to 15 minutes.

BETA-BLOCKERS

Beta-blockers (β-blockers) are widely used in the management of hypertension, ischemic heart disease, and cardiac dysrhythmias, and they may be taken in overdose by patients with underlying cardiovascular disease. The severity of an overdose depends not only on the dose ingested but also on the presence of underlying cardiac disease, co-ingestants, and the particular agent. Propranolol is the most toxic β-blocker.

The toxic mechanism that is common to all β-blockers is excessive beta-adrenergic blockade, which leads to decreased intracellular cyclic adenosine monophosphate (cAMP); negative inotropic, chronotropic, and dromotropic

effects on the heart; and peripheral vasoconstriction. In addition, some agents, such as propranolol, have quinidinelike effects (i.e., membrane stabilization).

The principal clinical effects of β-blocker overdose are cardiovascular, with hypotension and bradycardia the most common. Atrioventricular (AV) block, intraventricular conduction disturbances, cardiogenic shock, and asystole can occur in more severe cases. A QRS widening may be seen with propranolol. CNS toxicity occurs with the more lipid-soluble agents (such as propranolol) and may manifest as drowsiness, coma, and respiratory depression. Bronchospasm and hypoglycemia occur rarely.

Many patients with β-blocker overdose (particularly young, healthy subjects) are asymptomatic or minimally symptomatic and require only decontamination and observation. Specific therapy is required for cases in which there is evidence of more significant cardiotoxicity. Atropine should be administered if the heart rate is less than 60 beats/minute, but such a response occurs less than 25% of the time. Hypotension should initially be managed with volume expansion. If these interventions produce an inadequate response, glucagon should be administered as an IV bolus of 5 mg (which may be repeated) followed by a continuous infusion of 2 to 5 mg/hour. Glucagon is a specific antidote that bypasses beta-receptor blockade and acts to elevate intracellular cAMP levels directly. If the patient does not respond to glucagon, isoproterenol and epinephrine infusions should be added in sequence, and a pulmonary artery catheter should be inserted. In cases that remain unresponsive, the insertion of a pacemaker or circulatory assist device needs to be considered.

BUTTON BATTERY INGESTION

Forty-four percent of all button batteries that are ingested are done so by children who ingest hearing aid batteries from their own hearing aid. Another 40% of button battery ingestions occur immediately following removal from products such as watches, games, and toys.

If button battery ingestion is suspected, an x-ray examination should be obtained to determine the location of the battery. If the battery is seen in the esophagus, it should be immediately removed by endoscopy. Unless the ingested battery is a 15.6 mm mercuric oxide cell or a 15 mm battery in a child younger than 6 years of age, subsequent x-ray examinations are unnecessary if the patient is asymptomatic.

If the type of battery ingested is unknown, the type may be determined with the imprint code of a duplicate battery, by measuring the battery compartment within the product, or by checking the packaging. If the battery is greater than 15 mm in diameter, the presence of mercuric oxide may be determined from the packaging instructions or from the imprint code by calling the local poison center or the National Button Battery Ingestion Hotline at (202) 625-3333. Blood and mercury levels should be obtained if the battery splits in the GI tract.

Batteries located in the GI tract beyond the esophagus do not need to be removed unless the patient is symptomatic or unless a 15 mm battery does not pass within 48 hours in a child younger than 6 years of age.

CALCIUM CHANNEL BLOCKERS

Calcium channel blockers are widely used in the management of ischemic heart disease, hypertension, and cardiac dysrhythmias. As with β-blockers, overdose is commonly seen in the context of underlying cardiovascular pathology.

Calcium channel blockers slow the influx of calcium across the slow channels of cell membranes. This effect results in reduced cardiac contractility, slowed AV nodal conduction, depressed sinus node activity, and a fall in peripheral vascular resistance.

The principal clinical manifestations of intoxication with calcium channel blockers are hypotension and bradycardia. The bradycardia may be sinus, reflect second- or third-degree AV block, or reflect sinus arrest with junctional escape. The QRS duration is not affected. Noncardiac manifestations of toxicity include abnormal mental status and hyperglycemia.

Management of the symptomatic overdose centers on aggressive and early hemodynamic monitoring and support and may involve the insertion of a pulmonary artery catheter to guide fluid and inotrope administration. Inotropic agents should be titrated until an adequate response is achieved, with no one inotropic agent being superior to another. A 10% solution of calcium chloride 10 ml IV may reverse depression of cardiac contractility but is usually not effective for other manifestations of toxicity. Glucagon should be given according to the regimen described for β-blocker overdose, but its efficacy is not as well established in treating overdoses of calcium channel blockers.

CAUSTIC SUBSTANCES

Caustic substances, most commonly acids or alkalis, are found in a large number of household products. Accidental ingestion is most common in children under 4 years of age, whereas ingestion by older individuals may be a result of an attempted suicide or of self-mutilation. Immediate complications include upper airway obstruction, GI hemorrhage, and perforation of the esophagus, which leads to mediastinitis. Delayed complications include stricture of the esophagus or stomach.

The nature of the ingestion must be defined. Alkalis cause liquefactive necrosis, which results in more significant damage than the coagulative necrosis associated with acid ingestion. Liquid alkalis may cause widespread esophageal and gastric injury without evidence of oropharyngeal injury, whereas solid alkali preparations tend to produce a patchy distribution of upper esophageal and oropharyngeal injuries. The volume and concentration of the caustic substance are the major determinants of injury severity.

Management initially focuses on assessing the adequacy of the airway and ventilation and relieving any obstruction. The physical examination includes evaluating the patient for drooling; respiratory distress; oral or pharyngeal burns; and abdominal pain, guarding, or tenderness. An absence of oropharyngeal burns never excludes the possibility of esophageal injury. Esophageal injury is most common in the presence of two of the following: vomiting, drooling, and stridor. Chest and abdominal x-ray films may be needed to evaluate the complications.

Inducing emesis, performing a gastric lavage, or administering activated charcoal is contraindicated. Activated charcoal does not bind caustics, may cause vomiting, and interferes with subsequent endoscopy. Steroids are often used with alkali burns, but their efficacy is unclear. Antibiotics are indicated only if an esophageal perforation is suspected. An esophagoscopy to assess the extent of injury is indicated in patients with oropharyngeal burns or a history or symptoms of significant ingestion. The esophagoscopy should be performed within 24 to 48 hours.

CARBON MONOXIDE

Carbon monoxide (CO) poisoning is the most common toxin-induced cause of death. Accidental poisoning occurs during fires or where combustion of hydrocarbons has taken place in a confined or poorly ventilated space. Deliberate intoxication with suicidal intent also occurs.

Carbon monoxide binds to hemoglobin 210 times more avidly than does oxygen, which results in reduced oxyhemoglobin saturation and impaired oxygen delivery to the periphery. In addition, CO appears to directly inhibit cytochrome oxidase and may cause lipid peroxidation in the central nervous system, which further disrupts cellular function.

Acute signs and symptoms of CO poisoning reflect a primary dysfunction of those organs with the highest oxygen consumption (i.e., the brain and heart) and include headache, dizziness, nausea, a decreased level of consciousness, convulsions, chest pain, and cardiac dysrhythmias. In addition, a delayed syndrome of neuropsychologic dysfunction may be seen in as many as 30% of the survivors.

Carboxyhemoglobin (COHb) levels are useful in confirming the diagnosis of CO poisoning but do not always accurately reflect the severity of the poisoning. Levels as high as 10% may be seen in nonexposed smokers. Management should always be based on the clinical findings and not on an isolated COHb level.

Initial management consists of removing the individual from the exposure and providing appropriate supportive care together with the administration of high-flow oxygen. Oxygen is the specific antidote for this type of poisoning and should be delivered either via a tight-fitting mask in the conscious patient or via an endotracheal tube if intubation is indicated on clinical grounds. Oxygen therapy should be continued for at least 6 hours or until the patient is asymptomatic. Patients should be monitored for dysrhythmias, and a 12-lead ECG should be obtained to determine if there is evidence of myocardial ischemia.

Hyperbaric oxygen therapy greatly enhances the elimination of CO and should be considered if an equipped facility is readily available and there is a history of loss of consciousness, coma, abnormal mental status, any ECG abnormalities, or if the patient is pregnant (fetal hemoglobin preferentially binds CO).

Concomitant methemoglobinemia, cyanide poisoning, or irritant gas injury should always be considered in the fire victim.

COCAINE

Cocaine is a widely used drug of abuse. It may be inhaled, ingested, injected intravenously, or smoked as freebase ("crack"). Maximum effects are seen within several minutes after injection or smoking but may be delayed as long as 30 minutes after ingestion or nasal insufflation.

Cocaine intoxication results in a state of euphoria together with sympathetic and CNS stimulation. The CNS manifestations include anxiety, delirium, psychosis, hyperactivity, and seizures. Cardiovascular manifestations include tachycardia, ventricular dysrhythmias, hypertension, and peripheral vasoconstriction. Myocardial, cerebral, or intestinal infarction can occur. Other potential complications include intracranial hemorrhage or aortic dissection resulting from hypertension, hyperthermia from increased heat production, renal failure, pneumothorax, and pneumomediastinum.

Management is essentially supportive and includes monitoring for complications. Decontamination is indicated only after oral ingestion. Whole-bowel irrigation may be considered to decontaminate a patient who has swallowed cocaine-containing packages ("body packers" and "body stuffers").

CYCLIC ANTIDEPRESSANTS

Cyclic antidepressants share a common tricyclic structure that consists of a central seven-member amine ring flanked by two benzene rings. They are a major cause of poisoning admissions and deaths. Some of the newer agents (e.g., maprotiline, amoxapine) are structurally different and have different toxicologic profiles (see the box above).

Toxic mechanisms include anticholinergic effects, fast sodium-channel blockade of the cardiac-conducting tissue (quinidinelike effect), peripheral alpha-blockade, and blockade of neu-

CYCLIC ANTIDEPRESSANTS

Tricyclic agents
  Amitriptyline
  Desipramine
  Doxepin
  Imipramine
  Nortriptyline
  Protriptyline
  Trimipramine
Tricyclic dibenzoxazepines
  Amoxapine
Tetracyclic agents
  Maprotiline
Related, chemically distinct agents
  Trazodone

ronal norepinephrine uptake. These effects manifest primarily as cardiovascular and CNS toxicity.

Anticholinergic effects of poisoning with cyclic antidepressants consist of delirium, sedation, mydriasis, sinus tachycardia, ileus, urinary retention, hyperthermia, and myoclonic jerking.

Apart from the sinus tachycardia, cardiovascular toxicity includes prolongation of the PR, QRS, and QT intervals on the ECG; hypotension; and ventricular dysrhythmias. The QRS prolongation reflects fast sodium-channel blockade, and a duration of >0.12 msec is predictive of potential major cardiovascular or CNS toxicity. Hypotension may be a result of peripheral vasodilatation but in severe cases reflects direct myocardial depression.

Apart from drowsiness and coma, CNS toxicity may manifest as seizures, which are often difficult to control. Amoxapine toxicity in particular is characterized by severe, recurrent seizure activity that is refractory to standard management.

Death from tricyclic antidepressant (TCA) toxicity usually occurs within hours of ingestion and is a result of cardiovascular complications or respiratory arrest. Ingestion of a dose greater than 10 mg/kg is associated with severe toxicity. A rapid, often unheralded, deterioration in clinical status during the first few hours is characteristic of TCA toxicity.

Cyclic antidepressant toxicity should be suspected in any patient with a decreased level of consciousness or seizures associated with prolongation of the QRS complexes on the ECG. However, amoxapine may produce severe CNS toxicity that is unaccompanied by ECG changes.

Any acute overdose of cyclic antidepressants should be managed with rapid institution of appropriate supportive care and monitoring. Such management is likely to include attention to airway, ventilation, cardiac rhythm, hypotension, seizures, and hyperthermia. Respiratory acidosis is to be avoided because it exacerbates toxicity. Gastric lavage and the administration of activated charcoal should be performed. Obtaining specific drug levels is unhelpful in acute management.

Sodium bicarbonate is the specific antidote for cyclic antidepressant toxicity. There is a direct beneficial effect of an alkaline serum pH on fast sodium-channel function and further benefit from the elevation of extracellular sodium ion concentration. The administration of sodium bicarbonate is indicated for seizures, hypotension, or significant QRS prolongation (>0.12 msec). A bolus of 100 mEq should be administered followed by a continuous infusion and further boluses as needed to maintain an arterial pH between 7.45 and 7.55. Frequent ABGs are necessary to monitor pH and prevent overalkalinization.

Physostigmine, once advocated as an antidote to cyclic antidepressant toxicity, is now contraindicated. It may aggravate the conduction disturbances and precipitate asystole and seizures.

Asymptomatic patients who have been decontaminated in the emergency department should be observed for at least 6 hours after ingestion. If they remain asymptomatic at the end of that period, have normal vital signs, active bowel sounds, and a normal ECG, they may be safely discharged following a psychiatric evaluation. The symptomatic patient requires admission for supportive care and monitoring. Following discontinuation of sodium bicarbonate, cardiac monitoring should be continued for 24 hours after the ECG has normalized.

DIGITALIS

The cardiac glycosides are naturally occurring substances that are found in a number of plants, including foxglove, oleander, and rhododendrons. Digoxin and digitoxin are used therapeutically to enhance cardiac contractility and slow AV conduction. Digoxin, the most widely used form of the cardiac glycosides, is well absorbed orally, has a relatively large volume of distribution, and is primarily excreted unchanged by the kidney with an elimination half-life of 36 hours.

The cardiac glycosides inhibit the function of the sodium-potassium-adenosinetriphosphatase-dependent ion transport system and also enhance vagal tone. Toxicity is associated with a high mortality resulting from cardiac dysrhythmia.

Two distinct clinical presentations of toxicity occur: acute and chronic. Patients with an acute overdose usually have nausea and vomiting, hyperkalemia, and sinus and AV block. Ventricular dysrhythmias occur in severe cases. Chronically intoxicated patients have nausea and vomiting, visual disturbances, weakness, and confusion; the most common dysrhythmias are ventricular and atrial ectopic beats, paroxysmal atrial tachycardia with block, accelerated junctional rhythm, and ventricular dysrhythmias. Hyperkalemia is not characteristic of chronic toxicity. In fact, patients with chronic toxicity are often hypokalemic because of concomitant diuretic therapy. The clinical picture in the patient with chronic toxicity is often complicated by the presence of underlying cardiac disease.

The diagnosis of chronic digoxin toxicity is often missed but should be considered in any patient who is taking digoxin and has GI or CNS symptoms or a characteristic cardiac dysrhythmia. Digoxin levels should be obtained in any patient with suspected toxicity; a level higher than 2 ng/mL is consistent with chronic toxicity. Falsely elevated levels are seen during the first 6 to 12 hours following an acute ingestion and before tissue redistribution.

Hypokalemia exacerbates many digoxin-toxic dysrhythmias and should be slowly corrected. Atropine should be administered for hemodynamically significant bradycardia, and if necessary, cardiac pacing should be instituted. Phenytoin or lidocaine are the antidysrhythmics of choice for enhanced automaticity or ventricular dysrhythmias. Class 1a antidysrhythmics should be avoided because they may depress AV node conduction and exacerbate digoxin-toxic dysrhythmias.

Digoxin-specific Fab fragments (Digibind) are the specific antidote for digoxin toxicity; they are extremely safe. Commonly accepted indica-

---

INDICATIONS FOR THE USE OF DIGOXIN-SPECIFIC FAB FRAGMENTS

Significant cardiac dysrhythmias
   Ventricular dysrhythmias
   High-grade AV block
   Rapid atrial dysrhythmias
Hyperkalemia (K^+ >5 mEq/L)
Potentially life-threatening dose (>10 mg in an adult) and **any** signs of cardiotoxicity
Postdistribution serum digoxin >6 ng/mL
Cardiopulmonary arrest when digoxin toxicity is suspected

---

tions for administration are listed in the box below. The threshold for administration should be lower in elderly or very young patients or where underlying heart or lung disease is present. Fab fragments should also be administered in any case of cardiopulmonary arrest in which digoxin toxicity is suspected. Administration of these fragments may precipitate hypokalemia and, in a patient who is taking therapeutic digoxin, congestive heart failure or rapid atrial fibrillation. Serum potassium must be closely followed after administration. Serum digoxin concentrations rise significantly after Fab administration and therefore cannot be used to further monitor therapy.

HALLUCINOGENS

Hallucinogens cause perceptual distortions and consist of a wide variety of agents, including phencyclidine (PCP, angel dust), lysergic acid diethylamine (LSD, acid), and mescaline (buttons, peyote, cactus).

The clinical presentation of PCP use depends on the dose. Small doses result in a mildly intoxicated state that consists of agitation, excitement, disorganized thought processes, incoordination, a blank-stare appearance, drowsiness, and apathy. At higher doses hypertension, hyperthermia, muscular rigidity, myoclonus, nystagmus, diaphoresis, seizures, and coma may develop. Death may occur from self-destructive behavior or from complications of hyperthermia.

The effects of LSD last 4 to 12 hours, with an accompanying hallucinogenic state. Patients may have flashbacks months after the last ingestion.

Evaluation of hallucinogen use should include a confirmation of the ingestion and the exclusion of any accompanying poisoning, encephalopathy, or encephalitis. Treatment is supportive. Agitation and hallucinations may require reassurance and (rarely) sedation with benzodiazepines. Specific therapy may be required to manage complications, especially hyperthermia.

HYDROCARBONS

Hydrocarbons (petroleum distillates) are widely used organic compounds and are commonly found in both the home and the work place. Toxicity may involve direct injury from pulmonary aspiration or systemic toxicity after inhalation or ingestion.

The aspiration of a few milliliters of petroleum distillate can result in chemical pneumonitis, a potentially lethal complication. The risk of aspiration is greatest for those agents with low viscosity, including gasoline, kerosene, turpentine, petroleum naphtha, mineral seal oil, mineral spirits, and the halogenated and aromatic hydrocarbons. Conversely, the risk of aspiration is lowest for agents of high viscosity, such as lubricating oil, petroleum jelly, diesel oil, motor oil, paraffin wax, and mineral oil.

The initial symptoms of hydrocarbon aspiration appear early and involve gagging, choking, and coughing. In severe cases, there is a rapid progression to tachypnea, wheezing, and severe respiratory distress. Any patient who is symptomatic following a suspected hydrocarbon ingestion should be admitted for close observation, supplemental oxygen, and appropriate supportive care. Steroids and antibiotics are not beneficial. Patients who remain asymptomatic 4 hours after the suspected ingestion may be discharged.

Systemic toxicity may occur following the ingestion or inhalation of camphor, phenol, aromatic, and halogenated hydrocarbons. Systemic toxicity usually occurs only with large exposures and, with the exception of camphor, is rarely seen after small accidental ingestions in children. The systemic toxicity produced is variable but usually involves the central nervous system. Cardiac dysrhythmias and sudden death occur with certain halogenated hydrocarbons as a result of myocardial sensitization to circulating catecholamines. Patients with evidence of systemic toxicity need to be admitted for appropriate monitoring and supportive care.

Gastric decontamination is indicated only for large ingestions of hydrocarbons that have the potential to produce toxicity. For small ingestions or for large ingestions of agents that have not produced significant systemic toxicity, gastric decontamination is contraindicated because of the risk of pulmonary aspiration.

IRON

Potentially fatal poisoning from iron ingestion occurs most often in children. The risk of toxicity is related to the amount of elemental iron that has been ingested. This amount varies with the preparation and must be calculated for each ingestion. The ingestion of more than 40 mg/kg of elemental iron may result in serious toxicity, and more than 60 mg/kg may be fatal.

Body iron stores are controlled by the regulation of iron absorption from the GI tract. With an overdose, these regulatory mechanisms are overwhelmed, and large amounts of iron are absorbed and unable to be excreted. Once the iron-binding capacity of transferrin is exceeded, free iron accumulates and redistributes to the tissues, where by unknown mechanisms it acts as a powerful cellular toxin. In addition, iron has a direct corrosive affect on the GI mucosa.

Shortly after ingestion, victims of significant iron poisoning develop vomiting and diarrhea, which is often bloody and is a result of the direct corrosive effect of the iron. Massive GI fluid loss can occur, resulting in shock. An asymptomatic latent period may follow and last as long as 12 hours. This period may be followed by coma, shock, metabolic acidosis, and seizures. Delayed complications of iron poisoning include pyloric stenosis.

The initial management of iron poisoning centers on resuscitation and supportive care. Specific intervention directed toward coma, shock, acidosis, and seizures is required together with chelation with deferoxamine. Evaluation should include an abdominal radiograph, a complete blood count, electrolytes and creatinine, liver function tests, blood glucose, and a blood type and screen. A serum iron level should be measured between 4 and 6 hours after ingestion; a serum iron level that is obtained more than 6 hours after ingestion may be misleading because of tissue redistribution.

A gastric lavage should be performed as soon as possible after a potentially toxic iron ingestion. Activated charcoal does not adsorb iron and should be administered only if a significant co-ingestion is suspected. If an abdominal radiograph following the lavage reveals persistent radiopacities, more aggressive decontamination measures such as whole-bowel irrigation, endoscopy, or even gastrotomy should be considered.

A white blood cell count higher than 15,000 cells/mm^3 and a blood glucose level higher than 150 mg/dl are signs that are highly suggestive of significant iron toxicity. Obtaining the serum iron level within 4 to 6 hours provides a useful guide to therapy. A level greater than 500 μg/dl is very significant and warrants chelation therapy with deferoxamine. A level between 350 and 500 μg/dl warrants chelation only if the patient is symptomatic. An asymptomatic patient may be observed and discharged if a subsequent serum iron level is shown to be falling, which indicates that continued absorption is unlikely.

Deferoxamine is a specific chelating agent for iron. Its introduction into clinical practice has greatly reduced the mortality of iron poisoning. It should be administered at a rate of 15 mg/kg/hour by continuous IV infusion and should be continued until the serum iron level is less than 100 μg/dl. Deferoxamine may cause hypotension and should be administered only in an intensive care setting.

LITHIUM

Lithium carbonate is widely used in the treatment of bipolar disorders. Lithium, a cation, is well absorbed following oral administration and is slowly redistributed to the total body water, where it substitutes for sodium and potassium. It is eliminated entirely by glomerular filtration, but 70% of the filtered load is reabsorbed in the proximal tubule.

Lithium toxicity may occur following an acute overdose but is more common during chronic therapy, when an intercurrent illness results in a reduction in glomerular filtration rate or in sodium or water depletion, which leads to increased lithium reabsorption. Symptoms of lithium intoxication are predominantly neurologic and include weakness, lethargy, ataxia, and tremors; the symptoms progress to delirium, coma, and convulsions. Nonneurologic manifestations of acute intoxication include nausea, vomiting, and diarrhea. Cardiac conduction abnormalities and ST-T wave changes on the ECG may be seen in severe cases.

Manifestations of lithium toxicity are usually more severe in chronic rather than acute intoxications and are associated with minimally elevated serum levels (above the therapeutic range of 0.6 to 1.2 mEq/L). By contrast, with an acute overdose the patient may be asymptomatic despite very high serum levels. These levels fall rapidly, but symptoms may develop over the ensuing hours as lithium ions redistribute to the tissue compartments.

Water and sodium deficits need to be corrected by the administration of normal saline. Lavage is indicated following an acute overdose, and a whole-bowel irrigation should be considered, especially after the ingestion of sustained-release preparations. Charcoal does not bind lithium. All patients need close observation, supportive care, and an evaluation of serum lithium levels. Hemodialysis is the treatment of choice for the significantly intoxicated patient.

It is also indicated for any patient with severe neurologic or cardiovascular toxicity or for any symptomatic patient with a serum lithium level greater than 2.5 mEq/L in the setting of chronic toxicity. Serum lithium levels should be monitored after hemodialysis because a rebound effect associated with a redistribution from the tissues to the vascular compartment may occur. Administration of normal saline and the monitoring of serum lithium levels is adequate in a patient with less severe intoxication and normal renal function. Asymptomatic patients may be discharged if sequential serum lithium levels show a fall over a 4-hour period and if the predischarge level is less than 2 mEq/L.

NARCOTICS AND SEDATIVE-HYPNOTICS

Narcotics and sedative-hypnotics consistently produce CNS and respiratory depression along with the potential for hypotension. With a few

Table 65-2

NARCOTICS AND SEDATIVE-HYPNOTIC OVERDOSE: CLINICAL FINDINGS AND TREATMENT

	Narcotics	Sedative-Hypnotics	Barbiturates
Findings			
Neurologic			
Depressed/coma	Yes	Yes	Yes
Seizures (associated drugs)	Meperidine, propoxyphene	Methaqualone, meprobamate	Butabarbital, pentobarbital, secobarbital
Cardiovascular			
Hypotension/shock	Yes	Yes	Yes
Dysrhythmias	No	Chloral hydrate, haloperidol, meprobamate	No
Miosis	Yes (not meperidine)	Variable	Variable
Respiratory			
Depression	Yes	Yes	Yes
Pulmonary edema	Yes	Meprobamate, ethchlorvynol, paraldehyde	Yes
Anticholinergic	Lomotil (early)	Glutethimide, OTC sleep medications	No
Other	Analgesia (GI, GU motility; bronchoconstriction)	Paraldehyde—acute renal failure	Cutaneous bullae
Management			
Support	Yes	Yes	Yes
Gastric emptying	Yes	Yes	Yes
Antidote	Naloxone	No*	No
Diuresis	No	No	Phenobarbital (alkaline)
Dialysis	No	No	Phenobarbital

From Barkin RM, Rosen P: *Emergency pediatrics: a guide to ambulatory care*, ed 4, St Louis, 1994, Mosby.
*Flumazenil for benzodiazepines.

exceptions such as meperidine, narcotics commonly produce pinpoint pupils and, with an overdose, hypoventilation. The clinical distinctions between these classes of drugs are outlined in Table 65-2.

Supportive care is essential, and other causes of impaired mental status, including hypoglycemia, need to be excluded. For a narcotic overdose, naloxone 2 mg IV should be administered. As much as 10 mg may be given if only a partial response is noted, particularly with overdoses of partial agonists such as propoxyphene or pentazocine.

With a phenobarbital overdose, excretion may be enhanced by urinary alkalinization (see the section on salicylate toxicity) and by the administration of repeat doses of activated charcoal. Hemodialysis is effective for severe phenobarbital intoxication.

ORGANOPHOSPHATES AND CARBAMATES

Organophosphates and carbamates are pesticides that produce an acute cholinergic syndrome in the poisoned patient. The inhibition of acetylcholinesterase allows acetylcholine to accumulate in the central nervous system and at peripheral muscarinic and nicotinic receptors. The organophosphates and carbamates vary greatly in potency. Carbamates bind reversibly to acetylcholinesterase and do not cross the blood-brain barrier well, which causes a less severe syndrome that is of shorter duration than the organophosphates.

Organophosphates and carbamates are rapidly absorbed via the skin, GI tract, and respiratory tract. The onset of symptoms is usually rapid but may be delayed some hours following dermal exposure. Muscarinic effects include bradycardia, bronchorrhea, salivation, bronchospasm, sweating, miosis, nausea, vomiting, abdominal cramping, and diarrhea. Nicotinic effects include muscle weakness, fasciculation, and tremors. Central effects include agitation, seizures, and coma.

Initial management focuses on resuscitation. Acute respiratory deaths occur as a result of central respiratory depression, weakness of the muscles of respiration, and excessive respiratory secretions. Decontamination includes removing contaminated clothing and washing all exposed areas. Gastric decontamination by lavage and the administration of activated charcoal may be beneficial if performed within 1 hour of ingestion.

Specific antidotal therapy includes the administration of atropine, an antimuscarinic agent; and pralidoxime, an anticholinesterase reactivator. Atropine should be administered early and in large doses. A dose of 1 to 2 mg should be administered intravenously every 10 minutes until the drying of pulmonary secretions is observed. Massive doses may be required to achieve this endpoint, and repeat doses may be necessary because of the relatively short half-life of atropine. Pralidoxime should be given if there is any evidence of muscle weakness following organophosphate poisoning. Pralidoxime is most effective at reversing phosphorylation of acetylcholinesterase if administered during the first 24 hours.

Plasma and red blood cell acetylcholinesterase levels are useful to confirm exposure to organophosphates and carbamates. The plasma level is a more sensitive but less reliable indicator of exposure and returns to normal more quickly than the red blood cell level, which may remain depressed for weeks after the acute poisoning.

SALICYLATES (ASPIRIN)

Aspirin (acetylsalicylic acid, ASA) is found in a wide range of over-the-counter and prescription medications. Discrete syndromes of acute and chronic toxicity exist.

Aspirin is a weak acid with a pK_a of 3 and is rapidly absorbed from the stomach and hydrolyzed to form salicylic acid and acetic acid. In large overdoses, concretions may form in the stomach, which slows tablet dissolution and hence absorption. The volume of distribution is small (0.2 L/kg) but is increased by acidosis as a result of enhanced tissue penetration. Salicylic acid is eliminated primarily by hepatic metabolism, but all excretory mechanisms are saturable, and the half-life is greatly prolonged in overdose. Small amounts of salicylate are excreted unchanged in the urine, but this process is greatly enhanced in the presence of an alkaline urine because of "ion trapping."

The toxic effects of salicylate include central respiratory stimulation, which leads to respiratory alkalosis and a secondary metabolic acidosis; uncoupling of oxidative phosphorylation, which leads to an increased metabolic rate and cellular dysfunction; and interference with lipid and carbohydrate metabolism, which leads to metabolic acidosis.

A single ingestion of more than 300 mg/kg can lead to significant acute toxicity. Clinical features of toxicity include vomiting, hyper-

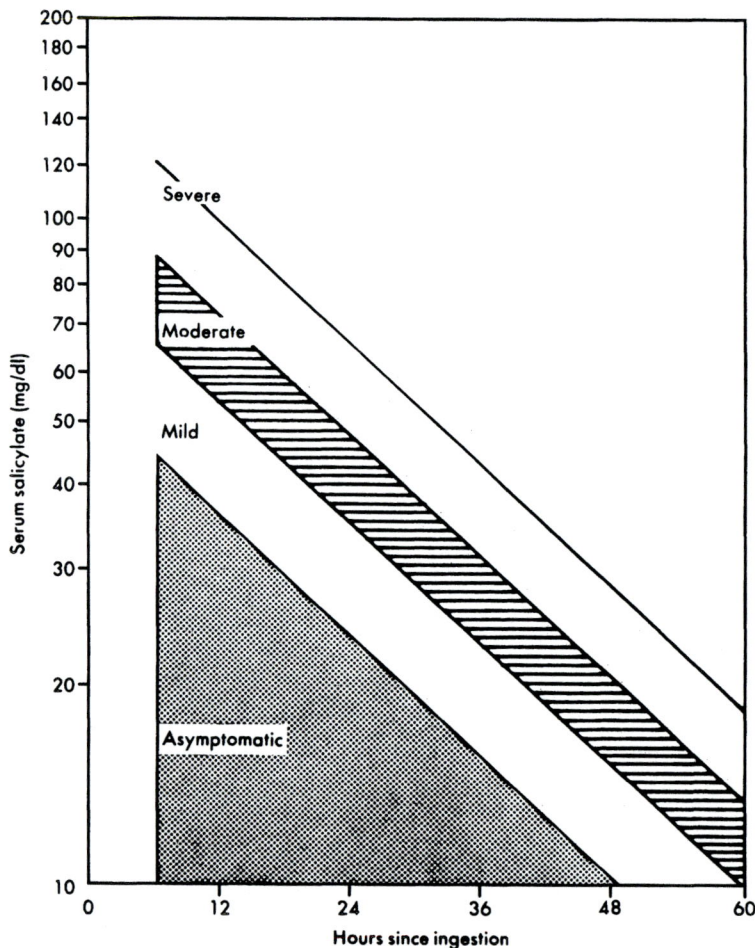

Fig 65-2   Done nomogram for salicylate poisoning. Note that this nomogram is not accurate for chronic ingestions. (From Done AK: Salicylate intoxication: significance of measurements of salicylate in blood in cases of acute intoxication, *Pediatrics* 26:800, 1960.)

pnea, tinnitus, respiratory alkalosis, anion-gap metabolic acidosis, dehydration, and altered mental status. Severe intoxications may result in coma, seizures, hyperthermia, hypoglycemia, and noncardiogenic pulmonary edema.

Chronic toxicity follows repeated overmedication, is associated with lower serum salicylate levels than acute toxicity, and has a worse prognosis. The clinical features of chronic toxicity are nonspecific and include confusion, dehydration, and metabolic acidosis; for this reason the diagnosis is often missed. In any patient who is using salicylates and is demonstrating an altered mental status, chronic toxicity should be suspected and a serum salicylate level should be checked.

Serum salicylate levels are useful but must be interpreted with care. The Done nomogram (Fig. 65-2) is used to predict the severity of intoxication but applies only to single acute ingestions in patients with normal renal function. Even in these circumstances the nomogram must be used with caution. A single serum level is never sufficient. When determining therapy, serial levels must be performed and considered in conjunction with the clinical status of the patient. The Done nomogram cannot be used to predict the severity of intoxication with chronic ingestions, in which much lower levels are associated with toxicity. A serum salicylate of 40 mg/dl may be associated with severe toxicity in this setting.

Initial assessment of salicylate toxicity should include electrolytes, ABGs, blood glucose, creatinine, a chest x-ray study, and calculation of the anion gap. Gastric lavage and activated charcoal should be administered to the acute overdose patient; activated charcoal alone should be given to the patient with chronic toxicity. Fluid and electrolyte deficits should be corrected. Acidosis should be aggressively corrected with IV sodium bicarbonate.

An asymptomatic patient who has decreasing serum salicylate levels may be discharged after 6 hours. Management of the symptomatic patient includes continuing supportive care and instituting measures to enhance salicylate excretion. Urinary alkalinization to a urine pH of 7.5 or greater enhances urinary excretion and is achieved by IV infusion of sodium bicarbonate (100 mEq in 1 L of 5% dextrose at 150 ml/hour). Potassium must be repleted to achieve urinary alkalinization, and ABGs must be monitored to avoid systemic alkalosis. Repeated doses of activated charcoal (25 to 50 g every 4 hours) enhances salicylate excretion by GI dialysis. Hemodialysis rapidly removes salicylate, corrects acid-base abnormalities, and is the method of choice in severe salicylate toxicity. The standard indications for hemodialysis are a serum salicylate level of greater than 100 mg/dl for an acute ingestion or 60 mg/dl for a chronic ingestion, severe acidosis, pulmonary edema, renal failure, significantly impaired mental status, or any clinical deterioration.

SULFONYLUREAS

Sulfonylureas are oral hypoglycemic agents and stimulate endogenous pancreatic insulin secretion. They are well absorbed orally, and metabolism and renal clearance vary with the individual agent. Active metabolites contribute to the wide variation in duration of effect.

The ingestion of excessive doses of sulfonylureas, whether accidental or deliberate, leads to hypoglycemia with commonly recognized clinical manifestations. The onset of effect may be delayed and the duration prolonged. The most common clinical presentation is that of altered mental status. The diagnosis is often made by measuring a low blood glucose level, but other toxic (β-blockers, ethanol, insulin) and nontoxic causes of hypoglycemia must be considered.

A bolus of 50 ml of 50% dextrose solution should be administered intravenously and repeated as necessary. A 5% to 10% dextrose solution as a continuous infusion together with repeat boluses may be required to maintain a blood glucose of greater than 100 mg/dl. Hospital admission is required until an adequate blood glucose is maintained without supplementation, which may require several days. In refractory cases, the administration of diazoxide may be indicated. All children with suspected sulfonylurea ingestion should be admitted to the hospital for 24 hours observation and serial glucose estimations.

THEOPHYLLINE

A methylxanthine widely used in the management of asthma, theophylline is often dispensed as a sustained-release preparation and has a low therapeutic index. Normal therapeutic levels are 10 to 20 mg/L, and toxicity may be seen at the upper level of this range. Toxicity occurs in the context of either an acute overdose or chronic administration. Acute and chronic intoxication should be regarded as distinct clinical syndromes.

Although theophylline is well absorbed orally, peak levels may not occur for as long as 16 hours following the ingestion of a sustained-release preparation. The volume of distribution is only 0.5 L/kg, and theophylline is metabolized via hepatic pathways that are saturable in overdose.

Acute toxicity may occur following the ingestion of as little as 10 mg/kg and is manifested by vomiting, tachycardia, tremulousness, and anxiety together with the characteristic metabolic effects of hypokalemia, hypophosphatemia, hyperglycemia, and metabolic acidosis. As serum levels rise, more serious manifestations occur, including supraventricular and ventricular dysrhythmias and seizures.

Sinus tachycardia is often seen with chronic overmedication, but GI effects are less common than in an acute overdose. Seizures may be the first manifestation of toxicity.

Diagnosis is made on clinical suspicion and confirmed by serum level. An acute theophylline overdose should be suspected in any patient presenting with status epilepticus and hypokalemia. Severe intoxication is associated with levels of >90 mg/L in acute overdose and >40 mg/L in chronic toxicity. Because of the possibility of bezoar formation or delayed absorption from sustained-release preparations, serum levels must be monitored until a consistent decline is noted.

Acute management requires initial resuscitation and the treatment of seizures, dysrhythmias, and hypotension (when present). Activated charcoal should always be administered. Emesis should never be induced because of the risk of seizures as toxicity progresses. Vital signs, serum electrolytes, cardiac rhythm, and serum theophylline levels need to be closely monitored. Cardiac dysrhythmias may respond to beta-blockade. Hypokalemia represents intracellular redistribution and rarely needs aggressive replacement therapy. Monitoring should continue for at least 16 hours following a significant overdose.

The enhanced elimination of theophylline by either hemoperfusion or repeat doses of activated charcoal is very effective because of the small volume of distribution of the drug. Hemoperfusion is the modality of choice for all cases of severe intoxication. Repeat doses of activated charcoal should be used for moderate intoxication. This therapeutic maneuver is usually complicated by emesis; therefore antiemetics will be necessary. Ondansetron is particularly effective in this setting.

||||||||KEY CONSIDERATIONS

WHAT IS THE LIFE THREAT?

Severe poisoning from the following substances can be lethal: acetaminophen, ethanol, methanol, ethylene glycol, anticholinergics, β-blockers, carbon monoxide, cocaine, cyclic antidepressants, digoxin, iron, lithium, narcotics, organophosphates, salicylates, and theophylline.

The aspiration of petroleum distillate may produce pneumonitis.

Ominous signs in cases of poisoning include hemodynamic instability, dysrhythmia, and seizure.

DOES THE PATIENT NEED ADMISSION?

Admit patients with altered sensorium or any life threats following a drug overdose. Admission may be necessary in asymptomatic patients who have elevated acetaminophen serum concentrations (as determined by the Rumack-Matthew nomogram) in order to administer *N*-acetylcysteine.

WHAT IS THE MOST SERIOUS DIAGNOSIS?

Patients with an overdose are at risk for continued absorption of toxins, which may cause coma, airway compromise, hypotension, and dysrhythmia.

HAVE I PERFORMED A THOROUGH WORK-UP?

Consider poisoning in comatose or obtunded patients, as well as those with dysrhythmia, acid-base disturbances, diaphoresis, nystagmus, agitation, or psychosis. Obtain and monitor the ECG, especially in cases of poisoning from cyclic antidepressants, β-blockers, digoxin, calcium channel blockers, cocaine, organophosphates, lithium, and theophylline. Evaluate and monitor the patient's oxygenation status, intubate the comatose patient, and assess ventilation. Obtain IV access and administer fluids or antidotes as needed to maintain blood pressure.

Patients who ingest a drug with suicidal intent should undergo psychiatric evaluation. Report poisonings to the regional poison control center, and seek their consultation for serious or unusual poisonings.

Recommended Reading

Burkhart KK et al: The other alcohols: methanol, ethylene glycol, and isopropanol, *Emerg Med Clin North Am* 8:913, 1990.

Ellenhorn MJ, Barceloux DG: *Medical toxicology: diagnosis and treatment of human poisoning*, New York, 1988, Elsevier Science Publishing.

Frommer DA et al: Tricyclic antidepressant overdose: a review, *JAMA* 257:521, 1987.

Goldfrank LR et al: *Goldfrank's toxicologic emergencies*, ed 5, Norwalk, 1994, Appleton & Lange.

Litovitz TL, Schmitz BF: Ingestion of cylindrical and button batteries: an analysis of 2382 cases, *Pediatrics* 89:747-757, 1992.

Olson KR et al: *Poisoning and drug overdose*, ed 2, Norwalk, 1994, Appleton & Lange.

Rosen P et al, editors: *Emergency medicine: concepts and clinical practice*, ed 3, St Louis, 1992, Mosby.

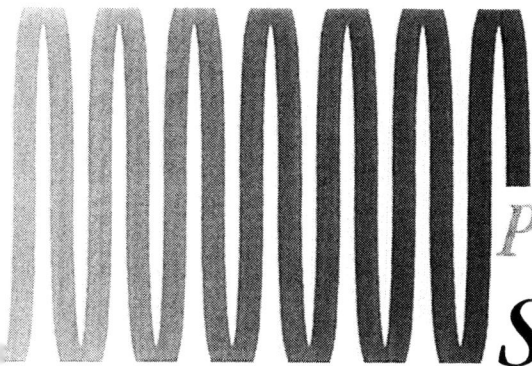

Part VI

SPECIAL PROBLEMS

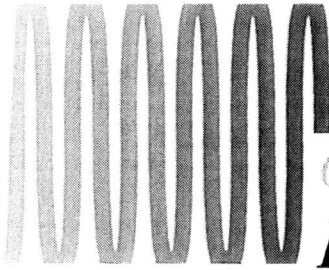

Chapter Sixty-six
PEDIATRIC EMERGENCIES

ANN M. DIETRICH

A pediatric patient is often a source of anxiety in the emergency department. Early recognition of clinical problems and stabilization are particularly important.

Pediatric emergencies that require resuscitation are primarily respiratory in origin and stem from a variety of conditions that result in upper or lower airway disease. These emergencies may result from obstruction and hypoxemia, which ultimately leads to cardiac arrest if left unrecognized and untreated. Other problems may progress to respiratory distress; if these problems are recognized early, the physician can avert such a progression and, ultimately, a serious illness. It is paramount in the care of children to identify potentially life-threatening problems, particularly respiratory compromise, that require intervention. The emergency physician, in addition, must recognize the relative environmental dependency of the child and the nonspecific nature of signs and symptoms.

GENERAL GUIDELINES

When approaching the pediatric patient, make every effort to respond to the uniqueness of the developing child while understanding the many parallels with older patients, who represent the vast majority of emergency department patients. Always consider size and age in pediatric management.

Developmental Stage

It is important to consider the developmental stage of the child when speaking to and assessing him or her and to provide explanations and support to the family (Table 66-1).

Vital Signs and Weight

Vital signs and weight vary by age (Table 66-2). Respiratory and pulse rates decrease with age, whereas blood pressure increases. An estimated normal systolic blood pressure can be obtained by adding twice the age in years to 80. The maximum effective resting heart rate in infants is 200 beats/minute; in preschool children, 150 beats/minute; and in older individuals, 120 beats/minute.

The average birth weight for a newborn is 3.3 kg. The weight of the infant normally doubles by 5 to 6 months of age and triples to an average of 10 kg by 1 year of age. An alternative method uses the length of the child to determine the appropriate equipment sizes and medication doses needed. A pediatric measurement tape (e.g., Broselow tape) is placed alongside the child in the supine position and read at the child's heel for the appropriate equipment sizes and medication doses. *Always administer drugs and fluids in a weight- (or length-) specific manner.*

Table **66-1**

AGES AND STAGES OF CHILDREN

	Birth–18 mo	19 mo–2 yr	3–5 yr	6–11 yr	12–18 yr
Theories of child development					
Erikson	Trust vs mistrust	Autonomy vs shame and doubt	Initiative vs guilt	Industry vs inferiority	Identify vs role confusion
Freud	Oral-sensory	Anal	Phallic	Latency	Genital
Piaget	Sensorimotor egocentrism	Preoperational, beginnings of perceptual constancy	Preoperational, prelogical reasoning	Concrete operations	Formal operations
Task mastery	Differentiate self and nonself	Toilet training	Use of language	Logic	Abstract thinking
Pain perception	Physical but possibly not cognitive pain perceived, in younger patients	Primarily egocentric: "Here and now" May see pain as punishment	Pain as punishment Overextension of causality Fear and fantasy	Beginning of understanding of true causality Fear of destruction and death	Concept of emotional and physical pain Understanding of root causes of pain

Suggested interventions				
1. Involve caretaker in care of child. 2. Keep child warm. 3. Keep room quiet. 4. Provide comfort measures (e.g., pacifier). 5. Keep child on caretaker's lap during physical examination. 6. Return child to caretaker as soon as possible after procedures; allow caretaker to comfort child.	1. Prepare caretaker for procedures. 2. Tell caretaker that he or she may assist in normal care. 3. Give child a familiar toy or blanket as a transitional object. 4. Use child's name. 5. Restrain child as little as possible. 6. Avoid covering child's face. 7. Describe sensations and talk with child during the procedures. 8. Praise, smile, and have a cheerful attitude.	1. Explain procedure *immediately before* performing it. 2. Allow child to see and touch samples of equipment. 3. Be honest: "This will sting." 4. Use simple distractions and talk to child. 5. Allow child to see under bandages. 6. Use praise, adhesive bandages, and small rewards.	1. Explain procedure beforehand. 2. Enlist cooperation. 3. Ask about simple preferences. 4. Give alternatives (e.g., child may yell but not move). 5. Identify sensations and personnel. 6. Use distraction and counting games. 7. Include child in discharge instructions. 8. Use rewards, stickers, badges, and praise.	1. Give *full* explanations. 2. Encourage child's participation. 3. Allow time for questions. 4. Provide *privacy.* Child may want to exclude parents. 5. Avoid teasing and embarrassing child. 6. Allow as much control as possible. 7. Provide discharge instructions to patient. 8. Reassure child that his or her behavior was appropriate.

From Seidel JS, Henderson DP: Approach to the pediatric patient in the emergency department. In Barkin RM, editor: *Pediatric emergency medicine*, St Louis, 1992, Mosby.

Table 66-2

VITAL SIGNS AND AIRWAY SUPPORT

Age	Weight (kg)	Heart Rate	Respiratory Rate	ET Tube Inner Diameter (mm)	Laryngoscope Blade	Suction cathether (Fr)
Premature	1	145	<40	2.5	0	6
Newborn	2-3	125	·	3.0	1	6-8
1 mo	4	120	24-35	3.5		
6 mo	7	130		3.5		
1 yr	10	125	20-30	4.0	1-2	8-10
2-3 yr	12-14	115		4.5		10
4-5 yr	16-18	100		5.0-6.0	2	
6-8 yr	20-26	100	12-25	6.0-6.5		
10-12 yr	32-42	75		7.0	2-3	12
>14 yr	>50	70	12-18	7.5-8.5	3	

Modified from Barkin RM, Rosen P: *Emergency pediatrics: a guide to ambulatory care,* ed 4, St Louis, 1994, Mosby. Modified from Nadas A: *Pediatric cardiology,* ed 3, Philadelphia, 1976, WB Saunders. From Vesmond HT et al: *Pediatrics* 67:607, 1981.

Venous Access

Venous access is often difficult in children and particularly in youngsters who are hypovolemic. The external jugular and scalp veins are valuable sites. If peripheral venous attempts are unsuccessful in a critically ill or injured child, intraosseous (IO) access is indicated. The IO access can be obtained rapidly and has been successfully used for volume expansion with crystalloids and blood products. Most medications may also be administered via this route.

Fluid Replacement

Cardiovascular signs of shock in a child include tachycardia, weak peripheral pulses, and delayed capillary refill (especially important because of the difficulty in measuring blood pressure). Remember that capillary refill may be inaccurate in children who are cold. Correlate the child's clinical findings with historical information (e.g., trauma, fever, vomiting, diarrhea).

Fluid replacement should be calculated on the basis of the patient's size; the average blood volume of a child is 70 to 90 ml/kg. Initiate fluid resuscitation with 20 ml/kg of normal saline or lactated Ringer's solution in a fluid-depleted child. Reassess the patient following each bolus. Repeated boluses may be necessary in a child who is severely hypovolemic.

For children with multiple trauma or an acute blood loss, administer 40 to 60 ml/kg of normal saline or lactated Ringer's solution. If the patient is still showing signs of shock, begin blood transfusions at a bolus rate of 10 ml/kg.

Tube Placement

Perform tube placement when required; use size-specific endotracheal (ET) and nasogastric (NG) tubes, urinary catheters, and others as appropriate. Two quick methods for estimating ET tube size include comparing the tube size to the child's little finger and estimating or measuring the nostril size. The NG tube and urinary catheter sizes are commonly 5 Fr for children under 6 months, 8 Fr for 1-year-olds, 10 Fr for 4- to 5-year-olds, and 12 Fr for adolescents. Continue to monitor the child during all interventions and procedures. Pediatric patients may become bradycardiac during intubation attempts (vagal stimulation) or NG tube placement. An oximeter may be particularly useful.

Psychologic Support

Psychologic support of the patient *and* the family is essential. Touching the child in a soothing manner and speaking in a calm and controlled tone may help win confidence and establish rapport. If emergent intervention is not required, taking a few early moments to establish rapport is often well worth the cooperation generated.

Allow the parent(s) to stay with the child whenever possible, which helps obtain cooperation from the youngster, provides important information, and maintains an intact family unit. Parents substantially affect care. If parents are unavailable, have a member of the health care team stay with the child to provide support as a surrogate parent. Be sure to continue to speak to the child and the family in an ongoing fashion, even if only briefly. Pediatric management involves continuing observation and monitoring for changes, and explaining this approach facilitates family cooperation and minimizes anger about time delays.

RESPIRATORY DISTRESS

The hallmarks of respiratory distress in pediatric patients are tachypnea, retractions, flaring, and grunting. Upper airway problems produce primarily ventilatory abnormalities associated with relative or absolute obstruction and stridor; lower airway disease may impair ventilation and perfusion. Inspiratory stridor is usually supraglottic; expiratory stridor stems from tracheal involvement. A diverse group of conditions causes lower airway disease, usually without associated stridor (see the box above).

Causes of respiratory distress in children

COMMON PEDIATRIC RESPIRATORY DISEASES	
Upper airway disease	**Lower airway disease**
Croup	Asthma
Epiglottitis	Pneumonia
Foreign body	Bronchiolitis
Bacterial tracheitis	Foreign body

under 2 years of age include pneumonia, asthma, bronchiolitis, croup, congenital heart disease, airway anomalies (laryngomalacia, tracheal web, cysts, lobar emphysema), foreign body aspiration, and nasopharyngeal obstruction (large tonsils and adenoids). *Older children* may experience asthma, pneumonia, bacterial tracheitis, foreign body aspiration, drowning, poisoning, and trauma.

Respiratory distress may also result from an increased oxygen demand generated by fever, sepsis, anemia, and shock. Interventions must focus on assessment and stabilization of the airway followed by ventilation as required.

Assessment

Children with upper airway disease typically have stridor. *It is essential to distinguish between croup and epiglottitis, particularly in the child who has stridor and signs of an upper airway infection. In the child with suspected epiglottitis, do not examine the neck or mouth without being prepared to intervene in airway stabilization on an emergent basis.* Children with epiglottitis classically have a rapid progression of respiratory distress and appear more toxic (Table 66-3). The incidence of epiglottitis has decreased over the last 5 years, which probably reflects the *Haemophilus influenzae* type b vaccine.

Although direct visualization under controlled conditions is often preferred because of its speed and relative infrequency of false-

*Table*66-3

DIFFERENTIATION BETWEEN CROUP AND EPIGLOTTITIS

	Croup	Epiglottitis
Age	6 mo-3 yr	Any age (peak 2-5 yr)
Season	Fall/winter	Any
Time of day	Night/early morning	Throughout day
Etiology	Viral	*H. influenzae*
Clinical onset	Insidious	Rapid
Upper respiratory tract infection	Yes	Rare
Fever	<103° F	High
Toxic	No	Yes
Sore throat	Variable	Yes
Drooling	No	Yes
Stridor	Inspiration and expiration	Inspiration
Position	Variable	Sitting
Epiglottis	Normal epiglottis	*Cherry red* epiglottis
Ancillary tests		
WBC	Normal	High
Blood culture	Negative	Positive
Arterial blood gas analysis	Variable	Variable
Lateral neck x-ray film	Normal (false-negative possible)	Enlarged epiglottis

Modified from Barkin RM, Rosen P: *Emergency pediatrics: a guide to ambulatory care,* ed 4, St Louis, 1994, Mosby.

negative results, many physicians obtain lateral neck x-ray films as a diagnostic adjunct (Figs. 66-1 and 66-2). If the patient is not in severe distress and no evidence of obstruction exists, the x-ray examination may substantiate the diagnosis of croup. However, false-negative results do occur. A clinician who is capable of intubating the patient must accompany the patient at all times with the appropriate equipment.

Differential Diagnosis

Differential considerations other than epiglottitis and croup must include bacterial tracheitis, foreign bodies of the airway, retropharyngeal or tonsillar abscesses, trauma, caustic ingestion, neoplasm, angioneurotic edema, or neurologic disease involving the vocal cords.

Bacterial tracheitis is commonly caused by *Staphylococcus aureus* or *H. influenzae,* with an accumulation of pus in the trachea causing a thick plug and ultimately leading to obstruction. Bacterial tracheitis often is associated with pneumonia and appears initially as a crouplike syndrome with toxicity and rapid progression. Active airway intervention combined with appropriate antibiotic coverage and aggressive pulmonary toilet is often necessary.

Management

Ensure that an adequate airway is present. Parents may be useful in calming the child. Do not agitate the child with unnecessary procedures and tests.

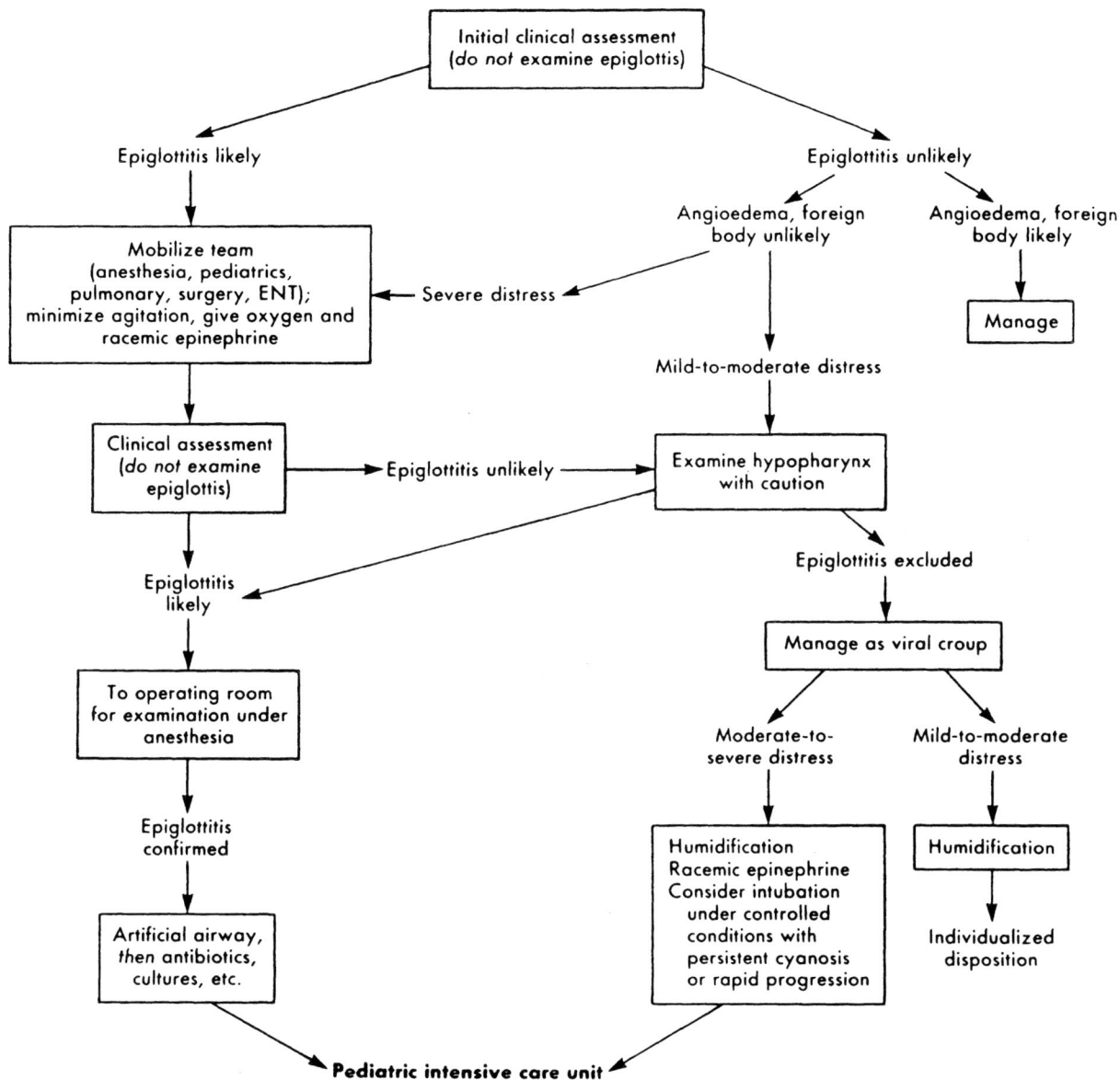

Fig.66-1 Optimal assessment and management of upper airway obstruction caused by epiglottitis or severe croup. Care must be individualized to reflect resources and logistic issues within a given institution.

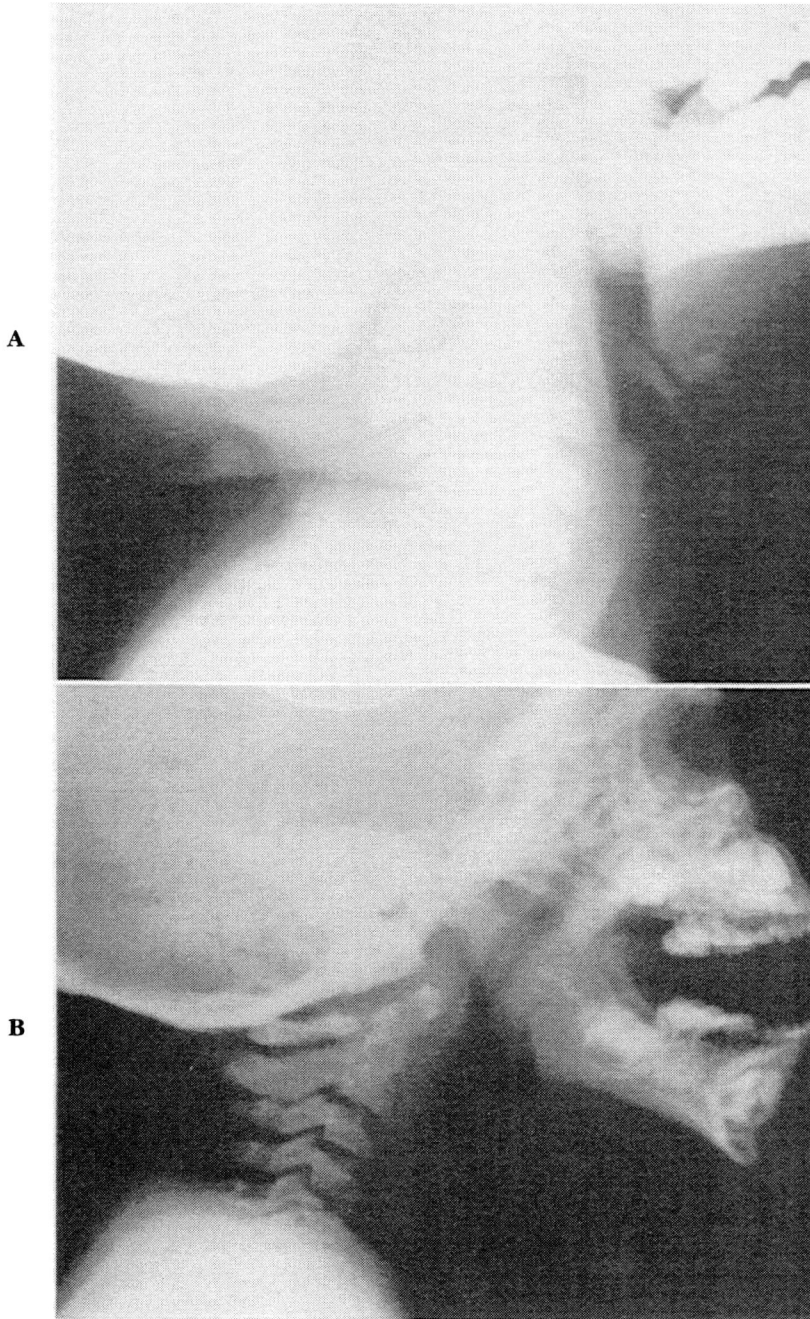

Fig. 66-2 Soft tissue lateral neck films. **A,** Normal. **B,** Markedly swollen epiglottis. Patients with epiglottitis have narrow valleculae and thick mass of tissue ("thumb" sign) extending from the valleculae to the arytenoids. (Courtesy Dr SZ Barkin, Denver, Colo.)

Unstable airway

If the patient's airway is nearly obstructed and the patient is in respiratory failure, diagnosing the underlying illness is less important than stabilizing the airway. Intubation may be required on an emergent basis. It is preferable to perform an intubation under controlled conditions in the operating room with equipment and personnel mobilized, but occasionally intubation may be required in the emergency department. A surgical airway is rarely required. If the patient's airway is obstructed before an airway is established, bag-mask positive pressure ventilation using a nonrebreathing bag with 100% oxygen may be temporarily effective.

Give oxygen and monitor the patient while mobilizing a team to visualize the epiglottis and stabilize the patient. Members of the team may include an otolaryngologist, anesthetist, and pediatric surgeon.

If *epiglottitis* is confirmed, perform an intubation and stabilize the patient before admission to an intensive care unit. Close intensive monitoring is essential and paramount to an optimal recovery. A tracheostomy is rarely indicated. After stabilizing the patient, obtain blood cultures and initiate antibiotics—cefotaxime 100 mg/kg/24 hours in 3 divided doses (every 8 hours) (or equivalent).

If *croup* is confirmed during intubation, initiate IV steroid therapy and admit the patient to the intensive care unit. If *bacterial tracheitis* is confirmed, proceed with antistaphylococcal antibiotics and aggressive suctioning.

Stable airway

Croup is usually diagnosed clinically on the basis of signs and symptoms and a normal appearance of the epiglottis. Active airway intervention is necessary in only 1% of the cases requiring hospital admission. Children with a history of previous airway manipulations or severe croup are particularly likely to have severe croup.

Croup can be managed without stridor with humidified air that is administered at home. Increasingly, physicians are also administering steroids (dexamethasone 0.6 mg/kg/dose IM, IV, or PO) in the emergency department and having them continued as home therapy for 1 to 3 days. Give specific instructions to the parents to watch for increasing stridor, breathing difficulties, cyanosis, onset of drooling, listlessness, agitation, or poor fluid intake.

Croup that occurs with stridor during rest may require hospitalization and management with racemic epinephrine and steroids. Racemic epinephrine is useful acutely in patients with respiratory distress. Administer racemic epinephrine by diluting the solution (2.25%) in normal saline to 5 ml. The standard dose is 0.25 ml per 5 kg to a maximum of 1.5 ml of racemic epinephrine. The improvement that occurs after administering racemic epinephrine may be short lived, with the patient's symptoms commonly returning within 4 to 6 hours. If the child improves following a single racemic epinephrine treatment and continues to be asymptomatic for 4 to 6 hours, he or she may be discharged with steroids and *mandatory* follow-up within 12 to 24 hours. If the child does not improve or requires multiple treatments, he or she should be admitted to an appropriate unit for observation. Helium-oxygen mixtures may be used occasionally for a severe case of croup by those experienced in its risks and benefits.

Foreign Body in the Airway

The clinical presentation of a foreign body in the airway depends on the acuteness and location of the obstruction. Laryngotracheal foreign bodies typically produce an acute obstruction, whereas bronchial foreign bodies produce a more subacute course. The peak age for foreign body aspiration is between 1 and 2 years, with the most commonly aspirated materials being food and vegetable matter.

Assessment

Acute obstruction caused by material in the laryngotracheal area results in life-threatening respiratory distress. Cyanosis, apnea, stridor, wheezing, cough, and dysphonia may be present. A subacute obstruction from bronchial foreign bodies and, rarely, a partial obstruction of the laryngotracheal segment produces air trapping, wheezing, cyanosis, a muffled voice, and coughing. Respiratory arrest and progressive complications of hypoxemia may occur. The absence of a positive history does not exclude a foreign body. With an acute bronchial obstruction, treatment and relief of obstruction obviously take priority over any diagnostic procedures.

If a bronchial foreign body may be present, a chest x-ray study, both inspiratory and expiratory, may suggest the necessity for further evaluation. X-ray films may also distinguish a foreign body in the trachea from one in the esophagus. Foreign bodies lie in the plane of least resistance. Flat foreign bodies, such as coins in the esophagus, lie in the frontal plane and appear as a full circle on the posteroanterior (PA) view, whereas those in the trachea rest in the sagittal plane and appear end-on in the PA chest x-ray film and flat on a lateral view.

Management

Unstable airway. In the patient with an obstructed airway, initiate efforts immediately to relieve the obstruction. A combination of maneuvers is more effective than any single method used alone, particularly in an infant under 1 year of age. In the infant the rapid increase in pressure that results from five back blows may expel or loosen the material. If the material is not expelled immediately, follow the back blows with five chest thrusts. In children and adolescents, use a manual abdominal thrust because of the reduced chest compliance. If the outcome is to be good, these procedures should be performed in the field. Attempt to remove any visible material in the pharynx. If

ventilation is unsuccessful, the foreign body may be removed by laryngoscopy and a forceps or clamp. Immediate bronchoscopy may also be helpful.

Stable airway. Patients who have a foreign body in the upper airway but can talk or cough are generally breathing adequately. If they are not in immediate respiratory failure, perform a bronchoscopy expeditiously. In patients who have smooth *bronchial* foreign bodies that have been present for fewer than 24 hours and in whom no marked respiratory distress exists, consult with ear, nose, and throat specialists or with general or thoracic surgeons for elective removal by bronchoscopy.

If the patient is in respiratory distress or if the object is intrinsically dangerous, such as a button battery, keep the child in a comfortable position and arrange for a bronchoscopy as soon as possible to remove the object.

Bronchiolitis

Bronchiolitis is an acute lower respiratory tract infection that produces inflammatory obstruction of the small airways. It occurs most commonly in children under 2 years of age during the winter months. The respiratory syncytial virus (RSV) accounts for 90% of the cases of bronchiolitis.

Assessment

Patients with bronchiolitis often have a preceding upper respiratory tract infection and develop marked tachypnea (often more than 60 breaths/minute) and diffuse wheezing. Most children are still alert and attentive. Accompanying otitis media or viral pneumonia may be present. Uncommonly, patients may develop respiratory distress and cyanosis, as well as dehydration, apnea (common in premature infants), bacterial pneumonia, or pneumothorax. A life-threatening illness is more likely to develop in infants who were born prematurely, in children with underlying heart or lung disease, or in infants less than 6 weeks of age. Pulse oximetry or an arterial blood gas analysis may be useful in assessing hypoxemia in the moderately to severely ill child. Chest x-ray films classically demonstrate hyperinflation that is often associated with a diffuse, patchy infiltrate or atelectasis.

Differential diagnosis

Differential considerations include other entities that cause wheezing, such as a foreign body, congestive heart failure, cystic fibrosis, a vascular ring, a neoplasm, and toxic or smoke inhalation.

Management

Initially ensure stability of the airway and ventilation. Admit the child if he or she has respiratory distress, hypoxemia, atelectasis, apnea, lethargy, poor oral intake, or inadequate follow-up.

Some children respond to inhaled bronchodilator therapy initiated in the emergency department. Administer albuterol 2.5 mg or terbutaline (1%) 0.03 ml/kg in 2 ml saline and repeat in response to clinical status. Theophylline and steroids, although used by some physicians, have not been shown to be of any benefit. Pulse oximetry and ongoing assessment are essential. Fluid intake may need to be supplemented with IV infusion.

Asthma

Asthma is usually defined as a bronchoconstriction from intrinsic mechanisms and is related to autonomic dysfunction or extrinsic sensitizing agents. Asthma may result from infection, allergens, irritants, stress, or intoxicants.

Assessment

Patients with asthma have wheezing, which often follows a viral illness or extrinsic exposure. The wheezing may be accompanied by respiratory distress (flaring, retracting, and grunting). Cyanosis, diaphoresis, agitation, somnolence, or pulsus paradoxus may occur with severe dis-

ease. Complications include respiratory failure, pneumothorax, pneumomediastinum, dehydration, and iatrogenic disease such as theophylline toxicity.

Differential diagnosis

Refer to the previous differential considerations for bronchiolitis.

The chest x-ray study usually demonstrates hyperinflation and occasionally an infiltrate. The x-ray study is required only for a child who is febrile or unresponsive to bronchodilatation and in children with respiratory failure. Arterial blood gas analysis may determine if hypoxemia or hypercapnia is present but is only required in children who are in impending or documented respiratory failure. Patients who are taking theophylline preparations require a serum theophylline level. Pulse oximetry measurement is helpful.

Management

Ensure an adequate airway and ventilation and then focus on bronchodilatation. Administer oxygen routinely. Follow with pulse oximetry monitoring.

Beta-adrenergic bronchodilators. Initially administer beta-adrenergic bronchodilator agents.

Nebulized therapy provides excellent bronchodilatation with few side effects. Albuterol and terbutaline are almost pure beta$_2$-agonists, and patients generally tolerate these agents with relatively few side effects. In the acute phase two aerosol treatments may be administered in a sequential manner or 20 minutes apart:

- Albuterol: 2.5 mg/3 ml saline every 3 to 4 hours
- Terbutaline: <2 yrs, 0.5 mg in 2.5 ml saline; 2 to 9 yrs, 1 mg in 2.5 ml saline; >9 yrs, 1.5 mg in 2.5 ml saline every 3 to 4 hours

Parenteral beta-agonists are less effective than inhaled therapy but may be used under specific circumstances in which logistics prevent the administration of inhaled agents. Because of the risk of undiagnosed cardiac disease that could be exacerbated by epinephrine use, the use of subcutaneous epinephrine should be avoided in children younger than 6 months of age who have no prior history of wheezing. The dosages are as follows:

- Epinephrine (1:1000): 0.01 ml/kg (maximum: 0.3 ml/dose) subcutaneously every 20 minutes as needed up to a total of three administrations
- Terbutaline: <12 yrs, 0.01 mg/kg (maximum: 0.4 mg/dose) subcutaneously every 20 minutes as needed up to a total of three doses

Theophylline. Theophylline is a bronchodilator that is no longer considered first-line therapy for acute asthma. However, theophylline continues to have a role in the management of chronic asthma and may play a limited role in children who are refractory to inhaled beta-agonists and corticosteroids and in those patients who have improved with the medication in the past.

Adjust the dose if the patient is taking other medications that will affect the metabolism. Decrease the dose if the patient has taken cimetidine or erythromycin or is ill. Children with viral illnesses may have a marked alteration in metabolism as recovery from the illness occurs. This change in metabolism requires a decrease in the amount of theophylline administered. Whenever possible, avoid the use of theophylline in children less than 1 year of age.

The loading dose of theophylline is 5 to 6 mg/kg. The maintenance dose varies from 0.5 mg/kg/hour for children 2 years of age to 0.8 mg/kg/hour IV for those over 10 years of age. Always monitor levels closely. The decision to use theophylline should be individualized for each patient and must be closely monitored.

Steroids. Corticosteroids are currently considered the most effective antiinflammatory drug available to manage asthma. Early initiation of steroids has been shown to decrease the rate of hospitalization and to decrease the need for further emergency department care. Stepwise therapy includes beginning a short course of oral steroids (before discharge from the emergency department) for all children who were on beta-agonist therapy at home or who have required multiple aerosols. The optimal duration for a oral steroid course has not been determined. Recommendations range from 1 to 2 mg/kg/day of prednisone divided every 6 to 12 hours for 5 to 10 days to tapers lasting longer than 10 days. All children who require hospitalization should have steroid therapy started as soon as possible; methylprednisolone (Solu-Medrol) 1 to 2 mg/kg IV every 6 hours is ideal.

Other considerations. Children who have had severe asthma episodes in the past are at risk for recurrent critical attacks. Several indicators that place a child at risk for fatal asthma include prior intubation or intensive care unit admission, more than two hospitalizations each year, hypoxemic seizures, frequent steroid use, psychiatric disease, and poor compliance.

Other potential interventions include continuous nebulized beta-agonists, beta-agonist infusions such as terbutaline or isoproterenol, the addition of an anticholinergic agent, management of respiratory failure and, if unavoidable, intubation. Very few children require intubation. The principle indication is patient fatigue. If at all possible the intubation should be performed in the operating room in the presence of an anesthesiologist who is skilled in the use of anesthetics with bronchodilating properties.

Discharging children with mild, responsive disease requires close follow-up to ensure that parents will return if breathing difficulty increases, if the patient's color changes, or if the patient becomes restless or agitated. Give instructions about medications. Hospitalize more seriously ill children and manage their treatment aggressively.

Pneumonia

Pneumonia is an acute infection of the lung parenchyma and causes an interstitial process involving the alveolar walls or alveoli. It is commonly caused by one of a number of organisms:

- Bacterial infections: *Streptococcus pneumonia* (most common bacterial cause), *H. influenzae* (primarily in children less than 9 years old), Group A streptococcus, and *S. aureus*
- Viral infections: RSV, influenza, parainfluenza, and adenovirus
- *Mycoplasma pneumoniae:* common in children over 5 years of age
- *Chlamydia* organisms: primarily children 2 to 12 weeks with an indolent lower respiratory infection characterized by cough, poor weight gain, hyperinflation, and conjunctivitis; usually of maternal origin; rales occur in more than 75%, conjunctivitis in 50%, and staccato cough in approximately 50%.

Assessment

Clinically, patients with pneumonia have a variety of signs and symptoms. *Bacterial* pneumonias are usually more rapid in onset and are associated with toxicity, tachypnea, high fevers, productive coughs, segmental consolidation, and sometimes with effusions.

In contrast, *viral* pneumonias are more insidious, with less toxicity and systemic illness. Chest radiographs usually demonstrate a diffuse interstitial process. Tachypnea may be an early sign of pneumonia, and most children do not have associated abnormalities on auscultation and percussion. Obtain cultures, including blood when possible; however, only a very low percentage of these cultures are positive.

Management

Initially evaluate the patient's respiratory status and administer oxygen whenever necessary. Because fever may increase respiratory rate, decrease the child's temperature with antipyretics. Stabilization involves administering antibiotics, assessing the respiratory status, and monitoring the child with oximetry. Any child with dehydration, persistent vomiting, ill appearance, or an oximetry reading less than 95% (oxygen require-

ment) should be admitted. The majority of these patients can be managed at home with oral antibiotics.

Management of children of different ages involves the following:

- *Children less than 2 months:* The child should receive parenteral antibiotics and be admitted to the hospital: ampicillin 100 to 200 mg/kg/day every 6 hours IV *and* cefotaxime (or equivalent) 100 to 150 mg/kg/day every 8 hours IV, or both.
- *Children 2 months to 9 years:* If it is a mild case, give oral amoxicillin (30 to 50 mg/kg/day every 8 hours PO) or equivalent; if moderate or severe, cefuroxime 200 mg/kg/day every 6 hours IV *or* cefotaxime (or equivalent) as above; if poor response, add nafcillin 100 mg/kg/day every 4 hours IV (or equivalent).
- *Children older than 9 years:* If mild, give oral erythromycin (30 to 50 mg/kg/day every 6 to 8 hours PO); if moderate or severe, administer cefuroxime as above; if response is poor, add nafcillin as above. Alter these dosages to reflect the sensitivity of cultures. Contact patients within 24 hours to ensure compliance and improvement if outpatient therapy is initiated. Generally, continue antibiotics for 10 days.

DEHYDRATION

In children, vomiting and diarrhea are the most common causes of dehydration. The underlying disease requires evaluation, but a specific treatment is rarely indicated.

Normal maintenance fluids reflect the need to replace daily water (Table 66-4) and electrolyte losses from the skin and the respiratory, urinary, and gastrointestinal tracts. These losses may be divided into insensible, urinary, and fecal components; they amount to 100 ml/kg/day up to the age of 1 year and decrease thereafter.

Beyond the newborn period, total body

Table 66-4

WATER REQUIREMENTS FOR CHILDREN AND ADULTS

Weight	Amount (per day)
Children under 10 kg	100 ml/kg
Children 11-20 kg	1000 ml plus 50 ml/kg for each kilogram over 10 kg
Children over 20 kg	1500 ml plus 20 ml/kg for each kilogram over 20 kg
Adult	2000-2400 ml

water accounts for approximately 60% of the body weight. Of this total body water, 40% is intracellular fluid (ICF) and the remaining 20% is extracellular fluid (ECF). The daily sodium requirement for children is approximately 3 mEq/kg (adult: 80 mEq) and the daily potassium need is 2 mEq/kg (adult: 50 mEq).

Assessment

The clinical assessment of dehydration determines the urgency and type of therapy required. The child may have mild, moderate, or severe dehydration (Table 66-5).

In the child with only mild dehydration (2% to 3%), a slight decrease in mucosal membrane moisture and a relative dryness and prominence of the papillae of the tongue may appear. In

Table 66-5

DEGREE OF DEHYDRATION

	Mild (<5%)	Moderate (10%)	Severe (15%)
Signs and Symptoms			
Dry mucous membrane	±	+	+
Reduced skin turgor	−	±	+
Depressed anterior fontanelle	−	+	+
Sunken eyeballs	−	+	+
Hyperpnea	−	±	+
Hypotension (orthostatic)	−	±	+
Increased pulse	−	+	+
Laboratory			
Urine			
Volume	Small	Oliguria	Oliguria/anuria
Specific gravity*	≤1.020[†]	>1.030	>1.035
Blood			
BUN	WNL[†]	Elevated	Very high
pH (arterial)	7.40-7.30[†]	7.30-7.00	<7.10

From Barkin RM, Rosen P: *Emergency pediatrics: a guide to ambulatory care*, ed 4, St Louis, 1994, Mosby.
+, Present; − absent; ±, variable.
*Specific gravity can provide evidence that confirms the physical assessment.
[†]Not usually indicated in mild dehydration.

younger children, information about the number and dampness of diapers during the day may be useful.

Determine the amount of fluid deficit by multiplying the percentage of dehydration by the weight of the child in kilograms. For example, a 10-kg child who is 10% dehydrated has a total deficit of 1000 ml. The electrolyte composition of this fluid depends on the rapidity of the progression of dehydration (normally 60% extracellular fluid and 40% intracellular fluid). The electrolyte composition of these compartments

Table 66-6

MANAGEMENT OF ISOTONIC DEHYDRATION

---

1. Initial Findings

Preillness weight: 10.0 kg (a 1-year-old)   Electrolytes
Degree of dehydration: moderate (10%) Na^+ 135 mEq/L Cl^- 115 mEq/L
Body weight on admission: 9.0 kg K^+ 5 mEq/L HCO_3^- 12 mEq/L

2. Summary of Fluid Requirements

	H_2O (ml)	Na^+ (mEq)	K^+ (mEq)
Maintenance	1000 (100 ml/kg)	30 (3 mEq/kg)	20 (2 mEq/kg)
Deficit (100 ml/kg)			
ECF (60%)	600	84 (140 mEq/L × 0.6)	—
ICF (40%)	400	—	30 (150 mEq/L × 0.4 × 50% correction)
Total	1000	84	30

3. Fluid Schedule

Phase	Calculation	Administered
I. 0-½ hour	20 ml/kg	200 ml NS or LR over 20 minutes
II. ½-9 hours	½ deficit: 500 ml D_5W with 42 mEq NaCl and 15 mEq KCl ⅓ maintenance: 333 ml D_5W with 10 mEq NaCl and 7 mEq KCl Total: 833 ml with 52 mEq NaCl and 22 mEq KCl	833 ml (~ 100 ml/hr) of D_5W 0.45% NS with 22 mEq KCl (~ 27 mEq/L) (this approximation facilitates care)
III. 9-25 hours	½ deficit ⅔ maintenance	1167 ml (~ 75 ml/hr) of D_5W 0.45% NS with 28 mEq KCl (~ 24 mEq/L) (this approximation facilitates care)

From Barkin RM: *Fluid and electrolyte balance.* In Barkin RM, editor: *Pediatric emergency medicine,* St Louis, 1992, Mosby.
Note: If the patient is acidotic with HCO_3 <11 mEq/L or pH <7.1 (on the basis of metabolic acidosis), ⅓ of the sodium is administered during phase II (½ = 9 hours) as $NaHCO_3$.

may be simplified as extracellular (140 mEq sodium/L) and intracellular (150 mEq potassium/L). The type of dehydration primarily reflects the sodium concentration. Isotonic dehydration is the most common form, with the sodium concentration being 130 to 150 mEq/L.

Management

Patients with severe dehydration require the immediate infusion of fluids. These patients require isotonic fluids to restore intravascular volume regardless of the cause of the dehydration. Normal saline or Ringer's lactate is given in 20 ml/kg fluid boluses over 15 to 30 minutes.

Reassess the child after the fluid bolus, and administer a second fluid bolus if the child requires it. Check the child's initial serum glucose. If it is low, administer 0.5 g/kg as a single bolus of 10% or 25% dextrose and recheck the serum glucose.

Specific therapeutic plans must reflect the degree and type of dehydration. Table 66-6 outlines the management of isotonic dehydration. Hypotonic dehydration is less common and requires, in addition to the calculations noted, a correction of the sodium deficit. Hypertonic dehydration therapy must replace the fluid deficit evenly over a 48-hour period.

SHOCK

Shock occurs when acute circulatory dysfunction is marked by the progressive impairment of blood flow to the skin, muscles, kidneys, mesentery, lungs, heart, and brain. In children, hypovolemia is the most common cause of shock. Compensatory mechanisms initially prevent function deterioration, but with the progression of shock, cellular metabolic changes occur and are marked by anaerobic metabolism, which leads to further injury and, eventually, cell death.

Compensated shock is associated with the maintenance of vital organ functions by intrinsic compensatory mechanisms. With volume loss, arteriolar constriction and fluid shifts from the interstitial to intravascular compartments increase. The effectiveness of these responses depends on the preexisting cardiac and pulmonary status and on the volume and rate of fluid loss. Orthostatic changes may be early indicators of volume status, and acidosis may be the earliest sign of impaired tissue perfusion.

Uncompensated shock is characterized by further impairment of microvascular perfusion, which leads to lowered perfusion pressures, increased precapillary arteriolar resistance, and contraction of venous capacitance. Hypotension, tachycardia, and decreased cardiac output progress to cardiovascular collapse and multiple-system failure with adult respiratory distress syndrome (ARDS), liver and pancreatic failure, coagulopathy, oliguria, renal failure, gastrointestinal bleeding, impaired mental status, acidosis, and ongoing cellular damage.

Three major classifications of shock may occur, and each requires different management approaches:

- *Hypovolemic shock* is caused by a reduction in circulatory volume, which commonly occurs as a result of fluid and electrolyte loss (vomiting or diarrhea) or trauma. Hypovolemic shock is by far the most common cause of shock in children.
- *Cardiogenic shock* is caused by depressed cardiac output from myocardial insufficiency or obstruction of venous return or cardiac outflow resulting from congenital, infectious, or vascular conditions.
- *Distributive shock* occurs when intravascular volume is abnormally distributed as a result of vasomotor paralysis and increased venous capacitance. Distributive shock is anaphylactic, septic, or neurogenic in origin.

Management

Initially focus on ensuring adequate oxygenation and ventilation. Because shock results in a impaired delivery of oxygen to the tissues, administer 100% oxygen, even to a child with a stable airway. Reassess cardiovascular status through heart rate, capillary refill, blood pressure, urine output, and mental alertness. Laboratory studies, including electrolytes and arterial blood gases, are important for assessing baseline status and monitoring ongoing therapy. Following stabilization, evaluate and manage the underlying process. Administer IV fluids following the insertion of IV lines, and monitor the child's response.

For hypovolemic shock, administer normal saline or lactated Ringer's solution at a rate of 20 ml/kg over 20 minutes. If there is no response, repeat the infusion once, with an ongoing evaluation of cardiovascular and ventilatory status. If possible, place a central venous pressure (CVP) line if there is no response to the initial infusions, and administer fluids while monitoring hemodynamic parameters.

If hemorrhage is the cause of hypovolemia, give type-specific or crossmatched blood following 40 to 60 ml/kg of crystalloid infusions. Whole blood is particularly useful for massive ongoing acute bleeding; however, packed red blood cells may be appropriate following the infusion of large amounts of crystalloid in an acute situation or in a more chronic process.

Cardiogenic shock may improve following an initial careful infusion of 5 ml/kg normal saline. Pressor agents are usually necessary once the patient is normovolemic. Carefully monitor the response, and maintain the CVP (or pulmonary capillary wedge pressure) at 15 mm Hg or less.

Patients with distributive shock may require a combination of fluid and pressor support, which again reflects the pathophysiology and clinical response.

Other considerations for treatment must include management with antidysrhythmic agents, vasodilators, and antibiotics, as well as the correction of hypothermia or hyperthermia, hypoglycemia, electrolyte abnormalities, acid-base problems, and coagulopathies.

NEUROLOGIC EMERGENCIES

Bacterial Meningitis

Bacterial meningitis is a significant concern in children with fever and an altered state of consciousness or behavior. The major determinant of bacterial etiology is the age of the child:

- Less than 1 month: *Escherichia coli,* group B streptococcus, *Listeria monocytogenes*
- 1 month to 2 months: *E. coli,* group B streptococcus, *L. monocytogenes, H. influenzae, Neisseria meningitidis, S. pneumoniae*
- 2 months to 9 years: *H. influenzae, Streptococcus pneumoniae, N. meningitidis*
- More than 9 years: *N. meningitidis, S. pneumoniae*

Considerations in the differential diagnosis must include viral meningitis (enteroviral most common) and a variety of fungal and mycobacterial agents.

Assessment

In younger children, the initial presentation of bacterial meningitis is nonspecific and includes fever, hypothermia, dehydration, bulging fontanelle, lethargy, irritability, anorexia, vomiting, seizures, respiratory distress, or cyanosis. Nuchal rigidity is often absent in children younger than 18 months of age. Older children often have the preceding problems, as well as the more classic adult findings of nuchal rigidity, Kernig sign, Brudzinski sign, and headache.

Children may have a concurrent infection, such as otitis media, but such an infection does not exclude the possibility that a child also has meningitis. Complications of meningitis include cerebral edema, shock, bacteremia, syndrome of inappropriate antidiuretic hormone (SIADH), subdural effusion, persistent fever, and neurologic findings. The lumbar puncture (LP) is the diagnostic test for meningitis. A low peripheral white blood cell count (WBC) does not exclude the diagnosis of meningitis; therefore the WBC should not be the basis for deciding if an LP is indicated.

Table 66-7

CEREBROSPINAL FLUID ANALYSIS IN CHILDREN

	Normal			*Bacterial*	*Viral*
	Preterm	*Term*	*>6 mo*		
Cell count (WBC/mm³)*					
Mean	9	8	0	>500	<500
Range	0-25	0-22	0-4	80% polymorphonuclear neutrophil (PMN) leukocyte	PMN leukocyte initially; lymphocyte later
Predominant cell type	Lymph	Lymph	Lymph		
Glucose (mg/dl)					
Mean	50	52	>40	<40	>40
Range	24-63	24–119			
Protein (mg/dl)					
Mean	115	90	<40	>100	<100
Range	65-150	20-170			
CSF/blood glucose (%)					
Mean	74	81	50	<40	>40
Range	55-150	44-248	40-60		
Gram stain	Negative	Negative	Negative	Positive[†]	Negative
Bacterial culture	Negative	Negative	Negative	Positive[‡]	Negative

Modified from Sarff LD, Platt LH, McCracken GH Jr: CSF evaluation in neonates: comparison of high risk infants with and without meningitis, *J Pediatr* 88:473, 1976; Portnoy JM, Olson LC: Normal CSF values in children: another look, *Pediatrics* 75:484, 1985.

*Total WBC/mm³ by age in the normal child can be further delineated as follows (mean ± 2 SD): <6 wk, 3.7 ± 6.8; 6 wk-3 mo: 2.9 ± 5.7; 3-6 mo: 1.9 ± 4.0; 6-12 mo: 2.6 ± 4.9; >12 mo: 1.9 ± 5.4.

[†]If the Gram stain is negative, a methylene blue stain may distinguish intracellular bacteria from nuclear material.

[‡]85% of partially treated patients will have a positive Gram stain, and >95% have positive cultures. Counterimmunoelectrophoresis may be helpful if the culture is negative.

Analysis of the spinal fluid should include a cell count and differential, protein, glucose, a Gram stain, and cultures (Table 66-7). The cerebrospinal fluid (CSF) may also be sent for latex particle agglutination or counterimmunoelectrophoresis (CIE) if the child has been pretreated with antibiotics. Partial treatment with antibiotics before the LP rarely alters the CSF enough to interfere with an appropriate interpretation.

Bloody LPs pose a diagnostic dilemma. Although an attempt may be made to determine if an excessive number of WBCs exist with respect to the number of RBCs, this approach is not reliable. A culture remains the "gold standard."

If the child is unstable, do not attempt to perform an LP, and never compromise the infant's airway during an LP. This fact is particularly important in small infants who are held tightly, which potentially causes suffocation or impaired central venous return.

Obtain the following additional studies: blood cultures, complete blood count (CBC), electrolytes, and blood glucose. Counterimmunoelectrophoresis (CIE) for *H. influenzae* and *S. pneumoniae* may be useful adjunctive measures in determining the bacterial etiology.

Differential diagnosis

Considerations in the patient with a stiff neck include meningitis, adenitis, osteomyelitis, trauma with or without fracture, hematoma, muscle injury, tumor, oculogyric crisis from drugs such as phenothiazines, hysteria, and torticollis.

Management

Evaluate airway, ventilation, and circulation, and initiate the necessary interventions. Even though cerebral edema may be a complication of meningitis, adequate volume resuscitation should be administered to any child with signs of shock. If a child is hemodynamically stable, fluids may be restricted to two thirds of the daily maintenance.

Antibiotics are the crucial part of the management of bacterial meningitis (Table 66-8). Antibiotics vary with the child's age and should reflect the underlying disease, immunologic status, and allergies. Start with broad-spectrum antibiotics, which may be adjusted once the culture and sensitivity data become available. *H. influenzae* is commonly resistant to ampicillin. Give dexamethasone 0.15 mg/kg/dose q6h IV for 16 doses to reduce hearing loss. Monitor electrolytes closely as therapy is initiated and as care proceeds.

If the child is afebrile, the sutures are split, or evidence of excessive bruising is present, consider a CT scan of the head before an LP. In older children in which the sutures have fused and the fontanelle is closed, consider a head CT scan if the history suggests child abuse or if an intracranial mass is suspected. Administer antibiotics following blood cultures and before the CT scan.

Chemoprophylaxis is indicated for all intimate contacts of patients with *N. meningitidis* (rifampin 10 mg/kg/dose every 12 hours PO for

Table **66-8**

ANTIBIOTIC THERAPY FOR BACTERIAL MENINGITIS OF UNKNOWN ETIOLOGY

Patient Age	Antibiotic
<2 months	Ampicillin, 100-200 mg/kg/day q4-6h IV *and* cefotaxime (or equivalent) 100-150 mg/kg/day q8-12h IV; *or* ampicillin, as above *and* chloramphenicol 50-100 mg/kg/day q6h IV
2 months-9 years	Cefotaxime (or equivalent) 200 mg/kg/day q8h IV; *or* ampicillin 200-400 mg/kg/day q4h IV *and* chloramphenicol 100 mg/kg/day q6h IV
>9 years	Penicillin G 250,000 units/kg/day q4h IV; many use ampicillin until culture results are available

From Barkin R, Rosen P: *Emergency pediatrics: a guide to ambulatory care*, ed 4, St Louis, 1994, Mosby.
NOTE: Ampicillin is needed for treatment of *L. monocytogenes* in children <2 months.
NOTE: Equivalent third-generation cephalosporins include ceftriaxone 100 mg/kg/day q12h IV.

four doses; adult: 600 mg every 12 hours PO for four doses). Prophylactic drug therapy for exposures to *H. influenzae* has questionable efficacy but is commonly initiated.

Status Epilepticus

Children are in status epilepticus when they have continuous seizures for 20 to 30 minutes or have had two seizures without a lucid period.

Poor compliance with antiseizure medications is the most common cause of this condition, but other considerations must include infection, head trauma, drug interactions, intoxication, or an exacerbation of an underlying seizure disorder.

Assessment

Grand mal seizures are the most common manifestation of status epilepticus. Seizure activity, loss of consciousness, and cyanosis occur. Very young children may have focal findings that are associated with seizures of a metabolic etiology. Delineate the preexisting status of the child and focus on possible infections that produce seizures because of lowered threshold or that primarily involve the central nervous system as in meningitis. Note the history of trauma, ingestion, and prior seizures. Determine the patient's compliance with prescribed anticonvulsants, if any.

Obtain blood glucose, electrolytes, calcium, magnesium, and serum anticonvulsant levels, if appropriate. Perform a metabolic work-up as appropriate. An EEG and CT scan may also be useful in either acute or chronic cases of this condition.

Management

Of primary importance is determining whether any compromise of airway or ventilation exists. Children can usually be supported by clearing the airway with suction, positioning the child, and administering oxygen while protecting the child from injury.

Intubation may occasionally be required. In a child with a first-time seizure, follow the diagnostic approach in Fig. 66-3 to direct further evaluation and intervention. Consider metabolic and intoxication abnormalities. If such abnormalities are present or suspected, administer the following:

1. Glucose ($D_{25}W$ 0.5 to 1.0 g [2 to 4 ml]/kg/dose IV slowly), optimally after obtaining blood for later determination of the serum glucose and after determining that the Dextrostix or chemstrip is low (<40 mg/dl).
2. Naloxone (Narcan) 0.1 mg/kg/dose up to 0.8 mg IV.

Other metabolic abnormalities may include hyponatremia, hypernatremia, hypocalcemia, or hypomagnesemia. Hyponatremia is very common, especially in a child with a history of excessive water intake and vomiting or diarrhea. Consider using isotonic saline as an initial IV solution for all children with a first-time seizure (D_5W or D5.2 may exacerbate an underlying hyponatremia).

Consider using anticonvulsants, but use them only after stabilizing the airway and remembering that cerebral injury occurs after prolonged (longer than 15 minutes) seizures. Maintain adequate oxygenation.

Generally, use drugs in a sequential fashion until control is achieved. A benzodiazepine may be used initially (valium or lorazepam). Lorazepam provides rapid control with a longer duration. Following the administration of a benzodiazepine, several options are available. If the seizure has stopped, it is reasonable to monitor the child and not give any further medications. A decision may be made to give the child a longer-acting anticonvulsant and is usually indicated in situations in which the child is subtherapeutic on the current anticonvulsant or has required anticonvulsants before. If the level is subtherapeutic, give a partial loading dose and focus on increasing the maintenance dosage.

If the child has continued seizure activity, administer a loading dose of phenytoin (Dilantin) or phenobarbital. Phenobarbital may cause marked respiratory depression when combined with diazepam, particularly in children. Phenytoin has the advantage as the second drug because no synergistic respiratory depression occurs.

Maintenance medications include phenobarbital or phenytoin. The following medications may be used for status epilepticus:

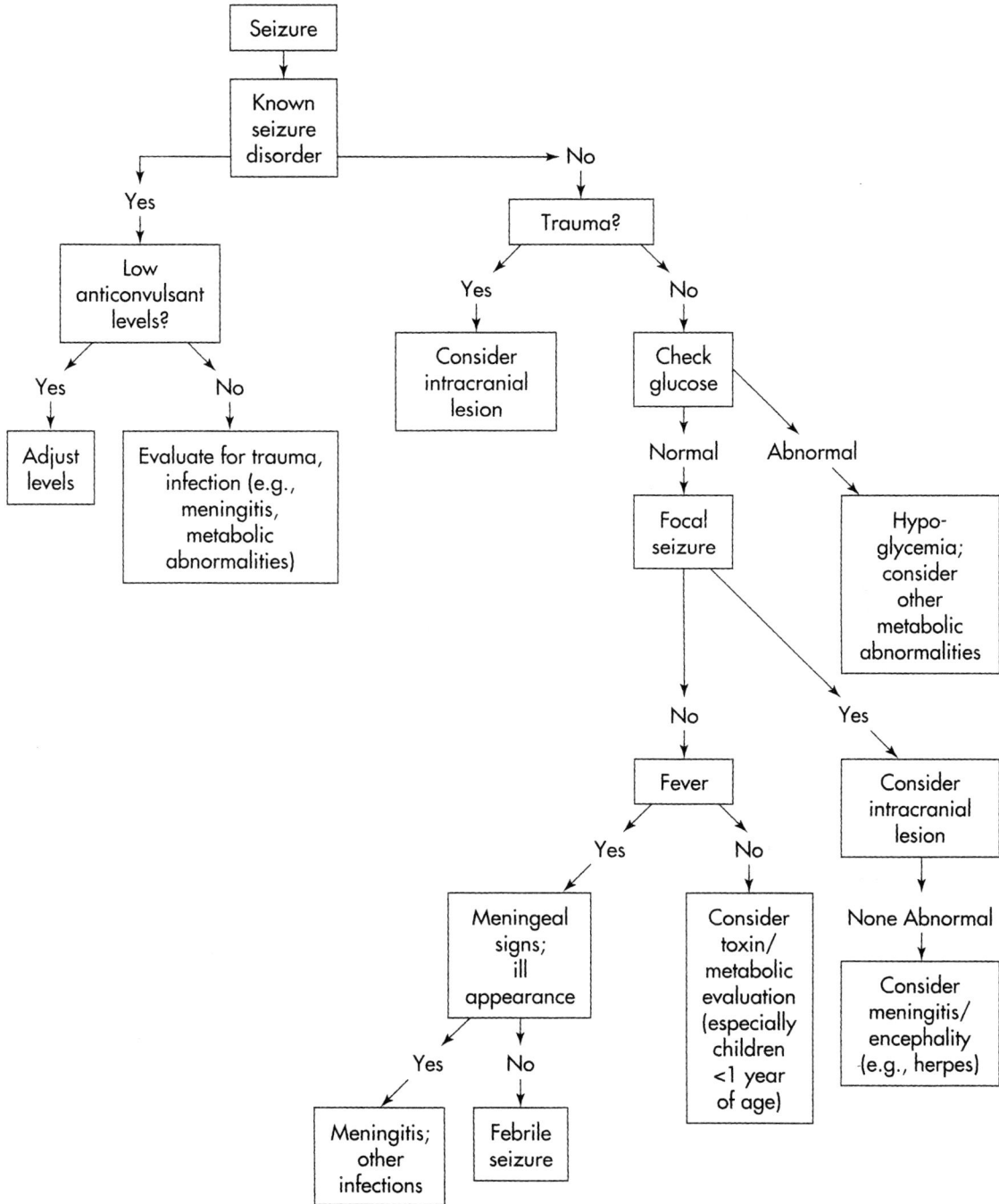

Fig.66-3 Algorithm for the evaluation of a seizure.

1. Diazepam (Valium). Administer 0.2 to 0.3 mg/kg/dose over 2 to 3 minutes at a rate not to exceed 1 mg/minute IV. Diazepam may also be given rectally (.5 mg/kg) if seizures continue and IV access is not obtained. The maximum total dose in children is 1.0 mg/kg. The peak effect occurs in 1 to 2 minutes, and the anticonvulsant effect lasts for 20 to 30 minutes.
2. Lorazepam (Ativan). Administer 0.1 mg/kg/dose IV. The onset is in 5 minutes, with a half-life of approximately 10 hours.
3. Phenobarbital. The loading dose is 10 to 20 mg/kg IV infusion, not to exceed 25 to 50 mg/minute. A second dose may be administered to a total dose of 40 mg/kg. The maintenance dose is 3 to 5 mg/kg/24 hr IV, IM, or PO. The therapeutic level is 10 to 25 μg/ml.
4. Phenytoin (Dilantin). The loading dose is 10 to 20 mg/kg IV infusion, not to exceed 50 mg/minute while monitoring the patient. The maintenance dose is 5 mg/kg/24 hr IV or PO. The therapeutic level is 10 to 20 μg/ml.

Hospitalization is usually indicated for patients who have seizures that are hard to control or for patients who have an underlying disease that needs management on an inpatient basis. Most children over 2 years of age who have an afebrile first-time seizure that requires no pharmacologic therapy and who have a negative work-up may be discharged to home with good follow-up.

Febrile Seizures

Generalized seizures commonly occur in children with febrile illness and do not specifically involve the central nervous system; as many as 2% to 5% of all children between 5 months and 5 years of age have febrile seizures. The peak age of incidence is between 8 and 20 months.

Underlying diseases that are commonly associated with febrile seizures include upper respiratory tract infections, gastroenteritis, and a host of less common infections in children.

Assessment

Typically the child has a generalized tonic-clonic seizure that is self-limited, lasts for as long as a few minutes, and is associated with a high fever. Most of these children are alert and without neurologic deficit shortly after the seizure. The neurologic examination is normal.

Obtain blood glucose levels, serum electrolytes, CBC, and other studies as appropriate. The LP is an important part of the evaluation, particularly for those under 1 year of age with a first febrile seizure or for those who remain irritable or lethargic after antipyretic therapy.

Management

As with any seizure, initial attention should be directed to the airway and ventilation to ensure that they are adequate. Because most febrile seizures are self-limited, active intervention beyond oxygen administration and head positioning is rarely required.

In patients who continue to have seizures after several minutes, consider anticonvulsant therapy; however, initiate this therapy in a deliberate fashion only with ongoing seizures.

In patients who are not actively seizing, evaluate for the underlying cause of the fever. Focus the questions on potential infectious sources, the history of seizures, neurologic deficits, developmental problems, family history, medications, precipitating events, and preceding illnesses. Treat these problems as indicated. Initiate aggressive antipyretic therapy early.

Long-term anticonvulsant therapy should be initiated only by, or in cooperation with, the physician who will be giving regular medical care to the child. Patients with two or more of the following risk factors may be candidates for long-term therapy:

- Abnormal neurologic or developmental history before the seizure
- Complex seizure: lasts longer than 15 minutes
- Seizure that is focal or followed by a transient or persistent neurologic abnormality
- Positive family history for afebrile seizures

It is imperative to discuss with the parents the high incidence of febrile seizures in healthy children and to emphasize the excellent prognosis and the less than 50% risk of recurrence. Children usually outgrow this type of seizure and have normal intelligence. Discuss aggressive antipyretic therapy with parents.

Breath-holding Spells

Breath-holding spells result from prolonged crying and produce cyanosis and ultimately a loss of consciousness. The spells are most common between 6 months and 4 years of age.

Assessment

Crying is often precipitated by a fall, an injury, or anger. The child develops cyanosis and unconsciousness and becomes limp. The episode is usually self-limited and lasts less than 1 minute. There may be some evidence of disturbance at home or in the maternal-child interaction.

Differential diagnosis

Distinguish breath-holding spells from seizures, which on rare occasions can accompany a breath-holding spell on a hypoxemic basis. A child who is cyanotic and then has a seizure usually has had a breath-holding spell, whereas with a seizure the child turns blue as a result of the seizure.

Management

Reassure and calm the parents. Because the episodes are usually self-limited, recognition is the hallmark of management. Minimize the events and factors that trigger the spells, and encourage parents to be firm and consistent with behavioral problems.

FEVER

Fevers in children are very common and are most often associated with a viral cause. The recognition of the unique pathophysiology of the child's condition as related to infection allows the physician to approach the patient in a logical, thorough fashion (see Chapter 7).

Assessment

Historically, parents usually report nonspecific observations related to behavior and associated signs and symptoms rather than those that permit an early focus on the involved system. However, make every effort to define the alterations in behavior, activity, and eating habits and to determine if respiratory, gastrointestinal, musculoskeletal, and dermatologic findings have developed. Urinary tract and CNS symptoms are reflected as behavioral changes, such as irritability and lethargy. Note recent exposures to children with similar complaints, as well as recent events such as diphtheria-pertussis-tetanus (DPT) immunizations.

Early antipyretic therapy is imperative in facilitating observation. Many children who initially are irritable and not interested in their environment improve markedly with aggressive antipyretic management. Administer acetaminophen (15 mg/kg/dose PO or rectally) to all children with temperatures higher than 39.4° C (102.9° F) on arrival to ensure optimal observation by reducing temperature and permitting a more accurate assessment of the child. The response to antipyretics does not predict the prevalence of bacteremia.

Systematically perform the physical examination to assess responsiveness; focus on carefully observing the child at play and encouraging the youngster to follow lights, bright objects, or a parent. Useful and reassuring components of this overall assessment include the following:

- The child looks at and focuses on the clinician and spontaneously explores the room.
- The child spontaneously makes sounds or talks in a playful manner.
- The child plays with and reaches for objects.
- The child smiles and interacts with the parent or clinician.
- The child quiets easily when held by parents.

While the child is distracted with play objects, define obvious physical abnormalities such as limitation of limb movement, a rash, and points of tenderness. Examination of the chest, heart, and abdomen require a gentle hand and patience. Tachypnea that is disproportionate to fever usually requires a chest x-ray study. After assessing these areas, perform a full examination of the ears, throat, and neck. Document in the chart the status of the child at the time examined, and record changes that occur during the time the child is observed (e.g., 1 hour following tylenol, child is playful and "mom says he acts normal").

Infants under 1 month of age

Infants under 1 month of age should receive a "complete septic evaluation," including a blood count, glucose, urine culture, blood culture, and LP. Admission is mandatory after antibiotics have been initiated (ampicillin 150 mg/kg/24 hour every 4 to 6 hours IV *and* gentamicin 5 to 7.5 mg/kg/24 hour every 8 hours IV); *or* ampicillin as above *and* a third-generation cephalosporin (cefotaxime 150 mg/kg/24 hour every 6 hours IV).

Infants between 1 and 3 months of age

Infants between 1 and 3 months of age require a more extensive evaluation than older children. The history is rarely more specific than the triad of fever, irritability, and poor feeding. The physical examination may fail to reveal specific focal findings despite the presence of systemic infections. Children under 3 months of age who have a temperature higher than 38.5° C have a greater than twentyfold risk of having a serious infection compared to older children with a similar temperature.

Current studies have divided febrile children into high risk vs low risk. A low-risk child is a child who appears well, has a WBC <20,000 cells/mm^3, a normal urinalysis, a stool sample without WBCs, and a normal CSF. These children should have blood, urine, and CSF cultures sent and should be given an IM or IV dose of ceftriaxone (50 mg/kg) and be followed up in 18 to 24 hours. A high-risk child is a child with a WBC >20,000 cells/mm^3, an abnormal urinalysis, WBCs in the stool, or an abnormal CSF. These children should receive parenteral antibiotics and be hospitalized.

In addition, any child who appears toxic or has an unstable social situation should be treated as high-risk, receive a full septic workup, and be admitted.

Immunocompromised children

Evaluate children who have a history of recurrent serious bacterial infections for immunodeficiency. Children who are undergoing cancer chemotherapy or who have a history of asplenia (from congenital or traumatic causes) are at risk. Those with sickle cell disease have 400 times the risk for pneumococcal septicemia if under 5 years of age and a fourfold risk of *H. influenzae* septicemia if under 9 years of age. Carefully question family members regarding the child's sickle cell status.

Children who are immunocompromised require an aggressive and anticipatory approach to potential infections. All of these children require a complete evaluation for the source of the fever. Children who are immunosuppressed by chemotherapy require hospitalization and IV antibiotics, particularly if they have a central line placed for ongoing therapy. All children with a chronic disease (e.g., sickle cell disease) should have a consultation with the specialist that cares for them.

Occult bacteremia

Although bacteremia occurs in association with a host of clinical entities, including meningitis, arthritis, epiglottitis, cellulitis, pneumonia, and kidney infections, approximately 6% of the patients who have fever without a defined focus have positive blood cultures. Occult bacteremia is a problem in children, and the following characteristics describe those at high risk:

CHILD APPEARS TOXIC?

Yes / No

Yes → Admit to Hospital
Sepsis work-up
Parenteral antibiotics

No → Temperature is 39.4°C or higher?

Yes / No

Yes:

1. Urine culture
   Males less than 6 months old
   Females less than 2 years old
2. Stool culture
   Blood and mucus in stool or 5
   or more WBCs/hpf in stool
3. Chest x-ray study
   Dyspnea, tachypnea, rales,
   or decreased breath sounds
4. Blood culture
   Option 1: All children with
   temperature of 39.4°C or more
   Option 2: Temperature of
   39.4°C or more and WBC count
   of 15,000/mm or more
5. Empiric antibiotic therapy
   Option 1: All children with
   temperature of 39.4°C or more
   Option 2: Temperature of
   39.4°C or more and WBC count
   of 15,000/mm or more
6. Acetaminophen
   15 mg/kg every 4 hours for
   temperature of 39.4°C or more
7. Follow-up in 24 to 48 hours
   Blood culture positive:
   Streptococcus pneumoniae:
   Persistent fever; admit for sepsis
   evaluation and parenteral antibiotics
   pending results; outpatient antibiotics
   it afebrile and well
   All others: Admit for sepsis
   evaluation and parenteral
   antibiotics pending results
   Urine culture positive:
   All organisms: Admit if
   febrile or ill appearing;
   outpatient antibiotics
   if afebrile and well

No:

1. No diagnostic tests or
   antibiotics
2. Acetaminophen: 15 mg/kg
   every 4 hours for fever
3. Return if fever persists
   more than 48 hours or
   if clinical condition
   deteriorates

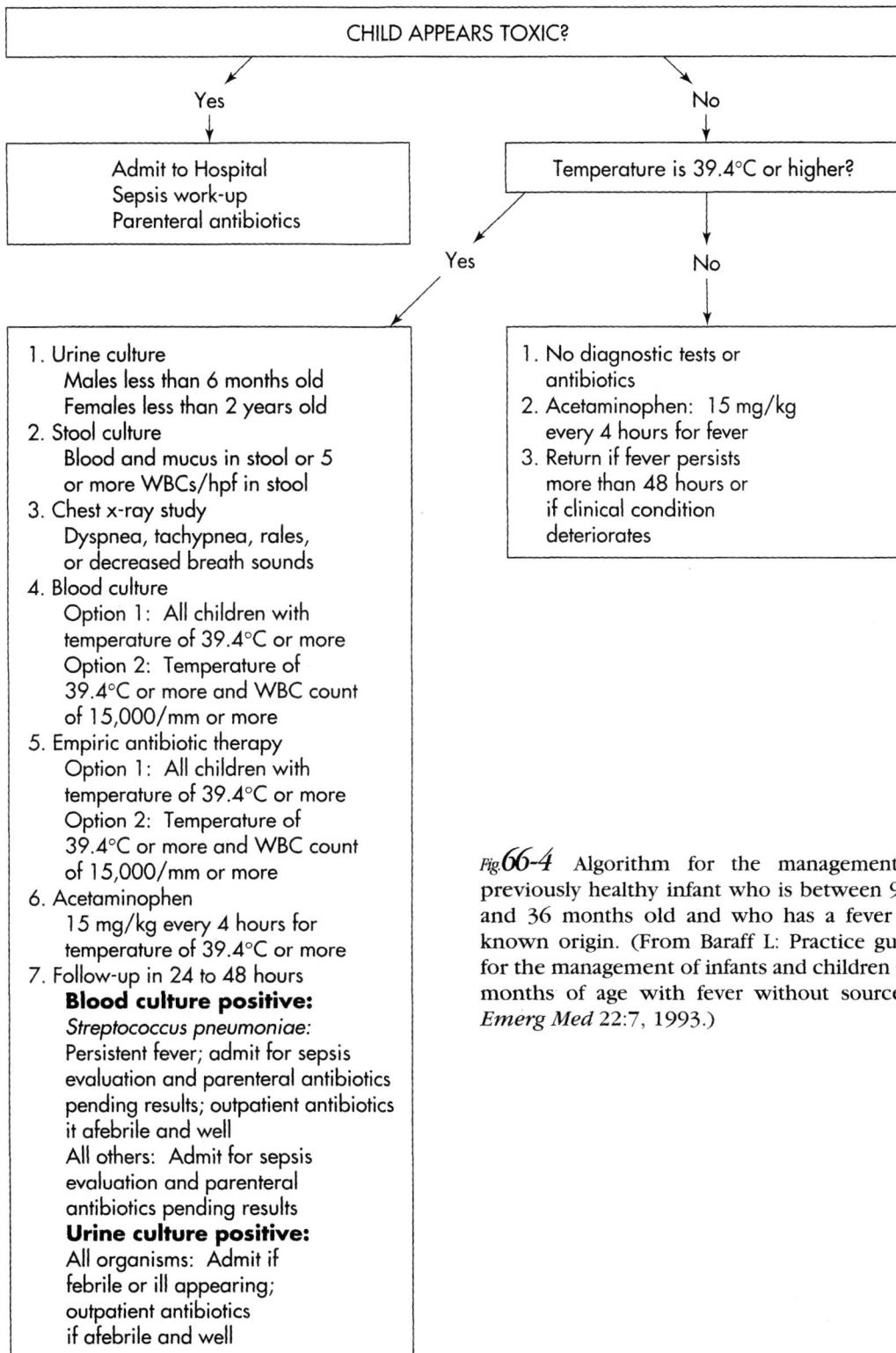

Fig.66-4 Algorithm for the management of a previously healthy infant who is between 91 days and 36 months old and who has a fever of unknown origin. (From Baraff L: Practice guideline for the management of infants and children 0 to 36 months of age with fever without source, *Ann Emerg Med* 22:7, 1993.)

- Age: ≤24 months
- Fever: ≥39.4° C
- WBC: ≥15,000 mm³ (differential does not increase prognostic value)

Always carefully evaluate the children in this high-risk group to be certain that there is no underlying disease such as pneumonia or meningitis. There is no conclusive evidence that performing an LP on a child with bacteremia increases the risk of subsequently developing meningitis.

Organisms commonly cultured include *S. pneumoniae, H. influenzae,* and *N. meningitidis.* Children less than 2 to 3 months of age may also have *E. coli* and *L. monocytogenes.*

General management

Consider meningitis in any febrile child who has a seizure. Perform an LP on children 12 months of age and younger, as well as on those who have altered behavior. Fig. 66-4 outlines management for a child who has a fever and is under 2 years of age.

If the fever has been present for fewer than 24 hours, if the child looks well on the basis of overall assessment and is more than 6 months old, and if no helpful history is detected, close follow-up in 6 to 12 hours may substitute for the laboratory evaluation. If the temperature remains elevated above 39.4° C at the follow-up appointment, proceed with the laboratory evaluation. Children who have a WBC greater than 15,000 mm³ and from whom blood cultures have been obtained may be treated with antibiotics with the potential to reduce complications. The most common regimen is ceftriaxone 50 mg/kg/day.

Follow-up is essential (usually in 12 to 24 hours) and depends on clinical and logistic constraints. If the cultures remain negative, antibiotics may be discontinued after 48 hours unless there was a specific focus initially or one develops. Continued follow-up is necessary until resolution of the illness occurs. If the culture is positive, which indicates bacteremia, reexamine

the patient and follow the recommendations in Fig. 66-4. If patients are febrile, have a toxic condition, or develop a focus, admit them for IV antibiotics and further evaluation.

RASHES

Many pediatric diseases are a reflection of infectious processes that cause accompanying rashes (see Chapter 49). Examine the rash and evaluate the associated systemic signs and symptoms to make the diagnosis. The distinction often is based on the morphology of the rash. The conditions often cause maculopapular or vesicular eruptions (Table 66-9). See the patient emergently if the lesions are purple or look like blood (purpura); do not blanch (petechiae); are burn-like (scalded skin); are red, blue, or tender to the touch (cellulitis); have red streaking; or are pustular.

GASTROINTESTINAL CONDITIONS REQUIRING SURGERY

A number of specific gastrointestinal entities have unique presentations in the pediatric age group and require early recognition and definitive lifesaving surgical management.

Appendicitis

Assessment

Crampy abdominal pain that occurs initially in the area of the umbilicus and gradually shifts to the right lower quadrant (McBurney's point) is typical in appendicitis. The abdomen demonstrates tenderness, rebound, and guarding. Tenderness may be present during a rectal examination. Accompanying vomiting, lethargy, and fever are common. The WBC is often slightly elevated, the urinalysis is normal, and the abdominal film is usually normal.

Table 66-9

ACUTE EXANTHEMS

	Macular	*Vesicular*	*Petechial or Purpuric*
Infection	Viral	Viral	Viral
	Measles	Chickenpox	Enterovirus
	Rubella	Herpes zoster	Hemorrhagic measles
	Roseola	Herpes simplex	Rubeola (atypical)
	Enterovirus	Enterovirus	Chickenpox
	Infectious	Hand-foot-and-mouth	
	mononucleosis	diseases	
	Pityriasis rosea	Herpangina	
		Molluscum contagiosum	
		Historical: smallpox	
	Other	Other	Other
	Scarlet fever	Impetigo	Meningococcemia
	Staphylococcal scalded	Rickettsialpox	*H. influenzae*
	skin	Candidiasis	Rocky Mountain
	Toxic shock syndrome	Staphylococcal scalded	spotted fever
	Kawasaki syndrome	skin syndrome	Sepsis (with
	Meningococcemia	Erythema multiforme	thrombocytopenia
	Mycoplasma		or DIC)
	pneumoniae		Gonococcemia
	Tick diseases		Endocarditis
	Rocky Mountain		Plague
	spotted fever		
	Typhus		
Intoxication	Ampicillin		
	Penicillin		
	Barbiturates		
	Anticonvulsants		
	Sulfonamides		
Other	Sunburn	Insect bites	Henoch-Schönlein purpura
	Juvenile rheumatoid		Idiopathic thrombocytopenia
	arthritis		Coagulation disorder
	Serum sickness		Trauma
			Tourniquet (distal)
			Coughing (head and neck)
			Leukemia
			Aplastic anemia

From Barkin R, Rosen P: *Emergency pediatrics: a guide to ambulatory care,* ed 4, St Louis, 1994, Mosby.

Management

Initially provide fluid resuscitation and surgical consultation. Initiate antibiotics, especially in children with evidence of perforation: ampicillin 100 to 200 mg/kg/day IV *and* clindamycin 30 to 40 mg/kg/day IV *and* gentamicin 5 to 7.5 mg/kg/day IV. Third-generation cephalosporins such as cefotaxime may be an excellent partial substitute.

Intussusception

Intussusception occurs when proximal bowel invaginates into distal bowel, which results in ischemia as well as possible infarction and gangrene of the inner bowel. The peak incidence occurs in children under 1 year of age.

Assessment

Patients with intussusception typically have an acute onset of intermittent episodes of intense pain with flexion of the legs and screaming. Vomiting, which is often bilious, and the passage of blood and mucus (currant jelly stools) via the rectum may occur. The abdomen is often distended and swollen. An altered mental status marked by lethargy, behavioral changes, irritability, and somnolence may occur.

An abdominal x-ray study may demonstrate decreased bowel gas, an abdominal mass, and air-fluid levels. A barium enema is both diagnostic and therapeutic. Obtain a CBC and type and crossmatch.

Management

Initiate fluid resuscitation in patients who are hypovolemic. Obtain a surgical consult immediately for a patient who has peritoneal signs. In stable patients, attempt hydrostatic reduction by using a cautiously performed barium enema; obtain a surgical consultation before doing the barium enema. Surgical intervention is indicated if the barium enema is unsuccessful or if the patient is hemodynamically unstable.

Pyloric Stenosis

Hypertrophy and hyperplasia of the circular antral and pyloric musculature result in gastric outlet obstruction. This condition commonly occurs in boys during the first few months of life.

Assessment

A gradual onset of vomiting that progresses from forceful to projectile nonbilious vomiting is typical with pyloric stenosis. Visible peristaltic waves and a palpable pylorus ("olive") may be present. Dehydration and hypokalemia are often present. An abdominal flat plate x-ray study may demonstrate gastric dilatation, and a barium swallow reveals a "string" sign and delayed gastric emptying. Abdominal ultrasonography has been found to be reliable. A CBC and electrolytes should be obtained. Fluid therapy with correction of any electrolyte abnormalities must be given before surgery.

Management

Initiate fluid therapy and IV rehydration. Following initial stabilization, confirm the diagnosis either by abdominal flat-plate x-ray studies or by ultrasonography. Perform a surgical pyloromyotomy.

Volvulus

Volvulus is a closed loop obstruction that results from the twisting of a section of the intestine on its own axis. This condition is unusual in children but may occur in the first few days of life and between 2 and 14 years of age.

Assessment

The sudden onset of crampy abdominal pain often greatest in the lower quadrants, is common. Intestinal obstruction with bilious vomiting often occurs. The rectum is empty of stool.

Abdominal flat-plate x-ray films show dilated gas-filled loops, often with air-fluid levels. With sigmoid volvulus, a barium enema demonstrates that the sigmoid colon has a circular pattern. Obtain a CBC and type and crossmatch.

Management

Stabilize and resuscitate the patient with fluids. Obtain a surgical consultation in cooperation with radiologic confirmation.

CHILD ABUSE AND SEXUAL ABUSE

Child Abuse

Abused children are those under 18 years of age who suffer nonaccidental trauma or a physical injury that threatens their health or welfare. Interpersonal dynamics form the basis for potential abuse and help identify those children who are at risk:

1. The abused child is usually under 4 years of age, may be handicapped, hyperactive, or temperamental, and has a "behavior" problem.
2. The abusive parent has low self-esteem and is depressed. Often abused as a child, the parent typically displays violent temper outbursts toward children. Expectations of the child are often rigid and unrealistic.
3. The family usually is isolated and mobile and has monetary, marital, or parenting problems.

A trigger specifically exacerbates the family and individual stresses. A family argument, discipline problems, substance abuse, job loss, eviction, an illness, and environmental stresses may all contribute to the abuse.

Assessment

With child abuse, the injury is inconsistent with the history, and the parents are reluctant to give information. Parents often bring in their children with complaints that are unrelated to the abuse; the purpose of the visit is to "ask for help." The parents often seek health care only after a delay.

Abused children commonly have bruises, burns, soft tissue injuries, fractures that are classically in various stages of healing (especially metaphyseal or chip fractures), retinal hemorrhages, acute abdominal injuries, or subdural hematomas. Explore any unexplained injury as possible child abuse.

X-ray studies of the long bones and skull are indicated for children under 5 years of age and in those over 5 years who have specific injuries or complaints. A bleeding screen is appropriate in children with a history of excessive or recurrent bruising.

Management

Begin by focusing on treating the specific problems that are medically detected. Evaluate the family and child's environment in a nonjudgmental and supportive fashion; social service personnel may expedite this process. Long-term follow-up and support are essential.

Contact the appropriate protective services worker immediately. *In all states physicians have a legal obligation to report suspected abuse.* Physicians are not liable for reporting suspected abuse, even if the injuries are proven not to be child abuse.

Hospitalization is indicated if it is medically appropriate, if there is an absence of alternative placement, and if the child cannot return home because of ongoing danger. A temporary crisis center may be an option. Maintain accurate and complete records. Often a picture or photograph of obvious injuries is helpful.

Sexual Abuse

Sexual assault—rape, molestation, or incest—may occur in any age group.

Assessment

Initially, establish confidence and rapport. Record a detailed history of the incident, and individualize the examination. Acute trauma may be demonstrated by perineal contusions or lacerations and by hymenal tears with bleeding, fissures, erythema, and discharge. Check for signs of sexually transmitted disease.

To maintain a chain of custody, submit cultures, the Venereal Disease Research Laboratories (VDRL) test, vaginal fluid, saliva (for ABO antigen testing), hair specimens, and related evidence to the appropriate officials.

Management

The key to the evaluation of sexual abuse is to be sensitive, thorough, and supportive. Specially trained support personnel often are available.

Careful documentation is essential. As with child abuse, all states require that physicians report sexual abuse to the appropriate protective services agency.

Prophylactic antibiotics may be indicated to prevent sexually transmitted disease, and a number of options exist to prevent pregnancy. Diethylstilbestrol (DES) 25 mg two times a day for 5 days within 48 hours of the incident may prevent pregnancy. Ovral is an alternative treatment. Treat the patient in conjunction with a gynecologic consultation. Long-term follow-up is essential.

SUDDEN INFANT DEATH SYNDROME

Sudden infant death syndrome (SIDS) is the sudden death of a child between 1 month and 1 year of age that is unexpected by history and in which a thorough postmortem examination fails to define an adequate cause of death. Multiple contributing factors lead to respiratory obstruction and central apnea with associated hypoxemia and death.

Assessment

SIDS is associated with irreversible cardiac and respiratory arrest. A patient with near-SIDS has variable vital signs.

Management

Initiate resuscitation if appropriate and the child is still potentially viable. If the child is dead, focus attention on supporting the family and friends. Notify the coroner. Ensure ongoing support through community resources. The local chapters of the National Sudden Infant Death Syndrome Foundation (1-800-221-7437) may be helpful.

NEWBORN EMERGENCIES

Giving careful attention to the complications that can occur during pregnancy, labor, and delivery can prevent many neonatal problems. Anticipation and preparation are essential.

Apnea and hypoventilation with associated cyanosis and hypoxemia may occur in the newborn. If not treated rapidly, tissue hypoxemia, acidosis, and resultant organ damage will occur.

Simple measures usually can resuscitate the patient; advanced life support is rarely required:

1. Provide tactile stimulation by drying and suctioning the oropharynx and nares. Slapping or flicking the soles of the feet or rubbing the infant's back may be useful.
2. In a radiant warmer, place the infant supine or on the side with the neck in the neutral position.
3. Use deep airway suction for no more than 3 to 5 seconds at a time. Do not perform this suction routinely because of reflex bradycardia.
4. Assess the infant's airway. Insert an oral airway if there is evidence of nasal obstruction or mandibular hypoplasia.
5. Administer oxygen.
6. If the infant is apneic and shows no response to stimulation, administer oxygen and begin bag-and-mask inflation. The bag should have an oxygen reservoir to deliver 100% oxygen. Positive-pressure ventilation is best achieved with the infant's head in the "sniffing" posi-

tion. If the response is poor, intubate the infant and continue to administer bag inflation.

7. Assess the infant's heart rate. If the infant is not readily responding, initiate closed chest massage.

8. Medications are usually not required. The response to ventilatory support is usually adequate. If ventilatory support is unsuccessful, routine routes as well as the umbilical vein can provide venous access. Volume resuscitation with solutions such as Plasmanate (5% albumin) or fresh-frozen plasma is preferred.

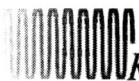

KEY CONSIDERATIONS

WHAT IS THE LIFE THREAT?

Respiratory distress is a life-threatening problem in children and is the most important early consideration in assessing the cause of cardiac arrest. Respiratory distress can be caused by pneumonia, asthma, bronchiolitis, congenital heart disease, airway abnormalities, croup, epiglottitis, foreign body aspiration, nasopharyngeal obstruction, poisoning, and trauma. Meningitis, dehydration, and sepsis are other serious life-threatening conditions.

DOES THE PATIENT NEED ADMISSION?

Admit a child who has respiratory distress that persists despite treatment.

Admit febrile newborn infants. Admit febrile infants and children between 3 months and 3 years old to the hospital if they appear toxic. If the child does not appear toxic, manage the patient as in Fig. 66-4. Meningitis and sepsis require inpatient management.

WHAT IS THE MOST SERIOUS DIAGNOSIS?

Respiratory distress, meningitis, sepsis, dehydration, surgical abdomen, and severe trauma are the most serious diagnoses.

HAVE I PERFORMED A THOROUGH WORK-UP?

Consider foreign body lodgement and upper airway obstruction in evaluating respiratory distress.

Consider dehydration, sepsis and meningitis in infants who are febrile, listless, irritable, or in those who feed poorly.

Assess febrile newborns and infants carefully with laboratory studies, cultures, and x-ray studies as outlined in Fig. 66-4.

In children, consider child abuse in cases of trauma or genital infections.

Recommended Reading

American Heart Association: Standards and guidelines for cardiopulmonary resuscitation (CPR) and emergency cardiac care (ECC), *JAMA* 268:2251, 1992.

Barkin RM, Rosen P, editors: *Emergency pediatrics: a guide to ambulatory care,* ed 3, St Louis, 1990, Mosby.

Chameides L: *Textbook of pediatric advanced life support,* Dallas, 1988, The American Heart Association.

Fleisher G, Ludwig S: *Textbook of pediatric emergency medicine,* ed 3, Baltimore, 1993, Williams & Wilkins.

Rosen P et al, editors: *Emergency medicine: concepts and clinical practice,* ed 3, St Louis, 1992, Mosby.

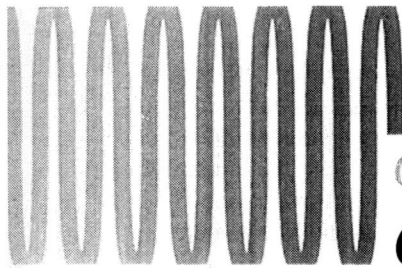

Chapter Sixty-seven
OTOLARYNGOLOGIC EMERGENCIES

THOMAS OSBORNE STAIR

OTITIS MEDIA

Acute otitis media is one of the most common emergency department diagnoses, particularly for children who are between 6 and 36 months of age. The condition usually appears as ear pain and fever, but infants may only be irritable, feed poorly, or pull at one ear. Otitis media usually begins with an upper respiratory infection with an adenovirus, enterovirus, influenza, parainfluenza, or respiratory syncytial virus. An inflamed eustachian tube prevents the equilibration of the negative pressure of the middle ear and produces a transudate that then becomes superinfected with *Streptococcus pneumoniae, Haemophilus influenzae,* group A streptococcus, or *Branhamella catarrhalis.* Although adult ear effusions do not always progress to bacterial superinfection, such a progression is so common and rapid for children that it is conventional for emergency physicians to prescribe antibiotics to children with ear pain, fever, and evidence of effusion.

The physical sign that is most diagnostic of otitis media is decreased mobility of the tympanic membrane in response to insufflation of the ear canal with a pneumatic otoscope. Acoustic otoscopes are available to measure the reflection of sound off the eardrum and to provide graphic or numeric outcome that is not so dependent on the experience of the examiner. Bullae on the tympanic membrane can be a sign of infection with *Mycoplasma pneumoniae* or other organisms that can also produce headache and coughing. The patient sometimes appears at the emergency department after rupturing the tympanic membrane with purulent drainage.

Uncomplicated otitis media in children may be treated with a 10-day course of oral amoxicillin, but increasing resistance among *Haemophilus* and *Moraxella* organisms may require the addition of clavulanate (Augmentin) or treatment with cefuroxime (Ceftin), erythromycin, and sulfisoxazole (Pediazole), or with trimethoprim and sulfamethoxazole (Bactrim). Pain and fever should be treated with acetaminophen or ibuprofen. Antihistamines are not helpful. Recurrences of infection may require tympanostomy until the eustachian tube matures.

OTITIS EXTERNA

External otitis may also appear as ear pain. This pain is worsened with movement of the tragus or by touching the ear canal with the otoscope. The ear canal may be full of pus from desquamated epithelium or may be swollen to the point of occlusion. The ear canal cleans and protects itself with a coat of waxy, acidic cerumen. Patients scratching or digging to remove ear wax with cotton swabs or fingernails can scratch through these defenses and cause cellulitis. Water that pools in the canal can macerate the skin and allow the breeding of *Pseudomonas* organisms, which are capable of dissolving intact skin and causing malignant otitis. Folliculitis, herpes zoster, and dermatitis can also cause otitis externa.

Treatment of otitis externa begins with a cleansing of the canal using a Frazier suction tube and instilling topical corticosteroid and antibiotic drops until the symptoms improve. If the canal is swollen shut and the medication cannot flow into the ear, insert a narrow wick of compressed cellulose into the ear. Wick insertion is painful, but analgesia is difficult to obtain. For long-term prophylaxis, 2% acetic acid can restore normal acidity and not allow selection of resistant organisms.

Pain that arises from infection in the mastoid air cells posteriorly or in the maxillary molars anteriorly can both be referred to the ear. Inflammation of the temporomandibular joint is a common affliction that can cause intermittent pain, tinnitus, muffling, or clicking sounds. Referred pain can cause the patient to scratch the ear canal and arrive at the emergency department with a secondary external otitis.

DECREASED HEARING

The most common cause of decreased hearing is impacted cerumen. The cerumen can be softened with detergents, removed with narrow swabs or special spoons, or irrigated out of the ear. Be careful not to scratch the skin of the canal or leave water that could cause external otitis to develop.

Another common cause of decreased hearing is an effusion in the middle ear. Children can have a serous or secretory otitis media as a sequela of treated infections. Serous otitis can cause a feeling of fullness, a muffling of sounds, or crackling from the movement of bubbles that can be seen through the tympanic membrane. Systemic sympathetic decongestants such as pseudoephedrine may help, especially in preventing compression of the middle ear when landing in an airplane.

Both cerumen impaction and effusion appear as a conduction hearing loss, which can be demonstrated by an abnormal Rinne test. In this test a vibrating tuning fork is allowed to fade to imperceptible when pressed against the mastoid (bone conduction) and is then listened for through the air (air conduction). Normally the tuning fork can be heard longer through the air than through the bone. Conduction loss also causes localization to the side of the lesion in the Weber test, in which the tuning fork is pressed to the midline of the forehead. The perceived vibration is stronger on the side of a conduction loss and sounds softer on the side of a sensory loss. The hearing loss may be insidious and noted, for example, only when the patient uses a telephone receiver. Sensory loss may be accompanied by tinnitus.

A loss of high-frequency sensation is common following exposure to a loud noise. A sudden unilateral sensory hearing loss may be evidence of brainstem ischemia. A bilateral sensory hearing loss may be caused by toxins or medications, including aminoglycosides, antibiotics, streptomycin, erythromycin, vancomycin, nonsteroidal antiinflammatory drugs, and furosemide. These drugs may also produce tinnitus and vertigo.

VERTIGO

Vertigo with vomiting and positional exacerbation tends to be caused by self-limiting viral infections of the peripheral nerve, and the symptoms may improve with diazepam or meclizine. Acoustic neuroma in the cerebellopontine angle and occlusion of the basilar artery are two other serious conditions that can appear as vertigo; their presentation usually includes defects of adjacent cranial nerve function. The nystagmus does not fatigue with repeat examination, and these conditions are less likely to manifest as acute, symptomatic vertigo.

EAR TRAUMA

Barotrauma, such as from a blow from an open hand, can rupture the tympanic membrane, which usually heals spontaneously in a month or two. However, warn the patient not to get water into the middle ear because doing so can be painful. Lacerations and hematomas of the pinna require special care in repair, drainage, and splinting because the cartilage is prone to ischemic necrosis and atrophy.

EPISTAXIS

Most nosebleeds originate in the vascular plexus of the anterior septum when the mucosal is lacerated by trauma or is irritated by dry, cold weather or an upper respiratory infection. The patient should be instructed to sit up and pinch the nose below the bridge for at least 5 minutes. The maneuver occludes the arteries of the Kiesselbach plexus and approximates the nasal mucosa, which encourages hemostasis. Ask the patient about medications, precipitating factors, recurrences, bleeding disorders, hypertension, and other illnesses. Hypertension can be lowered quickly with one capsule of nifedipine that is pierced, chewed, and swallowed.

If epistaxis continues, assemble lighting, a nasal speculum, bayonet forceps, a Frazier suction tube, and cotton pledgets soaked in cocaine (or a mixture of mucosal vasoconstrictor and anesthetic). It may be necessary to remove the new clot and restart the bleeding. Insert the medicated pledgets and press them against the mucosa for another 5 minutes. One blade of the nasal speculum should remain stationary on the floor of the nasal cavity while the other retracts the nares superiorly to allow inspection for bleeding sites. A small source of bleeding (less than 1 cm^2) can be cauterized with one silver nitrate stick, an injection of epinephrine, or electrocautery. Thrombocytopenia or other clotting disorders may not respond to cautery and require the application of a gelatin sponge (Gelfoam). Larger areas of bleeding require unilateral or bilateral packing. Use packing materials that are covered with antibiotic ointment and made from compressed cellulose, cotton gauze, or gauze-filled fingers from a rubber glove.

Less common sources of epistaxis may be diagnosed during the examination. Cocaine abuse can cause perforation of the septum. Angiofibromata and other tumors should not be probed or cauterized. Multiple telangiectasia may be hereditary. If bleeding from the nose has stopped but blood continues to flow down the posterior pharynx, the patient probably has posterior epistaxis.

Bleeding from the posterior choanae can be tamponaded with one or two balloon catheters designed for the purpose. A posterior nasal pack can be improvised with a Foley catheter that has been modified by cutting off the tip distal to the 5 ml balloon, passing it through the nose into the posterior pharynx, inflating it with 10 ml of saline, and applying traction forward. An anterior pack is then inserted.

Patients with anterior epistaxis may be discharged home after ½ hour of observation for reoccurrence. Posterior packing interferes with breathing and results in hypoxemia. Patients with posterior epistaxis are nearly always admitted to the hospital for humidified oxygen, sedation, blood pressure control, and surgical ligation when required. Because packing the nose causes iatrogenic sinusitis and toxic shock, patients with nasal packing packs that are left in longer than 1 day should be given prophylactic systemic antibiotics.

NASAL FRACTURE

When treating nasal fractures, any deformities that interfere with breathing must be reduced, and lacerations and bleeding should be handled as described elsewhere. Any hematoma of the septum represents a risk to the underlying cartilage and should be drained and packed; the patient should be given prophylactic antibiotics.

Radiographs of nasal bones are usually not necessary because diagnosing and reducing the nasal fracture is based on clinical appearance rather than bone alignment. If the nose is severely deformed but not yet too swollen to allow for assessment of reduction, anesthetize the nose with mucosal cocaine, grasp the septum with two padded forceps handles, distract, and reduce. If, as is usually the case, the nose is already swollen, apply ice and have the patient return for follow-up after 3 days (when the swelling has diminished) but before 7 days (when a bony callus has formed). A facial photograph taken before the injury should be brought in to help guide the repositioning.

PAROTITIS

The parotid gland sits in the cheek superficial to the molars and drains through Stensen's duct, which opens opposite the upper second molar. The infection of salivary glands may occur directly (e.g., mumps and other viruses), result from inoculation by retrograde oral bacteria (e.g., woodwind and brass players), occur when drainage of saliva is blocked (salivary stone or sublingual ranula), or occur in debilitated alcoholics. Sucking on lemon candy is a provacative diagnostic test because it stimulates salivation and therefore pain of salivary gland origin. The duct may be milked or probed to find stones or pus. Purulent drainage indicates suppurative parotitis, which requires systemic antibiotics.

KEY CONSIDERATIONS

WHAT IS THE LIFE THREAT?

If left untreated, otitis media can progress to mastoiditis or even a brain abscess. Uncontrolled bleeding from the nose or airway constitutes a life threat from blood loss or loss of airway.

DOES THE PATIENT NEED ADMISSION?

Posterior packing used to treat epistaxis can interfere with ventilation enough to cause hypoxemia. Such patients require admission and periodic monitoring of oxygen saturation.

WHAT IS THE MOST SERIOUS DIAGNOSIS?

Acoustic neuroma or vertebrobasilar artery occlusion are serious causes of vertigo. Blood dyscrasia and tumors are serious causes of epistaxis or oral bleeding. Suppurative parotitis, especially in elderly patients, can be a life-threatening infection.

HAVE I PERFORMED A THOROUGH WORK-UP?

In cases of epistaxis, evaluate the patient clinically for a bleeding disorder and hypertension. Look for septal hematoma in cases of trauma to the nose.

Recommended Reading

Bingham BJG, Hawke M, Kwok P: *Practical otolaryngology,* St Louis, 1992, Mosby.

Bluestone CD, Doyle WJ: Anatomy and physiology of eustachian tube and middle ear related to otitis media, *J Allerg Clin Immunol* 81:997, 1988.

Hartley C, Axon PR: The Foley catheter in epistaxis management: a scientific appraisal, *J Laryngol Otol* 108:399-402, 1994.

Jehle D, Cottington E: Acoustic otoscopy in the diagnosis of otitis media, *Ann Emerg Med* 18:396, 1989.

Josephson GD, Godley FA, Stierna P: Practical management of epistaxis, *Med Clin North Am* 75:1311-1320, 1991.

Kempthorne J, Giebink GS: Pediatric approach to the diagnosis and management of otitis media, *Otolaryngol Clin North Am* 24:905-929, 1991.

Ross GS, Bell J: Myocardial infarction associated with inappropriate use of topical cocaine as treatment for epistaxis, *Am J Emerg Med* 10:219, 1992.

Viducich RA, Blanda MP, Gerson LW: Posterior epistaxis: clinical features and acute complications, *Ann Emerg Med,* 25:592-596, 1995.

Zimmers T: Disposable noseclips used for temporary control of anterior nosebleeds, *Am J Emerg Med* 6:471, 1988.

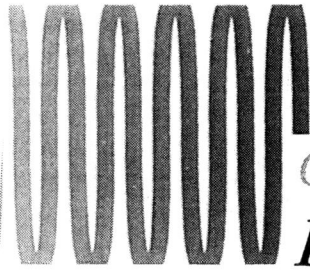

Chapter *Sixty-eight*
DISORDERS OF THE EYE

GERALYNN S. RENNER

The history of present illness for the patient with ocular complaints should include frequency; severity; rapidity of onset; and the duration and location of ocular symptoms such as pain, vision loss, photophobia, or a change in the appearance of the globe or surrounding structures. The presence of associated symptoms and the use of ophthalmic or systemic medications and drug allergies should be determined. In cases of trauma, a detailed mechanism of injury and tetanus immunization status should be obtained. Relevant elements of the past history include a past ocular disorder or injury, a preexisting vision reduction, and a medical illness that might have ophthalmic implications (e.g., hypertension or diabetes mellitus). Equipment that is useful in evaluating the patient with eye complaints is listed in the box on p. 828. The presence or absence of three cardinal symptoms should be assessed: loss of vision, change in the appearance of the eye, and ocular pain.

The ocular examination should include an ophthalmoscopy and an evaluation of visual acuity, external structures, pupils, ocular motility, intraocular pressure, visual fields. The visual acuity should be measured in each eye independently before performing a detailed examination. Standard Snellen notations should be used whenever possible using a conventional eye chart. If the patient did not bring corrective lenses, the visual acuity may be closely approximated using a pinhole occluder. Occasionally, vision is so impaired that conventional measurement is impossible. In such cases, visual acuity should be recorded as follows: finger counting, hand motion, light perception, or no light perception. The visual acuity of preschool children can be tested using "illiterate E" charts. In the extremely young child, noting that the child can fix his or her gaze on a light or can follow an object may indicate the presence of vision.

The external examination begins with the inspection and palpation of the periorbital soft tissues and orbital rim. A handheld light source is used to assess the lids, conjunctiva, corneal clarity, anterior chamber depth, and pupils. Eversion of the upper lid is mandatory if there is any suspicion of a foreign body or injury. The patient should first be instructed to look downward and avoid blinking. A cotton-tipped applicator is placed on the upper lid at the anatomic sulcus that overlies the upper border of the tarsal plate. The lashes are grasped firmly, and the lid is swung gently outward and upward while slight downward pressure is exerted on the applicator (Fig. 68-1). The lid will remain everted until the patient looks upward or blinks. Occasionally it is necessary to gain a clear view of the superior

Visual acuity cards and charts
Handheld light source
Cobalt blue lamp
Ophthalmoscope
Schiötz or other tonometer
Lid retractors
Foreign body spud
Cotton-tipped applicators
Eye patches
Fluorescein strips
Topical anesthetics
  Proparacaine (Ophthaine, Ophthetic) 0.5%
  Tetracaine (Pontocaine) 0.5%
Topical mydriatics/cycloplegics
  Phenylephrine 2.5%
  Cyclopentolate (Cyclogyl) 0.5%
  Tropicamide (Mydriacil) 0.5%

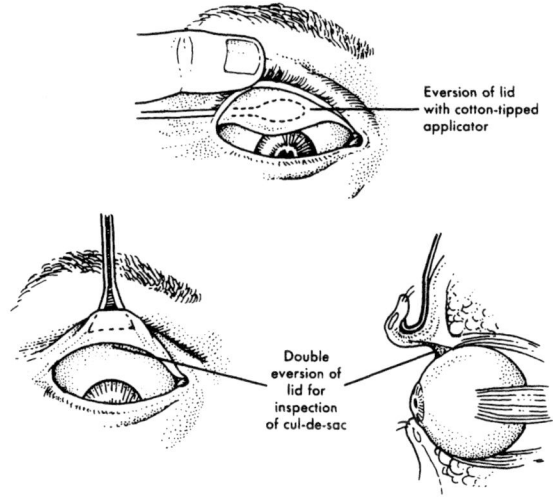

Fig. 68-1 Techniques of single and double eversion of upper lid.

cul-de-sac, which can be accomplished by everting the lid over the blade of a retractor. Once the lid is impinged on the edge of the retractor, outward and upward traction will provide good exposure of the superior cul-de-sac (see Fig. 68-1). The pupils should be inspected for equality, size, shape, and direct and consensual reaction to light. In addition, the "swinging flashlight" test is used to detect a defect in the afferent limb of the pupillary light reflex (Marcus Gunn pupil). Normally, the direct reaction is stronger than the consensual reaction; therefore as the light is swung back and forth in front of each eye, that pupil constricts slightly more. A Marcus Gunn pupil paradoxically dilates in response to direct illumination, whereas the consensual reaction is maintained.

Extraocular movements should be noted in all positions of gaze. A gross evaluation of visual fields may be made with confrontation testing of each eye and an individual comparison of the patient's field with that of the examiner. A handheld indirect ophthalmoscope should be used to systematically examine the fundi, including

clarity of the lens and media as well as the disc, retinal grounds, and vessels. A mydriatic solution (such as 2.5% phenylephrine) may be needed to ensure adequate fundus visualization. A mydriatic solution should not be instilled if the patient has a history of narrow-angle glaucoma or has a shallow angle on inspection.

A slit lamp provides the observer with a magnified stereoscopic view of the minute details of the external eye and anterior segment. It is an extremely useful tool for detecting corneal and conjunctival injuries, foreign bodies, and haziness of the anterior chamber. Schiötz tonometry provides a relatively accurate measurement of the intraocular pressure. The accurate but technically more difficult applanation tonometer is available on many slit lamps. A portable electronic tonometer is also manufactured. Intraocular pressure should be measured when there is a possibility of glaucoma. Normal intraocular pressure is 10 to 20 mm Hg. Any direct pressure on the globe, including tonometry, is contraindicated when perforating wounds of the cornea or sclera are suspected.

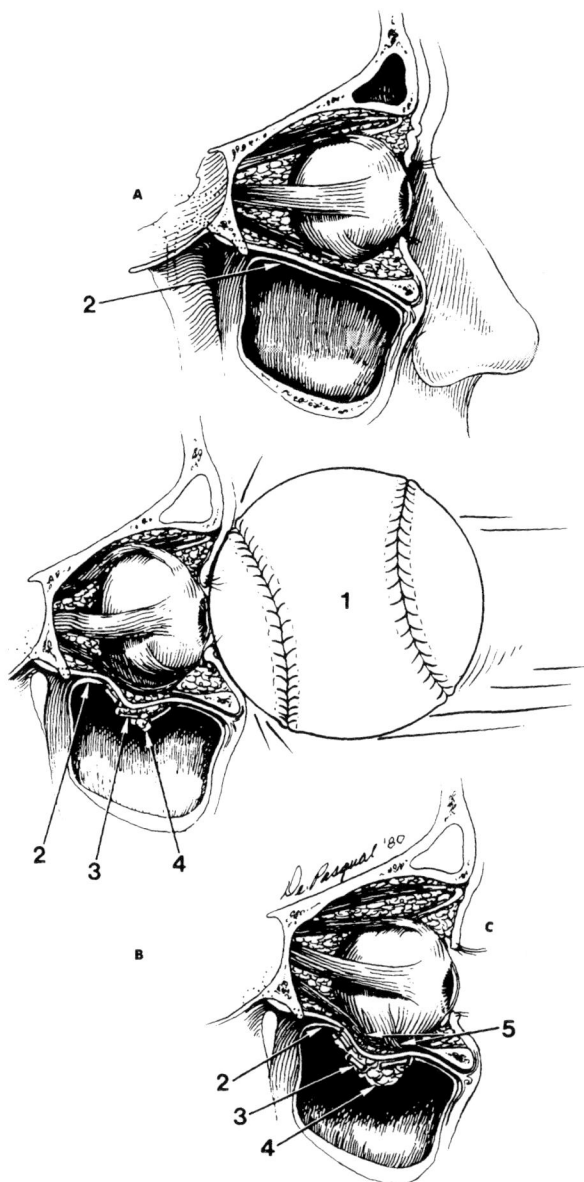

Fig. 68-2   Mechanism of injury; lateral view, sagittal section through orbit and associated structures. *1,* Force causing increased intraorbital pressure; *2,* posterior orbital floor; *3,* depressed orbital floor fragments; *4,* herniated periorbital fat; *5,* entrapment of inferior rectus and inferior oblique muscles. (From Gerlock AJ, McBride KL, Sinn DP: *Clinical and radiographic interpretation of facial fractures,* Boston, 1981, Little, Brown.)

Examination of the eye may be hindered by the presence of marked swelling of the lid or an inability of the lid to open voluntarily. Desmarres or paper clip retractors may be used to facilitate the evaluation in such circumstances.

TRAUMA

Lid Contusion

Clinical findings

Lid contusions can sometimes result in dramatic accumulations of blood and edema within the substance of the lid. If the patient is unable to open the eye voluntarily, retractors must be used to elevate the lid and assess the extent of injury. Lacerations of the cornea, a rupture of the globe, hyphema, and retinal detachment may be associated injuries.

Management

Management is conservative if no injuries beyond the lid hematoma are discovered. The intermittent application of cold packs for 24 hours after the injury helps reduce the swelling. Perform another examination when the swelling has subsided to ascertain that no injuries have been overlooked and that no late complications are present.

Orbital Blowout Fracture

Blunt forces to the globe are distributed to the entire contents of the orbit. If these forces are sufficiently powerful, the orbit fractures at its weakest point, usually the floor (Fig. 68-2, A). The inferior oblique and inferior rectus muscles may be driven downward through the fracture site along with orbital fat. Structures that herniate through the fracture site and into the maxillary antrum in this way can become entrapped.

Clinical findings

Herniation of orbital contents produces enophthalmos and slight ptosis. Entrapment of the inferior rectus and inferior oblique muscles may result in diplopia and paralysis of upward gaze (Fig. 68-2, **B**). If injury to the infraorbital nerve has occurred, anesthesia of the ipsilateral cheek and upper lip is present.

Plain orbital radiographs, including modified Waters views, are often sufficient to confirm the diagnosis of a blowout fracture. Conventional tomography, ultrasonography, and CT scans are all useful diagnostic adjuncts but are rarely necessary acutely.

Management

The initial management of blowout fractures is conservative. Because the fracture involves the paranasal sinuses, broad-spectrum antibiotic prophylaxis (e.g., amoxicillin) and decongestants are advisable. Nose blowing should be discouraged to prevent the development of orbital emphysema. A reexamination should occur in approximately 5 days, at which time a significant number of patients have a complete resolution of all symptoms and go on to a functionally and cosmetically acceptable outcome. If such a resolution does not occur, surgical intervention may be indicated.

Retrobulbar Hematoma

Blunt trauma may stretch and tear vessels of the rich orbital venous plexus and lead to a retrobulbar hematoma. An abrupt rise in intraorbital pressure may occur, which is transmitted to the globe and optic nerve.

Clinical findings

Exophthalmos as well as vision loss and afferent pupillary defects are seen. An orbital CT scan demonstrates the hematoma.

Management

Urgent ophthalmologic consultation is warranted for a retrobulbar hematoma. Surgical decompression is indicated for an acutely expanding hematoma with compromise of retinal blood flow.

Conjunctival Foreign Bodies
Clinical findings

Irritation and foreign body sensation are the most common complaints produced by conjunctival foreign bodies. The eye is red and the foreign body is usually apparent. Upper lid eversion and use of the slit lamp are recommended in the search for foreign bodies that are difficult to see.

Management

After topical 0.5% proparacaine (Ophthaine) or 1% tetracaine has been instilled, the foreign material can usually be irrigated away with sterile normal saline or swept out with a cotton-tipped applicator. Sawdust and similar material become translucent and almost invisible when wetted with tears. Occasionally, it may be necessary to gently sweep the anesthetized conjunctival surfaces of both lids with a cotton-tipped applicator to remove such material. An examination for associated corneal abrasions should follow.

Corneal Foreign Bodies
Clinical findings

The corneal epithelium is extremely sensitive, and therefore corneal foreign bodies are usually very painful. Foreign body sensation, tearing, pain, and conjunctival injection are all hallmarks of a corneal foreign body. Large foreign bodies can often be seen with the unaided eye, but smaller ones may require a slit lamp evaluation.

Management

Attempt to remove the foreign body by the most gentle means first. After instilling a topical anesthetic, irrigating the eye with sterile saline in a Luer-Lok syringe that has been fitted with a short teflon intravenous (IV) catheter may be successful. If this procedure fails, gently brush the cornea with a moistened cotton-tipped applicator to remove the particle. Lastly, attempt removal with a commercially available eye spud, or a 20-to-25 gauge sterile disposable hypodermic needle on a 1 to 3 ml syringe as a handle. This technique requires a cooperative and topically anesthetized patient and adequate magnification using a slit lamp or loupe.

After removing the foreign body, instill a topical ophthalmic antibiotic (such as 10% sulfacetamide sodium) and a cycloplegic (such as cyclopentolate), and apply a double patch. Patients who have had instrumentation of the cornea for the removal of foreign bodies should have a follow-up evaluation by an ophthalmologist within 24 hours. This follow-up should include the removal of corneal rust rings, which are the residue of a metallic corneal foreign body.

If there are multiple corneal foreign bodies involving the visual axis or if the object is deep and involves the stroma of cornea, initial removal of the object should be deferred to an ophthalmologic consultant.

Corneal Abrasion

Clinical findings

A history of injury to the eye, often with a foreign body or through the overwearing of contact lenses, is generally present in a corneal abrasion. Pain is the main feature. If the abrasion is particularly large or has been present for a long time, photophobia is also present. Visual acuity may be affected if the lesion lies within the visual axis.

A slit lamp examination with a fluorescein stain under cobalt blue illumination is the ideal method of examination, but many abrasions can be seen with a penlight or Wood ultraviolet (UV) light. Touching a moistened fluorescein strip to the lower conjunctival fornix deposits enough stain to reveal the abrasion. Damaged corneal epithelial cells stained with fluorescein fluoresce a bluish-green when viewed under cobalt blue illumination.

When foreign material is trapped on the tarsal plate beneath the upper lid, it will be dragged across the cornea with each blink or eye movement. This movement produces a characteristic pattern of fine vertical abrasions on the upper parts of the cornea.

Management

Topical anesthetic drops are useful in facilitating the examination. Any inciting foreign bodies on the tarsal plate must be removed. Patching is useful in the treatment of a corneal abrasion. The eye patch provides firm, even pressure against the closed lid, which prevents the lid margin from passing back and forth over the abraded area. A properly applied patch provides a large measure of comfort for the patient with an injured cornea. Apply the patch with the patient's eye closed firmly. Fold an oval eye pad, apply it over the closed lid, and cover it with a second unfolded pad. Apply multiple strips of tape diagonally over the pads, which produces some pressure on the patch. Instruct the patient to leave the patch in place for approximately 24 hours. Instill a broad-spectrum topical antibiotic into the eye before patching.

Photophobia and a deep, aching pain suggest a secondary iridocyclitis, and a drop of a short-acting cycloplegic such as 1% cyclopentolate (Cyclogyl) relieves most of the ciliary spasm producing these symptoms. Virtually all topical anesthetics inhibit wound healing and are toxic to the corneal epithelium. Moreover, repeated doses are increasingly less effective in producing anesthesia. Corneal lesions may result from the long-term use of topical anesthetics, and therefore these agents should never be dispensed for self-administration. The patient should be instructed not to drive while wearing the eye patch. The eye should be reevaluated in 12 to 24 hours.

Subconjunctival Hemorrhage

The rupture of a conjunctival vessel that leads to bleeding into the conjunctival space is a commonplace event and is most often the result of a blunt injury, sneezing, or coughing. It may also occur for no discernible reason. Rarely, it is associated with hypertension or a bleeding diathesis.

Clinical findings

The appearance of a subconjunctival hemorrhage is striking. The ordinarily white conjunctiva is blood red, flat, and smooth, and the blood may migrate freely over a large area. Despite its ominous appearance, this condition is usually asymptomatic unless there is an associated injury.

Management

Barring any other significant injury, the hemorrhage itself is benign, and the patient should be told that the blood will completely resorb over a period of approximately 2 weeks.

Traumatic Iritis

Blunt trauma to the globe may produce an intense inflammatory reaction of the iris and ciliary body, which in turn results in a spasm of the ciliary muscle and pupillary sphincter. The vessels of the iris and ciliary body become congested and more permeable to cells and protein, both of which leak into the anterior chamber.

Clinical findings

Inflammation and ciliary spasm produce a characteristic deep aching pain in the eye and eyebrow and is usually accompanied by photophobia. A deep ciliary flush may be seen around the limbus. A slit lamp examination using a narrow slit beam reveals "flare" in which, as a result of turbidity, the beam of light is visible as it passes through the normally clear aqueous humor.

Management

Prescribe cycloplegics to relieve the severe pain associated with photophobia and ciliary spasm. With this regimen, the majority of cases resolve within 1 week.

Hyphema

Contusing forces may rupture small vessels in the iris or ciliary body, which results in bleeding into the anterior chamber. The blood usually settles inferiorly.

Clinical findings

Visual acuity is reduced if the anterior chamber becomes clouded with blood. Most hyphemas can be detected with penlight illumination because gravity produces a layering of the red cells in a meniscus in the inferior portion of the anterior chamber (Fig. 68-3). A slit lamp examination may be necessary to detect small hyphemas. Pain is often present; in children, somnolence is also often present. The level of the meniscus should be noted carefully as a baseline to document any further bleeding.

Management

Conservative management of hyphema includes hospitalization, the placement of a protective Fox eye shield, and rest with the head of the bed elevated approximately 30 degrees. Sedation may be necessary. Aminocaproic acid is sometimes used to stabilize clot formation. Additional pharmacotherapy depends on the specific

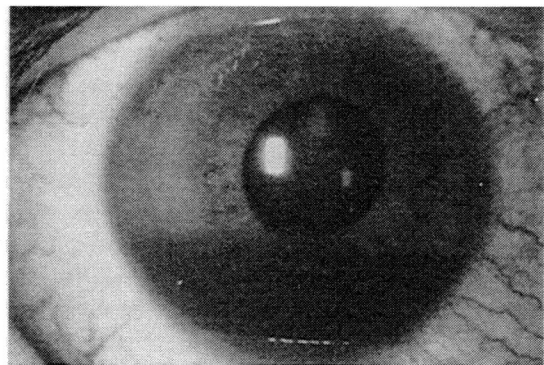

Fig. 68-3 Traumatic hyphema. (From Abrams D: *Ophthalmology in medicine: an illustrated clinical guide,* St Louis, 1990, Mosby.)

clinical situation and consulting ophthalmologist. Some ophthalmologists elect to manage smaller hyphemas on an outpatient basis.

Rebleeding is a distinct hazard. It often occurs between 3 and 5 days after the initial injury and is characteristically much more extensive than the original hemorrhage. The persistence of large amounts of blood in the anterior chamber can lead to secondary glaucoma and blood staining of the cornea.

Anterior Chamber Angle Recession

Contusing forces to the globe can drive the lens-iris diaphragm backward and result in a tearing of the trabecular meshwork and iris root. The trauma to the trabecular meshwork results in a restriction of aqueous outflow, which can cause an elevation of intraocular pressure. This elevation may occur within a few hours to a week or more after the initial injury.

Clinical findings

If elevation of the intraocular pressure is sudden or pronounced, the patient may complain of ocular pain, and corneal edema will result in reduced visual acuity and the perception of halos around lights. Lesser degrees of pressure elevation may be asymptomatic. A penlight or slit lamp examination demonstrates a deep anterior chamber compared with the uninjured eye. Tonometry should be performed in all cases in which anterior chamber recession is suspected.

Management

Acute glaucoma secondary to anterior chamber recession is managed like other acute glaucomas (see the section on acute-angle glaucoma).

Traumatic Mydriasis and Miosis

Blunt trauma to the globe may injure the pupillary sphincter and lead to mydriasis. Forces transmitted to the orbital contents may injure the ciliary ganglion, which also results in pupillary dilatation. Occasionally, however, blunt trauma produces miosis instead.

Clinical findings

Traumatic mydriasis results in a large, nonreactive pupil. The patient may be otherwise asymptomatic and have normal vision. Mydriasis may last for only a few hours or may be permanent. Traumatic miosis results in a small, nonreactive pupil; this condition usually resolves.

Management

No specific immediate treatment is indicated for traumatic mydriasis or miosis unless associated injuries are present, but refer the patient for an ophthalmologic follow-up.

Iridodialysis

Blunt injury to the globe may result in a stretching of the iris diaphragm that produces iridodialysis, a tearing of the iris at its root.

Clinical findings

Anisocoria is likely to be the first finding noted with this condition. Close inspection reveals the injured pupil to be D-shaped. The flattened portion of the D will be located at the point where the iris root has been ripped away from its attachment, and the dialysis will be seen as a blackened lentiform area (a "second pupil") at the periphery of the iris (Fig. 68-4). Large defects may cause monocular diplopia. A hyphema may be associated.

Management

All patients with iridodialysis require an ophthalmologic referral.

Traumatic Lens Subluxation and Dislocation

The lens is held in position by zonular fibers that originate from the ciliary muscle and insert

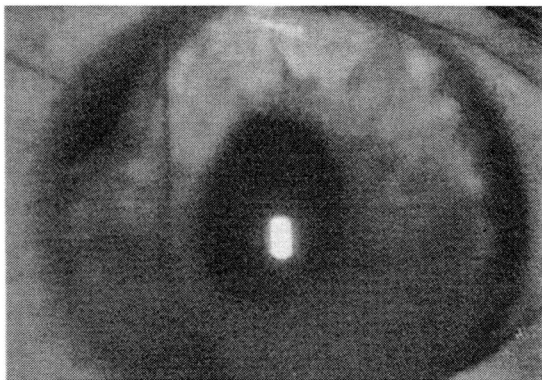

Fig. 68-4 Iridodialysis with bleeding producing hyphema. (From Ragge NK, Easty DL: *Immediate eye care: an illustrated manual,* St Louis, 1990, Mosby.)

on the equator of the lens capsule. Blunt trauma may rupture some or all of these fibers. The rupture of a significant fraction of the zonular fibers results in lens subluxation. If the fibers are completely disrupted, the lens dislocates either posteriorly into the vitreous or anteriorly into the anterior chamber.

Clinical findings

If the lens is subluxed, the patient may complain of visual distortion or monocular diplopia. Grossly blurred vision occurs if the lens has been completely dislocated. A trembling of the iris with head or eye movement (iridodonesis) should lead the observer to suspect either a subluxated or dislocated lens. If the lens has dislocated into the anterior chamber, it will be visible on close inspection and may precipitate acute glaucoma if aqueous flow through the pupil is blocked.

Management

An ophthalmologic consultation for surgical management is indicated for traumatic lens subluxation and dislocation.

Traumatic Cataract

The capsule of the lens may be disrupted by a blunt or penetrating injury. When this happens, the lens swells and clouds as a result of fluid penetration into the stroma. Irradiation or an electrical injury may also precipitate cataract formation. Cataract formation may occur acutely or may develop over months.

Clinical findings

The decrease in visual acuity is proportional to the density of the lens opacification. There is a loss of the red reflex, and the pupil appears hazy or white. Acute elevated intraocular pressure may occur if there is marked lens swelling.

Management

An ophthalmologic referral is indicated for a traumatic cataract.

Vitreous Hemorrhage

Bleeding into the vitreous body results from a vascular injury in the retinal or uveal tract. Spontaneous bleeding may occur in patients with sickle cell disease or diabetic retinopathy.

Clinical findings

Symptoms of a vitreous hemorrhage vary from "floaters" to markedly diminished visual acuity. The red reflex is decreased and the media is hazy with an inability to visualize the eye grounds with direct ophthalmoscopy.

Management

Indirect ophthalmoscopy or ultrasonography is useful in identifying a concurrent retinal injury. The head of the bed should be elevated to allow the blood to settle. Ophthalmologic consultation is warranted.

Retinal Detachment

Blunt trauma to the globe may cause a violent shifting of the vitreous body, which causes retinal tearing. A retinal detachment may occur. A spontaneous retinal detachment is seen most often in patients with diabetes or severe myopia.

Clinical findings

Retinal tears and detachments are painless, and the symptoms are visual. Vision is lost in the area of detachment, and the patient perceives a "veil" or "curtain" moving across the visual field as the retina detaches. "Floaters" may be seen as a result of bleeding, and a "flash of light" may be seen when the traction stimulates retinal neurons. If the detachment is sufficiently extensive, the red reflex is replaced by a gray reflection. Funduscopic examination may reveal the detachment as a blurred, gray elevation of the retina. Most tears occur in the retinal periphery and therefore are not visible with the direct ophthalmoscope.

Management

Management of a recent retinal detachment is usually surgical. Until an ophthalmologic consultation is obtained, vigorous physical activity should be avoided to prevent extension of the detachment.

Retinal Hemorrhage

Concussive forces can rupture the blood vessels that supply the retina. Bleeding can occur immediately in front of, beneath, or within the retina. A retinal hemorrhage may also be seen with diabetic retinopathy, blood dyscrasias, high-altitude illness, a subarachnoid hemorrhage, and the "shaken infant" syndrome.

Clinical findings

Preretinal (subhyaloid) hemorrhages are bright red with sharp borders. Hemorrhages in the superficial layers of the retina are flame shaped or striate, whereas deeper hemorrhages may have a more rounded shape and appear to be blue or gray. Vision is affected if the macula is involved.

Management

An ophthalmologist typically follows the retinal hemorrhage until it has cleared enough to permit the identification of a treatable lesion.

Rupture of the Globe

Sudden and extreme elevations of intraocular pressure as a result of blunt forces can rupture the globe. The sclera is thinnest under the insertions of the rectus muscles, and these sites are therefore common sites of rupture.

Clinical findings

Rupture of the globe often is not apparent on initial examination because the site of rupture is usually not visible. However, this condition should be suspected if a dramatic drop in visual acuity occurs following an injury, the eye is soft, the cornea is folded, the anterior chamber is distorted, or vitreous hemorrhage or bloody chemosis (hemorrhagic bulging of the bulbar conjunctiva) are present.

Management

Avoid any direct pressure on the globe and place a protective Fox metal eye shield over the eye. The patient should be kept NPO. Antiemetics are given if nausea is present to avert extrusion of intraocular contents during vomiting. Antibiotic prophylaxis is usually recommended. Although the outlook for this type of injury is generally poor, aggressive surgical management has yielded good results in select cases.

Optic Nerve Injury

The optic nerve or its blood supply may be damaged by a blunt or penetrating orbital injury or secondary to a basilar skull fracture that extends into the optic canal.

Clinical findings

Depending on the damage, visual field cuts or complete vision loss occurs with an optic nerve injury. An afferent pupillary defect is seen, and funduscopic findings are variable. An orbital CT scan is useful in delineating the injury.

Management

Although treatment for an optic nerve injury is usually expectant, an ophthalmologic referral is indicated.

Intraocular and Orbital Foreign Bodies

Intraocular and orbital foreign bodies may result from any perforating injury. Larger foreign bodies are usually obvious, but the entry site of an intraorbital foreign body may appear as a simple lid laceration. Small fragments that break off when metal is struck on metal can penetrate the lid or the globe so rapidly and painlessly that the event goes virtually unnoticed. The patient becomes aware of the injury only as an inflammatory reaction to the foreign body develops.

Clinical findings

The entire surface of the lids, conjunctiva, cornea, and iris should be systematically searched for a small entry site. The fundus should be examined for signs of a vitreous or retinal foreign body. Radiographs of the orbit may demonstrate the presence of a radiopaque foreign body, but a CT scan allows more precise localization. A magnetic resonance imaging (MRI) study or B-mode ultrasonography may reveal nonradiopaque objects.

Management

Once the presence of an intraorbital foreign body has been established, surgical removal rests with the ophthalmologist. Impaling objects such as knives or sticks should be left in place and removed only under operating room conditions.

Corneal and Scleral Lacerations

When the cornea is perforated, intraocular pressure may push aqueous out of the wound. This

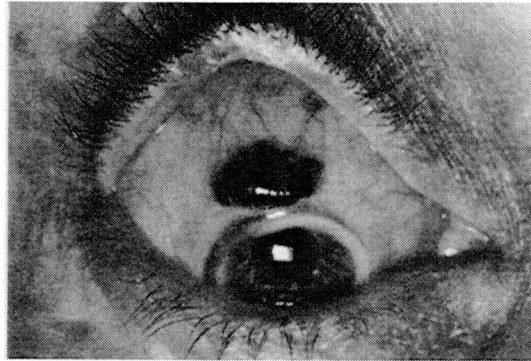

Fig. **68-5** Prolapse of iris at limbus. Note teardrop-shaped pupil. (From Abrams D: *Ophthalmology in medicine: an illustrated clinical guide,* St Louis, 1990, Mosby.)

phenomenon causes a forward surging of the lens-iris diaphragm and results in a shallow anterior chamber. Similarly, when the sclera is lacerated, vitreous may be lost, which leads to a softening of the eye and a deepening of the anterior chamber.

Clinical findings

Corneal and scleral lacerations are usually obvious, especially if a large protruding foreign body remains. Corneal lacerations may result in aqueous loss, a shallow anterior chamber, and prolapse of the iris through the wound (Fig. 68-5). Prolapse of the iris appears as a dark mass at the point of injury; the pupil becomes tear shaped, and the apex of the tear points toward the wound.

Full-thickness corneal lacerations are difficult to identify when they close spontaneously. A slit lamp examination is mandatory in all cases of suspected corneal laceration. Fluorescein stains the streaming aqueous a bright green and marks the area of an aqueous leak (Seidel test).

Scleral lacerations demonstrate the same signs and symptoms as a globe rupture. Ocular contents may protrude from a large wound, but small punctures may be self-sealing.

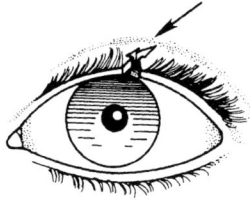

Fig. *68-6* Laceration of lid margin. Precise repair is necessary to avoid step-off or notching.

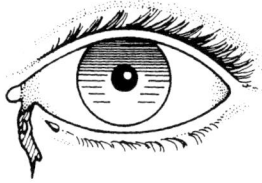

Fig. *68-7* Laceration of lacrymal canaliculus.

Management

An emergency ophthalmologic consultation and prompt surgical intervention are indicated for corneal and scleral lacerations.

Lid Lacerations

Clinical findings

Horizontal and oblique lacerations of the lids usually present no special diagnostic considerations, but the examiner must be assured that these lacerations have not violated the orbital septum or damaged the levator mechanism. The presence of concurrent perforating globe injuries or foreign bodies must be considered.

Management

Simple partial-thickness horizontal and oblique wounds are managed much like any other facial lacerations. Full-thickness lacerations that involve the lid margins (Fig. 68-6), lacerations that potentially involve the canalicular system (medial third of the lid) (Fig. 68-7), lacerations that involve the levator or canthal tendons, and punctures or lacerations that penetrate the or-

bital septum (which are heralded by a protrusion of [orbital] fat from the wound) should be referred to a plastic or ophthalmic surgeon for repair. The patient's tetanus immunization status should be addressed.

ENVIRONMENTAL AND CHEMICAL INJURIES

Ultraviolet Keratitis (Snow Blindness, Radiation Burn, Flash Burn)

The absorption of excessive amounts of UV radiation by the corneal epithelium produces edema, clouding, and desquamation. Sources of UV exposure include sun lamps, welder's arcs, and reflections from high-altitude snowy environments.

Clinical findings

With ultraviolet keratitis, there is usually a latent period of several hours between exposure and the appearance of symptoms. Even a slight swelling of the corneal epithelium is quite painful. Ocular pain and photophobia may be so severe that the patient is unable to open his or her eyes. Topical anesthetic drops may be used to facilitate the examination. Visual acuity is almost always reduced, and a slit lamp examination reveals a diffuse corneal edema that is most prominent centrally and in the inferior half of the cornea. Fluorescein staining displays a fine, stippled pattern on the corneal surface.

Management

Firm bilateral patching and potent systemic analgesics such as oxycodone are required. A short-acting cycloplegic such as cyclopentolate eases the pain caused by ciliary spasm. The problem usually resolves within 8 to 24 hours without sequelae.

Thermal Burns

Thermal burns usually affect the lids; reflexive blinking spares the globe. However, partial- and full-thickness lid burns may result in secondary globe injury as a result of exposure after tissue loss or contracture formation. Direct contact with a hot object can distort the cornea and cause visual impairment.

Clinical findings

The initial appearance of a burned cornea is opacification of the involved area. When the damaged epithelium sloughs, the underlying corneal stroma is usually clear, and the corneal epithelium rapidly regenerates to cover the defect.

Management

Superficial lid burns may be treated in essentially the same manner as a corneal abrasion, with irrigation, a topical ophthalmic antibiotic ointment, and patching. Deep partial- and full-thickness injuries should be covered with sterile plastic wrap to maintain corneal moisture pending an ophthalmic consultation.

Alkali Burns

Lye, lime, and ammonia are the most common alkaline substances that produce ocular burns. Corneal alkali burns are the most devastating of all chemical ocular injuries; these types of burns produce a liquefaction necrosis and penetrate deeply and rapidly into the cornea.

Clinical findings

Minor to moderately severe alkali burns of the eye produce a reddening of the lids and deep injection of the conjunctiva. The cornea may be partially or completely opacified, and the patient may be in severe pain. Severe alkali burns sclerose the conjunctival and scleral blood vessels, which causes secondary ischemic injury and opacification of the cornea. Perforation of the globe may occur.

Management

Immediate and thorough irrigation is mandatory, even if the patient has already irrigated the eye at the scene of the injury. Sweep the for-

nices to remove all particulate matter that may be a continuing source of alkaline contamination. Irrigate the injured eye with at least 2 L of sterile normal saline. After irrigation, the pH of the patient's tears should be tested by dipping indicator paper into the inferior conjunctival fornix. Irrigation should be repeated until the pH remains normal (7.4) for 10 minutes after irrigation has been stopped. Unless immediate irrigation is carried out, the prognosis for the severely chemically burned eye is very poor. Hospitalization is indicated for all but the most minor alkali burns.

Acid Burns

Unless highly concentrated acids are involved, acid burns are generally not as severe as alkaline burns. Acids produce a coagulation necrosis, with a denaturation of tissue proteins that limits the depth of penetration without persistant ongoing damage.

Clinical findings

Pain, photophobia, blepharospasm, conjunctival injection, and tearing are the principle symptoms and signs. A slit lamp examination usually reveals areas of denuded corneal epithelium.

Management

As with alkali burns, thorough eye irrigation is necessary. Remove particulate material to prevent further damage. Periodic pH testing with indicator paper provides some measure of the progress of irrigation. Lacrimal pH should be tested 10 minutes after a neutral reading to ensure complete acid removal. Minor injuries may be treated in the same way as a severe corneal abrasion, with topical antibiotics, cycloplegia, patching and systemic analgesics.

Other Chemical Injuries

Perfumes, organic solvents, and detergents are commonly splashed in the eye. Although they may be irritating, they are rarely destructive. Nevertheless, such injuries should initially be managed as alkali burns until a more detailed assessment can be made.

THE RED/PAINFUL EYE

Lids

Hordeolum (sty)

A typical external hordeolum involves a pustule at the lid margin (Fig. 68-8) that is usually caused by a staphylococcal infection of a lash follicle. Less commonly, an infection of a meibomian gland produces an internal hordeolum on the conjunctival surface of the tarsal plate. This type of sty is usually much more painful than an external sty. Treatment consists of the application of topical antibiotics, hot compresses, and incision and drainage.

Chalazion

A chalazion is a chronic granulomatous inflammation of a meibomian gland. A typical chalazion appears as a mass of the midportion of the upper lid (Fig. 68-9). It is differentiated from a hordeolum by the absence of acute inflamma-

tory signs. Many chalazia resolve spontaneously with conservative treatment. Large persistant lesions are treated with a surgical incision of the conjunctival surface and with curettage of the affected area.

Blepharitis

Blepharitis is a common chronic inflammation of the lid margins and may be either seborrheic, staphylococcal, or mixed in its cause. Symptoms include redness, itching, and crusting of the lid margins. Treatment includes cleaning the lid margins with baby shampoo and applying an antibiotic ointment daily.

Dacryocystitis

Dacryocystitis is an acute inflammation of the lacrimal sac and occurs secondary to nasolacrimal duct obstruction. Symptoms of this condition include tearing and tenderness, redness, and swelling below the inner canthus. Purulent drainage may be expressed from the punctum lacrimale by applying gentle pressure to the inflamed sac. Cellulitis of the overlying skin may also be present. Causative organisms include *Staphylococcus aureus*, *Streptococcus* organisms, and *Haemophilus* organisms. Treat-

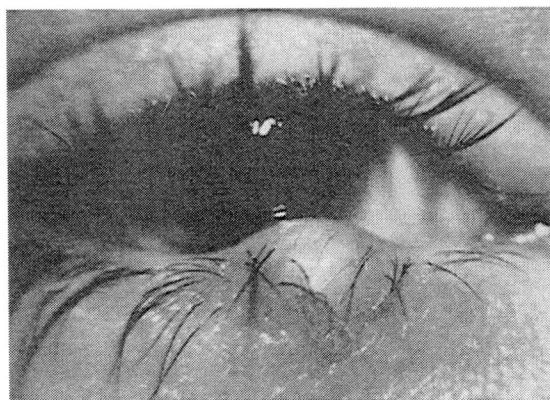

*Fig.*68-8 Acute hordeolum of lower eyelid. (From Newell FW: *Ophthalmology: principles and concepts,* ed 7, St Louis, 1992, Mosby.)

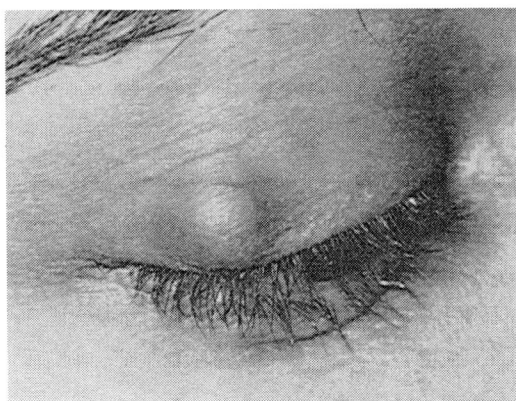

*Fig.*68-9 Chronic chalazion (lipogranuloma) of meibomian gland of upper eyelid. From Newell FW: *Ophthalmology: principles and concepts,* ed 7, St Louis, 1992, Mosby.)

ment consists of warm compresses and systemic antibiotics such as cephalexin.

Periorbital (preseptal) cellulitis

Infection of the periorbital soft tissues may occur following trauma such as a laceration or insect bite and is usually caused by staphylococci or streptococci. In young children, the infection is more often secondary to contiguous paranasal sinusitis, or hematogenous spread. In these cases, *Haemophilus influenzae* is a likely etiologic agent.

Clinical findings. The presenting signs and symptoms of periorbital cellulitis include erythema (often appearing violaceous with *H. influenzae*), edema, warmth, and perhaps tenderness of the lids and ocular adnexae. Vision and ocular motility are unaffected. Children with *H. influenzae* periorbital cellulitis may be toxic and have fever and bacteremia. Periorbital cellulitis may therefore lead to or coexist with other infected sites (lung, joints, meninges).

Management. Treatment for periorbital cellulitis consists of admission and IV antibiotics. Certain early cases may be treated with oral antibiotics and daily outpatient follow-up.

Conjunctiva

Inflammation or infection of the conjunctiva may be caused by bacteria, viruses, *Chlamydia* organisms, fungi, chemical irritants, and autoimmune or allergic disorders. Common signs and symptoms include diffuse hyperemia, discharge, and sometimes conjunctival edema (chemosis). Discomfort is usually minimal unless the cornea is involved (keratoconjunctivitis). Encouraging proper hygiene, including frequent handwashing, may prevent the spread of this condition to others.

Bacterial conjunctivitis

Acute bacterial conjunctivitis is extremely common and may be caused by a wide variety of organisms. Common causative bacteria are *S. aureus, Streptococcus pneumoniae,* and *Haemophilus* organisms. Although infrequent, *Neisseria gonorrhoeae* should be considered as a cause in sexually active individuals.

Clinical findings. The patient with bacterial conjunctivitis complains of mild ocular discomfort or a "gritty" sensation. A mucopurulent discharge with a crusting of the lashes is common. The conjunctival surface is diffusely injected, but the cornea usually remains clear. Gonococcal conjunctivitis progresses quickly to severe suppuration and may be destructive.

Management. Topical antibiotics usually clear the infection within 5 days; a drop every 2 hours during the waking hours is usually sufficient. Warm compresses clean the lash margins, increase comfort, and speed resolution. Gonococcal conjunctivitis also requires systemic antibiotics. A Gram stain of the exudate may be useful in elucidating the likely etiologic agent.

Viral conjunctivitis

A number of viruses can produce conjunctivitis, with adenoviruses being the most common. Conjunctivitis may also be produced by the herpes simplex virus.

Clinical findings. Viral conjunctivitis is characterized by a scant watery discharge and mild conjunctival irritation. The conjunctiva is injected peripherally, and the lid margins are often reddened. Conjunctival follicular hypertrophy and preauricular adenopathy may also be present.

Management. Viral conjunctivitis usually lasts for 2 to 3 weeks, and in most cases no specific treatment is warranted. Cool compresses may provide comfort. Topical antibiotics may be prescribed to prevent a secondary bacterial infection.

Inclusion conjunctivitis

Inclusion conjunctivitis caused by *Chlamydia trachomatis* usually occurs in sexually active young adults following oral-genital contact or through hand-to-eye transmission; it may have an acute or subacute onset. (A more chronic, insidious, scarring, potentially blinding form of chlamydial keratoconjunctivitis (Trachoma) is endemic in poorly developed areas of the world and is a leading cause of blindness.)

Clinical findings. In addition to redness and mucoid discharge, photophobia, pseudoptosis, preauricular adenopathy, and marked conjunctival follicular hypertrophy are common. Punctate keratitis may be seen in the superior cornea. Immunofluorescent antibody testing or Giemsa-stained smears may aid in the diagnosis.

Management. Treatment requires a 3-week course of oral tetracycline, doxycycline, or erythromycin.

Allergic conjunctivitis

Although not infectious, allergic conjunctivitis may mimic that of a viral etiology. Common inciting allergens include pollens, animal danders, drugs, or cosmetics.

Clinical findings. Itching and tearing are the prominent symptoms of allergic conjunctivitis. A stringy discharge may be present, and marked conjunctival edema may occur. Redness is usually mild. A conjunctival smear that shows eosinophilia is virtually diagnostic.

Management. Topical antihistamines and vasoconstrictors and cool compresses provide symptomatic relief for allergic conjunctivitis. Oral antihistamines may be of some value.

Cornea

Corneal ulcer

Most central corneal ulcers follow a mechanical trauma such as a contaminated corneal abrasion. The eye appears diffusely reddened, and close inspection under direct illumination reveals a corneal opacity. The ulcer crater is commonly filled with shaggy opaque debris. There is usually an associated iridocyclitis. Leukocytes and inflammatory debris often settle in the lower portion of the anterior chamber and form a meniscus (hypopyon). Many gram-positive and gram-negative bacteria have been implicated in the formation of corneal ulcers. *Pseudomonas* and *Acanthamoeba* organisms are often pathogens in corneal ulcers that are associated with soft (especially extended-wear) contact lenses. Fungal corneal ulcers are now seen more commonly since the introduction of corticosteroid drugs for use in ophthalmology. An ophthalmologic consultation and often hospitalization are indicated for the evaluation and treatment of corneal ulcers.

Herpes simplex keratitis

The patient with herpes simplex keratitis often complains of a foreign-body sensation, photophobia, pain, and tearing. The eye is diffusely reddened; a slit lamp examination usually reveals a dendritic pattern on the cornea (Fig. 68-10). The central area of the dendrite is anesthetic or hypoesthetic. Aggressive management with topical antiviral agents (e.g., idoxuridine or trifluridine) is indicated in consultation with an ophthalmologist. Most cases respond promptly to these agents.

Herpes zoster ophthalmicus

Recrudescence of the varicella-zoster virus in a partially immune person may affect the oph-

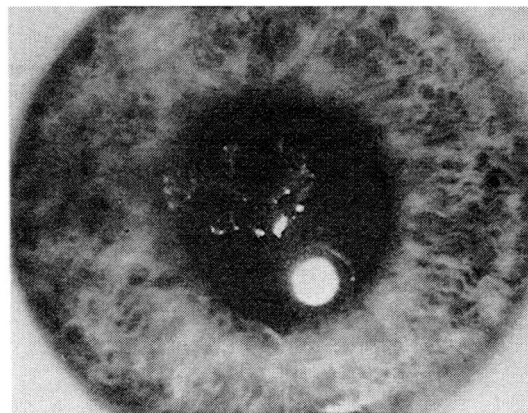

Fig. *68-10* Typical dendritic keratitis of herpes simplex. (From Arffa B: *Grayson's diseases of the cornea,* ed 3, St Louis, 1991, Mosby.

thalmic division of the trigeminal nerve with the same classic vesicular painful eruption that is seen in other dermatomes. Potential corneal involvement is heralded by the appearance of vesicles on the end of the nose because the nasociliary nerve branch supplies both areas. The uveal tract may also be involved. Ophthalmic consultation is warranted, and initial therapy involves high-dose oral acyclovir.

Globe and Orbit

Orbital cellulitis

In contrast to periorbital cellulitis, in which the infection is limited to the preseptal structures (external to the orbital septum), orbital cellulitis extends postseptally. Although the initial presentation may be similar, exophthalmos, headache, deep orbital pain, pain with extraocular muscle movement, and decreased visual acuity develop as the infection spreads to involve the deep orbital structures.

A CT scan or MRI study is useful for differentiating orbital from periorbital disease when the diagnosis is uncertain and for delineating the presence of an orbital abscess or foreign body. Potential complications of orbital cellulitis include extension into the cavernous sinus (with bilateral involvement of cranial nerves II to VI) or bony erosion into the cranial vault (brain abscess, meningitis). Admission and aggressive IV antibiotic therapy directed against *S. aureus* and *H. influenzae* are indicated. Surgical drainage of an abscess or sinus may be necessary.

Endophthalmitis

Endophthalmitis infection of the vitreous may occur following penetrating trauma, ocular surgery, or via hematogenous spread (immunocompromised patients, IV drug abuse). Symptoms include ocular pain and decreased vision. On funduscopic examination, the media are hazy. Intravenous as well an intravitreal antibiotics are given. A vitrectomy may be required, and the prognosis is often poor.

Miscellaneous Inflammatory Conditions

Episcleritis and scleritis

Episcleritis is a localized inflammation of the elastic membrane overlying the sclera and beneath the conjunctiva. It involves a localized area and presents with mild pain, tenderness, tearing and photophobia. Vision is unaffected. Most cases of this condition are idiopathic and self-limited. Treatment includes oral nonsteroidal antiinflammatory agents and, occasionally, topical steroids.

Scleritis is a deeper and destructive inflammation of the sclera itself. It may be diffuse or nodular and is often bilateral. Scleritis is usually associated with systemic illness such as autoimmune diseases, granulomatous diseases, or infections. Pain is severe, deep, and boring. Tearing and photophobia are common. Examination reveals engorged scleral vessels and a bluish hue. Posterior involvement may cause exophthalmos and vision loss. Treatment includes topical or systemic steroids and analgesics. Ophthalmologic consultation is warranted.

Uveal tract inflammation

Any portion of the middle coat of the eye (iris, ciliary body, or choroid) may be involved in an inflammatory process. Varying terminology is used and depends on the segment involved (e.g., anterior vs. posterior uveitis, iritis, iridocyclitis, chorioretinitis). Causes of uveal tract inflammation include infectious processes, autoimmune disorders, and trauma. Patients with anterior segment involvement have pain, injection, and photophobia. An examination reveals the presence of cells and flare in the anterior chamber and marked perilimbal injection. The initial treatment is cycloplegia pending an ophthalmic consultation. Patients with isolated posterior tract inflammation are more likely to have vision loss without redness. Chorioretinitis is common in patients with acquired immunodeficiency syndrome (AIDS), and the etiologic agents include cytomegalovirus, *Toxoplasma gondii*, *Mycobacterium avium-intracellulare*, and *Cryptococcus* organisms.

ACUTE ANGLE-CLOSURE GLAUCOMA

Primary acute angle-closure glaucoma occurs in eyes that have an abnormally shallow anterior chamber angle. Attacks of acute angle-closure glaucoma usually occur under conditions in which the pupil dilates and partially or completely occludes the chamber angle, which prevents the exit of aqueous humor. The ciliary body continues to produce aqueous humor, and the intraocular pressure rises. The elevated pressure causes corneal edema, and a prolonged pressure above 35 mm Hg paralyzes the pupillary sphincter. An attack of acute angle-closure glaucoma often typically begins in a darkened environment. Anticholinergic or sympathomimetic drugs may also cause this condition.

Secondary glaucoma may occur following any ocular condition in which the normal flow of aqueous humor is disrupted. (Although more common, primary open-angle glaucoma does not have emergent symptoms. The insidious loss of peripheral vision occurs as the only symptom. Abnormal enlargement of the optic cup is the only sign of this condition and is often an incidental finding.)

Clinical Findings

The patient with acute angle-closure glaucoma complains of severe eye pain, headache, blurred vision, seeing rainbow halos around lights, nausea, vomiting, and (occasionally) abdominal pain. The patient appears quite ill. The eye is deeply injected, the cornea is hazy, and the pupil is middilated and nonreactive to light. Visual acuity is dramatically reduced, and intraocular pressure is markedly elevated and is often higher than 50 mm Hg.

Management

The goals of management are to lower intraocular pressure in the affected eye and to prevent an attack of acute angle-closure glaucoma in the other eye. All aspects of therapy should be initiated promptly because optic nerve function may be lost rapidly at extremely high intraocular pressures.

A constriction of the pupil flattens the iris leaf and pulls the peripheral iris back from its anterior position, which reopens the angle and allows aqueous to escape in a normal fashion. Pilocarpine 2% should be administered, 1 drop every 15 to 30 minutes until the pupil constricts followed by 1 drop every 6 hours. The carbonic anhydrase inhibitor acetazolamide (Diamox) administered intravenously as an initial dose of 500 mg and followed by 250 mg orally every 4 hours reduces the production of aqueous by the ciliary body. Orally administered 50% glycerol given in a dose of 1 to 1.5 g/kg of body weight or oral isosorbide 50 to 100 g reduces the ocular volume and decreases the intraocular pressure; mannitol given in a dose of 0.5 to 2 g/kg IV over 30 to 60 minutes or until intraocular pressure falls accomplishes the same effect. Topical timolol drops (0.5%) in one dose and topical steroid (e.g., prednisolone acetate) 1% every 15 to 30 minutes × 4 doses (then hourly) are also used.

Following emergency treatment, laser or surgical iridotomy may be used to produce an aperture at the periphery of the iris that permits the free flow of aqueous humor from the posterior to the anterior chamber. This procedure will definitively prevent future attacks of acute angle-closure glaucoma.

ACUTE VISION LOSS

Central Retinal Artery Occlusion

A significant number of patients with central retinal artery occlusion have underlying atherosclerotic cardiovascular disease, hypertension, sickle cell disease, or diabetes mellitus. The immediate precipitating cause is usually from an embolus that originates from a carotid artery atherosclerotic plaque or from the cardiac valves. Occlusion may involve the central retinal artery or branch arteries. Branch artery occlusion produces sector defects in retinal arterial circulation. The result is ischemic retinal infarction and an abrupt loss of visual function in the affected areas.

Clinical findings

Occlusion of the central retinal artery results in a sudden, painless loss of vision in the affected eye. The pupil is dilated and nonreactive to direct light stimulation. Within a few minutes of occlusion, the retina begins to assume a milky appearance, with a pale disc and a residual cherry red spot in the macular area, where the intact choroidal vessels are visible and show through the thinner retinal layer at the fovea. There is emptying or attenuation of the retinal arterioles.

Management

Immediate attempts to dislodge the embolus involve globe massage, in which moderate digital pressure is applied and removed at 5-second intervals. Inhalation of carbogen, a mixture of 95% oxygen and 5% carbon dioxide, dilates the retinal arterioles and may induce the embolus to move peripherally. Paper bag rebreathing may be tried if carbogen is unavailable. Anterior chamber paracentesis rapidly drops intraocular pressure and may produce the same effect. Anticoagulants, thrombolytic agents, and low-molecular-weight dextran have also been tried as therapy for this condition, with reports of varying success. Immediate treatment is extremely important. The neuroretina tolerates anoxia poorly, and the prognosis for the return of vision is poor in most cases.

Central Retinal Vein Occlusion

Underlying causes of central retinal vein occlusion include atherosclerosis, diabetes, and hyperviscosity states.

Clinical findings

With this condition, painless loss of vision progresses over minutes to hours in the affected eye. Examination confirms a marked diminution of acuity, but it is often not as severe as that seen with central retinal artery occlusion. The pupil reacts sluggishly. On funduscopic examination, the retinal veins are engorged and tortuous, and there is a loss of venous pulsations. There is extensive retinal edema, and retinal hemorrhages are present diffusely throughout the fundus.

Management

The emergency department treatment of central retinal vein or branch vein occlusion is essentially the same as that for central retinal artery occlusion. Thrombolytics and anticoagulants are not indicated because of the retinal hemorrhage associated with this condition. Nevertheless, the prognosis for the return of vision is better than for arterial occlusion.

Temporal Arteritis

Temporal (giant cell) arteritis is an inflammatory process that is most common in patients over the age of 60 years. The superficial temporal, internal carotid, vertebral, and ophthalmic arteries are most commonly affected. Involvement of the central retinal artery by temporal arteritis can lead to arterial occlusion.

Clinical findings

Vision loss occurs in one third of the patients with temporal arteritis. The principal symptom is a sudden, painless, monocular loss of vision. There is usually a preceding history of unilateral temporal headache, malaise, and lethargy. Palpation of the temporal area may disclose a tender, tortuous temporal artery. Changes of retinal artery occlusion may be present on funduscopic examination. The erythrocyte sedimentation rate is markedly elevated (>70 mm/hour).

Management

Treatment includes corticosteroids—an initial dose of 100 mg/day of prednisone or an equivalent in any patient with a sudden vision loss resulting from temporal arteritis.

Optic Neuritis

Optic neuritis is an inflammation or demyelination of the optic nerve and may be intraocular (papillitis) or behind the eye (retrobulbar optic neuritis). Both conditions cause an acute onset of blurred vision that is sometimes associated with pain in the orbit or with eye movement. Examination reveals a relative afferent pupillary defect. On funduscopic examination, papillitis resembles papilledema, except that it is unilateral. With retrobulbar neuritis, the fundus appears normal despite severe decreased visual acuity (i.e., "The patient sees nothing and the doctor sees nothing"). Approximately one half of the cases are a result of multiple sclerosis, but any inflammatory condition that involves the central nervous system may be associated. The most common toxin that causes optic neuritis is methanol. Treatment depends on the underlying cause.

KEY CONSIDERATIONS

WHAT IS THE LIFE THREAT?

Trauma to the eye may be associated with concomitant trauma to the brain and surrounding structures. Injuries such as an epidural or subdural hematoma or other intracranial bleeding could be life threatening in such circumstances. Papilledema is a clinical sign of increasing intracranial pressure in unconscious patients. In children, *H. influenzae* presepital cellulitis may result in systemic bacteremia and severe illness.

DOES THE PATIENT NEED ADMISSION?

Admit patients with retrobulbar hematoma for surgical decompression. Obtain an ophthalmologic consultation for a traumatic injury to the lens or its attachments and for a rupture or laceration of the globe. Admit patients with severe periorbital and orbital cellulitis.

WHAT IS THE MOST SERIOUS DIAGNOSIS?

Conditions potentially resulting in a loss of sight include rupture of the globe, retrobulbar hematoma, vitreous hemorrhage, retinal arterial occlusion, central retinal vein occlusion, necrotizing scleritis, endophthalmitis, severe alkali burn, corneal ulcer, and untreated glaucoma. Temporal arteritis may also result in a loss of vision. A blowout fracture of the orbit may heal without sequelae or may involve entrapment of the inferior rectus or inferior oblique muscles, which can result in diplopia.

HAVE I PERFORMED A THOROUGH WORK-UP?

Evert the upper lid for inspection, and examine the eye with a slit lamp and a penlight for a suspected foreign body, corneal abrasion, or chemical burn. Thoroughly irrigate any eye that has been exposed to irritating chemicals. Serious alkali burns require at least 2 L irrigation, and irrigation continues until the pH remains less than 7.4 for at least 10 minutes after the irrigation is stopped.

Measure intraocular pressure in a patient who has severe eye pain, nausea, vomiting, headache, and blurred vision; such a patient may be experiencing acute angle-closure glaucoma. The cornea is typically "steamy" or hazy in such patients, and the pupil is typically nonreactive to light.

Recommended Reading

Catalano RA: *Ocular emergencies,* Philadelphia, 1992, WB Saunders.

Cinotti AA: *Handbook of ophthalmic emergencies,* ed 3, New York, 1985, Elsevier Science Publishing.

Cullom RD, Chang B: *The Wills eye manual: office and emergency room diagnosis and treatment of eye disease,* ed 2, Philadelphia, 1994, JB Lippincott.

Ghezzi K, Renner GS: Ophthalmologic disorders. In Rosen P et al, editors: *Emergency medicine: concepts and clinical practice,* ed 3, St Louis, 1992, Mosby.

Joondeph BC: Blunt ocular trauma, *Emerg Med Clin North Am* 6(1):147-167, 1988.

Lubeck D: Penetrating ocular injuries, *Emerg Med Clin North Am* 6(1):127-146, 1988.

Scott JL, Ghezzi KT: Emergency treatment of the eye, *Emerg Med Clin North Am* 13(3):521-700, 1995.

Vaughan DG, Asbury T, Riordan-Eva P: *General ophthalmology,* ed 14, East Norwalk, Conn, 1995, Appleton & Lange.

INDEX

A

AAA; see Abdominal aortic aneurysm
Abdominal aortic aneurysm, spinal pain
　　and, 315
Abdominal pain, 131-141
　　assessment of, 134-136
　　consultation in, 139
　　differential diagnosis of, 138, 139
　　disposition of patient with, 140
　　imaging of, 137-139
　　initial management of, 133-134
　　laboratory analysis of, 136-137
　　mesenteric vascular occlusion and, 484
　　neuroanatomy and perception of,
　　　131-133
　　referred, 132-133
　　somatic, 132
　　visceral, 131-132
Abdominal thrust for choking, 35-36
Abdominal trauma, 272-278
　　operative versus nonoperative
　　　management in, 274-275
Abduction test, 635
Abortion, 549-550
Abrasion, corneal, 831
Abruptio placentae, 552
Abscess
　　appendiceal or diverticular, radiography
　　　in, 161
　　Bartholin, 180-181
　　hepatic, 498-499, 738, 739
　　intracerebral, 97, 102
　　　amebiasis in, 742
　　　meningitis and encephalitis and, 620
　　　stroke versus, 603
　　orbital, 842
　　pancreatic, 504-505
　　perianal, 488-489
　　peritonsillar, 364
　　retropharyngeal, 364

Absence seizure, 204-205
Abuse
　　child, 819-820
　　sexual
　　　of child, 819-820
　　　pelvic pain and, 177
　　　straddle injury and, 279
　　substance, alcohol in; see Alcohol abuse
Acanthamoeba
　　in corneal infection, 841
　　in liver disease, 742
Access, vascular; see Vascular access
Accessory muscles of respiration, 106
　　assessment of, 115
Accidental hypothermia, 354
ACE inhibitors; see Angiotensin-converting
　　enzyme inhibitors
Acellular pertussis vaccine formulated with
　　diphtheria and tetanus toxoids, 703
Acetabular fracture, 316-317
Acetaminophen
　　with caffeine, 101
　　in fever, 78
　　　in child, 813, 815
　　　and seizures, 209
　　for headache, 101
　　hepatitis from, 723
　　in hyperthyroidism supportive therapy,
　　　694
　　liver toxicity of, 495, 497
　　in meningitis and encephalitis, 621
　　in otitis media, 822
　　in pancreatitis etiology, 503
　　in pharyngitis, 363
　　toxicity of, 771-772
Acetazolamide
　　in acute angle-closure glaucoma, 843
　　in hypokalemia, 676
　　in pseudotumor cerebri, 642
　　seizure and, 212-213

Acetic acid
　　in condyloma acuminatum, 184
　　in otitis externa, 823
Acetylcholine
　　botulism toxin and, 706
　　organophosphate toxicity and, 765, 783
Acetylcholinesterase inhibitors in
　　neuromuscular blockade, 214
N-Acetyl-L-cysteine in acetaminophen
　　overdose, 771
Acetylureas, 212-213
Achalasia, 475
Acid
　　burn from, 339
　　　eye, 840
　　uric, 190
Acid-base abnormality in comatose patient,
　　84-85
Acidosis
　　in comatose patient, 84-85
　　in hyperglycemic hyperosmolar
　　　nonketotic coma, 691
　　hyperkalemia and, 672
　　in ketoacidosis, 690-691
　　lactic
　　　diabetes and, 691
　　　drug poisoning and, 766
　　　vomiting and, 161
　　metabolic
　　　acute renal failure and, 531
　　　drug poisoning and, 765-766
　　　smoke inhalation burn and, 340
　　　vomiting and, 160
　　respiratory distress and, 106, 107
ACLS; see Advanced cardiac life support
Acoustic nerve, 609
Acoustic neuroma, 614
　　vertigo in, 823
Acquired immunodeficiency syndrome,
　　726-732

Acquired immunodeficiency syndrome—
    cont'd
  pneumonia in, 112
Acrocyanosis, 413, 418
Acrodermatitis chronica atrophicans, 753
Acromioclavicular separation, 313-314
ACTH
  adrenal failure and, 695, 696
  hypertension and, 433
Activated charcoal in poisoning, 767
  from methylxanthines, 786
Activated partial thromboplastin time,
    405-406
Acuity, visual, 237; see also Eye
Acute myocardial infarction; see Myocardial
    infarction
Acute psychosis; see Psychosis
Acyclovir
  in herpes simplex, 595, 717, 723
    genital, 180, 596
    in neuralgia, 633
  in herpes zoster
    of eye, 841
    in neuralgia, 633
    in varicella, 595, 597, 718, 722
  in meningitis and encephalitis, 624
  in postherpetic neuralgia, 633
Adaptic
  for burns, 337
  in wound care, 291
Addiction, cocaine and, 777
Addisonian crisis, 696
Adenoma sebaceum, 207
Adenosine
  in paroxysmal supraventricular
    tachycardia, 459-460
  in preexcitation syndromes, 467
Adenosine monophosphate, cyclic, 774
Adenosine triphosphatase inhibitors, 476
Adenosine triphosphate in shock, 50
Adenovirus, 716
  in otitis media, 822
  in pharyngitis, 361, 382
ADH; see Antidiuretic hormone
Adhesions, pelvic pain and, 174, 175
Adjunct physicians for trauma team, 61
Admission to hospital, 9
Adnexal torsion, 174-175
Adolescent, mononucleosis in, 722
Adrenal insufficiency, 695-696
Adrenergic agents
  in aortic trauma, 270
  in asthma, 801-802
  bradycardias from, 465
  in bronchitis, 366
  in cardiogenic shock, 56
  in chronic obstructive pulmonary disease,
    387
  classification of, 56
  in congestive heart failure, 446
  contraindicated
    in preexcitation syndromes, 467

Adrenergic agents—cont'd
  contraindicated—cont'd
    with verapamil, 460
  hyperkalemia and, 672
  in hyperthyroidism, 693, 694
  in ischemic heart disease, 430
  in syncope, 89
  in tetanus, 704
  in toxicology, 764, 768
Adult epiglottitis, 365; see also Epiglottitis
Adult respiratory distress syndrome, 109;
    see also Respiratory distress
Advanced cardiac life support, 36-40
Aerobid; see Flunisolide
Affect, suicidal behavior and, 657
Afferent fibers, visceral
  in abdominal pain, 132
  in vomiting, 153
African sleeping sickness, 742
Afrin; see Oxymetazoline spray
Afterload, optimizing, 450-451
Age
  of child, weight estimation and, 47
  venous thrombosis in, 400
Aged patient; see Elderly
Agitation in drug poisoning, 768-769
Agonal respirations, 82
Aides for trauma team, 61
AIDS; see Acquired immunodeficiency
    syndrome
Air in wound in pneumothorax, 259
Air cells, mastoid, 823
Air-fluid level in diaphragm injury, 260
Airway inflammation in asthma, 379
Airway management, 16-28
  assessment in, 19-21
  basic life support and, 30, 31, 32
  in burn, 334
  in child, 26-27
  in coma, 81-82
  cricothyrotomy and, 62
    in child, 66
  decision making in, 16-19
  in epiglottitis and croup, 799
  essential questions in, 17
  in facial trauma, 231
  foreign body and, 392, 800
  in gastrointestinal bleeding, 147
  in head injury, 223-224
  immediate, 21-26
  indications for, 16-19
    mandatory, 18
  in multiple trauma, 62
    in child, 66
  in oral injury, 239
  pediatric, 26-28, 45
    neonatal resuscitation and, 42, 820-821
  in peritonsillar abscess, 364
  in pulmonary burn, 340
  in smoke inhalation, 340
  in spinal injury, 245
  tracheostomy in, in child, 66

Airway management—cont'd
  in vomiting, 156, 161-162
Airway obstruction
  in diphtheria, 699
  hypoxemia and, 29
  in oral injury, 239
  respiratory distress versus, 107
Airway secretions in noisy breathing, 19
Akinetic seizures, 203, 204
Albendazole
  in amebiasis, 737
  in ascariasis, 737
  in enterobiasis, 738
  in hookworm infestations, 738, 741
  in hydatid cysts, 743
  in neurocysticercosis, 743
  in trichuriasis, 738
Albumin in hypovolemic shock, 53
Albuterol
  in asthma, 381, 382
    in child, 801
  in bronchiolitis, 801
  in hyperkalemia, 531, 537, 674
Alcohol
  abuse of; see Alcohol abuse
  in cluster headache, 99
  in sympatholytic syndrome, 765
  toxicity of, 772-773
  in vertigo, 610
Alcohol abuse
  coma in, 83
  esophageal varices in, 143
  gastric bleeding in, 144, 147
  hepatic disease in, 495-498
  hypocalcemia in, 680, 681
  hypomagnesemia in, 684-685
  hyponatremia in, 671
  immunosuppression in, 75
  pancreatitis in, 502
  peripheral neuropathies in, 629
  spinal injury in, 243
  suicidal behavior in, 656, 657
  toxicity and, 763, 772-773
  withdrawal seizures in, 204
    treatment of, 209
Aldactone; see Spironolactone
Aldosterone antagonists, hyperkalemia and,
    673
Alkali
  burn from, 339
    eye, 838
  ingestion of, 775-776
Alkalosis in septic shock, 57
Alkylating agents in polycythemia, 560
Allen test for arterial disease, 414
Allergy
  anesthetics and, 285-288
  in atopic dermatitis, 585
  in conjunctivitis, 841
  in contact dermatitis, 592-593
  in urticaria, 589
Allopurinol, 383

Aloe vera cream in frostbite, 357
Alpha-adrenergic agents; *see also*
    Adrenergic agents
    in tetanus, 704
    in toxicology, 764, 768
Alpha$_1$-antitrypsin deficiency disease, 110
Alpha-fetoprotein in hepatocellular cancer,
    500
Altered mental status, 80-86; *see also*
    Mental status
Alveolar bone fracture, 241
Alveolar-arterial oxygen gradient, 116
    in pulmonary embolism, 127
Amantadine
    in influenza, 718
    in Parkinson syndrome, 645
Ambulance team, 60-61
Amebiasis, 736-739
    in cerebral abscess, 742
    in meningitis and encephalitis, 618
Amebic cysts, 739
American Psychiatric Association Diagnostic
    and Statistical Manual of Mental
    Disorders, 647, 653
AMI; *see* Myocardial infarction, acute
Amicar; *see* Aminocaproic acid
Amides, wound closure and, 285
Amiloride
    congestive heart failure and, 449
    in hyperkalemia, 673
Aminocaproic acid
    after thrombolysis in pulmonary
        embolism or deep venous
        thrombosis, 408
    in coagulation disorders, 568
    in hyphema, 832
Aminoglycosides
    in abdominal pain, 134
    acute renal failure from, 530
    hearing loss from, 823
    in hepatic abscess, 499
    in tumor infection emergencies, 573
    in vascular access infection, 540
    in vertigo, 610, 613
Aminophylline
    in asthma, 382-383
    in chronic obstructive pulmonary disease,
        387
    in hypokalemia, 676
Amiodarone, liver toxicity of, 497
Amitriptyline
    in postherpetic neuralgia, 633
    toxicity of, 777
Amniotic membrane rupture, 554
Amoxapine, toxicity of, 777
Amoxicillin
    in bronchitis, 366, 388
    in chlamydial cervicitis, 181
    with clavulinic acid
        in bronchitis, 388
        in otitis media, 822
        in urinary tract infection in child, 513

Amoxicillin—cont'd
    in fever, 77
    in Lyme disease, 194, 753
    in orbital blowout fracture, 830
    in otitis media, 822
    in pneumonia in child, 803
    resistance to, 168
    in urinary tract infection, 510, 511, 513
Amphetamines
    in drug poisoning, 768
    in toxic syndromes, 764
Amphotericin B
    in AIDS and HIV, 730
    in hypokalemia, 676
    in hypomagnesemia, 685
    in leishmaniasis, 745
    liver toxicity of, 497
    in meningitis and encephalitis, 624
Ampicillin
    in abdominal pain, 134
    in appendicitis in child, 818
    in diarrhea, 172
    in fever in child, 814
    in hepatic abscess, 499
    in meningitis and encephalitis, 624, 625
        in child, 809
    in pneumonia in child, 803
    resistance to, 168
    in urinary tract infection, 510, 511, 514
        in child, 513
    pregnancy and, 512
Amputation
    after frostbite, 357
    of digits, 291-292
Amrinone
    in cardiogenic shock, 56
    in heart failure, 451, 452
    in pulmonary edema, 452, 453
Amylase
    lavage, in abdominal trauma, 274
    serum
        in abdominal pain, 137
        in abdominal trauma, 273
        in pancreatitis, 502
Amyotrophic lateral sclerosis, 643
Anabolic steroids, liver toxicity of, 497
Anaerobic organisms, 370, 374
Anal bleeding, 145
Anal fissure, 488
    rectal bleeding and, 145
Analgesics
    in abdominal pain, 134
    in burns, 336
    in cardiogenic shock, 56
    in cholelithiasis, 500
    in headache, 100
    in rib fracture, 255
    in trigeminal neuralgia, 104
Ancillary procedures in shock, 56-57
Ancylostoma braziliense, 745
Ancylostoma duodenale, 738, 741
    in pulmonary disorders, 743

Anectine; *see* Succinylcholine
Anemias, 556-558
    causes of, 557
    gastrointestinal bleeding and, 147
    headache and, 101
    hemolytic, 559-560
    history and physical examination in, 558
    iron deficiency, 558
    microcytic, 558
    sickle cell, 557, 559-560
Anesthesia, psychogenic, 635-636
Anesthetics
    in intubation, 22, 23, 24
    local
        in epistaxis, 824
        in facial laceration suturing, 236
        in nasal fracture, 825
        in wound closure, 285-288
        in wrist injury, 304
    in oral injury, 239
    topical
        in conjunctival foreign body removal,
            830
        in corneal abrasion, 831
        in corneal foreign body removal, 831
        in eye examination, 828
        in tendinitis, 192
Aneurysm
    aortic
        dissecting, 442-443
        spinal pain and, 315
    false
        fistula with, 420
        physical examination in, 414
    headache and, 102
    peripheral vascular, 416-417
        physical examination in, 414
Anger, 11-12
Angina
    duration of, 123
    hypertension and, 440-441
    ischemia in, 421
    Ludwig's, 365
    respiratory distress in, 113
    stable, 427-428
    unstable, 428
        diagnostic tests for, 126, 127
Angiodysplasia, 144
Angiography
    aortic transection and, 257
    in arterial disease, 415
    in gastrointestinal bleeding, 149, 150
    in ischemic heart disease, 431
    in pulmonary embolism, 128, 401, 405
    in vertigo, 612
Angiotensin-converting enzyme inhibitors,
    450-451
Angle-closure glaucoma, 843
Angulation in finger fracture, 303
Anhidrotic heat exhaustion, 349
Animal bite, rabies and, 724
Anion gap in drug poisoning, 765

Anisocoria
  iridodialysis and, 833
  subacute subdural hematoma and, 228
Ankle
  injury to, 323-329
  splinting of, 299
Ankylosing spondylitis, 578
Anopheles mosquito, 733
Anorectal disease, 488-489
Anoscopy, 147
Anovulatory menstrual cycle, 179
Anoxia, headache and, 96, 100-101
Antacids
  in gastrointestinal bleeding, 148
  in metabolic complications of renal
    failure, 531
  in peptic ulcer, 476
Antagonist, opiate, 83
Anterior chamber angle recession, 833
Anterior cord syndrome, 249, 250
Anterior cruciate ligament tear, 320-322
Antibiotics
  in abdominal pain, 134
  acute renal failure from, 530
  in AIDS and HIV, 728-729, 730
  in appendicitis in child, 818
  in bronchitis, 366
  in burn patient, 337-338
  in cellulitis, 585
  in child, 77
  in cholangitis, 501
  in chronic obstructive pulmonary disease,
    388
  in conjunctival infection, 840
  in corneal abrasion, 831
  in corneal foreign body, 831
  in corneal infection, 841
  in cystitis, 510
  in deep respiratory tract infection, 364,
    365
  in diarrhea, 168, 170, 172
  in diphtheria, 700
  in endophthalmitis, 842
  in epiglottitis, 799
  in fever, 77, 78
    in child, 813-816
  in foreign body aspiration, 393
  hearing loss from, 823
  in hydrocarbon poisoning, 780
  in impetigo, 599
  in inclusion conjunctivitis, 840-841
  in Lyme disease, 194, 750, 753-754
  in meningitis and encephalitis, 624, 625,
    809
  in meningococcemia, 711
  in near-drowning, 347
  in orbital blowout fracture, 830
  in otitis externa, 823
  in parotitis, 825
  in pelvic inflammatory disease, 184
  in pharyngitis, 363, 364
  in pneumococcemia, 709

Antibiotics—cont'd
  in pneumonia, 375
    in child, 803
  prophylactic, 288-289
  in pyelonephritis, 510-511
  in rheumatic fever, 195
  in Rocky Mountain spotted fever, 590
  in scarlet fever, 591-592
  in septic arthritis, 192
  sexual abuse of child and, 820
  in sinusitis, 365
  theophylline clearance and, 383
  topical
    in eye burns, 838
    in wound care, 288
  in toxic shock syndrome, 714
  tumor emergencies and, 572-573
  in urinary tract infection, 510-511, 512,
    514
    in child, 513
  in vertigo, 610
Anticholinergics
  in asthma, 381
  in cholelithiasis, 500
  in chronic obstructive pulmonary disease,
    387
  in Parkinson syndrome, 645
  toxicity of, 765, 773-774
  in vertigo, 615
  in vomiting, 162-164
Anticoagulants
  in central retinal artery occlusion, 846
  coagulation disorders and, 564
  in deep venous thrombosis, 396, 405-407
  in interstitial renal disease, 528
  in pulmonary embolism, 405-407
  in stroke, 604, 605
Anticonvulsants, 202-203, 208-210
  brain injury and, 225
  in febrile seizures, 812
  hypocalcemia and, 681
  loading dose of, 209
  in status epilepticus, 211-214
    in child, 810-812
Antidepressants
  in migraine, 100
  in postherpetic neuralgia, 633
  in syncope, 89
  toxicity of, 774, 777-778
    dysrhythmias from, 768
Antidiarrheal agents, 168, 170, 172
Antidiuretic hormone
  in cerebral edema, 625
  fluid balance and, 666-667
  hypernatremia and, 668
  hyponatremia and, 670
  syndrome of inappropriate, 666-667
Antidysrhythmics
  in ischemic heart disease, 430
  in syncope, 89
Antiemetics, 162-164
  in abdominal pain, 134

Antiemetics—cont'd
  in hyperemesis gravidarum, 551
  in methylxanthine toxicity, 786
  in vomiting, 473
Antifungal agents, 584
Antigen, hepatitis, 492
Anti-HB$_S$s, 723
Antihistamines
  in atopic dermatitis, 588
  in conjunctivitis, 841
  in drug eruptions, 588
  in herpes simplex, 595
  toxicity of, 765, 774
  in urticaria, 588
  in varicella, 595
  in vertigo, 615
  in vomiting, 162-164
Antihypertensives, 438-439
  in hypertensive encephalopathy, 436-437
  in intrarenal vascular disease, 529
Antiinflammatory agents
  in ankle sprains, 324
  for headache, 100, 101
  nonsteroidal; *see* Nonsteroidal anti-
    inflammatory agents
  in sacral fracture, 316
  for spinal pain, 315
Antinuclear antibodies
  in giant cell arteritis, 580
  in polymyalgia rheumatica, 578
  in systemic lupus erythematosus, 581
Antipruritics in urticaria, 588
Antipyretic therapy
  aspirin versus acetaminophen in, 78
  in child, 813
Antithrombin III
  deep venous thrombosis and, 396
  in proteinuria, 525
Antitoxins, diphtheria and, 700
Antivert; *see* Meclizine
Antiviral agents
  acyclovir as; *see* Acyclovir
  in AIDS and HIV, 730
  in herpes simplex keratitis, 841
  in herpes zoster ophthalmicus, 842
Anuria, hyperkalemia and, 673
Aortic aneurysm, spinal pain and, 315
Aortic arch, blunt injuries to major arterial
    branches of, 270
Aortic counterpulsation balloon, 41
Aortic dissection
  diagnostic tests for, 126, 128
  hypertension and, 442-443
  physical findings in, 125
  risk factors in, 123-124
Aortic rupture, 268-270
Aortic stenosis, 88, 91
Aortic transection, 257-258
Aortic trauma, 268-271
Aortography
  in aortic dissection, 128, 443
  in aortic trauma, 269

Aortoiliac occlusive disease, 412
Apathetic hyperthyroidism, 692
Aphasia in stroke, 603
Aplastic anemia, 557
Apnea, 82
Apneustic breathing, 82
Appendage, testicular, 516
Appendiceal abscess, radiography in, 161
Appendicitis, 482-483, 484
  in child, 816-818
  symptoms of, 133
Appendicolith, 133
Apresoline; *see* Hydralazine
APTT; *see* Activated partial thromboplastin
    time
Arboviruses, 618, 619-620
ARDS; *see* Adult respiratory distress
    syndrome
Arrest
  cardiac, 29-49; *see also* Cardiac arrest
  respiratory, 16, 17
Arterial blood gas analysis; *see* Blood gas
    analysis
Arterial embolism, peripheral, 410, 411,
    416
Arterial insufficiency, chronic, 412, 415-416
Arterial occlusion, acute, 411, 416
Arterial oxygen tension, 116
  in asthma, 382, 383
Arterial thrombosis, 416
Arteriolar dilator, 450, 451
Arteriosclerosis obliterans, 415
Arteriovascular disease, 410-420; *see also*
    Peripheral arteriovascular disease
Arteriovenous fistula, 420
  created for hemodialysis, 540
  physical examination in, 414
Arteriovenous malformation, 101-102
  gastrointestinal bleeding from, 144
  physical examination in, 414
Arteritis, giant cell or temporal, 418,
    579-580, 844-845
  headache and, 103
Arthritis
  gonococcal, 193, 194, 197
  Lyme disease, 193-194, 197, 750, 753-754
  regional enteritis and, 485
  rheumatoid, 192, 197, 577-578
  septic, 191-192, 196
  viral, 195, 197
Articular surface, fracture and, 295
Artificial graft for hemodialysis access, 540
Ascariasis, 737, 739-740, 742
  in pulmonary disorders, 743
Ascites, 498
L-asparaginase, 503
Aspergillus, 572
Aspiration
  of foreign material, 391-394
  knee, 320
Aspirin
  in chickenpox, 721

Aspirin—cont'd
  in fever, 78
  in headache, 101
  in ischemic heart disease, 429
  in Kawasaki syndrome, 712
  in pharyngitis, 363
  in thrombotic stroke, 605
  toxicity of, 783-785
    coagulation disorders and, 564
    respirations and, 762
    vomiting and, 161
Asplenia, 75
Assisted ventilation; *see* Ventilation
Asthma
  in adult, 379-384
  airway assessment in, 21, 23
  chest injury and, 255
  in child, 801-802
  respiratory distress and, 111
Asymptomatic bacteriuria in pregnancy, 512
Asystole, 39, 40
  in lightning injury, 343
Atarax; *see* Hydroxyzine
Ataxia in vertigo, 611, 612
Atheroembolus, 416
Atherosclerosis, 410; *see also* Peripheral
    arteriovascular disease
Athletic dental injury, 240
Atlantoaxial joint, subluxation of, 577
Atonic seizures, 204
Atopic dermatitis, 585-588
ATP; *see* Adenosine triphosphate
Atrial contraction, premature, 456-457
Atrial fibrillation, 462-463
Atrial flutter, 461
Atrial myxoma, 88
Atrial tachycardia with block, 461-462
Atrioventricular block; *see* Heart block
Atrophy, progressive spinal muscular, 643
Atropine
  as antidote in organophosphate and
    carbamate toxicity, 783
  in asystole, 40
  in atrioventricular heart block, 469
  in cardiac arrest, 37
  in chronic obstructive pulmonary disease,
    387
  diphenoxylate with, 172
  facial laceration suturing and, 236
  in intubation, 24
  in pediatric resuscitation, 46
  in pulseless electrical activity, 40
  toxicity of, 765, 774
Attendants for trauma team, 61
Augmentin; *see* Amoxicillin, with clavulinic
    acid
Auscultation
  of abdomen
    in pain, 136
    in vomiting, 157
  in airway assessment, 21
  in chest pain, 125

Autoimmune hemolytic anemia, 557
Automatisms, 205
Autonomic nervous system, peripheral
    neuropathies and, 629-630
Aveeno baths, 588
AVM; *see* Arteriovenous malformation
Avulsion
  of finger, 291-292
  of fracture, 295
    of ankle, 324
    of metatarsal, 329
    of tibia, 323
  of tooth, 241
Awake oral intubation, 21
Axid; *see* Nizatidine
Axillary aneurysm, 417
Axillary temperature, 71
Azathioprine
  in rheumatoid arthritis, 578
  toxicity of
    liver, 497
    pancreatic, 503
Azidothymidine; *see* Zidovudine
Azithromycin
  in bronchitis, 388
  in chlamydial cervicitis, 181
  in cryptosporidiosis, 739
  in urethritis, 512
  in urinary tract infection, 512
Azmacort; *see* Triamcinolone
Azotemia; *see also* Renal failure
  approach to patient with, 530-532
  prerenal, 526, 527
  urinary findings in, 522
AZT; *see* Zidovudine
Aztreonam, 511

B

Babesiosis, 751, 758-759
Babinski reflex, 85
  in Parkinson syndrome, 644
Bacillus organisms
  in diarrhea, 169
  in meningitis and encephalitis, 618
Back blows for foreign body removal, 800
Back pain, 195-199; *see also* Joint, pain in
  differential diagnosis in, 195
Bacteremia
  fever and, 75
  in child, 814-816
  in pneumococcemia, 707-709
Bacterial infection, 698-715
  cancer and, 572
  in chronic bronchitis, 385
  in conjunctiva, 840
  in cystitis, 512
  in diarrhea, 167-170, 172
  in diphtheria, 698-700
  in fever, 78
  in gonococcal arthritis, 193
  in meningitis and encephalitis, 618-619
    in child, 807-809

Bacterial infection—cont'd
  in meningitis and encephalitis—cont'd
    versus viral meningitis, 620
  in nongonococcal septic arthritis,
      191-192
  in peritonitis, 498
  in pharyngitis, 361-363
  in pneumonia
    in child, 803
    respiratory distress and, 112
  in prostatitis, 514
  in sinusitis, 365-366
  in tracheitis, 796, 799
  in urinary tract, 507-515
  in vaginosis, 182-183
Bacteriuria, 507-508, 509
  in pregnancy, asymptomatic, 512
Bacteroides in pelvic inflammatory disease,
    183
Bag-valve-mask ventilation
  in basic life support, 33
  in pediatric resuscitation, 45
  of neonate, 42
Balloon catheter in epistaxis, 824
Balloon counter pulsation, intraaortic, 56-57
Ball-valve thrombus, 88
Bandage for acromioclavicular separation,
    314
Barbiturates
  acidosis from, 766
  in seizures, 212-213
  toxicity of, 782-783
    respiratory center and, 762
    in sympatholytic syndrome, 765
  in ventricular tachycardia, 38
  in vertigo, 610
Barium enema
  appendicitis and, 483
  Hirschsprung disease and, 487
  intussusception of colon and, 486
Barotrauma, 824
Barrier dressings for wound closure, 288
Bartholin abscess, 180-181
Barton fracture, 305, 306
Basic life support, 30-36
Basilar artery, occlusion of, 823-824
Bath in heat stroke, 351-354
Battery ingestion, disk, 774
Beclomethasone, 384
Beclovent; *see* Beclomethasone
Bed rest in hip fracture, 299
Bell palsy, 631-632
  stroke versus, 603
Bell phenomenon, 637
Belladonna alkaloids
  in headache, 100
  toxicity of, 774
Benadryl; *see* Diphenhydramine
Benign early repolarization, 424, 425
Benign paroxysmal positional vertigo, 613
Benign prostatic hypertrophy, 516-517
Benzathine penicillin, 591-592

Benzathine penicillin—cont'd
  in rheumatic fever, 195
Benzocaine, 285
Benzodiazepines
  in burns, 336
  in chemical restraint, 662
  in muscle cramps, 545
  in pregnancy-induced hypertension, 553
  respiratory center and, 762
  in seizures, 208, 209, 212-213, 767-768
  in shivering from rapid cooling, 354
  in status epilepticus in child, 810, 812
  in sympatholytic syndrome, 765
  in tetanus, 704
Benzoin tincture, 184
Benztropine mesylate
  in Parkinson syndrome, 645
  toxicity of, 774
Berlin edema, 238
Beta-adrenergic agents
  in aortic trauma, 270
  in asthma, 381, 801-802
  bradycardias from, 465
  in bronchitis, 366
  in cardiogenic shock, 56
  in chronic obstructive pulmonary disease,
      387
  in congestive heart failure, 446
  contraindicated
    in preexcitation syndromes, 467
    with verapamil, 460
  in dysrhythmias from poisoning, 768
  hyperkalemia and, 672
  in hypertensive encephalopathy, 437
  in hyperthyroidism, 693, 694
  in ischemic heart disease, 430
  in migraine, 100
  in syncope, 89
  in tetanus, 704
  toxicity of, 764, 774
Betadine; *see* Povidone-iodine
Beta-hemolytic streptococcal infection,
    591-592
  in impetigo, 597-599
Beta-hydroxybutyrate, 689
Beta-lactam/beta-lactamase inhibitors, 376,
    377
Bicarbonate
  serum, in abdominal trauma, 273
  sodium
    in antidepressant overdose, 778
    in cardiac arrest, 37
    in dysrhythmias from poisoning, 768
    in hyperkalemia, 531, 537, 674
    in ketoacidosis, 690, 698
    in metabolic complications of renal
        failure, 531, 537
    in neonatal resuscitation, 44
    in pediatric resuscitation, 46
    of neonate, 44
    in postresuscitation care, 41
    in pulseless electrical activity, 40

Bicarbonate—cont'd
  sodium—cont'd
    in ventricular fibrillation, 38
    wound closure and, 288
Bier block, 303, 304
Biliary disease, physical findings in, 125
Biliary tract, 500-502
Bilious vomiting, 155
Biot breathing, 82
Bipap; *see* Nasal biphasic airway pressure
Bismuth-containing compounds, 476
Bites, rabies and, 724
Bladder
  disorders of
    schistosomiasis in, 741, 744-745
    urinary tract infection and, 507
  trauma to, 281
    in pelvic fracture, 316
Blastomyces species, 618
Bleeding; *see also* Hemorrhage
  anemia and, 556, 557
  in aortic transection, 257
  in arteriovenous malformations, 102
  in diverticular disease, 488
  dysfunctional uterine, 179-180
  in ear injury, 238-239
  in epidural hematoma, 228
  epistaxis; *see* Epistaxis
  evaluation of, 563, 564
  in female genital trauma, 279
  in femoral shaft fracture, 318
  in frenulum injury, 239
  gastrointestinal, 142-152, 477; *see also*
      Gastrointestinal tract, bleeding in
  in hematologic disorder, 556-571; *see
      also* Hematologic disorders
  hematoma and; *see* Hematoma
  in hematuria, 519
  in hemophilia, 566-567
  in hemothorax, 260
  in hyphema, 832-833
  in hypovolemic shock, 52, 53
  initial control of, 283
  intracranial
    computed tomography in, 222-223
    hypertension and, 440
  in maxillary fractures, 232
  in mesenteric vascular occlusion, 484
  in multiple trauma, 62-64
  in oral injury, 239
  in orbital fracture, 234
  ovarian, 175-176
  patterns of, 562
  in pregnancy, 548, 550, 551-552, 553
  retinal, 835
  in shock, 50-59; *see also* Shock
  in soft tissue trauma; *see* Soft tissue,
      trauma to
  subarachnoid; *see* Subarachnoid
      hemorrhage
  subconjunctival, 831-832
Blepharitis, 839

Blind nasotracheal intubation, 21-23
Blindness
   in giant cell arteritis, 579
   nonorganic, 636
Blister in pemphigus vulgaris, 594-596
Block
   beta-adrenergic; *see* Beta-adrenergic
      agents
   calcium channel; *see* Calcium channel
      blockers
   heart; *see* Heart block
   nerve; *see* Nerve block
Blood
   disorders of, 556-571; *see also*
      Hematologic disorders
   loss of; *see* Bleeding; Hemorrhage
   swallowed, 145
   at vaginal introitus in genital trauma, 279
Blood cells
   red; *see* Red blood cells
   in spinal fluid, in child, 808
   white; *see* White blood cells
Blood chemistry; *see* Blood studies
Blood culture in meningitis, 624
Blood factors
   deep venous thrombosis and, 396
   disorders of; *see* Coagulation disorders
   vitamin K–dependent, 407
Blood gas analysis
   in AIDS and HIV, 728
   in bronchiolitis, 801
   in chest pain decisions, 128, 129
   in chronic obstructive pulmonary disease,
      385
   in comatose patient, 82, 85
   in congestive heart failure, 448
   in drug poisoning, 766
   in electrical injury, 344
   in foreign body aspiration, 393
   in hypothermia, 355
   in near-drowning, 346
   in postresuscitation care, 41
   in pulmonary embolism, 127
   in respiratory distress, 116
   in smoke inhalation burn, 340
Blood pressure
   in cardiogenic shock, 54, 55
   in chest injury, 255
   in child, 434
   in coma, 82
   in headache, 100-101
   hypertension and, 433-444; *see also*
      Hypertension
   hypotension and; *see* Hypotension
   in multiple trauma, 63
   pregnancy and elevation of, 552-554
   shock and, 54, 55
Blood studies
   in abdominal trauma, 273
   in appendicitis, 483
   in gastrointestinal bleeding, 146-147, 150
   in headache, 97-98

Blood studies—cont'd
   in heat stroke, 354
   in hematuria, 524
   in hemophilia, 568
   in hypothermia, 355
   in joint pain, 188-190
Blood transfusions
   in ectopic pregnancy, 549
   in esophageal bleeding, 148
   in gastric bleeding, 148, 477
   in gastrointestinal bleeding, 148, 477
   in hypovolemic shock, 53-54
   in multiple trauma, 64
Blood urea nitrogen
   abdominal pain and, 137
   in chronic renal failure, 535
   in diarrhea, 172
   in gastrointestinal bleeding, 146-147
   in prerenal azotemia, 526
   in renal failure, 521
   in vomiting, 161
Blowout fracture, orbital, 234, 829-830
BLS; *see* Basic life support
Blue bloater, 110
Blue toe syndrome, 416
Blunt trauma
   of abdomen, 272-275
   Brown-Sequard syndrome and, 249, 250
   cardiovascular, 264-271; *see also*
      Cardiovascular system, trauma to
   of carotid artery, 239
   of chest
      in aortic transection, 257-258
      in cardiac tamponade, 261-262
      in diaphragm injury, 260-261
      in esophageal injury, 262
      in flail chest and pulmonary contusion,
         256-257
      in hemothorax, 260
      in myocardial contusion, 258
      in pneumothorax, 258-260
      in rib fracture, 255-256
   of diaphragm, 260-261
   of esophagus, 262
   in head injury, 219
   iritis in, 832
   lens subluxation in, 833-834
   in male genital tract, 279
   mydriasis and miosis in, 833
   in rupture of globe of eye, 835
   in tension pneumothorax, 259
   in urinary tract, 280
B-mode ultrasonography in arterial disease,
   415; *see also* Ultrasonography
BNTI; *see* Blind nasotracheal intubation
Body fluids, 664-671; *see also* Fluid
Body lice, 745-746
Body temperature; *see* Temperature
Boerhaave syndrome, 128, 476
Bohler angle, 329
Bone marrow, tibial, 44
Bonine; *see* Meclizine

Bony crepitus in humeral fracture, 310
Borderline hypertension, 433
Bordetella genus, 701
Borrelia organisms
   in Lyme disease, 193, 748-754
   in relapsing fever, 750, 754-755
Botulism, 705-707
Bouchard nodes, 192
Boutonniere deformity, 301, 302
Bowel; *see also* Gastrointestinal tract
   intussusception of, 818
   obstruction of, 480-482
      lesions responsible for, 481
      mechanical causes of, 482
   sexual activity and infections of, 488-489
Bowel sounds, bowel obstruction and,
   480-481
Boxer's fracture, 303
BPH; *see* Benign prostatic hypertrophy
Brachial artery, 310
Brachial plexus
   clavicular fracture and, 313
   in thoracic outlet syndrome, 419
Bradycardia, 465-466
   general assessment of, 456
   pericardial tamponade and, 267
Bradypnea in coma, 82
Brain; *see also* Neurologic disorder
   abscess of; *see* Abscess, intracerebral
   in cerebral aneurysm, 102
   coma and, 80-81
   headache and, 101-102
   herniation of, 575
   in hypertensive encephalopathy, 436-437
   in meningitis, 617
   trauma to, 219-230; *see also* Head injury
      contusions and, 226-227
      in electrical injury, 343
      posttraumatic syndromes and, 229
      swelling in, 219-220
   tumor of, 575
      parkinsonism from, 644
      stroke versus, 603
Brain death, 29
Brainstem
   ischemia of, vertigo in, 614
   ventilation and, 106
Branhamella catarrhalis, 822
Breath smell in coma, 84-85
Breath sounds
   airway assessment and, 20-21
   in pneumothorax, 259
   in respiratory distress, 115
Breath-holding spells, 813
Breathing
   apneustic, 82
   basic life support and, 30-33
   Biot, 82
   in burn, 334
   coma and, 82, 84-85
   in multiple trauma, 62
   in neonatal resuscitation, 42

Bretylium
  in cardiac arrest, 37
  in pediatric resuscitation, 46
  in ventricular fibrillation, 38
  in ventricular tachycardia, 39, 465
Brief psychotic disorder, 654
Bromocriptine, 645
Bronchial foreign body, 391
  in child, 799-800
Bronchiolitis, 718-719
Bronchitis, 366
  chronic, 385-389
  in chronic obstructive pulmonary disease,
      110
  diagnosis of, 128
  respiratory distress and, 109
Bronchoconstriction in asthma, 801-802
Bronchodilators
  in asthma, 381, 382, 383
    in child, 801-802
  in bronchiolitis, 801
  in bronchitis, 366
Bronchoscopy
  in foreign body aspiration, 393
  in pneumonia, 375
Bronchospasm in congestive heart failure,
    107-108
Brown macule, 584, 585
Brudzinski sign, 807
Bruising in cerebral contusion, 226-227
Bruit
  in clavicular fracture, 313
  in peripheral arteriovascular disease, 413
Buck traction, 318
Buerger disease, 415-416
Buerger sign, 414
Bulbar palsy, progressive, 643
Bulla, 584
  in pemphigus vulgaris, 594-596
Bullet wound, abdominal; *see* Gunshot
      wound
Bullous impetigo, 598
Bumetanide, 448-449
  in pancreatitis etiology, 503
  in pulmonary edema, 452-453, 538
Bundle branch block, 425, 426
Bupivacaine
  in chest injury, 255
  wound closure and, 285, 288
  in wrist injury, 304
Burn, 333-340
  chemical, 338-340
  death of patient from, 333
  degree of, 333-334
  in electrical injury, 342, 343
  estimation of size of, 334, 335
  eye, 837-838
    flash, 837
  general measures for, 336-337
  laboratory and x-ray studies in, 337
  management of, 334-336
    admission to burn unit in, 338

Burn—cont'd
  management of—cont'd
    outpatient, 337-338
  pathophysiology of, 333-334
  smoke inhalation in, 340
Burn unit, 338
Burow's solution
  in atopic dermatitis, 588
  in candidiasis, 585
  in contact dermatitis, 593
Bursa, 298
Bursitis, 192, 196
Butalbital, 101
Butoconazole, 183
Butterfly pattern rash, 580
Buttocks, perianal abscess and, 488
Button battery ingestion, 774-775
Butyrophenones
  in chemical restraint, 662
  parkinsonism from, 643, 645
  toxicity of, 774

C

C fibers, syncope and, 86
Cadmium, 681
Cafe coronary, 477
Caffeine in headache, 100, 101
Calamine lotion in varicella, 595
Calcaneal fracture, 325
Calcitonin in hypercalcemia, 680
Calcium, 677-683
  hypercalcemia and, 677-680
    in tumors, 574
  hypocalcemia and, 680-683
  magnesium and, 683, 684, 686
  in metabolic complications of renal
      failure, 531
Calcium ascorbate, 682
Calcium channel blockers
  in migraine, 100
  toxicity of, 775
    bradycardias from, 465
    in congestive heart failure, 446
    hyperkalemia and, 672
Calcium chloride
  in cardiac arrest, 37
  in hyperkalemia, 531, 537
  in hypocalcemia, 682, 683
  in multiple trauma, 64
  in pediatric resuscitation, 46
Calcium gluceptate, 682
Calcium gluconate
  in hydrofluoric acid burn, 339
  in hyperkalemia, 531, 537
  in hypocalcemia, 682, 683
Calcium lactate, 682
Calcium oxide burn, 339
Calcium pyrophosphate crystals, 189
Calculus
  in gallstones, 500
  salivary, 825
  urinary, 517-519

Calymmatobacterium granulomatis, 184
Camphor, toxicity of, 780
Campylobacter; see Helicobacter pylori
Canaliculi, lacrimal, lacerations of, 837
Cancer; *see* Malignancy
Candida albicans
  in AIDS and HIV, 730
  in esophagitis, 476
  in meningitis and encephalitis, 618
  in pharyngitis, 362
  in skin lesions, 585
  tumors and, 572
  in vaginal infection, 183
Cannon a waves, 91
CAPD; *see* Chronic ambulatory peritoneal
      dialysis
Capillary refill, 414
Capillary wedge pressure, pulmonary, 55
  in pulmonary edema, 109
Capital femoral epiphysis, slipped, 317
Capoten; *see* Captopril
Captain of trauma team, 61
Captopril
  in heart failure, 450, 451
  hyperkalemia and, 672
  in hypertension, 439
Caput medusae, 498
Carafate; *see* Sucralfate
Carbamate toxicity, 783
Carbamazepine
  in seizures, 211, 212-213
  theophylline clearance and, 383
  toxicity of
    liver, 497
    pancreatic, 503
  in trigeminal neuralgia, 104
Carbenicillin
  hypomagnesemia and, 685
  in tumor infection emergencies, 573
Carbenoxolone, 676
Carbidopa, 645
Carbogen, 844
Carbolic acid burn, 339
Carbon dioxide
  in respiratory distress, 116
  retinal artery and, 844
Carbon dioxide narcosis, 21
Carbon monoxide poisoning, 340, 776
  headache in, 96
  in smoke inhalation burn, 340
Carbonic anhydrase inhibitor, 843
Carboxyhemoglobin
  poisoning from, 776
  in smoke inhalation burn, 340
Carboxylic acid, 212-213
Carcinoid, 504
Carcinoma; *see also* Malignancy
  anorectal, 489
  bladder, 745
  in bowel obstruction, 480
  cervical, 179
  emergencies and, 572-576

Carcinoma—cont'd
  gastrointestinal, bleeding in, 144
  of liver, 499-500
  of pancreas, 505
  respiratory distress in, 113
  testicular, 516
  of uterus, 179
  vaginal bleeding in, 179
Cardiac arrest, 29-49
  in child, 45-48
  in drug poisoning, 768
  in electrical injury, 343, 344
  etiology of, 29-30
  in infant, 41-49
  life support for
    advanced, 36-40
    basic, 30-36
  in respiratory arrest, 16
Cardiac death, sudden, 429
Cardiac defects, anemia and, 557
Cardiac disease; *see* Heart
Cardiac enzymes
  in acute myocardial infarction, 428
  in ischemic heart disease, 427
Cardiac function, shock and, 54
Cardiac output
  neonatal resuscitation and, 42
  optimizing, 450-451
  in septic shock, 57
Cardiac pump, inadequate, 29
Cardiac sonography, 427
Cardiac tamponade; *see* Pericardial
    tamponade
Cardiac valves
  prosthetic, anemia and, 557
  syncope and, 88
Cardiac workload, 448
Cardiogenic causes of syncope, 88
Cardiogenic shock
  in child, 806
  drug therapy in, 55-56
  management of, 54-57
  in myocardial contusion, 265
  pathophysiology of, 50, 51, 54
Cardiomegaly, 447-448
Cardiomyopathies, respiratory distress and,
    113
Cardiopulmonary bypass in aortic trauma,
    270
Cardiopulmonary resuscitation
  in drug poisoning, 768
  life support in
    advanced, 36-40
    basic, 30-36
  postresuscitation care after, 41
  in spinal injury, 245
Cardiovascular system, 395-471
  arteriovascular disease in, 410-420;
    see also Peripheral arteriovascular
    disease
  deep venous thrombosis and, 395-409;
    see also Deep venous thrombosis

Cardiovascular system—cont'd
  dysrhythmias in, 455-471; *see also*
    Dysrhythmias
  heart failure in, 445-454; *see also* Heart
    failure
  hypertension in, 433-444; *see also*
    Hypertension
  ischemic heart disease in, 421-432; *see*
    also Ischemic heart disease
  Kawasaki syndrome and, 711, 712
  parasitic infestation in, 743-744
  procedures concerning, cardiopulmonary
    resuscitation in, 30-40
  pulmonary embolism and, 395-409; *see*
    also Pulmonary embolism
  in renal failure, 535
  trauma to, 264-271
    aortic trauma in, 268-270
    myocardial contusion in, 258, 264-265
    myocardial rupture in, 265-266
    pericardial tamponade in, 266-268
Cardioversion, 463, 465
  in pediatric resuscitation, 47
Cardizem; *see* Diltiazem
Carotid artery
  auscultation of pulse in, 413
  blunt trauma to, 239
  in giant cell arteritis, 579
  stenosis of, altered mental status and, 90
Carotid bodies, 106
Carotid endarterectomy
  in thrombotic stroke, 604
  in transient ischemic attacks, 604
Carotid sinus massage, atrial flutter and, 461
Carotid sinus syndrome, 87-88
Cast
  in ankle sprain, 324-325
  complications of, 299
  upper extremity and, 299
  in wrist fracture-dislocation, 303, 304
Catapres; *see* Clonidine
Cataract, traumatic, 834
Catgut suture, 286
Cathartics
  in drug poisoning, 767
  for foodborne botulism, 707
Catheter
  Foley
    in acute obstructive renal failure, 580
    in epistaxis, 824
    in esophageal foreign body, 478
    in urinary retention, 517
  in pericardial space in pericardial
    tamponade, 267
  pulmonary artery, in cardiogenic shock,
    54-55
  Tenckhoff, 542, 543
  urinary
    in burn patient, 336
    infection with, 512
    in multiple trauma, 64
Cation, potassium as, 671-672

Cation exchange resin, 674, 675
Cauda equina syndrome, 198, 199, 415
Caustic substance ingestion, 775-776
CD4 T-cells in AIDS and HIV, 727, 728
Cecal volvulus, 486-487
Cefaclor
  in bronchitis, 388
  in fever, 77
Cefazolin, 512
Cefixime
  in bronchitis, 388
  in gonorrheal cervicitis, 181
Cefoperazone, 625
Cefotaxime
  in epiglottitis, 799
  in fever in child, 814
  in gonococcal arthritis, 193
  in meningitis, 625
    in child, 809
  in pneumonia in child, 803
  in urinary tract infection in child, 513
Cefotetan, 184
Cefoxitin
  in abdominal pain, 134
  in pelvic inflammatory disease, 184
Cefpodoxime proxetil, 510
Ceftazidime, 573
Ceftizoxime, 193
Ceftriaxone
  in child, 77, 814, 815
  in epididymitis, 514
  in fever, 77
    in child, 814, 815
  in gonococcal arthritis, 193
  in gonorrheal cervicitis, 181
  in Lyme disease, 194, 750, 753
  in meningitis and encephalitis, 624, 625
  in pelvic inflammatory disease, 184
  in urinary tract infection, 510, 511
Cefuroxime
  in bronchitis, 388
  in Lyme disease, 753
  in meningitis, 625
  in otitis media, 822
  in pneumonia in child, 803
Cellular effects in shock, 50-51
Cellulitis, 585
  orbital, 842
  periorbital, 840
Central chemoreceptors, 106-107
  in chronic obstructive pulmonary disease,
    110
Central cord syndrome, 249, 250
Central nervous system; *see also* Brain;
    Neurologic disorder; Spine
  in AIDS and HIV, 729-730
  alcohol toxicity and, 772-773
  cardiac arrest and, 30
  coma and, 80-81
  hypomagnesemia and, 686
  in meningitis and encephalitis; *see*
    Meningitis and encephalitis

Central nervous system—cont'd
 parasitic infestation of, 742-743
 sinus headache and, 104
 syncope and, 89
 tumors and, 575
 ventilation and, 107
Central pontine myelinolysis, 671
Central retinal vessel occlusion, 843-844
Central venous line, 64
Central venous pressure
 in burn patient, 336
 hypovolemic shock and, 53
 in multiple trauma, 64
 of pericardial tamponade, 266
 in shock, 53
Cephalexin
 in impetigo, 599
 in urinary tract infection in pregnancy,
  512
Cephalic tetanus, 703-704
Cephalization of vessels, heart failure and,
 447
Cephalosporins
 in appendicitis in child, 818
 in bronchitis, 366
 in cellulitis, 585
 in diarrhea, 172
 in epiglottitis in adult, 364
 in fever in child, 814
 in hepatic abscess, 499
 in meningitis and encephalitis, 624, 625
 in meningococcemia, 711
 in pneumonia, 376, 377
 in tumor infection emergencies, 573
 in urinary tract infection, 510, 511
 in wound infection, 289
Cercariae, 741
Cerebellar hemorrhage
 management of, 605
 physical findings in, 601
 in vertigo, 614-615
Cerebral artery in stroke, 600, 601
Cerebral blood flow in head injury, 220
Cerebral disorder; see also Brain
 aneurysm in, 102
 contusion in, 226-227
 herniation in, 575
 hypertensive encephalomyopathy in,
  436-437
Cerebral edema in meningitis, 624-625
Cerebral hemangioma, seizures and, 207
Cerebral hemorrhage
 coma and, 80
Cerebrospinal fluid, 623
 in brain injury, 222
 in Guillian-Barré syndrome, 630
 in meningitis, 617, 622-624, 807-808
 in pseudotumor cerebri, 642
 trophozoites in, 742
Cerebrovascular accident, 600-607
 assessment in, 602-603
 clinical presentation of, 600-602

Cerebrovascular accident—cont'd
 differential diagnosis in, 603
 heat, 350-351
 hemorrhagic, 602
  management in, 605-606
  Hunt and Hess classification of, 605, 606
 in hypertension, 440
 ischemic, 600-602
  management in, 604-605
 management in, 603-606
 physical findings in, 601
 venous thrombosis in, 399
Cerumen, impacted, 823
Cervical lymph nodes in Kawasaki
  syndrome, 711
Cervical spine
 arthritis and, 577
 cross section of cord in, 249
 head injury and, 222, 223
 headache and, 104
 immobilization of, 243-245
  in near-drowning, 347
 injury to, 315-316
  in child, 65
  nonfracture, 314-315
Cervix, uterine
 carcinoma of, 179
 cervicitis and
  gonorrheal, 181
  herpes simplex, 596
 polyps of, 179
 strawberry, 744
Chagas disease, 743-744
Chagoma, 743
Chalazion, 839
Chamber angle recession, 833
Chaotic atrial rhythm, 463
Charcoal as poison antidote, 767, 786
Charting, 12-13
Chemicals
 in burns, 338-340; see also Thermal and
  chemical injury
 of eye, 838-839
 peripheral neuropathies from, 628, 629
Chemoprophylaxis; see Prophylaxis
Chemoreceptor trigger-zone, 153
Chemoreceptors, central, 106-107
 in chronic obstructive pulmonary disease,
  110
Chemotherapy; see also specific agent
 in fever in child, 814, 815
 herpetic neuralgia and herpes zoster and,
  633
 in superior vena cava syndrome, 573
 venous thrombosis in, 399
Chest compression, external, 33, 34-35
Chest pain, 120-129
 aggravating and alleviating factors in, 123
 in cardiogenic shock, 54-55
 character of, 122
 chronology of, 122-123
 clinical assessment of, 120-125

Chest pain—cont'd
 diagnostic tests for, 125-128
 differential diagnosis in, 120, 121
 in gastrointestinal disorders, 475-476
 history of patient with, 122-124
 in ischemic heart disease, 421
 location and radiation of, 122
 in myocardial infarction, 120, 122, 123,
  428
 patient management in, 129
 risk factors in, 123-124
 symptoms with, 123, 155
 in systemic lupus erythematosus, 580
Chest radiography; see Radiography
Chest thrusts for foreign body removal, 800
Chest trauma, 254-263
 blunt, 255-261
  aortic transection and, 257-258
  cardiac tamponade in, 261-262
  diaphragmatic injury and, 260-261
  esophageal, 262
  flail chest and pulmonary contusion in,
   256-257
  hemothorax in, 260
  myocardial contusion in, 258
  pneumothorax in, 258-260
  rib fracture in, 255-256
 cardiovascular trauma in, 264-271;
  see also Cardiovascular system,
  trauma to
 initial assessment and management in,
  254-255
 penetrating, 261-262
 wound closure for, 292
Chest wall, injury to, 255
Chewing in zygomatic fracture, 232-233
Cheyne-Stokes respirations, 82
CHF; see Heart failure
Chickenpox, 718, 719, 721-722
 skin rash in, 595, 596-597
 tumors and, 572
Chigger mites, 746
Chilblains, 356
Child, 791-821; see also Infant
 abdominal pain in, 131
 abuse of; see Child abuse
 airway management in, 26-27
  tube sizes for, 27
 appendicitis in, 483
 atopic dermatitis in, 588
 blood pressure in, 434
 bronchiolitis in, 800-801
 cardiac massage in, 47
 cardiopulmonary resuscitation in, 41-49
 dehydration in, 803-806
 disk battery ingestion in, 774-775
 epiglottitis in, 112-113
 epiphyseal injury in, 296, 297
 facial cellulitis in, 585
 fever in, 75-78, 813-816
 gastrointestinal system of, 816-819
  bleeding of, 477

Child—cont'd
general treatment guidelines for, 791-795
hypertension in, 434-435
meningitis and encephalitis in, 618, 620-621
multiple trauma in, 65-66
neurologic emergencies in, 807-809
nursemaid's elbow in, 308
pityriasis rosea in, 594
respiratory distress in, 795-803
retropharyngeal abscess in, 364
roseola infantum in, 590
shock in, 806-807
straddle injury in, 279
urinary tract infection in, 512-513
viral infections of, 720-722
vomiting in, 157-160
weight estimation of, by age, 47
Child abuse, 819-820
drug poisoning in, 769
sexual, 819-820
pelvic pain and, 177
straddle injury in, 279
subdural hematoma in infant from, 228
Chin lift, 30
Chlamydia organisms
in anorectal infection, 489
in Bartholin abscess, 180
in cervicitis, 181
in conjunctivitis, 842
in lymphogranuloma venereum, 185
in pelvic inflammatory disease, 182
in pharyngitis, 362
in pneumonia, 369, 370, 376, 377
in child, 803
in urethritis, 512
in urinary tract infections, 508, 512, 514
Chloral hydrate, 782
Chloramphenicol
in Eastern spotted fever, 758
in meningitis and encephalitis, 624, 625
in meningococcemia, 711
in Q fever, 751, 758
in Rocky Mountain spotted fever, 590, 751, 757
in vertigo, 610
Chloroquine
in amebiasis, 737
in malaria, 734-736
Chloroquine-resistant malaria, 734
Chlorpromazine
in headache, 100
liver toxicity of, 497
in vomiting, 164
Chlorthalidone, 449
in hypokalemia, 676
Chocolate cyst, 176
Choking, 35-36
Cholangitis, 501-502
Cholecystitis, 500-501
Cholelithiasis, 500

Cholesteatoma, 613
Cholesterol gallstones, 500
Cholinergics, toxicity of, 765
Chorionic gonadotropin, human, 547, 548
Chorioretinitis, 842
Choroid, inflammation of, 842
Christmas disease, 567
Chronic ambulatory peritoneal dialysis, 542-545
Chronic disease, anemia in, 557
Chronic obstructive pulmonary disease, 384-389
chest injury and, 255
indications for admission in, 388
respiratory distress and, 109-110
Chvostek sign, 682, 686
Ciliary body, inflammation of, 842
Ciliary spasm, 832
Cimetidine
in gastrointestinal bleeding, 148
in pancreatitis etiology, 503
in peptic bleeding, 476
theophylline clearance and, 383
Ciprofloxacin
in bronchitis, 388
in diarrhea, 168, 172
in epididymitis, 514
in gonorrheal cervicitis, 181
in pneumonia, 377
in urinary tract infection, 510, 511, 514
in pregnancy, 512
in wound infection, 289
Circulation
in burn, 334, 335-336
in coma, 82
in resuscitation
basic life support and, 33, 34-35
of child, 45-47
of neonate, 42, 43
in spinal injury, 245-246
Circumferential burn, 336
Cirrhosis, 495-498
Cisapride, 163, 164
Cisplatin
hypomagnesemia and, 685
liver toxicity of, 497
in pancreatitis etiology, 503
Cladosporium species, 618
Classic migraine, 99
Claudication
in giant cell arteritis, 579
intermittent, 412
arteriosclerosis obliterans and, 415
Clavicle
fracture of, 313
splinting of, 299
Clavulanate, amoxicillin with
in bronchitis, 388
in otitis media, 822
in urinary tract infection in child, 513
Cleansing of wound, facial, 235
Clicking in knee, 320

Clindamycin
in abdominal pain, 134
in appendicitis in child, 818
in babesiosis, 751
in bacterial vaginosis, 183
in ehrlichiosis, 751, 759
in hepatic abscess, 499
in malaria, 735
in pelvic inflammatory disease, 184
Clinical death, 29
Clonazepam for seizure, 211, 212-213
Clonic seizures, 204
Clonidine, 438
in pancreatitis etiology, 503
Closed chest cardiac compression, 45-47
Closed fracture, 295
of tibial shaft, 323
Clostridium botulinum, 705-707
Clostridium difficile, 165, 169
Clostridium perfringens, 169
Clostridium tetani, 703, 705
Closure, wound, 285-288
Clot, menstrual bleeding and, 177
Clotrimazole
in candidiasis, 585
in fungal infection, 584
in vaginal infection, 182, 183
Clotting factors
deep venous thrombosis and, 396
disorders of; *see* Coagulation disorders
vitamin K-dependent, 407
Cluster headache, 99
Coagulation disorders, 563-568; *see also* Disseminated intravascular coagulation
epistaxis in, 824
in septic shock, 57
venous thrombosis in, 400
deep, 396
Coagulation pathway, 561, 562, 567-568
Coagulopathy; *see* Coagulation disorders
Cobalt blue slit lamp examination, 831
Cocaine
abuse of, 777
in drug poisoning, 768
in epistaxis, 824
in nasal fracture, 825
toxicity of, 764, 777
wound closure and, 285
Coccidioides species
in AIDS and HIV, 729
in meningitis and encephalitis, 618
Coffee bean sign, 481
Coin in esophagus, 478
Colchicine
in gout, 190
in hypercalcemia, 681
in pancreatitis etiology, 503
Cold therapy in ankle sprains, 324
Cold water stimulation test in coma, 84
Colds, 716

Colic
  in cholecystitis, 501
  in gallstones, 500
  renal, 517-519
  ureteral, 133
Colitis
  in amebiasis, 739
  ulcerative, 485
Collagen vascular disease, platelet disorders
    in, 563
Collapsed lung, 158-160
  reexpansion of, 109
Collar, cervical, 315
Collateral ligament sprain, 320
Colles fracture, 304, 305
Colloidal compresses in drug eruptions, 588
Colloids in shock, 53
Colon
  bleeding from, 144
  carcinoma of, in intestinal obstruction,
    480
  motility disorders of, 487-488
  structural disorders of, 486-487
Colonoscopy in gastrointestinal bleeding,
    149
Color of patient, 20
Colorado tick fever, 751, 759
Coma, 80-86
  acid-base abnormality and, 84-85
  blood gas analysis and, 82, 85
  Glasgow score in; *see* Glasgow Coma
    Scale
  hyperglycemic hyperosmolar nonketotic,
    691
  myxedema, 694-695
  psychogenic, 637
Common migraine, 99
Communication of prehospital-care team
    with hospital, 60-61
Compartment syndrome
  from casts, 299
  forearm fracture and, 306
Compartmental changes, intracranial, 81
Compazine; *see* Prochlorperazine
Compensated shock
  in child, 806
  mechanisms in, 50-51
Complete blood count, 558
  in toxicology, 765
Complete fracture, 295
Complete heart block, 469-470
Complete spinal cord lesion, 249, 250
Completed miscarriage, 550
Complex absence seizures, 204-205
Complex partial seizures, 205-206
  treatment of, 211
Compound fracture, 295
Compression
  of chest in cardiopulmonary resuscitation
    in basic life support, 33, 34-35
    of child, 45-47
    of neonate, 42, 43

Compression—cont'd
  of fracture, 295, 299
    forearm fracture and, 306
  spinal tumor and, 575
  thoracic outlet syndrome and, 418-420
  of vertebrae, 199
Computerized tomography
  in AIDS and HIV, 729
  in altered mental status, 85, 86
  in aortic dissection, 128, 443
  in aortic trauma, 269
  in back pain, 199
  in brain injury, 222-223
  in comatose patient, 85-86
  in intracerebral abscess, 102
  in intraocular and orbital foreign bodies,
    836
  in kidney trauma, 280
  in liver disease in pregnancy, 499
  in orbital blowout fracture, 830
  in orbital cellulitis, 842
  in pain diagnosis, 138-139
  in pseudotumor cerebri, 102, 642
  in renal failure, 522
  in seizures, 208
  in spinal injury, 246, 250
  in stroke, 604
  in subarachnoid hemorrhage, 98, 102
  in subdural hematoma, 227, 228
  in trauma, 272, 274, 277
  in vertigo, 612
Concussion, 225-226
  myocardial, 264
Conduction hearing loss, 823
Condyle fracture, tibial, 322-323
Condyloma acuminatum, 184
Confusional state, protracted, 207
Congenital disorder
  cardiac, respiratory distress in, 113
  Hirschsprung disease and, 487
  intestinal obstruction and, 480
Congenital heart disease, respiratory
    distress and, 113
Congenital lobar emphysema, 110
Congestive heart failure; *see* Heart failure
Coning syndrome, 227, 228
Conjunctiva
  foreign body in, 830
  infection of, 840-841
Conjunctivitis, 840-841
Connective tissue diseases, 577-583
  ankylosing spondylitis and, 578
  arthritis and, 192, 197, 577-578
  giant cell arteritis in, 579-580
  polymyalgia rheumatica and, 578-579
  systemic lupus erythematosus in, 580-582
Consciousness; *see also* Mental status
  coma and, 80-86
  concussion and, 225-226
  psychogenic disorders of, 637
  syncope and, 86-92
Constipation in hypocalcemia, 679

Consultations in abdominal pain, 139
Contact dermatitis, 592-593
Continuous positive airway pressure
  in near-drowning, 346
  in pulmonary edema, 453
Contraceptive steroids, liver toxicity of, 497
Contraction
  cardiac
    premature atrial, 456-457
    premature ventricular, 457-459
  muscle
    electrical injury and, 342
    headache and, 101
Contrast media, acute renal failure from,
    530
Contusion
  cerebral, 226-227
  eyelid and, 829
  hyphema and, 832
  male genital tract and, 279
  myocardial, 258, 264-265
  pulmonary, 256-257
  scalp wound and, 289
Conversion reaction, hysteria, or disorder,
    634
Cooling
  in fever, 78
  in heat illness, 351-354
COPD; *see* Chronic obstructive pulmonary
    disease
Copper, deficiency of, 557
Copper sulfate in phosphorus burns, 339
Cord
  spinal, trauma to, 243-253; *see also* Spinal
    injury
  testicular torsion and, 515-516
Core rewarming, 355-356
  in near-drowning, 347
Cornea
  abrasion of, 831
  examination of, in vertigo, 612
  foreign body in, 830-831
  herpetic infection of, 841-842
  infection of, 841
  laceration of, 836
  rust rings in, 831
  thermal burn of, 837-838
  ulcer of, 841
Coronary angiography, 431
Coronary arteries
  Kawasaki syndrome and, 711, 712
  in myocardial contusion, 258
Coronavirus pharyngitis, 362
Corpus luteum cyst, 175
Corticosteroids; *see also* Steroids
  in asthma, 381, 382, 383-384
    in child, 802
  in atopic dermatitis, 588
  in Bell palsy, 632
  in contact dermatitis, 593
  in giant cell arteritis, 580
  in gout, 190

Corticosteroids—cont'd
in herpes zoster, 597
in multiple sclerosis, 641
in otitis externa, 823
in pancreatitis etiology, 503
in pemphigus vulgaris, 596
in pertussis, 702
in polymyalgia rheumatica, 579
in pseudotumor cerebri, 642
in rheumatoid arthritis, 578
in systemic lupus erythematosus, 581
in temporal arteritis, 103, 844
in toxic epidermal necrolysis, 588
Cortisol, plasma, 696
Corynebacterium diphtheria, 699, 700
tumors and, 572
Cosmesis in wound repair, 283
Costochondral junction tenderness, 422
Costochondritis, chest pain in, 122
Cosyntropin stimulation tests, 696
Co-trimoxazole, 503
Cotton suture, 287
Cough
assessment of, 115
in asthma, 380
in bronchitis, 366
in pertussis, 701-703
syncope and, 89
Cough suppressants in bronchitis, 366
Coumadin; *see* Warfarin
Countercurrent immunoelectrophoresis, 624
Countershock
in ventricular fibrillation, 36-38
in ventricular tachycardia, 38-39
COWS mnemonic, 84
Coxiella burnetti, 751, 758
Coxsackie viruses A and B, 716
CPD-MB; *see* Creatine phosphokinase-MB
Crackles, 115
Cramps
heat, 349-350
in hypomagnesemia, 686
menstrual, 177
Cranial nerves
Bell palsy and, 631-632
comatose patient and, 85
facial injury and, 232
headache and, 97
herpetic neuralgia and, 633
in meningitis, 621
optic or second; *see* Optic nerve
peripheral neuropathies and, 628
stroke and, 602
in tetanus, 703
vertigo and, 609, 612
Craniofacial separation, 232
Creatine kinase, 427
Creatine phosphokinase-MB, 126-127
Creatinine
in renal failure, 521
in vomiting, 161

Creeping eruption, 745
Crepitus, bony, 310
Cribriform plate fracture
airway management in, 223-224
in oral injury, 231
Cricoarytenoid joint, arthritis of, 577
Cricopharyngeal muscle, 472
Cricothyrotomy
in child, 27
in multiple trauma, 62, 66
needle, in pediatric airway management, 27
in spinal injury, 245
Critical illness polyneuropathy, 630
Crohn disease, 484-485
Crotamiton, 594, 746
Croup, 113, 716-718, 795-799
assessment of, 797
Cruciate ligament tear, 320-322
Crutches for angle sprain, 325
Crying, breath-holding spells and, 813
Cryoprecipitate
after thrombolysis in pulmonary
embolism or deep venous
thrombosis, 408
in hematologic disorders in renal failure, 532
Cryptococcal organisms
in AIDS and HIV, 729
in meningitis and encephalitis, 618
tumors and, 572
in uveal tract inflammation, 842
Cryptosporidiosis, 739
in diarrhea, 170
Crystal
calcium pyrophosphate, 189
uric acid, 190
Crystalline challenge in multiple trauma, 64
Crystalloids
in chest trauma, 255
in gastrointestinal bleeding, 148, 150, 477
in heat exhaustion, 350
in heat illnesses, 349
in hyperemesis gravidarum, 551
in hypovolemic shock, 53
in multiple trauma, 64
in pneumococcemia, 709
in septic shock, 57
in shock in child, 807
in syncope, 92
in toxic shock syndrome, 714
Cuff, rotator, tear of, 314
Culdocentesis
in ectopic pregnancy, 549
in vaginal bleeding, 178
Cullen sign, 502
Cultures
in fever, 73
in meningitis, 624
in pharyngitis, 363
in septic arthritis, 192
in septic shock, 57

Cultures—cont'd
in urinary tract infection, 509
Currant jelly stool, 145
Current, electrical, 342-344
Cutaneous diphtheria, 698, 699, 700
Cutaneous larva migrans, 745
Cutaneous lesions, 594-599; *see also* Skin
CVA; *see* Cerebrovascular accident
Cyanide poisoning, 340
Cyclic adenosine monophosphate, beta-
blocker toxicity and, 774
Cyclic antidepressants; *see* Antidepressants
Cyclobenzaprine
in back pain, 199
toxicity of, 774
Cyclogyl; *see* Cyclopentolate
Cyclooxygenase, 395-396
Cyclopentolate
in corneal abrasion, 831
in corneal foreign body removal, 831
in eye examination, 828
in ultraviolet keratitis, 837
Cyclophosphamide
liver toxicity of, 497
in systemic lupus erythematosus, 581
Cycloplegics
in corneal abrasion, 831
in corneal foreign body removal, 831
in traumatic iritis, 832
Cyclosporine in pancreatitis etiology, 503
Cyst
amebic, 739
chocolate, 176
Giardia, 736
hydatid, 743
in pulmonary disorders, 743
ovarian, 175-176
Cysticercosis, 743
Cysticercus cellulosae, 743
Cystitis, 507, 509
acute bacterial, 512
in male patient, 513-514
Cystography, retrograde, 281
Cytarabine, 503
Cytomegalovirus, 717, 723
in AIDS and HIV, 729
tumors and, 572
in uveal tract inflammation, 842
Cytotoxic agents in systemic lupus
erythematosus, 581

D

Dacron suture; *see* Monofilament plastic
sutures
Dacryocystitis, 839-840
Dapsone, 730
Datril; *see* Acetaminophen
DDAVP; *see* Desmopressin acetate
ddC, adverse effects of, 730
ddI; *see* Dideoxyinosine
DDL, adverse effects of, 730
Deafness, psychogenic, 636

Death, 29
  fetal, 550
  grieving and, 13-15
  hydrocarbon inhalation and, 779
  from myocardial contusion, 258
  in stroke, 600
  sudden cardiac, 429
  in sudden infant death syndrome, 820
    resuscitation termination and, 47-48
  from suicide, 656
  in tension pneumothorax, 259
Debridement of wound, 284
  in facial injury, 235
Deceleration injury
  in aortic trauma, 268-271
  in myocardial contusion, 264
Deciduous tooth, fracture of, 240-241
Decompression
  optic nerve sheath, in pseudotumor
    cerebri, 642
  in pericardial tamponade, 267
  of urinary bladder, 517
Decongestants, 365-366
  in drug poisoning, 768
  in middle ear effusions, 823
  in orbital blowout fracture, 831
  in toxic syndromes, 764
Deep frostbite, 357
Deep respiratory infection, 364-365
Deep tendon reflexes
  in meningitis, 621
  in spinal injury, 247-250
  in spinal pain, 315
  in stroke, 602
Deep venous thrombosis, 395-409
  clinical presentation of, 396-397
  diagnosis of, 400-401
  history of prior, 400
  pathophysiology of, 395-396
  risk factors for, 399
  thrombogenic and hypercoagulable states
    and, 399-400
  treatment of, 405-408
Deet; see Diethyltoluamide
Defecation, muscles of, 488
Defecation syncope, 89
Deferoxamine, 781
Defibrillation
  in pediatric resuscitation, 47
  protocol for, 36-40
Degenerative joint disease, 192
Degloving injury of penis, 279
Dehydration, 667-668
  in child, 803-806
    degree of, 804
  isotonic, 805
  in pyloric stenosis, 818
  in vomiting, 160, 162
Dehydroemetine, 737
Deltoid ligament sprain, 325
Delusional disorders, 652-654
Demeclocycline, 575

Dementia in Parkinson syndrome, 644
DEMENTIA mnemonic, 649
Demerol; see Meperidine
Demyelinating disease, 638-641
Demyelinating syndrome, osmotic, 671
Dendritic herpes simplex keratitis, 841
Dental injury, 232, 240-241
Dentin, 240-241
Deoxybarbiturates, 212-213
Deoxycorticosterone, 676
Depression
  of fracture fragment, 296
  in Parkinson syndrome, 644
  suicide and, 656-659
Dermacentor andersoni, 751, 756, 759
Dermacentor organisms, 750, 751, 755,
  756, 759
Dermacentor variabilis, 750, 751, 755, 756
Dermatitis
  atopic, 585-588
  contact, 592-593
  gonococcal, 598, 599
Dermatologic disorder, 584-599
  macular lesions in, 584-592
  papular lesions in, 592-594
  parasitic infestation of, 745
  pustular lesions as, 597-599
  in renal failure, 535
  vesicular lesions as, 594-597
Dermatomes, 248
  abdominal pain and, 132
Dermis
  sutures for, 135
  in wound repair, 283
Desipramine, toxicity of, 777
Desmopressin acetate
  in coagulation disorders, 568
  in hematologic disorders in renal failure,
    532
Detachment, retinal, 834-835
Detergents, eye injury from, 838-839
Developmental stages, 791, 792-793
Dexamethasone
  in Addisonian crisis, 696
  in croup, 799
  in meningitis, 626
    in child, 809
Dexatrim; see Phenylpropanolamine
Dexon suture; see Polyglycolic suture
Dextran
  in hypovolemic shock, 53
  low-molecular-weight, in central retinal
    artery occlusion, 844
Dextrose
  in Addisonian crisis, 696
  in coma, 83
  in hyperemesis gravidarum, 551
  in hypoglycemia, 692
  in hypothyroidism, 695
  in intoxications, 763
  in meningitis and encephalitis, 624
  and normal saline

Dextrose—cont'd
  and normal saline—cont'd
    in hypothermia, 355
    in vomiting, 162
  in sulfonylurea poisoning, 785-786
    in vomiting, 162
DHE-45, 100
Diabetes insipidus, 666
  hypernatremia and, 668-669
Diabetes mellitus, 688-689
  hypomagnesemia and, 685
  immunosuppression and, 75
  ketoacidosis in, 672, 690-691
  lactic acidosis in, 691
  peripheral neuropathies in, 629
Diagnosis
  most serious, 9
  peritoneal lavage in abdominal trauma
    for, 272, 273-274, 277
  renal staging in, 280
  support of, by evidence, 9
*Diagnostic and Statistical Manual of
  Mental Disorders,* 647, 653
Dialysis, 539-545
  in alcohol intoxication, 773
  complications of, 540-542
  in drug poisoning, 767, 781, 785
  hemodialysis in, 539-542
  in hyperkalemia, 537
  hypermagnesemia and, 684
  indications for, 539
  peritoneal, 542-545
    in hypothermia, 356
Diamond-Blackfan anemia, 557
Diaphoresis in asthma, 380
Diaphragm
  injury to, 260-261
    in abdominal trauma, 273, 275
  thoracotomy and, 260
Diarrhea
  in AIDS and HIV, 730
  in fecal impaction, 489
  in gastroenteritis, 716
  infectious, 165-173
    amebiasis in, 736-739
    assessment of, 170-172
    in cryptosporidiosis, 739
    diagnosis of, 166
    etiologic agents in, 166-170
    giardiasis in, 736, 742
    management of, 172
    pathophysiology of, 165-166
    protozoan, 170, 736-742
    schistosomiasis in, 741
  noninfectious causes of, 165, 166
Diastolic blood pressure
  in heart failure, 446
  in hypertensive-emergencies of
    pregnancy, 441
Diazepam
  in facial laceration suturing, 236
  in head injury, 225

Diazepam—cont'd
  in intubation procedures, 22
  in paroxysmal supraventricular
    tachycardia, 459
  in pregnancy-induced hypertension, 442,
    553
  in seizures, 208-209, 212-213
    from drug poisoning, 767
    febrile, 209
    in status epilepticus, 214
  in shoulder dislocation, 311
  in spinal injury, 315
  in status epilepticus in child, 812
  in ventricular tachycardia, 38
  in vertigo, 615, 823
Diazoxide
  contraindicated
    in hypertensive encephalopathy, 437
    in renal failure, 441
  in hypertension with renal failure, 441
  in pancreatitis etiology, 503
  in sulfonylurea poisoning, 786
Dibenzoxazepines, toxicity of, 777
DIC; *see* Disseminated intravascular
    coagulation
Dicloxacillin
  in impetigo, 599
  for sinusitis, 366
  in toxic epidermal necrolysis, 588
Dideoxyinosine, 502
Diet, abdominal pain and, 140
Diethylstilbestrol, 820
Diethyltoluamide, 760
Digiband; *see* Digoxin-specific Fab fragments
Digit
  of foot, fracture of, 329
  of hand
    fracture of, 300-303
    splint for, 298
    trauma to, 290-292
Digitalis
  in atrial fibrillation, 463
  in atrial tachycardia with block, 461
  calcium and, 683
  in congestive heart failure, 446, 451, 452
  hyperkalemia and, 672
  hypomagnesemia and, 685
  in syncope, 89
  toxicity of, 778-779
Digitoxin, thrombocytopenia and, 563
Digoxin, 451, 452
  in atrial fibrillation, 463
  in atrial flutter, 461
  in atrial tachycardia with block, 461
  bradycardias from, 465
  contraindicated in Wolff-Parkinson-White
    syndrome, 467
  toxicity of, 765, 778-779
Digoxin-specific Fab fragments, 779
Dihydroergotamine for migraine, 100
1,25-Dihydroxycholecalciferol, 534
Dilantin; *see* Phenytoin

Diloxanide furoate, 737
Diltiazem
  in atrial fibrillation, 463
  in atrial flutter, 461
  in atrial tachycardia with block, 461
  in heart failure, 450, 451
Dimenhydrinate, 162-164
Dinitrophenol, 762
Diphenhydramine
  in drug eruptions, 588
  in herpes simplex, 595
  sedative effect of, in psychosis, 652
  in varicella, 595
  in vertigo, 615
  in vomiting, 162-164
Diphenoxylate with atropine, 172
Diphenylhydantoin; *see* Phenytoin
Diphosphonates in hypercalcemia, 680
Diphtheria, 698-700
  and tetanus toxoids, 702
Diplopia, psychogenic monocular, 636
Dipstick in urine protein, 520-521
Discharge
  conjunctival, in infection, 840
  instructions for concussion patient
    before, 226
  vaginal, 181
Disk battery ingestion, 774-775
Disk herniation, 198, 199
Dislocation, 296
  ankle, 323-324
  elbow, 307-308
  hip, 294, 317-318
  knee, 294, 322
  lens, 833-834
  lunate bone, 303-304
  metacarpal, 303
  patellar, 319
  of phalanx, 301
  shoulder, 311-313
  temporomandibular joint, 234
Displacement of fracture, 295
  of olecranon, 307
Disposition of patient, 9-10
Dissecting aortic aneurysm, 442-443
Disseminated intravascular coagulation,
    557, 568, 569-570; *see also*
    Coagulation disorders
  laboratory evaluation in, 568
  in meningitis and encephalitis, 621
Dissociation, electromechanical; *see*
    Pulseless electrical activity
Dissolved food, aspiration of, 391
Distal humerus fracture, 310-311
Distal phalangeal injury, 300-303
Distension in bowel obstruction, 481
Distributive shock, 50, 51, 57-58
  in child, 806
Diuretics
  in brain injury, 224
  in cardiogenic shock, 56
  in congestive heart failure, 446, 448-449, 450

Diuretics—cont'd
  hypercalcemia and, 677-678, 680
  hyperkalemia and, 537
  hypokalemia and, 675, 676
  hypomagnesemia and, 685
  hyponatremia and, 671
  in meningitis, 625
  in pulmonary edema, 538
  in renal failure, 441, 532
  in syncope, 89
  thiazide
    in heart failure, 448, 449
    in renal failure, 441
    in vertigo, 610
Diverticular abscess, radiography in, 161
Diverticular disease, 487-488
Diverticulosis
  bleeding in, 144
  Meckel diverticulum in, 144
Dizziness, 608; *see also* Vertigo
Dobutamine
  in cardiogenic shock, 55-56
  in heart failure, 452
  in pediatric resuscitation, 46
  in pulmonary edema, 453
Doll's eye, 84
Done nomogram, 784, 785
Donovan bodies, 184
Dopamine
  in cardiac arrest, 37
  in cardiogenic shock, 55-56
  in heart failure, 452
  parkinsonism and, 644
  in pediatric resuscitation, 46
  in postresuscitation care, 41
  in pulmonary edema, 453
  in renal failure, 580
  in septic shock, 57
Doppler ultrasonography
  in arterial disease, 414-415; *see also*
    Ultrasonography
  in testicular torsion, 515-516
Dorsal side of part, 296
Dorsal splint for wrist, 298
Doxepin, toxicity of, 777
Doxycycline
  in chlamydial cervicitis, 181
  in epididymitis, 514
  in granuloma inguinale, 184
  in inclusion conjunctivitis, 841
  in Lyme disease, 194, 750, 753
  in lymphogranuloma venereum, 185
  in pelvic inflammatory disease, 184
  in urethritis, 512
Drainage
  abscess, peritonsillar, 364
  cast and, 299
Dramamine; *see* Dimenhydrinate
Drawer sign, positive, 320
Dressings
  burn, 337-338
  for finger wound, 291

INDEX

Dressings—cont'd
  for scalp wound, 289
  Tubegauze, 291
  for wound closure, 288
Droperidol
  in chemical restraint, 662
  in vomiting, 164
Drowning, 345
Drug abuse, coma and, 83
Drug screening, 765
  suicide behavior and, 656
Drug therapy
  in advanced life support, 36, 37
  antibiotic; see Antibiotics
  in brain injury, 224-225
  in chronic obstructive pulmonary disease,
    387, 388
  in coma, 83
  in fever, 77, 78
  in pediatric resuscitation, 46, 47
    of neonate, 44-45
  in rheumatoid arthritis, 192
  in seizures, 208-210, 212-213
Drug-induced disorders
  anemias in, 557
  gastrointestinal bleeding in, 144
  hepatic injury in, 497
  hepatitis in, 495, 497
  hypomagnesemia in, 685
  in interstitial renal disease, 528
  in nephrotic syndrome, 525
  pancreatitis in, 502, 503
  parkinsonism in, 643, 645
  psychosis in, 649, 651
  skin eruption in, 588
  syncope in, 87, 89
  vertigo in, 610
Dry drowning, 345
DSM-IV; see Diagnostic and Statistical
    Manual of Mental Disorders
DTaP; see Acellular pertussis vaccine
    formulated with diphtheria and
    tetanus toxoids
DTP; see Diphtheria, and tetanus toxoids
DUB; see Dysfunctional uterine bleeding
Duct
  parotid, 237
  Stensen, 825
Duodenum
  bleeding in, 144
  pain and, 476-477
DVT; see Deep venous thrombosis
Dyrenium; see Triamterene
Dysarthria in stroke, 603
Dysesthesias in peripheral neuropathies, 629
Dysfunctional uterine bleeding, 179-180
Dysmenorrhea, 177
Dysphagia, 473-475
Dyspnea, 106
  abdominal pain and, 133
  in asthma, 380
  in congestive heart failure, 446

Dyspnea—cont'd
  differential diagnosis in, 107-115
  paroxysmal nocturnal, in heart failure,
    446-447
Dysrhythmias, 455-471
  in Addisonian crisis, 696
  atrioventricular block in, 467-470
  bradycardia in, 465-466
  in drug poisoning, 768
  in electrical injury, 343
  in hypercalcemia, 678
  in hypokalemia, 675
  in hypomagnesemia, 686
  in hypothermia, 354
  irregular beats in, 456-459
    premature atrial contractions and,
      456-457
    premature ventricular contractions
      and, 457-459
  in myocardial contusion, 258, 265
  preexcitation syndromes in, 466-467
  sick sinus syndrome in, 470
  in syncope, 87, 88
  tachycardias in
    irregular narrow-complex, 462-463,
      464
    regular narrow-complex, 458, 459-462
    wide-complex, 465, 466
  in tricyclic antidepressant toxicity, 768
Dysuria, 509-512
  in trichomoniasis, 744

E

Ear
  infection of, 822-823
  ototoxicity of diuretics and, 449
  trauma to, 238-239, 824
    electrical, 343
  in vertigo, 611, 823-824
  wound closure and, 289
Early repolarization, benign, 424, 425
EAST; see Elevated arm stress test
Eastern spotted fever, 758
Echinococcus granulosus, 742-743
Echocardiography, 127
  transesophageal, in aortic dissection, 128
Echoviruses, 716
Eclampsia, 441, 552-554
ECM; see Erythema chronicum migrans
Ectoparasites, 745-746
Ectopic endometrial tissue, 176
Ectopic focus in atrial tachycardia with
    block, 461-462
Ectopic pregnancy, 174, 547, 548-549
Edema; see also Swelling
  Berlin, 238
  in burn patient, 336
  cerebral; see Cerebral edema
  facial, 231
  heat, 349
  hyponatremia and, 669
  in pregnancy-induced hypertension, 441

Edema—cont'd
  in proteinuria, 524
  pulmonary; see Pulmonary edema
  in superior vena cava syndrome, 573
Effusion
  in knee sprain, 320
  middle ear, 823
  pleural, 447
    in esophageal perforation, 476
    in pulmonary embolism, 402
Ehlers-Danlos syndrome, 562, 581-582
Ehrlichiosis, 751, 758
Elasticity, arterial
  in giant cell arteritis, 579-580
  hypertension and, 433
Elbow
  arthritis in, 577
  fracture or dislocation of, 306-308
  splint for, 298
Elderly
  abdominal pain in, 131, 135
  appendicitis in, 483
  meningitis in, 618
  pain perception in, 135
  pelvic pain in, 177
  wrist dislocation in, 304
Electrical activity, pulseless, 40
Electrical alternans, 267
Electrical injury, 342-344
Electrocardiography
  in abdominal pain, 137
  in cardiogenic shock, 55
  in chronic renal failure, 535, 536
  in drug poisoning, 766
  in hypercalcemia, 678
  in hyperkalemia, 674
  in hypocalcemia, 682
  in hypokalemia, 675
  in hypomagnesemia, 686
  in irregular heart beat, 457, 458, 459
  in ischemic heart disease, 422-425, 426
  in myocardial contusion, 265
  in myocardial infarction, 126
  in pericardial tamponade, 267
  in pulmonary embolism, 127, 401-402
  in syncope, 91
  in unstable angina, 127
  in vertigo, 612
  wide-complex tachycardia in, 465, 466
Electrocautery in epistaxis, 824
Electroencephalogram, 208
Electrolytes
  abdominal pain and, 137
  calcium and, 677-683
  dehydration in child and, 804, 805
  in diarrhea, 172
  in drug screening, 765
  fluid and, 664-687; see also Fluid
    basal requirements for, 666
    distribution of, 664, 665
    regulatory mechanisms for, 666-671
  magnesium and, 683-687

Electrolytes—cont'd
  potassium and, 671-677
  sodium and, 666-671
  in vomiting, 161, 162
Electromechanical dissociation; *see*
    Pulseless electrical activity
Electroporation, 342
Elemental metals, burns from, 340
Elemental sodium, 339
Elevated arm stress test, 420
Elimite; *see* Permethrin
ELISA; *see* Enzyme-linked immunosorbent
    assay
Ellis classification of tooth fracture, 240-241
Embolic stroke, 600, 601; *see also*
    Cerebrovascular accident
  hypertension and, 440
  management of, 604
Embolism
  arterial disease and, 410, 411
    peripheral, 416
    searching for source of, 412-413
  pulmonary; *see* Pulmonary embolism
Emergency medical technicians, 60
Emergency medicine
  history of, as specialty, 3-4
  interfaces of, with other specialties, 5
  medical student education and, 5
  research in, 5
  residency training in, 4-5
Emergency patient
  initial priorities for, 7-8
  subjective and objective improvement in,
    10-11
  work-up for, 10
Emesis, 154, 472-473; *see also* Vomiting
Eminence, malar, 232
Emphysema, 20, 21
  in chronic obstructive pulmonary disease,
    385
  congenital lobar, 110
  respiratory distress and, 109
  subcutaneous, in orbital fracture, 234
EMTs; *see* Emergency medical technicians
Enalapril, 450, 451
  in pancreatitis etiology, 503
Encephalitis; *see* Meningitis and
    encephalitis
Encephalopathy
  hypertensive, 436-437
  tumor and, 575
Endarterectomy
  in thrombotic stroke, 604
  in transient ischemic attacks, 604
Endocarditis, diagnosis of, 128
Endocrine disorders, 688-697
  adrenal insufficiency in, 695-696
  diabetes in, 688-689
  hyperthyroidism in, 692-693
  hypothyroidism in, 694-695
  pancreatic tumors in, 504
  thyroid storm in, 693-694

Endometriosis, 176
Endophthalmitis, 842
Endoscopic retrograde
    cholangiopancreatography, 501
Endoscopy
  in esophageal dysphagia, 475
  in gastrointestinal bleeding, 148-149,
    150, 477
  in gastrointestinal foreign bodies, 478
Endotracheal intubation, 21-26; *see also*
    Intubation
  in asthma, 383
  in burn patient, 334
  in coma, 81
  in inhalation injury, 340
  in pediatric resuscitation, 26-27, 45
  in tetanus, 704
  tube for; *see* Endotracheal tube
Endotracheal tube
  in child, 794-795
  in multiple trauma, 63
  sizes of, 27
End-stage renal disease, 533
Enemas
  barium
    appendicitis and, 483
    Hirschsprung disease and, 487
    intussusception of colon and, 486
  for foodborne botulism, 707
Enophthalmos in orbital blowout fracture,
    829
Enoxacin, 510, 511
Entamoeba histolytica
  in brain abscess, 742
  in diarrhea, 170, 739, 742
Enteritis, regional, 484-485
Enterobacter organisms
  in meningitis and encephalitis, 618, 619
  in urinary tract infections, 514
Enterobiasis, 738, 740-741, 742
Enterobius vermicularis, 738, 740-741, 742
Enterococcus, 508, 511
Enterotoxin-induced diarrhea, 169-170
Enteroviruses, 587
  in meningitis and encephalitis, 618, 619
  in otitis media, 822
Entex LA; *see* Phenylpropanolamine
Entrapment of rectus muscle with orbital
    fracture, 233-234
Environmental injuries
  electric and lightning, 342-344
  of eye, 837-839
  heat- and cold-induced, 349-358
  near-drowning in, 345-348
  thermal and chemical, 333-341
Enzyme-linked immunosorbent assay
  in Lyme disease, 753
  in strongyloidiasis, 740
Enzymes, cardiac; *see* Cardiac enzymes
Ephedrine in wound repair, 288
Epidermal necrolysis, toxic, 588
Epidermal sutures, 236

Epidermis in wound cosmesis, 283
Epididymitis, 514-515
Epididymoorchitis, 515
Epidural hematoma, 228
Epidural spinal compression, 575
Epiglottitis
  in adult, 363, 365
  airway management in, 18
  in child, 795-799
  respiratory distress and, 112-113
Epilepsy, 201; *see also* Seizures
Epileptogenic focus, 205
Epinephrine
  in asthma in child, 802
  asystole and, 39, 40
  in beta-blocker toxicity, 774
  in cardiac arrest, 37
  in chronic obstructive pulmonary disease,
    387
  in croup, 799
  in epistaxis, 824
  in neonatal resuscitation, 44
  in pediatric resuscitation, 46
  in pulseless electrical activity, 40
  in ventricular fibrillation, 38
Epiphysis
  injury to, 296, 297
  slipped capital femoral, 317
Episcleritis, 842
Epistaxis, 824
  in gastrointestinal bleeding, 145
  in hemophilia, 566
  traumatic, 238
Epithelialization, 284
Epstein-Barr virus
  mononucleosis and, 722
  pharyngitis and, 362
    exudative, 361
Equilibrium, vertigo and, 608
ERCP; *see* Endoscopic retrograde
    cholangiopancreatography
Ergotamine
  migraine and, 99-100
  in pancreatitis etiology, 503
Erikson theory of development, 792
Erosions, gastric, 143
Eruption, drug, 588
Erysipelas, 585
Erythema chronicum migrans, 749-752
Erythema infectiosum, 587
Erythema multiforme, 593
Erythrocyte sedimentation rate, 73
  in giant cell arteritis, 580
  in polymyalgia rheumatica, 578
Erythrocytic stage schizonts, 733
Erythromelalgia, 418
Erythromycin
  in bronchitis, 366, 388
  in chlamydial cervicitis, 181
  in diphtheria, 700
  hearing loss from, 823
  in impetigo, 599

Erythromycin—cont'd
    in inclusion conjunctivitis, 841
    liver toxicity of, 497
    in Lyme disease, 753
    in lymphogranuloma venereum, 185
    in otitis media, 822
    in pelvic inflammatory disease, 184
    in pharyngitis, 363
    in pneumonia, 376
        in child, 803
    in relapsing fever, 750, 754
    in rheumatic fever, 195
    in scarlet fever, 592
    in urethritis, 512
    in urinary tract infection, 512
    in vertigo, 610
    in wound infection, 289
Escharotomy, 336-337
Escherichia coli
    in Bartholin abscess, 180
    diarrhea from, 165, 169, 170
    in infected aneurysm, 417
    in meningitis in child, 807
    tumors and, 572
    in urinary tract infections, 510, 511, 512,
        514
        in child, 513
Esmolol
    in aortic trauma, 270
    in atrial fibrillation, 463
    in atrial flutter, 461
    in atrial tachycardia with block, 461
    contraindicated in Wolff-Parkinson-White
        syndrome, 467
    in multifocal atrial tachycardia, 463
    in tetanus, 704
Esophagitis
    in AIDS and HIV, 730
    bleeding in, 144
    chest pain in, 122, 476
Esophagoscopy in caustic burns, 776
Esophagus, 472
    bleeding from, 145, 476
    caustic burn of, 775-776
    chest pain and, 475-476
    coin in, 478
    dysphagia and, 474-475
    injury to, 262
    intubation of, accidental, 26
    nutcracker, 475
    perforation of, 262, 476
        from foreign bodies, 478
    reflux in, 475
    spasm of, 475
        chest pain in, 122, 475-476
ESRD; *see* End-stage renal disease
Essential hypertension, 433
Estrogens
    in hypercalcemia, 678
    in pancreatitis etiology, 503
    venous thrombosis in, 400

Ethacrynic acid
    hazards of, 538
    in hypokalemia, 675, 676
    in pancreatitis etiology, 503
    in vertigo, 610
Ethambutol, 729
Ethanol toxicity, 772
    hepatitis from, 723
Ethchlorvynol, 782
Ethosuximide for seizures, 211, 212-213
Ethyl chloride spray, 633
Ethylene glycol
    acidosis from, 766
    toxicity of, 772, 773
Eurax; *see* Crotamiton
Eutrombicular alfreddugèsi, 746
Eutrombicular splendens, 746
Evisceration in abdominal trauma, 275, 276
Exanthem, macular, 586-587, 589-592
Exhaustion, heat, 349, 350, 351
Exotoxins
    diphtheria and, 698-699
    in toxic shock syndrome, 713
Expectorants in pneumonia, 375
Expiration, flail chest and, 256
Extensor mechanism in hand wound, 291
External cardiac massage in child, 47
External chest compression, 33, 34-35
External cooling for fever, 78
External hemorrhoids, 488
External otitis, 822-823
External rewarming, 355
External sphincter, 488
Extracellular fluid, 664, 665
    calcium and, 684
    dehydration in child and, 804
    magnesium and, 683, 684
    osmolarity of, 665
    potassium and, 672, 673
Extraocular movements, 828
    in coma, 84
    in stroke, 602
Extrapyramidal system, parkinsonism and, 644
Extremity
    arterial disease and, 410-420
    arteriosclerosis obliterans and, 415
    embolism and, 410, 411, 416
    in Kawasaki syndrome, 711
    lower; *see* Lower extremity
    thromboangiitis obliterans and, 415-416
    upper; *see* Upper extremity
Exudative pharyngitis, 361
Eye, 827-846
    acute vision loss in, 843-845
    central retinal vessel occlusion and, 843-844
    comatose patient and, 84
    electrical injury and, 343
    examination of, 827-829
        equipment for, 828
    fluorescein examination of, 831
    foreign body in
        conjunctival, 830

Eye—cont'd
    foreign body in—cont'd
        corneal, 830-831
        intraocular, 836
    glaucoma and, 843
    headache and, 97
    history of disorder of, 827
    infections of, 839-842
    injury to, 237-238, 829-839
        anterior chamber angle recession in, 833
        cataract in, 834
        conjunctival foreign bodies in, 830
        corneal abrasion in, 831
        corneal foreign bodies in, 830-831
        corneal lacerations in, 836-837
        environmental and chemical, 837-839
        globe rupture in, 835
        hyphema in, 832-833
        intraocular and orbital foreign bodies
            in, 836
        iridodialysis in, 833
        lens subluxation and dislocation in,
            833-834
        lid contusion in, 829
        lid lacerations in, 837
        mydriasis and miosis in, 833
        optic nerve, 835-836
        orbital blowout fracture in, 829-830
        retrobulbar hematoma in, 830
        scleral lacerations in, 836-837
        subconjunctival hemorrhage in, 831-832
        vitreous hemorrhage in,834
    ophthalmoplegic migraine, 99
    orbital fracture and, 233-234
    painful, 839-843
    patching of; *see* Patching of eye
    red, 839-843
    retina and; *see* Retina
    sclera of
        laceration of, 836-837
        orbital fracture and, 234
    stroke and, 602
    temporal arteritis and, 103, 844
    vertigo and, 608, 609, 611
    visual impulses of, 608, 609
Eyebrow injury, 235
Eyelid, 827-828
    examination of, 828
        after contusion, 829
    infection of, 839-840
    injury to, 238
        contusion in, 829
        laceration in, 837

F

Facial cellulitis, 585
Facial nerve in tetanus, 703
Facial trauma, 231-242
    dental injury in, 240-241
    eye injury and, 829-839; *see also* Eye,
        injury to
    fractures in, 232-234, 235

Facial trauma—cont'd
  general considerations for, 231-232
  mandibular fractures in, 234, 235
  maxillary fractures in, 232, 233
  ophthalmic injury in, 237-238
  orbital fractures in, 233-234
  otolaryngologic injury in, 238-240
  soft tissue injury in, 235-237
  zygomatic fractures in, 232-233
Facial weakness, stroke and, 602
Factor, coagulation, 563-567
  disorders of, 567-568
  replacement of
    in coagulation disorders, 568
    in disseminated intravascular
      coagulation, 570
Failure
  heart; *see* Heart failure
  renal; *see* Renal failure
  respiratory, 16, 17, 106; *see also*
    Respiratory distress
  in flail chest, 257
Fallopian tube
  pregnancy in, 135, 174
  torsion of, 174-175
  trauma to, 278-281
Family, grieving, 13-15
Famotidine, 476
Fanconi syndrome, 557
Fascia, abdominal wound and, 292
Fat pad sign, 306-307
Febrile seizures, 204, 812-813
  treatment of, 209-210
Fecal impaction, 489
Feet, arthritis in, 577
Feldene; *see* Piroxicam
Female patient
  genital tract trauma and, 278-281
  urinary tract infection and, 509-512
Femoral artery
  aneurysm of, 416-417
  auscultation of pulse in, 413
Femoral epiphysis, slipped capital, 317
Femur, fracture of, 317-319
Ferritin, serum, 558
Fetus
  abruptio placentae and, 552
  death of, 550
FEV_1; *see* Forced expiratory flow in 1
  second
Fever, 71-79
  arthritis and
    gonococcal, 193
    septic, 191
  assessment of, 71-74
  in child, 75-78, 813-816
  Colorado tick, 751, 759
  disposition of patient with, 74-75
  Eastern spotted, 758
  headache and, 96-97, 100
  in Kawasaki syndrome, 711-712
  laboratory evaluation in, 73-74

Fever—cont'd
  management of, 78
  Mediterranean coast, 758
  in meningitis, 807
  normal body temperature and, 71
  Q, 371
  relapsing, 750, 754-755
  rheumatic, acute, 194-195
  Rocky Mountain spotted, 589-590
  scarlet, 587, 591-592
  seizures and, 812-813
  thermoregulation and, 71
  tumors and, 572-573
  vomiting and, 156
FEV_1/FVC ratio, 116
Fibrillation
  atrial, 462-463
  in electrical injury, 343
  hypomagnesemia and, 686
  ventricular, protocol for, 38
Fibrinogen
  in hematologic disorders, 562, 564
  in pregnancy, 551
Fibrinolysis, 396, 400
Fibroblasts, 283, 284
Fibroids, uterine, 176-177
Fibula
  ankle sprain and, 325
  fracture of, 323
Fifth cranial nerve, herpetic neuralgia and,
    633
Fifth disease, 587
Finger
  arthritis in, 577
  labeling of, 296
  mallet, 300
  trauma to, 290-292
Fingernail, laceration through, 291
Fingerstick glucose test, coma and, 82
Fiorinal; *see* Butalbital
First-degree atrioventricular block, 467-469
First-degree burn, 333
Fissures, anal, 488
Fistula, arteriovenous, 420
  created for hemodialysis, 540
  physical examination in, 414
Fitz-Hugh-Curtis syndrome, 183
Flaccidity of rectal sphincter, 246
Flagyl; *see* Metronidazole
Flail chest, 256-257
  in chest trauma, 255
  in myocardial contusions, 258
Flaps in facial trauma, 236
Flash burn of eye, 837
Flexeril, 199
Flexor mechanism in hand wound, 291
Floaters, 834-835
Flu, 371, 375, 718-720
Fluconazole
  in bacterial vaginosis, 183
  in esophagitis in AIDS and HIV, 730
Fluid; *see also* Electrolytes

Fluid—cont'd
  amniotic, 554
  antidiuretic hormone and balance of,
    666-667
  aspiration of, 391
  basal requirements for, 666
  body distribution of, 664, 665
  calcium and, 677-683
  cerebrospinal
    in brain injury, 222
    in meningitis, 807-808
  culdocentesis and, 549
  distribution of, 664, 665
  impaired intake of, in hypovolemic
    shock, 52
  magnesium and, 683-687
  osmolarity of, 664-665
  potassium and, 671-677
  sodium regulation and, 666-671
  synovial
    classification of, 189
    in differential diagnosis, 190
    in pseudogout, 190-191
    in septic arthritis, 189, 190
  water regulation and, 666-671
Fluid retention, heart failure and, 448-449
Fluid therapy
  in abdominal pain, 133-134
  basic requirements for, 666
  in brain injury, 224
  in burns, 335-336
  in cardiogenic shock, 55
  in child, 794, 803-806
  in ectopic pregnancy, 549
  in heat illness, 351
  in hypovolemic shock, 53-54
  in intoxications, 762-763
  in ketoacidosis, 690-691
  in meningitis, 625
  in pulmonary trauma, 255
  in pyloric stenosis, 818
  in septic shock, 57
  in status epilepticus, 211
Flunisolide, 384
Fluorescein examination of eye, 831
  in corneal lacerations, 836
5-Fluorocytosine, 624
Fluphenazine decanoate, 633
Focal neurologic deficits
  in multiple sclerosis, 639-641
  in stroke, 601
Folate deficiency, 557
Foley catheter; *see* Catheter, Foley
Follicular cyst rupture, 175
Fontanelle, bulging, 72
Food
  aspiration of, 391, 392
  in headache, 101
  undigested, in vomiting, 155
Foodborne disease
  botulism as, 705-706
  diarrhea as, 736, 738

Foot
  gout in, 190, 191
  injury of, 325-329
  tinea pedis of, 584
  wound closure in, 292
Forced expiratory flow in 1 second
  in asthma, 380, 381, 382
  in chronic obstructive pulmonary disease,
    110, 386, 389
  in renal failure, 523
Forced expiratory volume, 116
Forced vital capacity, 116
  in chronic obstructive pulmonary disease,
    386
Forchheimer sign, 720
Forearm fracture, 306
Foreign body
  aspiration of, 391-394
    in child, 799-800
    pediatric resuscitation in, 45
  basic life support and, 35-36
  esophageal or tracheal, 477-478
    in child, 799-800
    in pediatric resuscitation, 45
  in eye, 836
    in conjunctiva, 830
    in cornea, 830-831
    intraocular and orbital, 836
  food as, 391
  in foot, 292
  in hand, 291
  ingestion of, 477-478
  rectal, 489
  in soft tissue injury, 284
  in stomach, 477-478
  urinary tract infection and, 507
  vaginal, 177
Foscarnet
  in cytomegalovirus, 717
  in herpes simplex, 717
Fourth-degree burn, 334
Fox eye shield
  in hyphema, 832
  in rupture of globe, 835
Fractionated low-molecular-weight heparin,
  405-406
Fracture
  alveolar bone, 241
  cast complications and, 299
  communication and definitions in,
    295-296
  cribriform plate, 223-224
  facial, 232-234, 235
  lower extremity, 316-329
    acetabular, 316-317
    of ankle, 323-324
    of femoral shaft, 318-319
    of foot, 325-329
    hip in, 317
    of knee, 319-322
    of leg, 322-323
    pelvic, 279, 316

Fracture—cont'd
  lower extremity—cont'd
    sacral, 316
    sciatic nerve injury in, 317
    of tibia, 322-323
  nasal, 238, 825
  orbital blowout, 829-830
  rib, 255-256
    flail chest and, 256-257
  skull, 219, 226
    epidural hematoma and, 228
  terms to describe, 295
  tooth, 240-241
  treatment methods for, 298-299
  upper extremity, 300-314
    of elbow, 306-307
    of forearm, 306
    of hand, 300-303
    of humerus, 308-313
    of shoulder and clavicle, 313-314
    of wrist, 303-306
Francisella tularensis, 368, 372, 750, 755
Frazier suction tube
  in epistaxis, 824
  in otitis externa, 823
Free erythrocyte protoporphyrin, 558
Free-basing of cocaine, 777
Freezing in Parkinson syndrome, 644
Frenulum injury, 239
Fresh frozen plasma
  after thrombolysis in pulmonary
    embolism or deep venous
    thrombosis, 408
  in gastrointestinal bleeding, 148
  in hypovolemic shock, 53
  in multiple trauma, 64
Freshwater drowning, 345
Freud theory of development, 792
Frostbite, 357
Fulminant meningococcemia, 709
Functional mental disorders, 647, 648, 649
  violence and, 660
Fundoscopy
  in comatose patient, 84
  in headache, 97
  in stroke, 603
Fungal infection
  macular lesion in, 584, 585
  in meningitis and encephalitis, 618, 620,
    621
  in pneumonia, 375, 376, 377
  tumors and, 572
Furazolidone, 170
  in giardiasis, 738
Furosemide
  in brain injury, 224
  in cardiogenic shock, 56
  in congestive heart failure, 448-449
  hearing loss from, 823
  in hypercalcemia, 680
  in hyperkalemia, 674
  in hypermagnesemia, 684

Furosemide—cont'd
  in hypertension, 438
  in hypokalemia, 675, 676
  in hypomagnesemia, 685
  in intracerebral hemorrhage, 605
  in meningitis, 625
  in pancreatitis etiology, 503
  in pulmonary edema, 452, 453, 538
  in renal failure, 580
    from electrical injury, 343
  in syndrome of inappropriate antidiuretic
    hormone secretion, 671
  in vertigo, 610
  in water intoxication, 671
Fusiform swelling in lupus erythematosus,
  580
FVC; see Forced vital capacity

G

Gait disturbances, 611, 612
  in Parkinson syndrome, 644
  in psychogenic weakness or paralysis,
    635
Galeazzi fracture, 306
Gallbladder, 500-502
Gallop, cardiac, 447
Gallstones, 500
Gamma globulin
  in hepatitis, 493
  in Kawasaki syndrome, 712
Ganciclovir
  adverse effects of, 730
  in cytomegalovirus infection, 717, 722
Gantanol; see Sulfamethoxazole
Gantrisin; see Sulfisoxazole
Gardnerella vaginitis, 182
Gas, blood; see Blood gas analysis
Gaseous distension in bowel obstruction,
  481
Gasoline sniffing, 780
Gastric erosions, bleeding from, 143
Gastric juice aspiration, 391
Gastric lavage
  in bleeding, 147
  in iron poisoning, 781
  in poisoning, 767
Gastric pain, 475-476
Gastrinoma, 504
Gastritis
  bleeding in, 144
  pain in, 476-477
Gastroenteritis, 716
  acute, 473
  differential diagnosis in, 12
  toxin-induced, 169-170
Gastroesophageal reflux, 157-160
Gastrointestinal tract
  in AIDS and HIV complications, 730
  bleeding in, 142-152, 477
    in abdominal trauma, 275
    admission criteria in, 150
    in carcinoma, 144

Gastrointestinal tract—cont'd
  bleeding in—cont'd
    clinical presentation of, 145
    etiology of, 142-145
    evaluation of, 145-147
    in hemodialysis, 541
    history of, 146
    indications for emergency procedures
      in, 150
    laboratory tests for, 146-147
    in lower tract, 144-145
    management guidelines for, 150-152
    physical findings in, 146
    posture in, 146
    surgery for, 149-150
    treatment of, 147-150
    in upper tract, 142-144, 477
  in child, 816-819
  intestinal motility and, 165-166
  lower, 480-490
    anorectal disease in, 488-489
    appendicitis and, 482-483, 484
    bleeding in, 144-145
    colon disorders and, 486-487
    hernia in, 485-486
    mesenteric vascular occlusion and,
      483-484
    obstruction and; *see* Gastrointestinal
      tract, obstruction of
    regional enteritis and, 484-485
    ulcerative colitis and, 485
  obstruction of, 480-482
    lesions responsible for, 481
    mechanical causes of, 482
    vomiting in, 155, 157, 161
  parasitic infestation of, 736-742
  in renal failure, 532, 535
  upper, 472-479
    bleeding in, 142-144, 477
Gastroparesis, 154, 473
Gauze for burns, 337
Gaze in comatose patient, 84
GCS; *see* Glasgow Coma Scale
Gelatin sponge in epistaxis, 824
Generalized seizures, 202-205
  convulsive, 203-204
  nonconvulsive, 204-205
Genitourinary system disorders, 507-555
  acute, 507-519
    general principles of infections in,
      507-509
    hematuria in, 519
    infections in; *see* Genitourinary system
      disorders, infection in
    pelvic fracture in, 316
    scrotal mass in, 515-516
    trauma in, 278-281
    urinary lithiasis in, 517-519
    urinary retention in, 516-517
  infection in, 180-185, 507-515
    in females, 509-512
    herpes simplex and, 596

Genitourinary system disorders—cont'd
  infection in—cont'd
    in males, 513-515
    parasitic infestation in, 744-745
    pediatric, 512-513
    pelvic pain and, 174
    pregnancy and, 547-555
      first half of, 547-551
      second half of, 551-554
    renal failure and dialysis in, 520-546; *see*
      also Renal failure
Gentamicin
  in fever in child, 814
  in meningitis, 625
  in pelvic inflammatory disease, 184
  in tumor infection emergencies, 573
  in urinary tract infection, 510, 511
    in child, 513
German measles, 586, 591, 720-721
Gestational diabetes, 689
Gestational trophoblastic disease, 550
GFR; *see* Glomerular filtration rate
Giant cell arteritis, 418, 579-580, 844
  headache and, 103
Giardia, 736, 738, 742
  in diarrhea, 170
Gingival trauma, 240
Glands
  adrenal, 695-696
  meibomian lipogranuloma of, 839
  parotid
    laceration of, 236, 237
    parotitis and, 825
  thyroid, 692-694
    pharyngitis and, 362
Glasgow Coma Scale, 221
  airway assessment and, 16
  airway management and, 223
  in cerebral contusions, 226
  in comatose patient, 82
  in head injury, 221
    with paralysis, 225
  in penetrating cranial injury, 229
  in prehospital care team checking, 60
  in subacute subdural hematoma, 228
Glass in wound
  of face, 236
  of hand, 291
Glaucoma
  acute angle-closure, 843
  headache and, 97, 104
  intraocular pressure in, 828
Gliomas, seizures and, 207
Globe of eye
  injury to, 237-238, 833
    penetrating, 237, 238, 239
  rupture of, 835
Globulin, gamma, 493
Glomerular disease, 527-528
Glomerular filtration rate, 520
Glomerular proteinuria, 524
Glomerulonephritis, acute, 527-528

Glossina, 742
Glossopharyngeal neuralgia, 88
Glucagon
  in beta-blocker toxicity, 774
  in calcium channel blocker toxicity, 775
  in diabetes, 688
  hyperkalemia and, 672
  in hypoglycemia, 692
Glucagonoma, 504
Glucocorticoids
  in adrenal failure, 695-696
  in hypertension, 433
  in pemphigus vulgaris, 596
Glucose
  in dehydration in child, 806
  in diabetes, 688-689
  in hyperglycemic hyperosmolar
    nonketotic coma, 691
  in hyperkalemia, 674
  in hypoglycemia
    in coma, 81, 82-83
    in diabetes, 691-692
  in hyponatremia, 669, 670
  in hypothermia, 355
  intolerance to, 688-689
  in ketoacidosis, 690
  in neonatal resuscitation, 44
  in status epilepticus in child, 810
Glutethimide, 782
Glycerol
  in glaucoma, 843
  in pseudotumor cerebri, 642
Glycopyrrolate
  in cholelithiasis, 500
  in chronic obstructive pulmonary disease,
    387
Glycosylated hemoglobin, diabetes and, 689
Glycyrrhizic acid, 676
Goiter, 692-693
Gold salts
  liver toxicity of, 497
  in rheumatoid arthritis, 192, 578
Golytely in drug poisoning, 767
Gonadotropin, human chorionic, 547, 548
Gonococcal arthritis, 193, 194, 197
Gonococcal conjunctivitis, 841
Gonococcal dermatitis, 598, 599
Gonococcal urethritis, 514
Gonococcemia, 194
Gout, 190, 196
Grafts
  for burns, 337
  for hemodialysis access, 540
Gram-negative organisms
  cancer and, 572
  disseminated intravascular coagulation
    and, 568
  in fever, 73-74
  in meningitis and encephalitis, 618, 619,
    625
  in meningococcemia, 709-711
  in pneumonia, 376, 377

Gram-negative organisms—cont'd
  in urinary tract infection, 508
Gram-positive organisms
  cancer and, 572
  disseminated intravascular coagulation
      and, 568
  in fever, 73-74
  in meningitis and encephalitis, 618, 619
Grand mal seizures, 203
  in child, 809-812
Granulation, toxic, 73
Granulation in wound repair, 285
Granulocytopenia, tumors and, 572
Granuloma inguinale, 184
Graves disease, 692-693
Greenstick fracture, 296
Grey Turner sign, 502
Grief, 13-15
Griseofulvin, 584
Group A beta-hemolytic streptococcal
      infection
  in impetigo, 597-599
  in pharyngitis, 362, 363
  in pneumonia, 367, 372
  in rheumatic fever, 194
  in scarlet fever, 591
Guaiac test, 146
Guaifenesin, 366
Guillain-Barré syndrome, 630-631
Guilt feelings, 14
Gum, trauma to, 240
Gunshot wound
  abdominal, 277-278, 292
    computed tomography in, 278
    diagnostic peritoneal lavage and, 278
  in cardiovascular injuries to chest and
      neck, 270
Gyne-Lotrimin; see Clotrimazole

H

Haemophilus influenzae
  cellulitis and, 585
    periorbital, 840
  in child, 795, 796, 807, 809
  in conjunctivitis, 840
  in fever, 75
  meningitis and encephalitis and, 618,
      619, 621
    pediatric, 807, 809
    therapy for, 624, 625, 626
  in otitis media, 822
  in pharyngitis, 362
  in pneumonia, 368, 372, 376, 377
  in sickle cell disease, 559, 560
  in tracheitis, 796
Hallucinations in psychosis, 652, 653, 654
Hallucinogens, 779-780
Hallux, fracture of, 329
Halofantrine, 735
Haloperidol
  in chemical restraint, 662
  in psychosis, 652

Haloperidol—cont'd
  toxicity of, 497, 774, 782
Halothane, liver toxicity of, 495
Hamman sign, 125, 262
Hampton's hump, 402
Hand, arthritis in, 577
Hanging cast technique, 310
HAPE; see High-altitude pulmonary edema
Hard palate trauma, 239
Hare long-leg splint, 318
Hazardous materials team, 338
HAZMAT teams; see Hazardous materials team
HBcAg; see Hepatitis B surface antigen
HBeAg, 723
HBIg; see Hepatitis B immune globulin
HBsAg; see Hepatitis B surface antigen
HCG; see Human chorionic gonadotropin
HDCV; see Human diploid cell rabies vaccine
Head
  scalp of; see Scalp
  skull of; see Skull
Head injury, 219-230; see also Facial trauma
  assessment of, 220-223
  in child, 220
  concussion in, 225-226
  contusions in, 226-227
  hemorrhage in
    intracerebral, 229
    intracranial, 227-229
  management of, 223-225
  other injuries with, 220
  pathophysiology of, 219-220
  penetrating cranial, 229
  posttraumatic syndromes in, 229
  scalp in
    lacerations of, 225
    wound closure of, 289
  skull fracture in, 226
  in vertigo, 615
Headache, 94-105
  assessment of, 94-98
  of cervical origin, 104
  in giant cell arteritis, 579
  in glaucoma, 104
  inflammatory cause of, 103
  mechanisms of, 94
  in meningitis, 621
  migraine; see Migraine
  muscle contraction in, 101
  sinus, 104
  temporal relationships of, 94-95, 103
  traction, 101-103
  in trigeminal neuralgia, 95, 97, 103-104
  vascular, 98-101
Head-tilt lifts, 30, 31
Hearing, decreased, 823
Heart
  blunt trauma to chest and, 264-271;
      see also Cardiovascular system,
      trauma to
  cardiac arrest and, 29-49; see also
      Cardiac arrest

Heart—cont'd
  cardiogenic shock and, 54
  congenital disorders of, respiratory
      distress in, 113
  congestive heart failure and, 445-454; see
      also Heart failure
  contusions of, 258, 264-265
  dysrhythmias and, 455-471; see also
      Dysrhythmias
  in electrical injury, 343
  examination of, 125
  in heart block; see Heart block
  hypercalcemia and, 678, 679
  hypermagnesemia and, 684
  hypernatremia and, 669
  hypokalemia and, 675
  hypomagnesemia and, 686
  ischemic disease of, 421-432; see also
      Ischemic heart disease
  in Kawasaki syndrome, 711, 712
  in lightning injury, 343
  Lyme disease and, 750, 753
  myocardial infarction and; see Myocardial
      infarction
  in pericardial tamponade, 266-268
  potassium and, 672, 675-676
  respiratory distress and, 113
  shock management and, 54-57
  syncope and, 87, 88
Heart attack, 29-49; see also Cardiac
      arrest
Heart block, 467-470
  atrial tachycardia with, 461-462
  atrioventricular, 467-470
    in hypercalcemia, 678
    in syncope, 88, 91
  bundle branch, 425, 426
  complete, 469-470
    in myocardial contusion, 265
    in syncope, 88, 91
Heart failure, 445-454
  acute, 445-446
  chronic, 446
  high-output, 445
  hypertension in, 435, 440-441
  left-sided, 446
  low-output, 445
  physical findings in, 125
  pulmonary edema in, 452-453
  respiratory distress and, 107-109
  right-sided, 446
Heart murmur, fever and, 72
Heart rate
  congestive heart failure and, 447
  dysrhythmia and; see Dysrhythmias
  neonatal resuscitation and, 42
Heat
  body, in burn patient, 336
  in heat exhaustion, 349, 350, 351
  illness from, 349-354
  injury or illness from, 349-354; see also
      Hyperthermia

Heat—cont'd
injury or illness from—cont'd
predisposing factors for, 350
loss of, 349
Heatstroke, 350-351
Heavy metals, peripheral neuropathies in, 629
Heberden nodes, 192
Heimlich maneuver
choking and, 35-36
in foreign body aspiration, 393
Helicobacter pylori, 476
in diarrhea, 167, 168
Hemangioma
anemia and, 557
cerebral, seizures and, 207
Hemarthrosis in hemophilia, 567
Hematemesis, 145, 477
from swallowed blood, 145
Hematochezia, 145, 477
Hematocrit, 146, 150
in abdominal trauma, 273
in anemia, 557, 558
in pregnancy, 551
in sickle cell disease, 560
in vaginal bleeding, 178
Hematologic disorders, 556-571
anemia in, 556-558
hemolytic, 559-560
coagulation; *see* Coagulation disorders
disseminated intravascular, 568, 569-570
meningitis and encephalitis and, 621
hemostatic, 560-570
leukocytosis and leukopenia in, 570
platelet, 563-567
polycythemia in, 560
red blood cell disorders in, 556-560
in renal failure, 532, 535
sickle cell disease in, 559-560
vascular, 562-563
white blood cell, 570
Hematoma
elbow fracture and, 307
epidural, 228
eyelid contusion and, 829
in hemophilia, 566
intubation methods in, 22
nasal septal, 238
retrobulbar, 830
stroke versus, 603
subchondral, 238-239
subdural, 227-228
headache and, 102-103
Hematosalpinx, 174
Hematuria, 519
causes of, 523-524
in hemophilia, 567
in renal failure, 523-524
Heme in urine in renal failure, 520
Hemidiaphragm, 260-261
Hemiplegic migraine, 99
Hemoccult test, 146

Hemodialysis, 539-542
in alcohol intoxication, 773
in chronic renal failure, 536
in drug poisoning, 767, 781, 785
Hemodynamic instability, 455
dysrhythmias in, 455
management of, 456
foreign body aspiration in, 393
Hemoglobin
in anemia, 556, 558
cardiac arrest and, 29
concentrations of, 557
by age, 556
mean corpuscular, 557
in red blood cell indices, 557
sickle cell, 559, 560
in vaginal bleeding, 178
Hemoglobinuria in acute renal failure, 529
Hemolysis, anemia and, 560
Hemolytic-uremic syndrome, 557
Hemoperfusion in drug poisoning, 767
Hemophilia, 564, 566-568
complications of, 568
Hemorrhage
in abdominal trauma, 275
anemia from, 560
in aortic tear, 268-270; *see also* Bleeding
cerebellar
management of, 605
physical findings in, 601
coma and, 80
in gonococcal arthritis, 193
intracerebral, 229, 600; *see also*
Cerebrovascular accident
management of, 605
physical findings in, 601
radiography of, 223
intracranial, 227-229
hypertension and, 440
in myocardial rupture, 265-266
in pregnancy, 548, 550, 551-552, 553
retinal, 835
in subdural hematoma in infant, 228
in shock, 52, 600
clinical presentation of, 601, 602
management of, 605-606
in soft tissue injury, 284
subarachnoid; *see* Subarachnoid
hemorrhage
subconjunctival, 831-832
subscleral, 234
in telangiectasia, 562
vitreous, 834
Hemorrhoids, 488
bleeding, 145
Hemostasis, 562
venous thrombosis and, 395-396
Hemostatic disorders, 560-570
Hemothorax, 260
Henoch-Schönlein purpura, 564
Heparin
coagulation disorders and, 564

Heparin—cont'd
in disseminated intravascular coagulation, 570
in embolic stroke, 604
fractionated low–molecular-weight, 405-406
hyperkalemia and, 672
in ischemic heart disease, 429
in pulmonary embolism or deep venous thrombosis, 405-407
thrombocytopenia and, 406, 563
in transient ischemic attacks, 604
Hepatic abscess, 498-499, 738, 739
Hepatic disease, 491-500
ketoacidosis versus, 691
Hepatitis, 491-495, 496, 717, 719, 722
immunization for, 492-493, 496
in meningitis and encephalitis, 618
nonviral causes of, 495
serum, 723; *see also* Hepatitis B
Hepatitis A, 722
Hepatitis B, 717, 719, 723
in viral arthritis, 195
Hepatitis B antigens, 492, 493, 494
Hepatitis B immune globulin, 723
Hepatitis B surface antigen, 723
Hepatitis C, 717
Hepatitis E virus, 491, 493
Hepatorenal syndrome, 498
Hepatotoxins, hepatitis from, 723
Heredity
Reiter syndrome and, 193
urticaria and, 589
Herniation
brain
coma in, 81
tumor and, 575
disk, 198
gastrointestinal tract, 485-486
orbital blowout fracture and, 829-830
Heroin in intoxication, 763
Herpes simplex virus, 717-718, 723
in corneal infection, 841, 842
genital, 180
in meningitis and encephalitis, 618, 619
in skin infection, 595, 596
tumors and, 572
Herpes zoster, 595, 597
in corneal infection, 841
neurologic disorders in, 632-633, 721
Herpes zoster ophthalmicus, 841-842
Herpetic neuralgia, 632-633
High-altitude pulmonary edema, 109
High-output congestive heart failure, 445
Hip
dislocation of, 294, 317-318
fracture of, 317
immobilization of, 299
Hirschsprung disease, 487
Histamine H$_2$ antagonists
in esophageal spasm, 475
in gastrointestinal bleeding, 148

Histamine H$_2$ antagonists—cont'd
  in peptic ulcer, 476
Histamine headache, 99
Histoplasma species
  in AIDS and HIV, 729
  in meningitis and encephalitis, 618
  tumors and, 572
History
  of emergency medicine as specialty, 3-4
  of patient
    with coma, 83
    in respiratory distress, 115
    with syncope, 89-90
  of peripheral arteriovascular disease,
    410-412
  of vertigo, 610-611
Hives, 588
Hollenhorst plaques, 413
Homatropine, toxicity of, 774
Hookworm infestations, 738, 741
  cutaneous, 745
  pulmonary, 743
Hoover sign, 635
Hordeolum, 839
Hormone
  antidiuretic
    fluid balance and, 666-667
    hyponatremia and, 670
    in dysfunctional uterine bleeding,
      179-180
    postmenopausal woman and, 177
    thyroid, 692-694
Horner syndrome, 246
Hospital
  admission to, 9
  discharge from, instructions for
    concussion patient and, 226
  prehospital-care team communication
    with, 60-61
Hospital attendants for trauma team, 61
HSV; *see* Herpes simplex virus
Human chorionic gonadotropin, 547, 548
Human diploid cell rabies vaccine, 724
Human immunodeficiency virus, 726-732
  altered mental status and, 85
  in esophagitis, 476
  herpetic neuralgia and herpes zoster and,
    633
  meningitis and encephalitis and, 621
Human tetanus immune globulin, 704-705
Humerus
  dislocation of, 296
  fracture of, 308-313
Hunt and Hess classification of
    subarachnoid stroke, 605, 606
HVS; *see* Hyperviscosity syndrome
Hydantoins, 212-213
Hydatid cysts, 743
Hydatidiform mole, 550
Hydralazine
  in congestive heart failure, 450, 451
  in heart failure, 450, 451

Hydralazine—cont'd
  in hypertension, 438
  in pregnancy, 442, 553
Hydration; *see* Fluid therapy
Hydrocarbon, toxicity of, 780
Hydrocephalus, normal pressure, 642-643
Hydrochlorothiazide, 448, 449
  hypokalemia from, 675
Hydrocortisone
  in Addisonian crisis, 696
  in hypothyroidism, 695
Hydrofluoric acid burn, 339
Hydrogen peroxide, 284
  in facial wounds, 237
Hydrosalpinx, 174
Hydroxyethyl starch, 53
5-Hydroxytryptamine, 100
Hydroxyzine
  in urticaria, 588
  in vomiting, 163, 164
Hygroton; *see* Chlorthalidone
Hymenal penetration in straddle injury, 279
Hyperadrenalism, 434-435
Hyperbaric oxygen
  in carbon monoxide poisoning, 340
  in multiple sclerosis, 641
Hypercalcemia, 677-680
  tumor and, 574
Hypercapnia in respiratory distress, 106
Hypercoagulable state in pregnancy, 551
Hyperemesis gravidarum, 550-551
Hyperglycemia
  in diabetes, 688
  hyponatremia and, 669
Hyperglycemic hyperosmolar nonketotic
    coma, 691
Hyperkalemia, 672-675
  in acute renal failure, 531
  in chronic renal failure, 536-538
Hypermagnesemia, 684
  in acute renal failure, 531
Hypernatremia, 668-669
  coma and, 81
Hyperosmolar nonketotic coma,
    hyperglycemic, 691
Hyperphosphatemia in acute renal failure,
    531
Hyperpnea, dyspnea versus, 106
Hypersensitivity, carotid sinus, 87-88
Hypertension, 433-444
  angina and, 440-441
  aortic dissection and, 442-443
  in aortic trauma, 269, 270
  arteries and, 433
  causes of, 434
  cerebrovascular accident and, 440-441
  coma and, 83
  congestive heart failure and, 440-441
  in drug poisoning, 768
  emergencies in; *see* Hypertensive
    emergencies
  emergency department assessment in, 435

Hypertension—cont'd
  encephalopathy and, 436-437, 440
  headache and, 100-101
  intracranial
    airway placement and, 82
    coma and, 81, 82
    idiopathic, 641-642
  in intrarenal vascular disease, 529
  malignant, 437-440
  portal, anemia in, 557
  in pregnancy, 441-442
  pregnancy-induced, 552-554
  pulmonary edema and, 440
  renal failure and, 441
  in scleroderma, 581
  in superior vena cava syndrome, 573
Hypertensive emergencies, 435-443
  in aortic dissection, 442-443
  with cerebrovascular accident, 440
  with congestive heart failure and angina,
    440-441
  encephalopathy in, 436-437
  malignant hypertension in, 437-440
  of pregnancy, 441-442, 552-554
  with pulmonary edema, 440
  with renal failure, 441
  stroke and, 603
Hyperthermia
  coma and, 81
  in drug poisoning, 764, 769
  fever and; *see* Fever
  in heat illnesses, 349-354
  in toxic syndromes, 764
Hyperthyroidism, 692-693
Hypertonic saline, 671
Hypertrophic subaortic stenosis, 88
Hyperuricemia
  gout and, 190
  tumors and, 574
Hyperventilation
  in brain injury, 224
  in intracerebral hemorrhage, 605
  with metabolic acidemia, 106
  psychogenic, 20, 113
Hyperviscosity syndrome, 574
  tumor, 574
Hyphema, 832
  iridodialysis with, 833
Hypnotics
  overdose of, 782-783
  in syncope, 89
  toxicity of, 782-783
    respiratory center and, 762
    in sympatholytic syndrome, 765
Hypocalcemia, 680-683
  in acute renal failure, 531
Hypoglycemia
  diabetes and, 691-692
  stroke versus, 603
  in syncope, 88-89
Hypokalemia, 675-677
  in vomiting, 160

Hypomagnesemia, 684-687
Hyponatremia, 669-671
  dehydration and, 668
Hypoperfusion in shock, 50
Hypopyon, 841
Hypotension
  abdominal pain and, 135-136
  in cardiogenic shock, 54, 55
  in chest injury, 255
  in chest trauma, 255
  in coma, 83
  in dehydration, 668
  in drug poisoning, 768
  in hemodialysis, 541
  in hypermagnesemia, 684
  in pericardial tamponade, 267
  in pregnancy, 551
  pulmonary edema and, 452, 453
  in spinal injury, 243, 246
  in toxic shock syndrome, 714
Hypothalamic control of body temperature,
    71
Hypothenar hammer syndrome, 417
Hypothermia, 354-358
  coma and, 81
  in drug poisoning, 765, 769
  factors predisposing to, 352
  in near-drowning, 347
  physiology of, 353
  in toxic syndromes, 765
Hypothyroidism, 694-695
  anemia in, 557
Hypovolemia
  in foreign body aspiration, 393
  in multiple trauma in pregnancy, 66
  pulseless electrical activity and, 40
  vomiting and, 156
Hypovolemic shock, 51, 52-54
  in child, 806
  in pelvic fractures, 316
Hypoxemia, 29
  airway management in, 19
  in coma, 81
  in foreign body aspiration, 393
  in near-drowning, 347
  in neonatal resuscitation, 44
  in respiratory distress, 106
  tissue, smoke inhalation and, 340
Hysteria malingering, 634

I

IABP; *see* Intraaortic balloon counterpulsation
Iatrogenic disorders
  esophageal perforation in, 262
  hypoglycemia in diabetes in, 691
  pericardial tamponade in, 266
Ibuprofen
  in dysmenorrhea, 177
  in fever, 78
  in frostbite, 357
  in otitis media, 822
  in pharyngitis, 363

Ice chips in rapid cooling for heat illness, 351
Ice packs in ankle sprains, 324
Ictal characteristics in febrile seizures, 204
IDA; *see* Technetium 99m-labeled
    iminodiacetic acid
Idiopathic intracranial hypertension, 641-642
Idiopathic thrombocytopenic purpura,
    563-565
Idoxuridine, 718, 843
IHD; *see* Ischemic heart disease
Ileus
  in burn patient, 336
  vomiting in, 156-157
Imaging; *see* Computerized tomography;
    Radiography
Iminostilbenes, 212-213
Imipenem-cilastatin
  in pneumonia, 377
  in urinary tract infection, 511
Imipramine, toxicity of, 777
Immersion syndrome, 345
Immobilization
  in ankle sprains, 324-325
  in femoral shaft fracture, 318-319
  in rotator cuff tear, 314
  in spinal injury, 243-245
    in near-drowning, 347
Immune globulin
  in cytomegalovirus infection, 717
  in hepatitis, 493, 722
  in rabies, 724
  in varicella-zoster, 595, 722
Immune thrombocytopenia, 563-566
Immunization
  for diphtheria, 698
  for hepatitis, 492-493, 496, 722, 723
  for pertussis, 702-703
  in pneumococcemia, 709
  for polio, 724
  for rabies, 724
Immunoelectrophoresis, 624
Immunoglobulins in Lyme disease, 753
Immunologic disorders
  peripheral neuropathies in, 628, 629
  in renal failure, 535
Immunosuppressed patient
  cryptosporidiosis in, 739
  fever in, 74-75
    in child, 814
  herpetic neuralgia and herpes zoster in,
    633
  meningitis and, 621
  multiple sclerosis and, 641
Imodium; *see* Loperamide
Impaction
  cerumen, 823
  fecal, 489
  of fracture, 295
Impetigo, 597-599
IN SAD CAGES mnemonic, 656
Inactivated poliovirus vaccine, 724
Inapsine; *see* Droperidol

Inclusion conjunctivitis, 840-841
Incomplete miscarriage, 550
Inderal; *see* Propranolol
Index finger fracture, 303
Indomethacin
  in gout, 190
  in pancreatitis etiology, 503
Indwelling catheter, urinary tract infection
    and, 512; *see also* Catheter
Inevitable miscarriage, 550
Infant; *see also* Child; Neonate
  atopic dermatitis in, 588
  blood pressure in, 434-435
  botulism in, 715
  cardiopulmonary resuscitation in, 41-49,
    820-821
  fever in, 75, 76, 814
  Hirschsprung disease of, 487
  hypermagnesemia in, 684
  hypertension in, 434-435
  lumbar puncture in, 808
  meningitis and encephalitis in, 618,
    620-621
  streptococcal infection in, 361
  subdural hematoma in, 228
  sudden infant death syndrome in, 820
  tetanus in, 704
  urinary tract infection in, 512-513
Infarction
  cerebellar
    management of, 605
    physical findings in, 601
  coma and, 80
  myocardial; *see* Myocardial infarction
  vertebrobasilar, 601, 605
Infection, 698-761
  in acquired immunodeficiency syndrome,
    726-732
  AIDS and HIV in, 726-732
  of aneurysm, 417
  anorectal, 488-489
  in arthritis, 191-192
  bacterial, 698-715; *see also* Bacterial
    infection
  in botulism, 705-707
  bronchiolitis and, 800-801
  in burns, 337
  in cholangitis, 501-502
  in cirrhosis, 498
  in croup, 795-796, 797
  in diarrhea, 165-173
  in diphtheria, 698-700
  in disseminated intravascular coagulation,
    568
  in ear, 822-823
  in eye, 839-843
  genital, 180-185
    pelvic pain and, 174
  human immunodeficiency virus and,
    726-732
  in Kawasaki syndrome, 711-712
  in Lyme disease, 748-754

Infection—cont'd
  in meningitis, 617-627, 807-809; *see also*
    Meningitis and encephalitis
  in meningococcemia, 709-711
  in mononucleosis, 722
  in orchitis, 515
  parasitic disease in, 733-747
  in peritoneal dialysis, 543-544
  in pertussis, 701-703
  in pneumococcemia, 707-709
  in pneumonia, 367-374, 375, 376-377
    in child, 802-803
  in polio, 724
  in prostatitis, 514
  in rabies, 724
  in renal failure, 538-539
  respiratory tract, 361-378
    bronchitis in, 366
    lower, 366-378
    pneumonia in, 367-374, 375, 376-377
    upper, 361-366
  in shock, 57-58
  in sickle cell disease, 559-560
  in tetanus, 703-705
  tickborne, 748-761; *see also* Tickborne
    illnesses
  in toxic shock syndrome, 713-714
  tumors and, 572-573
  of vascular access, 540
  viral, 716-725; *see also* Viral infection
  vomiting with, 155
  wound, 288-289
Inferior myocardial infarction, 428
Inflammatory disorders
  anemia in, 557
  in appendicitis, 482-483, 484
  in arthritis, 192-195, 196-197, 577-578
  in atopic dermatitis, 585-588
  of bowel
    in diverticular disease, 487-488
    venous thrombosis in, 400
  coma and, 81
  in cystitis, 512, 513-514
  in epididymitis, 514-515
  of eye, 839-843
    in blepharitis, 839
    in conjunctivitis, 840-841
    in cornea, 841-842
    in dacryocystitis, 839-840
    in episcleritis and scleritis, 842
    in globe and orbit, 842
    in periorbital cellulitis, 840
    in traumatic iritis, 832
    in uveal tract, 842
  in headache, 103
  intrascrotal, 514-515
  of meibomian gland, 839
  in odynophagia, 475
  in orchitis, 515
  in prostatitis, 514
  referred pain and, 133
  in Reiter syndrome, 193

Inflammatory disorders—cont'd
  in relapsing polychondritis, 582
  in sinusitis, 365-366
  in tendinitis, 192, 196
  in urethritis, 512, 514
  in uveal tract, 842
  in vascular disease, 413
Influenza virus, 371, 375, 718-720
  in otitis media, 822
  in pharyngitis, 362
Infraorbital nerve injury, 829
Infrapopliteal arterial occlusion, 416
Ingestion of foreign body, 477-478
Inguinal hernia, 485-486
Inhalation injury
  in carbon monoxide poisoning, 776
  hydrocarbons and, 780
  smoke, 340
Initial priorities for emergency patient, 7-8
Initial survey
  for multiple trauma, 64-65
  of wound, 283
Inoculum, aspiration of, 391
Inotropic agent
  in calcium channel blocker toxicity, 775
  congestive heart failure and, 451-452
Insecticide toxicity, 765
Inspection
  of abdomen in vomiting, 156-157
  of nose and throat in airway assessment, 20
Inspiration, flail chest and, 256
Insulin
  in diabetes, 688, 689
  in hyperglycemic hyperosmolar
    nonketotic coma, 691
  in hyperkalemia, 531, 674
  in hypomagnesemia, 685
  in ketoacidosis, 690
Insulinoma, 504
Intercostal nerve block, 255
Intercostal vessel in rib fracture, 255
Interferons in hepatitis, 717
Intermittent claudication, 412
  in arteriosclerosis obliterans, 415
Internal hemorrhoids, 488
Internal sphincter, 488
International Classification of Epileptic
    Seizures, 203
Internuclear ophthalmoplegia, 640
Interphalangeal joints, arthritis of, 577
Interstitial fluid, 664, 665
Interstitial nephritis, 527
Intestine; *see* Gastrointestinal tract
Intoxication
  alcohol, 772-773
  coma and, 81
  initial stabilization in, 762-763; *see also*
    Toxicology
  water, furosemide in, 671
Intraaortic balloon counterpulsation, 56-57
Intracellular cation, 671-672
Intracellular fluid, 664, 665

Intracellular fluid—cont'd
  dehydration in child and, 804
  osmolarity of, 665
  potassium and, 672
Intracerebral abscess, 97, 102
  amebiasis and, 742
  in meningitis and encephalitis, 620
  stroke versus, 603
Intracerebral hemorrhage; *see* Hemorrhage,
    intracerebral
Intracranial hemorrhage, 227-229
  hypertension and, 440
Intracranial hypertension, idiopathic,
    641-642
Intracranial pressure
  airway placement and, 82
  brain injury and, 220
  coma and, 81, 82
  in meningitis and encephalitis, 622
  in subarachnoid hemorrhage, 606
Intraocular foreign body, 836
Intraocular pressure in glaucoma, 828, 843
Intraosseous puncture, 44
Intrarenal vascular disease, 528-529
Intrascrotal inflammatory disorders, 514-515
Intrauterine device in ectopic pregnancy,
    548
Intravenous access
  in abdominal pain, 133-134
  advanced life support and, 36
  burn area and, 336
  in chest pain management, 129
  in gastrointestinal bleeding, 148
  multiple trauma and, 62-64, 65
Intravenous fluid therapy; *see also* Fluid
    therapy
  in brain injury, 227
  cardiac arrest and, 37
  in ectopic pregnancy, 549
  in gastrointestinal bleeding, 148
  in hyperemesis gravidarum, 551
  in hypothermia, 355
  in hypovolemic shock, 53-54
  in vomiting, 162
Intravenous pyelography
  in kidney trauma, 280, 281
  in lithiasis, 518
  in renal failure, 522
Intrinsic acute renal failure, 527-530
Intubation
  airway management and, 21-26
  complications of, 26
  in child, 26-27, 45-47, 794-795
  endotracheal; *see* Endotracheal intubation
  in head injury, 223-224
  indications for difficult, 22
  nasotracheal
    blind, 21
    in child, 26-27
    coma and, 82
  oral
    awake, 21, 22

Intubation—cont'd
  oral—cont'd
    complications of, 25-26
    cribriform plate fracture and, 223-224
    in trauma, 231
  orotracheal, spinal injury and, 245
  rapid sequence, 23-25
  tracheal, near-drowning and, 346
Intussusception, 145, 160, 486, 818
Invagination of bowel, 486, 818
Iodoquinol, 737
Ipratropium
  in asthma, 381
  in chronic obstructive lung disease, 387
IPV; *see* Inactivated poliovirus vaccine
Iridocyclitis, 842
Iridodialysis, 833
Iridotomy, 843
Iris
  in blunt injury to globe, 833
  inflammation of, 842
  prolapse of, at limbus, 836
Iritis, traumatic, 238, 832
Iron
  in pregnancy, 551
  serum, 558
  toxicity of, 767, 780-781
Iron deficiency anemia, 558
Iron saturation, 558
Irregular heartbeat, 456-459
  premature atrial contractions in, 445-457
  premature ventricular contractions and,
    457-459
  tachycardia in
    irregular narrow-complex, 462-463, 464
    regular narrow-complex, 458, 459-462
    wide-complex, 465, 466
Irregular narrow-complex tachycardia,
    462-463, 464
Irregular wide-complex tachycardia, 465, 466
Irrigation of eye in chemical burns
  acid, 838
  alkali, 838
  thermal, 838
Ischemia
  in arterial disease, 410, 412
  brainstem, vertigo in, 614
  in mesenteric vascular occlusion, 484
  myocardial, 421-432; *see also* Ischemic
    heart disease
  stroke and, 440
Ischemic attack, transient, 601
  management of, 604
  in syncope, 88
Ischemic heart disease, 421-432; *see also*
    Myocardial infarction
  assessment in, 421-427
  cardiac enzymes in, 427
  cardiac sonography in, 427
  chest pain in, 122
  chest radiography in, 427
  clinical presentation of, 427-429

Ischemic heart disease—cont'd
  differential diagnosis in, 427
  history of, 421-422
  management of, 429-431
  pain in, 421
  physical examination in, 422
Ischemic stroke, 600-602
  hemorrhagic, 602
    management in, 605-606
  management in, 604-605
Isoenzymes, pancreatic, 273
Isoniazid
  liver toxicity of, 495, 497
  in pancreatitis etiology, 503
  in tuberculosis with AIDS and HIV, 729
Isopropyl alcohol toxicity, 772-773
Isoproterenol
  in asthma in child, 802
  in beta-blocker toxicity, 774
  theophylline clearance and, 383
Isordil; *see* Isosorbide
Isoretinoin, 503
Isosorbide, 451
Isotonic dehydration, 805
IUD; *see* Intrauterine device
Ivermectin, 738
Ixodes dammini, 748, 749, 750, 751, 758
Ixodes pacificus, 749, 750

J

J wave, electrocardiographic, 354
Jacksonian epilepsy, 205
Jarisch-Herxheimer–type reaction, 754
Jaundice
  in hepatitis, 496
  in liver disease in pregnancy, 499
Jaw thrust, 30, 32
Jimsonweed poisoning, 765, 774
Joint
  arthritis in, 190-195, 196-197, 577
  pain in, 187-200
    assessment of, 187-190
    lumbosacral, 195-199
    monoarticular arthritis in, 190-192,
      196-197
    pathophysiology in, 187, 188
    polyarticular arthritis in, 192-195,
      196-197
Jones fracture, 329
Jugular venous pressure in heart failure, 447

K

Kaopectate, 595
Kawasaki syndrome, 711-712
Kayexalate; *see* Sodium polystyrene sulfonate
Kehr sign, referred pain and, 133
Keratitis
  herpes simplex, 841
  ultraviolet, 837
Keratoconjunctivitis
  chlamydial, 841
  in newborn, 723

Kerlex dressings for burns, 337
Kerley A and B lines, 447
Kernig sign, 621
  in meningitis in child, 807
Ketamine
  in facial laceration suturing, 236
  in intubation, 23, 383
Ketoacidosis, 690-691
  hyperkalemia and, 672
  hypomagnesemia and, 685
  vomiting and, 161
Ketoconazole
  liver toxicity of, 497
  in meningitis and encephalitis, 624
Ketone testing, 689, 690
Ketorolac, 518
Kidney, ureter, and bladder examination, 281
Kidney failure; *see* Renal failure
Kidney pain, 133
Kidney trauma, 279-281
Kirschner wire in metacarpal fracture, 303
Klebsiella, 368, 372
  tumors and, 572
  in urinary tract infections, 510, 511, 514
Kling dressings for burns, 337
Knee
  dislocation of, 294, 322
  fracture of, 319
  hip dislocation and, 318
  splinting of, 299
  sprains of, 319-322
Knife injury to chest, 261
KOH; *see* Potassium hydroxide
Koplik spot in measles, 589, 720
KUB examination; *see* Kidney, ureter, and
    bladder examination
Kussmaul respirations, 82
  in ketoacidosis, 690
Kwell, 594
K-Y jelly in hydrofluoric acid burn, 339

L

Labetalol in hypertension, 439
  with encephalopathy, 437
  in pregnancy, 442, 553-554
Labored respirations, 20
Labyrinth disorders, 613, 615
Labyrinthitis, 613, 615
Laceration
  dental injury and, 240-241
  of ear, 239
  in eye trauma, 837
  of eyelid, 238
  facial, 235-237
  of foot, 292
  of hand, 290-292
  of mouth and lips, 289-290
  of penis, 279
  of scalp, 225, 289
    closure in, 289
  soft tissue; *see* Soft tissue, trauma to
Lactate dehydrogenase in AIDS and HIV, 728

Lactated Ringer's solution; see Ringer's lactate
Lactic acidosis
  diabetes and, 691
  in drug poisoning, 766
  vomiting and, 161
Lactulose in constipation from antacids, 545
Laparoscopy, 277
Laparotomy
  adnexal torsion after, 174
  clinical indications for, 272-273
Larva migrans, cutaneous, 745
Larvae, Trichinella spiralis, 744
Laryngotracheal foreign body, 392
  in child, 799-800
Laryngotracheobronchitis, 113
Larynx
  in diphtheria, 698-699, 700
  injury to, 240
Laser therapy in cirrhosis, 498
Lasix; see Furosemide
Lateral sclerosis, primary, 643
Lavage
  esophageal perforation and, 262
  gastric
    in bleeding, 147
    in iron poisoning, 781
    in poisoning, 767
  peritoneal
    in abdominal trauma, 272, 273-274, 277
    in diaphragm injury, 261
Lavage amylase in abdominal trauma, 274
Lavage lipase in abdominal trauma, 274
LDH; see Lactate dehydrogenase
L-dopa; see Levodopa
Lead poisoning, 557
LeFort fracture, 232, 233
Left-sided heart failure, 108, 446
Legionella pneumophila, 369, 373, 376, 377
Leiomyoma, uterine, 176-177, 178
Leishmaniasis, 745
Lens, subluxation of, 833-834
Lethargy, 80
Leukocyte esterase test, 508
Leukocytes
  in cerebrospinal fluid, 623
  polymorphonuclear, 73
Leukocytosis, 570
  in pertussis, 702
  in pneumococcemia, 708
Leukopenia, 570
  in septic shock, 57
Levodopa, 644, 645
Levothyroxine, 695
Lhermitte sign, 639
Lice, 593-594, 745-746, 750
Lid; see Eyelid
Lidocaine
  in cardiac arrest, 37
  in dysrhythmias from poisoning, 768
  in herpes simplex, 595
  in intubation, 24
  in ischemic heart disease, 430

Lidocaine—cont'd
  in pediatric resuscitation, 46
  in premature ventricular contractions,
    457-459
  in status epilepticus, 214
  in ventricular fibrillation, 38
  in ventricular tachycardia, 38, 39, 465
  wound closure and, 285, 288
Life support
  advanced, 36-40
  basic, 30-36
  in penetrating brain injury, 229
Life threat, 8-9
Ligament
  ankle sprains and, 324-325
  knee injury and, 320-322
  of Treitz, 483
Light reflex, pupillary, 84, 828
Lightning injury, 342-344
Limb; see Extremity
Lime, burn from, 339
Lindane, 594, 746
Linton tube, 149
Lip
  laceration of, 235-237
  vermilion border of, 290
  wound closure for, 289-290
Lipase
  lavage, in abdominal trauma, 274
  serum
    in abdominal trauma, 273
    in pancreatitis, 502
Lipid aspiration, 391
Lipogranuloma of meibomian gland, 839
Liquiprin; see Acetaminophen
Lisfranc fracture dislocation, 325
Lisinopril, 450, 451
Listeria monocytogenes, 618, 619, 621,
    624, 625
  in child, 807
Lithiasis; see Stones
Lithium
  in hypercalcemia, 678
  in migraine, 100
  toxicity of, 767, 781-782
    burns and, 339, 340
Little finger fracture, 303
Live attenuated oral poliovirus vaccine, 724
Liver disease, 491-500
  abscess in, 498-499, 738, 739
  alcoholic, 495-498
  cancer in, 499-500
  cirrhosis in, 498
  drug-induced, 495, 497
  hepatitis in, 491-495, 496
  in pregnancy, 499
Liver functions in abdominal trauma, 273
Livido reticularis, 413, 418
LMWH; see Fractionated low–molecular-
    weight heparin
Local anesthetics
  in oral injury, 239

Local anesthetics—cont'd
  in wound closure, 285-288
    of face, 236
  in wrist injury, 304
Löffler syndrome, 740
Lomefloxacin, 510, 511
Lomotil; see Diphenoxylate with atropine
Long finger fracture, 303
Long-leg splints, 318
Loniten; see Minoxidil
Loop diuretics, 448-449
  in cardiogenic shock, 56
Loperamide, 172
Lorazepam, 810, 812
  in chemical restraint, 662
  in psychosis, 652
  in seizures, 209
    from drug poisoning, 767
Loss of consciousness, 220-221; see also
    Coma; Mental status, altered
  in spinal injury, 243
Louse infestation, 593-594
Lovastatin, liver toxicity of, 497
Lower back pain, 315
Lower esophageal dysphagia, 474
Lower extremity; see also Extremity
  arterial aneurysm in, 416-417
  injury to, 316-329
    ankle in, 323-325
    femoral shaft fracture in, 318-319
    foot in, 325-329
    hip in, 317-318
    knee in, 319-322
    pelvic fracture in, 316
    sacral fracture in, 316
    tibial fracture in, 322-323
  splinting of, 299
  thromboangiitis obliterans and, 415-416
  wound closure in, 292
Lower gastrointestinal tract; see
    Gastrointestinal tract, lower
Lower respiratory tract
  in child, 795, 800-803
  infection of, 366-379, 718-720
    bronchitis in, 366
    pneumonia in, 367-374, 375, 376-377
Lower urinary tract infection, 509-515
Low-molecular-weight dextran in central
    retinal artery occlusion, 844
Low-output congestive heart failure, 445
LSD; see Lysergic acid diethylamide
Ludwig's angina, 365
Lugol solution, 693
Lumbar back pain, 195-199
Lumbar disk disease, 198, 199
Lumbar puncture
  in AIDS and HIV, 729
  altered mental status and, 85
  in child, 807-808
  in fever, 77-78
  headache and, 98, 103
  in meningitis, 622-624

Lumbar puncture—cont'd
  in pseudotumor cerebri, 642
  in stroke, 604
Lumbosacral spinal injury, 314-315
Lunate bone dislocation, 303-304
Lund and Browder chart for burn
    estimation, 335
Lung; *see also* Pulmonary disorders;
    Respiratory distress
  carcinoma of, respiratory distress in, 113
  collapsed, 158-160
    reexpansion of, 109
  examination of, 125
  flail chest and, 256-257
  in pneumothorax, 258-260
  in smoke inhalation burn, 340
Lupus erythematosus, systemic, 580-582
Lye, ingestion of, 775-776
Lyme disease, 193-194, 197, 748-754
Lymph node in Kawasaki syndrome, 711
Lymphadenopathy, fever and, 72
Lymphocytosis in pertussis, 702
Lymphogranuloma venereum, 185
Lysergic acid diethylamide, 779-780
Lysis, tumor, 573-574

M

Maceration of scalp wound, 289
Macrolide antibiotics
  in pneumonia, 376, 377
  theophylline clearance and, 383
Macular exanthems, 586-587, 589-592
Macular lesion, 584-592
MADFOCS mnemonic, 648
Mafenide acetate, 337
Magnesium, 683-687
  in atrial tachycardia with block, 461
  in cathartics, hazards of, 707
  conversions for, 683
  functions of, 683
  hypocalcemia and, 681
  in multifocal atrial tachycardia, 463
Magnesium sulfate
  in asthma, 381
  in chronic obstructive pulmonary disease,
    387
  in hypomagnesemia, 687
  in pregnancy-induced hypertension, 442,
    553
Magnetic resonance imaging
  in intraocular and orbital foreign bodies, 836
  in orbital cellulitis, 842
  in pseudotumor cerebri, 642
Maissonneuve fracture, 324
Malar fracture, 232
Malaria, 733-736
  cerebral, 742
Malathion, 746
Male patient
  genital trauma in, 279
  urinary tract infection in, 513-515

Malignancy
  anemias in, 557
  anorectal, 489
  bleeding in
    cervical, 179
    vaginal, 178-179
  bowel obstruction and, 480
  emergencies related to, 572-576
  headache and, 101
  liver and, 499-500
  pancreatic, 505
  testicular, 516
  tumor lysis syndrome and, 573-574
  venous thrombosis in, 399
Malignant hypertension, 437-440
  in intrarenal vascular disease, 529
Mallet finger, 300
Mallory-Weiss tear, 143, 147
Mandibular fracture, 234, 235
Mannitol
  in acute renal failure, 580-581
  in head injury, 224
  in intracerebral hemorrhage, 605
  in renal failure from electrical injury, 343
Manometry
  in esophageal spasm, 475
  in odynophagia or achalasia, 475
Maprotiline, toxicity of, 777
Marcaine; *see* Bupivacaine
Marcus Gunn pupil, 828
Marfan syndrome, 581
Marijuana, theophylline clearance and, 383
Marrow, bone, tibial, 44
Mass
  adnexal torsion and, 174-175
  intracranial, headache and, 101
  ovarian, 175-176
  scrotal or testicular, 515-516
Massage, external cardiac, 47
MAST; *see* Military antishock trousers
Mastication in zygomatic fracture, 232-233
Mastoid air cells, 823
MAT; *see* Multifocal atrial tachycardia
Mature liver stage schizonts, 733
Maxillary fracture, 232, 233
McBurney point, 483
McMurry sign, 320
MCP; *see* Metacarpophalangeal joint
MDI; *see* Metered-dose inhaler
Mean corpuscular hemoglobin, 557, 558
Mean corpuscular hemoglobin
    concentration, 557
Mean corpuscular volume, 557, 558
Measles, 586, 589, 719, 720
Measles, mumps, rubella vaccine, 721
Mebendazole
  in amebiasis, 737
  in ascariasis, 737, 740
  in enterobiasis, 738, 741
  in hookworm infestations, 738, 741
  in *Trichinella spiralis* infestations, 744
  in trichuriasis, 738, 740

Mechanical ventilation; *see* Ventilation
Meclizine
  in vertigo, 615, 823
  in vomiting, 163, 164
Mediastinal shift, 256
Medical student education, 5
Mediterranean coast fever, 758
Medullary chemoreceptors, 106-107
  in chronic obstructive pulmonary disease,
    110
Mefenamic acid, 503
Mefloquine, 735
Megacolon
  Hirschsprung disease and, 487
  toxic, 485
Meibomian gland, lipogranuloma of, 839
Melena, 145
Membrane
  amniotic, rupture of, 554
  diphtheritic, 699
  tympanic
    bubbles seen through, 823
    rupture of, 822, 824
Ménière disease, 613
Meningitis and encephalitis, 617-627
  altered mental status in, 85
  assessment of, 621-624
  in child, 618, 814-816
  clinical presentation of, 620-621
  cryptococcal, in AIDS and HIV, 729
  etiology of, 618-620
  headache in, 97
  host factors in, 619
  laboratory tests for, 86
  management of, 624-626
  pathophysiology in, 617-618
  postinfectious, 620
  in sickle cell disease, 560
Meningococcemia, 589, 709-711
  chronic, 709
Meniscal tear of knee, 320-322
Menopause, pelvic pain after, 177
Menorrhagia, 179
Menstrual cycle
  dysfunctional uterine bleeding and, 179
  dysmenorrhea and, 177
  normal, 178
Mental status
  altered, 80-86
    approach to patient with, 81-86
    etiology of, 80-81
    examinations for, 83-86
    history of patient with, 83
    monitoring of, 85
    therapy for, 86
  in concussions, 226
  in fever, 72
  in hypernatremia, 669
  in intussusception of colon, 486
  in meningitis, 621
  in psychosis, 649, 650
  in spinal injury, 243, 245

Mental status—cont'd
  in suicidal behavior, 657
Meperidine
  in headache, 100
  in pancreatitis, 504
  in toxicology, 763, 782
  in urinary stone disease, 518
Mephenytoin, 211, 212-213
Mephobarbital, 212-213
Meprobamate, 782
Merozoites, 733, 734
Mescaline, 779-780
Mesenteric artery, superior, 483-484
Mesenteric vascular occlusion, 483-484
Metabolic acidosis
  in acute renal failure, 531
  in drug poisoning, 765-766
  in smoke inhalation burn, 340
  in vomiting, 160
Metabolic demands in airway management,
    20-21
Metabolic disorders, 664-697
  coma and, 81
  in diabetes mellitus, 689
  endocrine disorders in, 688-697
  fluids and electrolytes in, 664-687; *see
      also* Electrolytes; Fluid
  renal failure and
    acute, 531-532
    chronic, 534
  syncope and, 88-89
  vertigo and, 615
  vomiting and, 473
Metabolites, coma and, 81
Metacarpal injuries, 303
Metacarpophalangeal joint, arthritis of, 577
Metals
  elemental, burn from, 340
  heavy, peripheral neuropathies in, 628
Metastasis, brain, 575
Metatarsal fracture, 325-329
Metered-dose inhaler, 383
Methanol toxicity, 772, 773
  acidosis from, 766
Methocarbamol, 315
Methotrexate
  liver toxicity of, 497
  in rheumatoid arthritis, 192, 578
Methoxyflurane, liver toxicity of, 497
Methsuximide, 211, 212-213
Methylated spirits in phenol burn, 339
Methylated xanthine foods in headache, 101
Methyldopa
  liver toxicity of, 497
  in pancreatitis etiology, 503
Methylparaben, allergic reaction to, 285
Methylprednisolone
  in asthma in child, 802
  in chronic obstructive pulmonary disease,
      387
Methylxanthine toxicity, 786
Methysergide, 100

Metoclopramide
  in esophageal spasm, 475
  in headache, 100
  in vomiting, 163, 164
Metolazone, 448, 449
Metoprolol
  in ischemic heart disease, 430
  in multifocal atrial tachycardia, 463
Metronidazole
  in amebiasis, 737
  in bacterial vaginosis, 183
  contraindicated in pregnancy, 736, 745
  in diarrhea, 170
  Giardia lamblia and, 736, 738
  in hepatic abscess, 499
  in pancreatitis etiology, 503
  in pelvic inflammatory disease, 184
  in *Trichomonas vaginalis* infestations,
      182, 744-745
Metrorrhagia, 179
MFAT; *see* Multifocal atrial tachycardia
Miconazole, 584
  in candidiasis, 585
  in meningitis and encephalitis, 624
  in vaginitis, 183
Microcytic anemia, 558
Microgametocytes, 734
MicroNephrin; *see* Epinephrine
Micturition syncope, 89
Midamor; *see* Amiloride
Midazolam
  in intubation procedures, 22
  in paroxysmal supraventricular
      tachycardia, 459
  shoulder dislocation and, 311
  in ventricular tachycardia, 38
Middle ear effusions, 823
Middle phalangeal injury, 301
Migraine, 98-100
  family history of, 96
  stroke versus, 603
Migraine equivalents, 99
Migrainous neuralgia, 99
Military antishock trousers
  in hypovolemic shock, 54
  in pelvic fracture, 316
Milrinone, 451, 452
Mini-Mental Status Examination, 649, 650
  in suicidal behavior, 657
Minipress; *see* Prazosin
Minocycline, 610
Minor burn, 337-338
Minoxidil
  in congestive heart failure, 450
  in hypertension, 439
Miosis, traumatic, 833
Miracidia, 741
Miscarriage, 549-550
Missed abortion, 550
Missile injury
  to abdomen, 277-278
  in chest, 261

Mite infestation, 594, 745-746
Mithramycin, 680, 681
Mittelschmerz, 175
Mixed cholinergic syndrome, 765
Mnemonics
  COWS, 84
  DEMENTIA, 649
  MADFOCS, 648
  PET VICTIMS, 81
  IN SAD CAGES, 656
  SLUD, 765
  WHHHIMP, 648
Mobiluncus organism vaginosis,
    182-183
Mobitz atrioventricular blocks, 468, 469
Mole, hydatidiform, 550
Monistat; *see* Miconazole
Monitoring
  in chest pain management, 129
  in multiple trauma, 64
Monoarticular arthritis, 190-192
  overview of, 196-197
Monocular diplopia, psychogenic, 636
Monofilament plastic sutures, 287
Mononeuropathy, 628
Mononeuropathy multiplex, 628
Mononucleosis, 722
Monospot test, 722
Monteggia fracture, 306
Mood, suicidal behavior in, 657
Mood disorders, 654
Moraxella organisms, 376, 377, 822
Morphine
  in cardiogenic shock, 56
  in intoxication, 763
  in ischemic heart disease, 430
  in pulmonary edema, 452, 453, 538
  in urinary stone disease, 518
Motility
  colonic, 487-488
  diarrhea and, 165-166
Motility disorders, vomiting in, 154
Motor activity in spinal injury, 246-247
Motor function
  in dysphagia, 473
  in hand wound, 291
  in headache, 97
  in stroke, 602
  in subacute neuropathies, 629
Mouth
  bleeding from, 145
  trauma to, 239
  wound closure in, 289
Mouth-to-mask ventilation, 33
Mouth-to-mouth ventilation
  in basic life support, 30-33
  in pediatric resuscitation, 45
Mouth-to-nose ventilation, 30-33
Movement in coma, 84
MPTP, parkinsonism from, 645
Mucocutaneous herpes, primary, 723; *see
    also* Herpes simplex

Mucocutaneous lesions in leishmaniasis, 745
Mucosa, ulcerative colitis and, 485
Mucosal suture, 236
Multifocal atrial tachycardia, 463-464
Multiple sclerosis, 638-641
Multiple trauma, 60-68
  airway assessment in, 62, 63
  airway management in, 18-19
  assessment of, 61-62
  in child, 65-66
  diagnostic tests for, 65
  initial injury survey in, 64-65
  management of, 65
  in pregnancy, 66
  priorities in, 66-67
  resuscitation in, 62-64
  special concerns in, 65-66
  transfer of patients in, 67
  trauma team for, 60-61
Mumps, 719, 721
  in meningitis and encephalitis, 618, 619
Mupirocin, 599
Murmur, heart, fever and, 72
Murphy sign, 501
Muscle
  of defecation, 488
  headache and, 101
  hypernatremia and, 669
  hypokalemia and, 675
  hypomagnesemia and, 686
  tetanus and, 703-705
Muscle contraction headache, 101
Muscle relaxants
  in back pain, 199
  in migraine, 100
Muscle spasm; *see* Spasm
Muscular atrophy, progressive spinal, 643
Musculoskeletal disorders
  in Lyme disease, 753
  in renal failure, 535, 545
  rheumatologic and connective tissue
    diseases and, 577-583
  spinal injury in, 252
Mushroom poisoning, 765, 774
Mutilating trauma of penis, 279
Mycobacterium avium-intracellulare, 842
Mycobacterium tuberculosis, 371, 377
  in AIDS and HIV, 729
  in meningitis and encephalitis, 618
Mycoplasma organisms, 371, 374, 375, 377
  in meningitis and encephalitis, 618
  in pharyngitis, 362
  in pneumonia, 374, 375, 376, 377
    in child, 803
  in sickle cell disease, 560
  tuberculosis and, 371, 377
  in vaginosis, 182-183
Mycotic aneurysm, 417
Mydriacil; *see* Tropicamide
Mydriasis, traumatic, 833
Mydriatics, 828
Myelinolysis, central pontine, 671

Myelitis, transverse, 640
Myerson sign, 644
Myocardial concussion, 264
Myocardial contusion, 258, 264-265
Myocardial infarction, 421
  acute, 428-429
    anterior wall, 428
    venous thrombosis in, 400
  cardiac enzymes in, 427
  chest pain in, 120, 122, 421
    duration of, 123
  chest radiography in, 427
  cocaine and, 777
  diagnostic tests for, 126-127
  electrocardiography in, 422-425, 426
  in hemodialysis, 541-542
  ischemia in, 421; *see also* Ischemic heart
    disease
  Kawasaki syndrome and, 712
  management of, 429-431
  physical findings in, 125
  risk factors in, 123-124
  sudden death in, 429
  traumatic, 264
  unstable angina and, 428
Myocardial mechanoreceptors, syncope
  and, 86
Myocardial rupture, 264, 265-266
Myocarditis, *Trichinella spiralis* in, 744
Myocardium
  in cardiogenic shock, 54, 55
  contusions of, 258, 264-265
  electrical injury and, 343
  ischemia of, 421-432; *see also* Ischemic
    heart disease
Myoglobin, 427
  in myocardial infarction, 126
Myoglobinuria, 519
  in acute renal failure, 529
Mysoline; *see* Primidone
Myxedema coma, 694-695
Myxoma, atrial, 88

N

NAC; *see* N-Acetyl-L-cysteine
NADH; *see* Nicotinamide adenine
  dinucleotide
Naegleria, 742
Nafcillin
  in cellulitis, 585
  in meningitis, 625
  in pneumonia in child, 803
  in staphylococcal scalded skin syndrome,
    588
  in toxic epidermal necrolysis, 588
  in tumor infection emergencies, 573
Naloxone
  coma and, 83
  in meningitis and encephalitis, 624
  narcotic overdose and, 763, 783
  in neonatal resuscitation, 44
  status epilepticus in child and, 810

Naproxen, 177
Narcan; *see* Naloxone
Narcosis, carbon dioxide, 21
Narcotics
  in abdominal pain, 141
  antagonists to; *see* Naloxone
  bradycardias from, 465
  for burn patients, 336
  in headache, 100, 101
  in herpetic neuralgia and herpes zoster, 633
  in ischemic heart disease, 430
  respiratory center and, 762, 763, 782
  toxicity of, 762, 763, 782-783
Nares, inspection of, 20
Narrow-complex tachycardia
  irregular, 462-463, 464
  regular, 458, 459-462
Nasal biphasic airway pressure, 388
  in pulmonary edema, 453
Nasal bleeding, 824
  traumatic, 238
Nasal fracture, 238, 825
Nasal speculum in epistaxis, 824
Nasogastric tube
  in abdominal pain, 134
  in child, 794-795
  in esophageal injury, 262
  in gastric bleeding, 147
Nasopharyngeal airway, 30
Nasopharyngeal infection, 361-364
Nasotracheal intubation
  in child, 26-27
  in coma, 82
Nausea, 472
  in pregnancy, 550-551
  and vomiting, 154
    in renal failure, 545
Navicular fracture of wrist, 303
Near-drowning, 345-348
  hypothermia in, 347
Necator americanus, 738, 741
  in pulmonary disorders, 743
Neck; *see also* Cervical spine
  femoral, fracture of, 317
  headache and, 104
  injury to
    cardiovascular, 270
    laryngeal, 240
  nuchal rigidity and
    headache and, 97
    meningitis and, 621, 807
    retropharyngeal abscess and, 364
  wound closure for, 290
Necrolysis, toxic epidermal, 588
Necrotizing vasculitides, 418
Neisseria gonorrhoeae
  in Bartholin abscess, 180
  in cervicitis, 181
  in conjunctivitis, 840
  in pelvic inflammatory disease, 183
  in pharyngitis, 362
  in urinary tract infections, 514

Neisseria meningitidis, 618, 619
  in child, 807
  in meningococcemia, 709-710
  therapy for, 624, 625, 626
Neonate; *see also* Infant
  cardiopulmonary resuscitation of, 41-49,
    820-821
  cytomegalovirus in, 722
  gastroesophageal reflux in, 157-160
  herpes infection in, 180, 723
  hypermagnesemia and, 684
  tetanus in, 704
  urinary tract infection in, 512-513
  vomiting in, 160
Neoplasm; *see* Malignancy
Neosporin, 288
Neostigmine in neuromuscular blockade, 214
Nephritis, interstitial, 528
Nephrostomy, percutaneous, 580
Nephrotic syndrome, 524-525
Nephrotomography, 280
Nerve
  facial injury and, 232
  hand wound and, 291
  shoulder dislocation and, 311
Nerve blocks; *see also* Neuromuscular
    blockade
  Bier, 303
    in wrist injury, 304
  intercostal, 255
  in postherpetic neuralgia, 633
  in rib fracture, 255
Nerve roots
  compression of, 198
  spinal, 628
Nervous system
  central; *see* Central nervous system
  viral infection of, 724
Neuralgia
  glossopharyngeal, 88
  herpetic, 632-633
  migrainous, 99
  postherpetic, 633
  trigeminal, 103-104
    headache and, 95, 97
Neurinoma, acoustic, 614
Neuritis
  optic, 845
    in multiple sclerosis, 640
  retrobulbar, in multiple sclerosis, 640
Neurocysticercosis, 743
Neurofibromas, seizures and, 207
Neurogenic hypotension in spinal injury,
    246
Neurologic disorders, 600-646
  amyotrophic lateral sclerosis in, 643
  Bell palsy in, 631-632
  in child, 807-809
  demyelinating disease in, 638-641
  in diphtheria, 699
  diseases of, in AIDS and HIV, 729-730
  electrical injury and, 343

Neurologic disorders—cont'd
  Guillain-Barré in, 630-631
  in hemodialysis complications, 542
  herpes zoster in, 632-633, 721-722
  herpetic neuralgia in, 632-633
  in lightning injury, 343
  in Lyme disease, 750, 752-753
  meningitis and encephalitis in, 617-627;
    see also Meningitis and encephalitis
  normal pressure hydrocephalus in, 642-643
  Parkinson syndrome in, 643-645
  peripheral neuropathy in, 628-630
  in pertussis, 702
  pseudotumor cerebri in, 641-642
  psychogenic, 633-638
  in renal failure, 532, 534-535
  in sacral fracture, 316
  shingles in, 632-633
  in spinal injury, 243
  in spinal pain, 314-315
  stroke in, 600-607; *see also*
    Cerebrovascular accident
  in syndrome of inappropriate antidiuretic
    hormone, 667
  in tumors, 575
  vertigo in, 608-616; *see also* Vertigo
Neurologic examination
  in coma, 85
  in head injury, 220, 221-222
  in headache, 97
  in spinal injury, 243, 246-250
Neurologic problems; *see* Neurologic
    disorders
Neuroma, acoustic, 823
Neuromuscular blockade; *see also* Nerve blocks
  in intubation, 22, 23, 24
  in spinal injury, 245
  in status epilepticus, 214
Neuromuscular system
  dysphagia and, 474
  hypokalemia and, 675
Neuronitis, vestibular, 613-614
Neuropathy
  diabetes and, 689
  peripheral, 628-630
  subacute sensory motor, 629
Neurotoxin, 703
Neurotransmitters
  in migraine, 100
  parkinsonism and, 644
Neurotrauma, venous thrombosis in, 399
Neutropenia, 570
  in malignancy, 573-573
Neutrophils in fever, 73
Nevi, vascular, 207
Newborn; *see* Neonate
Nicotinamide adenine dinucleotide, liver
    toxicity and, 497
Nifedipine
  in heart failure, 450, 451
  in hypertension, 439
    and encephalopathy, 436-437

Nifedipine—cont'd
  in hypertension—cont'd
    in malignant hypertension, 440
    in pregnancy, 442, 553
Nifurtimox, 744
Nimodipine, 606
Nitrates
  in congestive heart failure, 450, 451
  in ischemic heart disease, 429
  in syncope, 89
Nitrofurantoin
  in pancreatitis etiology, 503
  in urinary tract infection, 510
  in pregnancy, 512
Nitrogen, blood urea; *see* Blood urea nitrogen
Nitroglycerin
  in angina with hypertension, 441
  in cardiogenic shock, 56
  in cluster headache, 99
  in congestive heart failure, 450, 451
  in ischemic heart disease, 429
  in pulmonary edema, 453, 538
  in volume disturbances in renal failure, 532
Nitroprusside
  in aortic trauma, 270
  in cardiogenic shock, 56
  in chest pain management, 129
  in hypertension
    with aortic dissection, 443
    with cerebrovascular accident, 440
    with congestive heart failure and
      angina, 441, 450
    with encephalopathy, 436
    in pregnancy, 442
    with renal failure, 441
  in pulmonary edema, 440, 538
  in renal failure, 441
  in tetanus, 704
Nits, 594
Nizatidine, 476
Noise, hearing loss from, 823
Nomogram, Done, 784, 785
Non-A, non-B hepatitis virus, 491, 493
Nonaccidental trauma to child, 819-820
Noncardiogenic pulmonary edema, 109
Nonconvulsive neurotoxin, 703
Nonconvulsive seizure, 204-205
Nongonococcal septic arthritis, 191-192
Nongonococcal urethritis, 514
Nonimmune thrombocytopenia, 565
Nonketotic coma, hyperglycemic
    hyperosmolar, 691
Nonmigrainous vascular headache, 100-101
Nonorganic blindness, 636
Non-staphylococci-induced toxic epidermal
    necrolysis, 588
Nonsteroidal antiinflammatory agents; *see*
    also Antiinflammatory agents
  in back pain, 199
  in bursitis and tendinitis, 192
  in cholelithiasis, 500
  in dysmenorrhea, 177

Nonsteroidal antiinflammatory agents—
    cont'd
  in gout, 190
  hearing loss from, 823
  in hypercalcemia, 680
  hyperkalemia and, 672
  in interstitial renal disease, 528
  in migraine, 100, 101
  in polymyalgia rheumatica, 579
  in Reiter syndrome, 193
  in rheumatoid arthritis, 578
Norfloxacin
  in diarrhea, 172
  in urinary tract infection, 510, 511
Normal pressure hydrocephalus, 642-643
Normal saline; *see* Saline
Normodyne; *see* Labetalol
North Asian tick typhus, 758
Nortriptyline, toxicity of, 777
Norwalk virus, 716
Nose
  epistaxis and, 145, 824
    traumatic, 238
  wound closure for, 289
Nosebleed; *see* Epistaxis
Noxious stimulants, abdominal pain and, 135
Nuchal rigidity
  meningitis and, 621
    in child, 807
  retropharyngeal abscess and, 364
Nuclear medicine studies, 127
  in cholecystitis, 501
  in pulmonary embolism, 401
Numbness, psychogenic, 635-636
Nurse for trauma team, 61
Nursemaid's elbow, 308
Nutcracker esophagus, 475
Nylon suture, 287
Nystagmus
  in coma, 84
  drugs causing, 610
  optokinetic, test for, 636
  physical examination for, 611-612
  in vertigo, 608, 609, 610
Nystatin, 585

O

Oatmeal baths, 588
Obesity, venous thrombosis in, 400
Oblique popliteal ligament, 322
Obstetrics; *see* Pregnancy
Obstruction
  in acute renal failure, 526-527
  airway; *see also* Airway management
    in child, 800
    epiglottitis and, 799
    foreign body aspiration and, 392, 393,
      800
    oral injury and, 239
    respiratory distress versus, 107
  intestinal, 480-482
    Hirschsprung disease and, 487

Obstruction—cont'd
  intestinal—cont'd
    lesions responsible for, 481
    mechanical causes of, 482
    pain and, 481, 482
    vomiting in, 155, 157, 161, 480
  superior vena cava syndrome and, 573
  urinary retention and, 516-517
  urinary tract infection and, 507
Obtundation, 80
Obturator dislocation, 318
Obturator sign, 483
Occlusion
  acute arterial, 411, 416
  of basilar artery, 823-824
  in cerebrovascular accident; *see*
    Cerebrovascular accident
  mesenteric vascular, 483-484
  retinal artery and, 843-844
  retinal vein and, 844
  stroke and, 600; *see also* Cerebrovascular
    accident
Occlusive disease, aortoiliac, 412
Occult bacteremia, 814-816
Octreotide, 739
Oculocephalogyric maneuver, 84
Odynophagia, 475
Ofloxacin
  in cervicitis, 181
  in pelvic inflammatory disease, 184
  in urethritis, 512
  in urinary tract infections, 510, 511, 512
Ointments, polysporin, 237
Olecranon fracture, 307
Oliguria, hyperkalemia and, 673
Omeprazole, 476
Oncologic emergencies, 572-576; *see also*
    Malignancy
Ondansetron
  in methylxanthine toxicity, 786
  in vomiting, 163, 164, 473
On-off phenomenon in Parkinson
    syndrome, 644
Oocysts, 739
Open fracture
  of ankle, 324
  definition of, 295
  of femoral shaft, 319
  nasal, 238
  of tibial shaft, 323
Open pneumothorax, 259-260
Ophthaine; *see* Proparacaine
Ophthalmic injury, 237-238
Ophthalmoplegia, internuclear, 640
Ophthalmoplegic migraine, 99
Ophthalmoscopy, 827
  in vitreous hemorrhage, 834
Ophthetic; *see* Proparacaine
Opiates
  antagonists to; *see* Naloxone
  in cholelithiasis, 500
  in ischemic heart disease, 430

Opiates—cont'd
  in pancreatitis etiology, 503
  in sympatholytic syndrome, 765
  toxicity of, 782-783
Opisthotonos in tetanus, 703
Optic nerve
  decompression of, 642
  injury of, 835-836
  neuritis of, 845
    in multiple sclerosis, 640
Optokinetic nystagmus test, 636
OPV; *see* Oral poliovirus vaccine
Oral estrogens, venous thrombosis in, 400
Oral intubation, 21-26
  awake, 21
  in child, 26-27
  complications of, 26
  cribriform plate fracture and, 223
  in head injury, 223-224
  oral injury and, 231
Oral poliovirus vaccine, 724
Oral temperature, 71
Oral trauma, 239; *see also* Facial trauma
Orbital cellulitis, 842
Orbital foreign body, 836
Orbital fracture, 233-234
  blowout, 829-830
Orbivirus organisms, 751, 759
Orchitis, 515
  mumps, 721
Organic mental disorders, 647, 648, 649
  physical examination in, 649-651
  treatable causes of, 651
  violence and, 660
Organophosphate toxicity, 765, 783
Ornithodoros organisms, 750, 754
Ornithosis, 370
Oropharyngeal airway, 30
Oropharyngeal dysphagia, 474
Oropharynx
  alkali burn of, 775-776
  infection of, 361-364
Orotracheal intubation in spinal injury, 245
Orthopedic trauma, 294-330
  communication and definitions in, 295-298
    for fractures, 295-296
    for sprains and strains, 296-298
  fracture in, 298-314; *see also* Fracture
  general principles for, 294
  of lower extremity, 316-329; *see also*
    Lower extremity
  spinal injury in, 314-315; *see also* Spine,
    injury to
Orthopnea, 107
  in congestive heart failure, 446
  respiratory distress and, 107
Orthostatic syncope, 86
Os calcis fracture, 325
Osborn wave, 354
Osmolal gap, 766, 772
Osmolality, serum, in hyperglycemic
    hyperosmolar nonketotic coma, 691

Osmolarity of body fluids, 664-665
  calculated or measured, 766, 772
  drug poisoning and, 766
Osmotic demyelinating syndrome, 671
Osmotic diarrhea, 165
Osmotic diuretics in head injury, 224
Osteoarthritis, 192, 196
Osteogenesis imperfecta, 562, 582
Osteomyelitis
  septic arthritis from, 191
  tibial shaft fracture and, 323
Otic injury, 238-239
Otitis externa, 822-823
Otitis media, 822
  retropharyngeal abscess and, 364
  secretory, 823
Otolaryngologic emergencies, 238-240, 822-826
Otologic damage, electrical injury and, 343
Otorrhea, blood in ear in, 239
Ototoxicity of diuretics, 449
Ovary
  bleeding from, in vaginal bleeding, 179
  cyst of, 175-176
  torsion of, 174-175
  trauma to, 278-281
Overdose
  of acetaminophen, 771-772
  barbiturate, 782-783
  cyclic antidepressant, 777-778
  salicylate, 783-785
  theophylline, 786
Overflow proteinuria, 524
Oxacillin, 573
Oxamniquine, 738
Oxazolidinediones, 212-213
Oximetry, 116
  in chest pain, 128
  coma and, 82
Oxycodone, 837
Oxygen
  in carbon monoxide poisoning, 340, 776
  cardiac arrest and, 29
  in chronic obstructive pulmonary disease,
    387
  coma and, 81, 83
  in hydrocarbon poisoning, 780
  hyperbaric, 340
    in multiple sclerosis, 641
  in hypothermia, 355
  intubation and, 21
  in ischemic heart disease, 429
  in near-drowning, 346
  neonatal resuscitation and, 44, 820-821
  pneumonia and, in child, 803
  in poisoning, 762
  respiratory distress and, 116
  retinal artery and, 844
  in shock, 53, 55
  in smoke inhalation burn, 340
Oxygen gradient, alveolar-arterial, 116
Oxygen tension in chronic obstructive
  pulmonary disease, 388

Oxymetazoline spray, 366

P

P wave, 456, 457
PAC; see Premature atrial contraction
Pacemaker
  in atrioventricular heart block, 469, 470
  bradycardias from, 465
  in Chagas disease, 744
Packed red blood cells
  in gastrointestinal bleeding, 477
  in multiple trauma, 64
Packing in epistaxis, 824
Pain
  abdominal; see Abdominal pain
  in acute arterial occlusion, 410
  in appendicitis, 483
  back, 195-199; see also Joint, pain in
  in Bell palsy, 631
  in bowel obstruction, 480
  cast and, 299
  chest
    esophageal disorders and, 475-476
    gastrointestinal disorders and, 476-477
    in ischemic heart disease, 421
  in chest injury, 255
  in ectopic pregnancy, 548
  eye, 839-842
  in headache, 94-105; see also Headache
  in intussusception of colon, 486
  joint, 187-200; see also Joint, pain in
  kidney, 133
  in mesenteric vascular occlusion, 484
  in odynophagia, 475
  in pancreatitis, 502
  pelvic, 174-180
  perception of, in child, 792-793
  in postherpetic neuralgia, 633
  in rotator cuff tear, 314
  in spinal injury, 243, 314-315
  in testicular torsion, 515
  in trigeminal neuralgia, 95, 97, 103-104
  in ultraviolet keratitis, 837
  in volvulus, 818
  in vomiting, 155
  wound repair and, 285-288
Palate, 239
Pallor in acute arterial occlusion, 410
Palpation
  of abdomen in vomiting, 157
  in abdominal pain, 136
Palsy
  bell, 631-632
  progressive bulbar, 643
Pancreatic abscess, 504-505
Pancreatic cancer, 505
Pancreatic disease, 502-505
Pancreatic endocrine tumors, 504
Pancreatic isoenzymes in abdominal trauma,
  273
Pancreatic pseudocyst, 504-505
Pancreatic tumor, 505

Pancreatitis, 502-504
  radiography in, 161
Pancuronium, 24
  in head injury, 224
  in status epilepticus, 214
Paper tape in wound closure, 287
Papilledema, 84
  in stroke, 602
Papillitis, 845
Papillomavirus, 184
Papular lesion, 584, 592-594
  in tularemia, 755
Paracoccidioides species, 618
Paradoxical chest wall movement in chest
  injury, 255
Parainfluenza viruses, 716
  in otitis media, 822
Paraldehyde, 782
Paralysis
  in acute arterial occlusion, 410, 411
  in botulism, 706
  in giant cell arteritis, 580
  in Guillain-Barré syndrome, 630
  in polio, 724
  postictal, stroke versus, 603
  psychogenic, 634-635
  of seventh cranial nerve, 631-632
  in status epilepticus, 245
  in stroke, 601, 602, 603
  tick, 751, 759-760
Paralytic agents
  in intubation, 22, 23, 24
    in head injury, 224
  in tetanus, 704
Paramethadione, 211, 212-213
Paranasal sinus, 104
Parapharyngeal infection, 365
Paraplegia in aortic transection, 258, 443
Parasites, 733-747
  in cardiovascular system, 743-744
  in central nervous system, 742-743
  dermatologic, 745
  ectoparasitic, 745-746
  gastrointestinal, 736-742
  genitourinary, 744-745
  malaria from, 733-736
  in meningitis and encephalitis, 618
  pulmonary, 743
Parathyroid hormone, hypercalcemia and, 677
Paresthesia
  in acute arterial occlusion, 410, 411
  in peripheral neuropathies, 629
Parietal peritoneum in abdominal pain, 132
Parkinson syndrome, 643-645
Paromomycin
  in amebiasis, 737
  in cryptosporidiosis, 739
  in giardiasis, 738
Parotid duct, 237
Parotid gland, facial lacerations and, 236, 237
Parotitis, 825
  mumps, 721

Paroxysmal nocturnal dyspnea, 107
  in heart failure, 446-447
Paroxysmal positional vertigo, benign, 613
Paroxysmal supraventricular tachycardia,
    459-460
  preexcitation syndromes and, 466-467
Partial pressure of oxygen, 116
Partial seizures, 205-206
  treatment of, 211
Partial spinal cord lesion, 249, 250
Partial thromboplastin time, 562, 567-568
Particulate matter aspiration, 391-392, 393
Passive external rewarming, 355
Passive immunization in hepatitis, 722, 723
Passive rewarming in myxedema coma, 695
Pasteurella, 369, 373
Patching of eye
  in corneal abrasions, 831
  in corneal foreign bodies, 831
  in penetrating trauma, 238
  in ultraviolet keratitis, 837
Patella, injury to, 319
Patient disposition, 9-10
PCP; *see* Phencyclidine
PCWP; *see* Pulmonary capillary wedge
    pressure
PE; *see* Pulmonary embolism
Peak expiratory flow rate in asthma, 380,
    381, 382
Peak expiratory flow reserve in chronic
    obstructive pulmonary disease, 386
Pediatric patient; *see* Child
Pediculosis, 593-594
Pediculus humanus, 746
PEEP; *see* Positive end-expiratory pressure
PEFR; *see* Peak expiratory flow rate
Pelvic fracture, 279, 316
Pelvic inflammatory disease, 183-184
  indications for hospitalization in, 184
Pelvic pain, 174-180
Pemphigus vulgaris, 594-596
Penetrating trauma
  of abdomen, 274-278
    wound closure and, 292
  of bladder, 281
  of brain, 219, 229
  chest, 261-262
  diaphragmatic, 260-261
  esophageal, 262
  of eye, 237, 238
  of genital tract, 278-279
  of kidney, 280-281
  pericardial tamponade after, 266-268
  in urinary tract, 280-281
Penicillamine in rheumatoid arthritis, 192, 578
Penicillin
  in cellulitis, 585
  in diphtheria, 700
  in epiglottitis in adult, 364
  in gonococcal arthritis, 193
  in interstitial renal disease, 528
  in Lyme disease, 194, 753

Penicillin—cont'd
  in meningitis and encephalitis, 624
    in child, 809
  in meningococcemia, 711
  in rheumatic fever, 195
  in scarlet fever, 591-592
  in tumor infection emergencies, 573
  in wound infection, 289
Penicillin G
  in Lyme disease, 753
  in meningitis, 624, 625
  in meningococcemia, 711
  in pneumococcemia, 709
Penicillin G benzathine
  in diphtheria, 700
  in pharyngitis, 363
Penicillin V potassium in pharyngitis, 363
Penicillinase-resistant penicillin
  in epiglottitis in adult, 364
  in toxic shock syndrome, 714
Penis, trauma to, 279
Pentamidine
  in African sleeping sickness, 742
  in AIDS and HIV, 729, 730
  in pancreatitis etiology, 503
Pentazocine, 783
Pepcid; *see* Famotidine
Peptic ulcer disease
  anemia and, 557
  bleeding in, 143
  pain in, 476-477
  physical findings in, 125
  vomiting in, 154, 156
Peptococcus, 183
Peptostreptococcus, 183
Percussion of abdomen
  in pain, 136
  in vomiting, 157
Percutaneous nephrostomy, 580
Perforation
  esophageal, 262, 476
    from foreign bodies, 478
  peptic ulcer, 476-477
Perfumes, eye injury from, 838-839
Perianal abscess, 488-489
Pericardial friction rub, 262
Pericardial space, catheter in, 267
Pericardial tamponade, 261-262, 266-268
  in chest injury, 261-262
  diagnosis of, 128
  physical findings in, 125
  in pulseless electrical activity, 40
  in tumors, 574-575
Pericardiocentesis, pericardial tamponade
    and, 267
Pericarditis
  electrocardiography and, 425
  in renal failure, 532
Periorbital cellulitis, 840
Peripheral arterial aneurysm, 416-417
  physical examination in, 414
Peripheral arterial embolism, 416-417

Peripheral arterial embolism—cont'd
  physical examination in, 414
Peripheral arteriovascular disease, 410-420
  acute arterial occlusion in, 411, 416
  aneurysms in, 416-417
  arteriovenous fistulae in, 420
  chronic arterial insufficiency in, 415-416
  necrotizing vasculitides in, 418
  pathophysiology of, 410
  physical examination in, 412-415
  thoracic outlet syndrome in, 418-420
  vascular history of, 410-412
  vasospastic disorders in, 417-418
Peripheral arteriovenous fistulae, 420
Peripheral blood smear, 558
Peripheral cold injuries, 356-357
Peripheral neuropathy, 628-630
Peripheral resistance of pericardial
    tamponade, 266
Peripheral vascular occlusive disease,
    physical findings in, 125
Peritoneal cavity
  in abdominal trauma, 275-277
  signs of, 275
Peritoneal dialysis, 542-545
  hypothermia and, 356
Peritoneal lavage
  in abdominal trauma, 272, 273-274, 277
  in diaphragmatic injury, 261
Peritoneum
  irritation of, in abdominal trauma, 272
  parietal, in abdominal pain, 132
  violation of, in abdominal trauma, 275-277
Peritonitis
  bacterial, spontaneous, 498
  from peritoneal dialysis, 543-544
  in vomiting, 155
Peritonsillar abscess, 364
Permanent tooth, avulsion of, 241
Permethrin, 594, 746, 760
Pernio, 356
Peroxide in peritoneal dialysis site
    cleansing, 544
Perphenazine, 633
Pertussis, 701-703
PET VICTIMS mnemonic, 81
Petit mal seizures, 205
  status epilepticus and, 206
Petroleum distillates, 780
Phalangeal fracture, 300-303
Pharmacologic causes of syncope, 88-89
Pharyngitis, 361-364
Pharynx
  diphtheria and, 698-699, 700
  exudate from, in fever, 72
Phenacemide, 212-213
Phenaphen; *see* Acetaminophen, with
    caffeine
Phencyclidine
  toxicity of, 769, 779-780
  in vertigo, 610
Phenergan; *see* Promethazine

Phenformin, 503
Phenobarbital
  in brain injury, 225
  in drug poisoning, activated charcoal for, 767
  liver toxicity of, 497
  in pregnancy-induced hypertension, 442
  in seizures, 211, 212-213
  in status epilepticus, 214
    in child, 810, 812
  theophylline clearance and, 383
Phenol
  burn from, 339
  toxicity of, 780
Phenothiazines
  parkinsonism from, 643, 645
  in postherpetic neuralgia, 633
  in syncope, 89
  toxicity of, 774
Phenoxymethyl penicillin, 585
Phensuximide for seizures, 212-213
Phentolamine, 768
Phenurone; see Phenacemide
Phenylephrine in eye examination, 828
Phenylpropanolamine
  in sinusitis, 366
  in toxicology, 768
Phenytoin, 211, 212-213
  in atrial tachycardia with block, 461
  contraindicated in Wolff-Parkinson-White
    syndrome, 467
  in dysrhythmias from poisoning, 768
  in head injury, 225
  hypocalcemia and, 681
  liver toxicity of, 497
  in seizures with syndrome of inappropriate
    antidiuretic hormone, 575
  in status epilepticus, 211-214
    in child, 810, 812
  in subarachnoid hemorrhage, 606
  theophylline clearance and, 383
  thrombocytopenia and, 563
  in vertigo, 610
Pheochromocytoma, 434
Phlebotomus, 745
Phlebotomy, 560
Phosphodiesterase inhibitors, 446, 451, 452
Phosphorus
  burn from, 339
  radioactive, in polycythemia, 560
Photophobia
  in corneal abrasion, 831
  in episcleritis, 842
Phthirus pubis, 746
Phycomycetes, tumors and, 572
Physician
  anger in, 11-12
  charting by, 12-13
  grief and, 13-15
  preparation of, for soft tissue trauma care,
    284
Physostigmine
  anticholinergic toxicity and, 773-774

Physostigmine—cont'd
  in tricyclic antidepressant toxicity, 778
Piaget theory of development, 792
PID; see Pelvic inflammatory disease
Pigment gallstones, 500
Pigment-induced acute renal failure, 529
Pigskin graft for burns, 337
Pink puffer, 20
  in chronic obstructive pulmonary disease,
    110
Pinna, trauma to, 824
Pinpoint unreactive pupil, 84
Pinworm, 738, 740-741
PIP; see Proximal interphalangeal joint
Piperacillin, 573
Piperonyl bromide, pyrethrins with, 746
Piroxicam, 234
  in pancreatitis etiology, 503
Pityriasis rosea, 594
Pizotifen, 100
Placenta previa, 552
Plaque, 584
  Hollenhorst, 413
  in multiple sclerosis, 639
Plasma, fresh frozen; see Fresh frozen plasma
Plasma cortisol in adrenal disorders, 696
Plasma proteins in pregnancy, 551
Plasmapheresis
  in Guillain-Barré syndrome, 630
  in multiple sclerosis, 641
Plasmin, deep venous thrombosis and, 396
Plasminogen activator/inhibitor after
    thrombolysis in pulmonary embolism
    or deep venous thrombosis, 408
Plasmodium species, 733, 734, 742
Plate, cribriform
  fracture of, 223-224
  in oral injury, 231
Plateau, tibial, fracture of, 322-323
Platelets
  in deep venous thrombosis, 395
  disorders of, 563-567
  in gastrointestinal bleeding, 146-147, 148
  in hypovolemic shock, 53
Pleura in chest trauma, 261
Pleural effusion, 447
  chest pain in, 122
  in esophageal perforation, 476
  pulmonary embolism, 402
  respiratory distress in, 113
Pleural friction rub, 125
Pleurisy, chest pain in, 122
Plexopathy, 628
Plexus, brachial
  clavicular fracture and, 313
  in thoracic outlet syndrome, 419
PND; see Paroxysmal nocturnal dyspnea
Pneumococcal pneumonia, 375
Pneumococcal vaccine, 709
Pneumococcemia, 707-709
Pneumocystis carinii pneumonia, 112, 375
  tumors and, 572

Pneumomediastinum, 125
Pneumonia, 367-374, 375, 376-377
  in AIDS and HIV, 727-729
  chest pain in, 122
  in child, 802-803
  diagnosis of, 128
  physical findings in, 125
  respiratory distress and, 112
Pneumonitis, roundworm and, 743
Pneumoperitoneum in abdominal trauma,
    272-273
Pneumothorax, 258-260
  auscultation and, 21, 125
  in chest trauma, 255, 261
  pulseless electrical activity and, 40
  respiratory distress and, 111-112
  risk factors in, 123-124
  tension; see Tension pneumothorax
Podophyllum resin, 184
PO_2/FiO_2 ratio, 116
Poisoning, 762-787; see also Toxicology
  coma and, 81
  cyanide, 340
  history and, 763
  initial stabilization in, 762-763
  laboratory tests and, 765-766
  peripheral neuropathies in, 628, 629
  physical examination and, 763-764
  smoke inhalation and, 340
  syndromes and, 764-766
  treatment of, 766-769
Polio, 719, 724
Polyarteritis nodosa, 628
Polyarticular arthritis, 192-195
  osteoarthritis in, 192
  overview of, 196-197
  rheumatoid, 192
Polychondritis, relapsing, 582
Polycythemia, 560
  venous thrombosis in, 400
Polyethylene glycol in phenol burn, 339
Polyglycolic suture, 286
Polymorphonuclear leukocytes, 73
  in diarrhea, 167, 172
  in meningitis, 710
  in rheumatoid arthritis, 192
  tumors and, 572
Polymyalgia rheumatica, 578-579
Polyneuritis, Guillain-Barré syndrome as,
    630-631
Polyneuropathy, 628
  critical illness, 630
  Guillain-Barré syndrome as, 630-631
Polyps, cervical, 179
Polysporin ointment, 237
Polytef pledgets, 268
Pontine myelinolysis, central, 671
Pontocaine; see Tetracaine
Popliteal aneurysms, 416
Popliteal ligament, oblique, 322
Popliteal vessel, knee dislocation and, 294,
    322

Popping in knee, 320
Pork tapeworm, 742-743
Portal hypertension, anemia in, 557
Positioning
  in facial trauma, 231
  of finger fracture, 301, 302
  in pediatric resuscitation, 45
  of neonate, 42, 43
Positive drawer sign, 320
Positive end-expiratory pressure
  in cardiogenic shock, 55
  in foreign body aspiration, 393
Postherpetic neuralgia, 633
Postictal paralysis, stroke versus, 603
Postinfectious encephalitis, 620
Post-lumbar puncture headache, 103
Postmenopausal pelvic pain, 177
Postoperative state, venous thrombosis in, 400
Postrenal acute renal failure, 526-527
Postresuscitation care, 41
Posttraumatic infected aneurysm, 417
Posttraumatic syndrome after head injury, 229
Potassium, 671-677
  burns from, 339, 340
  dehydration and, 804, 805
  in hyponatremia, 671
Potassium chloride in ketoacidosis, 690
Potassium hydroxide
  in scabies, 746
  vaginosis and, 182
Potassium iodide in thyroid storm, 693
Potassium-sparing diuretics, 449
Povidone-iodine, 284
  in peritoneal dialysis site cleansing, 544
Pralidoxime, 783
Praziquantel
  in neurocysticercosis, 743
  in schistosomiasis, 738, 741
Prazosin
  in congestive heart failure, 450
  in hypertension, 439
Prednisone
  in asthma, 381
    in child, 802
  in Bell palsy, 632
  in cluster headache, 100
  in gout, 190
  in pemphigus vulgaris, 596
  in pharyngitis, 363
  in postherpetic neuralgia, 633
  in temporal arteritis, 103, 847
Preeclampsia, 551, 553
Preexcitation syndromes, 466-467
Pregnancy, 547-555
  appendicitis versus, 135
  asthma in, 384
  ectopic, 547, 548-549
  electrical injury in, 343
  genitourinary system in, 547-555
    first half of, 547-551
    second half of, 551-554
  hemorrhage in, 548, 550, 551-552, 553

Pregnancy—cont'd
  herpes infection and, 180
  hypertension and, 441-442, 552-554
  migraine in, 99
  pelvic pain during, 177
  physiologic changes in, 551
  trauma in, 66
  tubal, 174
    abdominal pain in, 135
  urinary tract infection in, 512
  venous thrombosis in, 400
Pregnancy test, 137
Prehospital care team, 60-61
Preload, optimizing, 450-451
Premature atrial contractions, 456-457
Premature rupture of membranes, 554
Premature ventricular contraction, 457-459
  in myocardial contusion, 265
Prepubertal pelvic pain, 177
Prerenal azotemia, 526, 527
Preretinal hemorrhage, 835
Preseptal cellulitis, 840
Pressor agents in shock in child, 807
Pressure
  blood; *see* Blood pressure
  cast and, 299
  intracranial; *see* Intracranial pressure
  intraocular, 828
  systemic venous, 447
Prevertebral space infection, 364-365
Prickly heat, 349
Prilosec; *see* Omeprazole
Primaquine phosphate, 735
Primary lateral sclerosis, 643
Primary repair of wound, 285
Primary spinal injury, 251
Primary survey of wound, 283
Primidone
  hypocalcemia and, 681
  in seizures, 211, 212-213
Priorities for emergency patient, 7-8
Probenecid, 184
Procainamide
  in atrial fibrillation, 463
  in atrial flutter, 461
  in cardiac arrest, 37
  in pancreatitis etiology, 503
  in preexcitation syndromes, 467
  in premature ventricular contractions, 459
  in ventricular tachycardia, 38, 39, 465
  in Wolff-Parkinson-White syndrome, 467
Procaine, wound closure and, 285
Procardia; *see* Nifedipine
Prochlorperazine in vomiting, 163, 164, 473
  in renal failure, 545
Proctosigmoidoscopy, 147
Progesterone
  in pregnancy, 551
  in uterine bleeding, 180
Progressive bulbar palsy, 643
Progressive spinal muscular atrophy, 643
Projectile vomiting, 155

Prolapse
  of iris at limbus, 836
  rectal, 489
PROM; *see* Premature rupture of membranes
Promethazine
  in vertigo, 615
  in vomiting, 163, 164, 473
Proparacaine, 237, 828, 831
Prophylaxis
  antibiotics in, 288-289
  hepatitis and, 493
  meningitis and, 626, 809
  sexual abuse of child and, 820
  tumor lysis syndrome and, 574
Propoxyphene, 783
Propranolol
  in aortic dissection, 443
  in atrial fibrillation, 463
  in atrial flutter, 461
  in atrial tachycardia with block, 461
  contraindicated
    in hyperthyroidism, 694
    in Wolff-Parkinson-White syndrome, 467
  in hypertension, 438
  in hyperthyroidism, 694
  in migraine, 100
  theophylline clearance and, 383
  toxicity of, 774
Proprioceptors, 608
Propulsid; *see* Cisapride
Propylthiouracil, 693
Prostatic hypertrophy, benign, 516-517
Prostatitis, 514
Prosthetic heart valves, 557
Protein C, 396, 407
Protein S, 396, 407
Proteinuria
  in hypertensive emergencies of pregnancy, 441, 442
  in renal failure, 520-521, 524-525
Proteus
  in Bartholin abscess, 180
  in urinary tract infections, 510, 511, 514
    in child, 513
Prothrombin time, 562, 567-568
  in gastrointestinal bleeding, 146
Protoporphyrin, free-erythrocyte, 558
Protozoan infection, 736-744; *see also* Parasites
  in diarrhea, 170, 736-742
Provocative tests in psychogenic coma, 637
Proximal fibular fracture, 323
Proximal humeral fracture, 308
Proximal interphalangeal joint, arthritis of, 577
Proximal phalangeal fracture or injury, 301-303
Pseudoaneurysm
  fistula with, 420
  physical examination in, 414
Pseudocyst, pancreatic, 504-505
Pseudoephedrine
  in secretory otitis media, 823

Pseudoephedrine—cont'd
in sinusitis, 366
Pseudogout, 190-191, 196
Pseudomonas
in corneal infection, 841
in otitis externa, 823
tumors and, 572
in urinary tract infections, 508, 511, 514
Pseudoseizures, 636-637
Pseudotumor
of bowel, 481
cerebral, 102, 641-642
heart failure and, 447
Psittacosis, 370
Psoas sign, 483
PSVT; *see* Paroxysmal supraventricular
tachycardia
Psychiatric emergency, 647-663
acute psychosis in, 647-655; *see also*
Psychosis
coma and, 81
suicide in, 656-659
violence in, 660-663
Psychogenic breathlessness, 113
Psychogenic coma, 637
Psychogenic emesis, 473
Psychogenic hyperventilation, 20, 113
Psychogenic neurologic disorders, 633-638
disposition of patients with, 638
Psychogenic numbness, 635-636
Psychogenic vision loss, 636
Psychologic factors in grief, 13-15
Psychologic support for child, 793, 795
Psychomotor seizures, 205
status epilepticus and, 206
treatment of, 211
Psychosis, 647-655
approach to patient with, 647-648, 649
disposition of patient with, 652
laboratory and radiographic examination
in, 651, 652
life-threatening causes of, 648
mental status in, 649, 650
physical examination in, 649-651
reversible causes of, 649
rules of thumb in evaluation of, 649
thought disorders in, 652-654
treatment of, 652
violence and, 660
Psychosomatic causes of syncope, 89
Psychotropic drugs, parkinsonism from,
643, 645
Ptosis in orbital blowout fracture, 829
Pubic louse, 746
Puborectalis muscle, 488
Puerperium, venous thrombosis in, 400
Pulmonary angiography in pulmonary
embolism, 128, 401, 405
Pulmonary artery catheter in cardiogenic
shock, 54-55
Pulmonary capillary wedge pressure
in cardiogenic shock, 55

Pulmonary capillary wedge pressure—
cont'd
in pulmonary edema, 109
Pulmonary contusion, 256-257
Pulmonary disorders
chronic obstructive; *see* Chronic
obstructive pulmonary disease
in chronic renal failure, 534, 538
parasitic infestation in, 743
in rheumatic diseases, 582
Pulmonary edema
in chronic renal failure, 538
in congestive heart failure, 108-109, 447,
452-453
high-altitude, 109
in hypertension, 440
intubation in, 23
in respiratory distress, 115
respiratory distress and, 109
in upper airway obstruction, 113
Pulmonary embolism, 395-409
chest pain in, 120, 122
clinical presentation of, 398-399
deep venous thrombosis and; *see* Deep
venous thrombosis
diagnosis of, 401-405
physical findings in, 125
tests for, 126, 127-128
respiratory distress and, 111
risk factors for, 123-124, 399-400
signs and symptoms of, 398
thrombogenic and hypercoagulable states
and, 399-400
treatment of, 405-408
Pulmonary function
hypoxemia and, 29
near-drowning and, 345-346
Pulmonary infarction, 111
Pulmonary stenosis, 88
Pulmonary trauma in burns, 340
Pulp, dental, 240-241
Pulse
in acute arterial occlusion, 410
in arterial disease, 410, 412-413
comatose patient and, 82
Pulse oximeter
in chest pain, 128
coma and, 82
in respiratory distress, 82
Pulseless electrical activity, 40
Pulsus alternans
in heart failure, 447
in pericardial tamponade, 267
Pulsus paradoxus
in asthma, 380
in pericardial tamponade, 267
Puncture, lumbar; *see* Lumbar puncture
Pupil
in acute angle-closure glaucoma, 843
in comatose patient, 84
iridodialysis and, 833
light reflex of, 84, 828

Pupil—cont'd
second, 833
in stroke, 602
in subacute subdural hematoma, 228
in traumatic mydriasis and miosis, 833
Purpura, thrombocytopenic, 563-565
Pustule, 597-599
in gonococcal arthritis, 193
PVC; *see* Premature ventricular contraction
Pyelography
in kidney trauma, 280, 281
in lithiasis, 518
in renal failure, 522, 523
Pyelonephritis, 507, 509
acute, 512
antibiotics in, 510-511
in men, 513-514
Pyloric stenosis, 160, 473, 818
Pyloromyotomy, 473
Pyogenic liver abscess, 498-499
Pyogenic material, aspiration of, 391
Pyosalpinx, 174
Pyrantel pamoate
in amebiasis, 737
in ascariasis, 737
in enterobiasis, 738
in hookworm infestations, 738, 741
Pyrazinamide, 729
Pyrethrins with piperonyl bromide in lice, 746
Pyridoxine
deficiency of, 557
in seizures, 768
Pyrimethamine, 734

Q

Q fever, 371, 751, 758
Q wave, 424-425
QRS complex
in paroxysmal supraventricular
tachycardia, 466, 467
in premature atrial contraction, 457
in premature ventricular contraction, 457, 459
Quadriceps tendon, 319, 320
Queensland tick typhus, 758
Quidinine in malaria, 734, 735
Quinacrine, 738
Quinidine
in dysrhythmias from poisoning, 768
liver toxicity of, 497
thrombocytopenia and, 563
in vertigo, 610
Quinine
in babesiosis, 751
in ehrlichiosis, 759
in malaria, 734, 735
in muscle cramps, 545
thrombocytopenia and, 563
in vertigo, 610

R

Rabies, 719, 724
Rabies immune globulin, 724

Racemic epinephrine, 799
Radial head, 308
    displacement or communition of, 307-308
Radial nerve in humeral fracture, 310
Radial side of part, 296
Radiation burn of eye, 837
Radiation therapy in superior vena cava
        syndrome with tumors, 573
Radioactive phosphorus, 560
Radiography
    in abdominal pain, 137-139
    in acromioclavicular separation, 313
    in aortic dissection, 128
    in aortic transection, 257, 258
    in aortic trauma, 269
    in appendicitis, 483
    in asthma, 111
        in child, 801
    in back pain, 199
    in bowel obstruction, 481
    in brain injury, 222-223
    in burn patient, 337
    in cardiac tamponade, 575
    in chest pain, 128
    in child abuse, 819
    in chronic obstructive pulmonary disease,
        385
    in comatose patient, 85-86
    in congestive heart failure, 447
    in croup, 796, 798
    in diaphragmatic injury, 260
    in diverticular disease, 488
    in elbow fracture, 306-307
    in epiglottitis, 796, 798
    in esophageal injury, 262
    in flail chest, 257
    of foot, 326, 327, 328
    in foreign body aspiration
        airway and, 392-393, 800
        in child, 800
        gastrointestinal tract and, 478
    in hemothorax, 260
    in hip dislocation, 318
    in hip fracture, 317
    in Hirschsprung disease, 487
    in humeral fracture, 310
    in intraocular foreign body, 837
    in intussusception, 486
        in child, 818
    in lunate bone dislocation, 303
    in mandibular fracture, 234, 235
    in multiple trauma, 65
        in pregnancy, 66
    of nasal bones, 825
    in near-drowning, 346
    in odynophagia or achalasia, 475
    in orbital blowout fracture, 830
    in orthopedic trauma, 294
    in pelvic fractures, 316
    in pericardial tamponade, 267
    in pneumonia in child, 803
    in pneumothorax, 112, 259

Radiography—cont'd
    in psychosis, 651, 652
    in pulmonary contusion, 257
    in pulmonary disorders, 128
    in pulmonary embolism, 127, 402
    in pyloric stenosis, 473
    in renal stones, 518
    in retropharyngeal abscess, 364
    in shoulder dislocation, 311, 312, 313
    in sinusitis, 365
    in slipped capital femoral epiphysis, 296
    in spinal injury, 250-251
    in superior vena cava syndrome, 573
    in systemic lupus erythematosus, 581
    in urinary trauma, 280-281
    in volvulus, 486
        in child, 818-819
    in vomiting, 161
    in zygomatic fracture, 233
Radionuclide studies
    in back pain, 199
    in gastrointestinal bleeding, 149
    in pulmonary embolism, 401
Radius
    fracture of, 306
    wrist fractures and, 305
Rales, 115
Ranitidine, 476
Ranula, sublingual, 825
Rapid sequence intubation, 23-25
Rash
    in child, 816
    ectoparasitic, 745-746
    fever and, 72
    in Kawasaki syndrome, 711
    in Lyme disease, 193, 749-752
    macular, 584-592
    in measles, 720
    pustular lesions and, 584, 597-599
    scaly papule and, 594
    in systemic lupus erythematosus, 580
Ratios
    FEV$_1$/FVC, 116
    PO$_2$/FiO$_2$, 116
Raynaud disease, 417-418
    physical examination in, 413-414
Raynaud phenomenon, 418
Rebound headache, 101
Rebound tenderness, 136, 157
Recession, anterior chamber angle, 833
Recklinghausen disease, seizures and, 207
Recombinant tissue plasminogen activator,
        431
Reconstituted packed red blood cells, 64
Recording on chart, 12-13
Rectal examination
    in abdominal pain, 136
    in appendicitis, 483
    in brain injury, 222
Rectal prolapse, 489
Rectal sphincter tone in spinal injury, 246, 250
Rectal temperature, 71

Rectocolitis, 739
Rectum
    anorectal disease of, 488-489
    bleeding from, 145
    foreign body in, 489
Red blood cells
    in abdominal trauma, 273
    disorders of, 556-560
    enzyme deficiency and, 557
    gastrointestinal bleeding and, 148
    indices for, 557, 558
    in multiple trauma, 64
    in penetrating abdominal trauma, 277
    in urine in pregnancy-induced
        hypertension, 442
Red eye, 841-845
Red macule, 585-592
Red papule, 592-594
Reduction in dislocations
    of hip, 318
    of patella, 319
    of shoulder, 311-313
Referred pain
    abdominal, 132-133, 139
    neuroanatomy and, 131
Reflex
    Babinski, 85
        in Parkinson syndrome, 644
    deep tendon; see Deep tendon reflexes
    pupillary, 84, 828
Reflux
    esophageal, 475
        chest pain and, 475-476
        dysphagia and, 474-475
    gastroesophageal, in neonate and child,
        157-160
    urinary tract infection and, 507
Regional enteritis, 484-485
Reglan; see Metoclopramide
Regular narrow-complex tachycardia, 458,
        459-462
Regurgitation, 155; see also Vomiting
Reimplantation of finger, 291-292
Reiter syndrome, 193, 197
Relapsing fever, 750, 754-755
Relapsing polychondritis, 582
Renal artery in aortic dissection, 443
Renal colic, 517-519
Renal disease, anemia in, 557
Renal failure, 520-546
    acute, 525-530
        approach to patient with, 530-532
    chronic, 532-539
        reversible factors in, 536
    coagulation disorders in, 564
    constipation in, 545
    dialysis and, 539-545
    emergency department diagnostics in,
        520-523
    hematuria in, 523-524
    hyperkalemia and, 673
    hypertension and, 441

Renal failure—cont'd
  hypertension and—cont'd
    malignant, 437
    intractable nausea and vomiting in, 545
    muscle cramps in, 545
    proteinuria in, 524-525
Renal insufficiency, chronic, 533
Renal staging, diagnostic, 280
Renal system
  electrical injury and, 343
  fluid balance and, 666
  hypernatremia and, 669
  hypomagnesemia and, 685
  trauma to, 279-281
Repolarization, benign early, 424, 425
Reporting of child abuse, 819
Rescue breathing, 30-33
Research in emergency medicine, 5
Residency training in emergency medicine, 4-5
Respirations
  agonal, 82
  in chest injury, 254-255
  in coma, 82, 83-84
  in head injury, 220
  labored, 20
  in neonatal resuscitation, 42
  in poisoning, 762
  vomiting and, 156
Respiratory alkalosis in septic shock, 57
Respiratory arrest, 16, 17
Respiratory distress, 106-119
  adult, syndrome of, 109
  algorithm for, 114
  diagnostic approach in, 114, 115-117
  differential diagnosis in, 107-115
  management of, 117
    algorithm for, 114
  in toxic shock syndrome, 714
Respiratory effort in chest trauma, 255
Respiratory failure, 16, 17, 106; see also
    Respiratory distress
  in flail chest, 257
Respiratory syncytial virus, 718
  in bronchiolitis, 718
  in otitis media, 822
Respiratory system; see also Pulmonary entries
  in AIDS and HIV, 729-730
  in aspirations, 391-394
  in asthma, 379-384
  in child, 795-803
  in chronic obstructive pulmonary disease,
    384-389
  foreign bodies in, 391-394
  in hypermagnesemia, 684
  infection of, 361-378
    bronchitis in, 366
    lower, 366-375, 376-377
    pneumonia in, 367-374, 375, 376-377
    upper, 361-366
  in near-drowning, 345-346
  in pulmonary edema; see Pulmonary
    edema

Respiratory system—cont'd
  in respiratory distress, 106-119; see also
    Respiratory distress
Respiratory viruses in pneumonia, 376, 377
Rest pain in arteriosclerosis obliterans, 415
Restraint of violent patient, 662
Resuscitation
  cardiopulmonary; see Cardiopulmonary
    resuscitation
  fluid; see also Fluid therapy
    in burn patient, 335-336
    in electrical injury, 343
    in hypothermia, 355
    in multiple trauma, 62-64
    in child, 66
  Retching, 154, 472; see also Vomiting
Retention
  of fluid, heart failure and, 448-449
  urinary, 516-517
Reticulocytes
  count of, 558
  in sickle cell disease, 560
Retina
  hemorrhage of, 835
    in subdural hematoma in infant, 228
  swelling of, 238
  traumatic detachment of, 834-835
  vessel occlusion in, 843-844
Retinal artery, occlusion of, 843-844
Retinal vein, occlusion of, 844
Retinopathy, diabetic, 689
Retractions, 21
Retrobulbar hematoma, 830
Retrobulbar optic neuritis, 845
  in multiple sclerosis, 640
Retrograde cystogram, 281
Retroperitoneal space, 315
Retropharynx, abscess of, 364
Revascularization procedures in ischemic
    heart disease, 431
Rewarming in hypothermia, 355-356
  in near-drowning, 347
  protocol for, 357
Reye syndrome, fever and, 78
Rhabdomyolysis in acute renal failure,
    529, 530
Rheumatic fever, acute, 194-195, 197
Rheumatoid arthritis, 192, 197, 577-578
Rheumatoid disease, 577-583
  ankylosing spondylitis in, 578
  arthritis in, 192, 197, 577-578
  giant cell arteritis in, 579-580
  polymyalgia rheumatica in, 578-579
  sites and types of, 188
  systemic lupus erythematosus in, 580-582
Rheumatoid factor in giant cell arteritis, 580
Rhinorrhea
  in oral injury, 232
  in sinusitis, 365
Rhinoviruses, 362, 716
Rhythm, cardiac, 455-471; see also
    Dysrhythmias

Rib
  fracture of, 255-256
  pathology of, chest pain in, 122
Ribavirin, 718
Rickettsia, 751, 756-758
Rickettsia burnetti, 371, 377
Rickettsia rickettsii, 751, 756-758
Rifampin
  in meningitis, 626, 809
  in meningococcemia prophylaxis, 711
  in pancreatitis etiology, 503
  theophylline clearance and, 383
  in tuberculosis with AIDS and HIV, 729
Right-sided heart failure, 446
Rigidity, nuchal
  headache and, 97
  in meningitis, 621
    in child, 807
  in retropharyngeal abscess, 364
Rimantadine, 718
Ringer's lactate
  in abdominal pain, 134
  in burn patient, 336
  in dehydration in child, 806
  in drug poisoning, 768
  in multiple trauma, 64
  in shock in child, 807
Rinne test, 823
Risk factors, abdominal pain and, 133
Robaxin; see Methocarbamol
Rocky Mountain spotted fever, 589-590,
    751, 756-758
Roentgenography; see Radiography
Roseola, 586, 590-591
Rotator cuff tear, 314
Rotaviruses, 716
Roundworm, 737, 739-740
RSI; see Rapid sequence intubation
rt-PA; see Recombinant tissue plasminogen
    activator
Rubella, 586, 591, 719
  in viral arthritis, 195
Rubella vaccine, 721
Rubeola; see Measles
Rule of nines, 334
Rumack-Matthew nomogram, 772
Rupture
  aortic, 268-270
  of diaphragm, 260
  of endometrioma, 176
  of globe of eye, 835
  myocardial, 264, 265-266
  of ovarian cyst, 175
  of quadriceps tendon, 319, 320

S

S_3 gallop, 447, 452
S_4 gallop, 447
Sacral fracture, 316
Sacral sparing, 246
SAD PERSONS scale, 658
Safety glass, 236

Salicylates
  respirations and, 762
  in rheumatoid arthritis, 578
  toxicity of, 497, 783-785
    acidosis in, 766
    pancreatitis and, 503
    vertigo and, 610
Saline
  in abdominal pain, 134
  in Addisonian crisis, 696
  in bronchiolitis, 801
  in dehydration in child, 806
  in drug poisoning, 768, 782
  in enemas for foodborne botulism, 707
  in eye irrigation, 830
  in facial wounds, 237
  in gastrointestinal bleeding, 148, 152
  in heat illnesses, 351
  in hyperglycemic hyperosmolar
    nonketotic coma, 691
  in hyponatremia, 671
  in ketoacidosis, 690
  in multiple trauma, 64
  in shock
    in child, 807
    hypovolemic, 53
  in vomiting, 473
Salivary stone, 825
Salivation, lacrimation, spontaneous
  urination, and defecation, 765
Salmeterol, 384
Salmonella
  in diarrhea, 165, 167
  in infected aneurysm, 417
  in sickle cell disease, 560
Salpingitis, abdominal pain in, 135
Salter-Harris classification of epiphyseal
  injury, 296, 297
Saltwater drowning, 345
Sandflies, 745
Sarcoidosis, 677
Sarcoptes scabiei, 746
SBP; *see* Spontaneous bacterial peritonitis
Scabies, 594, 746
Scalded skin syndrome, staphylococcal, 588
Scalene muscle, 106
Scalp
  fungal infection of, 584
  laceration of, 225
  wound closure of, 289
Scaly papule, 594
Scaphoid bone fracture, 303
Scapular fracture, 314
Scarlet fever, 587, 591-592
Scarring, facial, 235-237
Schiötz tonometry, 828
Schistosoma haematobium, 741-742
  in genitourinary infestations, 741,
    744-745
Schistosoma japonicum, 738, 741-742
Schistosoma mansoni, 738, 741-742
Schizoaffective disorders, 654

Schizonts, 733-734
Schizophrenia, 652-654
Schizophreniform disorder, 654
Sciatic nerve injury, 317
  in femoral shaft fracture, 318
Scintigraphy in pulmonary embolism, 401;
    see also Radionuclide studies
Sclera
  laceration of, 836-837
  in orbital fracture, 234
Scleritis, 842
Scleroderma, 581
  in intrarenal vascular disease, 529
Sclerosis, lateral
  amyotrophic, 643
  primary, 643
Sclerotherapy
  in cirrhosis, 498
  in gastrointestinal bleeding, 477
Scombroid in diarrhea, 169
Scopolamine
  toxicity of, 765, 774
  vertigo and, 615
  in vomiting, 164
Screening, toxicologic, 765; *see also* Toxicology
Scrotum
  in epididymitis, 514-515
  mass in, 515-516
  trauma to, 279
Seborrhea in Parkinson syndrome, 644
Seclusion, environmental, 662
Second pupil, 833
Secondary drowning, 345
Secondary repair of wound, 285
Secondary spinal injury, 251
Second-degree atrioventricular block, 468, 469
Second-degree burn, 333-334
  fluid therapy in, 336
  percentage of areas affected by, 335
Secretions, airway, in noisy breathing, 19;
    see also Airway management
Secretory diarrhea, 165
Secretory otitis media, 823
Sedation
  in abdominal pain, 134
  in spinal injury, 245
Sedatives
  in headache, 100, 101
  in intubation, 22, 23
  psychologic emergency and, 662
  toxicity of, 782-783
    respiratory center and, 762
    in sympatholytic syndrome, 765
Seidel test, 836
Seizures, 201-216
  altered mental status and, 85
  in brain tumors, 575
  classification of, 201-206
  coma and, 81, 86
  diagnosis of, 206-208
  disposition in, 214
  drug therapy for, head injury and, 225

Seizures—cont'd
  in eclampsia, 553
  etiology of, 201, 202
  febrile, 812-813
  in hypernatremia, 669
  in meningitis, 621, 625
  near-drowning and, 346
  in poisoning, 767-768
  posttraumatic, 229
  prognosis in, 214
  in status epilepticus, 206
    in child, 809-812
    head injury and, 225
    management of, 211-215
  in subacute subdural hematoma, 228
  in syncope, 88
  term of, 201
  treatment of, 208-215
    anticonvulsants in, 208-210, 212-213
    long-term, 210-211, 212-213
    status epilepticus, 211-215
Sengstaken-Blakemore tube, 149, 150
Sensation
  in hand wound, 291
  psychogenic impairment of, 635-636
Sensory dermatome, 248
Sensory examination
  in chest pain, 122
  in headache, 97
  in shoulder dislocation, 311
  in spinal injury, 247-250
  in stroke, 602
Sensory neuropathies, subacute, 629
Separation
  acromioclavicular, 313-314
  craniofacial, 232
Sepsis
  coma and, 81
  sickle cell disease and, 559-560
Septal deformity, nasal, 238
Septic arthritis, 191-192, 196
Septic shock, 57-58
Septicemia in botulism, 707
Serevent; *see* Salmeterol
Seroheptadine, 100
Serotonin in deep venous thrombosis, 395
Serotonin inhibitors in headache, 100
Serratia, 511
Serum, examination of
  in abdominal trauma, 273
  in hematuria, 524
  in renal failure, 521-522
Serum amylase
  in abdominal pain, 137
  in abdominal trauma, 273
  in pancreatitis, 502
Serum bicarbonate in abdominal trauma, 273
Serum ferritin, 558
Serum hepatitis, 723; *see also* Hepatitis B
Serum iron, 558
Serum lipase
  in abdominal trauma, 273

Serum lipase—cont'd
in pancreatitis, 502
Serum osmolality in hyperglycemic
hyperosmolar nonketotic coma, 691
Seventh cranial nerve
Bell palsy of, 631-632
facial injury and, 232
Sexual abuse of child, 819-820
pelvic pain in, 177
straddle injury in, 279
Sexually transmitted disease, 723-724
in anorectal infection, 488-489
bowel syndrome in, 488-489
chlamydial; see *Chlamydia* organisms
in epididymitis, 514-515
in herpes simplex, 596, 717-718, 723
Trichomonas vaginalis as, 744
in urethritis, 512
Shaft fracture
femoral, 318-319
humeral, 308-310
tibial, 323
Shigella
diarrhea from, 165, 167-168
management of, 168
Shingles, 632-633, 721-722
skin problems in, 595, 597
Shock, 50-59
in child, 806-807
compensated and uncompensated, 50-51
complications of, 58
in ectopic pregnancy, 548
etiologic classification of, 51
evaluation and management of, 52-58
in head injury, 220
laboratory evaluation in, 52
pathophysiology of, 50-51
spinal, 245
in toxic shock syndrome, 589, 713-714
vomiting and, 156
Shortness of breath, 106
in congestive heart failure, 107-109
Shoulder
dislocation of, 311-313
fracture of, 313-314
splint for, 299
Shunt, meningitis and, 621
SIADH; see Syndrome of inappropriate
antidiuretic hormone
Sick sinus syndrome, 470
syncope and, 88
syncope in, 88
Sickle cell disease, 557, 559-560
Sideroblastic anemia, 557
Sigmoid volvulus, 486
Signs
Babinski, 644
Chvostek, 682, 686
Cullen, 502
Forchheimer, 720
Grey Turner, 502
Hoover, 635

Signs—cont'd
Kernig, 621
Lhermitte, 639
Murphy, 501
Myerson, 644
obturator, 483
psoas, 483
Trousseau, 682, 686
vital; see Vital signs
Silk suture, 287
Silvadene, 237-238
Silver fork deformity, 304
Silver nitrate, 237
Simple absence seizure, 204-205
Simple fracture, 295
Simple partial seizures, 205
treatment of, 211
Simple pneumothorax, 259
Sinus
inflammation of, 365-366
in periorbital cellulitis, 840
sphenoid, 104
transillumination of, 365
Sinus bradycardia, 465-466
Sinus headache, 104
Sinus node dysfunction, 88, 470
Sinus tachycardia, 458, 459
Sinusitis, 365-366
in periorbital cellulitis, 840
SK; see Streptokinase
Skeletal injury; see Orthopedic trauma
Skin, 584-599
burns of; see Burn
in child abuse, 819
in diphtheria, 698, 699, 700
electrical injury to, 342, 343
in gonococcemia, 194
in Lyme disease, 193, 749-752
parasitic infestation and, 745
Skull
computed tomography of, 222-223
conventional x-ray studies of, 223
fracture of, epidural hematoma and, 228
Sleeping sickness, 742
Sling for acromioclavicular separation, 314
Slipped capital femoral epiphysis, 317
Slitlamp examination, 828
corneal
in abrasions, 831
in lacerations, 836
keratitis and
herpes simplex, 841
ultraviolet, 837
in traumatic iritis, 832
SLUD mnemonic, 765
Small bowel
bleeding from, 145
obstruction of, 480-482
Small finger fracture, 303
Small intestine; see Gastrointestinal tract
Smallpox, 719
Smith fracture, 305

Smoke inhalation, 340
Snow blindness, 837
Sodium
dehydration and, 804, 805
elemental, burns from, 339, 340
excess; see Hypernatremia
in fluid balance, 664, 665, 666-671
fractional excretion of, 522, 523
losses of, in vomiting, 160
in syndrome of inappropriate antidiuretic
hormone, 575
urine, 522
Sodium bicarbonate; see Bicarbonate, sodium
Sodium iodide, 693
Sodium nitroprusside; see Nitroprusside
Sodium polystyrene sulfonate, 531, 674, 675
Sodium sulfacetamide, 831
Sodium-potassium pump, shock and, 50
Soft palate, 239
Soft tissue
in respiratory tract infection, 364-365
suturing of; see Suture
trauma to, 283-293
dressings in, 288
facial, 235-237
hemorrhage control in, 284
history of injury in, 283
in peripheral cold injuries, 356-357
physician preparation and, 284
prophylactic antibiotics in, 288-289
suturing in; see Suture
terminology of, 296-298
wound anatomy and physiology in,
283-284
wound closure in, 285-288
wound infections in, 288-289
wound preparation in, 284
Solvents
eye injury from, 838-839
peripheral neuropathies in, 628, 629
Somatic pain, 132
Somatostatinoma, 504
Sorbitol
with activated charcoal in poisoning,
767
in constipation from antacids, 545
in hyperkalemia, 675
Sore, pressure, 299
Sore throat, 361-364
Sounds
bowel, in obstruction, 480-481
breath
airway assessment and, 20-21
in pneumothorax, 259
in respiratory distress, 115
Space
pericardial, catheter in, 267
prevertebral, 364-365
retroperitoneal, 315
Spasm
ciliary, 832
esophageal, 475

Spasm—cont'd
  esophageal—cont'd
    chest pain in, 122
  in shoulder dislocation, 311
  in tetanus, 703
Spectinomycin
  in gonococcal arthritis, 193
  in gonorrheal cervicitis, 181
  in tularemia, 750, 756
Speech
  assessment of, in stroke, 603
  psychogenic disorders of, 637-638
Sphenoid sinus, 104
Sphincter
  anal, 488
  rectal, in spinal injury, 246, 250
Spinal artery in aortic dissection, 443
Spinal cord
  abdominal pain and, 132
  ankylosing spondylitis and, 578
  cross section of cervical, 249
  rheumatoid arthritis and, 577
Spinal fluid; *see* Cerebrospinal fluid
Spinal injury
  airway management in, 245
  in aortic trauma, 270
  circulatory support in, 245-246
  general approach in, 243, 244
  immobilization in, 243-245
    in near-drowning, 347
  injuries associated with, 246
  musculoskeletal, 252
  neurologic evaluation in, 246-250
  nonfracture, 314-315
  prioritization in, 243
  radiography of, 250-251
  rectal sphincter tone and, 246
  secondary, 251
  spinal cord, 249, 250, 251-252; *see also*
    Spinal cord
  surgery in, 251-252
  treatment and disposition in, 251-252
Spinal muscular atrophy, progressive, 643
Spinal nerve roots, 628
Spinal precautions, 243-245
Spinal shock, 245
Spine
  cervical; *see* Cervical spine
  injury to, 243-253; *see also* Spinal injury
  tumor compression of, 575
Spiral fracture of humerus, 310
Spirochetes
  Borrelia burgdorferi as, 748-754
  in relapsing fever, 754
Spirometry, 116
  in chronic obstructive pulmonary disease,
    385-386
Spironolactone
  in congestive heart failure, 449
  hyperkalemia and, 672, 673
  in hypertension, 438
Splenomegaly, fever and, 72

Splint
  lower extremity
    in ankle sprain, 324-325
    in femoral shaft fracture, 319
    in foot trauma, 292
    in hip sprain, 318
  upper extremity, 298
    in elbow injury, 307
    in humeral injury, 308
    in phalangeal fracture, 300
    in shoulder fracture, 314
    sugar-tong, 309, 310
Spondylitis, ankylosing, 578
Spontaneous bacterial peritonitis, 498
Spontaneous miscarriage, 549-550
Spontaneous pneumothorax, 111-112
Sporozoites, 739
Spots, Koplik, 589
Sprain, 296-298
  ankle, 324-325
  definition of, 296
  knee, 319-322
Spray, oxymetazoline, 366
Sputum in pneumonia, 367-374
ST segment elevation, 424, 425
Stab wound
  abdominal, 275-277, 292
  chest, 261
Stable angina, 427-428
Stage of development, 791, 792-793
Staphylococcal infection
  in aneurysm, 417
  in cellulitis, 585
  in child, 796
  in conjunctivitis, 840
  in diarrhea, 169
  in impetigo, 597-599
  in meningitis and encephalitis, 618, 619,
    625
  in orbital cellulitis, 842
  in peritoneal dialysis, 543
  in pneumonia, 367, 372, 376, 377
  in scalded skin syndrome, 588
  in sickle cell disease, 560
  in toxic shock syndrome, 713-714
  in tracheitis, 796
  tumors and, 572, 573
  in urinary tract, 508, 510, 511, 512
    in child, 513
Staples in wound closure, 287
Starvation ketosis, vomiting and, 161
Stasis of urine, 507
Status epilepticus, 206
  in brain injury, 225
  in child, 809-812
  management of, 211-215
Stenosis
  aortic, altered mental status and, 91
  cardiac valve, 88
  pyloric, 160, 473, 818
Stensen's duct, parotitis and, 825
Sternocleidomastoid muscle, 106

Steroids; *see also* Corticosteroids
  adverse effects of, in head injury, 224
  anabolic, liver toxicity of, 497
  in asthma, 381, 382, 383, 384
    in child, 802
  in atopic dermatitis, 588
  in Bell palsy, 632
  in bronchiolitis, 801
  in bronchitis, 366
  in caustic burns, 776
  in chronic obstructive pulmonary disease,
    387
  in cluster headache, 100
  contraceptive, liver toxicity of, 497
  in croup, 799
  glucocorticoid
    adrenal failure and, 695-696
    hypertension and, 433
  in herpes zoster, 597
  in hydrocarbon poisoning, 780
  in hypercalcemia, 680
  in hypertension, 433
  in meningitis, 625-626
  in multiple sclerosis, 641
  in pemphigus vulgaris, 596
  in pertussis, 702
  in pseudotumor cerebri, 642
  in rheumatoid arthritis, 192
  in scleritis, 842
  in temporal arteritis, 103, 844
  in tendinitis, 192
  in toxic epidermal necrolysis, 588
  in *Trichinella spiralis* infestations, 744
Stevens-Johnson syndrome, 593
Stibogluconate sodium in leishmaniasis,
  745
Stiff neck
  in meningitis, 621
    in child, 807
  in retropharyngeal abscess, 364
Stimulation
  in comatose patient, 84
  in neonatal resuscitation, 42
  in toxic syndromes, 764
Stomach, bleeding from, 145; *see also*
    Gastric *entries;* Gastrointestinal tract,
    bleeding in
Stones
  gallstones as, 500
  salivary, 825
  urinary, 517-519
Stool in diarrhea, 165, 166
Storage diseases, anemias in, 557
Straddle injury
  in child, 279
  vaginal bleeding and, 179
Strain, 296-298
  definition of, 296
Strangulation, bowel, 481
Stravudine, 730
Strawberry cervix, 744
Strawberry tongue, 712

Street drugs, parkinsonism from, 645
Streptococcal infection
    in cellulitis, 585
    in conjunctivitis, 840
    diagnosis of acute infection with, 194
    in fever, 75
    in impetigo, 597-599
    in meningitis and encephalitis, 618, 619
        in child, 807
        therapy for, 624, 625, 626
    in otitis media, 822
    in pharyngitis, 361-363, 362
    in pneumococcemia, 707-709
    in pneumonia, 367, 372, 375, 376, 377
        in child, 803
    in rheumatic fever, 194
    in scarlet fever, 591
    in sickle cell disease, 559, 560
Streptokinase, 430-431
Streptomycin
    hearing loss from, 823
    in tuberculosis with AIDS and HIV, 729
Stress testing, 127
Stridor, 19
    assessment of, 115
    in croup, 795-796, 799
    in upper airway obstruction, 113
Stroke; *see* Cerebrovascular accident
Strongyloides stercoralis, 740, 742
    in pulmonary disorders, 743
Strongyloidiasis, 738, 740
Stubbing of toe, 329
Stupor, 80
Sty, 839
Subacute sensory motor neuropathies, 629
Subacute subdural hematoma, 227-228
Subaortic stenosis, hypertrophic, 88
Subarachnoid hemorrhage, 600, 602
    altered mental status in, 85
    in coma, 86
    headache in, 102
    management of, 605-606
    physical findings in, 600
    in syncope, 89
Subarachnoid stroke, Hunt and Hess
        classification of, 605, 606
Subchondral hematoma, 238-239
Subclavian artery
    aneurysm of, 417
    clavicular fracture and, 313
    in thoracic outlet syndrome, 419
Subclavian steal syndrome in syncope, 88,
        614
Subclavian-axillary aneurysm, 417
Subconjunctival hemorrhage, 831-832
Subcutaneous emphysema, 234
Subdiaphragmatic abdominal thrust, 35-36
    in child, 45
Subdural hematoma, 227-228
    acute, 227-228
    chronic, 228
    headache in, 102-103

Subhyaloid hemorrhage, 835
Sublingual ranula, 825
Subluxation
    of atlantoaxial joint, 577
    definition of, 296
    of elbow, 307-308
    lens, 833-834
    of radial head, 308
    tooth, 241
Subscleral hemorrhage, 234
Succinimides, 212-213
Succinylcholine
    hyperkalemia and, 672
    in intubation, 23, 24
Succussion splash, 157
Sucralfate
    in esophageal spasm, 475
    in peptic ulcers, 476
Suction
    in neonatal resuscitation, 42
    in oral injury, 231
Sudden cardiac death, 429
    in child, 47-48
    in myocardial contusion, 258
Sudden infant death syndrome, 820
Sugar-tong splint, 309, 310
Suicide, 656-659
    indications for hospitalization and, 658, 659
    predicting likelihood of, 658
Sulbactam, 134
Sulfacetamide sodium, 831
Sulfadoxine, 734
Sulfamethoxazole; *see also* Trimethoprim,
        with sulfamethoxazole
    in AIDS and HIV, 728-729, 730
    in otitis media, 822
    in urinary tract infection, in child, 513
Sulfisoxazole
    in chlamydial cervicitis, 181
    in otitis media, 822
Sulfonamides
    in pancreatitis etiology, 503
    for seizures, 212-213
    thrombocytopenia and, 563
Sulfonylureas
    hypoglycemia secondary to, 692
    toxicology of, 765, 785-786
Sulindac, 503
Sumatriptan, 100
Superior mesenteric artery, 483-484
Superior vena cava syndrome, 573
Supine hypotension in pregnancy, 551
Suppressants, cough, 366
Suppurative parotitis, 825
Supracondylar fracture, 310
Supraventricular tachycardia
    with aberrancy, 465
    paroxysmal, 459-460
    in syncope, 88
Suramin sodium, 742
Surgery, anemia and, 557

Surgical airway
    cricothyrotomy for; *see* Cricothyrotomy
    tracheostomy for, in child, 66
Survey, multiple trauma, 64-65
Suture
    for dermis, 135
    dressings for, 288
    epidermal, 236
    in facial trauma, 235-236
    materials for, 286-287
    in nasal fracture, 238
    in neck wound, 290
    in nose wound, 289
    placement of, 288
    removal of, 288
    in scalp repair, 289
    for special areas, 289-292
SVCS; *see* Superior vena cava syndrome
Swallowed blood, 145
Swallowing
    dysphagia and, 473-475
    syncope and, 89
Swan-Ganz catheter in burn patient, 336
Swelling; *see also* Edema
    in elbow dislocation, 307-308
    in oral injury, 239
    in orbital fracture, 234
    of retina, 238
    in sinusitis, 365
    in sprains, 298
    in testicular trauma, 279
    in uvula injury, 239
Sympatholytic syndrome, 765
Sympathomimetics in headache, 101
Syncope, 86-92
    heat, 349
    situational causes of, 89
Syndrome of inappropriate antidiuretic
        hormone, 666-667
    in meningitis in child, 807
    tumors and, 575
Synovial fluid
    classification of, 189
    in differential diagnosis, 190
    in pseudogout, 190-191
    septic arthritis and, 189, 190
Syphilis
    in AIDS and HIV, 729
    anorectal infection and, 488
Systemic lupus erythematosus, 580-582
Systemic vascular resistance in distributive
        shock, 57
Systemic venous pressure in heart failure, 447
Systemic viral infection, 722-723
Systolic blood pressure
    in heart failure, 446
    in hypertensive-emergencies of
        pregnancy, 441

T

T wave, 458
    hyperacute, 422-424

Tachycardia
  in asthma, 380
  general assessment in, 455-456
  in hypomagnesemia, 685-686, 687
  in myocardial contusion, 265
  narrow-complex
    irregular, 462-463, 464
    regular, 458, 459-462
  in pulmonary embolism, 125
  supraventricular, in syncope, 88
  in syncope, 88
  ventricular
    protocol for, 38-39
    in syncope, 88
  wide-complex, 465, 466
Tachydysrhthmias in syncope, 88
Tachypnea
  assessment of, 115, 116
  in asthma, 380
  dyspnea versus, 106
  in pulmonary embolism, 125
Tactile stimulation of neonate, 42, 819
Taenia solium, 742-743
Tagamet; *see* Cimetidine
Tamponade, pericardial; *see* Pericardial
    tamponade
Tapeworms in central nervous system,
    742-743; *see also* Parasites
Task mastery, 792
Td; *see* Tetanus and diphtheria toxoid
Team, trauma, 60-61
Team captain, 61
Tear
  ankle ligament, 324-325
  aortic, 268-270
  knee ligament, 320-322
  rotator cuff, 314
  subdural hematoma and, 227-228
  testicular, 279
Technetium 99m-labeled iminodiacetic acid,
    501
Technicians for trauma team, 61
Teeth, trauma and, 240-241
  of face, 232
Telangiectasia, epistaxis in, 824
Temperature
  abdominal pain and, 136
  in cold-induced injuries, 352-353, 354-358
  coma and, 81, 83
  in drug poisoning, 769
  in fever, 71-79; *see also* Fever
  in heat illnesses, 349-354
  importance of, 8
  in multiple trauma in child, 65
Temporal arteritis, 418, 579-580, 844
  headache and, 103
Temporal lobe seizure, 205-206
Temporomandibular joint, 234
  arthritis and, 577
Tempra; *see* Acetaminophen
TEN; *see* Toxic epidermal necrolysis
Tenckhoff catheter, 542, 543

Tenderness
  in ectopic pregnancy, 548-549
  in tendinitis, 192, 196
Tendinitis, 192, 196
Tendon
  in hand wound, 291
  inflammation of, 192, 196
  in knee injury, 320-322
Tendon reflexes, deep; *see* Deep tendon
    reflexes
TENS in postherpetic neuralgia, 633
Tension, arterial oxygen, 116
Tension pneumothorax, 259
  pericardial tamponade versus, 267
  in pulseless electrical activity, 40
  respiratory distress and, 112
Terbutaline
  in asthma in child, 801, 802
  in bronchiolitis, 801
  in chronic obstructive pulmonary disease,
    387
Terconazole, 183
Tertiary repair of wound, 285
Testis
  orchitis and, 515
  trauma to, 279
Tetanolysin, 703
Tetanospasmin, 703
Tetanus, 703-705
  prophylaxis for, 704-705
    in burn patient, 336
Tetanus and diphtheria toxoid, 705
Tetanus immune globulin, 704-705
Tetany, heat, 349
Tetracaine
  in conjunctival foreign body removal, 830
  in eye examination, 828
  wound closure and, 285
Tetracycline
  in bronchitis, 388
  in Eastern spotted fever, 758
  in ehrlichiosis, 758
  in inclusion conjunctivitis, 841
  liver toxicity of, 497
  in malaria, 735
  in pancreatitis etiology, 503
  in pneumonia, 376
  in Q fever, 751, 758
  in relapsing fever, 750, 754
  in Rocky Mountain spotted fever, 590,
    751, 757-758
  in tularemia, 750, 756
Tetraiodothyronine, 692, 693
Thalassemia syndromes, 557
THC; *see* Transhepatic cholangiography
Theophylline
  in asthma in child, 802
  in bronchiolitis, 801
  in chronic obstructive pulmonary disease,
    389
  clearance of, 382-383
  in drug poisoning, 765

Theophylline—cont'd
  in drug poisoning—cont'd
    activated charcoal for, 767
  toxicity of, 786
Theories of child development, 792-793
Thermal and chemical injury, 333-341; *see
    also* Burn
  chemicals in, 338-340
  in eye burns, 837-838
  general considerations for, 333
  laboratory and x-ray studies of, 337
  management of, 334-336
    admission to burn unit in, 338
    general measures in, 336-337
    outpatient, 337-338
  pathophysiology of, 333-334
  smoke inhalation in, 340
Thermoregulation, 71, 349
Thiabendazole
  in cutaneous larva migrans, 745
  in strongyloidiasis, 738
  theophylline clearance and, 383
Thiamine
  for comatose patient, 83
  in meningitis and encephalitis, 624
Thiazide diuretics
  in heart failure, 448, 449
  in hypercalcemia, 677-678
  in hypertension, 438
  hypokalemia and, 675, 676
  hypomagnesemia and, 685
  in pancreatitis etiology, 503
  in renal failure, 441
Thigh, femoral fracture and, 318
Thionamides, 693
Thioridazine, 633
Third-degree atrioventricular block, 469-470
Third-degree burn, 334
  fluid therapy in, 336
  percentage of area affected by, 335
Thirst, 666
Thomas long-leg splint, 318
Thoracic cavity trauma, 254-263; *see also*
    Chest trauma
Thoracic outlet syndrome, 418-420
Thoracic spinal injury, 315
  nonfracture, 314-315
Thoracostomy
  in chest injury, 254, 261
  in pneumothorax, 260
  tube; *see* Tube thoracostomy
Thoracotomy, 260
  in cardiovascular injuries to chest and
    neck, 270
  in myocardial rupture, 266
  in pericardial tamponade, 267
Thorax; *see* Chest *entries*
Thorazine; *see* Chlorpromazine
Thought disorders, 652-654
Threatened miscarriage, 550
Throat
  bleeding from, 145

Throat—cont'd
  diphtheria and, 698-699
  pharyngitis and, 361-364
Thrombectomy
  in pulmonary embolism or deep venous
    thrombosis, 407-408
  in thrombotic stroke, 604
Thrombin time, 568
Thromboangiitis obliterans, 415-416
Thrombocytopenia, 563-567
  epistaxis in, 824
  heparin-associated, 406
Thrombocytopenic purpura, 563-565
Thrombocytosis, 565-567
  venous thrombosis in, 400
Thrombolysis
  in central retinal artery occlusion, 844
  contraindications to, 430
  in ischemic heart disease, 430-431
  in postresuscitation care, 41
  in pulmonary embolism or deep venous
    thrombosis, 407-408
Thrombosis; *see* Thrombus
Thrombotic stroke, 600, 601
  in hypertension, 440
  management of, 604-605
Thromboxane
  in deep venous thrombosis, 395
  topical, inhibition of, in frostbite, 357
Thrombus
  arterial, 416
    in acute occlusion, 410
  ball-valve, 88
  deep vein; *see* Deep venous thrombosis
  in-situ, 410, 411
    physical examination in, 412-413
  physical findings in, 125
  in stroke; *see* Thrombotic stroke
Thrust
  abdominal, in choking, 35-36
  jaw, 30, 32
Thumb fracture, 303
Thyroid disorder, 692-694
  hypercalcemia in, 677
Thyroid hormone
  in myxedema coma, 695
  in thyrotoxicosis, 692-693
Thyroid storm, 693-694
Thyroidectomy in hypocalcemia, 680
Thyroiditis, 362
Thyrotoxicosis, hypercalcemia in, 677
Thyroxin
  hypomagnesemia and, 685
  in myxedema coma, 695
TIA; *see* Transient ischemic attack
Tibial bone marrow, 44
Tibial fracture, 322-323
Tibial veins in deep venous thrombosis,
  397
Ticarcillin
  with clavulanate in urinary tract infection,
    511

Ticarcillin—cont'd
  in tumor infection emergencies, 573
Tick paralysis, 751, 759-760
Tickborne illnesses, 748-761
  babesiosis in, 751, 758-759
  Colorado tick fever in, 751, 759
  Eastern spotted fever in, 758
  ehrlichiosis in, 751, 758
  Lyme disease in, 748-754
  paralysis in, 751, 759-760
  prevention of, 760
  Q fever in, 751, 758
  relapsing fever in, 750, 754-755
  Rocky Mountain spotted fever in, 750,
    756-758
  tick life cycle in, 748
  tularemia in, 750, 755-756
Ticlopidine, 605
TIG; *see* Human tetanus immune globulin
Tigan; *see* Trimethobenzamide
Timolol, 843
Tinactin; *see* Tolnaftate
Tincture of benzoin, 184
Tinea, 584, 585
Tinidazole
  in amebiasis, 737
  in giardiasis, 738
Tinnitus with vomiting, 155
Tioconazole, 183
Tissue hypoxemia, smoke inhalation and, 340
Tissue plasminogen activator, 431
Tobramycin
  in pelvic inflammatory disease, 184
  in tumor infection emergencies, 573
  in vascular access infection, 540
Todd paralysis, 207
  stroke versus, 603
Toe
  splinting of, 298, 299
  stubbing of, 329
  wound closure and, 292
Tolnaftate, 584
o-Toluidine test, 146
Tomography
  computerized; *see* Computerized tomography
  in orbital blowout fracture, 830
Tongue
  injury to, 239
  relaxed, 30
Tonic-clonic seizures, 203
Tonometry, Schiötz, 828
Tooth
  avulsion of, 241
  fracture of, 240-241
Topical anesthetics
  for eye, 828
    in conjunctival foreign body removal, 830
    in corneal abrasion, 831
    in corneal foreign body removal, 831
  in tendinitis, 192
Topical antibiotics
  in conjunctivitis, 840-841

Topical antibiotics—cont'd
  in wound care, 288
Topical antiviral agents in corneal infections,
  841
Toradol; *see* Ketorolac
Torque injury to phalanx, 301-303
Torsion
  adnexal, 174-175
  testicular, 515-516
  of testicular appendage, 516
Torus fracture, 296
Total body water, 664
  dehydration and, 667-668
  in hyponatremia, 669, 671
  osmolarity and, 665
Total iron binding capacity, 558
Total peripheral resistance of pericardial
  tamponade, 266
Toxic epidermal necrolysis, 588
Toxic granulation in neutrophils, 73
Toxic megacolon, 485
Toxic nodular goiter, 692
Toxic shock syndrome, 589, 713-714
Toxic syndromes, 764-766
Toxicity, digitalis, 451
Toxicologic screen, 765
Toxicology, 762-787; *see also* Poisoning
  acetaminophen in, 771-772
  of alcohol; *see* Alcohol abuse
  principles in, 762-770
    history and, 763
    initial stabilization in, 762-763
    laboratory tests and, 765-766
    physical examination and, 763-764
    syndromes and, 764-766
    treatment, 766-769
Toxidromes, 764
Toxins
  botulism and, 706-707
  coma and, 81
  diarrhea from, 169, 170
  hearing loss from, 823
  peripheral neuropathies in, 628, 629
  in tetanus, 703, 705
Toxoid, diphtheria and tetanus, 702-703, 705
Toxoplasmosis
  in AIDS and HIV, 729
  in uveal tract inflammation, 842
t-PA; *see* Tissue plasminogen activator
Tracheal intubation, near-drowning and, 346
Tracheitis, bacterial, 796, 799
Tracheobronchial diphtheria, 699, 700
Tracheostomy in child, 27, 66
Trachoma, 841
Traction in hip dislocation, 318
Traction headache, 101-103
Tranquilizers
  in chemical restraint, 662
  in headache, 100, 101
  in psychosis, 652
Transcutaneous electrical nerve stimulation
  in postherpetic neuralgia, 633

Transcutaneous oximetry, 113
in chest pain, 128
in coma, 82
Transection, aortic, 268-270
Transesophageal echocardiography, 128
Transfer of patient in multiple trauma, 67
Transfusion, blood; *see* Blood transfusion
Transhepatic cholangiography, 501
Transient erythroblastopenia of childhood,
557
Transient focal paresis, 207
Transient ischemic attack, 601
management of, 604
in syncope, 88
Transillumination of sinus, 365
Transverse myelitis, 640
Trauma; *see also* Wound *entries*
abdominal, 272-278
operative versus nonoperative
management of, 273-274
airway management in, 18, 20, 25
anemia and, 557
blunt; *see* Blunt trauma
cardiovascular, 264-271
chest, 254-263; *see also* Chest trauma
coma and, 81
electrical, 342-344
eye
cataract from, 834
hyphema from, 832-833
iridodialysis in, 833
iritis from, 832
mydriasis and miosis from, 833
facial, 231-242; *see also* Facial trauma
eye and, 829-839; *see also* Eye, injury to
fracture and; *see* Fracture
genitourinary tract, 278-281
head, 219-230; *see also* Head injury
intubation and, 18-19, 25
from lightning, 342-344
multiple, 60-68
intubation in, 18-19
orthopedic, 294-330; *see also* Orthopedic
trauma
pharyngitis and, 362
soft tissue, 283-293; *see also* Soft tissue,
trauma to
spinal; *see* Spine, injury to
thermal, 333-341; *see also* Burn; Thermal
and chemical injury
in vaginal bleeding, 179
Trauma team, 60-61
Trazodone, toxicity of, 777
Treitz ligament, 483
Tremor
differential diagnosis in, 645
in Parkinson syndrome, 644, 645
Treponema pallidum in meningitis and
encephalitis, 618
Triage, 8
Triamcinolone
in asthma, 384

Triamcinolone—cont'd
in dermatitis, 588
Triamterene
in heart failure, 449
in hyperkalemia, 673
in hypertension, 439
Trichinella spiralis, 744
Trichomonas vaginalis, 181-182
in genitourinary infestations, 744-745
Trichomoniasis, 181-182
Trichuriasis, 738, 740
Tricyclic antidepressants in migraine, 100
Trifluridine, 718, 723, 843
Trigeminal neuralgia, 95, 97, 103-104
Trihexyphenidyl, 645
Triiodothyronine, 692, 693
Trimalleolar fracture, 323-324
Trimethadione, 211, 212-213
Trimethobenzamide in vomiting, 163, 164,
473
in renal failure, 545
Trimethoprim
with sulfamethoxazole
in AIDS and HIV, 728-729, 730
in bronchitis, 388
in diarrhea, 168, 172
in otitis media, 822
in urinary tract infection, 510, 511,
513, 514
in urinary tract infection, 510, 511, 514
in child, 513
Trimipramine, toxicity of, 777
Trismus, 232, 233
in tetanus, 703
Trophozoites, 739, 742
Tropicamide, 828
Trousseau sign, 682, 686
Trypanosoma cruzi, 743-744
Trypanosoma gambiense, 742
Trypanosoma rhodesiense, 742
Tsetse fly, 742
Tubal pregnancy, 174
abdominal pain in, 135
Tube
endotracheal; *see* Endotracheal intubation
fallopian
pregnancy in, 135, 174
torsion of, 174-175
trauma to, 278-281
Tube thoracostomy
in diaphragmatic injury, 260
in hemothorax, 260
in multiple trauma, 62
in pneumothorax, 259, 260
Tubegauze dressings, 291
Tuberculosis
in AIDS and HIV, 729
in meningitis and encephalitis, 618, 621
Tuberous sclerosis, seizures and, 207
Tubular necrosis, acute, 526
intrinsic renal failure from, 527, 529-530
urinary findings in, 522

Tularemia, 750, 755-756
Tumor, 572-576; *see also* Malignancy
anorectal, 489
coma and, 80
headache and, 101
liver and, 499-500
pancreatic, 504, 505
testicular, 516
Tumor lysis syndrome, 573-574
Tylenol; *see* Acetaminophen
Tympanic membrane
bubbles seen through, 823
rupture of
in barotrauma, 824
in otitis media, 822
Tympanostomy, 822
Typhus, North Asian or Queensland tick, 758
Tzanck test, 180, 721

U

Ulcer
bleeding from, 143
chest pain and, 475-476
corneal, 841
cutaneous, in leishmaniasis, 745
vomiting and, 154, 156
Ulcerative colitis, 485
Ulna, fracture of, 306
Ulnar artery, aneurysm of, 417
Ulnar nerve, injury to, 308
Ulnar side of part, 296
Ultrasonography
in abdominal pain, 137-138
in abdominal trauma, 274
in aortic dissection, 443
in arterial disease, 414-415
cardiac, 427
in cholangitis, 501
in cholecystitis, 501
in deep venous thrombosis, 400-401
in intraocular and orbital foreign bodies, 836
in orbital blowout fracture, 830
in ovarian cyst, 176
in pericardial tamponade, 267
in pregnancy, 547-548
ectopic, 549
in pyloric stenosis, 473
in renal stones, 518
in testicular torsion, 515-516
in vaginal bleeding, 178
in vitreous hemorrhage, 834
Ultraviolet keratitis, 837
U_{Na}; *see* Sodium, fractional excretion of
Uncompensated shock, 50-51, 806
Undigested food in vomiting, 155
Unmonitored cardiac arrest, 36
Unreactive pupil, 84
Unresponsiveness, 81
Unstable angina, 428
diagnostic tests for, 126, 127
Upper airway obstruction, 107, 112-113
Upper esophageal dysphagia, 473-474

Upper extremity; *see also* Extremity
aneurysms of, 417
fracture of, 300-314
elbow, 306-307
forearm, 306
hand, 300-303
humeral, 308-313
shoulder and clavicle, 313-314
wrist, 303-306
shoulder and
dislocation of, 311-313
splint for, 314
thoracic outlet syndrome of, 418-420
wound closure for, 290
Upper gastrointestinal tract, 472-479
bleeding from, 142-144
Upper respiratory tract
in child, 795-800
infection of, 361-366, 716-718
Upper urinary tract
infection of, 507, 509
trauma to, 279-281
Urea nitrogen; *see* Blood urea nitrogen
Uremia; *see* Renal failure
Ureteral colic, 133, 517-519
Urethra, pelvic fracture and, 316
Urethritis, 512, 514
Uric acid
in gout, 190
tumor and, 574
Urinalysis; *see also* Urine
in abdominal pain, 137
in pyelonephritis, 514
in renal failure, 520-521
in urinary tract infection, 508
in child, 513
Urinary bladder
disorders of
schistosomiasis in, 741, 744-745
urinary tract infection in, 507
trauma to, 281
Urinary catheter; *see* Catheter
Urinary retention, 516-517
Urinary symptoms in adnexal torsion, 174
Urinary tract
infection of, 507-515
catheter-associated, 512
complicated, 507, 508-509, 511
definitions in, 507
low count, 507
in pelvic fracture, 316
trauma to, 279-281
Urination, syncope and, 89
Urine; *see also* Urinalysis
cultures of, in urinary tract infection, 508, 509
in diabetes, 689
hematuria and, 519
in hypertensive-emergencies of
pregnancy, 441, 442
in hyponatremia, 670
microscopic examination of, in renal
failure, 521

Urine—cont'd
sodium excretion in, 522, 523
stasis of, urinary tract infection and, 507
volume of, in renal failure, 520, 531-532
Urticaria, 589
Uterine bleeding, dysfunctional, 179-180
Uterus
carcinoma of, 179
cervix and; *see* Cervix, uterine
leiomyoma of, 176-177
bleeding from, 178
trauma to, 278-281
pregnancy and, 66
Uveitis, 842
Uvula, 239

V

Vaccine
measles, mumps, rubella, 721
in pertussis, 701, 702-703
pneumococcal, 709
polio, 724
rabies, 724
rubella, 721
Vaginal bleeding, 178-180
Vaginal discharge, 181-185
Vaginal foreign body, 177
Vaginal introitus in genital trauma, 279
Vaginitis, herpes simplex, 596
Vaginosis, bacterial, 182-183
Valgus deformity, 296
Valium; *see* Diazepam
Valproic acid, 211, 212-213
liver toxicity of, 497
in pancreatitis etiology, 503
Valsalva maneuver, atrial flutter and, 461
Valve, cardiac
prosthetic, anemia and, 557
syncope and, 88
Vanceril; *see* Beclomethasone
Vancomycin
hearing loss from, 823
in meningitis, 625
in tumor infection emergencies, 573
in vascular access infection, 540
in vertigo, 610
Varicella-zoster immune globulin, 595, 722
Varicella-zoster virus, 718, 719, 721-722
in corneal infection, 841
in neurologic disorders, 632-633
in skin disorders, 595, 596-597, 597
tumors and, 572
Varices, esophageal or gastric, 143, 149
bleeding from, 477
Vascular access
in advanced life support, 36
in burn patient, 336
in child, 794
in resuscitation, 42-44, 47
complications of, 540
in multiple trauma, 62-64, 65
in neonate, 42-44

Vascular headache, 94, 98-101
Vascular nevi, seizures and, 207
Vascular resistance, systemic, 57
Vascular system; *see also* Veins
cephalization of, heart failure and, 447
disorders of, 562-563
coma and, 81
hematologic, 562-563
intrarenal, 528-529
in syncope, 88
vertigo in, 614
in elbow dislocation, 307
in humeral shaft fracture, 310
Kawasaki syndrome and, 711, 712
in knee dislocation, 322
in mesenteric occlusion, 483-484
in orthopedic trauma, 294
Vasculitis
in giant cell arteritis, 579
in headache, 103
necrotizing, 418
Vasoconstrictors
in allergic conjunctivitis, 841
in epistaxis, 824
Vasodepressor syncope, 86
Vasodilation in migraine, 99
Vasodilators
in cardiogenic shock, 56
in congestive heart failure, 450, 451
in pregnancy-induced hypertension, 553
in pulmonary edema, 453
in syncope, 89
Vasogenic shock, 50, 51, 57-58
Vasoocclusive crisis of sickle cell disease, 559
Vasopressin
in coagulation disorders, 568
in gastrointestinal bleeding, 149, 150
Vasopressors
in cardiogenic shock, 55-56
in septic shock, 57
in toxic shock syndrome, 714
Vasospasm
disorders of, 417-418
physical examination in, 413-414
in subarachnoid hemorrhage, 605-606
Vasovagal syncope, 86
Vecuronium, 24
Vegetable matter, aspiration of, 392
Veins
retinal, occlusion of, 844
in subdural hematoma, 227-228
Velpeau bandage, 308
in shoulder fracture, 314
Vena cava
in pregnancy, 66
in superior vena cava syndrome, 573
Venereal warts, 184
Venodilators
in congestive heart failures, 450, 451
in pulmonary edema, 454-453
Venous access in child, 794; *see also*
Vascular access

Venous hypertension, 573
Venous pressure
central; *see* Central venous pressure
systemic, in heart failure, 447
Venous thrombosis
deep; *see* Deep venous thrombosis
physical findings in, 125
Ventilation
in asthma, 383
brainstem and, 106
central nervous system and, 107
mouth-to-mask, 33
mouth-to-mouth, 30-33
mouth-to-nose, 30-33
in multiple trauma, 63
in myxedema coma, 695
in pediatric resuscitation, 45
of neonate, 42
in pulmonary edema, 453
in shock management, 53
Ventilation-perfusion scan, 116
in pulmonary embolism, 127-128, 401, 404
Ventilatory insufficiency
in flail chest, 257
in hypoxemia, 29
in respiratory distress, 116
Ventricular failure, 108
Ventricular fibrillation
in drug poisoning, 768
in electrical injury, 343
protocol for, 38
Ventricular tachycardia
in hypomagnesemia, 685-686, 687
protocol for, 38-39
in syncope, 88
in wide-complex tachycardia, 465, 466
Ventriculoperitoneal shunt, meningitis and, 621
Verapamil
in atrial fibrillation, 463
in atrial flutter, 461
in atrial tachycardia with block, 461
contraindicated
in preexcitation syndromes, 467
in Wolff-Parkinson-White syndrome, 467
liver toxicity of, 497
in multifocal atrial tachycardia, 463
in paroxysmal supraventricular tachycardia, 460
Vermilion border of lip, 290
Versed; *see* Midazolam
Vertebral compression, 199
Vertebrobasilar artery insufficiency, 611, 614, 616
Vertebrobasilar syndrome, 601
management of, 605
Vertigo, 608-616, 823-824
benign paroxysmal positional, 613
diagnosis in, 610-612
differential, 613-615
drugs causing, 610
history of, 610-611

Vertigo—cont'd
management of, 615-616
pathophysiology of, 608-610
with vomiting, 155
Vesicular lesions, 584, 594-597
Vessels; *see* Vascular system
Vestibular apparatus, 609
Vestibular neuronitis, 613-614
Vestibulospinal tract, lateral, 610
Vestibulotoxicity of drugs, 610
Vestigial appendage in scrotum, 516
Vibrio, diarrhea from, 165, 167, 169
Vicryl suture; *see* Polyglycolic suture
Vidarabine
in chickenpox, 722
in herpes simplex, 717, 718, 723
in varicella, 718
Violence, 660-663
diagnoses and conditions associated with, 661
recognition of impending, 660-661
VIPoma, 504
Viral infection, 716-725
in acquired immunodeficiency syndrome, 726-732
arthritis and, 195, 197
of childhood, 720-722
conjunctival, 840
in diarrhea, 166-167
Epstein-Barr; *see* Epstein-Barr virus
gastroenteritis in, 716
in hepatitis, 491-495, 496
in herpes simplex, 596
genital, 180
in meningitis and encephalitis, 618-620, 624, 807
in mononucleosis, 722
of nervous system, 724
in orchitis, 515
in parotitis, 825
in pharyngitis, 362
in pneumonia, 371, 374, 375, 376, 377
in child, 803
sexually transmitted, 723-724; *see also* Sexually transmitted disease
systemic, 722-723
tumors and, 572
upper respiratory tract, 716-718
Visceral afferent fibers
in abdominal pain, 132
in vomiting, 153
Visceral pain, 131-132
afferents in, 122
Viscosity
synovial fluid and, 189
tumor and, 574
Vision; *see also* Eye
eye injury and, 237-238
loss of
acute, 843-844
psychogenic, 636
orbital fracture and, 234

Vision—cont'd
temporal arteritis and, 103
visual acuity, measurement of, 827
Vistaril; *see* Hydroxyzine
Visual impulses, 608, 609
Vital capacity, forced, 116
Vital signs
in abdominal trauma, 275
ancillary ventilatory support and, 63
in bowel obstruction, 480
in child, 791, 794
in coma, 83-84
in fever, 72
in gastrointestinal bleeding, 146
in headache, 96
importance of, 8
in multiple trauma, 63
in vomiting, 156
Vitamin A in hypercalcemia, 678
Vitamin B_1 for comatose patient, 83
Vitamin B_6
deficiency of, 557
in seizures, 768
Vitamin B_{12}, deficiency of, 557
Vitamin D
in chronic renal failure, 534
in hypercalcemia, 678
Vitamin E, deficiency of, 557
Vitamin K
coagulation and, 407
in liver disease in pregnancy, 499
in warfarin reversal, 407
Vitamin K–dependent clotting factors, 407
Vitrectomy, 842
Vitreous
hemorrhage in, 834
infection of, 842
Voice in airway assessment, 19-20
Volar Barton fracture, 305-306
Volar side of part, 296
Volar splint, 298
in wrist injury, 304
Volume replacement; *see also* Blood transfusions; Crystalloids
in burn patients, 335-336
in neonatal resuscitation, 44
Volume depletion in vomiting, 160, 162
Volvulus, 486-487
in child, 818-819
radiography in, 161
Vomiting, 153-164
abdominal pain and, 135
antiemetics in, 162-164
of blood, 145
in bowel obstruction, 480
chemoreceptor trigger-zone and, 153
in child, 157-160
rehydration and, 162
diagnostic work-up in, 160-161
differential diagnosis in, 157-160, 171
etiology and assessment of, 154-160
in gastroenteritis, 716

Vomiting—cont'd
  history of, 154-156
  intussusception of colon and, 486
  management of, 161-164
  mechanism of, 154
  in neonate and infant, 160
    rehydration in, 162
  physical findings in, 156-157
  in pregnancy, 550-551
  projectile, 155
  in pyloric stenosis, 818
  vomiting center in, 153-154
Vomiting center, 153-154
von Recklinghausen disease, seizures and,
    207
von Willebrand disease, 564, 565
VT; see Ventricular tachycardia
VZIg; see Varicella-zoster immune globulin

W

Wall of chest, flail chest and, 256-257
Wandering atrial tachycardia, 463
Warfarin
  in coagulation disorders, 564
  in venous thrombosis, 407
Warts, venereal, 184
Water intoxication, furosemide in, 671
Waterhouse-Friderichsen syndrome, 709
Wave
  P, 456, 457
  T, 458
Weakness
  psychogenic, 634-635
  in stroke, 601, 602
Weapon, patient with, 662
Weber test, 823
Wedge pressure, pulmonary capillary
  in cardiogenic shock, 55
  in pulmonary edema, 109
Weight of child, 791, 794
  age in estimation of, 47

Wernicke syndrome, coma and, 83
Westermark's sign, 402
Wheezing
  in airway assessment, 21, 115
  in asthma, 111, 380
    in child, 801
  in respiratory distress, 115
WHHHIMP mnemonic, 648
Whipworm, 738, 740
White blood cells
  in abdominal pain, 136
  in abdominal trauma, 273
  in anemia, 558
  in cerebrospinal fluid, 623
  in child, 816
  disorders of, 570
    in iron poisoning, 781
  in fever, 73, 816
  noninfectious causes of alterations in,
    73
  in pneumococcemia, 708
  in sickle cell disease, 560
Whooping cough, 701-703
Wide-complex tachycardia, 465, 466
Windshield, facial trauma and, 236
Wire suture, 286
Withdrawal
  alcohol, hypomagnesemia and, 686
  seizures in, 204
    treatment of, 209
Wolff-Parkinson-White syndrome, 88,
    466-467
  tachycardia in
    narrow-complex, 459
    paroxysmal supraventricular, 459
    wide-complex, 465
Wood light, 746
Wood ultraviolet light, 831
Workload, cardiac, 448
Work-up for emergency patient, 10

Wound
  burn, 337-338
  closure of, 285-288; see also Suture
  dressings for, 288
  electrical injury and, 342, 343
  facial, covering of, 236-237
  infections of, 288-289
  initial or primary survey of, 283
  primary, secondary, and tertiary repair of,
    285
  requiring initial open management, 285
  scalp, 289
  soft tissue, 283-293; see also Soft tissue,
    trauma to
  stab, abdominal, 275-277
  tetanus and, 703
Wrist
  arthritis in, 577
  fracture or dislocations of, 303-306
  splint for, 298

X

Xanthines in headache, 101
Xenograft, 337

Y

Yellow fever, 719
Yersinia
  in diarrhea, 167, 168-19
  in pneumonia, 369, 373

Z

Zaroxolyn; see Metolazone
Zidovudine, 730
Zofran; see Ondansetron
Zoster; see Varicella-zoster virus
Zoster immune globulin, 595
Zovirax; see Acyclovir
Zygomatic fracture, 232-233